3rd Edition

HARRISON'S™

GASTROENTEROLOGY AND HEPATOLOGY

Derived from Harrison's Principles of Internal Medicine, 19th Edition

Editors

DENNIS L. KASPER, MD
William Ellery Channing Professor of Medicine and Professor of Microbiology and Immunobiology, Division of Immunology, Department of Microbiology and Immunobiology, Harvard Medical School, Boston, Massachusetts

ANTHONY S. FAUCI, MD
Chief, Laboratory of Immunoregulation; Director, National Institute of Allergy and Infectious Diseases, National Institutes of Health, Bethesda, Maryland

STEPHEN L. HAUSER, MD
Robert A. Fishman Distinguished Professor and Chairman, Department of Neurology, University of California, San Francisco, San Francisco, California

DAN L. LONGO, MD
Professor of Medicine, Harvard Medical School; Senior Physician, Brigham and Women's Hospital; Deputy Editor, *New England Journal of Medicine*, Boston, Massachusetts

J. LARRY JAMESON, MD, PhD
Robert G. Dunlop Professor of Medicine; Dean, Perelman School of Medicine at the University of Pennsylvania; Executive Vice-President, University of Pennsylvania for the Health System, Philadelphia, Pennsylvania

JOSEPH LOSCALZO, MD, PhD
Hersey Professor of the Theory and Practice of Medicine, Harvard Medical School; Chairman, Department of Medicine, and Physician-in-Chief, Brigham and Women's Hospital, Boston, Massachusetts

3rd Edition

HARRISON'S™

GASTROENTEROLOGY AND HEPATOLOGY

EDITORS

Dennis L. Kasper, MD
William Ellery Channing Professor of Medicine and Professor of Microbiology and Immunobiology, Division of Immunology, Department of Microbiology and Immunobiology, Harvard Medical School, Boston, Massachusetts

Anthony S. Fauci, MD
Chief, Laboratory of Immunoregulation; Director, National Institute of Allergy and Infectious Diseases, National Institutes of Health, Bethesda, Maryland

Stephen L. Hauser, MD
Robert A. Fishman Distinguished Professor and Chairman, Department of Neurology, University of California, San Francisco, San Francisco, California

Dan L. Longo, MD
Professor of Medicine, Harvard Medical School; Senior Physician, Brigham and Women's Hospital; Deputy Editor, *New England Journal of Medicine,* Boston, Massachusetts

J. Larry Jameson, MD, PhD
Robert G. Dunlop Professor of Medicine; Dean, Perelman School of Medicine at the University of Pennsylvania; Executive Vice-President, University of Pennsylvania for the Health System, Philadelphia, Pennsylvania

Joseph Loscalzo, MD, PhD
Hersey Professor of the Theory and Practice of Medicine, Harvard Medical School; Chairman, Department of Medicine, and Physician-in-Chief, Brigham and Women's Hospital, Boston, Massachusetts

ASSOCIATE EDITOR

Carol A. Langford, MD, MHS
Harold C. Schott Chair; Associate Professor of Medicine; Director, Center for Vasculitis Care and Research, Department of Rheumatic and Immunologic Diseases, Cleveland Clinic, Cleveland, Ohio

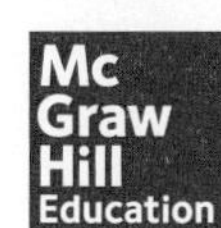

New York Chicago San Francisco Athens London Madrid Mexico City
Milan New Delhi Singapore Sydney Toronto

Harrison's Gastroenterology and Hepatology, Third Edition

Dr. Fauci's work as an editor and author was performed outside the scope of his employment as a U.S. government employee. This work represents his personal and professional views and not necessarily those of the U.S. government.

1 2 3 4 5 6 7 8 9 DOW 21 20 19 18 17 16

ISBN 978-1-259-83584-1
MHID 1-259-83584-7

This book was set in Minion Pro by Cenveo® Publisher Services. The editors were James F. Shanahan and Kim J. Davis. The production supervisor was Catherine H. Saggese. Project management was provided by Srishti Malasi of Cenveo Publisher Services. The cover design was by Dreamit, Inc.

RR Donnelley was the printer and binder.

Library of Congress Cataloging-in-Publication Data

Title: Harrison's gastroenterology and hepatology / editors, Dennis L. Kasper, Anthony S. Fauci, Stephen L. Hauser, Dan L. Longo, J. Larry Jameson, Joseph Loscalzo; associate editor, Carol A. Langford.
Other titles: Gastroenterology and hepatology | Abridgement of (expression): Harrison's principles of internal medicine. 19th edition.
Description: Third edition. | New York : McGraw-Hill Education Medical, [2017] | This book is aimed at bringing together the chapters of the current and 19th edition of Harrison's Principles of internal medicine related to gastroenterology and hepatology in a conveniently sized book for a focused study of this medical subspecialty. | Includes index.
Identifiers: LCCN 2016015940 (print) | LCCN 2016017234 (ebook) | ISBN 9781259835841 (pbk. : alk. paper) | ISBN 1259835847 (pbk. : alk. paper) | ISBN 9781259835858 (ebook) | ISBN 1259835855 (ebook)
Subjects: | MESH: Gastrointestinal Diseases | Liver Diseases
Classification: LCC RC801 (print) | LCC RC801 (ebook) | NLM WI 140 | DDC 616.3/3—dc23
LC record available at https://lccn.loc.gov/2016015940

CONTENTS

SECTION X
NUTRITION

SECTION XI
OBESITY AND EATING DISORDERS

CONTRIBUTORS

Numbers in brackets refer to the chapter(s) written or cowritten by the contributor.

Manal F. Abdelmalek, MD, MPH
Associate Professor of Medicine, Division of Gastroenterology and Hepatology, Duke University, Durham, North Carolina [43]

Rizwan Ahmed, MD
General Surgery Resident, Department of General Surgery, Johns Hopkins Hospital, Baltimore, Maryland [20, 21]

Rosa M. Andrade, MD
Department of Medicine, Division of Infectious Diseases, University of California, San Diego, San Diego, California [33]

John C. Atherton, MD, FRCP
Professor of Gastroenterology and Dean of the School of Medicine, University of Nottingham, Nottingham, United Kingdom [27]

Bruce R. Bacon, MD
James F. King, MD Endowed Chair in Gastroenterology; Professor of Internal Medicine, Saint Louis University Liver Center, Saint Louis University School of Medicine, St. Louis, Missouri [44, 46]

Peter A. Banks, MD
Professor of Medicine, Harvard Medical School; Senior Physician, Division of Gastroenterology, Brigham and Women's Hospital, Boston, Massachusetts [49, 50]

Miriam Baron Barshak, MD
Assistant Professor, Harvard Medical School; Associate Physician, Massachusetts General Hospital, Boston, Massachusetts [26]

Jean Bergounioux, MD, PhD, PhC
Pediatric Intensive Care Unit, Hôpital Raymond-Poincaré, Université de Versailles-Saint Quentin, Garches, France [29]

Atul K. Bhan, MD, MBBS
Professor of Pathology, Harvard Medical School, Department of Pathology, Massachusetts General Hospital, Boston, Massachusetts [45]

Henry J. Binder, MD
Professor Emeritus of Medicine, Senior Research Scientist, Yale University, New Haven, Connecticut [16, 17]

Bruce R. Bistrian, MD, PhD, MPH
Professor of Medicine, Harvard Medical School; Chief, Clinical Nutrition, Beth Israel Deaconess Medical Center, Boston, Massachusetts [59]

Martin J. Blaser, MD
Muriel and George Singer Professor of Medicine; Professor of Microbiology; Director, Human Microbiome Program, New York University Langone Medical Center, New York, New York [27, 30]

Richard S. Blumberg, MD
Chief, Division of Gastroenterology, Hepatology and Endoscopy, Brigham and Women's Hospital, Harvard Medical School, Boston, Massachusetts [18]

Cynthia D. Brown, MD
Associate Professor of Clinical Medicine, Division of Pulmonary, Critical Care, Sleep and Occupational Medicine, Indiana University, Indianapolis, Indiana [Review and Self-Assessment]

Stephen B. Calderwood, MD
Morton N. Swartz, MD Academy Professor of Medicine (Microbiology and Immunobiology), Harvard Medical School; Chief, Division of Infectious Diseases, Massachusetts General Hospital, Boston, Massachusetts [24]

Michael Camilleri, MD
Atherton and Winifred W. Bean Professor; Professor of Medicine, Pharmacology, and Physiology, Mayo Clinic College of Medicine, Rochester, Minnesota [6]

Brian I. Carr, MD, PhD, FRCP
IRCCS de Bellis National Center for GI Diseases, Castellana Grotte, BA, Italy [53]

Raymond T. Chung, MD
Associate Professor of Medicine, Harvard Medical School; Director of Hepatology and Liver Center; Vice Chief, Gastroenterology, Massachusetts General Hospital, Boston, Massachusetts [48]

Darwin L. Conwell, MD, MS
Professor of Medicine, The Ohio State University College of Medicine; Director, Division of Gastroenterology, Hepatology and Nutrition; The Ohio State University Wexner Medical Center, Columbus, Ohio [49, 50]

Kathleen E. Corey, MD, MPH
Clinical and Research Fellow, Harvard Medical School; Fellow, Gastrointestinal Unit, Massachusetts General Hospital, Boston, Massachusetts [9]

David Cunningham, MD, MB, ChB, FRCP
Professor, Head of Gastrointestinal/Lymphoma Unit; Director of Clinical Research, Royal Marsden NHS Trust, London, United Kingdom [54]

John Del Valle, MD
Professor and Senior Associate Chair of Medicine, Department of Internal Medicine, University of Michigan School of Medicine, Ann Arbor, Michigan [15]

Anna Mae Diehl, MD
Florence McAlister Professor of Medicine; Chief, Division of Gastroenterology, Duke University, Durham, North Carolina [43]

Jules L. Dienstag, MD
Carl W. Walter Professor of Medicine and Dean for Medical Education, Harvard Medical School; Physician, Gastrointestinal Unit, Department of Medicine, Massachusetts General Hospital, Boston, Massachusetts [39-41, 45, 48]

David F. Driscoll, PhD
Associate Professor of Medicine, University of Massachusetts Medical School, Worchester, Massachusetts [59]

Samuel C. Durso, MD, MBA
Mason F. Lord Professor of Medicine; Director, Division of Geriatric Medicine and Gerontology, Johns Hopkins University School of Medicine, Baltimore, Maryland [2, 3]

Johanna Dwyer, DSc, RD
Jean Mayer USDA Human Nutrition Research Center on Aging; Professor, Tufts Medical Center and Director, Frances Stern Nutrition Center, Tufts Medical Center, Boston, Massachusetts [56]

Robert H. Eckel, MD
Professor of Medicine, Division of Endocrinology, Metabolism and Diabetes, Division of Cardiology; Professor of Physiology and Biophysics, Charles A. Boettcher, II Chair in Atherosclerosis, University of Colorado School of Medicine, Anschutz Medical Campus, Director Lipid Clinic, University of Colorado Hospital, Aurora, Colorado [63]

Jeffrey S. Flier, MD
Caroline Shields Walker Professor of Medicine and Dean, Harvard Medical School, Boston, Massachusetts [60]

Lawrence S. Friedman, MD
Professor of Medicine, Harvard Medical School; Professor of Medicine, Tufts University School of Medicine; Assistant Chief of Medicine, Massachusetts General Hospital, Boston, Massachusetts; Anton R. Fried, MD Chair, Department of Medicine, Newton-Wellesley Hospital, Newton, Massachusetts [9]

Sonia Friedman, MD
Associate Professor of Medicine, Harvard Medical School; Associate Physician, Brigham and Women's Hospital, Boston, Massachusetts [18]

Susan L. Gearhart, MD
Associate Professor, Surgery, Johns Hopkins Medical Institutions, Baltimore, Maryland [20]

Dale N. Gerding, MD
Professor of Medicine, Department of Medicine, Loyola University Chicago Stritch School of Medicine, Maywood, Illinois; Research Physician, Edward Hines Jr. Veterans Affairs Hospital, Hines, Illinois [25]

Marc G. Ghany, MD, MHSc
Staff Physician, Liver Diseases Branch, National Institute of Diabetes and Digestive and Kidney Diseases, National Institutes of Health, Bethesda, Maryland [36]

Roger I. Glass, MD, PhD
Director, Fogarty International Center, Bethesda, Maryland [32]

Norton J. Greenberger, MD
Clinical Professor of Medicine, Harvard Medical School; Senior Physician, Division of Gastroenterology, Brigham and Women's Hospital, Boston, Massachusetts [47, 49, 50]

William L. Hasler, MD
Professor, Division of Gastroenterology, University of Michigan Health System, Ann Arbor, Michigan [5, 11]

Douglas C. Heimburger, MD, MS
Professor of Medicine, Associate Director for Education and Training, Vanderbilt Institute for Global Health, Vanderbilt University School of Medicine, Nashville, Tennessee [58]

Ikuo Hirano, MD
Professor of Medicine, Division of Gastroenterology, Northwestern University Feinberg School of Medicine, Chicago, Illinois [4, 14]

L. John Hoffer, MD, PhD
Professor, Faculty of Medicine, McGill University; Senior Physician, Divisions of Internal Medicine and Endocrinology, Lady Davis Institute for Medical Research, Jewish General Hospital, Montreal, Quebec, Canada [59]

Jay H. Hoofnagle, MD
Director, Liver Diseases Research Branch, National Institute of Diabetes and Digestive and Kidney Diseases, National Institutes of Health, Bethesda, Maryland [36]

Brian Houston, MD
Division of Cardiology, Department of Medicine, Johns Hopkins Hospital, Baltimore, Maryland [Review and Self-Assessment]

Danny O. Jacobs, MD, MPH, FACS
Executive Vice President, Provost, and Dean of the School of Medicine; Thomas N. and Gleaves T. James Distinguished Chair, The University of Texas Medical Branch at Galveston, Galveston, Texas [1, 22, 23]

J. Larry Jameson, MD, PhD
Robert G. Dunlop Professor of Medicine; Dean, Perelman School of Medicine at the University of Pennsylvania; Executive Vice President, University of Pennsylvania for the Health System, Philadelphia, Pennsylvania [10]

Robert T. Jensen, MD
Chief, Cell Biology Section, National Institutes of Diabetes, Digestive and Kidney Diseases, National Institutes of Health, Bethesda, Maryland [55]

Savio John, MD
Assistant Professor of Medicine, Division of Gastroenterology and Hepatology, State University of New York Upstate Medical University, Syracuse, New York [8]

Stuart Johnson, MD
Associate Professor of Medicine, Loyola University Chicago Stritch School of Medicine; Staff Physician, Edward Hines Jr. VA Hospital, Hines, Illinois [25]

Peter J. Kahrilas, MD
Gilbert H. Marquardt Professor of Medicine, Feinberg School of Medicine, Northwestern University, Chicago, Illinois [4, 14]

Dennis L. Kasper, MD, MA
William Ellery Channing Professor of Medicine, Professor of Microbiology and Immunobiology, Department of Microbiology and Immunobiology, Harvard Medical School; Division of Infectious Diseases, Brigham and Women's Hospital, Boston, Massachusetts [26]

Robert F. Kushner, MD, MS
Professor of Medicine, Northwestern University Feinberg School of Medicine, Chicago, Illinois [61]

Loren Laine, MD
Professor of Medicine, Yale University School of Medicine, New Haven, Connecticut; VA Connecticut Healthcare System, West Haven, Connecticut [7]

Regina C. LaRocque, MD, MPH
Assistant Professor of Medicine, Harvard Medical School; Assistant Physician, Massachusetts General Hospital, Boston, Massachusetts [24]

William M. Lee, MD
Professor of Internal Medicine; Meredith Mosle Chair in Liver Diseases, University of Texas Southwestern Medical Center at Dallas, Dallas, Texas [40]

Mark E. Mailliard, MD
Frederick F. Paustian Professor; Chief, Division of Gastroenterology and Hepatology, Department of Internal Medicine, University of Nebraska College of Medicine, Omaha, Nebraska [42]

Mahmoud Malas, MD, MHS, FACS
Associate Professor of Surgery, Johns Hopkins University; Director of Endovascular Surgery; Director of The Vascular and Endovascular Clinical Research Center, Johns Hopkins Bayview Medical Center, Baltimore, Maryland [21]

Eleftheria Maratos-Flier, MD
Professor of Medicine, Harvard Medical School; Division of Endocrinology, Beth Israel Deaconess Medical Center, Boston, Massachusetts [60]

Robert J. Mayer, MD
Faculty Vice President for Academic Affairs, Dana-Farber Cancer Institute; Stephen B. Kay Family Professor of Medicine, Harvard Medical School, Boston, Massachusetts [51, 52]

Samuel I. Miller, MD
Professor, Departments of Microbiology, Medicine and Genome Sciences, University of Washington, Seattle, Washington [28]

Joseph A. Murray, MD
Professor of Medicine, Departments of Internal Medicine and Immunology, Mayo Clinic, Rochester, Minnesota [6]

Thomas B. Nutman, MD
Head, Helminth Immunology Section, Head, Clinical Parasitology Unit, Laboratory of Parasitic Diseases, National Institute of Allergy and Infectious Diseases, National Institutes of Health, Bethesda, Maryland [35]

Chung Owyang, MD
H. Marvin Pollard Professor of Internal Medicine; Chief, Division of Gastroenterology, University of Michigan Health System, Ann Arbor, Michigan [11, 19]

Umesh D. Parashar, MBBS, MPH
Lead, Viral Gastroenteritis Epidemiology Team, Division of Viral Diseases, National Center for Immunization and Respiratory Diseases, Centers for Disease Control and Prevention, Atlanta, Georgia [32]

Gustav Paumgartner, MD
Professor Emeritus of Medicine, University of Munich, Munich, Germany [47]

David A. Pegues, MD
Professor of Medicine, Division of Infectious Diseases, Perelman School of Medicine, University of Pennsylvania, Philadelphia, Pennsylvania [28]

Daniel S. Pratt, MD
Assistant Professor of Medicine, Harvard Medical Center; Massachusetts General Hospital, Boston, Massachusetts [8, 37]

Sharon L. Reed, MD, MSCTM, D(ABMM)
Professor of Pathology and Medicine; Director, Microbiology Laboratory, University of California, San Diego School of Medicine, La Jolla, California [33]

Victor I. Reus, MD
Department of Psychiatry, University of California, San Francisco School of Medicine; Langley Porter Neuropsychiatric Institute, San Francisco, California [62]

Russell G. Robertson, MD
Professor of Family Medicine, Chicago Medical School, Rosalind Franklin University of Medicine and Science, Chicago, Illinois [10]

Robert M. Russell, MD
Professor Emeritus of Medicine and Nutrition, Tufts University, Boston, Massachusetts; Office of Dietary Supplements, National Institutes of Health, Bethesda, Maryland [57]

Edward T. Ryan, MD, FACP, FIDSA, FASTMH
Professor of Medicine, Harvard Medical School; Professor of Immunology and Infectious Diseases, Harvard School of Public Health; Director, Global Infectious Diseases, Division of Infectious Diseases, Massachusetts General Hospital, Boston, Massachusetts [24, 31]

Philippe J. Sansonetti, MD
Professor, Collège de France; Institut Pasteur, Paris, France [29]

William Silen, MD
Johnson and Johnson Professor Emeritus of Surgery, Harvard Medical School, Auburndale, Massachusetts [1]

Elizabeth Smyth, MB BAO, MSc
Department of Gastrointestinal Oncology, Royal Marsden NHS Foundation Trust, London and Sutton, United Kingdom [54]

Michael F. Sorrell, MD
Robert L. Grissom Professor of Medicine, Department of Internal Medicine, University of Nebraska Medical Center, Omaha, Nebraska [42]

Paolo M. Suter, MD, MS
Professor, Clinic and Policlinic of Internal Medicine, University Hospital, Zurich, Switzerland [57]

Mark Topazian, MD
Professor of Medicine, Mayo Clinic, Rochester, Minnesota [12, 13]

Matthew K. Waldor, MD, PhD
Edward H. Kass Professor of Medicine, Channing Laboratory, Brigham and Women's Hospital; Harvard Medical School and Howard Hughes Medical Institute, Boston, Massachusetts [31]

Peter F. Weller, MD
Chief, Infectious Disease Division; Chief, Allergy and Inflammation Division; Beth Israel Deaconess Medical Center, Boston, Massachusetts [34, 35]

Charles M. Wiener, MD
Vice President of Academic Affairs, Johns Hopkins Medicine International, Professor of Medicine and Physiology, Johns Hopkins School of Medicine, Baltimore, Maryland [Review and Self-Assessment]

Allan W. Wolkoff, MD
The Herman Lopata Chair in Liver Disease Research; Professor of Medicine and Anatomy and Structural Biology; Associate Chair of Medicine for Research; Chief, Division of Gastroenterology and Liver Diseases; Director, Marion Bessin Liver Research Center, Albert Einstein College of Medicine and Montefiore Medical Center, Bronx, New York [38]

Louis Michel Wong Kee Song, MD
Associate Professor, Division of Gastroenterology and Hepatology, Mayo Clinic College of Medicine, Rochester, Minnesota [12, 13]

Janet A. Yellowitz, DMD, MPH
Associate Professor; Director, Geriatric Dentistry, University of Maryland Dental School, Baltimore, Maryland [3]

PREFACE

Harrison's Principles of Internal Medicine (HPIM) has long been a major source of information related to the principles and practice of medicine for many practitioners and trainees. Yet, in its aim to cover the broad spectrum of medicine, the book has become more than 3000 pages in length and is pushing the envelope of "portability." *HPIM* has spawned several offspring tailored to diverse uses for sources of medical information. The entire book plus a large cache of supplemental visual and textual information are available as *Harrison's Online*, a component of McGraw-Hill's Access Medicine offering. In addition, the 19th edition of *HPIM* is now available on iPad. A condensed version of *HPIM*, called *Harrison's Manual of Medicine,* has been published in print format suitable for carrying in a white coat pocket and in several electronic formats (PDA, Blackberry, iPhone). A companion to *HPIM* that serves as a study guide for standardized tests in medicine, *HPIM Self-Assessment and Board Review*, is an effective teaching tool that highlights important areas of medicine discussed in *HPIM*. All of these products retain the broad spectrum of topics presented in the *HPIM* "mother book" in variable degrees of depth.

In 2006, for the first time, the Editors of *HPIM* experimented with extracting portions of *HPIM* that were focused on a specific subspecialty of internal medicine. The products of that effort, *Harrison's Endocrinology, Harrison's Rheumatology,* and *Harrison's Neurology*, were very well-received by audiences keenly interested in the respective subspecialties of internal medicine. Accordingly, we extended the concept of sectional publication 2009 with the publication of books in other internal medicine subspecialties including *Harrison's Gastroenterology and Hepatology* based on the 17th edition of *HPIM*. These volumes, too, appeared to serve the needs of many readers. Therefore, we are continuing the publication of books with a subspecialty focus.

According to a report from the National Institute of Diabetes and Digestive and Kidney Diseases, for every 100 residents of the United States, there were 35 ambulatory care contacts and 5 overnight hospital stays at which a digestive disease diagnosis was noted. In 2004, digestive diseases accounted for more than 236,000 deaths. Thus, training in the disciplines of gastroenterology and hepatology are essential to any primary care physician or general internist and even to practitioners of other internal medicine subspecialties.

This book is aimed at bringing together the chapters of the current and 19th edition of *HPIM* related to gastroenterology and hepatology in a conveniently sized book for a focused study of this medical subspecialty. The book is organized into 63 chapters and eleven sections: (I) Cardinal Manifestations of Gastrointestinal Disease; (II) Evaluation of the Patient with Alimentary Tract Symptoms; (III) Disorders of the Alimentary Tract; (IV) Infections of the Alimentary Tract; (V) Evaluation of the Patient with Liver Disease; (VI) Disorders of the Liver and Biliary Tree; (VII) Liver Transplantation; (VIII) Disorders of the Pancreas; (IX) Neoplastic Diseases of the Gastrointestinal System; (X) Nutrition; and (XI) Obesity and Eating Disorders.

The information presented here is contributed by physician/authors who have personally made notable advances in the fields of their expertise. The chapters reflect authoritative analyses by individuals who have been active participants in the extraordinary surge of new information on genetics, cell biology, pathophysiology, and treatment that has characterized all of medicine in the last 20 years. In addition to the didactic value of the chapters, a section of test questions, answers, and an explanation of the correct answers is provided to facilitate learning and assist the reader in preparing for standardized examinations.

Gastroenterology and hepatology, like many other areas of medicine, are changing rapidly. Novel technologies of imaging, development of new drugs, and the application of molecular pathogenesis information to detect disease early and prevent disease in people at risk are just a few of the advances that have made an impact on the practice of gastroenterology. Physicians are now applying endoscopic techniques in ways that were once unimaginable including performing operations successfully without an incision; operations that once required major surgery with attendant morbidity and expense. The pace of discovery demands that physicians undertake nearly continuous self-education. It is our hope that this book will help physicians in this process.

We are grateful to Kim Davis and James Shanahan at McGraw-Hill for their help in producing this book.

We thank Chung Owyang, MD, from the University of Michigan, Jay Hoofnagle, MD, from the National Institutes of Health, and Dennis Kasper, MD, from Harvard Medical School, for helpful discussions in shaping the content of this volume.

Dan L. Longo, MD
Anthony S. Fauci, MD

NOTICE

Medicine is an ever-changing science. As new research and clinical experience broaden our knowledge, changes in treatment and drug therapy are required. The authors and the publisher of this work have checked with sources believed to be reliable in their efforts to provide information that is complete and generally in accord with the standards accepted at the time of publication. However, in view of the possibility of human error or changes in medical sciences, neither the authors nor the publisher nor any other party who has been involved in the preparation or publication of this work warrants that the information contained herein is in every respect accurate or complete, and they disclaim all responsibility for any errors or omissions or for the results obtained from use of the information contained in this work. Readers are encouraged to confirm the information contained herein with other sources. For example and in particular, readers are advised to check the product information sheet included in the package of each drug they plan to administer to be certain that the information contained in this work is accurate and that changes have not been made in the recommended dose or in the contraindications for administration. This recommendation is of particular importance in connection with new or infrequently used drugs.

Review and self-assessment questions and answers were taken from Wiener CM, Brown CD, Houston B (eds). *Harrison's Self-Assessment and Board Review*, 19th ed. New York, McGraw-Hill, 2017, ISBN 978-1-259-64288-3.

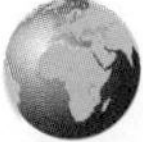

The global icons call greater attention to key epidemiologic and clinical differences in the practice of medicine throughout the world.

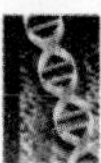

The genetic icons identify a clinical issue with an explicit genetic relationship.

SECTION I

CARDINAL MANIFESTATIONS OF GASTROINTESTINAL DISEASE

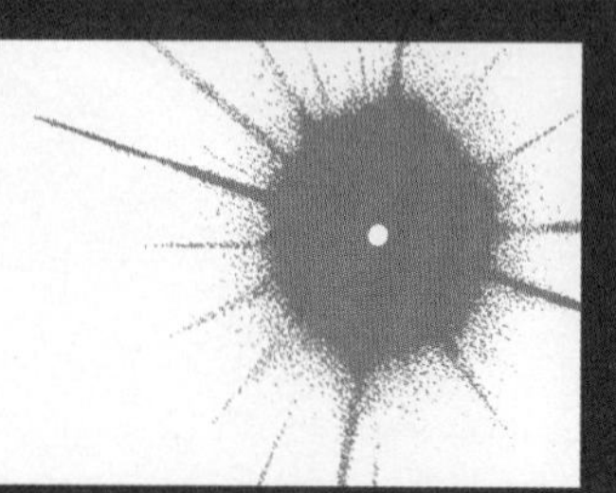

CHAPTER 1
ABDOMINAL PAIN

Danny O. Jacobs ■ William Silen

Correctly interpreting acute abdominal pain can be quite challenging. Few clinical situations require greater judgment, because the most catastrophic of events may be forecast by the subtlest of symptoms and signs. In every instance, the clinician must distinguish those conditions that require urgent intervention from those that do not and can best be managed nonoperatively. A meticulously executed, detailed history and physical examination are critically important for focusing the differential diagnosis, where necessary, and allowing the diagnostic evaluation to proceed expeditiously (Table 1-1).

The etiologic classification in Table 1-2, although not complete, provides a useful framework for evaluating patients with abdominal pain.

The most common causes of abdominal pain on admission are acute appendicitis, nonspecific abdominal pain, pain of urologic origin, and intestinal obstruction. A diagnosis of "acute or surgical abdomen" is not acceptable because of its often misleading and erroneous connotations. Most patients who present with acute abdominal pain will have self-limited disease processes. However, it is important to remember that pain severity does not necessarily correlate with the severity of the underlying condition. The most obvious of "acute abdomens" may not require operative intervention, and the mildest of abdominal pains may herald an urgently correctable lesion. Any patient with abdominal pain of recent onset requires early and thorough evaluation and accurate diagnosis.

TABLE 1-1

SOME KEY COMPONENTS OF THE PATIENT'S HISTORY
Age
Time and mode of onset of the pain
Pain characteristics
Duration of symptoms
Location of pain and sites of radiation
Associated symptoms and their relationship to the pain
Nausea, emesis, and anorexia
Diarrhea, constipation, or other changes in bowel habits
Menstrual history

SOME MECHANISMS OF PAIN ORIGINATING IN THE ABDOMEN

Inflammation of the parietal peritoneum

The pain of parietal peritoneal inflammation is steady and aching in character and is located directly over the inflamed area, its exact reference being possible because it is transmitted by somatic nerves supplying the parietal peritoneum. The intensity of the pain is dependent on the type and amount of material to which the peritoneal surfaces are exposed in a given time period. For example, the sudden release into the peritoneal cavity of a small quantity of *sterile* acid gastric juice causes much more pain than the same amount of grossly contaminated neutral feces. Enzymatically active pancreatic juice incites more pain and inflammation than does the same amount of sterile bile containing no potent enzymes. Blood is normally only a mild irritant and the response to urine can be bland, so exposure of blood and urine to the peritoneal cavity may go unnoticed unless it is sudden and massive. Bacterial contamination, such as may occur with pelvic inflammatory disease or perforated distal intestine, causes low-intensity pain until multiplication causes a significant amount of inflammatory mediators to be released. Patients with perforated upper gastrointestinal ulcers may present entirely differently depending on how quickly gastric juices enter the peritoneal cavity. Thus, the rate at which any inflammatory material irritates the peritoneum is important.

The pain of peritoneal inflammation is invariably accentuated by pressure or changes in tension of the peritoneum, whether produced by palpation or by movement such as with coughing or sneezing. The patient

TABLE 1-2

SOME IMPORTANT CAUSES OF ABDOMINAL PAIN

Pain Originating in the Abdomen	
Parietal peritoneal inflammation	Vascular disturbances
Bacterial contamination	Embolism or thrombosis
Perforated appendix or other perforated viscus	Vascular rupture
Pelvic inflammatory disease	Pressure or torsional occlusion
Chemical irritation	Sickle cell anemia
Perforated ulcer	Abdominal wall
Pancreatitis	Distortion or traction of mesentery
Mittelschmerz	Trauma or infection of muscles
Mechanical obstruction of hollow viscera	Distension of visceral surfaces, e.g., by hemorrhage
Obstruction of the small or large intestine	Hepatic or renal capsules
Obstruction of the biliary tree	Inflammation
Obstruction of the ureter	Appendicitis
	Typhoid fever
	Neutropenic enterocolitis or "typhlitis"
Pain Referred from Extraabdominal Source	
Cardiothoracic	Pleurodynia
Acute myocardial infarction	Pneumothorax
Myocarditis, endocarditis, pericarditis	Empyema
Congestive heart failure	Esophageal disease, including spasm, rupture, or inflammation
Pneumonia (especially lower lobes)	Genitalia
Pulmonary embolus	Torsion of the testis
Metabolic Causes	
Diabetes	Acute adrenal insufficiency
Uremia	Familial Mediterranean fever
Hyperlipidemia	Porphyria
Hyperparathyroidism	C1 esterase inhibitor deficiency (angioneurotic edema)
Neurologic/Psychiatric Causes	
Herpes zoster	Spinal cord or nerve root compression
Tabes dorsalis	Functional disorders
Causalgia	Psychiatric disorders
Radiculitis from infection or arthritis	
Toxic Causes	
Lead poisoning	
Insect or animal envenomation	
Black widow spider bites	
Snake bites	
Uncertain Mechanisms	
Narcotic withdrawal	
Heat stroke	

with peritonitis characteristically lies quietly in bed, preferring to avoid motion, in contrast to the patient with colic, who may be thrashing in discomfort.

Another characteristic feature of peritoneal irritation is tonic reflex spasm of the abdominal musculature, localized to the involved body segment. Its intensity depends on the integrity of the nervous system, the location of the inflammatory process, and the rate at which it develops. Spasm over a perforated retrocecal appendix or perforation into the lesser peritoneal sac may be minimal or absent because of the protective effect of overlying viscera. Catastrophic abdominal emergencies may be associated with minimal or no detectable pain or muscle spasm in obtunded, seriously ill, debilitated, immunosuppressed, or psychotic patients. A slowly developing process also often greatly attenuates the degree of muscle spasm.

Obstruction of hollow viscera

Intraluminal obstruction classically elicits intermittent or colicky abdominal pain that is not as well localized as the pain of parietal peritoneal irritation. However, the absence of cramping discomfort should not be misleading because distention of a hollow viscus may also produce steady pain with only rare paroxysms.

Small-bowel obstruction often presents as poorly localized, intermittent periumbilical or supraumbilical pain. As the intestine progressively dilates and loses muscular tone, the colicky nature of the pain may diminish. With superimposed strangulating obstruction, pain may spread to the lower lumbar region if there is traction on the root of the mesentery. The colicky pain of colonic obstruction is of lesser intensity, is commonly located in the infraumbilical area, and may often radiate to the lumbar region.

Sudden distention of the biliary tree produces a steady rather than colicky type of pain; hence, the term *biliary colic* is misleading. Acute distention of the gallbladder usually causes pain in the right upper quadrant with radiation to the right posterior region of the thorax or to the tip of the right scapula, but it is also not uncommonly found near the midline. Distention of the common bile duct often causes epigastric pain that may radiate to the upper lumbar region. Considerable variation is common, however, so that differentiation between these may be impossible. The typical subscapular pain or lumbar radiation is frequently absent. Gradual dilatation of the biliary tree, as can occur with carcinoma of the head of the pancreas, may cause no pain or only a mild aching sensation in the epigastrium or right upper quadrant. The pain of distention of the pancreatic ducts is similar to that described for distention of the common bile duct but, in addition, is very frequently accentuated by recumbency and relieved by the upright position.

Obstruction of the urinary bladder usually causes dull, low-intensity pain in the suprapubic region. Restlessness without specific complaint of pain may be the only sign of a distended bladder in an obtunded patient. In contrast, acute obstruction of the intravesicular portion of the ureter is characterized by severe suprapubic and flank pain that radiates to the penis, scrotum, or inner aspect of the upper thigh. Obstruction of the ureteropelvic junction manifests as pain near the costovertebral angle, whereas obstruction of the remainder of the ureter is associated with flank pain that often extends into the same side of the abdomen.

Vascular disturbances

A frequent misconception is that pain due to intraabdominal vascular disturbances is sudden and catastrophic in nature. Certain disease processes, such as embolism or thrombosis of the superior mesenteric artery or impending rupture of an abdominal aortic aneurysm, can certainly be associated with diffuse, severe pain. Yet, just as frequently, the patient with occlusion of the superior mesenteric artery only has mild continuous or cramping diffuse pain for 2 or 3 days before vascular collapse or findings of peritoneal inflammation appear. The early, seemingly insignificant discomfort is caused by hyperperistalsis rather than peritoneal inflammation. Indeed, absence of tenderness and rigidity in the presence of continuous, diffuse pain (e.g., "pain out of proportion to physical findings") in a patient likely to have vascular disease is quite characteristic of occlusion of the superior mesenteric artery. Abdominal pain with radiation to the sacral region, flank, or genitalia should always signal the possible presence of a rupturing abdominal aortic aneurysm. This pain may persist over a period of several days before rupture and collapse occur.

Abdominal wall

Pain arising from the abdominal wall is usually constant and aching. Movement, prolonged standing, and pressure accentuate the discomfort and associated muscle spasm. In the case of hematoma of the rectus sheath, now most frequently encountered in association with anticoagulant therapy, a mass may be present in the lower quadrants of the abdomen. Simultaneous involvement of muscles in other parts of the body usually serves to differentiate myositis of the abdominal wall from other processes that might cause pain in the same region.

REFERRED PAIN IN ABDOMINAL DISEASE

Pain referred to the abdomen from the thorax, spine, or genitalia may present a vexing diagnostic challenge because diseases of the upper part of the abdominal cavity such as acute cholecystitis or perforated ulcer may be associated with intrathoracic complications. A most important, yet often forgotten, dictum is that the possibility of intrathoracic disease must be considered in every patient with abdominal pain, especially if the pain is in the upper abdomen.

Systematic questioning and examination directed toward detecting myocardial or pulmonary infarction, pneumonia, pericarditis, or esophageal disease (the intrathoracic diseases that most often masquerade as abdominal emergencies) will often provide sufficient clues to establish the proper diagnosis. Diaphragmatic pleuritis resulting from pneumonia or pulmonary infarction may cause pain in the right upper quadrant and pain in the supraclavicular area, the latter radiation to be distinguished from the referred subscapular pain caused by acute distention of the extrahepatic biliary tree. The ultimate decision as to the origin of abdominal pain may require deliberate and planned observation over a period of several hours, during which repeated questioning and examination will provide the diagnosis or suggest the appropriate studies.

Referred pain of thoracic origin is often accompanied by splinting of the involved hemithorax with respiratory lag and decrease in excursion more marked than that seen in the presence of intraabdominal disease. In addition, apparent abdominal muscle spasm caused by referred pain will diminish during the inspiratory phase of respiration, whereas it persists throughout both respiratory phases if it is of abdominal origin. Palpation over the area of referred pain in the abdomen also does not usually accentuate the pain and, in many instances, actually seems to relieve it.

Thoracic disease and abdominal disease frequently coexist and may be difficult or impossible to differentiate. For example, the patient with known biliary tract disease often has epigastric pain during myocardial infarction, or biliary colic may be referred to the precordium or left shoulder in a patient who has suffered previously from angina pectoris.

Referred pain from the spine, which usually involves compression or irritation of nerve roots, is characteristically intensified by certain motions such as cough, sneeze, or strain and is associated with hyperesthesia over the involved dermatomes. Pain referred to the abdomen from the testes or seminal vesicles is generally accentuated by the slightest pressure on either of these organs. The abdominal discomfort experienced is of dull, aching character and is poorly localized.

METABOLIC ABDOMINAL CRISES

Pain of metabolic origin may simulate almost any other type of intraabdominal disease. Several mechanisms may be at work. In certain instances, such as hyperlipidemia, the metabolic disease itself may be accompanied by an intraabdominal process such as pancreatitis, which can lead to unnecessary laparotomy unless recognized. C1 esterase deficiency associated with angioneurotic edema is often associated with episodes of severe abdominal pain. Whenever the cause of abdominal pain is obscure, a metabolic origin always must be considered. Abdominal pain is also the hallmark of familial Mediterranean fever.

The problem of differential diagnosis is often not readily resolved. The pain of porphyria and of lead colic is usually difficult to distinguish from that of intestinal obstruction, because severe hyperperistalsis is a prominent feature of both. The pain of uremia or diabetes is nonspecific, and the pain and tenderness frequently shift in location and intensity. Diabetic acidosis may be precipitated by acute appendicitis or intestinal obstruction, so if prompt resolution of the abdominal pain does not result from correction of the metabolic abnormalities, an underlying organic problem should be suspected. Black widow spider bites produce intense pain and rigidity of the abdominal muscles and back, an area infrequently involved in intraabdominal disease.

IMMUNOCOMPROMISE

Evaluating and diagnosing causes of abdominal pain in immunosuppressed or otherwise immunocompromised patients is very difficult. This includes those who have undergone organ transplantation; who are receiving immunosuppressive treatments for autoimmune diseases, chemotherapy, or glucocorticoids; who have AIDS; and who are very old. In these circumstances, normal physiologic responses may be absent or masked. In addition, unusual infections may cause abdominal pain where the etiologic agents include cytomegalovirus, mycobacteria, protozoa, and fungi. These pathogens may affect all gastrointestinal organs, including the gallbladder, liver, and pancreas, as well as the gastrointestinal tract, causing occult or overtly symptomatic perforations of the latter. Splenic abscesses due to *Candida* or *Salmonella* infection should also be considered, especially when evaluating patients with left upper quadrant or left flank pain. Acalculous cholecystitis is a relative common complication in patients with AIDS, where it is often associated with cryptosporidiosis or cytomegalovirus infection.

Neutropenic enterocolitis is often identified as a cause of abdominal pain and fever in some patients with bone marrow suppression due to chemotherapy. Acute graft-versus-host disease should be considered. Optimal management of these patients may require meticulous follow-up including serial examinations to be certain that surgical intervention is not required to treat an underlying disease process.

NEUROGENIC CAUSES

Diseases that injure sensory nerves may cause causalgic pain. It has a burning character and is usually limited to the distribution of a given peripheral nerve. Normal nonpainful stimuli such as touch or a change in temperature may be causalgic and may frequently be present even at rest. The demonstration of irregularly spaced cutaneous pain spots may be the only indication that an old nerve injury exists. Even though the pain may be precipitated by gentle palpation, rigidity of the abdominal muscles is absent, and the respirations are not disturbed. Distention of the abdomen is uncommon, and the pain has no relationship to the intake of food.

Pain arising from spinal nerves or roots comes and goes suddenly and is of a lancinating type. It may be caused by herpes zoster, impingement by arthritis, tumors, a herniated nucleus pulposus, diabetes, or syphilis. It is not associated with food intake, abdominal distention, or changes in respiration. Severe muscle spasm, as in the gastric crises of tabes dorsalis, is common but is either relieved or not accentuated by abdominal palpation. The pain is made worse by movement of the spine and is usually confined to a few dermatomes. Hyperesthesia is very common.

Pain due to functional causes conforms to none of the aforementioned patterns. Mechanisms of disease are not clearly established. Irritable bowel syndrome (IBS) is a functional gastrointestinal disorder characterized by abdominal pain and altered bowel habits. The diagnosis is made on the basis of clinical criteria **(Chap. 19)** and after exclusion of demonstrable structural abnormalities. The episodes of abdominal pain are often brought on by stress, and the pain varies considerably in type and location. Nausea and vomiting are rare. Localized tenderness and muscle spasm are inconsistent or absent. The causes of IBS or related functional disorders are not known.

APPROACH TO THE PATIENT: Abdominal Pain

Few abdominal conditions require such urgent operative intervention that an orderly approach need be abandoned, no matter how ill the patient. Only patients with exsanguinating intraabdominal hemorrhage (e.g., ruptured aneurysm) must be rushed to the operating room immediately, but in such instances, only a few minutes are required to assess the critical nature of the problem. Under these circumstances, all obstacles must be swept aside, adequate venous access for fluid replacement obtained, and the operation begun. Many of these patients have died in the radiology department or the emergency room while awaiting unnecessary examinations such as electrocardiograms or computed tomography (CT) scans. *There are no contraindications to operation when massive intraabdominal hemorrhage is present.* Fortunately, this situation is relatively rare. This statement does not necessarily apply to patients with intraluminal gastrointestinal hemorrhage, who can often be managed by other means **(Chap. 7)**. Nothing will supplant an orderly, painstakingly *detailed history,* which is far more valuable than any laboratory or radiographic examination. This kind of history is laborious and time-consuming, making it not especially popular, even though a reasonably accurate diagnosis can be made on the basis of the history alone in the majority of cases.

In cases of *acute* abdominal pain, a diagnosis is readily established in most instances, whereas success is not so frequent in patients with *chronic* pain. IBS is one of the most common causes of abdominal pain and must always be kept in mind **(Chap. 19)**. The location of the pain can assist in narrowing the differential diagnosis (Table 1-3); however, the *chronological sequence of events* in the patient's history is often more important than the pain's location. If the examiner is sufficiently open-minded and unhurried, asks the proper questions, and listens, the patient will usually provide the diagnosis. Careful attention should be paid to the extraabdominal regions. Narcotics or analgesics should *not* be withheld until a definitive diagnosis or a definitive plan has been formulated; obfuscation of the diagnosis by adequate analgesia is unlikely.

An accurate menstrual history in a female patient is essential. It is important to remember that normal anatomic relationships can be significantly altered by the gravid uterus. Abdominal and pelvic pain may occur during pregnancy due to conditions that do not require surgery. Lastly, some otherwise noteworthy laboratory values (e.g., leukocytosis) may represent the normal physiologic changes of pregnancy.

In the examination, simple critical inspection of the patient, e.g., of facies, position in bed, and respiratory activity, provides valuable clues. The amount of information to be gleaned is directly proportional to the *gentleness* and thoroughness of the examiner. Once a patient with peritoneal inflammation has been examined brusquely, accurate assessment by the next examiner becomes almost impossible. Eliciting rebound tenderness by sudden release of a deeply palpating hand in a patient with suspected peritonitis is cruel and unnecessary. The same information can be obtained by gentle percussion of the abdomen (rebound tenderness on a miniature scale), a maneuver that can be far more precise and localizing. Asking the patient to cough will elicit true rebound tenderness without the need for placing a hand on the abdomen. Furthermore, the forceful demonstration of rebound tenderness will startle and induce protective spasm in a nervous or worried patient in whom true rebound tenderness is not present. A palpable gallbladder will be missed if palpation is so aggressive that voluntary muscle spasm becomes superimposed on involuntary muscular rigidity. As with history taking, sufficient time should be spent in the examination. Abdominal signs may be minimal but nevertheless, if accompanied by consistent symptoms, may be exceptionally meaningful. Abdominal signs may be virtually or totally absent in cases of pelvic peritonitis, so careful *pelvic and rectal examinations are mandatory in every patient with abdominal pain.* Tenderness on pelvic or rectal examination in the absence of other abdominal signs can be caused by operative indications such as perforated appendicitis, diverticulitis, twisted ovarian cyst, and many others. Much attention has been paid to the presence or absence of peristaltic sounds, their quality, and their frequency. Auscultation of the abdomen is one of the least

TABLE 1-3

DIFFERENTIAL DIAGNOSES OF ABDOMINAL PAIN BY LOCATION

Right Upper Quadrant	Epigastric	Left Upper Quadrant
Cholecystitis Cholangitis Pancreatitis Pneumonia/empyema Pleurisy/pleurodynia Subdiaphragmatic abscess Hepatitis Budd-Chiari syndrome	Peptic ulcer disease Gastritis GERD Pancreatitis Myocardial infarction Pericarditis Ruptured aortic aneurysm Esophagitis	Splenic infarct Splenic rupture Splenic abscess Gastritis Gastric ulcer Pancreatitis Subdiaphragmatic abscess
Right Lower Quadrant	**Periumbilical**	**Left Lower Quadrant**
Appendicitis Salpingitis Inguinal hernia Ectopic pregnancy Nephrolithiasis Inflammatory bowel disease Mesenteric lymphadenitis Typhlitis	Early appendicitis Gastroenteritis Bowel obstruction Ruptured aortic aneurysm	Diverticulitis Salpingitis Inguinal hernia Ectopic pregnancy Nephrolithiasis Irritable bowel syndrome Inflammatory bowel disease
Diffuse Nonlocalized Pain		
Gastroenteritis Mesenteric ischemia Bowel obstruction Irritable bowel syndrome Peritonitis Diabetes	Malaria Familial Mediterranean fever Metabolic diseases Psychiatric disease	

Abbreviation: GERD, gastroesophageal reflux disease.

revealing aspects of the physical examination of a patient with abdominal pain. Catastrophes such as a strangulating small intestinal obstruction or perforated appendicitis may occur in the presence of normal peristaltic sounds. Conversely, when the proximal part of the intestine above obstruction becomes markedly distended and edematous, peristaltic sounds may lose the characteristics of borborygmi and become weak or absent, even when peritonitis is not present. It is usually the severe chemical peritonitis of sudden onset that is associated with the truly silent abdomen.

Laboratory examinations may be valuable in assessing the patient with abdominal pain, yet, with few exceptions, they rarely establish a diagnosis. Leukocytosis should never be the single deciding factor as to whether or not operation is indicated. A white blood cell count >20,000/μL may be observed with perforation of a viscus, but pancreatitis, acute cholecystitis, pelvic inflammatory disease, and intestinal infarction may also be associated with marked leukocytosis. A normal white blood cell count is not rare in cases of perforation of abdominal viscera. The diagnosis of anemia may be more helpful than the white blood cell count, especially when combined with the history.

The urinalysis may reveal the state of hydration or rule out severe renal disease, diabetes, or urinary infection. Blood urea nitrogen, glucose, and serum bilirubin levels may be helpful. Serum amylase levels may be increased by many diseases other than pancreatitis, e.g., perforated ulcer, strangulating intestinal obstruction, and acute cholecystitis; thus, elevations of serum amylase do not rule out the need for an operation.

Plain and upright or lateral decubitus radiographs of the abdomen may be of value in cases of intestinal obstruction, perforated ulcer, and a variety of other conditions. They are usually unnecessary in patients with acute appendicitis or strangulated external hernias. In rare instances, barium or water-soluble contrast study of the upper part of the gastrointestinal tract may demonstrate partial intestinal obstruction that may elude diagnosis by other means. If there is any question of obstruction of the colon, oral administration of barium sulfate should be avoided. On the other hand, in cases of suspected colonic obstruction (without perforation), a contrast enema may be diagnostic.

In the absence of trauma, peritoneal lavage has been replaced as a diagnostic tool by CT scanning and laparoscopy. Ultrasonography has proved to be useful in detecting an enlarged gallbladder or pancreas, the presence of gallstones, an enlarged ovary, or a tubal pregnancy. Laparoscopy is especially helpful in diagnosing pelvic conditions, such as ovarian cysts, tubal pregnancies, salpingitis, and acute appendicitis.

Radioisotopic hepatobiliary iminodiacetic acid scans (HIDAs) may help differentiate acute cholecystitis or biliary colic from acute pancreatitis. A CT scan may demonstrate an enlarged pancreas, ruptured spleen, or thickened colonic or appendiceal wall and streaking of the mesocolon or mesoappendix characteristic of diverticulitis or appendicitis.

Sometimes, even under the best circumstances with all available aids and with the greatest of clinical skill, a definitive diagnosis cannot be established at the time of the initial examination. Nevertheless, even in the absence of a clear anatomic diagnosis, it may be abundantly clear to an experienced and thoughtful physician and surgeon that operation is indicated on clinical grounds alone. Should that decision be questionable, watchful waiting with repeated questioning and examination will often elucidate the true nature of the illness and indicate the proper course of action.

CHAPTER 2

ORAL MANIFESTATIONS OF DISEASE

Samuel C. Durso

As primary care physicians and consultants, internists are often asked to evaluate patients with disease of the oral soft tissues, teeth, and pharynx. Knowledge of the oral milieu and its unique structures is necessary to guide preventive services and recognize oral manifestations of local or systemic disease **(Chap. 3)**. Furthermore, internists frequently collaborate with dentists in the care of patients who have a variety of medical conditions that affect oral health or who undergo dental procedures that increase their risk of medical complications.

DISEASES OF THE TEETH AND PERIODONTAL STRUCTURES

Tooth formation begins during the sixth week of embryonic life and continues through 17 years of age. Teeth start to develop in utero and continue to develop until after the tooth erupts. Normally, all 20 deciduous teeth have erupted by age 3 and have been shed by age 13. Permanent teeth, eventually totaling 32, begin to erupt by age 6 and have completely erupted by age 14, though third molars ("wisdom teeth") may erupt later.

The erupted tooth consists of the visible *crown* covered with enamel and the root submerged below the gum line and covered with bonelike *cementum. Dentin*, a material that is denser than bone and exquisitely sensitive to pain, forms the majority of the tooth substance, surrounding a core of myxomatous *pulp* containing the vascular and nerve supply. The tooth is held firmly in the alveolar socket by the *periodontium*, supporting structures that consist of the gingivae, alveolar bone, cementum, and periodontal ligament. The periodontal ligament tenaciously binds the tooth's cementum to the alveolar bone. Above this ligament is a collar of attached gingiva just below the crown. A few millimeters of unattached or free gingiva (1–3 mm) overlap the base of the crown, forming a shallow sulcus along the gum-tooth margin.

Dental caries, pulpal and periapical disease, and complications

Dental caries usually begin asymptomatically as a destructive infectious process of the enamel. Bacteria—principally *Streptococcus mutans*—colonize the organic buffering biofilm (*plaque*) on the tooth surface. If not removed by brushing or by the natural cleansing and antibacterial action of saliva, bacterial acids can demineralize the enamel. Fissures and pits on the occlusal surfaces are the most frequent sites of early decay. Surfaces between the teeth, adjacent to tooth restorations and exposed roots, are also vulnerable, particularly as individuals age. Over time, dental caries extend to the underlying dentin, leading to cavitation of the enamel. Without management, the caries will penetrate to the tooth pulp, producing *acute pulpitis*. At this stage, when the pulp infection is limited, the tooth may become sensitive to percussion and to hot or cold, and pain resolves immediately when the irritating stimulus is removed. Should the infection spread throughout the pulp, *irreversible pulpitis* occurs, leading to *pulp necrosis*. At this later stage, pain can be severe and has a sharp or throbbing visceral quality that may be worse when the patient lies down. Once pulp necrosis is complete, pain may be constant or intermittent, but cold sensitivity is lost.

Treatment of caries involves removal of the softened and infected hard tissue and restoration of the tooth structure with silver amalgam, glass ionomer, composite resin, or gold. Once irreversible pulpitis occurs, root canal therapy becomes necessary; removal of the contents of the pulp chamber and root canals is followed by thorough cleaning and filling with an inert material. Alternatively, the tooth may be extracted.

Pulpal infection leads to *periapical abscess* formation, which can produce pain on chewing. If the infection is mild and chronic, a *periapical granuloma* or eventually a *periapical cyst* forms, either of which produces radiolucency at the root apex. When unchecked, a periapical abscess can erode into the alveolar bone, producing osteomyelitis; penetrate and drain through the gingivae, producing a parulis (gumboil); or track along deep fascial planes, producing virulent cellulitis (Ludwig's angina) involving the submandibular space and floor of the mouth. Elderly patients, patients with diabetes mellitus, and patients taking glucocorticoids may experience little or no pain or fever as these complications develop.

Periodontal disease

Periodontal disease and dental caries are the primary causes of tooth loss. Like dental caries, chronic infection of the gingiva and anchoring structures of the tooth begins with formation of bacterial plaque. The process begins at the gum line. Plaque and *calculus* (calcified plaque) are preventable by appropriate daily oral hygiene, including periodic professional cleaning. Left undisturbed, chronic inflammation can ensue and produce hyperemia of the free and attached gingivae (*gingivitis*), which then typically bleed with brushing. If this issue is ignored, severe *periodontitis* can develop, leading to deepening of the physiologic sulcus and destruction of the periodontal ligament. Gingival pockets develop around the teeth. As the periodontium (including the supporting bone) is destroyed, the teeth loosen. A role for chronic inflammation due to chronic periodontal disease in promoting coronary heart disease and stroke has been proposed. Epidemiologic studies have demonstrated a moderate but significant association between chronic periodontal inflammation and atherogenesis, though a causal role remains unproven.

Acute and aggressive forms of periodontal disease are less common than the chronic forms described above. However, if the host is stressed or exposed to a new pathogen, rapidly progressive and destructive disease of the periodontal tissue can occur. A virulent example is *acute necrotizing ulcerative gingivitis*. Stress and poor oral hygiene are risk factors. The presentation includes sudden gingival inflammation, ulceration, bleeding, interdental gingival necrosis, and fetid halitosis. *Localized juvenile periodontitis*, which is seen in adolescents, is particularly destructive and appears to be associated with impaired neutrophil chemotaxis. *AIDS-related periodontitis* resembles acute necrotizing ulcerative gingivitis in some patients and a more destructive form of adult chronic periodontitis in others. It may also produce a gangrene-like destructive process of the oral soft tissues and bone that resembles *noma*, an infectious condition seen in severely malnourished children in developing nations.

Prevention of tooth decay and periodontal infection

Despite the reduced prevalences of dental caries and periodontal disease in the United States (due in large part to water fluoridation and improved dental care, respectively), both diseases constitute a major public health problem worldwide, particularly in certain groups. The internist should promote preventive dental care and hygiene as part of health maintenance. Populations at high risk for dental caries and periodontal disease include those with hyposalivation and/or xerostomia, diabetics, alcoholics, tobacco users, persons with Down syndrome, and those with gingival hyperplasia. Furthermore, patients lacking access to dental care (e.g., as a result of low socioeconomic status) and patients with a reduced ability to provide self-care (e.g., individuals with disabilities, nursing home residents, and persons with dementia or upper-extremity disability) suffer at a disproportionate rate. It is important to provide counseling regarding regular dental hygiene and professional cleaning, use of fluoride-containing toothpaste, professional fluoride treatments, and (for patients with limited dexterity) use of electric toothbrushes and also to instruct persons caring for those who are not capable of self-care. Cost, fear of dental care, and differences in language and culture create barriers that prevent some people from seeking preventive dental services.

Developmental and systemic disease affecting the teeth and periodontium

In addition to posing cosmetic issues, *malocclusion*, the most common developmental oral problem, can interfere with mastication unless corrected through orthodontic and surgical techniques. Impacted third molars are common and can become infected or erupt into an insufficient space. Acquired prognathism due to *acromegaly* may also lead to malocclusion, as may deformity of the maxilla and mandible due to *Paget's disease* of the bone. Delayed tooth eruption, a receding chin, and a protruding tongue are occasional features of *cretinism* and *hypopituitarism*. Congenital syphilis produces tapering, notched (*Hutchinson's*) incisors and finely nodular (*mulberry*) molar crowns. *Enamel hypoplasia* results in crown defects ranging from pits to deep fissures of primary or permanent teeth. Intrauterine infection (syphilis, rubella), vitamin deficiency (A, C, or D), disorders of calcium metabolism (malabsorption, vitamin D–resistant rickets, hypoparathyroidism), prematurity, high fever, and rare inherited defects (*amelogenesis imperfecta*) are all causes. Tetracycline, given in sufficiently high doses during the first 8 years of life, may produce enamel hypoplasia and discoloration. Exposure to endogenous pigments can discolor developing teeth; etiologies include *erythroblastosis fetalis* (green or bluish-black), congenital liver disease (green or yellow-brown), and porphyria (red or brown that fluoresces with ultraviolet light). *Mottled enamel* occurs if excessive fluoride is ingested during development. Worn enamel is seen with age, bruxism, or excessive acid exposure (e.g., chronic gastric reflux or bulimia). Celiac disease is associated with nonspecific enamel defects in children but not in adults.

Total or partial tooth loss resulting from periodontitis is seen with cyclic neutropenia, Papillon-Lefévre syndrome, Chédiak-Higashi syndrome, and leukemia. Rapid focal tooth loosening is most often due to infection, but rarer causes include Langerhans cell histiocytosis, Ewing's sarcoma, osteosarcoma, and Burkitt's lymphoma. Early loss of primary teeth is a feature of *hypophosphatasia*, a rare congenital error of metabolism.

Pregnancy may produce gingivitis and localized *pyogenic granulomas*. Severe periodontal disease occurs in uncontrolled diabetes mellitus. *Gingival hyperplasia* may be caused by phenytoin, calcium channel blockers (e.g., nifedipine), and cyclosporine, though excellent daily oral care can prevent or reduce its occurrence. *Idiopathic familial gingival fibromatosis* and several syndrome-related disorders cause similar conditions. Discontinuation of the medication may reverse the drug-induced form, though surgery may be needed to control both of the latter entities. *Linear gingival erythema* is variably seen in patients with advanced HIV infection and probably represents immune deficiency and decreased neutrophil activity. Diffuse or focal gingival swelling may be a feature of early or late acute myelomonocytic leukemia as well as of other lymphoproliferative disorders. A rare but pathognomonic sign of granulomatosis with polyangiitis is a red-purplish, granular gingivitis (*strawberry gums*).

DISEASES OF THE ORAL MUCOSA

Infections

Most oral mucosal diseases involve microorganisms (Table 2-1).

Pigmented lesions

See Table 2-2.

Dermatologic diseases

See Tables 2-1, 2-2, and 2-3.

Diseases of the tongue

See Table 2-4.

HIV disease and AIDS

See Tables 2-1, 2-2, 2-3, and 2-5.

Ulcers

Ulceration is the most common oral mucosal lesion. Although there are many causes, the host and the pattern of lesions, including the presence of organ system features, narrow the differential diagnosis (Table 2-1). Most acute ulcers are painful and self-limited. Recurrent aphthous ulcers and herpes simplex account for the majority. Persistent and deep aphthous ulcers can be idiopathic or can accompany HIV/AIDS. Aphthous lesions are often the presenting symptom in *Behçet's syndrome*. Similar-appearing, though less painful, lesions may occur in reactive arthritis, and aphthous ulcers are occasionally present during phases of *discoid* or *systemic lupus erythematosus*. Aphthous-like ulcers are seen in *Crohn's disease* **(Chap. 18)**, but, unlike the common aphthous variety, they may exhibit granulomatous inflammation on histologic examination. Recurrent aphthae are more prevalent in patients with *celiac disease* and have been reported to remit with elimination of gluten.

Of major concern are chronic, relatively painless ulcers and mixed red/white patches (erythroplakia and leukoplakia) of >2 weeks' duration. Squamous cell carcinoma and premalignant dysplasia should be considered early and a diagnostic biopsy performed. This awareness and this procedure are critically important because early-stage malignancy is vastly more treatable than late-stage disease. High-risk sites include the lower lip, floor of the mouth, ventral and lateral tongue, and soft palate–tonsillar pillar complex. Significant risk factors for oral cancer in Western countries include sun exposure (lower lip), tobacco and alcohol use, and human papillomavirus infection. In India and some other Asian countries, smokeless tobacco mixed with betel nut, slaked lime, and spices is a common cause of oral cancer. Rarer causes of chronic oral ulcer, such as tuberculosis, fungal infection, granulomatosis with polyangiitis, and midline granuloma may look identical to carcinoma. Making the correct diagnosis depends on recognizing other clinical features and performing a biopsy of the lesion. The syphilitic chancre is typically painless and therefore easily missed. Regional lymphadenopathy is invariably present. The syphilitic etiology is confirmed with appropriate bacterial and serologic tests.

Disorders of mucosal fragility often produce painful oral ulcers that fail to heal within 2 weeks. *Mucous membrane pemphigoid* and *pemphigus vulgaris* are the major acquired disorders. While their clinical features are often distinctive, a biopsy or immunohistochemical examination should be performed to diagnose these

TABLE 2-1

VESICULAR, BULLOUS, OR ULCERATIVE LESIONS OF THE ORAL MUCOSA

CONDITION	USUAL LOCATION	CLINICAL FEATURES	COURSE
Viral Diseases			
Primary acute herpetic gingivostomatitis (HSV type 1; rarely type 2)	Lip and oral mucosa (buccal, gingival, lingual mucosa)	Labial vesicles that rupture and crust, and intraoral vesicles that quickly ulcerate; extremely painful; acute gingivitis, fever, malaise, foul odor, and cervical lymphadenopathy; occurs primarily in infants, children, and young adults	Heals spontaneously in 10–14 days; unless secondarily infected, lesions lasting >3 weeks are not due to primary HSV infection
Recurrent herpes labialis	Mucocutaneous junction of lip, perioral skin	Eruption of groups of vesicles that may coalesce, then rupture and crust; painful to pressure or spicy foods	Lasts ~1 week, but condition may be prolonged if secondarily infected; if severe, topical or oral antiviral treatment may reduce healing time
Recurrent intraoral herpes simplex	Palate and gingiva	Small vesicles on keratinized epithelium that rupture and coalesce; painful	Heals spontaneously in ~1 week; if severe, topical or oral antiviral treatment may reduce healing time
Chickenpox (VZV)	Gingiva and oral mucosa	Skin lesions may be accompanied by small vesicles on oral mucosa that rupture to form shallow ulcers; may coalesce to form large bullous lesions that ulcerate; mucosa may have generalized erythema	Lesions heal spontaneously within 2 weeks
Herpes zoster (VZV reactivation)	Cheek, tongue, gingiva, or palate	Unilateral vesicular eruptions and ulceration in linear pattern following sensory distribution of trigeminal nerve or one of its branches	Gradual healing without scarring unless secondarily infected; postherpetic neuralgia is common; oral acyclovir, famciclovir, or valacyclovir reduces healing time and postherpetic neuralgia
Infectious mononucleosis (Epstein-Barr virus)	Oral mucosa	Fatigue, sore throat, malaise, fever, and cervical lymphadenopathy; numerous small ulcers usually appear several days before lymphadenopathy; gingival bleeding and multiple petechiae at junction of hard and soft palates	Oral lesions disappear during convalescence; no treatment is given, though glucocorticoids are indicated if tonsillar swelling compromises the airway
Herpangina (coxsackievirus A; also possibly coxsackievirus B and echovirus)	Oral mucosa, pharynx, tongue	Sudden onset of fever, sore throat, and oropharyngeal vesicles, usually in children <4 years old, during summer months; diffuse pharyngeal congestion and vesicles (1–2 mm), grayish-white surrounded by red areola; vesicles enlarge and ulcerate	Incubation period of 2–9 days; fever for 1–4 days; recovery uneventful
Hand-foot-and-mouth disease (most commonly coxsackievirus A16)	Oral mucosa, pharynx, palms, and soles	Fever, malaise, headache with oropharyngeal vesicles that become painful, shallow ulcers; highly infectious; usually affects children under age 10	Incubation period 2–18 days; lesions heal spontaneously in 2–4 weeks
Primary HIV infection	Gingiva, palate, and pharynx	Acute gingivitis and oropharyngeal ulceration, associated with febrile illness resembling mononucleosis and including lymphadenopathy	Followed by HIV seroconversion, asymptomatic HIV infection, and usually ultimately by HIV disease
Bacterial or Fungal Diseases			
Acute necrotizing ulcerative gingivitis ("trench mouth")	Gingiva	Painful, bleeding gingiva characterized by necrosis and ulceration of gingival papillae and margins plus lymphadenopathy and foul breath	Debridement and diluted (1:3) peroxide lavage provide relief within 24 h; antibiotics in acutely ill patients; relapse may occur
Prenatal (congenital) syphilis	Palate, jaws, tongue, and teeth	Gummatous involvement of palate, jaws, and facial bones; Hutchinson's incisors, mulberry molars, glossitis, mucous patches, and fissures at corner of mouth	Tooth deformities in permanent dentition irreversible

(*continued*)

TABLE 2-1

VESICULAR, BULLOUS, OR ULCERATIVE LESIONS OF THE ORAL MUCOSA (*CONTINUED*)

CONDITION	USUAL LOCATION	CLINICAL FEATURES	COURSE
Primary syphilis (chancre)	Lesion appearing where organism enters body; may occur on lips, tongue, or tonsillar area	Small papule developing rapidly into a large, painless ulcer with indurated border; unilateral lymphadenopathy; chancre and lymph nodes containing spirochetes; serologic tests positive by third to fourth weeks	Healing of chancre in 1–2 months, followed by secondary syphilis in 6–8 weeks
Secondary syphilis	Oral mucosa frequently involved with mucous patches, which occur primarily on palate and also at commissures of mouth	Maculopapular lesions of oral mucosa, 5–10 mm in diameter with central ulceration covered by grayish membrane; eruptions occurring on various mucosal surfaces and skin, accompanied by fever, malaise, and sore throat	Lesions may persist from several weeks to a year
Tertiary syphilis	Palate and tongue	Gummatous infiltration of palate or tongue followed by ulceration and fibrosis; atrophy of tongue papillae produces characteristic bald tongue and glossitis	Gumma may destroy palate, causing complete perforation
Gonorrhea	Lesions may occur in mouth at site of inoculation or secondarily by hematogenous spread from a primary focus	Most pharyngeal infection is asymptomatic; may produce burning or itching sensation; oropharynx and tonsils may be ulcerated and erythematous; saliva viscous and fetid	More difficult to eradicate than urogenital infection, though pharyngitis usually resolves with appropriate antimicrobial treatment
Tuberculosis	Tongue, tonsillar area, soft palate	Painless, solitary, 1- to 5-cm, irregular ulcer covered with persistent exudate; ulcer has firm undermined border	Autoinoculation from pulmonary infection is usual; lesions resolve with appropriate antimicrobial therapy
Cervicofacial actinomycosis	Swellings in region of face, neck, and floor of mouth	Infection may be associated with extraction, jaw fracture, or eruption of molar tooth; in acute form, resembles acute pyogenic abscess, but contains yellow "sulfur granules" (gram-positive mycelia and their hyphae)	Typically, swelling is hard and grows painlessly; multiple abscesses with draining tracts develop; penicillin first choice; surgery usually necessary
Histoplasmosis	Any area of the mouth, particularly tongue, gingiva, or palate	Nodular, verrucous, or granulomatous lesions; ulcers are indurated and painful; usual source hematogenous or pulmonary, but may be primary	Systemic antifungal therapy necessary
Candidiasis[a]			
Dermatologic Diseases			
Mucous membrane pemphigoid	Typically produces marked gingival erythema and ulceration; other areas of oral cavity, esophagus, and vagina may be affected	Painful, grayish-white collapsed vesicles or bullae of full-thickness epithelium with peripheral erythematous zone; gingival lesions desquamate, leaving ulcerated area	Protracted course with remissions and exacerbations; involvement of different sites develops slowly; glucocorticoids may temporarily reduce symptoms but do not control disease
EM minor and EM major (Stevens-Johnson syndrome)	Primarily oral mucosa and skin of hands and feet	Intraoral ruptured bullae surrounded by inflammatory area; lips may show hemorrhagic crusts; "iris" or "target" lesion on skin is pathognomonic; patient may have severe signs of toxicity	Onset very rapid; usually idiopathic, but may be associated with trigger such as drug reaction; condition may last 3–6 weeks; mortality rate for untreated EM major is 5–15%

(*continued*)

TABLE 2-1

VESICULAR, BULLOUS, OR ULCERATIVE LESIONS OF THE ORAL MUCOSA (*CONTINUED*)

CONDITION	USUAL LOCATION	CLINICAL FEATURES	COURSE
Pemphigus vulgaris	Oral mucosa and skin; sites of mechanical trauma (soft/hard palate, frenulum, lips, buccal mucosa)	Usually (>70%) presents with oral lesions; fragile, ruptured bullae and ulcerated oral areas; mostly in older adults	With repeated occurrence of bullae, toxicity may lead to cachexia, infection, and death within 2 years; often controllable with oral glucocorticoids
Lichen planus	Oral mucosa and skin	White striae in mouth; purplish nodules on skin at sites of friction; occasionally causes oral mucosal ulcers and erosive gingivitis	White striae alone usually asymptomatic; erosive lesions often difficult to treat, but may respond to glucocorticoids
Other Conditions			
Recurrent aphthous ulcers	Usually on nonkeratinized oral mucosa (buccal and labial mucosa, floor of mouth, soft palate, lateral and ventral tongue)	Single or clustered painful ulcers with surrounding erythematous border; lesions may be 1–2 mm in diameter in crops (herpetiform), 1–5 mm (minor), or 5–15 mm (major)	Lesions heal in 1–2 weeks but may recur monthly or several times a year; protective barrier with benzocaine and topical glucocorticoids relieve symptoms; systemic glucocorticoids may be needed in severe cases
Behçet's syndrome	Oral mucosa, eyes, genitalia, gut, and CNS	Multiple aphthous ulcers in mouth; inflammatory ocular changes, ulcerative lesions on genitalia; inflammatory bowel disease and CNS disease	Oral lesions often first manifestation; persist several weeks and heal without scarring
Traumatic ulcers	Anywhere on oral mucosa; dentures frequently responsible for ulcers in vestibule	Localized, discrete ulcerated lesions with red border; produced by accidental biting of mucosa, penetration by foreign object, or chronic irritation by dentures	Lesions usually heal in 7–10 days when irritant is removed, unless secondarily infected
Squamous cell carcinoma	Any area of mouth, most commonly on lower lip, lateral borders of tongue, and floor of mouth	Red, white, or red and white ulcer with elevated or indurated border; failure to heal; pain not prominent in early lesions	Invades and destroys underlying tissues; frequently metastasizes to regional lymph nodes
Acute myeloid leukemia (usually monocytic)	Gingiva	Gingival swelling and superficial ulceration followed by hyperplasia of gingiva with extensive necrosis and hemorrhage; deep ulcers may occur elsewhere on mucosa, complicated by secondary infection	Usually responds to systemic treatment of leukemia; occasionally requires local irradiation
Lymphoma	Gingiva, tongue, palate, and tonsillar area	Elevated, ulcerated area that may proliferate rapidly, giving appearance of traumatic inflammation	Fatal if untreated; may indicate underlying HIV infection
Chemical or thermal burns	Any area in mouth	White slough due to contact with corrosive agents (e.g., aspirin, hot cheese) applied locally; removal of slough leaves raw, painful surface	Lesion heals in several weeks if not secondarily infected

[a]See Table 2-3.
Abbreviations: CNS, central nervous system; EM, erythema multiforme; HSV, herpes simplex virus; VZV, varicella-zoster virus.

entities and to distinguish them from *lichen planus* and drug reactions.

Hematologic and nutritional disease

Internists are more likely to encounter patients with acquired, rather than congenital, bleeding disorders. Bleeding should stop 15 min after minor trauma and within an hour after tooth extraction if local pressure is applied. More prolonged bleeding, if not due to continued injury or rupture of a large vessel, should lead to investigation for a clotting abnormality. In addition to bleeding, petechiae and ecchymoses are prone to occur at the vibrating line between the soft and hard palates in patients with platelet dysfunction or thrombocytopenia.

TABLE 2-2

PIGMENTED LESIONS OF THE ORAL MUCOSA

CONDITION	USUAL LOCATION	CLINICAL FEATURES	COURSE
Oral melanotic macule	Any area of mouth	Discrete or diffuse, localized, brown to black macule	Remains indefinitely; no growth
Diffuse melanin pigmentation	Any area of mouth	Diffuse pale to dark-brown pigmentation; may be physiologic ("racial") or due to smoking	Remains indefinitely
Nevi	Any area of mouth	Discrete, localized, brown to black pigmentation	Remains indefinitely
Malignant melanoma	Any area of mouth	Can be flat and diffuse, painless, brown to black; or can be raised and nodular	Expands and invades early; metastasis leads to death
Addison's disease	Any area of mouth, but mostly buccal mucosa	Blotches or spots of bluish-black to dark-brown pigmentation occurring early in disease, accompanied by diffuse pigmentation of skin; other symptoms of adrenal insufficiency	Condition controlled by adrenal steroid replacement
Peutz-Jeghers syndrome	Any area of mouth	Dark-brown spots on lips, buccal mucosa, with characteristic distribution of pigment around lips, nose, and eyes and on hands; concomitant intestinal polyposis	Oral pigmented lesions remain indefinitely; gastrointestinal polyps may become malignant
Drug ingestion (neuroleptics, oral contraceptives, minocycline, zidovudine, quinine derivatives)	Any area of mouth	Brown, black, or gray areas of pigmentation	Gradually disappears following cessation of drug intake
Amalgam tattoo	Gingiva and alveolar mucosa	Small blue-black pigmented areas associated with embedded amalgam particles in soft tissues; may show up on radiographs as radiopaque particles in some cases	Remains indefinitely
Heavy metal pigmentation (bismuth, mercury, lead)	Gingival margin	Thin blue-black pigmented line along gingival margin; rarely seen except in children exposed to lead-based paint	Indicative of systemic absorption; no significance for oral health
Black hairy tongue	Dorsum of tongue	Elongation of filiform papillae of tongue, which become stained by coffee, tea, tobacco, or pigmented bacteria	Improves within 1–2 weeks with gentle brushing of tongue or (if due to bacterial overgrowth) discontinuation of antibiotic
Fordyce spots	Buccal and labial mucosa	Numerous small yellowish spots just beneath mucosal surface; no symptoms; due to hyperplasia of sebaceous glands	Benign; remains without apparent change
Kaposi's sarcoma	Palate most common, but may occur at any other site	Red or blue plaques of variable size and shape; often enlarge, become nodular, and may ulcerate	Usually indicative of HIV infection or non-Hodgkin's lymphoma; rarely fatal, but may require treatment for comfort or cosmesis
Mucous retention cysts	Buccal and labial mucosa	Bluish, clear fluid–filled cyst due to extravasated mucus from injured minor salivary gland	Benign; painless unless traumatized; may be removed surgically

TABLE 2-3

WHITE LESIONS OF ORAL MUCOSA

CONDITION	USUAL LOCATION	CLINICAL FEATURES	COURSE
Lichen planus	Buccal mucosa, tongue, gingiva, and lips; skin	Striae, white plaques, red areas, ulcers in mouth; purplish papules on skin; may be asymptomatic, sore, or painful; lichenoid drug reactions may look similar	Protracted; responds to topical glucocorticoids
White sponge nevus	Oral mucosa, vagina, anal mucosa	Painless white thickening of epithelium; adolescence/early adulthood onset; familial	Benign and permanent
Smoker's leukoplakia and smokeless tobacco lesions	Any area of oral mucosa, sometimes related to location of habit	White patch that may become firm, rough, or red-fissured and ulcerated; may become sore and painful but is usually painless	May or may not resolve with cessation of habit; 2% of patients develop squamous cell carcinoma; early biopsy essential
Erythroplakia with or without white patches	Floor of mouth commonly affected in men; tongue and buccal mucosa in women	Velvety, reddish plaque; occasionally mixed with white patches or smooth red areas	High risk of squamous cell cancer; early biopsy essential
Candidiasis	Any area in mouth	*Pseudomembranous type* ("thrush"): creamy white curdlike patches that reveal a raw, bleeding surface when scraped; found in sick infants, debilitated elderly patients receiving high-dose glucocorticoids or broad-spectrum antibiotics, and patients with AIDS	Responds favorably to antifungal therapy and correction of predisposing causes where possible
		Erythematous type: flat, red, sometimes sore areas in same groups of patients	Course same as for pseudomembranous type
		Candidal leukoplakia: nonremovable white thickening of epithelium due to *Candida*	Responds to prolonged antifungal therapy
		Angular cheilitis: sore fissures at corner of mouth	Responds to topical antifungal therapy
Hairy leukoplakia	Usually on lateral tongue, rarely elsewhere on oral mucosa	White areas ranging from small and flat to extensive accentuation of vertical folds; found in HIV carriers (all risk groups for AIDS)	Due to Epstein-Barr virus; responds to high-dose acyclovir but recurs; rarely causes discomfort unless secondarily infected with *Candida*
Warts (human papillomavirus)	Anywhere on skin and oral mucosa	Single or multiple papillary lesions with thick, white, keratinized surfaces containing many pointed projections; cauliflower lesions covered with normal-colored mucosa or multiple pink or pale bumps (focal epithelial hyperplasia)	Lesions grow rapidly and spread; squamous cell carcinoma must be ruled out with biopsy; excision or laser therapy; may regress in HIV-infected patients receiving antiretroviral therapy

TABLE 2-4

ALTERATIONS OF THE TONGUE

TYPE OF CHANGE	CLINICAL FEATURES
Size or Morphology	
Macroglossia	Enlarged tongue that may be part of a syndrome found in developmental conditions such as Down syndrome, Simpson-Golabi-Behmel syndrome, or Beckwith-Wiedemann syndrome; may be due to tumor (hemangioma or lymphangioma), metabolic disease (e.g., primary amyloidosis), or endocrine disturbance (e.g., acromegaly or cretinism); may occur when all teeth are removed
Fissured ("scrotal") tongue	Dorsal surface and sides of tongue covered by painless shallow or deep fissures that may collect debris and become irritated

(*continued*)

TABLE 2-4

ALTERATIONS OF THE TONGUE (*CONTINUED*)

TYPE OF CHANGE	CLINICAL FEATURES
Median rhomboid glossitis	Congenital abnormality with ovoid, denuded area in median posterior portion of tongue; may be associated with candidiasis and may respond to antifungal treatment
Color	
"Geographic" tongue (benign migratory glossitis)	Asymptomatic inflammatory condition of tongue, with rapid loss and regrowth of filiform papillae leading to appearance of denuded red patches "wandering" across surface
Hairy tongue	Elongation of filiform papillae of medial dorsal surface area due to failure of keratin layer of papillae to desquamate normally; brownish-black coloration may be due to staining by tobacco, food, or chromogenic organisms
"Strawberry" and "raspberry" tongue	Appearance of tongue during scarlet fever due to hypertrophy of fungiform papillae as well as changes in filiform papillae
"Bald" tongue	Atrophy may be associated with xerostomia, pernicious anemia, iron-deficiency anemia, pellagra, or syphilis; may be accompanied by painful burning sensation; may be an expression of erythematous candidiasis and respond to antifungal treatment

TABLE 2-5

ORAL LESIONS ASSOCIATED WITH HIV INFECTION

LESION MORPHOLOGY	ETIOLOGIES
Papules, nodules, plaques	Candidiasis (hyperplastic and pseudomembranous)[a] Condyloma acuminatum (human papillomavirus infection) Squamous cell carcinoma (preinvasive and invasive) Non-Hodgkin's lymphoma[a] Hairy leukoplakia[a]
Ulcers	Recurrent aphthous ulcers[a] Angular cheilitis Squamous cell carcinoma Acute necrotizing ulcerative gingivitis[a] Necrotizing ulcerative periodontitis[a] Necrotizing ulcerative stomatitis Non-Hodgkin's lymphoma[a] Viral infection (herpes simplex, herpes zoster, cytomegalovirus infection) Infection caused by *Mycobacterium tuberculosis* or *M. avium-intracellulare* Fungal infection (histoplasmosis, cryptococcosis, candidiasis, geotrichosis, aspergillosis) Bacterial infection (*Escherichia coli, Enterobacter cloacae, Klebsiella pneumoniae, Pseudomonas aeruginosa*) Drug reactions (single or multiple ulcers)
Pigmented lesions	Kaposi's sarcoma[a] Bacillary angiomatosis (skin and visceral lesions more common than oral) Zidovudine pigmentation (skin, nails, and occasionally oral mucosa) Addison's disease
Miscellaneous	Linear gingival erythema[a]

[a]Strongly associated with HIV infection.

All forms of leukemia, but particularly *acute myelomonocytic leukemia*, can produce gingival bleeding, ulcers, and gingival enlargement. Oral ulcers are a feature of agranulocytosis, and ulcers and mucositis are often severe complications of chemotherapy and radiation therapy for hematologic and other malignancies. *Plummer-Vinson syndrome* (iron deficiency, angular stomatitis, glossitis, and dysphagia) raises the risk of oral squamous cell cancer and esophageal cancer at the postcricoidal tissue web. Atrophic papillae and a red, burning tongue may occur with pernicious anemia. Deficiencies in B-group vitamins produce many of these same symptoms as well as oral ulceration and cheilosis.

Consequences of *scurvy* include swollen, bleeding gums; ulcers; and loosening of the teeth.

NONDENTAL CAUSES OF ORAL PAIN

Most, but not all, oral pain emanates from inflamed or injured tooth pulp or periodontal tissues. Nonodontogenic causes are often overlooked. In most instances, toothache is predictable and proportional to the stimulus applied, and an identifiable condition (e.g., caries, abscess) is found. Local anesthesia eliminates pain originating from dental or periodontal structures, but not referred pains. The most common nondental source of pain is myofascial pain referred from muscles of mastication, which become tender and ache with increased use. Many sufferers exhibit *bruxism* (grinding of the teeth) secondary to stress and anxiety. *Temporomandibular joint disorder* is closely related. It affects both sexes, with a higher prevalence among women. Features include pain, limited mandibular movement, and temporomandibular joint sounds. The etiologies are complex; malocclusion does not play the primary role once attributed to it. *Osteoarthritis* is a common cause of masticatory pain. Anti-inflammatory medication, jaw rest, soft foods, and heat provide relief. The temporomandibular joint is involved in 50% of patients with *rheumatoid arthritis*, and its involvement is usually a late feature of severe disease. Bilateral preauricular pain, particularly in the morning, limits range of motion.

Migrainous neuralgia may be localized to the mouth. Episodes of pain and remission without an identifiable cause and a lack of relief with local anesthesia are important clues. *Trigeminal neuralgia* (*tic douloureux*) can involve the entire branch or part of the mandibular or maxillary branch of the fifth cranial nerve and can produce pain in one or a few teeth. Pain may occur spontaneously or may be triggered by touching the lip or gingiva, brushing the teeth, or chewing. *Glossopharyngeal neuralgia* produces similar acute neuropathic symptoms in the distribution of the ninth cranial nerve. Swallowing, sneezing, coughing, or pressure on the tragus of the ear triggers pain that is felt in the base of the tongue, pharynx, and soft palate and may be referred to the temporomandibular joint. *Neuritis* involving the maxillary and mandibular divisions of the trigeminal nerve (e.g., maxillary sinusitis, neuroma, and leukemic infiltrate) is distinguished from ordinary toothache by the neuropathic quality of the pain. Occasionally, *phantom pain* follows tooth extraction. Pain and hyperalgesia behind the ear and on the side of the face in the day or so before facial weakness develops often constitute the earliest symptom of *Bell's palsy*. Likewise, similar symptoms may precede visible lesions of herpes zoster infecting the seventh nerve (*Ramsey-Hunt syndrome*) or trigeminal nerve. *Postherpetic neuralgia* may follow either condition. *Coronary ischemia* may produce pain exclusively in the face and jaw; as in typical angina pectoris, this pain is usually reproducible with increased myocardial demand. Aching in several upper molar or premolar teeth that is unrelieved by anesthetizing the teeth may point to *maxillary sinusitis*.

Giant cell arteritis is notorious for producing headache, but it may also produce facial pain or sore throat without headache. Jaw and tongue claudication with chewing or talking is relatively common. Tongue infarction is rare. Patients with subacute thyroiditis often experience pain referred to the face or jaw before the tenderness of the thyroid gland and transient hyperthyroidism are appreciated.

"Burning mouth syndrome" (*glossodynia*) occurs in the absence of an identifiable cause (e.g., vitamin B_{12} deficiency, iron deficiency, diabetes mellitus, low-grade *Candida* infection, food sensitivity, or subtle xerostomia) and predominantly affects postmenopausal women. The etiology may be neuropathic. Clonazepam, α-lipoic acid, and cognitive behavioral therapy have benefited some patients. Some cases associated with an angiotensin-converting enzyme inhibitor have remitted when treatment with the drug was discontinued.

DISEASES OF THE SALIVARY GLANDS

Saliva is essential to oral health. Its absence leads to dental caries, periodontal disease, and difficulties in wearing dental prostheses, masticating, and speaking. Its major components, water and mucin, serve as a cleansing solvent and lubricating fluid. In addition, saliva contains antimicrobial factors (e.g., lysozyme, lactoperoxidase, secretory IgA), epidermal growth factor, minerals, and buffering systems. The major salivary glands secrete intermittently in response to autonomic stimulation, which is high during a meal but low otherwise. Hundreds of minor glands in the lips and cheeks secrete mucus continuously throughout the day and night. Consequently, oral function becomes impaired when salivary function is reduced. The sensation of a dry mouth (*xerostomia*) is perceived when salivary flow is reduced by 50%. The most common etiology is medication, especially drugs with anticholinergic properties but also alpha and beta blockers, calcium channel blockers, and diuretics. Other causes include Sjögren's syndrome, chronic parotitis, salivary duct obstruction, diabetes mellitus, HIV/AIDS, and radiation therapy that includes the salivary glands in the field (e.g., for Hodgkin's disease and for head and neck cancer). Management involves the elimination or limitation of drying medications, preventive dental care, and supplementation with oral liquid or salivary substitutes. Sugarless mints or chewing gum may stimulate salivary secretion if dysfunction is mild. When sufficient exocrine tissue remains, pilocarpine or cevimeline has been shown to increase secretions. Commercial saliva substitutes or gels relieve dryness. Fluoride supplementation is critical to prevent caries.

Sialolithiasis presents most often as painful swelling but in some instances as only swelling or only pain. Conservative therapy consists of local heat, massage, and hydration. Promotion of salivary secretion with mints or lemon drops may flush out small stones. Antibiotic treatment is necessary when bacterial infection in suspected. In adults, *acute bacterial parotitis* is typically unilateral and most commonly affects postoperative, dehydrated, and debilitated patients. *Staphylococcus aureus* (including methicillin-resistant strains) and anaerobic bacteria are the most common pathogens. Chronic bacterial *sialadenitis* results from lowered salivary secretion and recurrent bacterial infection. When suspected bacterial infection is not responsive to therapy, the differential diagnosis should be expanded to include benign and malignant neoplasms, lymphoproliferative disorders, Sjögren's syndrome, sarcoidosis, tuberculosis, lymphadenitis, actinomycosis, and granulomatosis with polyangiitis. Bilateral nontender parotid enlargement occurs with diabetes mellitus, cirrhosis, bulimia, HIV/AIDS, and drugs (e.g., iodide, propylthiouracil).

Pleomorphic adenoma comprises two-thirds of all salivary neoplasms. The parotid is the principal salivary gland affected, and the tumor presents as a firm, slow-growing mass. Although this tumor is benign, its recurrence is common if resection is incomplete. Malignant tumors such as mucoepidermoid carcinoma, adenoid cystic carcinoma, and adenocarcinoma tend to grow relatively fast, depending upon grade. They may ulcerate and invade nerves, producing numbness and facial paralysis. Surgical resection is the primary treatment. Radiation therapy (particularly neutron-beam therapy) is used when surgery is not feasible and as post-resection for certain histologic types with a high risk of recurrence. Malignant salivary gland tumors have a 5-year survival rate of ~68%.

DENTAL CARE FOR MEDICALLY COMPLEX PATIENTS

Routine dental care (e.g., uncomplicated extraction, scaling and cleaning, tooth restoration, and root canal) is remarkably safe. The most common concerns regarding care of dental patients with medical disease are excessive bleeding for patients taking anticoagulants, infection of the heart valves and prosthetic devices from hematogenous seeding by the oral flora, and cardiovascular complications resulting from vasopressors used with local anesthetics during dental treatment. Experience confirms that the risk of any of these complications is very low.

Patients undergoing tooth extraction or alveolar and gingival surgery rarely experience uncontrolled bleeding when warfarin anticoagulation is maintained within the therapeutic range currently recommended for prevention of venous thrombosis, atrial fibrillation, or mechanical heart valve. Embolic complications and death, however, have been reported during subtherapeutic anticoagulation. Therapeutic anticoagulation should be confirmed before and continued through the procedure. Likewise, low-dose aspirin (e.g., 81–325 mg) can safely be continued. For patients taking aspirin and another antiplatelet medication (e.g., clopidogrel), the decision to continue the second antiplatelet medication should be based on individual consideration of the risks of thrombosis and bleeding.

Patients at risk for bacterial endocarditis should maintain optimal oral hygiene, including flossing, and have regular professional cleanings. Currently, guidelines recommend that prophylactic antibiotics be restricted to those patients at high risk for bacterial endocarditis who undergo dental and oral procedures involving significant manipulation of gingival or periapical tissue or penetration of the oral mucosa. If unexpected bleeding occurs, antibiotics given within 2 h after the procedure provide effective prophylaxis.

Hematogenous bacterial seeding from oral infection can undoubtedly produce late prosthetic-joint infection and therefore requires removal of the infected tissue (e.g., drainage, extraction, root canal) and appropriate antibiotic therapy. However, evidence that late prosthetic-joint infection follows routine dental procedures is lacking. For this reason, antibiotic prophylaxis is not recommended before dental surgery for patients with orthopedic pins, screws, and plates. Antibiotic prophylaxis is recommended for patients within the first 2 years after joint replacement who have inflammatory arthropathies, immunosuppression, type 1 diabetes mellitus, previous prosthetic-joint infection, hemophilia, or malnourishment.

Concern often arises regarding the use of vasoconstrictors to treat patients with hypertension and heart disease. Vasoconstrictors enhance the depth and duration of local anesthesia, thus reducing the anesthetic dose and potential toxicity. If intravascular injection is avoided, 2% lidocaine with 1:100,000 epinephrine (limited to a total of 0.036 mg of epinephrine) can be used safely in patients with controlled hypertension and stable coronary heart disease, arrhythmia, or congestive heart failure. Precautions should be taken with patients taking tricyclic antidepressants and nonselective beta blockers because these drugs may potentiate the effect of epinephrine.

Elective dental treatments should be postponed for at least 1 month and preferably for 6 months after myocardial infarction, after which the risk of reinfarction is low provided the patient is medically stable (e.g., stable rhythm, stable angina, and no heart failure). Patients who have suffered a stroke should have elective dental care deferred for 6 months. In both situations, effective stress reduction requires good pain control, including the use of the minimal amount of vasoconstrictor necessary to provide good hemostasis and local anesthesia.

Bisphosphonate therapy is associated with *osteonecrosis* of the jaw. However, the risk with oral bisphosphonate therapy is very low. Most patients affected have received high-dose aminobisphosphonate therapy for multiple myeloma or metastatic breast cancer and have undergone tooth extraction or dental surgery. Intraoral lesions, of which two-thirds are painful, appear as exposed yellow-white hard bone involving the mandible or maxilla. Screening tests for determining risk of osteonecrosis are unreliable. Patients slated for aminobisphosphonate therapy should receive preventive dental care that reduces the risk of infection and the need for future dentoalveolar surgery.

HALITOSIS

Halitosis typically emanates from the oral cavity or nasal passages. Volatile sulfur compounds resulting from bacterial decay of food and cellular debris account for the malodor. Periodontal disease, caries, acute forms of gingivitis, poorly fitting dentures, oral abscess, and tongue coating are common causes. Treatment includes correcting poor hygiene, treating infection, and tongue brushing. Hyposalivation can produce and exacerbate halitosis. Pockets of decay in the tonsillar crypts, esophageal diverticulum, esophageal stasis (e.g., achalasia, stricture), sinusitis, and lung abscess account for some instances. A few systemic diseases produce distinctive odors: renal failure (ammoniacal), hepatic (fishy), and ketoacidosis (fruity). *Helicobacter pylori* gastritis can also produce ammoniacal breath. If a patient presents because of concern about halitosis but no odor is detectable, then pseudohalitosis or halitophobia must be considered.

AGING AND ORAL HEALTH

While tooth loss and dental disease are not normal consequences of aging, a complex array of structural and functional changes that occur with age can affect oral health. Subtle changes in tooth structure (e.g., diminished pulp space and volume, sclerosis of dentinal tubules, and altered proportions of nerve and vascular pulp content) result in the elimination or diminution of pain sensitivity and a reduction in the reparative capacity of the teeth. In addition, age-associated fatty replacement of salivary acini may reduce physiologic reserve, thus increasing the risk of hyposalivation. In healthy older adults, there is minimal, if any, reduction in salivary flow.

Poor oral hygiene often results when general health fails or when patients lose manual dexterity and upper-extremity flexibility. This situation is particularly common among frail older adults and nursing home residents and must be emphasized because regular oral cleaning and dental care reduce the incidence of pneumonia and oral disease as well as the mortality risk in this population. Other risks for dental decay include limited lifetime fluoride exposure. Without assiduous care, decay can become quite advanced yet remain asymptomatic. Consequently, much of a tooth—or the entire tooth—can be destroyed before the patient is aware of the process.

Periodontal disease, a leading cause of tooth loss, is indicated by loss of alveolar bone height. More than 90% of the U.S. population has some degree of periodontal disease by age 50. Healthy adults who have not had significant alveolar bone loss by the sixth decade of life do not typically experience significant worsening with advancing age.

Complete edentulousness with advanced age, though less common than in previous decades, still affects ~50% of the U.S. population ≥85 years of age. Speech, mastication, and facial contours are dramatically affected. Edentulousness may also exacerbate obstructive sleep apnea, particularly in asymptomatic individuals who wear dentures. Dentures can improve verbal articulation and restore diminished facial contours. Mastication can also be restored; however, patients expecting dentures to facilitate oral intake are often disappointed. Accommodation to dentures requires a period of adjustment. Pain can result from friction or traumatic lesions produced by loose dentures. Poor fit and poor oral hygiene may permit the development of candidiasis. This fungal infection may be either asymptomatic or painful and is suggested by erythematous smooth or granular tissue conforming to an area covered by the appliance. Individuals with dentures and no natural teeth need regular (annual) professional oral examinations.

CHAPTER 3

ATLAS OF ORAL MANIFESTATIONS OF DISEASE

Samuel C. Durso ■ Janet A. Yellowitz

The health status of the oral cavity is linked to cardiovascular disease, diabetes, and other systemic illnesses. Thus, examining the oral cavity for signs of disease is a key part of the physical exam. This chapter presents numerous outstanding clinical photographs illustrating many of the conditions discussed in **Chap. 2**, Oral Manifestations of Disease. Conditions affecting the teeth, periodontal tissues, and oral mucosa are all represented.

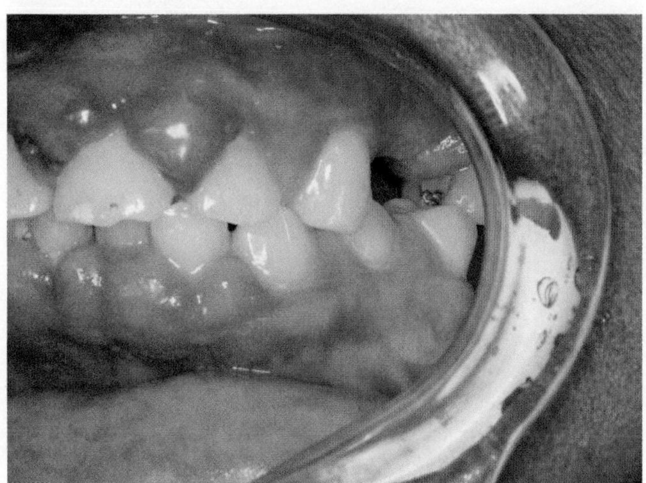

FIGURE 3-1
Gingival overgrowth secondary to calcium channel blocker use.

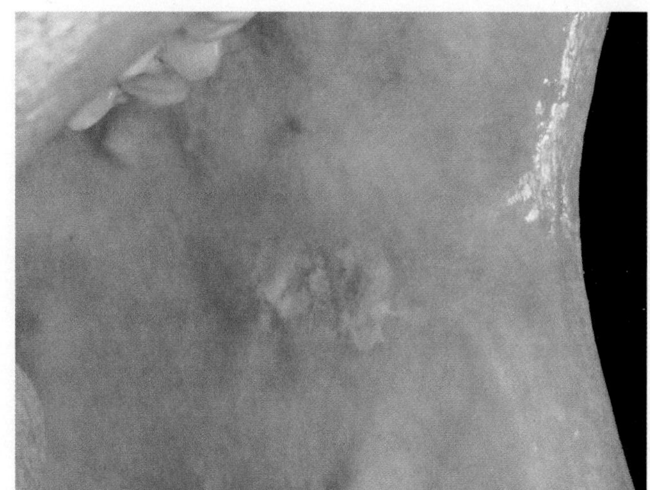

FIGURE 3-2
Oral lichen planus.

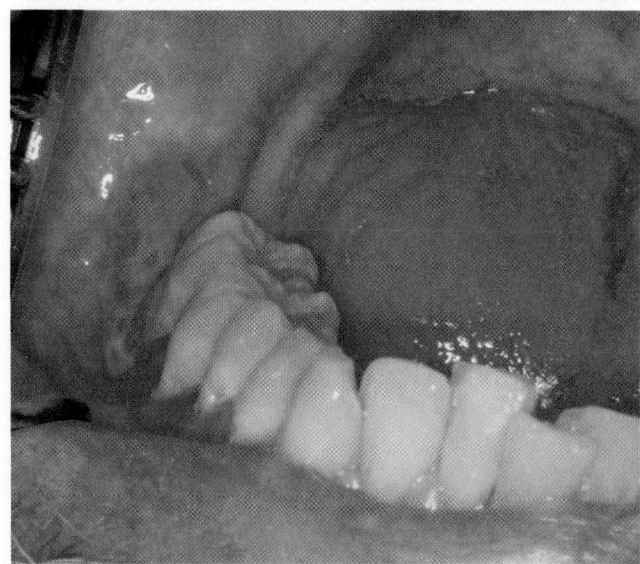

FIGURE 3-3
Erosive lichen planus.

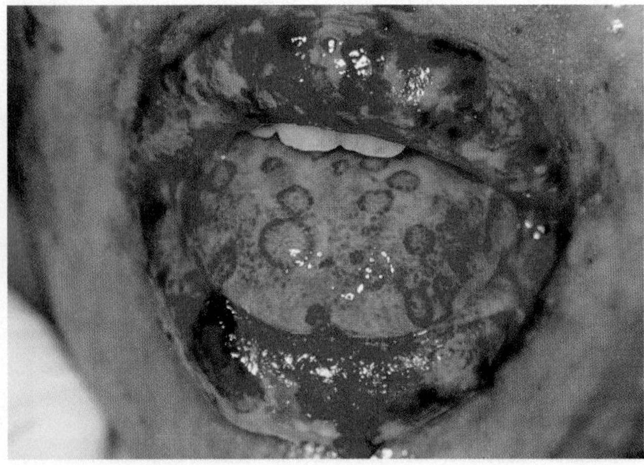

FIGURE 3-4
Stevens-Johnson syndrome—reaction to nevirapine.

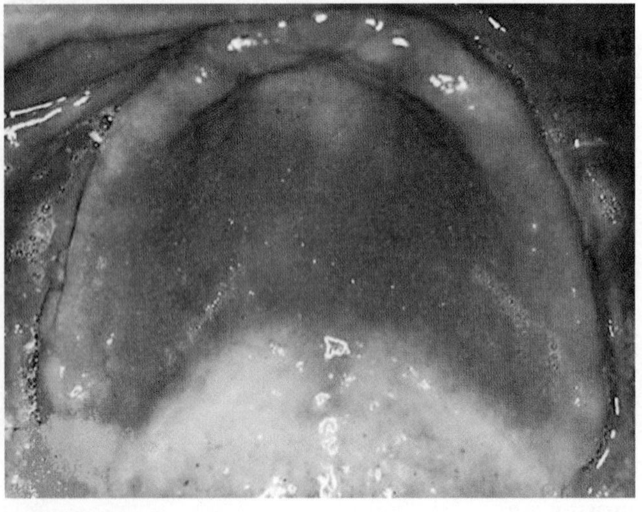

FIGURE 3-5
Erythematosus candidiasis under a denture (i.e., the patient should be treated for this fungal infection).

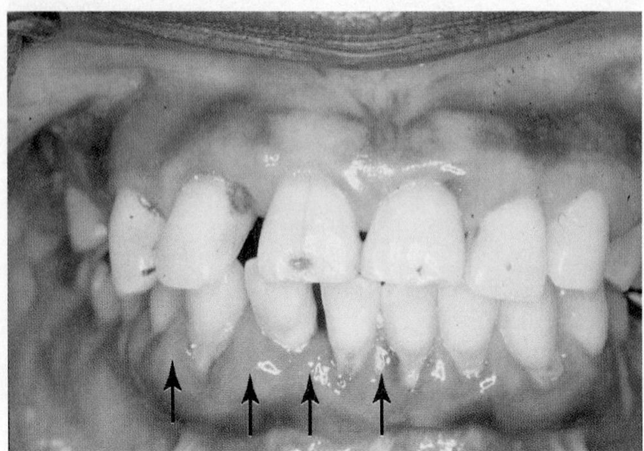

FIGURE 3-6
Severe periodontitis.

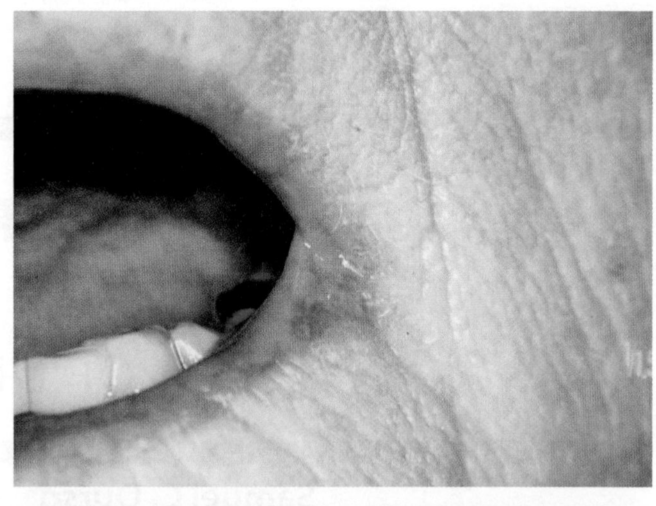

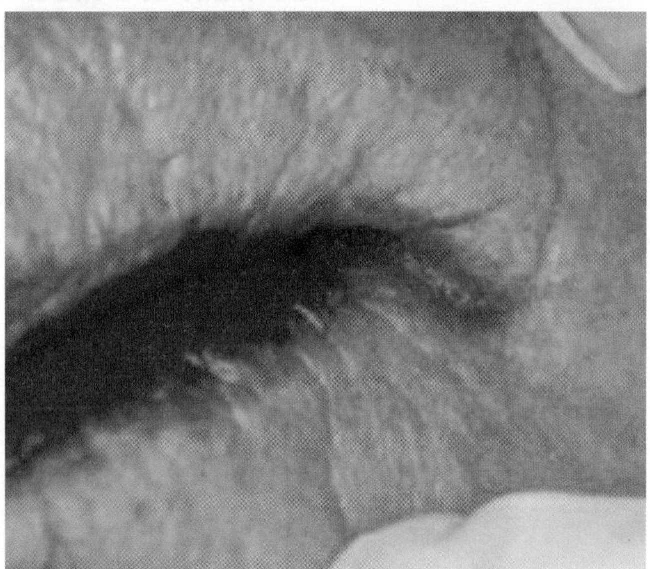

FIGURE 3-7
Angular cheilitis.

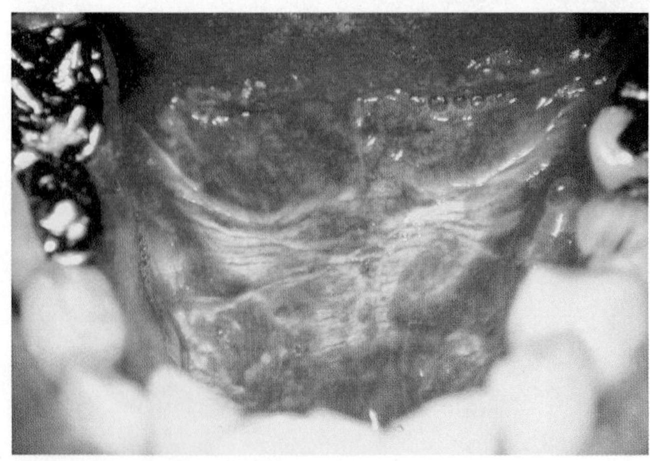

FIGURE 3-8
Sublingual leukoplakia.

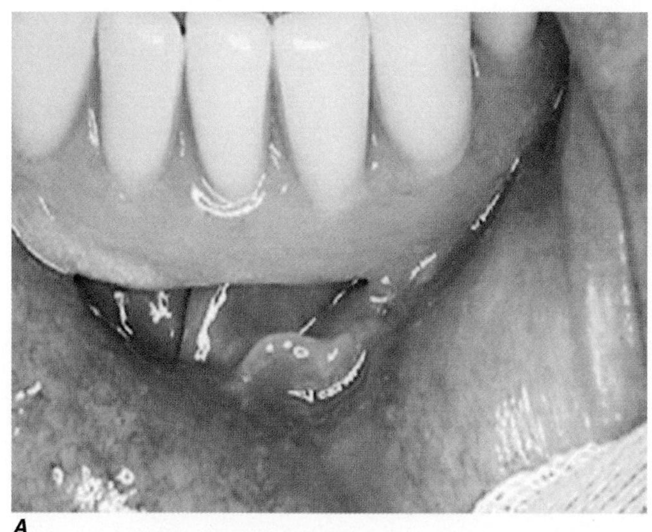
A

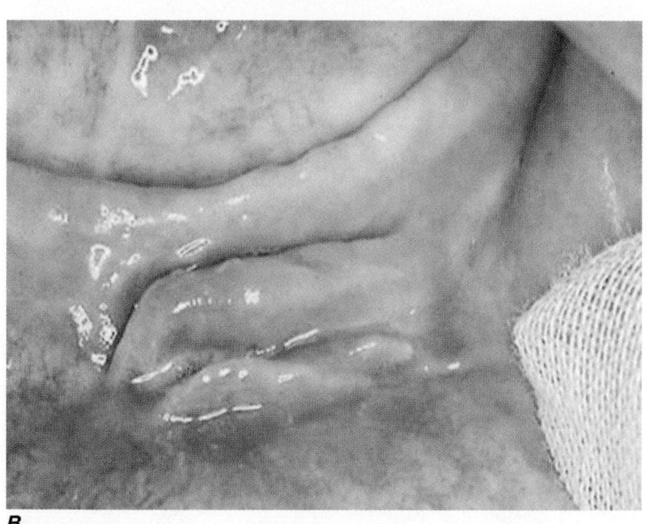
B

FIGURE 3-9
A. Epulis (gingival hypertrophy) under denture. ***B***. Epulis fissuratum.

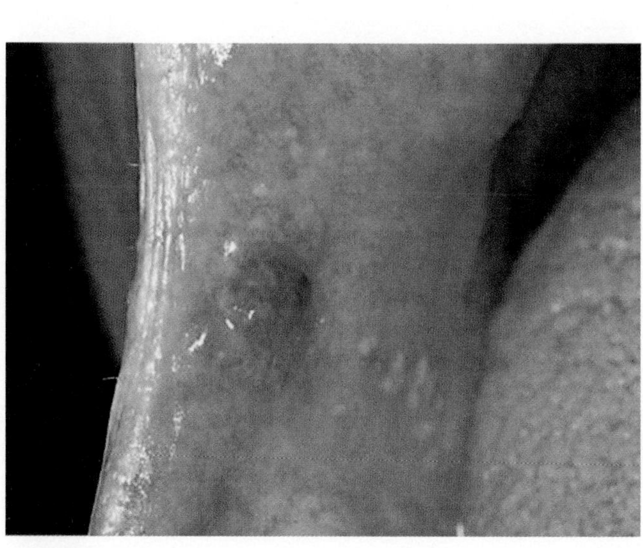

FIGURE 3-10
Traumatic lesion inside of cheek.

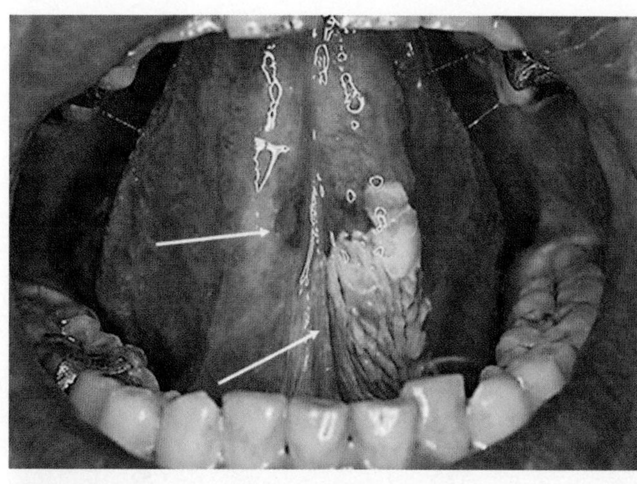

FIGURE 3-11
Oral leukoplakia, subtype homogenous leukoplakia.

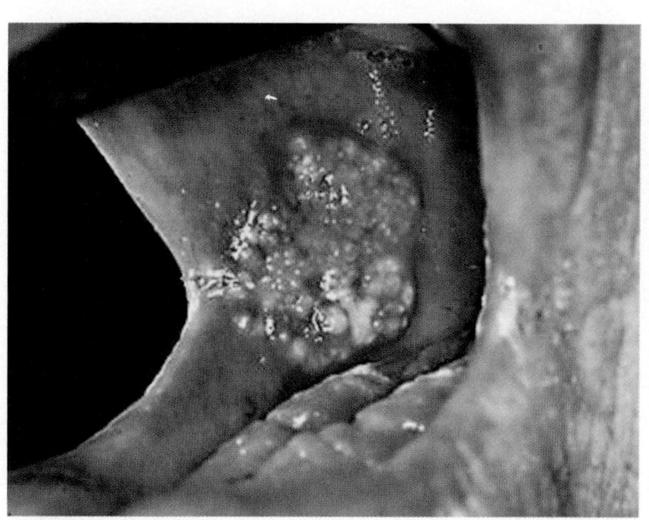

FIGURE 3-12
Oral carcinoma.

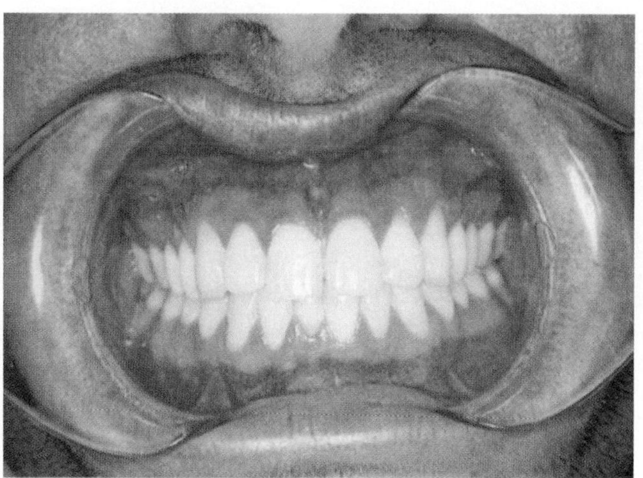

FIGURE 3-13
Healthy mouth.

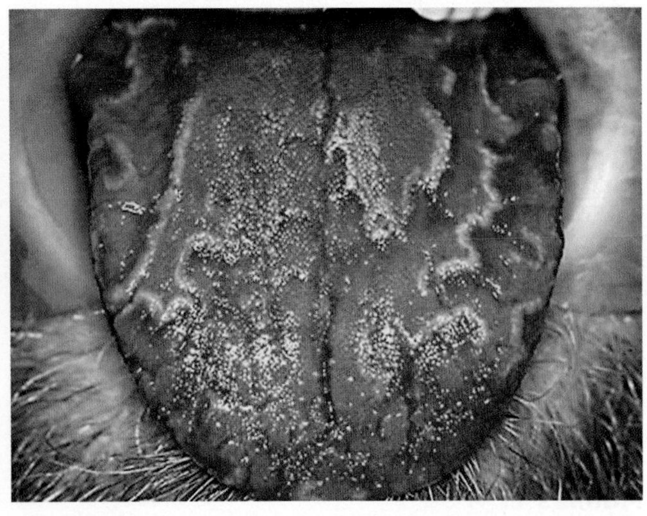

FIGURE 3-14
Geographic tongue.

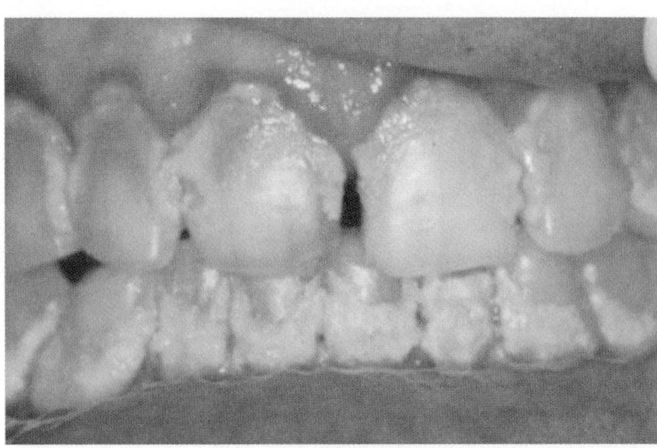

FIGURE 3-17
Heavy calculus and gingival inflammation.

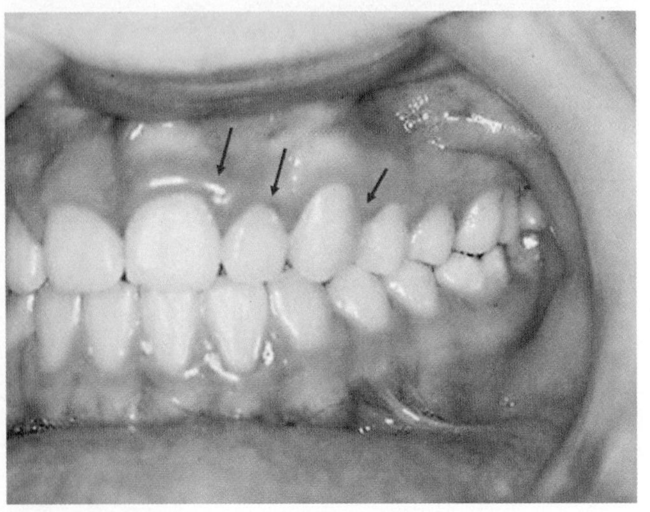

FIGURE 3-15
Moderate gingivitis.

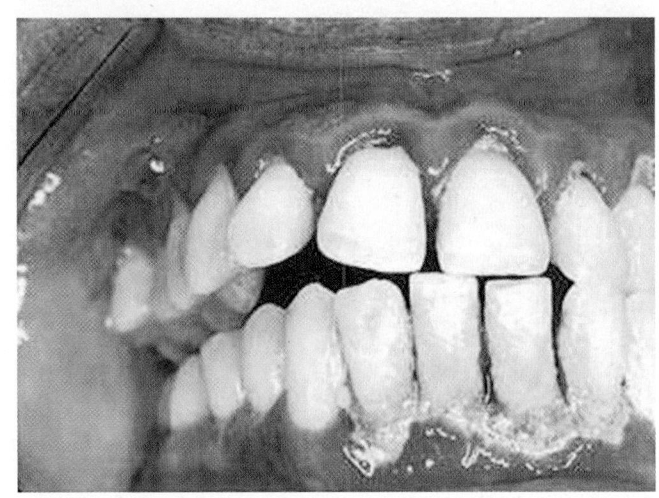

FIGURE 3-18
Severe gingival inflammation and heavy calculus.

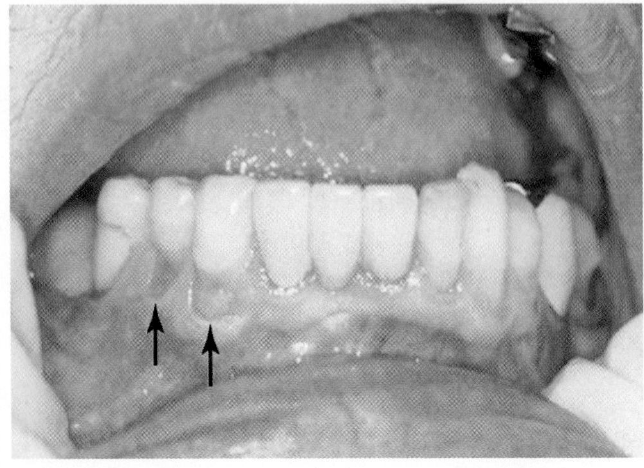

FIGURE 3-16
Gingival recession.

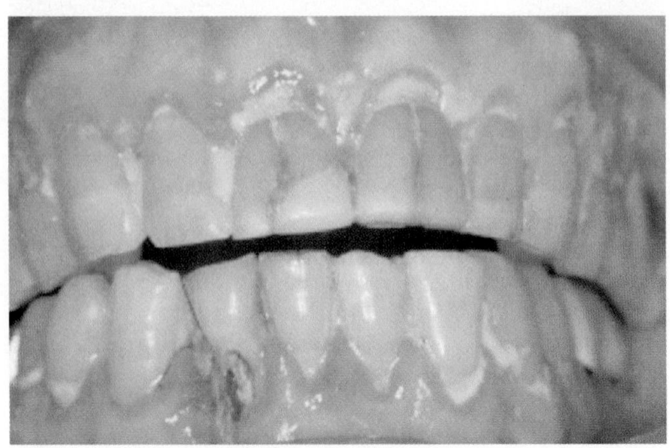

FIGURE 3-19
Root cavity in presence of severe periodontal disease.

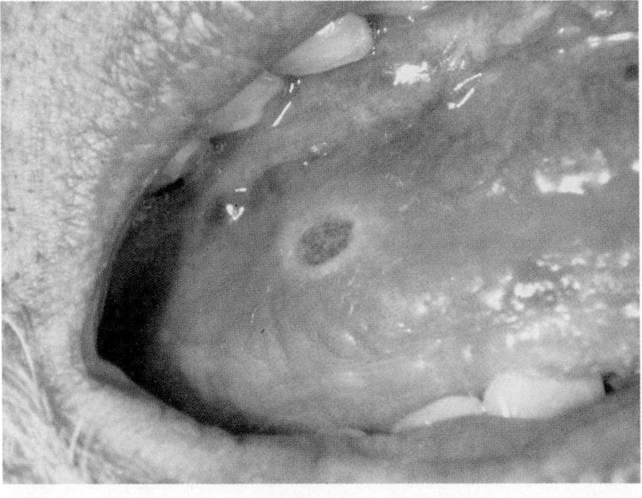

FIGURE 3-20
Ulcer on lateral border of tongue —potential carcinoma.

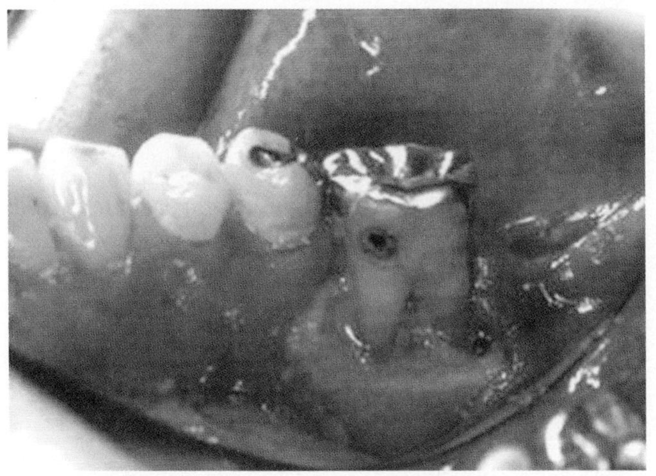

FIGURE 3-21
Osteonecrosis.

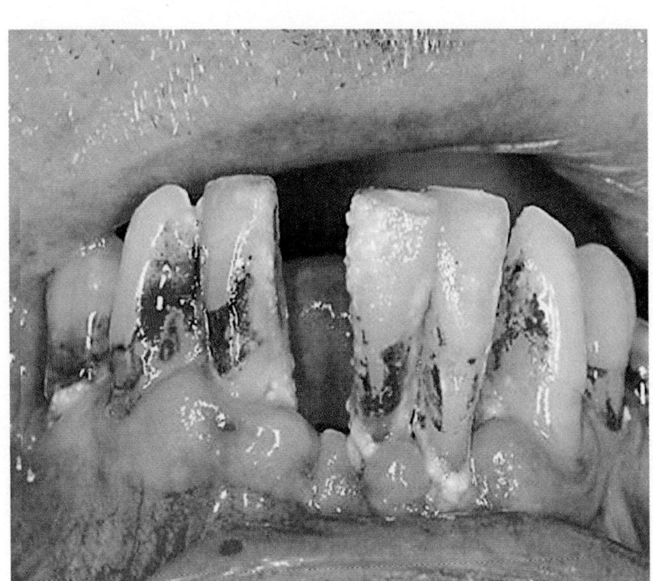

FIGURE 3-22
Severe periodontal disease, missing tooth, very mobile teeth.

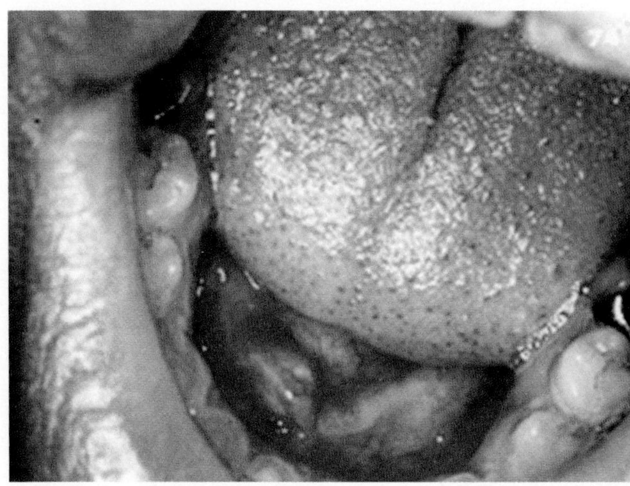

FIGURE 3-23
Salivary stone.

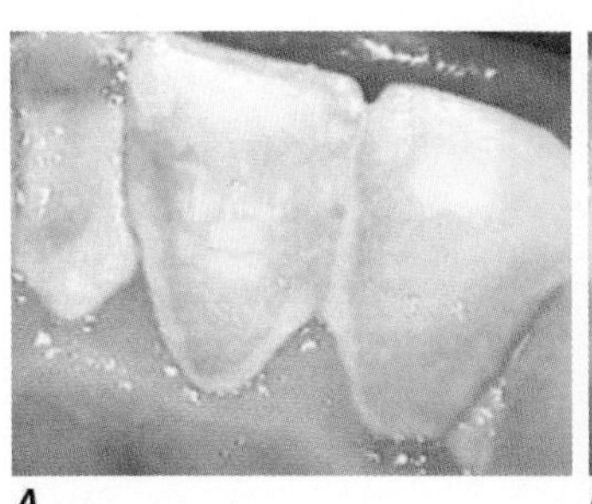

A *B*

FIGURE 3-24
A. Calculus. **B.** Teeth cleaned.

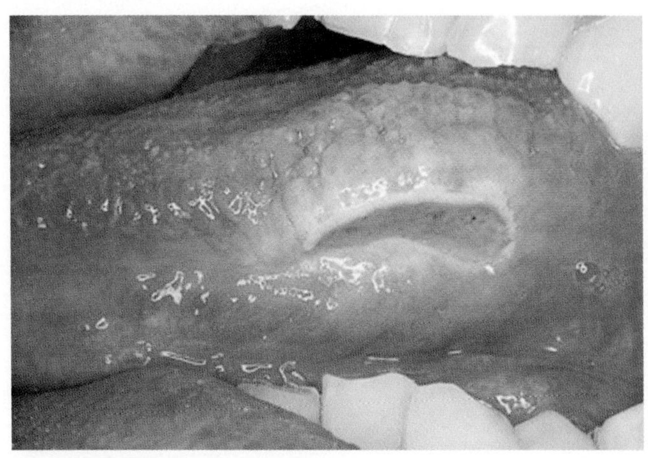

FIGURE 3-25
Traumatic ulcer.

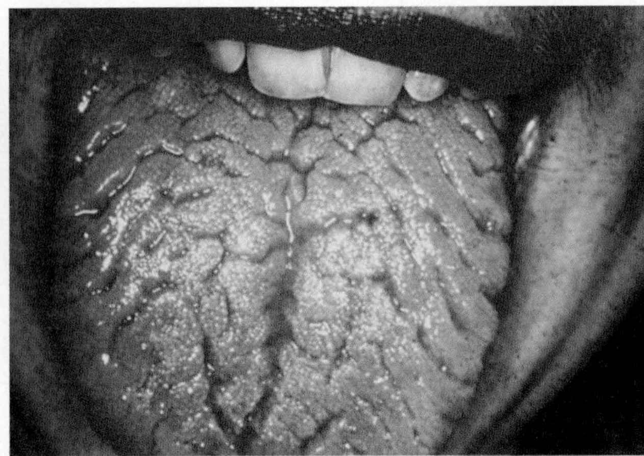

FIGURE 3-26
Fissured tongue.

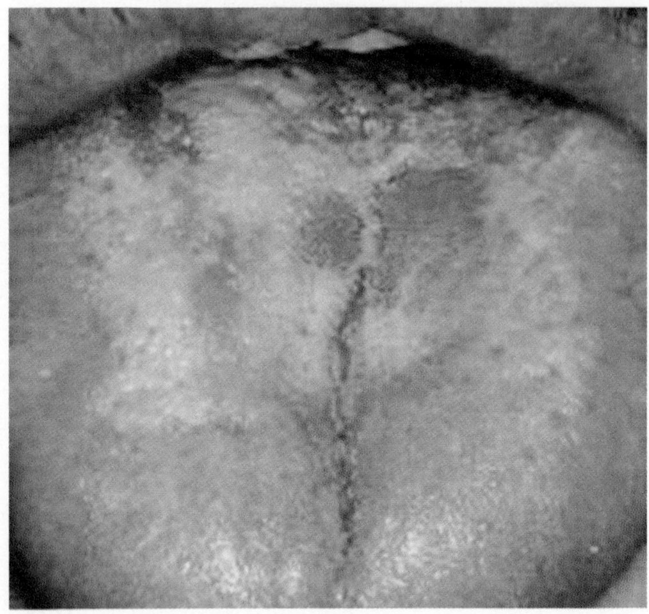

FIGURE 3-27
White coated tongue —likely candidiasis.

ACKNOWLEDGMENT

Dr. Jane Atkinson was a co-author of this chapter in the 17th edition of Harrison's Principles of Internal Medicine. Some of the materials have been carried over into this edition.

CHAPTER 4
DYSPHAGIA

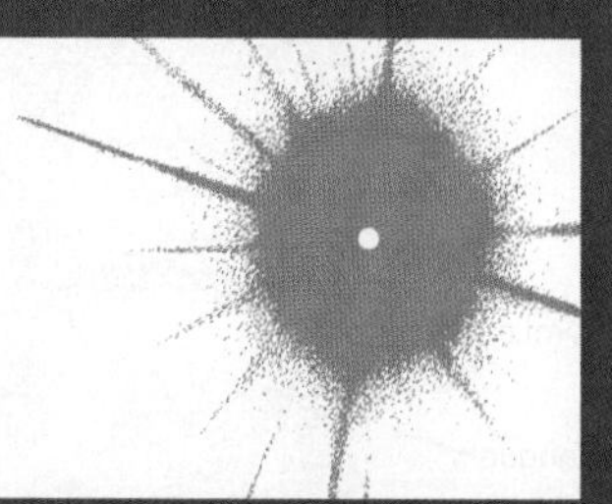

Ikuo Hirano ■ Peter J. Kahrilas

Dysphagia—difficulty with swallowing—refers to problems with the transit of food or liquid from the mouth to the hypopharynx or through the esophagus. Severe dysphagia can compromise nutrition, cause aspiration, and reduce quality of life. Additional terminology pertaining to swallowing dysfunction is as follows. *Aphagia* (inability to swallow) typically denotes complete esophageal obstruction, most commonly encountered in the acute setting of a food bolus or foreign body impaction. *Odynophagia* refers to painful swallowing, typically resulting from mucosal ulceration within the oropharynx or esophagus. It commonly is accompanied by dysphagia, but the converse is not true. *Globus pharyngeus* is a foreign body sensation localized in the neck that does not interfere with swallowing and sometimes is relieved by swallowing. *Transfer dysphagia* frequently results in nasal regurgitation and pulmonary aspiration during swallowing and is characteristic of oropharyngeal dysphagia. *Phagophobia* (fear of swallowing) and *refusal to swallow* may be psychogenic or related to anticipatory anxiety about food bolus obstruction, odynophagia, or aspiration.

PHYSIOLOGY OF SWALLOWING

Swallowing begins with a voluntary (oral) phase that includes preparation during which food is masticated and mixed with saliva. This is followed by a transfer phase during which the bolus is pushed into the pharynx by the tongue. Bolus entry into the hypopharynx initiates the pharyngeal swallow response, which is centrally mediated and involves a complex series of actions, the net result of which is to propel food through the pharynx into the esophagus while preventing its entry into the airway. To accomplish this, the larynx is elevated and pulled forward, actions that also facilitate upper esophageal sphincter (UES) opening. Tongue pulsion then propels the bolus through the UES, followed by a peristaltic contraction that clears residue from the pharynx and through the esophagus. The lower esophageal sphincter (LES) relaxes as the food enters the esophagus and remains relaxed until the peristaltic contraction has delivered the bolus into the stomach. Peristaltic contractions elicited in response to a swallow are called *primary peristalsis* and involve sequenced inhibition followed by contraction of the musculature along the entire length of the esophagus. The inhibition that precedes the peristaltic contraction is called *deglutitive inhibition*. Local distention of the esophagus anywhere along its length, as may occur with gastroesophageal reflux, activates *secondary peristalsis* that begins at the point of distention and proceeds distally. Tertiary esophageal contractions are nonperistaltic, disordered esophageal contractions that may be observed to occur spontaneously during fluoroscopic observation.

The musculature of the oral cavity, pharynx, UES, and cervical esophagus is striated and directly innervated by lower motor neurons carried in cranial nerves (Fig. 4-1). Oral cavity muscles are innervated by the fifth (trigeminal) and seventh (facial) cranial nerves; the tongue, by the twelfth (hypoglossal) cranial nerve. Pharyngeal muscles are innervated by the ninth (glossopharyngeal) and tenth (vagus) cranial nerves.

Physiologically, the UES consists of the cricopharyngeus muscle, the adjacent inferior pharyngeal constrictor, and the proximal portion of the cervical esophagus. UES innervation is derived from the vagus nerve, whereas the innervation to the musculature acting on the UES to facilitate its opening during swallowing comes from the fifth, seventh, and twelfth cranial nerves. The UES remains closed at rest owing to both its inherent elastic properties and neurogenically mediated contraction of the cricopharyngeus muscle. UES opening during swallowing involves both cessation of vagal excitation to the cricopharyngeus and simultaneous contraction of the suprahyoid and geniohyoid muscles that pull open the UES in conjunction with the upward and forward displacement of the larynx.

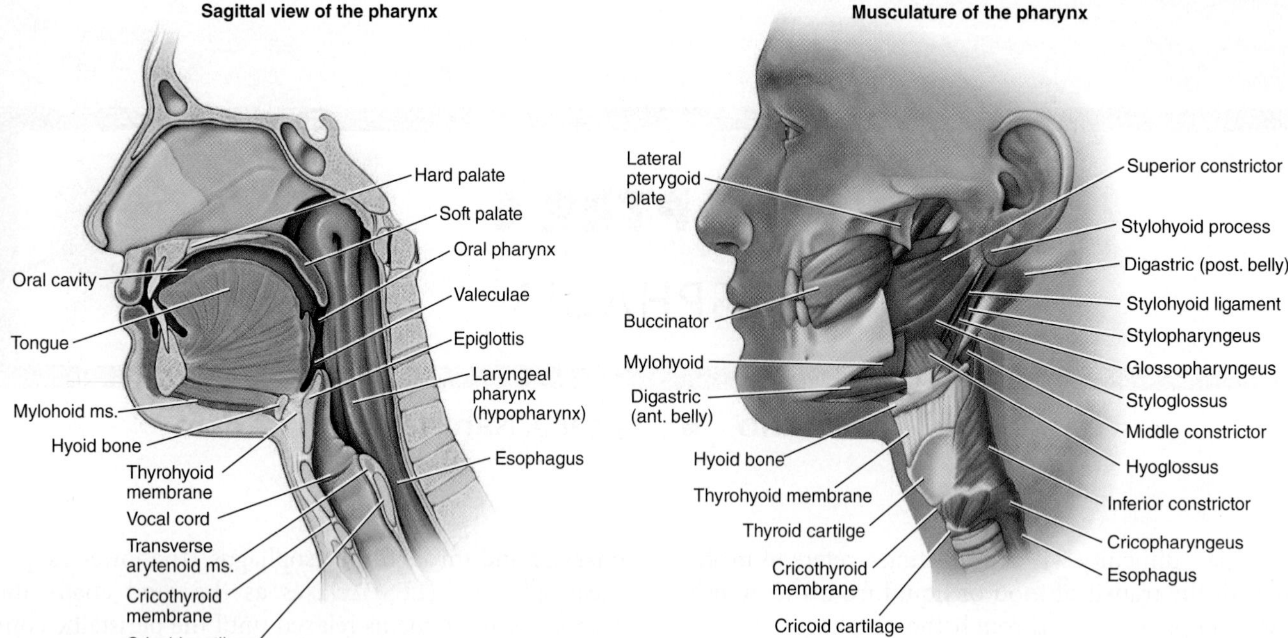

FIGURE 4-1

Sagittal and diagrammatic views of the musculature involved in enacting oropharyngeal swallowing. Note the dominance of the tongue in the sagittal view and the intimate relationship between the entrance to the larynx (airway) and the esophagus. In the resting configuration illustrated, the esophageal inlet is closed. This is transiently reconfigured such that the esophageal inlet is open and the laryngeal inlet closed during swallowing. *(Adapted from PJ Kahrilas, in DW Gelfand and JE Richter [eds]: Dysphagia: Diagnosis and Treatment. New York: Igaku-Shoin Medical Publishers, 1989, pp. 11–28.)*

The neuromuscular apparatus for peristalsis is distinct in proximal and distal parts of the esophagus. The cervical esophagus, like the pharyngeal musculature, consists of striated muscle and is directly innervated by lower motor neurons of the vagus nerve. Peristalsis in the proximal esophagus is governed by the sequential activation of the vagal motor neurons in the nucleus ambiguus. In contrast, the distal esophagus and LES are composed of smooth muscle and are controlled by excitatory and inhibitory neurons within the esophageal myenteric plexus. Medullary preganglionic neurons from the dorsal motor nucleus of the vagus trigger peristalsis via these ganglionic neurons during primary peristalsis. Neurotransmitters of the excitatory ganglionic neurons are acetylcholine and substance P; those of the inhibitory neurons are vasoactive intestinal peptide and nitric oxide. Peristalsis results from the patterned activation of inhibitory followed by excitatory ganglionic neurons, with progressive dominance of the inhibitory neurons distally. Similarly, LES relaxation occurs with the onset of deglutitive inhibition and persists until the peristaltic sequence is complete. At rest, the LES is contracted because of excitatory ganglionic stimulation and its intrinsic myogenic tone, a property that distinguishes it from the adjacent esophagus. The function of the LES is supplemented by the surrounding muscle of the right diaphragmatic crus, which acts as an external sphincter during inspiration, cough, or abdominal straining.

PATHOPHYSIOLOGY OF DYSPHAGIA

Dysphagia can be subclassified both by location and by the circumstances in which it occurs. With respect to location, distinct considerations apply to oral, pharyngeal, or esophageal dysphagia. Normal transport of an ingested bolus depends on the consistency and size of the bolus, the caliber of the lumen, the integrity of peristaltic contraction, and deglutitive inhibition of both the UES and the LES. Dysphagia caused by an oversized bolus or a narrow lumen is called *structural dysphagia*, whereas dysphagia due to abnormalities of peristalsis or impaired sphincter relaxation after swallowing is called *propulsive* or *motor dysphagia*. More than one mechanism may be operative in a patient with dysphagia. Scleroderma commonly presents with absent peristalsis as well as a weakened LES that predisposes patients to peptic stricture formation. Likewise, radiation therapy for head and neck cancer may compound the functional deficits in the oropharyngeal swallow attributable to the tumor and cause cervical esophageal stenosis.

Oral and pharyngeal (oropharyngeal) dysphagia

Oral-phase dysphagia is associated with poor bolus formation and control so that food has prolonged retention within the oral cavity and may seep out of the mouth. Drooling and difficulty in initiating swallowing are other characteristic signs. Poor bolus control also may lead to premature spillage of food into the hypopharynx with resultant aspiration into the trachea or regurgitation into the nasal cavity. Pharyngeal-phase dysphagia is associated with retention of food in the pharynx due to poor tongue or pharyngeal propulsion or obstruction at the UES. Signs and symptoms of concomitant hoarseness or cranial nerve dysfunction may be associated with oropharyngeal dysphagia.

Oropharyngeal dysphagia may be due to neurologic, muscular, structural, iatrogenic, infectious, and metabolic causes. Iatrogenic, neurologic, and structural pathologies are most common. Iatrogenic causes include surgery and radiation, often in the setting of head and neck cancer. Neurogenic dysphagia resulting from cerebrovascular accidents, Parkinson's disease, and amyotrophic lateral sclerosis is a major source of morbidity related to aspiration and malnutrition. Medullary nuclei directly innervate the oropharynx. Lateralization of pharyngeal dysphagia implies either a structural pharyngeal lesion or a neurologic process that selectively targeted the ipsilateral brainstem nuclei or cranial nerve. Advances in functional brain imaging have elucidated an important role of the cerebral cortex in swallow function and dysphagia. Asymmetry in the cortical representation of the pharynx provides an explanation for the dysphagia that occurs as a consequence of unilateral cortical cerebrovascular accidents.

Oropharyngeal structural lesions causing dysphagia include Zenker's diverticulum, cricopharyngeal bar, and neoplasia. Zenker's diverticulum typically is encountered in elderly patients, with an estimated prevalence between 1:1000 and 1:10,000. In addition to dysphagia, patients may present with regurgitation of particulate food debris, aspiration, and halitosis. The pathogenesis is related to stenosis of the cricopharyngeus that causes diminished opening of the UES and results in increased hypopharyngeal pressure during swallowing with development of a pulsion diverticulum immediately above the cricopharyngeus in a region of potential weakness known as Killian's dehiscence. A cricopharyngeal bar, appearing as a prominent indentation behind the lower third of the cricoid cartilage, is related to Zenker's diverticulum in that it involves limited distensibility of the cricopharyngeus and can lead to the formation of a Zenker's diverticulum. However, a cricopharyngeal bar is a common radiographic finding, and most patients with transient cricopharyngeal bars are asymptomatic, making it important to rule out alternative etiologies of dysphagia before treatment. Furthermore, cricopharyngeal bars may be secondary to other neuromuscular disorders.

Since the pharyngeal phase of swallowing occurs in less than a second, rapid-sequence fluoroscopy is necessary to evaluate for functional abnormalities. Adequate fluoroscopic examination requires that the patient be conscious and cooperative. The study incorporates recordings of swallow sequences during ingestion of food and liquids of varying consistencies. The pharynx is examined to detect bolus retention, regurgitation into the nose, or aspiration into the trachea. Timing and integrity of pharyngeal contraction and opening of the UES with a swallow are analyzed to assess both aspiration risk and the potential for swallow therapy. Structural abnormalities of the oropharynx, especially those which may require biopsies, also should be assessed by direct laryngoscopic examination.

Esophageal dysphagia

The adult esophagus measures 18–26 cm in length and is anatomically divided into the cervical esophagus, extending from the pharyngoesophageal junction to the suprasternal notch, and the thoracic esophagus, which continues to the diaphragmatic hiatus. When distended, the esophageal lumen has internal dimensions of about 2 cm in the anteroposterior plane and 3 cm in the lateral plane. Solid food dysphagia becomes common when the lumen is narrowed to <13 mm but also can occur with larger diameters in the setting of poorly masticated food or motor dysfunction. Circumferential lesions are more likely to cause dysphagia than are lesions that involve only a partial circumference of the esophageal wall. The most common structural causes of dysphagia are Schatzki's rings, eosinophilic esophagitis, and peptic strictures. Dysphagia also occurs in the setting of gastroesophageal reflux disease without a stricture, perhaps on the basis of altered esophageal sensation, distensibility, or motor function.

Propulsive disorders leading to esophageal dysphagia result from abnormalities of peristalsis and/or deglutitive inhibition, potentially affecting the cervical or thoracic esophagus. Since striated muscle pathology usually involves both the oropharynx and the cervical esophagus, the clinical manifestations usually are dominated by oropharyngeal dysphagia. Diseases affecting smooth muscle involve both the thoracic esophagus and the LES. A dominant manifestation of this, absent peristalsis, refers to either the complete absence of swallow-induced contraction or the presence of nonperistaltic, disordered contractions. Absent peristalsis and failure of deglutitive LES relaxation are the defining features of achalasia. In diffuse esophageal spasm (DES), LES function is normal, with the disordered motility restricted to the esophageal body. Absent peristalsis combined with severe weakness of the LES is a nonspecific pattern commonly found in patients with scleroderma.

APPROACH TO THE PATIENT: Dysphagia

Figure 4-2 shows an algorithm for the approach to a patient with dysphagia.

HISTORY The patient history is extremely valuable in making a presumptive diagnosis or at least substantially restricting the differential diagnoses in most patients. Key elements of the history are the localization of dysphagia, the circumstances in which dysphagia is experienced, other symptoms associated with dysphagia, and progression. Dysphagia that localizes to the suprasternal notch may indicate either an oropharyngeal or an esophageal etiology as distal dysphagia is referred proximally about 30% of the time. Dysphagia that localizes to the chest is esophageal in origin. Nasal regurgitation and tracheobronchial aspiration manifest by coughing with swallowing are hallmarks of oropharyngeal dysphagia. Severe cough with swallowing may also be a sign of a tracheoesophageal fistula. The presence of hoarseness may be another important diagnostic clue. When hoarseness precedes dysphagia, the primary lesion is usually laryngeal; hoarseness that occurs after the development of dysphagia may result from compromise of the recurrent laryngeal nerve by a malignancy. The type of food causing dysphagia is a crucial detail. Intermittent dysphagia that occurs only with solid food implies structural dysphagia, whereas constant dysphagia with both liquids and solids strongly suggests a motor abnormality. Two caveats to this pattern are that despite having a motor abnormality, patients with scleroderma generally develop mild dysphagia for solids only and, somewhat paradoxically, that patients with oropharyngeal dysphagia often have greater difficulty managing liquids than solids. Dysphagia that is progressive over the course of weeks to months raises concern for neoplasia. Episodic dysphagia to solids that is unchanged over years indicates a benign disease process such as a Schatzki's ring or eosinophilic esophagitis. Food impaction with a prolonged inability to pass an ingested bolus even with ingestion of liquid is typical of a structural dysphagia. Chest pain frequently accompanies dysphagia whether it is related to motor disorders, structural disorders, or reflux disease. A prolonged history of heartburn preceding the onset of dysphagia is suggestive of peptic stricture and, infrequently, esophageal adenocarcinoma. A history of prolonged nasogastric intubation, esophageal or head and neck surgery, ingestion of caustic agents or pills, previous radiation or chemotherapy, or associated mucocutaneous diseases may help isolate the cause of dysphagia. With accompanying odynophagia, which usually is indicative of

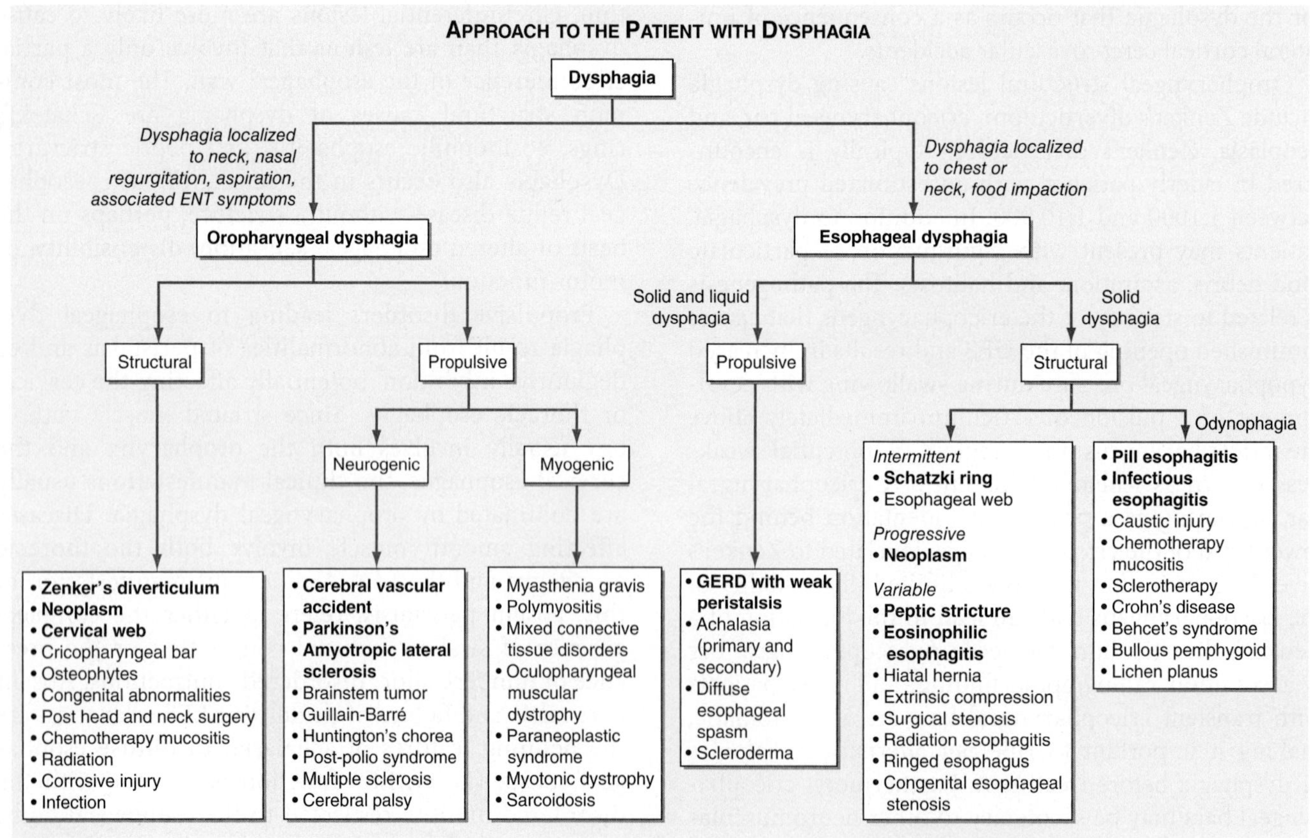

FIGURE 4-2

Approach to the patient with dysphagia. Etiologies in bold print are the most common. ENT, ear, nose, and throat; GERD, gastroesophageal reflux disease.

ulceration, infectious or pill-induced esophagitis should be suspected. In patients with AIDS or other immunocompromised states, esophagitis due to opportunistic infections such as *Candida*, herpes simplex virus, or cytomegalovirus and to tumors such as Kaposi's sarcoma and lymphoma should be considered. A strong history of atopy increases concerns for eosinophilic esophagitis.

PHYSICAL EXAMINATION Physical examination is important in the evaluation of oral and pharyngeal dysphagia because dysphagia is usually only one of many manifestations of a more global disease process. Signs of bulbar or pseudobulbar palsy, including dysarthria, dysphonia, ptosis, tongue atrophy, and hyperactive jaw jerk, in addition to evidence of generalized neuromuscular disease, should be elicited. The neck should be examined for thyromegaly. A careful inspection of the mouth and pharynx should disclose lesions that may interfere with passage of food. Missing dentition can interfere with mastication and exacerbate an existing cause of dysphagia. Physical examination is less helpful in the evaluation of esophageal dysphagia as most relevant pathology is restricted to the esophagus. The notable exception is skin disease. Changes in the skin may suggest a diagnosis of scleroderma or mucocutaneous diseases such as pemphigoid, lichen planus and epidermolysis bullosa, all of which can involve the esophagus.

DIAGNOSTIC PROCEDURES Although most instances of dysphagia are attributable to benign disease processes, dysphagia is also a cardinal symptom of several malignancies, making it an important symptom to evaluate. Cancer may result in dysphagia due to intraluminal obstruction (esophageal or proximal gastric cancer, metastatic deposits), extrinsic compression (lymphoma, lung cancer), or paraneoplastic syndromes. Even when not attributable to malignancy, dysphagia is usually a manifestation of an identifiable and treatable disease entity, making its evaluation beneficial to the patient and gratifying to the practitioner. The specific diagnostic algorithm to pursue is guided by the details of the history (Fig. 4-2). If oral or pharyngeal dysphagia is suspected, a fluoroscopic swallow study, usually done by a swallow therapist, is the procedure of choice. Otolaryngoscopic and neurologic evaluation also can be important, depending on the circumstances. For suspected esophageal dysphagia, upper endoscopy is the single most useful test. Endoscopy allows better visualization of mucosal lesions than does barium radiography and also allows one to obtain mucosal biopsies. Endoscopic or histologic abnormalities are evident in the leading causes of esophageal dysphagia: Schatzki ring, gastroesophageal reflux disease and eosinophilic esophagitis. Furthermore, therapeutic intervention with esophageal dilation can be done as part of the procedure if it is deemed necessary. The emergence of eosinophilic esophagitis as a leading cause of dysphagia in both children and adults has led to the recommendation that esophageal mucosal biopsies be obtained routinely in the evaluation of unexplained dysphagia even if endoscopically identified esophageal mucosal lesions are absent. For cases of suspected esophageal motility disorders, endoscopy is still the appropriate initial evaluation as neoplastic and inflammatory conditions can secondarily produce patterns of either achalasia or esophageal spasm. Esophageal manometry is done if dysphagia is not adequately explained by endoscopy or to confirm the diagnosis of a suspected esophageal motor disorder. Barium radiography can provide useful adjunctive information in cases of subtle or complex esophageal strictures, prior esophageal surgery, esophageal diverticula, or paraesophageal herniation. In specific cases, computed tomography (CT) examination and endoscopic ultrasonography may be useful.

TREATMENT Treatment of dysphagia depends on both the locus and the specific etiology. Oropharyngeal dysphagia most commonly results from functional deficits caused by neurologic disorders. In such circumstances, the treatment focuses on utilizing postures or maneuvers devised to reduce pharyngeal residue and enhance airway protection learned under the direction of a trained swallow therapist. Aspiration risk may be reduced by altering the consistency of ingested food and liquid. Dysphagia resulting from a cerebrovascular accident usually, but not always, spontaneously improves within the first few weeks after the event. More severe and persistent cases may require gastrostomy and enteral feeding. Patients with myasthenia gravis and polymyositis may respond to medical treatment of the primary neuromuscular disease. Surgical intervention with cricopharyngeal myotomy is usually not helpful, with the exception of specific disorders such as the idiopathic cricopharyngeal bar, Zenker's diverticulum, and oculopharyngeal muscular dystrophy. Chronic neurologic disorders such as Parkinson's disease and amyotrophic lateral sclerosis may manifest with severe oropharyngeal dysphagia. Feeding by a nasogastric tube or an endoscopically placed gastrostomy tube may be considered for nutritional support; however, these maneuvers do not provide protection against aspiration of salivary secretions or refluxed gastric contents.

Treatment of esophageal dysphagia is covered in detail in **Chap. 14**. The majority of causes of esophageal dysphagia are effectively managed by means of esophageal dilatation using bougie or balloon dilators. Cancer and achalasia are often managed surgically, although endoscopic techniques are available for both palliation and primary therapy, respectively. Infectious etiologies respond to antimicrobial medications or treatment of the underlying immunosuppressive state. Finally, eosinophilic esophagitis has emerged as an important cause of dysphagia that is amenable to treatment by elimination of dietary allergens or administration of swallowed, topically acting glucocorticoids.

CHAPTER 5

NAUSEA, VOMITING, AND INDIGESTION

William L. Hasler

Nausea is the subjective feeling of a need to vomit. *Vomiting* (emesis) is the oral expulsion of gastrointestinal contents due to contractions of gut and thoracoabdominal wall musculature. Vomiting is contrasted with *regurgitation,* the effortless passage of gastric contents into the mouth. *Rumination* is the repeated regurgitation of food residue, which may be rechewed and reswallowed. In contrast to emesis, these phenomena may exhibit volitional control. *Indigestion* is a term encompassing a range of complaints including nausea, vomiting, heartburn, regurgitation, and dyspepsia (the presence of symptoms thought to originate in the gastroduodenal region). Some individuals with dyspepsia report predominantly epigastric burning, gnawing, or pain. Others experience postprandial fullness, early satiety (an inability to complete a meal due to premature fullness), bloating, eructation (belching), and anorexia.

NAUSEA AND VOMITING

MECHANISMS

Vomiting is coordinated by the brainstem and is effected by responses in the gut, pharynx, and somatic musculature. Mechanisms underlying nausea are poorly understood but likely involve the cerebral cortex, as nausea requires conscious perception. This is supported by functional brain imaging studies showing activation of a range of cerebral cortical regions during nausea.

Coordination of emesis

Brainstem nuclei—including the nucleus tractus solitarius; dorsal vagal and phrenic nuclei; medullary nuclei regulating respiration; and nuclei that control pharyngeal, facial, and tongue movements—coordinate initiation of emesis. Neurokinin NK_1, serotonin $5\text{-}HT_3$, and vasopressin pathways participate in this coordination.

Somatic and visceral muscles respond stereotypically during emesis. Inspiratory thoracic and abdominal wall muscles contract, producing high intrathoracic and intraabdominal pressures that evacuate the stomach. The gastric cardia herniates above the diaphragm, and the larynx moves upward to propel the vomitus. Distally migrating gut contractions are normally regulated by an electrical phenomenon, the slow wave, which cycles at 3 cycles/min in the stomach and 11 cycles/min in the duodenum. During emesis, the slow wave is abolished and is replaced by orally propagating spikes that evoke retrograde contractions that assist in expulsion of gut contents.

Activators of emesis

Emetic stimuli act at several sites. Emesis evoked by unpleasant thoughts or smells originates in the brain, whereas cranial nerves mediate vomiting after gag reflex activation. Motion sickness and inner ear disorders act on the labyrinthine system. Gastric irritants and cytotoxic agents like cisplatin stimulate gastroduodenal vagal afferent nerves. Nongastric afferents are activated by intestinal and colonic obstruction and mesenteric ischemia. The area postrema, in the medulla, responds to bloodborne stimuli (emetogenic drugs, bacterial toxins, uremia, hypoxia, ketoacidosis) and is termed the *chemoreceptor trigger zone.*

Neurotransmitters mediating vomiting are selective for different sites. Labyrinthine disorders stimulate vestibular muscarinic M_1 and histaminergic H_1 receptors. Vagal afferent stimuli activate serotonin $5\text{-}HT_3$ receptors. The area postrema is served by nerves acting on $5\text{-}HT_3$, M_1, H_1, and dopamine D_2 subtypes. Cannabinoid CB_1 pathways may participate in the cerebral cortex. Optimal pharmacologic therapy of vomiting requires understanding of these pathways.

DIFFERENTIAL DIAGNOSIS

Nausea and vomiting are caused by conditions within and outside the gut as well as by drugs and circulating toxins (Table 5-1).

Intraperitoneal disorders

Visceral obstruction and inflammation of hollow and solid viscera may elicit vomiting. Gastric obstruction results from ulcers and malignancy, whereas small-bowel and colon blockage occur because of adhesions, benign or malignant tumors, volvulus, intussusception, or inflammatory diseases like Crohn's disease. The superior mesenteric artery syndrome, occurring after weight loss or prolonged bed rest, results when the duodenum is compressed by the overlying superior mesenteric artery. Abdominal irradiation impairs intestinal motor function and induces strictures. Biliary colic causes nausea by acting on local afferent nerves. Vomiting with pancreatitis, cholecystitis, and appendicitis is due to visceral irritation and induction of ileus. Enteric infections with viruses like norovirus or rotavirus or bacteria such as *Staphylococcus aureus* and *Bacillus cereus* often cause vomiting, especially in children. Opportunistic infections like cytomegalovirus or herpes simplex virus induce emesis in immunocompromised individuals.

Gut sensorimotor dysfunction often causes nausea and vomiting. *Gastroparesis* presents with symptoms of gastric retention with evidence of delayed gastric emptying and occurs after vagotomy or with pancreatic carcinoma, mesenteric vascular insufficiency, or organic diseases like diabetes, scleroderma, and amyloidosis. Idiopathic gastroparesis is the most common etiology. It occurs in the absence of systemic illness and may follow a viral illness, suggesting an infectious trigger. *Intestinal pseudoobstruction* is characterized by disrupted intestinal and colonic motor activity with retention of food residue and secretions; bacterial overgrowth; nutrient malabsorption; and symptoms of nausea, vomiting, bloating, pain, and altered defecation. Intestinal pseudoobstruction may be idiopathic, inherited as a familial visceral myopathy or neuropathy, result from systemic disease, or occur as a paraneoplastic consequence of malignancy (e.g., small-cell lung carcinoma). Patients with gastroesophageal reflux may report nausea and vomiting, as do some with irritable bowel syndrome (IBS) or chronic constipation.

Other functional gastroduodenal disorders without organic abnormalities have been characterized in adults. *Chronic idiopathic nausea* is defined as nausea without vomiting occurring several times a week. *Functional vomiting* is defined as one or more vomiting episodes weekly in the absence of an eating disorder or

TABLE 5-1

CAUSES OF NAUSEA AND VOMITING

INTRAPERITONEAL	EXTRAPERITONEAL	MEDICATIONS/METABOLIC DISORDERS
Obstructing disorders	Cardiopulmonary disease	Drugs
Pyloric obstruction	Cardiomyopathy	Cancer chemotherapy
Small-bowel obstruction	Myocardial infarction	Antibiotics
Colonic obstruction	Labyrinthine disease	Cardiac antiarrhythmics
Superior mesenteric artery syndrome	Motion sickness	Digoxin
Enteric infections	Labyrinthitis	Oral hypoglycemics
Viral	Malignancy	Oral contraceptives
Bacterial	Intracerebral disorders	Endocrine/metabolic disease
Inflammatory diseases	Malignancy	Pregnancy
Cholecystitis	Hemorrhage	Uremia
Pancreatitis	Abscess	Ketoacidosis
Appendicitis	Hydrocephalus	Thyroid and parathyroid disease
Hepatitis	Psychiatric illness	Adrenal insufficiency
Altered sensorimotor function	Anorexia and bulimia nervosa	Toxins
Gastroparesis	Depression	Liver failure
Intestinal pseudoobstruction	Postoperative vomiting	Ethanol
Gastroesophageal reflux		
Chronic idiopathic nausea		
Functional vomiting		
Cyclic vomiting syndrome		
Cannabinoid hyperemesis syndrome		
Rumination syndrome		
Biliary colic		
Abdominal irradiation		

psychiatric disease. *Cyclic vomiting syndrome* presents with periodic discrete episodes of relentless nausea and vomiting in children and adults and shows an association with migraine headaches, suggesting that some cases may be migraine variants. Some adult cases have been described in association with rapid gastric emptying. A related condition, *cannabinoid hyperemesis syndrome*, presents with cyclical vomiting with intervening well periods in individuals (mostly men) who use large quantities of cannabis over many years and resolves with its discontinuation. Pathologic behaviors such as taking prolonged hot baths or showers are associated with the syndrome. *Rumination syndrome*, characterized by repetitive regurgitation of recently ingested food, is often misdiagnosed as refractory vomiting.

Extraperitoneal disorders

Myocardial infarction and congestive heart failure may cause nausea and vomiting. Postoperative emesis occurs after 25% of surgeries, most commonly laparotomy and orthopedic surgery. Increased intracranial pressure from tumors, bleeding, abscess, or blockage of cerebrospinal fluid outflow produces vomiting with or without nausea. Patients with psychiatric illnesses including anorexia nervosa, bulimia nervosa, anxiety, and depression often report significant nausea that may be associated with delayed gastric emptying.

Medications and metabolic disorders

Drugs evoke vomiting by action on the stomach (analgesics, erythromycin) or area postrema (opiates, antiparkinsonian drugs). Other emetogenic agents include antibiotics, cardiac antiarrhythmics, antihypertensives, oral hypoglycemics, antidepressants (selective serotonin and serotonin norepinephrine reuptake inhibitors), smoking cessation drugs (varenicline, nicotine), and contraceptives. Cancer chemotherapy causes vomiting that is acute (within hours of administration), delayed (after 1 or more days), or anticipatory. Acute emesis from highly emetogenic agents (e.g., cisplatin) is mediated by 5-HT_3 pathways, whereas delayed emesis is less dependent on 5-HT_3 mechanisms. Anticipatory nausea may respond to anxiolytic therapy rather than antiemetics.

Metabolic disorders elicit nausea and vomiting. Pregnancy is the most prevalent endocrinologic cause, and nausea affects 70% of women in the first trimester. Hyperemesis gravidarum is a severe form of nausea of pregnancy that produces significant fluid loss and electrolyte disturbances. Uremia, ketoacidosis, adrenal insufficiency, and parathyroid and thyroid disease are other metabolic etiologies.

Circulating toxins evoke emesis via effects on the area postrema. Endogenous toxins are generated in fulminant liver failure, whereas exogenous enterotoxins may be produced by enteric bacterial infection. Ethanol intoxication is a common toxic etiology of nausea and vomiting.

APPROACH TO THE PATIENT: Nausea and Vomiting

HISTORY AND PHYSICAL EXAMINATION The history helps define the etiology of nausea and vomiting. Drugs, toxins, and infections often cause acute symptoms, whereas established illnesses evoke chronic complaints. Gastroparesis and pyloric obstruction elicit vomiting within an hour of eating. Emesis from intestinal blockage occurs later. Vomiting occurring within minutes of meal consumption prompts consideration of rumination syndrome. With severe gastric emptying delays, the vomitus may contain food residue ingested hours or days before. Hematemesis raises suspicion of an ulcer, malignancy, or Mallory-Weiss tear. Feculent emesis is noted with distal intestinal or colonic obstruction. Bilious vomiting excludes gastric obstruction, whereas emesis of undigested food is consistent with a Zenker's diverticulum or achalasia. Vomiting can relieve abdominal pain from a bowel obstruction, but has no effect in pancreatitis or cholecystitis. Profound weight loss raises concern about malignancy or obstruction. Fevers suggest inflammation. An intracranial source is considered if there are headaches or visual field changes. Vertigo or tinnitus indicates labyrinthine disease.

The physical examination complements the history. Orthostatic hypotension and reduced skin turgor indicate intravascular fluid loss. Pulmonary abnormalities raise concern for aspiration of vomitus. Abdominal auscultation may reveal absent bowel sounds with ileus. High-pitched rushes suggest bowel obstruction, whereas a succussion splash upon abrupt lateral movement of the patient is found with gastroparesis or pyloric obstruction. Tenderness or involuntary guarding raises suspicion of inflammation, whereas fecal blood suggests mucosal injury from ulcer, ischemia, or tumor. Neurologic disease presents with papilledema, visual field loss, or focal neural abnormalities. Neoplasm is suggested by palpation of masses or adenopathy.

DIAGNOSTIC TESTING For intractable symptoms or an elusive diagnosis, selected screening tests can direct clinical care. Electrolyte replacement is indicated for hypokalemia or metabolic alkalosis. Iron-deficiency anemia mandates a search for mucosal injury. Pancreaticobiliary disease is indicated by abnormal pancreatic or liver biochemistries, whereas endocrinologic, rheumatologic, or paraneoplastic etiologies are suggested by hormone or serologic abnormalities. If bowel obstruction is suspected, supine and upright abdominal radiographs may show intestinal air-fluid levels with reduced colonic air. Ileus is characterized by diffusely dilated air-filled bowel loops.

Anatomic studies may be indicated if initial testing is nondiagnostic. Upper endoscopy detects ulcers, malignancy, and retained gastric food residue in gastroparesis. Small-bowel barium radiography or computed tomography (CT) diagnoses partial bowel obstruction. Colonoscopy or contrast enema radiography detects colonic obstruction. Ultrasound or CT defines intraperitoneal inflammation; CT and magnetic resonance imaging (MRI) enterography provide superior definition of inflammation in Crohn's disease. CT or MRI of the head can delineate intracranial disease. Mesenteric angiography, CT, or MRI is useful for suspected ischemia.

Gastrointestinal motility testing may detect an underlying motor disorder when anatomic abnormalities are absent. Gastroparesis commonly is diagnosed by gastric scintigraphy, by which emptying of a radiolabeled meal is measured. Isotopic breath tests and wireless motility capsule methods are alternatives tests to define gastroparesis in different regions of the world. Intestinal pseudoobstruction often is suggested by abnormal barium transit and luminal dilation on small-bowel contrast radiography. Delayed small-bowel transit also may be detected by wireless capsule techniques. Small-intestinal manometry can confirm the diagnosis and further characterize the motor abnormality as neuropathic or myopathic based on contractile patterns. Such investigation can obviate the need for surgical intestinal biopsy to evaluate for smooth muscle or neuronal degeneration. Combined ambulatory esophageal pH/impedance testing and high-resolution manometry can facilitate diagnosis of rumination syndrome.

TREATMENT Nausea and Vomiting

GENERAL PRINCIPLES Therapy of vomiting is tailored to correcting remediable abnormalities if possible. Hospitalization is considered for severe dehydration, especially if oral fluid replenishment cannot be sustained. Once oral intake is tolerated, nutrients are restarted with low-fat liquids, because lipids delay gastric emptying. Foods high in indigestible residue are avoided because these prolong gastric retention. Controlling blood glucose in poorly controlled diabetics can reduce hospitalizations in gastroparesis.

ANTIEMETIC MEDICATIONS The most commonly used antiemetic agents act on central nervous system sites (Table 5-2). Antihistamines like dimenhydrinate and meclizine and anticholinergics like scopolamine act on labyrinthine pathways to treat motion sickness and inner ear disorders. Dopamine D_2 antagonists treat emesis evoked by area postrema stimuli and are used for medication, toxic, and metabolic etiologies. Dopamine antagonists cross the blood-brain barrier and cause anxiety, movement disorders, and hyperprolactinemic effects (galactorrhea, sexual dysfunction).

Other classes exhibit antiemetic properties. 5-HT_3 antagonists such as ondansetron and granisetron can prevent postoperative vomiting, radiation therapy–induced symptoms, and cancer chemotherapy–induced emesis, but also are used for other causes of emesis with limited evidence for efficacy. Tricyclic antidepressant agents provide symptomatic benefit in patients with chronic idiopathic nausea and functional vomiting as well as in long-standing diabetic patients with nausea and vomiting. Other antidepressants such as mirtazapine and olanzapine also may exhibit antiemetic effects.

GASTROINTESTINAL MOTOR STIMULANTS Drugs that stimulate gastric emptying are used for gastroparesis (Table 5-2). Metoclopramide, a combined 5-HT_4 agonist and D_2 antagonist, is effective in gastroparesis, but antidopaminergic side effects, such as dystonias and mood and sleep disturbances, limit use in ~25% of cases. Erythromycin increases gastroduodenal motility by action on receptors for motilin, an endogenous stimulant of fasting motor activity. Intravenous erythromycin is useful for inpatients with refractory gastroparesis, but oral forms have some utility. Domperidone, a D_2 antagonist not available in the United States, exhibits prokinetic and antiemetic effects but does not cross into most brain regions; thus, anxiety and dystonic reactions are rare. The main side effects of domperidone relate to induction of hyperprolactinemia via effects on pituitary regions served by a porous blood-brain barrier.

Refractory motility disorders pose significant challenges. Intestinal pseudoobstruction may respond to the somatostatin analogue octreotide, which induces propagative small-intestinal motor complexes. Acetylcholinesterase inhibitors such as pyridostigmine are also observed to benefit some patients with small-bowel dysmotility. Pyloric injections of botulinum toxin are reported in uncontrolled studies to reduce gastroparesis symptoms, but small controlled trials observe benefits no greater than sham treatments. Surgical pyloroplasty has improved symptoms in case series. Placing a feeding jejunostomy reduces hospitalizations and improves overall health in some patients with drug-refractory gastroparesis. Postvagotomy gastroparesis may improve with near-total gastric resection; similar operations are now being tried for other gastroparesis etiologies. Implanted gastric electrical stimulators may reduce symptoms, enhance nutrition, improve quality of life, and decrease health care expenditures in medication-refractory gastroparesis, but small controlled trials do not report convincing benefits.

SAFETY CONSIDERATIONS Safety concerns about selected antiemetics have been emphasized. Centrally acting antidopaminergics, especially metoclopramide, can cause irreversible movement disorders such as tardive dyskinesia, particularly in older patients. This complication should be carefully explained and documented in the medical record. Some agents with antiemetic properties including domperidone,

TABLE 5-2
TREATMENT OF NAUSEA AND VOMITING

TREATMENT	MECHANISM	EXAMPLES	CLINICAL INDICATIONS
Antiemetic agents	Antihistaminergic	Dimenhydrinate, meclizine	Motion sickness, inner ear disease
	Anticholinergic	Scopolamine	Motion sickness, inner ear disease
	Antidopaminergic	Prochlorperazine, thiethylperazine	Medication-, toxin-, or metabolic-induced emesis
	5-HT_3 antagonist	Ondansetron, granisetron	Chemotherapy- and radiation-induced emesis, postoperative emesis
	NK_1 antagonist	Aprepitant	Chemotherapy-induced nausea and vomiting
	Tricyclic antidepressant	Amitriptyline, nortriptyline	Functional vomiting, chronic idiopathic nausea, cyclic vomiting syndrome, ?gastroparesis
	Other antidepressant	Mirtazapine, olanzapine	?Functional vomiting, ?chronic idiopathic nausea, ?gastroparesis
Prokinetic agents	5-HT_4 agonist and antidopaminergic	Metoclopramide	Gastroparesis
	Motilin agonist	Erythromycin	Gastroparesis, ?intestinal pseudoobstruction
	Peripheral antidopaminergic	Domperidone	Gastroparesis
	Somatostatin analogue	Octreotide	Intestinal pseudoobstruction
	Acetylcholinesterase inhibitor	Pyridostigmine	?Small-intestinal dysmotility/pseudoobstruction
Special settings	Benzodiazepines	Lorazepam	Anticipatory nausea and vomiting with chemotherapy
	Glucocorticoids	Methylprednisolone, dexamethasone	Chemotherapy-induced emesis
	Cannabinoids	Tetrahydrocannabinol	Chemotherapy-induced emesis

Note: ?, indication is uncertain.

erythromycin, tricyclics, and 5-HT_3 antagonists can induce dangerous cardiac rhythm disturbances, especially in those with QTc interval prolongation on electrocardiography (ECG). Surveillance ECG testing has been advocated for some of these agents.

SELECTED CLINICAL SETTINGS Some cancer chemotherapies are intensely emetogenic. Combining a 5-HT_3 antagonist, an NK_1 antagonist, and a glucocorticoid provides significant control of both acute and delayed vomiting after highly emetogenic chemotherapy. Unlike other drugs in the same class, the 5-HT_3 antagonist palonosetron exhibits efficacy at preventing delayed chemotherapy-induced vomiting. Benzodiazepines such as lorazepam can reduce anticipatory nausea and vomiting. Miscellaneous therapies with benefit in chemotherapy-induced emesis include cannabinoids, olanzapine, and alternative therapies like ginger. Most antiemetic regimens produce greater reductions in vomiting than in nausea.

Clinicians should exercise caution in managing pregnant patients with nausea. Studies of the teratogenic effects of antiemetic agents provide conflicting results. Few controlled trials have been performed in nausea of pregnancy. Antihistamines such as meclizine and doxylamine, antidopaminergics such as prochlorperazine, and antiserotonergics such as ondansetron demonstrate limited efficacy. Some obstetricians offer alternative therapies such as pyridoxine, acupressure, or ginger.

Managing cyclic vomiting syndrome is a challenge. Prophylaxis with tricyclic antidepressants, cyproheptadine, or β-adrenoceptor antagonists can reduce the severity and frequency of attacks. Intravenous 5-HT_3 antagonists combined with the sedating effects of a benzodiazepine like lorazepam are a mainstay of treatment of acute flares. Small studies report benefits with antimigraine agents, including the 5-HT_1 agonist sumatriptan, as well as selected anticonvulsants such as zonisamide and levetiracetam.

INDIGESTION

MECHANISMS

The most common causes of indigestion are gastroesophageal reflux and functional dyspepsia. Other cases are a consequence of organic illness.

Gastroesophageal reflux

Gastroesophageal reflux results from many physiologic defects. Reduced lower esophageal sphincter (LES) tone contributes to reflux in scleroderma and pregnancy and may be a factor in some patients without systemic illness. Others exhibit frequent transient LES relaxations (TLESRs) that cause bathing of the esophagus by acid or nonacidic fluid. Overeating and aerophagia override the barrier function of the LES, whereas reductions in esophageal body motility or salivary secretion prolong fluid exposure. Increased intragastric pressure promotes gastroesophageal reflux in obesity. The role of hiatal hernias is controversial—most reflux patients have hiatal hernias, but most with hiatal hernias do not have excess heartburn.

Gastric motor dysfunction

Disturbed gastric motility may contribute to gastroesophageal reflux in up to one-third of cases. Delayed gastric emptying is also found in ~30% of functional dyspeptics. Conversely, some dyspeptics exhibit rapid gastric emptying. The relation of these defects to symptom induction is uncertain; studies show poor correlation between symptom severity and degrees of motor dysfunction. Impaired gastric fundus relaxation after eating (i.e., accommodation) may underlie selected dyspeptic symptoms like bloating, nausea, and early satiety in ~40% of patients.

Visceral afferent hypersensitivity

Disturbed gastric sensation is another pathogenic factor in functional dyspepsia. Visceral hypersensitivity was first reported in IBS with demonstration of heightened perception of rectal balloon inflation without changes in compliance. Similarly, ~35% of dyspeptic patients note discomfort with fundic distention to lower pressures than healthy controls. Others with dyspepsia exhibit hypersensitivity to chemical stimulation with capsaicin or with acid or lipid exposure in the duodenum. Some individuals with functional heartburn without increased acid or nonacid reflux are believed to have heightened perception of normal esophageal pH and volume.

Other factors

Helicobacter pylori has a clear etiologic role in peptic ulcer disease, but ulcers cause a minority of dyspepsia cases. *H. pylori* is a minor factor in the genesis of functional dyspepsia. Functional dyspepsia is associated with chronic fatigue, produces reduced physical and mental well-being, and is exacerbated by stress. Anxiety, depression, and somatization may have contributing roles in some cases. Functional MRI studies show increased activation of several brain regions, emphasizing contributions from central nervous system factors. Analgesics cause dyspepsia, whereas nitrates, calcium channel blockers, theophylline, and progesterone promote gastroesophageal reflux. Other stimuli that induce reflux include ethanol, tobacco, and caffeine via LES relaxation. Genetic factors may promote development of reflux and dyspepsia.

DIFFERENTIAL DIAGNOSIS

Gastroesophageal reflux disease

Gastroesophageal reflux disease (GERD) is prevalent. Heartburn is reported once monthly by 40% of Americans and daily by 7–10%. Most cases of heartburn occur because of excess acid reflux, but reflux of nonacidic fluid produces similar symptoms. Alkaline reflux esophagitis produces GERD-like symptoms most often in patients who have had surgery for peptic ulcer disease. Ten percent of patients with heartburn exhibit normal esophageal acid exposure and no increase in nonacidic reflux (functional heartburn).

Functional dyspepsia

Nearly 25% of the populace has dyspepsia at least six times yearly, but only 10–20% present to clinicians. Functional dyspepsia, the cause of symptoms in >60% of dyspeptic patients, is defined as ≥3 months of bothersome postprandial fullness, early satiety, or epigastric pain or burning with symptom onset at least 6 months before diagnosis in the absence of organic cause. Functional dyspepsia is subdivided into postprandial distress syndrome, characterized by meal-induced fullness, early satiety, and discomfort, and epigastric pain syndrome, which presents with epigastric burning pain unrelated to meals. Most cases follow a benign course, but some with *H. pylori* infection or on nonsteroidal anti-inflammatory drugs (NSAIDs) develop ulcers. As with idiopathic gastroparesis, some cases of functional dyspepsia result from prior infection.

Ulcer disease

In most GERD patients, there is no destruction of the esophagus. However, 5% develop esophageal ulcers, and some form strictures. Symptoms cannot distinguish nonerosive from erosive or ulcerative esophagitis. A minority of cases of dyspepsia stem from gastric or duodenal ulcers. The most common causes of ulcer disease are *H. pylori* infection and use of NSAIDs. Other rare causes of gastroduodenal ulcers include Crohn's disease **(Chap. 18)** and Zollinger-Ellison syndrome **(Chap. 15)**, resulting from gastrin overproduction by an endocrine tumor.

Malignancy

Dyspeptic patients often seek care because of fear of cancer, but few cases result from malignancy.

Esophageal squamous cell carcinoma occurs most often with long-standing tobacco or ethanol intake. Other risks include prior caustic ingestion, achalasia, and the hereditary disorder tylosis. Esophageal adenocarcinoma usually complicates prolonged acid reflux. Eight to 20% of GERD patients exhibit esophageal intestinal metaplasia, termed *Barrett's metaplasia,* a condition that predisposes to esophageal adenocarcinoma **(Chap. 51)**. Gastric malignancies include adenocarcinoma, which is prevalent in certain Asian societies, and lymphoma.

Other causes

Opportunistic fungal or viral esophageal infections may produce heartburn but more often cause odynophagia. Other causes of esophageal inflammation include eosinophilic esophagitis and pill esophagitis. Biliary colic is in the differential diagnosis of unexplained upper abdominal pain, but most patients with biliary colic report discrete acute episodes of right upper quadrant or epigastric pain rather than the chronic burning, discomfort, and fullness of dyspepsia. Twenty percent of patients with gastroparesis report a predominance of pain or discomfort rather than nausea and vomiting. Intestinal lactase deficiency as a cause of gas, bloating, and discomfort occurs in 15–25% of whites of northern European descent but is more common in blacks and Asians. Intolerance of other carbohydrates (e.g., fructose, sorbitol) produces similar symptoms. Small-intestinal bacterial overgrowth may cause dyspepsia, often associated with bowel dysfunction, distention, and malabsorption. Eosinophilic infiltration of the duodenal mucosa is described in some dyspeptics, particularly with postprandial distress syndrome. Celiac disease, pancreatic disease (chronic pancreatitis, malignancy), hepatocellular carcinoma, Ménétrier's disease, infiltrative diseases (sarcoidosis, eosinophilic gastroenteritis), mesenteric ischemia, thyroid and parathyroid disease, and abdominal wall strain cause dyspepsia. Gluten sensitivity in the absence of celiac disease is reported to evoke unexplained upper abdominal symptoms. Extraperitoneal etiologies of indigestion include congestive heart failure and tuberculosis.

APPROACH TO THE PATIENT: Indigestion

HISTORY AND PHYSICAL EXAMINATION Care of the indigestion patient requires a thorough interview. GERD classically produces heartburn, a substernal warmth that moves toward the neck. Heartburn often is exacerbated by meals and may awaken the patient. Associated symptoms include regurgitation of acid or nonacidic fluid and water brash, the reflex release of salty salivary secretions into the mouth. Atypical symptoms include pharyngitis, asthma, cough, bronchitis, hoarseness, and chest pain that mimics angina. Some patients with acid reflux on esophageal pH testing do not report heartburn, but note abdominal pain or other symptoms.

Dyspeptic patients typically report symptoms referable to the upper abdomen that may be meal-related, as with postprandial distress syndrome, or independent of food ingestion, as in epigastric pain syndrome. Functional dyspepsia overlaps with other disorders including GERD, IBS, and idiopathic gastroparesis.

The physical exam with GERD and functional dyspepsia usually is normal. In atypical GERD, pharyngeal erythema and wheezing may be noted. Recurrent acid regurgitation may cause poor dentition. Dyspeptics may exhibit epigastric tenderness or distention.

Discriminating functional and organic causes of indigestion mandates excluding certain historic and exam features. Odynophagia suggests esophageal infection. Dysphagia is concerning for a benign or malignant esophageal blockage. Other alarm features include unexplained weight loss, recurrent vomiting, occult or gross bleeding, jaundice, palpable mass or adenopathy, and a family history of gastrointestinal neoplasm.

DIAGNOSTIC TESTING Because indigestion is prevalent and most cases result from GERD or functional dyspepsia, a general principle is to perform only limited and directed diagnostic testing of selected individuals.

Once alarm factors are excluded (Table 5-3), patients with typical GERD do not need further evaluation and are treated empirically. Upper endoscopy is indicated to exclude mucosal injury in cases with atypical symptoms, symptoms unresponsive to acid suppression, or alarm factors. For heartburn >5 years in duration, especially in patients >50 years old, endoscopy is advocated to screen for Barrett's metaplasia. The benefits and cost-effectiveness of this approach have not been validated in controlled studies. Ambulatory esophageal pH testing using a catheter method or a wireless capsule endoscopically attached to the esophageal wall is considered for drug-refractory

TABLE 5-3

ALARM SYMPTOMS IN GASTROESOPHAGEAL REFLUX DISEASE
Odynophagia
Unexplained weight loss
Recurrent vomiting
Occult or gross gastrointestinal bleeding
Jaundice
Palpable mass or adenopathy
Family history of gastrointestinal malignancy

symptoms and atypical symptoms like unexplained chest pain. High-resolution esophageal manometry is ordered when surgical treatment of GERD is considered. A low LES pressure predicts failure of drug therapy and provides a rationale to proceed to surgery. Poor esophageal body peristalsis raises concern about postoperative dysphagia and directs the choice of surgical technique. Nonacidic reflux may be detected by combined esophageal impedance-pH testing in medication-unresponsive patients.

Upper endoscopy is recommended as the initial test in patients with unexplained dyspepsia who are >55 years old or who have alarm factors because of the purported elevated risks of malignancy and ulcer in these groups. However, endoscopic findings in unexplained dyspepsia include erosive esophagitis in 13%, peptic ulcer in 8%, and gastric or esophageal malignancy in only 0.3%. Management of patients <55 years old without alarm factors depends on the local prevalence of *H. pylori* infection. In regions with low *H. pylori* prevalence (<10%), a 4-week trial of an acid-suppressing medication such as a proton pump inhibitor (PPI) is recommended. If this fails, a "test and treat" approach is most commonly applied. *H. pylori* status is determined with urea breath testing, stool antigen measurement, or blood serology testing. Those who are *H. pylori* positive are given therapy to eradicate the infection. If symptoms resolve on either regimen, no further intervention is required. For patients in areas with high *H. pylori* prevalence (>10%), an initial test and treat approach is advocated, with a subsequent trial of an acid-suppressing regimen offered for those in whom *H. pylori* treatment fails or for those who are negative for the infection. In each of these patient subsets, upper endoscopy is reserved for those whose symptoms fail to respond to therapy.

Further testing is indicated in some settings. If bleeding is noted, a blood count can exclude anemia. Thyroid chemistries or calcium levels screen for metabolic disease, whereas specific serologies may suggest celiac disease. Pancreatic and liver chemistries are obtained for possible pancreaticobiliary causes. Ultrasound, CT, or MRI is performed if abnormalities are found. Gastric emptying testing is considered to exclude gastroparesis for dyspeptic symptoms that resemble postprandial distress when drug therapy fails and in some GERD patients, especially if surgical intervention is an option. Breath testing after carbohydrate ingestion detects lactase deficiency, intolerance to other carbohydrates, or small-intestinal bacterial overgrowth.

TREATMENT Indigestion

GENERAL PRINCIPLES For mild indigestion, reassurance that a careful evaluation revealed no serious organic disease may be the only intervention needed. Drugs that cause gastroesophageal reflux or dyspepsia should be stopped, if possible. Patients with GERD should limit ethanol, caffeine, chocolate, and tobacco use due to their effects on the LES. Other measures in GERD include ingesting a low-fat diet, avoiding snacks before bedtime, and elevating the head of the bed. Patients with functional dyspepsia also may be advised to reduce intake of fat, spicy foods, caffeine, and alcohol.

Specific therapies for organic disease should be offered when possible. Surgery is appropriate for biliary colic, whereas diet changes are indicated for lactase deficiency or celiac disease. Peptic ulcers may be cured by specific medical regimens. However, because most indigestion is caused by GERD or functional dyspepsia, medications that reduce gastric acid, modulate motility, or blunt gastric sensitivity are used.

ACID-SUPPRESSING OR -NEUTRALIZING MEDICATIONS 'Drugs that reduce or neutralize gastric acid are often prescribed for GERD. Histamine H_2 antagonists like cimetidine, ranitidine, famotidine, and nizatidine are useful in mild to moderate GERD. For severe symptoms or for many cases of erosive or ulcerative esophagitis, PPIs such as omeprazole, lansoprazole, rabeprazole, pantoprazole, esomeprazole, or dexlansoprazole are needed. These drugs inhibit gastric H^+, K^+-ATPase and are more potent than H_2 antagonists. Up to one-third of GERD patients do not respond to standard PPI doses; one-third of these patients have nonacidic reflux, whereas 10% have persistent acid-related disease. Furthermore, heartburn typically responds better to PPI therapy than regurgitation or atypical GERD symptoms. Some individuals respond to doubling of the PPI dose or adding an H_2 antagonist at bedtime. Infrequent complications of long-term PPI therapy include infection, diarrhea (from *Clostridium difficile* infection or microscopic colitis), small-intestinal bacterial overgrowth, nutrient deficiency (vitamin B_{12}, iron, calcium), hypomagnesemia, bone demineralization, interstitial nephritis, and impaired medication absorption (e.g., clopidogrel). Many patients started on a PPI can be stepped down to an H_2 antagonist or be switched to an on-demand schedule.

Acid-suppressing drugs are also effective in selected patients with functional dyspepsia. A meta-analysis of eight controlled trials calculated a risk ratio of 0.86, with a 95% confidence interval of 0.78–0.95, favoring PPI therapy over placebo. H_2 antagonists also reportedly improve symptoms in functional dyspepsia; however, findings of trials of this drug class likely are influenced by inclusion of large numbers of GERD patients.

Antacids are useful for short-term control of mild GERD but have less benefit in severe cases unless given at high doses that cause side effects (diarrhea and constipation with magnesium- and aluminum-containing agents, respectively). Alginic acid combined with antacids forms a floating barrier to reflux in patients with upright symptoms. Sucralfate, a salt of aluminum hydroxide and sucrose octasulfate that buffers acid and binds pepsin and bile salts, shows efficacy in GERD similar to H_2 antagonists.

***HELICOBACTER PYLORI* ERADICATION** *H. pylori* eradication is definitively indicated only for peptic ulcer and mucosa-associated lymphoid tissue gastric lymphoma. The utility of eradication therapy in functional dyspepsia is limited, although some cases (particularly with the epigastric pain syndrome subtype) relate to this infection. A meta-analysis of 18 controlled trials calculated a relative risk reduction of 10%, with a 95% confidence interval of 6–14%, favoring *H. pylori* eradication over placebo. Most drug combinations **(Chap. 27)** include 10–14 days of a PPI or bismuth subsalicylate in concert with two antibiotics. *H. pylori* infection is associated with reduced prevalence of GERD, especially in the elderly. However, eradication of the infection does not worsen GERD symptoms. No consensus recommendations regarding *H. pylori* eradication in GERD patients have been offered.

AGENTS THAT MODIFY GASTROINTESTINAL MOTOR ACTIVITY Prokinetics like metoclopramide, erythromycin, and domperidone have limited utility in GERD. The γ-aminobutyric acid B (GABA-B) agonist baclofen reduces esophageal exposure to acid and nonacidic fluids by reducing TLESRs by 40%; this drug is proposed for refractory acid and nonacid reflux. Several studies have promoted the efficacy of motor-stimulating drugs in functional dyspepsia, but publication bias and small sample sizes raise questions about reported benefits of these agents. Some clinicians suggest that patients with the postprandial distress subtype may respond preferentially to prokinetic drugs. The 5-HT_1 agonist buspirone may improve some functional dyspepsia symptoms by enhancing meal-induced gastric accommodation. Acotiamide promotes gastric emptying and augments accommodation by enhancing gastric acetylcholine release via muscarinic receptor antagonism and acetylcholinesterase inhibition. This agent is approved for functional dyspepsia in Japan and is in testing elsewhere.

OTHER OPTIONS Antireflux surgery (fundoplication) to increase LES pressure may be offered to GERD patients who are young and require lifelong therapy, have typical heartburn and regurgitation, are responsive to PPIs, and show evidence of acid reflux on pH monitoring. Surgery also is effective for some cases of nonacidic reflux. Individuals who respond less well to fundoplication include those with atypical symptoms or who have esophageal body motor disturbances. Dysphagia, gas-bloat syndrome, and gastroparesis are long-term complications of these procedures; ~60% develop recurrent GERD symptoms over time. The utility and safety of endoscopic therapies (radiofrequency ablation, transoral incisionless fundoplication) to enhance gastroesophageal barrier function have unproved durable benefits for refractory GERD.

Some patients with functional heartburn and functional dyspepsia refractory to standard therapies may respond to antidepressants in tricyclic and selective serotonin reuptake inhibitor classes, although studies are limited. Their mechanism of action may involve blunting of visceral pain processing in the brain. Gas and bloating are among the most troubling symptoms in some patients with indigestion and can be difficult to treat. Dietary exclusion of gas-producing foods such as legumes and use of simethicone or activated charcoal provide benefits in some cases. Low FODMAP (fermentable oligosaccharide, disaccharide, monosaccharide, and polyol) diets and therapies to modify gut flora (nonabsorbable antibiotics, probiotics) reduce gaseous symptoms in some IBS patients. The utility of low-FODMAP diets, antibiotics, and probiotics in functional dyspepsia is unproven. Herbal remedies such as STW 5 (Iberogast, a mixture of nine herbal agents) are useful in some dyspeptic patients. Psychological treatments (e.g., behavioral therapy, psychotherapy, hypnotherapy) may be offered for refractory functional dyspepsia, but no convincing data confirm their efficacy.

CHAPTER 6

DIARRHEA AND CONSTIPATION

Michael Camilleri ■ Joseph A. Murray

Diarrhea and constipation are exceedingly common and, together, exact an enormous toll in terms of mortality, morbidity, social inconvenience, loss of work productivity, and consumption of medical resources. Worldwide, >1 billion individuals suffer one or more episodes of acute diarrhea each year. Among the 100 million persons affected annually by acute diarrhea in the United States, nearly half must restrict activities, 10% consult physicians, ~250,000 require hospitalization, and ~5000 die (primarily the elderly). The annual economic burden to society may exceed $20 billion. Acute infectious diarrhea remains one of the most common causes of mortality in developing countries, particularly among impoverished infants, accounting for 1.8 million deaths per year. Recurrent, acute diarrhea in children in tropical countries results in environmental enteropathy with long-term impacts on physical and intellectual development.

Constipation, by contrast, is rarely associated with mortality and is exceedingly common in developed countries, leading to frequent self-medication and, in a third of those, to medical consultation. Population statistics on chronic diarrhea and constipation are more uncertain, perhaps due to variable definitions and reporting, but the frequency of these conditions is also high. United States population surveys put prevalence rates for chronic diarrhea at 2–7% and for chronic constipation at 12–19%, with women being affected twice as often as men. Diarrhea and constipation are among the most common patient complaints presenting to internists and primary care physicians, and they account for nearly 50% of referrals to gastroenterologists.

Although diarrhea and constipation may present as mere nuisance symptoms at one extreme, they can be severe or life-threatening at the other. Even mild symptoms may signal a serious underlying gastrointestinal lesion, such as colorectal cancer, or systemic disorder, such as thyroid disease. Given the heterogeneous causes and potential severity of these common complaints, it is imperative for clinicians to appreciate the pathophysiology, etiologic classification, diagnostic strategies, and principles of management of diarrhea and constipation, so that rational and cost-effective care can be delivered.

NORMAL PHYSIOLOGY

While the primary function of the small intestine is the digestion and assimilation of nutrients from food, the small intestine and colon together perform important functions that regulate the secretion and absorption of water and electrolytes, the storage and subsequent transport of intraluminal contents aborally, and the salvage of some nutrients that are not absorbed in the small intestine after bacterial metabolism of carbohydrate allows salvage of short-chain fatty acids. The main motor functions are summarized in Table 6-1. Alterations in fluid and electrolyte handling contribute significantly to diarrhea. Alterations in motor and sensory functions of the colon result in highly prevalent syndromes such as irritable bowel syndrome (IBS), chronic diarrhea, and chronic constipation.

TABLE 6-1

NORMAL GASTROINTESTINAL MOTILITY: FUNCTIONS AT DIFFERENT ANATOMIC LEVELS
Stomach and Small Bowel
Synchronized MMC in fasting
Accommodation, trituration, mixing, transit
Stomach ~3 h
Small bowel ~3 h
Ileal reservoir empties boluses
Colon: Irregular Mixing, Fermentation, Absorption, Transit
Ascending, transverse: reservoirs
Descending: conduit
Sigmoid/rectum: volitional reservoir

Abbreviation: MMC, migrating motor complex.

NEURAL CONTROL

The small intestine and colon have intrinsic and extrinsic innervation. The *intrinsic innervation*, also called the enteric nervous system, comprises myenteric, submucosal, and mucosal neuronal layers. The function of these layers is modulated by interneurons through the actions of neurotransmitter amines or peptides, including acetylcholine, vasoactive intestinal peptide (VIP), opioids, norepinephrine, serotonin, adenosine triphosphate (ATP), and nitric oxide (NO). The myenteric plexus regulates smooth-muscle function through intermediary pacemaker-like cells called the interstitial cells of Cajal, and the submucosal plexus affects secretion, absorption, and mucosal blood flow. The enteric nervous system receives input from the extrinsic nerves, but it is capable of independent control of these functions.

The *extrinsic innervations* of the small intestine and colon are part of the autonomic nervous system and also modulate motor and secretory functions. The parasympathetic nerves convey visceral sensory pathways from and excitatory pathways to the small intestine and colon. Parasympathetic fibers via the vagus nerve reach the small intestine and proximal colon along the branches of the superior mesenteric artery. The distal colon is supplied by sacral parasympathetic nerves (S_{2-4}) via the pelvic plexus; these fibers course through the wall of the colon as ascending intracolonic fibers as far as, and in some instances including, the proximal colon. The chief excitatory neurotransmitters controlling motor function are acetylcholine and the tachykinins, such as substance P. The sympathetic nerve supply modulates motor functions and reaches the small intestine and colon alongside their arterial vessels. Sympathetic input to the gut is generally excitatory to sphincters and inhibitory to non-sphincteric muscle. Visceral afferents convey sensation from the gut to the central nervous system (CNS); initially, they course along sympathetic fibers, but as they approach the spinal cord they separate, have cell bodies in the dorsal root ganglion, and enter the dorsal horn of the spinal cord. Afferent signals are conveyed to the brain along the lateral spinothalamic tract and the nociceptive dorsal column pathway and are then projected beyond the thalamus and brainstem to the insula and cerebral cortex to be perceived. Other afferent fibers synapse in the prevertebral ganglia and reflexly modulate intestinal motility, blood flow, and secretion.

INTESTINAL FLUID ABSORPTION AND SECRETION

On an average day, 9 L of fluid enter the gastrointestinal (GI) tract, ~1 L of residual fluid reaches the colon, and the stool excretion of fluid constitutes about 0.2 L/d. The colon has a large capacitance and functional reserve and may recover up to four times its usual volume of 0.8 L/d, provided the rate of flow permits reabsorption to occur. Thus, the colon can partially compensate for excess fluid delivery to the colon that may result from intestinal absorptive or secretory disorders.

In the small intestine and colon, sodium absorption is predominantly electrogenic (i.e., it can be measured as an ionic current across the membrane because there is not an equivalent loss of a cation from the cell), and uptake takes place at the apical membrane; it is compensated for by the export functions of the basolateral sodium pump. There are several active transport proteins at the apical membrane, especially in the small intestine, whereby sodium ion entry is coupled to monosaccharides (e.g., glucose through the transporter SGLT1, or fructose through GLUT-5). Glucose then exits the basal membrane through a specific transport protein, GLUT-5, creating a glucose concentration gradient between the lumen and the intercellular space, drawing water and electrolytes passively from the lumen. A variety of neural and nonneural mediators regulate colonic fluid and electrolyte balance, including cholinergic, adrenergic, and serotonergic mediators. Angiotensin and aldosterone also influence colonic absorption, reflecting the common embryologic development of the distal colonic epithelium and the renal tubules.

SMALL-INTESTINAL MOTILITY

During the fasting period, the motility of the small intestine is characterized by a cyclical event called the migrating motor complex (MMC), which serves to clear nondigestible residue from the small intestine (the intestinal "housekeeper"). This organized, propagated series of contractions lasts, on average, 4 min, occurs every 60–90 min, and usually involves the entire small intestine. After food ingestion, the small intestine produces irregular, mixing contractions of relatively low amplitude, except in the distal ileum where more powerful contractions occur intermittently and empty the ileum by bolus transfers.

ILEOCOLONIC STORAGE AND SALVAGE

The distal ileum acts as a reservoir, emptying intermittently by bolus movements. This action allows time for salvage of fluids, electrolytes, and nutrients. Segmentation by haustra compartmentalizes the colon and facilitates mixing, retention of residue, and formation of solid stools. There is increased appreciation of the intimate interaction between the colonic function and the luminal ecology. The resident microorganisms, predominantly anaerobic bacteria, in the colon are necessary for the digestion of unabsorbed carbohydrates that reach the colon even in health, thereby providing a vital source of nutrients to the mucosa. Normal colonic flora also keeps pathogens at bay by a variety of mechanisms. In health, the ascending and transverse regions of colon function as reservoirs (average transit time, 15 h), and the descending colon acts as a conduit (average transit time, 3 h). The colon is efficient at conserving sodium and water, a function that is particularly important in sodium-depleted patients in whom the small intestine alone is unable to maintain sodium balance. Diarrhea or constipation may result from alteration in the reservoir function of the proximal colon or the propulsive function of the left colon. Constipation may also result from disturbances of the rectal or sigmoid reservoir, typically as a result of dysfunction of the pelvic floor, the anal sphincters, the coordination of defecation, or dehydration.

COLONIC MOTILITY AND TONE

The small intestinal MMC only rarely continues into the colon. However, short duration or phasic contractions mix colonic contents, and high-amplitude (>75 mmHg) propagated contractions (HAPCs) are sometimes associated with mass movements through the colon and normally occur approximately five times per day, usually on awakening in the morning and postprandially. Increased frequency of HAPCs may result in diarrhea or urgency. The predominant phasic contractions in the colon are irregular and non-propagated and serve a "mixing" function.

Colonic tone refers to the background contractility upon which phasic contractile activity (typically contractions lasting <15 s) is superimposed. It is an important cofactor in the colon's capacitance (volume accommodation) and sensation.

COLONIC MOTILITY AFTER MEAL INGESTION

After meal ingestion, colonic phasic and tonic contractility increase for a period of ~2 h. The initial phase (~10 min) is mediated by the vagus nerve in response to mechanical distention of the stomach. The subsequent response of the colon requires caloric stimulation (e.g., intake of at least 500 kcal) and is mediated, at least in part, by hormones (e.g., gastrin and serotonin).

DEFECATION

Tonic contraction of the puborectalis muscle, which forms a sling around the rectoanal junction, is important to maintain continence; during defecation, sacral parasympathetic nerves relax this muscle, facilitating the straightening of the rectoanal angle (Fig. 6-1). Distention of the rectum results in transient relaxation of the internal anal sphincter via intrinsic and reflex sympathetic innervation. As sigmoid and rectal contractions, as well as straining (Valsalva maneuver), which increases intraabdominal pressure, increase the pressure within the rectum, the rectosigmoid angle opens by >15°. Voluntary relaxation of the external anal

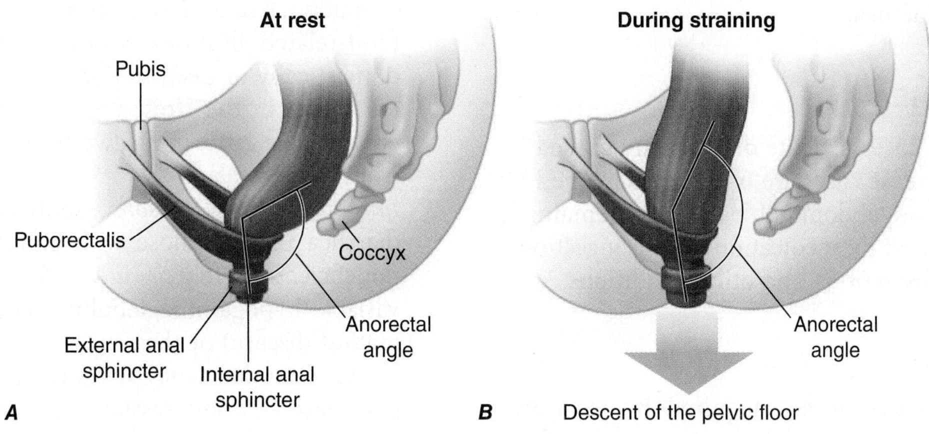

FIGURE 6-1
Sagittal view of the anorectum (*A*) at rest and (*B*) during straining to defecate. Continence is maintained by normal rectal sensation and tonic contraction of the internal anal sphincter and the puborectalis muscle, which wraps around the anorectum, maintaining an anorectal angle between 80° and 110°. During defecation, the pelvic floor muscles (including the puborectalis) relax, allowing the anorectal angle to straighten by at least 15°, and the perineum descends by 1–3.5 cm. The external anal sphincter also relaxes and reduces pressure on the anal canal. *(Reproduced with permission from A Lembo, M Camilleri: N Engl J Med 349:1360, 2003.)*

sphincter (striated muscle innervated by the pudendal nerve) in response to the sensation produced by distention permits the evacuation of feces. Defecation can also be delayed voluntarily by contraction of the external anal sphincter.

DIARRHEA

DEFINITION

Diarrhea is loosely defined as passage of abnormally liquid or unformed stools at an increased frequency. For adults on a typical Western diet, stool weight >200 g/d can generally be considered diarrheal. Diarrhea may be further defined as *acute* if <2 weeks, *persistent* if 2–4 weeks, and *chronic* if >4 weeks in duration.

Two common conditions, usually associated with the passage of stool totaling <200 g/d, must be distinguished from diarrhea, because diagnostic and therapeutic algorithms differ. *Pseudodiarrhea*, or the frequent passage of small volumes of stool, is often associated with rectal urgency, tenesmus, or a feeling of incomplete evacuation, and accompanies IBS or proctitis. *Fecal incontinence* is the involuntary discharge of rectal contents and is most often caused by neuromuscular disorders or structural anorectal problems. Diarrhea and urgency, especially if severe, may aggravate or cause incontinence. Pseudodiarrhea and fecal incontinence occur at prevalence rates comparable to or higher than that of chronic diarrhea and should always be considered in patients complaining of "diarrhea." Overflow diarrhea may occur in nursing home patients due to fecal impaction that is readily detectable by rectal examination. A careful history and physical examination generally allow these conditions to be discriminated from true diarrhea.

ACUTE DIARRHEA

More than 90% of cases of acute diarrhea are caused by infectious agents; these cases are often accompanied by vomiting, fever, and abdominal pain. The remaining 10% or so are caused by medications, toxic ingestions, ischemia, food indiscretions, and other conditions.

Infectious agents

Most infectious diarrheas are acquired by fecal-oral transmission or, more commonly, via ingestion of food or water contaminated with pathogens from human or animal feces. In the immunocompetent person, the resident fecal microflora, containing >500 taxonomically distinct species, are rarely the source of diarrhea and may actually play a role in suppressing the growth of ingested pathogens. Disturbances of flora by antibiotics can lead to diarrhea by reducing the digestive function or by allowing the overgrowth of pathogens, such as *Clostridium difficile* **(Chap. 25)**. Acute infection or injury occurs when the ingested agent overwhelms or bypasses the host's mucosal immune and nonimmune (gastric acid, digestive enzymes, mucus secretion, peristalsis, and suppressive resident flora) defenses. Established clinical associations with specific enteropathogens may offer diagnostic clues.

In the United States, five high-risk groups are recognized:

1. *Travelers*. Nearly 40% of tourists to endemic regions of Latin America, Africa, and Asia develop so-called traveler's diarrhea, most commonly due to enterotoxigenic or enteroaggregative *Escherichia coli* as well as to *Campylobacter*, *Shigella*, *Aeromonas*, norovirus, *Coronavirus*, and *Salmonella*. Visitors to Russia (especially St. Petersburg) may have increased risk of *Giardia*-associated diarrhea; visitors to Nepal may acquire *Cyclospora*. Campers, backpackers, and swimmers in wilderness areas may become infected with *Giardia*. Cruise ships may be affected by outbreaks of gastroenteritis caused by agents such as norovirus.
2. *Consumers of certain foods*. Diarrhea closely following food consumption at a picnic, banquet, or restaurant may suggest infection with *Salmonella*, *Campylobacter*, or *Shigella* from chicken; enterohemorrhagic *E. coli* (O157:H7) from undercooked hamburger; *Bacillus cereus* from fried rice or other reheated food; *Staphylococcus aureus* or *Salmonella* from mayonnaise or creams; *Salmonella* from eggs; *Listeria* from uncooked foods or soft cheeses; and *Vibrio* species, *Salmonella*, or acute hepatitis A from seafood, especially if raw. State departments of public health issue communications regarding food-related illnesses, which may have originated domestically or been imported, but ultimately cause epidemics in the United States (e.g., the *Cyclospora* epidemic of 2013 in midwestern states that resulted from bagged salads).
3. *Immunodeficient persons*. Individuals at risk for diarrhea include those with either primary immunodeficiency (e.g., IgA deficiency, common variable hypogammaglobulinemia, chronic granulomatous disease) or the much more common secondary immunodeficiency states (e.g., AIDS, senescence, pharmacologic suppression). Common enteric pathogens often cause a more severe and protracted diarrheal illness, and, particularly in persons with AIDS, opportunistic infections, such as by *Mycobacterium* species, certain viruses (cytomegalovirus, adenovirus, and herpes simplex), and protozoa (*Cryptosporidium*, *Isospora belli*, Microsporida, and *Blastocystis hominis*) may also play a role. In patients with AIDS, agents

transmitted venereally per rectum (e.g., *Neisseria gonorrhoeae*, *Treponema pallidum*, *Chlamydia*) may contribute to proctocolitis. Persons with hemochromatosis are especially prone to invasive, even fatal, enteric infections with *Vibrio* species and *Yersinia* infections and should avoid raw fish.

4. *Daycare attendees and their family members*. Infections with *Shigella*, *Giardia*, *Cryptosporidium*, rotavirus, and other agents are very common and should be considered.
5. *Institutionalized persons*. Infectious diarrhea is one of the most frequent categories of nosocomial infections in many hospitals and long-term care facilities; the causes are a variety of microorganisms but most commonly *C. difficile*. *C. difficile* can affect those with no history of antibiotic use and may be acquired in the community.

The pathophysiology underlying acute diarrhea by infectious agents produces specific clinical features that may also be helpful in diagnosis (Table 6-2). Profuse, watery diarrhea secondary to small-bowel hypersecretion occurs with ingestion of preformed bacterial toxins, enterotoxin-producing bacteria, and enteroadherent pathogens. Diarrhea associated with marked vomiting and minimal or no fever may occur abruptly within a few hours after ingestion of the former two types; vomiting is usually less, abdominal cramping or bloating is greater, and fever is higher with the latter. Cytotoxin-producing and invasive microorganisms all cause high fever and abdominal pain. Invasive bacteria and *Entamoeba histolytica* often cause bloody diarrhea (referred to as *dysentery*). *Yersinia* invades the terminal ileal and proximal colon mucosa and may cause especially severe abdominal pain with tenderness mimicking acute appendicitis.

Finally, infectious diarrhea may be associated with systemic manifestations. Reactive arthritis (formerly known as Reiter's syndrome), arthritis, urethritis, and conjunctivitis may accompany or follow infections

TABLE 6-2

ASSOCIATION BETWEEN PATHOBIOLOGY OF CAUSATIVE AGENTS AND CLINICAL FEATURES IN ACUTE INFECTIOUS DIARRHEA

PATHOBIOLOGY/AGENTS	INCUBATION PERIOD	VOMITING	ABDOMINAL PAIN	FEVER	DIARRHEA
Toxin producers					
Preformed toxin					
Bacillus cereus, Staphylococcus aureus, Clostridium perfringens	1–8 h 8–24 h	3-4+	1-2+	0–1+	3–4+, watery
Enterotoxin					
Vibrio cholerae, enterotoxigenic *Escherichia coli, Klebsiella pneumoniae, Aeromonas* species	8–72 h	2-4+	1-2+	0–1+	3–4+, watery
Enteroadherent					
Enteropathogenic and enteroadherent *E. coli*, *Giardia* organisms, cryptosporidiosis, helminths	1–8 d	0–1+	1–3+	0–2+	1–2+, watery, mushy
Cytotoxin producers					
C. difficile	1–3 d	0–1+	3–4+	1–2+	1–3+, usually watery, occasionally bloody
Hemorrhagic *E. coli*	12–72 h	0–1+	3–4+	1–2+	1–3+, initially watery, quickly bloody
Invasive organisms					
Minimal inflammation					
Rotavirus and norovirus	1–3 d	1–3+	2–3+	3–4+	1–3+, watery
Variable inflammation					
Salmonella, Campylobacter, and *Aeromonas* species, *Vibrio parahaemolyticus, Yersinia*	12 h–11 d	0–3+	2–4+	3–4+	1–4+, watery or bloody
Severe inflammation					
Shigella species, enteroinvasive *E. coli, Entamoeba histolytica*	12 h–8 d	0–1+	3–4+	3–4+	1–2+, bloody

Source: Adapted from DW Powell, in T Yamada (ed): *Textbook of Gastroenterology and Hepatology*, 4th ed. Philadelphia, Lippincott Williams & Wilkins, 2003.

by *Salmonella*, *Campylobacter*, *Shigella*, and *Yersinia*. Yersiniosis may also lead to an autoimmune-type thyroiditis, pericarditis, and glomerulonephritis. Both enterohemorrhagic *E. coli* (O157:H7) and *Shigella* can lead to the *hemolytic-uremic syndrome* with an attendant high mortality rate. The syndrome of postinfectious IBS has now been recognized as a complication of infectious diarrhea. Similarly, acute gastroenteritis may precede the diagnosis of celiac disease or Crohn's disease. Acute diarrhea can also be a major symptom of several systemic infections including *viral hepatitis*, *listeriosis*, *legionellosis*, and *toxic shock syndrome*.

Other causes

Side effects from medications are probably the most common noninfectious causes of acute diarrhea, and etiology may be suggested by a temporal association between use and symptom onset. Although innumerable medications may produce diarrhea, some of the more frequently incriminated include antibiotics, cardiac antidysrhythmics, antihypertensives, nonsteroidal anti-inflammatory drugs (NSAIDs), certain antidepressants, chemotherapeutic agents, bronchodilators, antacids, and laxatives. Occlusive or nonocclusive *ischemic colitis* typically occurs in persons >50 years; often presents as acute lower abdominal pain preceding watery, then bloody diarrhea; and generally results in acute inflammatory changes in the sigmoid or left colon while sparing the rectum. Acute diarrhea may accompany colonic *diverticulitis* and *graft-versus-host disease*. Acute diarrhea, often associated with systemic compromise, can follow ingestion of toxins including organophosphate insecticides; amanita and other mushrooms; arsenic; and preformed environmental toxins in seafood, such as ciguatera and scombroid. Acute anaphylaxis to food ingestion can have a similar presentation. Conditions causing chronic diarrhea can also be confused with acute diarrhea early in their course. This confusion may occur with inflammatory bowel disease (IBD) and some of the other inflammatory chronic diarrheas that may have an abrupt rather than insidious onset and exhibit features that mimic infection.

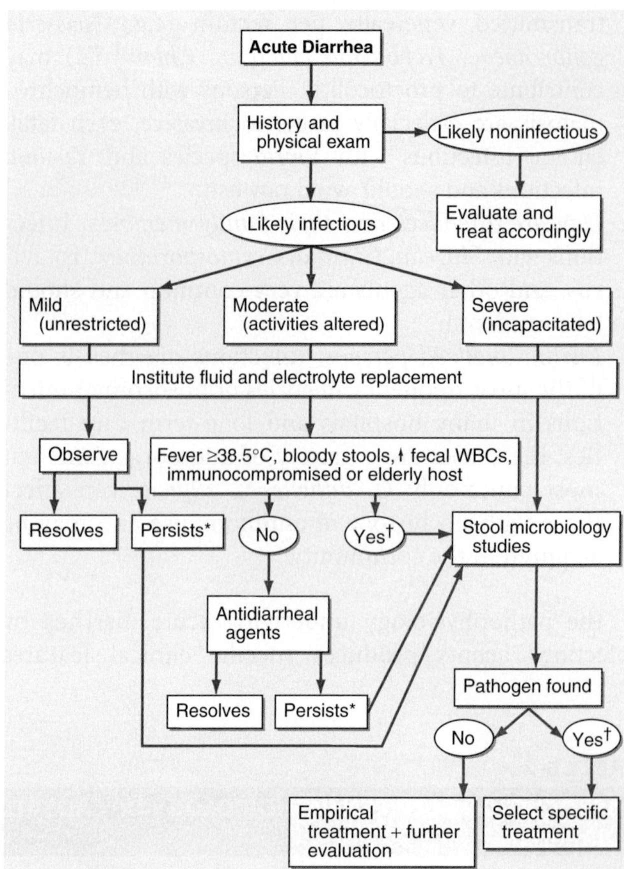

FIGURE 6-2

Algorithm for the management of acute diarrhea. Consider empirical treatment before evaluation with (*) metronidazole and with (†) quinolone. WBCs, white blood cells.

APPROACH TO THE PATIENT: Acute Diarrhea

The decision to evaluate acute diarrhea depends on its severity and duration and on various host factors (Fig. 6-2). Most episodes of acute diarrhea are mild and self-limited and do not justify the cost and potential morbidity rate of diagnostic or pharmacologic interventions. Indications for evaluation include profuse diarrhea with dehydration, grossly bloody stools, fever ≥38.5°C (≥101°F), duration >48 h without improvement, recent antibiotic use, new community outbreaks, associated severe abdominal pain in patients >50 years, and elderly (≥70 years) or immunocompromised patients. In some cases of moderately severe febrile diarrhea associated with fecal leukocytes (or increased fecal levels of the leukocyte proteins, such as calprotectin) or with gross blood, a diagnostic evaluation might be avoided in favor of an empirical antibiotic trial (see below).

The cornerstone of diagnosis in those suspected of severe acute infectious diarrhea is microbiologic analysis of the stool. Workup includes cultures for bacterial and viral pathogens, direct inspection for ova and parasites, and immunoassays for certain bacterial toxins (*C. difficile*), viral antigens (rotavirus), and protozoal antigens (*Giardia*, *E. histolytica*). The aforementioned clinical and epidemiologic associations may assist in focusing the evaluation. If a particular pathogen or set of possible pathogens is so implicated, then either the whole panel of routine studies may not be necessary or, in some instances, special cultures may be appropriate as for enterohemorrhagic and other types of *E. coli*, *Vibrio* species, and *Yersinia*. Molecular diagnosis of pathogens in stool can be made by identification of unique DNA sequences; and evolving microarray technologies have led to more rapid, sensitive, specific, and cost-effective diagnosis.

Persistent diarrhea is commonly due to *Giardia* **(Chap. 33)**, but additional causative organisms that should be considered include *C. difficile* (especially if antibiotics had been administered), *E. histolytica*, *Cryptosporidium*, *Campylobacter*, and others. If stool studies are unrevealing, flexible sigmoidoscopy with biopsies and upper endoscopy with duodenal aspirates and biopsies may be indicated. Brainerd diarrhea is an increasingly recognized entity characterized by an abrupt-onset diarrhea that persists for at least 4 weeks, but may last 1–3 years, and is thought to be of infectious origin. It may be associated with subtle inflammation of the distal small intestine or proximal colon.

Structural examination by sigmoidoscopy, colonoscopy, or abdominal computed tomography (CT) scanning (or other imaging approaches) may be appropriate in patients with uncharacterized persistent diarrhea to exclude IBD or as an initial approach in patients with suspected noninfectious acute diarrhea such as might be caused by ischemic colitis, diverticulitis, or partial bowel obstruction.

TREATMENT Acute Diarrhea

Fluid and electrolyte replacement are of central importance to all forms of acute diarrhea. Fluid replacement alone may suffice for mild cases. Oral sugar-electrolyte solutions (isoosmolar sport drinks or designed formulations) should be instituted promptly with severe diarrhea to limit dehydration, which is the major cause of death. Profoundly dehydrated patients, especially infants and the elderly, require IV rehydration.

In moderately severe nonfebrile and nonbloody diarrhea, antimotility and antisecretory agents such as loperamide can be useful adjuncts to control symptoms. Such agents should be avoided with febrile dysentery, which may be exacerbated or prolonged by them. Bismuth subsalicylate may reduce symptoms of vomiting and diarrhea but should not be used to treat immunocompromised patients or those with renal impairment because of the risk of bismuth encephalopathy.

Judicious use of antibiotics is appropriate in selected instances of acute diarrhea and may reduce its severity and duration (Fig. 6-2). Many physicians treat moderately to severely ill patients with febrile dysentery empirically without diagnostic evaluation using a quinolone, such as ciprofloxacin (500 mg bid for 3–5 d). Empirical treatment can also be considered for suspected giardiasis with metronidazole (250 mg qid for 7 d). Selection of antibiotics and dosage regimens are otherwise dictated by specific pathogens, geographic patterns of resistance, and conditions found **(Chaps. 24 and 28–196)**. Antibiotic coverage is indicated, whether or not a causative organism is discovered, in patients who are immunocompromised, have mechanical heart valves or recent vascular grafts, or are elderly. Bismuth subsalicylate may reduce the frequency of traveler's diarrhea. Antibiotic prophylaxis is only indicated for certain patients traveling to high-risk countries in whom the likelihood or seriousness of acquired diarrhea would be especially high, including those with immunocompromise, IBD, hemochromatosis, or gastric achlorhydria. Use of ciprofloxacin, azithromycin, or rifaximin may reduce bacterial diarrhea in such travelers by 90%, though rifaximin is not suitable for invasive disease, but rather as treatment for uncomplicated traveler's diarrhea. Finally, physicians should be vigilant to identify if an outbreak of diarrheal illness is occurring and to alert the public health authorities promptly. This may reduce the ultimate size of the affected population.

CHRONIC DIARRHEA

Diarrhea lasting >4 weeks warrants evaluation to exclude serious underlying pathology. In contrast to acute diarrhea, most of the causes of chronic diarrhea are noninfectious. The classification of chronic diarrhea by pathophysiologic mechanism facilitates a rational approach to management, although many diseases cause diarrhea by more than one mechanism (Table 6-3).

Secretory causes

Secretory diarrheas are due to derangements in fluid and electrolyte transport across the enterocolonic mucosa. They are characterized clinically by watery, large-volume fecal outputs that are typically painless and persist with fasting. Because there is no malabsorbed solute, stool osmolality is accounted for by normal endogenous electrolytes with no fecal osmotic gap.

Medications

Side effects from regular ingestion of drugs and toxins are the most common secretory causes of chronic diarrhea. Hundreds of prescription and over-the-counter medications (see earlier section, "Acute Diarrhea, Other Causes") may produce diarrhea. Surreptitious or habitual use of stimulant laxatives (e.g., senna, cascara, bisacodyl, ricinoleic acid [castor oil]) must also be considered. Chronic ethanol consumption may cause a secretory-type diarrhea due to enterocyte injury with impaired sodium and water absorption as well as rapid transit and other alterations. Inadvertent ingestion of certain environmental toxins (e.g., arsenic) may lead to chronic rather than acute forms of diarrhea. Certain bacterial infections may occasionally persist and be associated with a secretory-type diarrhea.

TABLE 6-3

MAJOR CAUSES OF CHRONIC DIARRHEA ACCORDING TO PREDOMINANT PATHOPHYSIOLOGIC MECHANISM

Secretory Causes
- Exogenous stimulant laxatives
- Chronic ethanol ingestion
- Other drugs and toxins
- Endogenous laxatives (dihydroxy bile acids)
- Idiopathic secretory diarrhea or bile acid diarrhea
- Certain bacterial infections
- Bowel resection, disease, or fistula (↓ absorption)
- Partial bowel obstruction or fecal impaction
- Hormone-producing tumors (carcinoid, VIPoma, medullary cancer of thyroid, mastocytosis, gastrinoma, colorectal villous adenoma)
- Addison's disease
- Congenital electrolyte absorption defects

Osmotic Causes
- Osmotic laxatives (Mg^{2+}, PO_4^{-3}, SO_4^{-2})
- Lactase and other disaccharide deficiencies
- Nonabsorbable carbohydrates (sorbitol, lactulose, polyethylene glycol)
- Gluten and FODMAP intolerance

Steatorrheal Causes
- Intraluminal maldigestion (pancreatic exocrine insufficiency, bacterial overgrowth, bariatric surgery, liver disease)
- Mucosal malabsorption (celiac sprue, Whipple's disease, infections, abetalipoproteinemia, ischemia, drug-induced enteropathy)
- Postmucosal obstruction (1° or 2° lymphatic obstruction)

Inflammatory Causes
- Idiopathic inflammatory bowel disease (Crohn's, chronic ulcerative colitis)
- Lymphocytic and collagenous colitis
- Immune-related mucosal disease (1° or 2° immunodeficiencies, food allergy, eosinophilic gastroenteritis, graft-versus-host disease)
- Infections (invasive bacteria, viruses, and parasites, Brainerd diarrhea)
- Radiation injury
- Gastrointestinal malignancies

Dysmotile Causes
- Irritable bowel syndrome (including postinfectious IBS)
- Visceral neuromyopathies
- Hyperthyroidism
- Drugs (prokinetic agents)
- Postvagotomy

Factitial Causes
- Munchausen
- Eating disorders

Iatrogenic Causes
- Cholecystectomy
- Ileal resection
- Bariatric surgery
- Vagotomy, fundoplication

Abbreviation: FODMAP, fermentable oligosaccharides, disaccharides, monosaccharides, and polyols.

Bowel resection, mucosal disease, or enterocolic fistula

These conditions may result in a secretory-type diarrhea because of inadequate surface for reabsorption of secreted fluids and electrolytes. Unlike other secretory diarrheas, this subset of conditions tends to worsen with eating. With disease (e.g., Crohn's ileitis) or resection of <100 cm of terminal ileum, dihydroxy bile acids may escape absorption and stimulate colonic secretion (cholerheic diarrhea). This mechanism may contribute to so-called *idiopathic secretory diarrhea or bile acid diarrhea (BAD)*, in which bile acids are functionally malabsorbed from a normal-appearing terminal ileum. This *idiopathic bile acid malabsorption (BAM)* may account for an average of 40% of unexplained chronic diarrhea. Reduced negative feedback regulation of bile acid synthesis in hepatocytes by fibroblast growth factor 19 (FGF-19) produced by ileal enterocytes results in a degree of bile-acid synthesis that exceeds the normal capacity for ileal reabsorption, producing BAD. An alternative cause of BAD is a genetic variation in the receptor proteins (β-klotho and fibroblast growth factor 4) on the hepatocyte that normally mediate the effect of FGF-19. Dysfunction of these proteins prevents FGF-19 inhibition of hepatocyte bile acid synthesis.

Partial bowel obstruction, ostomy stricture, or fecal impaction may paradoxically lead to increased fecal output due to fluid hypersecretion.

Hormones

Although uncommon, the classic examples of secretory diarrhea are those mediated by hormones. *Metastatic gastrointestinal carcinoid tumors* or, rarely, *primary bronchial carcinoids* may produce watery diarrhea alone or as part of the carcinoid syndrome that comprises episodic flushing, wheezing, dyspnea, and right-sided valvular heart disease. Diarrhea is due to the release into the circulation of potent intestinal secretagogues including serotonin, histamine, prostaglandins, and various kinins. Pellagra-like skin lesions may rarely occur as the result of serotonin overproduction with niacin depletion. *Gastrinoma*, one of the most common neuroendocrine tumors, most typically presents with refractory peptic ulcers, but diarrhea occurs in up to one-third of cases and may be the only clinical manifestation in 10%. While other secretagogues released with gastrin may play a role, the diarrhea most often results from fat maldigestion owing to pancreatic enzyme inactivation by low intraduodenal pH. The watery diarrhea hypokalemia achlorhydria syndrome, also called *pancreatic cholera*, is due to a non-β cell pancreatic adenoma, referred to as a *VIPoma*, that secretes VIP and a host of other peptide hormones including pancreatic polypeptide, secretin, gastrin, gastrin-inhibitory polypeptide (also called glucose-dependent insulinotropic peptide), neurotensin, calcitonin, and prostaglandins.

The secretory diarrhea is often massive with stool volumes >3 L/d; daily volumes as high as 20 L have been reported. Life-threatening dehydration; neuromuscular dysfunction from associated hypokalemia, hypomagnesemia, or hypercalcemia; flushing; and hyperglycemia may accompany a VIPoma. *Medullary carcinoma of the thyroid* may present with watery diarrhea caused by calcitonin, other secretory peptides, or prostaglandins. Prominent diarrhea is often associated with metastatic disease and poor prognosis. *Systemic mastocytosis,* which may be associated with the skin lesion urticaria pigmentosa, may cause diarrhea that is either secretory and mediated by histamine or inflammatory due to intestinal infiltration by mast cells. Large *colorectal villous adenomas* may rarely be associated with a secretory diarrhea that may cause hypokalemia, can be inhibited by NSAIDs, and are apparently mediated by prostaglandins.

Congenital defects in ion absorption

Rarely, defects in specific carriers associated with ion absorption cause watery diarrhea from birth. These disorders include defective Cl^-/HCO_3^- exchange (*congenital chloridorrhea*) with alkalosis (which results from a mutated *DRA* [down-regulated in adenoma] gene) and defective Na^+/H^+ exchange (*congenital sodium diarrhea),* which results from a mutation in the *NHE3* (sodium-hydrogen exchanger) gene and results in acidosis.

Some hormone deficiencies may be associated with watery diarrhea, such as occurs with adrenocortical insufficiency (Addison's disease) that may be accompanied by skin hyperpigmentation.

Osmotic causes

Osmotic diarrhea occurs when ingested, poorly absorbable, osmotically active solutes draw enough fluid into the lumen to exceed the reabsorptive capacity of the colon. Fecal water output increases in proportion to such a solute load. Osmotic diarrhea characteristically ceases with fasting or with discontinuation of the causative agent.

Osmotic laxatives

Ingestion of magnesium-containing antacids, health supplements, or laxatives may induce osmotic diarrhea typified by a stool osmotic gap (>50 mosmol/L): serum osmolarity (typically 290 mosmol/kg) − (2 × [fecal sodium + potassium concentration]). Measurement of fecal osmolarity is no longer recommended because, even when measured immediately after evacuation, it may be erroneous because carbohydrates are metabolized by colonic bacteria, causing an increase in osmolarity.

Carbohydrate malabsorption

Carbohydrate malabsorption due to acquired or congenital defects in brush-border disaccharidases and other enzymes leads to osmotic diarrhea with a low pH. One of the most common causes of chronic diarrhea in adults is *lactase deficiency*, which affects three-fourths of nonwhites worldwide and 5–30% of persons in the United States; the total lactose load at any one time influences the symptoms experienced. Most patients learn to avoid milk products without requiring treatment with enzyme supplements. Some sugars, such as sorbitol, lactulose, or fructose, are frequently malabsorbed, and diarrhea ensues with ingestion of medications, gum, or candies sweetened with these poorly or incompletely absorbed sugars.

Wheat and fodmap intolerance

Chronic diarrhea, bloating, and abdominal pain are recognized as symptoms of nonceliac gluten intolerance (which is associated with impaired intestinal or colonic barrier function) and intolerance of fermentable oligosaccharides, disaccharides, monosaccharides, and polyols (FODMAPs). The latter's effects represent the interaction between the GI microbiome and the nutrients.

Steatorrheal causes

Fat malabsorption may lead to greasy, foul-smelling, difficult-to-flush diarrhea often associated with weight loss and nutritional deficiencies due to concomitant malabsorption of amino acids and vitamins. Increased fecal output is caused by the osmotic effects of fatty acids, especially after bacterial hydroxylation, and, to a lesser extent, by the neutral fat. Quantitatively, steatorrhea is defined as stool fat exceeding the normal 7 g/d; rapid-transit diarrhea may result in fecal fat up to 14 g/d; daily fecal fat averages 15–25 g with small-intestinal diseases and is often >32 g with pancreatic exocrine insufficiency. Intraluminal maldigestion, mucosal malabsorption, or lymphatic obstruction may produce steatorrhea.

Intraluminal maldigestion

This condition most commonly results from pancreatic exocrine insufficiency, which occurs when >90% of pancreatic secretory function is lost. *Chronic pancreatitis,* usually a sequel of ethanol abuse, most frequently causes pancreatic insufficiency. Other causes include *cystic fibrosis*; *pancreatic duct obstruction*; and, rarely, *somatostatinoma.* Bacterial overgrowth in the small intestine may deconjugate bile acids and alter micelle formation, impairing fat digestion; it occurs with stasis from a blind-loop, small-bowel diverticulum or dysmotility and is especially likely in the elderly. Finally, cirrhosis or biliary obstruction may lead to mild steatorrhea due to deficient intraluminal bile acid concentration.

Mucosal malabsorption

Mucosal malabsorption occurs from a variety of enteropathies, but it most commonly occurs from *celiac disease*. This gluten-sensitive enteropathy affects all ages and is characterized by villous atrophy and crypt hyperplasia in the proximal small bowel and can present with fatty diarrhea associated with multiple nutritional deficiencies of varying severity. Celiac disease is much more frequent than previously thought; it affects ~1% of the population, frequently presents without steatorrhea, can mimic IBS, and has many other GI and extraintestinal manifestations. *Tropical sprue* may produce a similar histologic and clinical syndrome but occurs in residents of or travelers to tropical climates; abrupt onset and response to antibiotics suggest an infectious etiology. *Whipple's disease,* due to the bacillus *Tropheryma whipplei* and histiocytic infiltration of the small-bowel mucosa, is a less common cause of steatorrhea that most typically occurs in young or middle-aged men; it is frequently associated with arthralgias, fever, lymphadenopathy, and extreme fatigue, and it may affect the CNS and endocardium. A similar clinical and histologic picture results from *Mycobacterium avium-intracellulare* infection in patients with AIDS. *Abetalipoproteinemia* is a rare defect of chylomicron formation and fat malabsorption in children, associated with acanthocytic erythrocytes, ataxia, and retinitis pigmentosa. Several other conditions may cause mucosal malabsorption including infections, especially with protozoa such as *Giardia*; numerous medications (e.g., olmesartan, mycophenolate mofetil, colchicine, cholestyramine, neomycin); amyloidosis; and chronic ischemia.

Postmucosal lymphatic obstruction

The pathophysiology of this condition, which is due to the rare *congenital intestinal lymphangiectasia* or to *acquired lymphatic obstruction* secondary to trauma, tumor, cardiac disease or infection, leads to the unique constellation of fat malabsorption with enteric losses of protein (often causing edema) and lymphocytopenia. Carbohydrate and amino acid absorption are preserved.

Inflammatory causes

Inflammatory diarrheas are generally accompanied by pain, fever, bleeding, or other manifestations of inflammation. The mechanism of diarrhea may not only be exudation but, depending on lesion site, may include fat malabsorption, disrupted fluid/electrolyte absorption, and hypersecretion or hypermotility from release of cytokines and other inflammatory mediators. The unifying feature on stool analysis is the presence of leukocytes or leukocyte-derived proteins such as calprotectin. With severe inflammation, exudative protein loss can lead to anasarca (generalized edema). Any middle-aged or older person with chronic inflammatory-type diarrhea, especially with blood, should be carefully evaluated to exclude a colorectal tumor.

Idiopathic inflammatory bowel disease

The illnesses in this category, which include *Crohn's disease* and *chronic ulcerative colitis*, are among the most common organic causes of chronic diarrhea in adults and range in severity from mild to fulminant and life-threatening. They may be associated with uveitis, polyarthralgias, cholestatic liver disease (primary sclerosing cholangitis), and skin lesions (erythema nodosum, pyoderma gangrenosum). *Microscopic colitis*, including both lymphocytic and *collagenous colitis*, is an increasingly recognized cause of chronic watery diarrhea, especially in middle-aged women and those on NSAIDs, statins, proton pump inhibitors (PPIs), and selective serotonin reuptake inhibitors (SSRIs); biopsy of a normal-appearing colon is required for histologic diagnosis. It may coexist with symptoms suggesting IBS or with celiac sprue or drug-induced enteropathy. It typically responds well to anti-inflammatory drugs (e.g., bismuth), to the opioid agonist loperamide, or to budesonide.

Primary or secondary forms of immunodeficiency

Immunodeficiency may lead to prolonged infectious diarrhea. With selective IgA deficiency or common variable *hypogammaglobulinemia*, diarrhea is particularly prevalent and often the result of giardiasis, bacterial overgrowth, or sprue.

Eosinophilic gastroenteritis

Eosinophil infiltration of the mucosa, muscularis, or serosa at any level of the GI tract may cause diarrhea, pain, vomiting, or ascites. Affected patients often have an atopic history, Charcot-Leyden crystals due to extruded eosinophil contents may be seen on microscopic inspection of stool, and peripheral eosinophilia is present in 50–75% of patients. While hypersensitivity to certain foods occurs in adults, true food allergy causing chronic diarrhea is rare.

Other causes

Chronic inflammatory diarrhea may be caused by *radiation enterocolitis*, *chronic graft-versus-host disease*, *Behçet's syndrome*, and *Cronkhite-Canada syndrome*, among others.

Dysmotility causes

Rapid transit may accompany many diarrheas as a secondary or contributing phenomenon, but primary dysmotility is an unusual etiology of true diarrhea. Stool features often suggest a secretory diarrhea, but mild steatorrhea of up to 14 g of fat per day can be produced by maldigestion from rapid transit alone. *Hyperthyroidism*, *carcinoid syndrome*, and certain drugs (e.g., prostaglandins, prokinetic agents) may produce hypermotility with resultant diarrhea. Primary visceral neuromyopathies or idiopathic acquired intestinal pseudoobstruction may lead to stasis with secondary bacterial overgrowth causing diarrhea. *Diabetic diarrhea*, often accompanied by peripheral and generalized autonomic neuropathies, may occur in part because of intestinal dysmotility.

The exceedingly common IBS (10% point prevalence, 1–2% per year incidence) is characterized by disturbed intestinal and colonic motor and sensory responses to various stimuli. Symptoms of stool frequency typically cease at night, alternate with periods of constipation, are accompanied by abdominal pain relieved with defecation, and rarely result in weight loss.

Factitial causes

Factitial diarrhea accounts for up to 15% of unexplained diarrheas referred to tertiary care centers. Either as a form of *Munchausen syndrome* (deception or self-injury for secondary gain) or *eating disorders*, some patients covertly self-administer laxatives alone or in combination with other medications (e.g., diuretics) or surreptitiously add water or urine to stool sent for analysis. Such patients are typically women, often with histories of psychiatric illness, and disproportionately from careers in health care. Hypotension and hypokalemia are common co-presenting features. The evaluation of such patients may be difficult: contamination of the stool with water or urine is suggested by very low or high stool osmolarity, respectively. Such patients often deny this possibility when confronted, but they do benefit from psychiatric counseling when they acknowledge their behavior.

APPROACH TO THE PATIENT: Chronic Diarrhea

The laboratory tools available to evaluate the very common problem of chronic diarrhea are extensive, and many are costly and invasive. As such, the diagnostic evaluation must be rationally directed by a careful history, including medications, and physical examination (Fig. 6-3*A*). When this strategy is unrevealing, simple triage tests are often warranted to direct the choice of more complex investigations (Fig. 6-3*B*). The history, physical examination (Table 6-4), and routine blood studies should attempt to characterize the mechanism of diarrhea, identify diagnostically helpful associations, and assess the patient's fluid/electrolyte and nutritional status. Patients should be questioned about the onset, duration, pattern, aggravating (especially diet) and relieving factors, and stool characteristics of their diarrhea. The presence or absence of fecal incontinence, fever, weight loss, pain, certain exposures (travel, medications, contacts with diarrhea), and common extraintestinal manifestations (skin changes, arthralgias, oral aphthous ulcers) should be noted. A family history of IBD or sprue may indicate those possibilities. Physical findings may offer clues such as a thyroid mass, wheezing, heart murmurs, edema, hepatomegaly, abdominal masses, lymphadenopathy, mucocutaneous abnormalities, perianal fistulas, or anal sphincter laxity. Peripheral blood leukocytosis, elevated sedimentation rate, or C-reactive protein suggests inflammation; anemia reflects blood loss or nutritional deficiencies; or eosinophilia may occur with parasitoses, neoplasia, collagen-vascular disease, allergy, or eosinophilic gastroenteritis. Blood chemistries may demonstrate electrolyte, hepatic, or other metabolic disturbances. Measuring IgA tissue transglutaminase antibodies may help detect celiac disease. Bile acid diarrhea is confirmed by a scintigraphic radiolabeled bile acid retention test; however, this is not available in many countries. Alternative approaches are a screening blood test (serum C4 or FGF-19), measurement of fecal bile acids, or a therapeutic trial with a bile acid sequestrant (e.g., cholestyramine or colesevelam).

A therapeutic trial is often appropriate, definitive, and highly cost-effective when a specific diagnosis is suggested on the initial physician encounter. For example, chronic watery diarrhea, which ceases with fasting in an otherwise healthy young adult, may justify a trial of a lactose-restricted diet; bloating and diarrhea persisting since a mountain backpacking trip may warrant a trial of metronidazole for likely giardiasis; and postprandial diarrhea persisting following resection of terminal ileum might be due to bile acid malabsorption and be treated with cholestyramine or colesevelam before further evaluation. Persistent symptoms require additional investigation.

Certain diagnoses may be suggested on the initial encounter (e.g., idiopathic IBD); however, additional focused evaluations may be necessary to confirm the diagnosis and characterize the severity or extent of disease so that treatment can be best guided. Patients suspected of having IBS should be initially evaluated with flexible sigmoidoscopy with colorectal biopsies to exclude IBD, or particularly microscopic colitis, which is clinically indistinguishable from IBS with diarrhea; those with normal findings might be reassured and, as indicated, treated empirically with antispasmodics, antidiarrheals, or antidepressants (e.g., tricyclic agents). Any patient who presents with chronic diarrhea and hematochezia should be evaluated with stool microbiologic studies and colonoscopy.

In an estimated two-thirds of cases, the cause for chronic diarrhea remains unclear after the initial encounter, and further testing is required. Quantitative stool collection and analyses can yield important objective data that may establish a diagnosis or characterize the type of diarrhea as a triage for focused additional studies (Fig. 6-3*B*). If stool weight is >200 g/d, additional stool analyses should be performed that might include electrolyte concentration, pH, occult blood testing, leukocyte

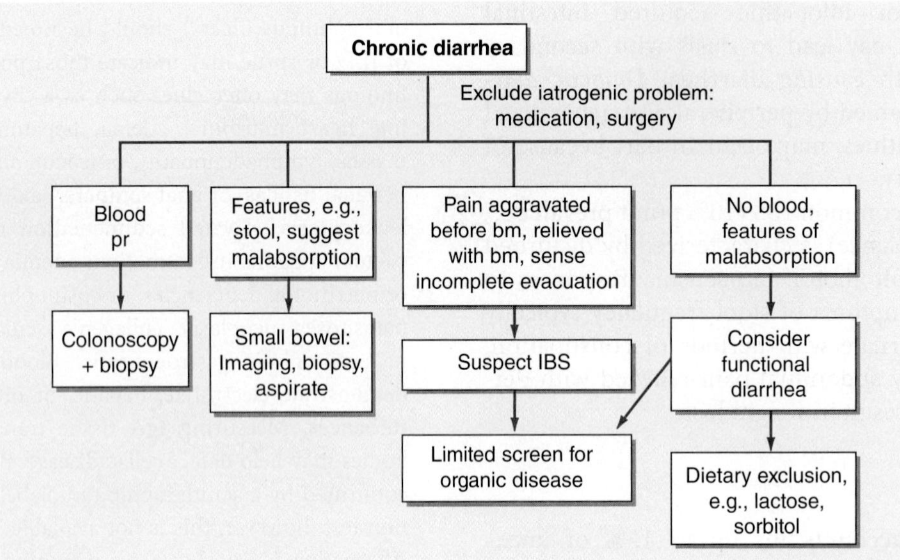

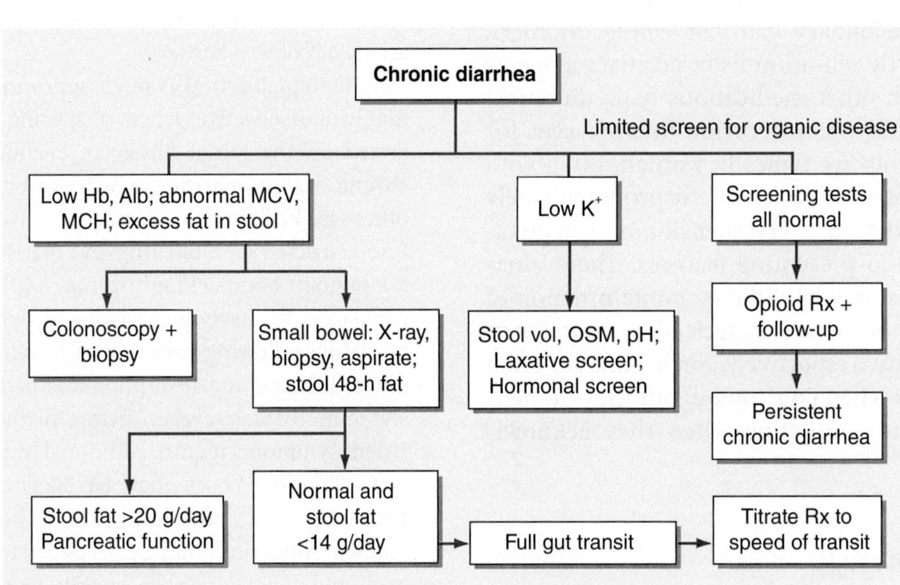

FIGURE 6-3

Chronic diarrhea. *A.* Initial management based on accompanying symptoms or features. ***B.*** Evaluation based on findings from a limited age-appropriate screen for organic disease. Alb, albumin; bm, bowel movement; Hb, hemoglobin; IBS, irritable bowel syndrome; MCH, mean corpuscular hemoglobin; MCV, mean corpuscular volume; OSM, osmolality; pr, per rectum. *(Reprinted from M Camilleri: Clin Gastroenterol Hepatol. 2:198, 2004.)*

inspection (or leukocyte protein assay), fat quantitation, and laxative screens.

For secretory diarrheas (watery, normal osmotic gap), possible medication-related side effects or surreptitious laxative use should be reconsidered. Microbiologic studies should be done including fecal bacterial cultures (including media for *Aeromonas* and *Plesiomonas*), inspection for ova and parasites, and *Giardia* antigen assay (the most sensitive test for giardiasis). Small-bowel bacterial overgrowth can be excluded by intestinal aspirates with quantitative cultures or with glucose or lactulose breath tests involving measurement of breath hydrogen, methane, or other metabolite. However, interpretation of these breath tests may be confounded by disturbances of intestinal transit. Upper endoscopy and colonoscopy with biopsies and small-bowel x-rays (formerly barium, but increasingly CT with enterography or magnetic resonance with enteroclysis) are helpful to rule out structural or occult inflammatory disease. When suggested by history or other findings, screens for peptide hormones should

TABLE 6-4

PHYSICAL EXAMINATION IN PATIENTS WITH CHRONIC DIARRHEA

1. Are there general features to suggest malabsorption or inflammatory bowel disease (IBD) such as anemia, dermatitis herpetiformis, edema, or clubbing?
2. Are there features to suggest underlying autonomic neuropathy or collagen-vascular disease in the pupils, orthostasis, skin, hands, or joints?
3. Is there an abdominal mass or tenderness?
4. Are there any abnormalities of rectal mucosa, rectal defects, or altered anal sphincter functions?
5. Are there any mucocutaneous manifestations of systemic disease such as dermatitis herpetiformis (celiac disease), erythema nodosum (ulcerative colitis), flushing (carcinoid), or oral ulcers for IBD or celiac disease?

be pursued (e.g., serum gastrin, VIP, calcitonin, and thyroid hormone/thyroid-stimulating hormone, urinary 5-hydroxyindolacetic acid, histamine).

Further evaluation of osmotic diarrhea should include tests for lactose intolerance and magnesium ingestion, the two most common causes. Low fecal pH suggests carbohydrate malabsorption; lactose malabsorption can be confirmed by lactose breath testing or by a therapeutic trial with lactose exclusion and observation of the effect of lactose challenge (e.g., a liter of milk). Lactase determination on small-bowel biopsy is not generally available. If fecal magnesium or laxative levels are elevated, inadvertent or surreptitious ingestion should be considered and psychiatric help should be sought.

For those with proven fatty diarrhea, endoscopy with small-bowel biopsy (including aspiration for *Giardia* and quantitative cultures) should be performed; if this procedure is unrevealing, a small-bowel radiograph is often an appropriate next step. If small-bowel studies are negative or if pancreatic disease is suspected, pancreatic exocrine insufficiency should be excluded with direct tests, such as the secretin-cholecystokinin stimulation test or a variation that could be performed endoscopically. In general, indirect tests such as assay of fecal elastase or chymotrypsin activity or a bentiromide test have fallen out of favor because of low sensitivity and specificity.

Chronic inflammatory-type diarrheas should be suspected by the presence of blood or leukocytes in the stool. Such findings warrant stool cultures; inspection for ova and parasites; *C. difficile* toxin assay; colonoscopy with biopsies; and, if indicated, small-bowel contrast studies.

TREATMENT Chronic Diarrhea

Treatment of chronic diarrhea depends on the specific etiology and may be curative, suppressive, or empirical. If the cause can be eradicated, treatment is curative as with resection of a colorectal cancer, antibiotic administration for Whipple's disease or tropical sprue, or discontinuation of a drug. For many chronic conditions, diarrhea can be controlled by suppression of the underlying mechanism. Examples include elimination of dietary lactose for lactase deficiency or gluten for celiac sprue, use of glucocorticoids or other anti-inflammatory agents for idiopathic IBDs, bile acid sequestrants for bile acid malabsorption, PPIs for the gastric hypersecretion of gastrinomas, somatostatin analogues such as octreotide for malignant carcinoid syndrome, prostaglandin inhibitors such as indomethacin for medullary carcinoma of the thyroid, and pancreatic enzyme replacement for pancreatic insufficiency. When the specific cause or mechanism of chronic diarrhea evades diagnosis, empirical therapy may be beneficial. Mild opiates, such as diphenoxylate or loperamide, are often helpful in mild or moderate watery diarrhea. For those with more severe diarrhea, codeine or tincture of opium may be beneficial. Such antimotility agents should be avoided with severe IBD, because toxic megacolon may be precipitated. Clonidine, an α_2-adrenergic agonist, may allow control of diabetic diarrhea, although the medication may be poorly tolerated because it causes postural hypotension. The 5-HT_3 receptor antagonists (e.g., alosetron) may relieve diarrhea and urgency in patients with IBS diarrhea. For all patients with chronic diarrhea, fluid and electrolyte repletion is an important component of management (see "Acute Diarrhea," earlier). Replacement of fat-soluble vitamins may also be necessary in patients with chronic steatorrhea.

CONSTIPATION

DEFINITION

Constipation is a common complaint in clinical practice and usually refers to persistent, difficult, infrequent, or seemingly incomplete defecation. Because of the wide range of normal bowel habits, constipation is difficult to define precisely. Most persons have at least three bowel movements per week; however, low stool frequency alone is not the sole criterion for the diagnosis of constipation. Many constipated patients have a normal frequency of defecation but complain of excessive straining, hard stools, lower abdominal fullness, or a sense of incomplete evacuation. The individual patient's symptoms must be analyzed in detail to ascertain what is meant by "constipation" or "difficulty" with defecation.

Stool form and consistency are well correlated with the time elapsed from the preceding defecation. Hard, pellety stools occur with slow transit, whereas loose, watery stools are associated with rapid transit. Both small pellety or very large stools are more difficult to expel than normal stools.

The perception of hard stools or excessive straining is more difficult to assess objectively, and the need for enemas or digital disimpaction is a clinically useful way to corroborate the patient's perceptions of difficult defecation.

Psychosocial or cultural factors may also be important. A person whose parents attached great importance to daily defecation will become greatly concerned when he or she misses a daily bowel movement; some children withhold stool to gain attention or because of fear of pain from anal irritation; and some adults habitually ignore or delay the call to have a bowel movement.

CAUSES

Pathophysiologically, chronic constipation generally results from inadequate fiber or fluid intake or from disordered colonic transit or anorectal function. These result from neurogastroenterologic disturbance, certain drugs, advancing age, or in association with a large number of systemic diseases that affect the GI tract (Table 6-5). Constipation of recent onset may be a symptom of significant organic disease such as tumor or stricture. In *idiopathic constipation*, a subset of patients exhibit delayed emptying of the ascending and transverse colon with prolongation of transit (often in the proximal colon) and a reduced frequency of propulsive HAPCs. *Outlet obstruction to defecation* (also called *evacuation disorders*) accounts for about a quarter of cases presenting with constipation in tertiary care and may cause delayed colonic transit, which is usually corrected by biofeedback retraining of the disordered defecation. Constipation of any cause may be exacerbated by hospitalization or chronic illnesses that lead to physical or mental impairment and result in inactivity or physical immobility.

TABLE 6-5

CAUSES OF CONSTIPATION IN ADULTS

TYPES OF CONSTIPATION AND CAUSES	EXAMPLES
Recent Onset	
Colonic obstruction	Neoplasm; stricture: ischemic, diverticular, inflammatory
Anal sphincter spasm	Anal fissure, painful hemorrhoids
Medications	
Chronic	
Irritable bowel syndrome	Constipation-predominant, alternating
Medications	Ca^{2+} blockers, antidepressants
Colonic pseudoobstruction	Slow-transit constipation, megacolon (rare Hirschsprung's, Chagas' diseases)
Disorders of rectal evacuation	Pelvic floor dysfunction; anismus; descending perineum syndrome; rectal mucosal prolapse; rectocele
Endocrinopathies	Hypothyroidism, hypercalcemia, pregnancy
Psychiatric disorders	Depression, eating disorders, drugs
Neurologic disease	Parkinsonism, multiple sclerosis, spinal cord injury
Generalized muscle disease	Progressive systemic sclerosis

APPROACH TO THE PATIENT: Constipation

A careful history should explore the patient's symptoms and confirm whether he or she is indeed constipated based on frequency (e.g., fewer than three bowel movements per week), consistency (lumpy/hard), excessive straining, prolonged defecation time, or need to support the perineum or digitate the anorectum to facilitate stool evacuation. In the vast majority of cases (probably >90%), there is no underlying cause (e.g., cancer, depression, or hypothyroidism), and constipation responds to ample hydration, exercise, and supplementation of dietary fiber (15–25 g/d). A good diet and medication history and attention to psychosocial issues are key. Physical examination and, particularly, a rectal examination should exclude fecal impaction and most of the important diseases that present with constipation and possibly indicate features suggesting an evacuation disorder (e.g., high anal sphincter tone, failure of perineal descent, or paradoxical puborectalis contraction during straining to simulate stool evacuation).

The presence of weight loss, rectal bleeding, or anemia with constipation mandates either flexible sigmoidoscopy plus barium enema or colonoscopy alone, particularly in patients >40 years, to exclude structural diseases such as cancer or strictures. Colonoscopy alone is most cost-effective in this setting because it provides an opportunity to biopsy mucosal lesions, perform polypectomy, or dilate strictures. Barium enema has advantages over colonoscopy in the patient with isolated constipation because it is less costly and identifies colonic dilation and all significant mucosal lesions or strictures that are likely to present with constipation. Melanosis coli, or pigmentation of the colon mucosa, indicates the use of anthraquinone laxatives such as cascara or senna; however, this is usually apparent from a careful history. An unexpected disorder such as megacolon or cathartic colon may also be detected by colonic radiographs. Measurement of serum calcium, potassium, and thyroid-stimulating hormone levels will identify rare patients with metabolic disorders.

Patients with more troublesome constipation may not respond to fiber alone and may be helped by a bowel-training regimen, which involves taking an osmotic laxative (e.g., magnesium salts, lactulose, sorbitol, polyethylene glycol) and evacuating with enema or suppository

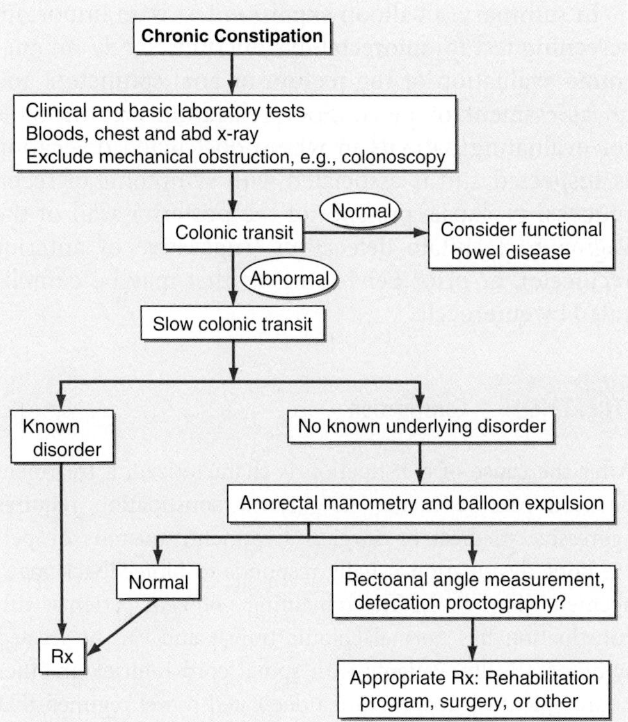

FIGURE 6-4

Algorithm for the management of constipation. abd, abdominal.

(e.g., glycerine or bisacodyl) as needed. After breakfast, a distraction-free 15–20 min on the toilet without straining is encouraged. Excessive straining may lead to development of hemorrhoids, and, if there is weakness of the pelvic floor or injury to the pudendal nerve, may result in obstructed defecation from descending perineum syndrome several years later. Those few who do not benefit from the simple measures delineated above or require long-term treatment or fail to respond to potent laxatives should undergo further investigation (Fig. 6-4). Novel agents that induce secretion (e.g., lubiprostone, a chloride channel activator, or linaclotide, a guanylate cyclase C agonist that activates chloride secretion) are also available.

INVESTIGATION OF SEVERE CONSTIPATION

A small minority (probably <5%) of patients have severe or "intractable" constipation; about 25% have evacuation disorders. These are the patients most likely to require evaluation by gastroenterologists or in referral centers. Further observation of the patient may occasionally reveal a previously unrecognized cause, such as an evacuation disorder, laxative abuse, malingering, or psychological disorder. In these patients, evaluations of the physiologic function of the colon and pelvic floor and of psychological status aid in the rational choice of treatment. Even among these highly selected patients with severe constipation, a cause can be identified in only about one-third of tertiary referral patients, with the others being diagnosed with normal transit constipation.

Measurement of colonic transit

Radiopaque marker transit tests are easy, repeatable, generally safe, inexpensive, reliable, and highly applicable in evaluating constipated patients in clinical practice. Several validated methods are very simple. For example, radiopaque markers are ingested; an abdominal flat film taken 5 days later should indicate passage of 80% of the markers out of the colon without the use of laxatives or enemas. This test does not provide useful information about the transit profile of the stomach and small bowel.

Radioscintigraphy with a delayed-release capsule containing radiolabeled particles has been used to noninvasively characterize normal, accelerated, or delayed colonic function over 24–48 h with low radiation exposure. This approach simultaneously assesses gastric, small bowel (which may be important in ~20% of patients with delayed colonic transit because they reflect a more generalized GI motility disorder), and colonic transit. The disadvantages are the greater cost and the need for specific materials prepared in a nuclear medicine laboratory.

Anorectal and pelvic floor tests

Pelvic floor dysfunction is suggested by the inability to evacuate the rectum, a feeling of persistent rectal fullness, rectal pain, the need to extract stool from the rectum digitally, application of pressure on the posterior wall of the vagina, support of the perineum during straining, and excessive straining. These significant symptoms should be contrasted with the simple sense of incomplete rectal evacuation, which is common in IBS.

Formal psychological evaluation may identify eating disorders, "control issues," depression, or post-traumatic stress disorders that may respond to cognitive or other intervention and may be important in restoring quality of life to patients who might present with chronic constipation.

A simple clinical test in the office to document a non-relaxing puborectalis muscle is to have the patient strain to expel the index finger during a digital rectal examination. Motion of the puborectalis posteriorly during straining indicates proper coordination of the pelvic floor muscles. Motion anteriorly with paradoxical contraction during simulated evacuation indicates pelvic floor dysfunction.

Measurement of perineal descent is relatively easy to gauge clinically by placing the patient in the left decubitus position and watching the perineum to detect inadequate descent (<1.5 cm, a sign of pelvic floor dysfunction) or perineal ballooning during straining relative to bony landmarks (>4 cm, suggesting excessive perineal descent).

A useful overall test of evacuation is the balloon expulsion test. A balloon-tipped urinary catheter is placed and inflated with 50 mL of water. Normally, a patient can expel it while seated on a toilet or in the left lateral decubitus position. In the lateral position, the weight needed to facilitate expulsion of the balloon is determined; normally, expulsion occurs with <200 g added or unaided within 2 min.

Anorectal manometry, when used in the evaluation of patients with severe constipation, may find an excessively high resting (>80 mmHg) or squeeze anal sphincter tone, suggesting anismus (anal sphincter spasm). This test also identifies rare syndromes, such as adult Hirschsprung's disease, by the absence of the rectoanal inhibitory reflex.

Defecography (a dynamic barium enema including lateral views obtained during barium expulsion or a magnetic resonance defecogram) reveals "soft abnormalities" in many patients; the most relevant findings are the measured changes in rectoanal angle, anatomic defects of the rectum such as internal mucosal prolapse, and enteroceles or rectoceles. Surgically remediable conditions are identified in only a few patients. These include severe, whole-thickness intussusception with complete outlet obstruction due to funnel-shaped plugging at the anal canal or an extremely large rectocele that fills preferentially during attempts at defecation instead of expulsion of the barium through the anus. In summary, defecography requires an interested and experienced radiologist, and abnormalities are not pathognomonic for pelvic floor dysfunction. The most common cause of outlet obstruction is failure of the puborectalis muscle to relax; this is not identified by barium defecography, but can be demonstrated by magnetic resonance defecography, which provides more information about the structure and function of the pelvic floor, distal colorectum, and anal sphincters.

Neurologic testing (electromyography) is more helpful in the evaluation of patients with incontinence than of those with symptoms suggesting obstructed defecation. The absence of neurologic signs in the lower extremities suggests that any documented denervation of the puborectalis results from pelvic (e.g., obstetric) injury or from stretching of the pudendal nerve by chronic, long-standing straining. Constipation is common among patients with spinal cord injuries, neurologic diseases such as Parkinson's disease, multiple sclerosis, and diabetic neuropathy.

Spinal-evoked responses during electrical rectal stimulation or stimulation of external anal sphincter contraction by applying magnetic stimulation over the lumbosacral cord identify patients with limited sacral neuropathies with sufficient residual nerve conduction to attempt biofeedback training.

In summary, a balloon expulsion test is an important screening test for anorectal dysfunction. Rarely, an anatomic evaluation of the rectum or anal sphincters and an assessment of pelvic floor relaxation are the tools for evaluating patients in whom obstructed defecation is suspected and is associated with symptoms of rectal mucosal prolapse, pressure of the posterior wall of the vagina to facilitate defecation (suggestive of anterior rectocele), or prior pelvic surgery that may be complicated by enterocele.

TREATMENT Constipation

After the cause of constipation is characterized, a treatment decision can be made. Slow-transit constipation requires aggressive medical or surgical treatment; anismus or pelvic floor dysfunction usually responds to biofeedback management (Fig. 40-4). The remaining ~60% of patients with constipation has normal colonic transit and can be treated symptomatically. Patients with spinal cord injuries or other neurologic disorders require a dedicated bowel regimen that often includes rectal stimulation, enema therapy, and carefully timed laxative therapy.

Patients with constipation are treated with bulk, osmotic, prokinetic, secretory, and stimulant laxatives including fiber, psyllium, milk of magnesia, lactulose, polyethylene glycol (colonic lavage solution), lubiprostone, linaclotide, and bisacodyl, or, in some countries, prucalopride, a 5-HT_4 agonist. If a 3-to 6-month trial of medical therapy fails, unassociated with obstructed defecation, the patients should be considered for laparoscopic colectomy with ileorectostomy; however, this should not be undertaken if there is continued evidence of an evacuation disorder or a generalized GI dysmotility. Referral to a specialized center for further tests of colonic motor function is warranted. The decision to resort to surgery is facilitated in the presence of megacolon and megarectum. The complications after surgery include small-bowel obstruction (11%) and fecal soiling, particularly at night during the first postoperative year. Frequency of defecation is 3–8 per day during the first year, dropping to 1–3 per day from the second year after surgery.

Patients who have a combined (evacuation and transit/motility) disorder should pursue pelvic floor retraining (biofeedback and muscle relaxation), psychological counseling, and dietetic advice first. If symptoms are intractable despite biofeedback and optimized medical therapy, colectomy and ileorectostomy could be considered as long as the evacuation disorder is resolved and optimized medical therapy is unsuccessful. In patients with pelvic floor dysfunction alone, biofeedback training has a 70–80% success rate, measured by the acquisition of comfortable stool habits. Attempts to manage pelvic floor dysfunction with operations (internal anal sphincter or puborectalis muscle division) or injections with botulinum toxin have achieved only mediocre success and have been largely abandoned.

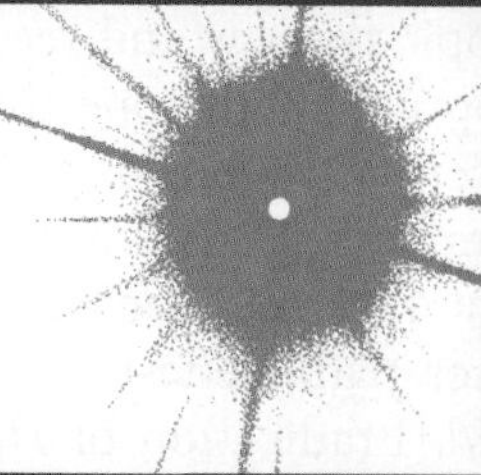

CHAPTER 7
GASTROINTESTINAL BLEEDING

Loren Laine

Gastrointestinal bleeding (GIB) accounts for ~150 hospitalizations per 100,000 population annually in the United States, with upper GIB (UGIB) ~1.5–2 times more common than lower GIB (LGIB) The incidence of GIB has decreased in recent decades, primarily due to a reduction in UGIB, and the mortality has also decreased to <5%. Patients today rarely die from exsanguination, but rather die due to decompensation of other underlying illnesses.

GIB presents as either overt or occult bleeding. *Overt GIB* is manifested by *hematemesis*, vomitus of red blood or "coffee-grounds" material; *melena*, black, tarry, foul-smelling stool; and/or *hematochezia*, passage of bright red or maroon blood from the rectum. *Occult GIB* may be identified in the absence of overt bleeding when patients present with *symptoms of blood loss or anemia* such as lightheadedness, syncope, angina, or dyspnea; or when routine diagnostic evaluation reveals iron deficiency anemia or a positive fecal occult blood test. GIB is also categorized by the site of bleeding as UGIB, LGIB, or obscure GIB if the source is unclear.

SOURCES OF GASTROINTESTINAL BLEEDING

Upper gastrointestinal sources of bleeding

(Table 7-1) Peptic ulcers are the most common cause of UGIB, accounting for ~50% of cases. Mallory-Weiss tears account for ~5–10% of cases. The proportion of patients bleeding from varices varies widely from ~5–40%, depending on the population. Hemorrhagic or erosive gastropathy (e.g., due to nonsteroidal anti-inflammatory drugs [NSAIDs] or alcohol) and erosive esophagitis often cause mild UGIB, but major bleeding is rare.

Peptic ulcers

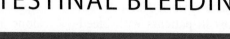

Characteristics of an ulcer at endoscopy provide important prognostic information. One-third of patients with active bleeding or a nonbleeding visible vessel have further bleeding that requires urgent surgery if they are treated conservatively. These patients benefit from endoscopic therapy with bipolar electrocoagulation, heater probe, injection therapy (e.g., absolute alcohol, 1:10,000 epinephrine), and/or clips with reductions in bleeding, hospital stay, mortality, and costs. In contrast, patients with clean-based ulcers have rates of recurrent bleeding approaching zero. If stable with no other reason for hospitalization, such patients may be discharged home after endoscopy. Patients without clean-based ulcers usually remain in the hospital for 3 days because most episodes of recurrent bleeding occur within 3 days.

Randomized controlled trials document that high-dose, constant-infusion IV proton pump inhibitor (PPI) (80-mg bolus and 8-mg/h infusion), designed to sustain intragastric pH >6 and enhance clot stability, decreases further bleeding and mortality in patients

TABLE 7-1

SOURCES OF BLEEDING IN PATIENTS HOSPITALIZED FOR UPPER GASTROINTESTINAL BLEEDING

SOURCES OF BLEEDING	PROPORTION OF PATIENTS, %
Ulcers	31–67
Varices	6–39
Mallory-Weiss tears	2–8
Gastroduodenal erosions	2–18
Erosive esophagitis	1–13
Neoplasm	2–8
Vascular ectasias	0–6
No source identified	5–14

Source: Data on hospitalizations from year 2000 onward from *Am J Gastroenterol* 98:1494, 2003; *Gastrointest Endosc* 57:AB147, 2003; 60;875, 2004; *Eur J Gastroenterol Hepatol* 16:177, 2004; 17:641, 2005; *J Clin Gastroenterol* 42:128, 2008; *World J Gastroenterol* 14:5046, 2008; *Dig Dis Sci* 54:333, 2009; Gut 60:1327, 2011; *Endoscopy* 44:998, 2012; *J Clin Gastroenterol* 48:113, 2014.

with high-risk ulcers (active bleeding, nonbleeding visible vessel, adherent clot) when given after endoscopic therapy. Patients with lower-risk findings (flat pigmented spot or clean base) do not require endoscopic therapy and receive standard doses of oral PPI. Approximately one-third of patients with bleeding ulcers will rebleed within the next 1–2 years if no preventive strategies are employed. Prevention of recurrent bleeding focuses on the three main factors in ulcer pathogenesis, *Helicobacter pylori*, NSAIDs, and acid. Eradication of *H. pylori* in patients with bleeding ulcers decreases rates of rebleeding to <5%. If a bleeding ulcer develops in a patient taking NSAIDs, the NSAIDs should be discontinued. If NSAIDs must be given, a cyclooxygenase 2 (COX-2) selective inhibitor (coxib) plus a PPI should be used. PPI co-therapy alone or a coxib alone is associated with an annual rebleeding rate of ~10% in patients with a recent bleeding ulcer, whereas the combination of a coxib and PPI provides a further significant decrease in recurrent ulcer bleeding. Patients with established cardiovascular disease who develop bleeding ulcers while taking low-dose aspirin should restart aspirin as soon as possible after their bleeding episode (1–7 days). A randomized trial showed that failure to restart aspirin was associated with no significant difference in rebleeding (5% vs. 10% at 30 days) but a significant increase in mortality at 30 days (9% vs. 1%) and 8 weeks (13% vs. 1%) compared with immediate reinstitution of aspirin. Patients with bleeding ulcers unrelated to *H. pylori* or NSAIDs should remain on PPI therapy indefinitely. **Peptic ulcers are discussed in Chap. 15.**

Mallory-Weiss tears

The classic history is vomiting, retching, or coughing preceding hematemesis, especially in an alcoholic patient. Bleeding from these tears, which are usually on the gastric side of the gastroesophageal junction, stops spontaneously in 80–90% of patients and recurs in only 0–10%. Endoscopic therapy is indicated for actively bleeding Mallory-Weiss tears. Angiographic therapy with embolization and operative therapy with oversewing of the tear are rarely required. **Mallory-Weiss tears are discussed in Chap. 14.**

Esophageal varices

Patients with variceal hemorrhage have poorer outcomes than patients with other sources of UGIB. Urgent endoscopy within 12 h is recommended in cirrhotics with UGIB, and if esophageal varices are present, endoscopic ligation is performed and an IV vasoactive medication (e.g., octreotide 50 μg bolus and 50 μg/h infusion) is given for 2–5 days. Combination endoscopic and medical therapy appears to be superior to either therapy alone in decreasing rebleeding. In patients with advanced liver disease (e.g., Child-Pugh class C with score 10–13), a transjugular intrahepatic portosystemic shunt (TIPS) should be strongly considered within the first 1–2 days of hospitalization because randomized trials show significant decreases in rebleeding and mortality compared with standard endoscopic and medical therapy. Over the long term, treatment with nonselective beta blockers plus endoscopic ligation is recommended because the combination of endoscopic and medical therapy is more effective than either alone in reduction of recurrent esophageal variceal bleeding.

In patients who have persistent or recurrent bleeding despite endoscopic and medical therapy, TIPS is recommended. Decompressive surgery (e.g., distal splenorenal shunt) may be considered instead of TIPS in patients with well-compensated cirrhosis.

Portal hypertension is also responsible for bleeding from gastric varices, varices in the small and large intestine, and portal hypertensive gastropathy and enterocolopathy. Bleeding gastric varices due to cirrhosis are treated with endoscopic injection of tissue adhesive (e.g., *n*-butyl cyanoacrylate), if available; if not, TIPS is performed.

Hemorrhagic and erosive gastropathy ("gastritis")

Hemorrhagic and erosive gastropathy, often labeled gastritis, refers to endoscopically visualized subepithelial hemorrhages and erosions. These are mucosal lesions and do not cause major bleeding due to the absence of arteries and veins in the mucosa. Erosions develop in various clinical settings, the most important of which are NSAID use, alcohol intake, and stress. Half of patients who chronically ingest NSAIDs have erosions, whereas up to 20% of actively drinking alcoholic patients with symptoms of UGIB have evidence of subepithelial hemorrhages or erosions.

Stress-related gastric mucosal injury occurs only in extremely sick patients, such as those who have experienced serious trauma, major surgery, burns covering more than one-third of the body surface area, major intracranial disease, or severe medical illness (i.e., ventilator dependence, coagulopathy). Severe bleeding should not develop unless ulceration occurs. The mortality rate in these patients is quite high because of their serious underlying illnesses.

The incidence of bleeding from stress-related gastric mucosal injury has decreased dramatically in recent years, most likely due to better care of critically ill patients. Pharmacologic prophylaxis for bleeding may be considered in the high-risk patients mentioned above. Meta-analyses of randomized trials indicate that PPIs are more effective than H_2 receptor antagonists in reduction of overt and clinically important UGIB without differences in mortality or nosocomial pneumonia.

Other causes

Other less frequent causes of UGIB include erosive duodenitis, neoplasms, aortoenteric fistulas, vascular lesions (including hereditary hemorrhagic telangiectasias [Osler-Weber-Rendu] and gastric antral vascular ectasia ["watermelon stomach"]), Dieulafoy's lesion (in which an aberrant vessel in the mucosa bleeds from a pinpoint mucosal defect), prolapse gastropathy (prolapse of proximal stomach into esophagus with retching, especially in alcoholics), and hemobilia or hemosuccus pancreaticus (bleeding from the bile duct or pancreatic duct).

Small-intestinal sources of bleeding

Small-intestinal sources of bleeding (bleeding from sites beyond the reach of the standard upper endoscope) are often difficult to diagnose and are responsible for the majority of cases of obscure GIB. Fortunately, small-intestinal bleeding is uncommon. The most common causes in adults are vascular ectasias, tumors (e.g., GI stromal tumor, carcinoid, adenocarcinoma, lymphoma, metastases), and NSAID-induced erosions and ulcers. Other less common causes in adults include Crohn's disease, infection, ischemia, vasculitis, small-bowel varices, diverticula, Meckel's diverticulum, duplication cysts, and intussusception.

Meckel's diverticulum is the most common cause of significant LGIB in children, decreasing in frequency as a cause of bleeding with age. In adults <40–50 years, small-bowel tumors often account for obscure GIB; in patients >50–60 years, vascular ectasias and NSAID-induced lesions are more commonly responsible.

Vascular ectasias should be treated with endoscopic therapy if possible. Although estrogen/progesterone compounds have been used for vascular ectasias, a large double-blind trial found no benefit in prevention of recurrent bleeding. Octreotide is also used, based on case series but no randomized trials. A randomized trial reported significant benefit of thalidomide and awaits further confirmation. Other isolated lesions, such as tumors, are generally treated with surgical resection.

Colonic sources of bleeding

Hemorrhoids are probably the most common cause of LGIB; anal fissures also cause minor bleeding and pain. If these local anal processes, which rarely require hospitalization, are excluded, the most common causes of LGIB in adults are diverticula, vascular ectasias (especially in the proximal colon of patients >70 years), neoplasms (primarily adenocarcinoma), colitis (ischemic, infectious, idiopathic inflammatory bowel disease), and postpolypectomy bleeding. Less common causes include NSAID-induced ulcers or colitis, radiation proctopathy, solitary rectal ulcer syndrome, trauma, varices (most commonly rectal), lymphoid nodular hyperplasia, vasculitis, and aortocolic fistulas. In children and adolescents, the most common colonic causes of significant GIB are inflammatory bowel disease and juvenile polyps.

Diverticular bleeding is abrupt in onset, usually painless, sometimes massive, and often from the right colon; chronic or occult bleeding is not characteristic. Clinical reports suggest that bleeding colonic diverticula stop bleeding spontaneously in ~80% of patients and, on long-term follow-up, rebleed in ~15–25% of patients. Case series suggest endoscopic therapy may decrease recurrent bleeding in the uncommon case when colonoscopy identifies the specific bleeding diverticulum. When diverticular bleeding is found at angiography, transcatheter arterial embolization by superselective technique stops bleeding in a majority of patients. If bleeding persists or recurs, segmental surgical resection is indicated.

Bleeding from right colonic vascular ectasias in the elderly may be overt or occult; it tends to be chronic and only occasionally is hemodynamically significant. Endoscopic hemostatic therapy may be useful in the treatment of vascular ectasias, as well as discrete bleeding ulcers and postpolypectomy bleeding. Surgical therapy is generally required for major, persistent, or recurrent bleeding from the wide variety of colonic sources of GIB that cannot be treated medically, angiographically, or endoscopically.

APPROACH TO THE PATIENT: Gastrointestinal Bleeding

INITIAL ASSESSMENT Measurement of the heart rate and blood pressure is the best way to initially assess a patient with GIB. Clinically significant bleeding leads to postural changes in heart rate or blood pressure, tachycardia, and, finally, recumbent hypotension. In contrast, the hemoglobin does not fall immediately with acute GIB, due to proportionate reductions in plasma and red cell volumes (i.e., "people bleed whole blood"). Thus, hemoglobin may be normal or only minimally decreased at the initial presentation of a severe bleeding episode. As extravascular fluid enters the vascular space to restore volume, the hemoglobin falls, but this process may take up to 72 h. Transfusion is recommended when the hemoglobin drops below 7 g/dL, based on a large randomized trial showing this restrictive transfusion strategy decreases rebleeding and death in acute UGIB compared with a transfusion threshold of 9 g/dL. Patients with slow, chronic GIB may have very low hemoglobin values despite normal blood pressure and heart rate. With the development of iron-deficiency anemia, the mean corpuscular volume will be low and red blood cell distribution width will increase.

DIFFERENTIATION OF UGIB FROM LGIB Hematemesis indicates an upper GI source of bleeding (above the ligament of Treitz). Melena indicates blood has been present in the GI tract for at least 14 h, and as long as 3–5 days. The more proximal the bleeding site, the more likely melena will occur. Hematochezia usually represents a lower GI source of bleeding, although an upper GI lesion may bleed so briskly that blood transits the bowel before melena develops. When hematochezia is the presenting symptom of UGIB, it is associated with hemodynamic instability and dropping hemoglobin. Bleeding lesions of the small bowel may present as melena or hematochezia. Other clues to UGIB include hyperactive bowel sounds and an elevated blood urea nitrogen (due to volume depletion and blood proteins absorbed in the small intestine).

A nonbloody nasogastric aspirate may be seen in up to ~18% of patients with UGIB, usually from a duodenal source. Even a bile-stained appearance does not exclude a bleeding postpyloric lesion because reports of bile in the aspirate are incorrect in ~50% of cases. Testing of aspirates that are not grossly bloody for occult blood is not useful.

EVALUATION AND MANAGEMENT OF UGIB At presentation, patients are generally stratified as higher or lower risk for further bleeding and death (Fig. 7-1). Baseline characteristics predictive of rebleeding and death include hemodynamic compromise (tachycardia or hypotension), increasing age, and comorbidities. PPI infusion may be considered at presentation: it decreases high-risk ulcer stigmata (e.g., active bleeding) and need for endoscopic therapy but does not improve clinical outcomes such as further bleeding, surgery, or death. Treatment to improve endoscopic visualization with the promotility agent erythromycin, 250 mg intravenously ~30 min before endoscopy, also may be considered: it provides a small but significant increase in diagnostic yield and decrease in second endoscopies but is not documented to decrease further bleeding or death. Cirrhotic patients presenting with UGIB should be placed on antibiotics (e.g., quinolone, ceftriaxone) and started on a vasoactive medication (octreotide, terlipressin, somatostatin, vapreotide) upon presentation, even before endoscopy. Antibiotics decrease bacterial infections, rebleeding, and mortality in this population, and vasoactive medications appear to improve control of bleeding in the first 12 h after presentation.

Upper endoscopy should be performed within 24 h in most patients with UGIB. Patients at higher risk (e.g., hemodynamic instability, cirrhosis) may benefit from more urgent endoscopy within 12 h. Early endoscopy is also beneficial in low-risk patients for management decisions. Patients with major bleeding and high-risk endoscopic findings (e.g., varices, ulcers with active bleeding or a visible vessel) benefit from endoscopic hemostatic therapy, whereas patients with low-risk lesions (e.g., clean-based ulcers, nonbleeding Mallory-Weiss tears, erosive or hemorrhagic gastropathy) who have stable vital signs and hemoglobin and no other medical problems can be discharged home.

EVALUATION AND MANAGEMENT OF LGIB Patients with hematochezia and hemodynamic instability should have upper endoscopy to rule out an upper GI source before evaluation of the lower GI tract (Fig. 7-2).

Colonoscopy after an oral lavage solution is the procedure of choice in most patients admitted with LGIB unless bleeding is too massive, in which case angiography is recommended. Sigmoidoscopy is used primarily in patients

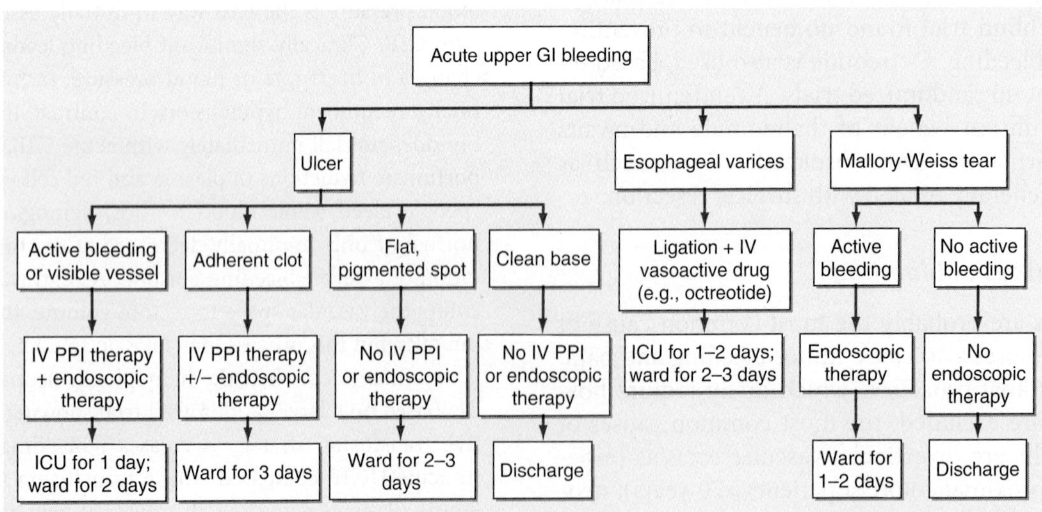

FIGURE 7-1
Suggested algorithm for patients with acute upper gastrointestinal (GI) bleeding. Recommendations on level of care and time of discharge assume patient is stabilized without further bleeding or other concomitant medical problems. ICU, intensive care unit; PPI, proton pump inhibitor.

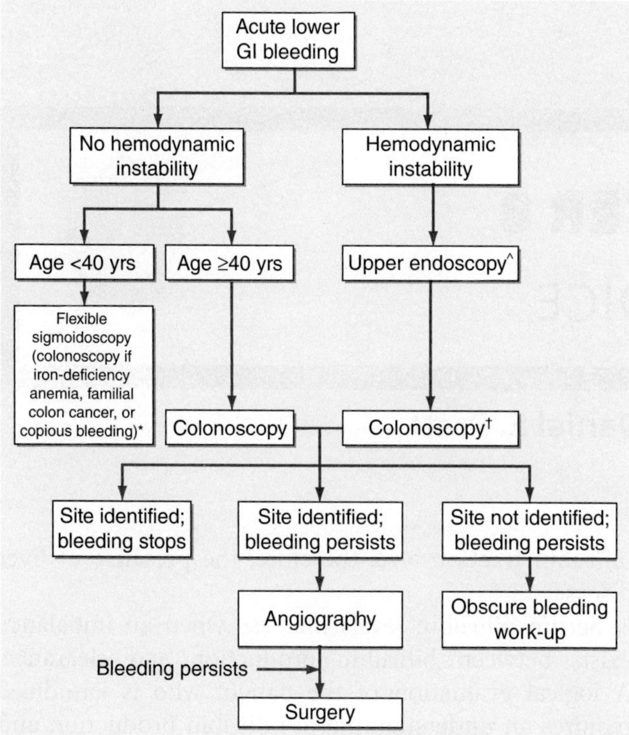

FIGURE 7-2

Suggested algorithm for patients with acute lower gastrointestinal (GI) bleeding.

*Some suggest colonoscopy for any degree of rectal bleeding in patients <40 years as well.

^If upper GI endoscopy reveals definite source, no further evaluation is needed.

†If massive bleeding does not allow time for colonic lavage, proceed to angiography.

<40 years old with minor bleeding. In patients with no source identified on colonoscopy, imaging studies may be employed. ^{99m}Tc-labeled red cell scan allows repeated imaging for up to 24 h and may identify the general location of bleeding. However, radionuclide scans should be interpreted with caution because results, especially from later images, are highly variable. Multidector computed tomography (CT) "angiography" is an increasingly used technique that is likely superior to nuclear scintigraphy. In active LGIB, angiography can detect the site of bleeding (extravasation of contrast into the gut) and permits treatment with embolization. Even after bleeding has stopped, angiography may identify lesions with abnormal vasculature, such as vascular ectasias or tumors.

EVALUATION AND MANAGEMENT OF OBSCURE GIB Obscure GIB is defined as persistent or recurrent bleeding for which no source has been identified by routine endoscopic and contrast x-ray studies; it may be overt (melena, hematochezia) or occult (iron-deficiency anemia). Current guidelines suggest angiography as the initial test for massive obscure bleeding, and video capsule endoscopy, which allows examination of the entire small intestine, for all others. Push enteroscopy, usually performed with a pediatric colonoscope, to inspect the entire duodenum and proximal jejunum also may be considered as an initial evaluation. A systematic review of 14 trials comparing push enteroscopy to capsule revealed "clinically significant findings" in 26% and 56% of patients, respectively. However, in contrast to enteroscopy, lack of control of the capsule prevents its manipulation and full visualization of the intestine; in addition, tissue cannot be sampled and therapy cannot be applied.

If capsule endoscopy is positive, management is dictated by the finding. If capsule endoscopy is negative, current recommendations suggest patients may either be observed or, if their clinical course mandates (e.g., recurrent bleeding, need for transfusions or hospitalization), undergo further testing. "Deep" enteroscopy (e.g., double-balloon, single-balloon, and spiral enteroscopy) is commonly the next test undertaken in patients with clinically important obscure GIB because it allows the endoscopist to examine, obtain specimens from, and provide therapy to much or all of the small intestine. CT and magnetic resonance enterography also are used to examine the small intestine. Other imaging techniques sometimes used in evaluation of obscure GIB include ^{99m}Tc-labeled red blood cell scintigraphy, multidetector CT "angiography," angiography, and ^{99m}Tc-pertechnetate scintigraphy for Meckel's diverticulum (especially in young patients). If all tests are unrevealing, intraoperative endoscopy is indicated in patients with severe recurrent or persistent bleeding requiring repeated transfusions.

POSITIVE FECAL OCCULT BLOOD TEST Fecal occult blood testing is recommended only for colorectal cancer screening and may be used beginning at age 50 in average-risk adults and beginning at age 40 in adults with a first-degree relative with colorectal neoplasm at ≥60 years or two second-degree relatives with colorectal cancer. A positive test necessitates colonoscopy. If evaluation of the colon is negative, further workup is not recommended unless iron-deficiency anemia or GI symptoms are present.

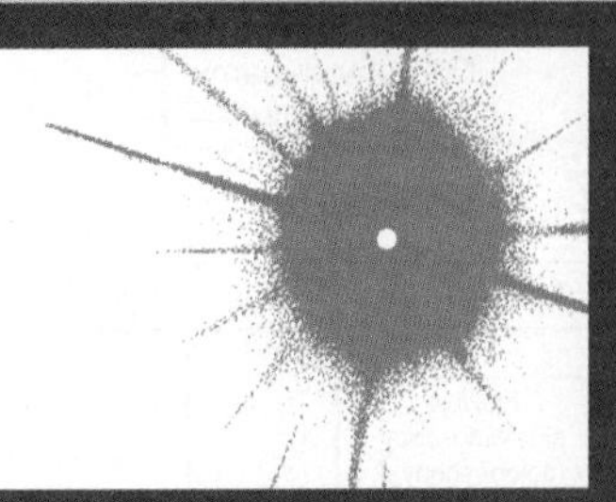

CHAPTER 8
JAUNDICE

Savio John ■ Daniel S. Pratt

Jaundice, or icterus, is a yellowish discoloration of tissue resulting from the deposition of bilirubin. Tissue deposition of bilirubin occurs only in the presence of serum hyperbilirubinemia and is a sign of either liver disease or, less often, a hemolytic disorder. The degree of serum bilirubin elevation can be estimated by physical examination. Slight increases in serum bilirubin level are best detected by examining the sclerae, which have a particular affinity for bilirubin due to their high elastin content. The presence of scleral icterus indicates a serum bilirubin level of at least 51 μmol/L (3 mg/dL). The ability to detect scleral icterus is made more difficult if the examining room has fluorescent lighting. If the examiner suspects scleral icterus, a second site to examine is underneath the tongue. As serum bilirubin levels rise, the skin will eventually become yellow in light-skinned patients and even green if the process is long-standing; the green color is produced by oxidation of bilirubin to biliverdin.

The differential diagnosis for yellowing of the skin is limited. In addition to jaundice, it includes carotenoderma, the use of the drug quinacrine, and excessive exposure to phenols. Carotenoderma is the yellow color imparted to the skin of healthy individuals who ingest excessive amounts of vegetables and fruits that contain carotene, such as carrots, leafy vegetables, squash, peaches, and oranges. In jaundice the yellow coloration of the skin is uniformly distributed over the body, whereas in carotenoderma the pigment is concentrated on the palms, soles, forehead, and nasolabial folds. Carotenoderma can be distinguished from jaundice by the sparing of the sclerae. Quinacrine causes a yellow discoloration of the skin in 4–37% of patients treated with it.

Another sensitive indicator of increased serum bilirubin is darkening of the urine, which is due to the renal excretion of conjugated bilirubin. Patients often describe their urine as tea- or cola-colored. Bilirubinuria indicates an elevation of the direct serum bilirubin fraction and, therefore, the presence of liver disease.

Serum bilirubin levels increase when an imbalance exists between bilirubin production and clearance. A logical evaluation of the patient who is jaundiced requires an understanding of bilirubin production and metabolism.

PRODUCTION AND METABOLISM OF BILIRUBIN

(See also Chap. 38) Bilirubin, a tetrapyrrole pigment, is a breakdown product of heme (ferroprotoporphyrin IX). About 70–80% of the 250–300 mg of bilirubin produced each day is derived from the breakdown of hemoglobin in senescent red blood cells. The remainder comes from prematurely destroyed erythroid cells in bone marrow and from the turnover of hemoproteins such as myoglobin and cytochromes found in tissues throughout the body.

The formation of bilirubin occurs in reticuloendothelial cells, primarily in the spleen and liver. The first reaction, catalyzed by the microsomal enzyme heme oxygenase, oxidatively cleaves the α bridge of the porphyrin group and opens the heme ring. The end products of this reaction are biliverdin, carbon monoxide, and iron. The second reaction, catalyzed by the cytosolic enzyme biliverdin reductase, reduces the central methylene bridge of biliverdin and converts it to bilirubin. Bilirubin formed in the reticuloendothelial cells is virtually insoluble in water due to tight internal hydrogen bonding between the water-soluble moieties of bilirubin—i.e., the bonding of the proprionic acid carboxyl groups of one dipyrrolic half of the molecule with the imino and lactam groups of the opposite half. This configuration blocks solvent access to the polar residues of bilirubin and places the hydrophobic residues on the outside. To be transported in blood, bilirubin must be solubilized. Solubilization is accomplished by the reversible, noncovalent binding of bilirubin to albumin. Unconjugated bilirubin bound to albumin is transported to the liver. There, the bilirubin—but not the albumin—is taken up by hepatocytes via a process that at least partly involves carrier-mediated membrane transport. No specific bilirubin transporter has yet been identified **(Chap. 38, Fig. 38-1)**.

After entering the hepatocyte, unconjugated bilirubin is bound in the cytosol to a number of proteins including proteins in the glutathione-S-transferase superfamily. These proteins serve both to reduce efflux of bilirubin back into the serum and to present the bilirubin for conjugation. In the endoplasmic reticulum, bilirubin is solubilized by conjugation to glucuronic acid, a process that disrupts the internal hydrogen bonds and yields bilirubin monoglucuronide and diglucuronide. The conjugation of glucuronic acid to bilirubin is catalyzed by bilirubin uridine diphosphate-glucuronosyl transferase (UDPGT). The now-hydrophilic bilirubin conjugates diffuse from the endoplasmic reticulum to the canalicular membrane, where bilirubin monoglucuronide and diglucuronide are actively transported into canalicular bile by an energy-dependent mechanism involving the multidrug resistance–associated protein 2 (MRP2).

The conjugated bilirubin excreted into bile drains into the duodenum and passes unchanged through the proximal small bowel. Conjugated bilirubin is not taken up by the intestinal mucosa. When the conjugated bilirubin reaches the distal ileum and colon, it is hydrolyzed to unconjugated bilirubin by bacterial β-glucuronidases. The unconjugated bilirubin is reduced by normal gut bacteria to form a group of colorless tetrapyrroles called *urobilinogens*. About 80–90% of these products are excreted in feces, either unchanged or oxidized to orange derivatives called *urobilins*. The remaining 10–20% of the urobilinogens are passively absorbed, enter the portal venous blood, and are re-excreted by the liver. A small fraction (usually <3 mg/dL) escapes hepatic uptake, filters across the renal glomerulus, and is excreted in urine.

MEASUREMENT OF SERUM BILIRUBIN

The terms *direct* and *indirect* bilirubin—i.e., conjugated and unconjugated bilirubin, respectively—are based on the original van den Bergh reaction. This assay, or a variation of it, is still used in most clinical chemistry laboratories to determine the serum bilirubin level. In this assay, bilirubin is exposed to diazotized sulfanilic acid and splits into two relatively stable dipyrrylmethene azopigments that absorb maximally at 540 nm, allowing photometric analysis. The direct fraction is that which reacts with diazotized sulfanilic acid in the absence of an accelerator substance such as alcohol. The direct fraction provides an approximation of the conjugated bilirubin level in serum. The *total* serum bilirubin is the amount that reacts after the addition of alcohol. The indirect fraction is the difference between the total and the direct bilirubin levels and provides an estimate of the unconjugated bilirubin in serum.

With the van den Bergh method, the normal serum bilirubin concentration usually is 17 μmol/L (<1 mg/dL). Up to 30%, or 5.1 μmol/L (0.3 mg/dL), of the total may be direct-reacting (conjugated) bilirubin. Total serum bilirubin concentrations are between 3.4 and 15.4 μmol/L (0.2 and 0.9 mg/dL) in 95% of a normal population.

Several new techniques, although less convenient to perform, have added considerably to our understanding of bilirubin metabolism. First, studies using these methods demonstrate that, in normal persons or those with Gilbert's syndrome, almost 100% of the serum bilirubin is unconjugated; <3% is monoconjugated bilirubin. Second, in jaundiced patients with hepatobiliary disease, the total serum bilirubin concentration measured by these new, more accurate methods is lower than the values found with diazo methods. This finding suggests that there are diazo-positive compounds distinct from bilirubin in the serum of patients with hepatobiliary disease. Third, these studies indicate that, in jaundiced patients with hepatobiliary disease, monoglucuronides of bilirubin predominate over diglucuronides. Fourth, part of the direct-reacting bilirubin fraction includes conjugated bilirubin that is covalently linked to albumin. This albumin-linked bilirubin fraction (*delta fraction,* or *biliprotein*) represents an important fraction of total serum bilirubin in patients with cholestasis and hepatobiliary disorders. The delta fraction (delta bilirubin) is formed in serum when hepatic excretion of bilirubin glucuronides is impaired and the glucuronides accumulate in serum. By virtue of its tight binding to albumin, the clearance rate of delta bilirubin from serum approximates the half-life of albumin (12–14 days) rather than the short half-life of bilirubin (about 4 h).

The prolonged half-life of albumin-bound conjugated bilirubin accounts for two previously unexplained enigmas in jaundiced patients with liver disease: (1) that some patients with conjugated hyperbilirubinemia do not exhibit bilirubinuria during the recovery phase of their disease because the bilirubin is covalently bound to albumin and therefore not filtered by the renal glomeruli, and (2) that the elevated serum bilirubin level declines more slowly than expected in some patients who otherwise appear to be recovering satisfactorily. Late in the recovery phase of hepatobiliary disorders, all the conjugated bilirubin may be in the albumin-linked form.

MEASUREMENT OF URINE BILIRUBIN

Unconjugated bilirubin is always bound to albumin in the serum, is not filtered by the kidney, and is not found in the urine. Conjugated bilirubin is filtered at the glomerulus, and the majority is reabsorbed by the proximal tubules; a small fraction is excreted in the urine. Any bilirubin found in the urine is conjugated bilirubin. The presence of bilirubinuria implies the presence of liver disease. A urine dipstick test (Ictotest) gives the same information as fractionation of the serum bilirubin and is very accurate. A false-negative result is possible in patients with prolonged cholestasis due to the predominance of delta bilirubin, which is covalently bound to albumin and therefore not filtered by the renal glomeruli.

APPROACH TO THE PATIENT: Jaundice

The goal of this chapter is not to provide an encyclopedic review of all of the conditions that can cause jaundice. Rather, the chapter is intended to offer a framework that helps a physician to evaluate the patient with jaundice in a logical way (Fig. 8-1).

Simply stated, the initial step is to perform appropriate blood tests in order to determine whether the patient has an isolated elevation of serum bilirubin. If so, is the bilirubin elevation due to an increased unconjugated or conjugated fraction? If the hyperbilirubinemia is accompanied by other liver test abnormalities, is the disorder

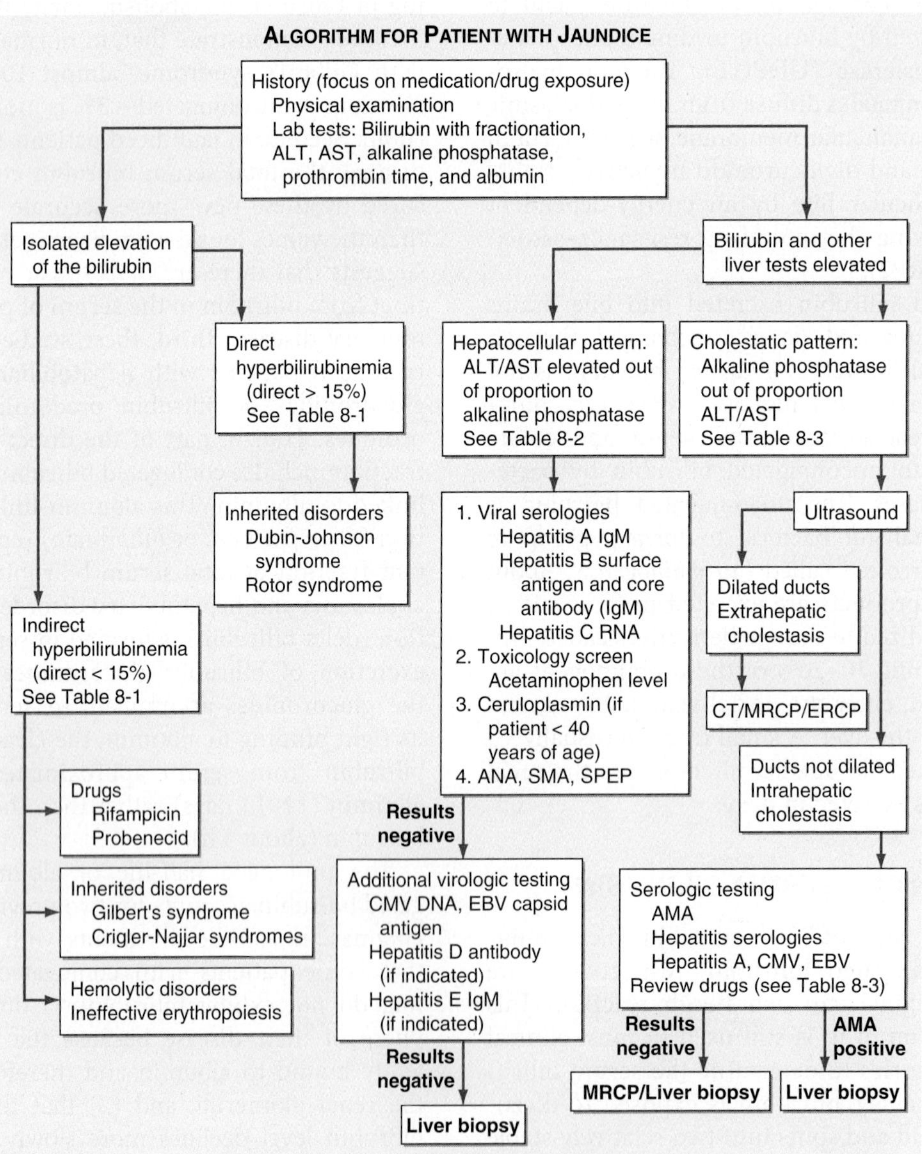

FIGURE 8-1

Evaluation of the patient with jaundice. ALT, alanine aminotransferase; AMA, antimitochondrial antibody; ANA, antinuclear antibody; AST, aspartate aminotransferase; CMV, cytomegalovirus; EBV, Epstein-Barr virus; LKM, liver-kidney microsomal antibody; MRCP, magnetic resonance cholangiopancreatography; SMA, smooth-muscle antibody; SPEP, serum protein electrophoresis.

hepatocellular or cholestatic? If cholestatic, is it intra- or extrahepatic? All of these questions can be answered with a thoughtful history, physical examination, and interpretation of laboratory and radiologic tests and procedures.

The bilirubin present in serum represents a balance between input from the production of bilirubin and hepatic/biliary removal of the pigment. Hyperbilirubinemia may result from (1) overproduction of bilirubin; (2) impaired uptake, conjugation, or excretion of bilirubin; or (3) regurgitation of unconjugated or conjugated bilirubin from damaged hepatocytes or bile ducts. An increase in unconjugated bilirubin in serum results from overproduction, impaired uptake, or conjugation of bilirubin. An increase in conjugated bilirubin is due to decreased excretion into the bile ductules or backward leakage of the pigment. The initial steps in evaluating the patient with jaundice are to determine (1) whether the hyperbilirubinemia is predominantly conjugated or unconjugated in nature and (2) whether other biochemical liver tests are abnormal.

The thoughtful interpretation of limited data permits a rational evaluation of the patient (Fig. 8-1). The following discussion will focus solely on the evaluation of the adult patient with jaundice.

ISOLATED ELEVATION OF SERUM BILIRUBIN

Unconjugated Hyperbilirubinemia The differential diagnosis of isolated unconjugated hyperbilirubinemia is limited (Table 8-1). The critical determination is whether the patient is suffering from a hemolytic process resulting in an overproduction of bilirubin (hemolytic disorders and ineffective erythropoiesis) or from impaired hepatic uptake/conjugation of bilirubin (drug effect or genetic disorders).

Hemolytic disorders that cause excessive heme production may be either inherited or acquired. Inherited disorders include spherocytosis, sickle cell anemia, thalassemia, and deficiency of red cell enzymes such as pyruvate kinase and glucose-6-phosphate dehydrogenase. In these conditions, the serum bilirubin level rarely exceeds 86 μmol/L (5 mg/dL). Higher levels may occur when there is coexistent renal or hepatocellular dysfunction or in acute hemolysis, such as a sickle cell crisis. In evaluating jaundice in patients with chronic hemolysis, it is important to remember the high incidence of pigmented (calcium bilirubinate) gallstones found in these patients, which increases the likelihood of choledocholithiasis as an alternative explanation for hyperbilirubinemia.

Acquired hemolytic disorders include microangiopathic hemolytic anemia (e.g., hemolytic-uremic syndrome), paroxysmal nocturnal hemoglobinuria, spur cell anemia, immune hemolysis, and parasitic infections (e.g., malaria and babesiosis). Ineffective erythropoiesis occurs in cobalamin, folate, and iron deficiencies. Resorption of hematomas and massive blood transfusions both can result in increased hemoglobin release and overproduction of bilirubin.

TABLE 8-1

CAUSES OF ISOLATED HYPERBILIRUBINEMIA

I. Indirect hyperbilirubinemia
    A. Hemolytic disorders
        1. Inherited
            a. Spherocytosis, elliptocytosis, glucose-6-phosphate dehydrogenase and pyruvate kinase deficiencies
            b. Sickle cell anemia
        2. Acquired
            a. Microangiopathic hemolytic anemias
            b. Paroxysmal nocturnal hemoglobinuria
            c. Spur cell anemia
            d. Immune hemolysis
            e. Parasitic infections
                (1) Malaria
                (2) Babesiosis
    B. Ineffective erythropoiesis
        1. Cobalamin, folate, and severe iron deficiencies
        2. Thalassemia
    C. Increased bilirubin production
        1. Massive blood transfusion
        2. Resorption of hematoma
    D. Drugs
        1. Rifampin
        2. Probenecid
        3. Ribavirin
    E. Inherited conditions
        1. Crigler-Najjar types I and II
        2. Gilbert's syndrome
II. Direct hyperbilirubinemia (inherited conditions)
    A. Dubin-Johnson syndrome
    B. Rotor syndrome

In the absence of hemolysis, the physician should consider a problem with the hepatic uptake or conjugation of bilirubin. Certain drugs, including rifampin and probenecid, may cause unconjugated hyperbilirubinemia by diminishing hepatic uptake of bilirubin. Impaired bilirubin conjugation occurs in three genetic conditions: Crigler-Najjar syndrome types I and II and Gilbert's syndrome. *Crigler-Najjar type I* is an exceptionally rare condition found in neonates and characterized by severe jaundice (bilirubin >342 μmol/L [>20 mg/dL]) and neurologic impairment due to kernicterus, frequently leading to death in infancy or childhood. These patients have a complete absence of bilirubin UDPGT activity, usually due to mutations in the critical 3′ domain of the *UDPGT* gene; are totally unable to conjugate bilirubin; and hence cannot excrete it.

Crigler-Najjar type II is somewhat more common than type I. Patients live into adulthood with serum bilirubin levels of 103–428 μmol/L (6–25 mg/dL). In these patients, mutations in the bilirubin *UDPGT* gene cause the reduction—but not the complete eradication—of the enzyme's activity. Bilirubin UDPGT activity can be induced by the administration of phenobarbital, which can reduce serum bilirubin levels in these patients. Despite marked jaundice, these patients usually survive into adulthood, although they may be susceptible to kernicterus under the stress of intercurrent illness or surgery.

Gilbert's syndrome is also marked by the impaired conjugation of bilirubin (to approximately one-third of normal) due to reduced bilirubin UDPGT activity. Patients with Gilbert's syndrome have mild unconjugated hyperbilirubinemia, with serum levels almost always <103 μmol/L (6 mg/dL). The serum levels may fluctuate, and jaundice is often identified only during periods of fasting. The molecular defect in Gilbert's syndrome is linked to a reduction in transcription of the bilirubin *UDPGT* gene due to mutations in the promoter and, rarely, in the coding region. Unlike both Crigler-Najjar syndromes, Gilbert's syndrome is very common. The reported incidence is 3–7% of the population, with males predominating over females by a ratio of 2–7:1.

Conjugated hyperbilirubinemia Elevated conjugated hyperbilirubinemia is found in two rare inherited conditions: *Dubin-Johnson syndrome* and *Rotor syndrome* (Table 8-1). Patients with either condition present with asymptomatic jaundice. The defect in Dubin-Johnson syndrome is the presence of mutations in the gene for MRP2. These patients have altered excretion of bilirubin into the bile ducts. Rotor syndrome may represent a deficiency of the major hepatic drug uptake transporters OATP1B1 and OATP1B3. Differentiating between these syndromes is possible but is clinically unnecessary due to their benign nature.

ELEVATION OF SERUM BILIRUBIN WITH OTHER LIVER TEST ABNORMALITIES The remainder of this chapter will focus on the evaluation of patients with conjugated hyperbilirubinemia in the setting of other liver test abnormalities. This group of patients can be divided into those with a primary hepatocellular process and those with intra- or extrahepatic cholestasis. This distinction, which is based on the history and physical examination as well as the pattern of liver test abnormalities, guides the clinician's evaluation (Fig. 8-1).

History A complete medical history is perhaps the single most important part of the evaluation of the patient with unexplained jaundice. Important considerations include the use of or exposure to any chemical or medication, whether physician-prescribed, over-the-counter, complementary, or alternative medicines (e.g., herbal and vitamin preparations) or other drugs such as anabolic steroids. The patient should be carefully questioned about possible parenteral exposures, including transfusions, intravenous and intranasal drug use, tattooing, and sexual activity. Other important points include recent travel history; exposure to people with jaundice; exposure to possibly contaminated foods; occupational exposure to hepatotoxins; alcohol consumption; the duration of jaundice; and the presence of any accompanying signs and symptoms, such as arthralgias, myalgias, rash, anorexia, weight loss, abdominal pain, fever, pruritus, and changes in the urine and stool. While none of the latter manifestations is specific for any one condition, any of them can suggest a particular diagnosis. A history of arthralgias and myalgias predating jaundice suggests hepatitis, either viral or drug-related. Jaundice associated with the sudden onset of severe right-upper-quadrant pain and shaking chills suggests choledocholithiasis and ascending cholangitis.

Physical examination The general assessment should include evaluation of the patient's nutritional status. Temporal and proximal muscle wasting suggests long-standing disease such as pancreatic cancer or cirrhosis. Stigmata of chronic liver disease, including spider nevi, palmar erythema, gynecomastia, caput medusae, Dupuytren's contractures, parotid gland enlargement, and testicular atrophy, are commonly seen in advanced alcoholic (Laennec's) cirrhosis and occasionally in other types of cirrhosis. An enlarged left supraclavicular node (Virchow's node) or a periumbilical nodule (Sister Mary Joseph's nodule) suggests an abdominal malignancy.

Jugular venous distention, a sign of right-sided heart failure, suggests hepatic congestion. Right pleural effusion in the absence of clinically apparent ascites may be seen in advanced cirrhosis.

The abdominal examination should focus on the size and consistency of the liver, on whether the spleen is palpable and hence enlarged, and on whether ascites is present. Patients with cirrhosis may have an enlarged left lobe of the liver, which is felt below the xiphoid, and an enlarged spleen. A grossly enlarged nodular liver or an obvious abdominal mass suggests malignancy. An enlarged tender liver could signify viral or alcoholic hepatitis; an infiltrative process such as amyloidosis; or, less often, an acutely congested liver secondary to right-sided heart failure. Severe right-upper-quadrant tenderness with respiratory arrest on inspiration (Murphy's sign) suggests cholecystitis. Ascites in the presence of jaundice suggests either cirrhosis or malignancy with peritoneal spread.

Laboratory tests A battery of tests are helpful in the initial evaluation of a patient with unexplained jaundice. These include total and direct serum bilirubin measurement with fractionation; determination of serum aminotransferase, alkaline phosphatase, and albumin concentrations; and prothrombin time tests. Enzyme tests (alanine aminotransferase [ALT], aspartate aminotransferase [AST], and alkaline phosphatase [ALP]) are helpful in differentiating between a hepatocellular process and a cholestatic process (**Table 37-1**; Fig. 8-1)—a critical step in determining what additional workup is indicated. Patients with a hepatocellular process generally have a rise in the aminotransferases that is disproportionate to that in ALP, whereas patients with a cholestatic process have a rise in ALP that is disproportionate to that of the aminotransferases. The serum bilirubin can be prominently elevated in both hepatocellular and cholestatic conditions and therefore is not necessarily helpful in differentiating between the two.

In addition to enzyme tests, all jaundiced patients should have additional blood tests—specifically, an albumin level and a prothrombin time—to assess liver function. A low albumin level suggests a chronic process such as cirrhosis or cancer. A normal albumin level is suggestive of a more acute process such as viral hepatitis or choledocholithiasis. An elevated prothrombin time indicates either vitamin K deficiency due to prolonged jaundice and malabsorption of vitamin K or significant hepatocellular dysfunction. The failure of the prothrombin time to correct with parenteral administration of vitamin K indicates severe hepatocellular injury.

The results of the bilirubin, enzyme, albumin, and prothrombin time tests will usually indicate whether a jaundiced patient has a hepatocellular or a cholestatic disease and offer some indication of the duration and severity of the disease. The causes and evaluations of hepatocellular and cholestatic diseases are quite different.

Hepatocellular conditions Hepatocellular diseases that can cause jaundice include viral hepatitis, drug or environmental toxicity, alcohol, and end-stage cirrhosis from any cause (Table 8-2). Wilson's disease occurs primarily in young adults. Autoimmune hepatitis is typically seen in young to middle-aged women but may affect men and women of any age. Alcoholic hepatitis can be differentiated from viral and toxin-related hepatitis by the pattern of the aminotransferases: patients with alcoholic hepatitis typically have an AST-to-ALT ratio of at least 2:1, and the AST level rarely exceeds 300 U/L. Patients with acute viral hepatitis and toxin-related injury severe enough to produce jaundice typically have aminotransferase levels >500 U/L, with the ALT greater than or equal to the AST. While ALT and AST values <8 times normal may be seen in either hepatocellular or cholestatic liver disease, values 25 times normal or higher are seen primarily in acute hepatocellular diseases.

TABLE 8-2

HEPATOCELLULAR CONDITIONS THAT MAY PRODUCE JAUNDICE

- Viral hepatitis
  - Hepatitis A, B, C, D, and E
  - Epstein-Barr virus
  - Cytomegalovirus
  - Herpes simplex virus
- Alcoholic hepatitis
- Drug toxicity
  - Predictable, dose-dependent (e.g., acetaminophen)
  - Unpredictable, idiosyncratic (e.g., isoniazid)
- Environmental toxins
  - Vinyl chloride
  - Jamaica bush tea—pyrrolizidine alkaloids
  - Kava Kava
  - Wild mushrooms—*Amanita phalloides, A. verna*
- Wilson's disease
- Autoimmune hepatitis

Patients with jaundice from cirrhosis can have normal or only slightly elevated aminotransferase levels.

When the clinician determines that a patient has a hepatocellular disease, appropriate testing for acute viral hepatitis includes a hepatitis A IgM antibody assay, a hepatitis B surface antigen and core IgM antibody assay, a hepatitis C viral RNA test, and, depending on the circumstances, a hepatitis E IgM antibody assay. Because it can take many weeks for hepatitis C antibody to become detectable, its assay is an unreliable test if acute hepatitis C is suspected. Studies for hepatitis D and E viruses, Epstein-Barr virus (EBV), and cytomegalovirus (CMV) may also be indicated. Ceruloplasmin is the initial screening test for Wilson's disease. Testing for autoimmune hepatitis usually includes an antinuclear antibody assay and measurement of specific immunoglobulins.

Drug-induced hepatocellular injury can be classified as either predictable or unpredictable. Predictable drug reactions are dose-dependent and affect all patients who ingest a toxic dose of the drug in question. The classic example is acetaminophen hepatotoxicity. Unpredictable or idiosyncratic drug reactions are not dose-dependent and occur in a minority of patients. A great number of drugs can cause idiosyncratic hepatic injury. Environmental toxins are also an important cause of hepatocellular injury. Examples include industrial chemicals such as vinyl chloride, herbal preparations containing pyrrolizidine alkaloids (Jamaica bush tea) or Kava Kava, and the mushrooms *Amanita phalloides* and *A. verna*, which contain highly hepatotoxic amatoxins.

Cholestatic conditions When the pattern of the liver tests suggests a cholestatic disorder, the next step is to determine whether it is intra- or extrahepatic cholestasis (Fig. 8-1). Distinguishing intrahepatic from extrahepatic cholestasis may be difficult. History, physical examination, and laboratory tests often are not helpful. The next appropriate test is an ultrasound. The ultrasound is inexpensive, does not expose the patient to ionizing radiation, and can detect dilation of the intra- and extrahepatic biliary tree with a high degree of sensitivity and specificity. The absence of biliary dilation suggests intrahepatic cholestasis, while its presence indicates extrahepatic cholestasis. False-negative results occur in patients with partial obstruction of the common bile duct or in patients with cirrhosis or primary sclerosing cholangitis (PSC), in which scarring prevents the intrahepatic ducts from dilating.

Although ultrasonography may indicate extrahepatic cholestasis, it rarely identifies the site or cause of obstruction. The distal common bile duct is a particularly difficult area to visualize by ultrasound because of overlying bowel gas. Appropriate next tests include CT, magnetic resonance cholangiopancreatography (MRCP), endoscopic retrograde cholangiopancreatography (ERCP), and endoscopic ultrasound (EUS). CT scanning and MRCP are better than ultrasonography for assessing the head of the pancreas and for identifying choledocholithiasis in the distal common bile duct, particularly when the ducts are not dilated. ERCP is the "gold standard" for identifying choledocholithiasis. Beyond its diagnostic capabilities, ERCP allows therapeutic interventions, including the removal of common bile duct stones and the placement of stents. MRCP has replaced ERCP as the initial diagnostic test in cases where the need for intervention is thought to be small. EUS displays sensitivity and specificity comparable to that of MRCP in the detection of bile duct obstruction. EUS also allows biopsy of suspected malignant lesions, but is invasive and requires sedation.

In patients with apparent *intrahepatic cholestasis*, the diagnosis is often made by serologic testing in combination with percutaneous liver biopsy. The list of possible causes of intrahepatic cholestasis is long and varied (Table 8-3). A number of conditions that typically cause a hepatocellular pattern of injury can also present as a cholestatic variant. Both hepatitis B and C viruses can cause cholestatic hepatitis (fibrosing cholestatic hepatitis). This disease variant has been reported in patients who have undergone solid organ transplantation. Hepatitis A and E, alcoholic hepatitis, and EBV or CMV infections may also present as cholestatic liver disease.

Drugs may cause intrahepatic cholestasis that is usually reversible after discontinuation of the offending agent, although it may take many months for cholestasis to resolve. Drugs most commonly associated with cholestasis are the anabolic and contraceptive steroids. Cholestatic hepatitis has been reported with chlorpromazine, imipramine, tolbutamide, sulindac, cimetidine, and erythromycin estolate. It also occurs in patients taking trimethoprim; sulfamethoxazole; and penicillin-based antibiotics such as ampicillin, dicloxacillin, and clavulanic acid. Rarely, cholestasis may be chronic and associated with progressive fibrosis despite early discontinuation of the offending drug. Chronic cholestasis has been associated with chlorpromazine and prochlorperazine.

Primary biliary cirrhosis is an autoimmune disease predominantly affecting middle-aged women and characterized by progressive destruction of interlobular bile ducts. The diagnosis is made by the detection of antimitochondrial antibody, which is found in 95% of patients. *Primary sclerosing cholangitis* is characterized by the destruction and fibrosis of larger bile ducts. The diagnosis of PSC is made with cholangiography (either MRCP or ERCP), which demonstrates the pathognomonic segmental strictures. Approximately 75% of patients with PSC have inflammatory bowel disease.

The *vanishing bile duct syndrome* and *adult bile ductopenia* are rare conditions in which a decreased number of bile ducts are seen in liver biopsy specimens. The histologic picture is similar to that in primary biliary cirrhosis. This picture is seen in patients who develop chronic

TABLE 8-3

CHOLESTATIC CONDITIONS THAT MAY PRODUCE JAUNDICE

I. Intrahepatic
  A. Viral hepatitis
    1. Fibrosing cholestatic hepatitis—hepatitis B and C
    2. Hepatitis A, Epstein-Barr virus infection, cytomegalovirus infection
  B. Alcoholic hepatitis
  C. Drug toxicity
    1. Pure cholestasis—anabolic and contraceptive steroids
    2. Cholestatic hepatitis—chlorpromazine, erythromycin estolate
    3. Chronic cholestasis—chlorpromazine and prochlorperazine
  D. Primary biliary cirrhosis
  E. Primary sclerosing cholangitis
  F. Vanishing bile duct syndrome
    1. Chronic rejection of liver transplants
    2. Sarcoidosis
    3. Drugs
  G. Congestive hepatopathy and ischemic hepatitis
  H. Inherited conditions
    1. Progressive familial intrahepatic cholestasis
    2. Benign recurrent cholestasis
  I. Cholestasis of pregnancy
  J. Total parenteral nutrition
  K. Nonhepatobiliary sepsis
  L. Benign postoperative cholestasis
  M. Paraneoplastic syndrome
  N. Veno-occlusive disease
  O. Graft-versus-host disease
  P. Infiltrative disease
    1. Tuberculosis
    2. Lymphoma
    3. Amyloidosis
  Q. Infections
    1. Malaria
    2. Leptospirosis
II. Extrahepatic
  A. Malignant
    1. Cholangiocarcinoma
    2. Pancreatic cancer
    3. Gallbladder cancer
    4. Ampullary cancer
    5. Malignant involvement of the porta hepatis lymph nodes
  B. Benign
    1. Choledocholithiasis
    2. Postoperative biliary strictures
    3. Primary sclerosing cholangitis
    4. Chronic pancreatitis
    5. AIDS cholangiopathy
    6. Mirizzi's syndrome
    7. Parasitic disease (ascariasis)

rejection after liver transplantation and in those who develop graft-versus-host disease after bone marrow transplantation. Vanishing bile duct syndrome also occurs in rare cases of sarcoidosis, in patients taking certain drugs (including chlorpromazine), and idiopathically.

There are also familial forms of intrahepatic cholestasis. The familial intrahepatic cholestatic syndromes include *progressive familial intrahepatic cholestasis* (PFIC) *types 1–3* and *benign recurrent cholestasis* (BRC). PFIC1 and BRC are autosomal recessive diseases that result from mutations in the *ATP8B1* gene that encodes a protein belonging to the subfamily of P-type ATPases; the exact function of this protein remains poorly defined. While PFIC1 is a progressive condition that manifests in childhood, BRC presents later and is marked by recurrent episodes of jaundice and pruritus; the episodes are self-limited but can be debilitating. PFIC2 is caused by mutations in the *ABCB11* gene, which encodes the bile salt export pump, and PFIC3 is caused by mutations in the multidrug-resistant P-glycoprotein 3. *Cholestasis of pregnancy* occurs in the second and third trimesters and resolves after delivery. Its cause is unknown, but the condition is probably inherited, and cholestasis can be triggered by estrogen administration.

Other causes of intrahepatic cholestasis include total parenteral nutrition (TPN); nonhepatobiliary sepsis; benign postoperative cholestasis; and a paraneoplastic syndrome associated with a number of different malignancies, including Hodgkin's disease, medullary thyroid cancer, renal cell cancer, renal sarcoma, T cell lymphoma, prostate cancer, and several gastrointestinal malignancies. The term *Stauffer's syndrome* has been used for intrahepatic cholestasis specifically associated with renal cell cancer. In patients developing cholestasis in the intensive care unit, the major considerations should be sepsis, ischemic hepatitis ("shock liver"), and TPN jaundice. Jaundice occurring after bone marrow transplantation is most likely due to veno-occlusive disease or graft-versus-host disease. In addition to hemolysis, sickle cell disease may cause intrahepatic and extrahepatic cholestasis. Jaundice is a late finding in heart failure caused by hepatic congestion and hepatocellular hypoxia. Ischemic hepatitis is a distinct entity of acute hypoperfusion characterized by an acute and dramatic elevation in the serum aminotransferases followed by a gradual peak in serum bilirubin.

Jaundice with associated liver dysfunction can be seen in severe cases of *Plasmodium falciparum* malaria. The jaundice in these cases is due to a combination of indirect hyperbilirubinemia from hemolysis and both cholestatic and hepatocellular jaundice. Weil's disease, a severe presentation of leptospirosis, is marked by jaundice with renal failure, fever, headache, and muscle pain.

Causes of *extrahepatic cholestasis* can be split into malignant and benign (Table 8-3). Malignant causes include pancreatic, gallbladder, and ampullary cancers as well as cholangiocarcinoma. This last malignancy is most commonly associated with PSC and is exceptionally difficult to diagnose because its appearance is often identical to that of PSC. Pancreatic and gallbladder tumors as well as cholangiocarcinoma are rarely resectable and have poor prognoses. Ampullary carcinoma has the highest surgical cure rate of all the tumors that present as painless jaundice. Hilar lymphadenopathy due to metastases from other cancers may cause obstruction of the extrahepatic biliary tree.

Choledocholithiasis is the most common cause of extrahepatic cholestasis. The clinical presentation can range from mild right-upper-quadrant discomfort with only minimal elevations of enzyme test values to ascending cholangitis with jaundice, sepsis, and circulatory collapse. PSC may occur with clinically important strictures limited to the extrahepatic biliary tree. IgG4-associated cholangitis is marked by stricturing of the biliary tree. It is critical that the clinician differentiate this condition from PSC as it is responsive to glucocorticoid therapy. In rare instances, chronic pancreatitis causes strictures of the distal common bile duct, where it passes through the head of the pancreas. AIDS cholangiopathy is a condition that is usually due to infection of the bile duct epithelium with CMV or cryptosporidia and has a cholangiographic appearance similar to that of PSC. The affected patients usually present with greatly elevated serum alkaline phosphatase levels (mean, 800 IU/L), but the bilirubin level is often near normal. These patients do not typically present with jaundice.

GLOBAL CONSIDERATIONS

While extrahepatic biliary obstruction and drugs are common causes of new-onset jaundice in developed countries, infections remain the leading cause in developing countries. Liver involvement and jaundice are observed with numerous infections, particularly malaria, babesiosis, severe leptospirosis, infections due to *Mycobacterium tuberculosis* and the *Mycobacterium avium* complex, typhoid fever, viral hepatitis secondary to infection with hepatitis viruses A–E, EBV and CMV infections, late phases of yellow fever, dengue hemorrhagic fever, schistosomiasis, fascioliasis, clonorchiasis, opisthorchiasis, ascariasis, echinococcosis, hepatosplenic candidiasis, disseminated histoplasmosis, cryptococcosis, coccidioimycosis, ehrlichiosis, chronic Q fever, yersiniosis, brucellosis, syphilis, and leprosy. Bacterial infections that do not necessarily involve the liver and bile ducts may also lead to jaundice, as in cholestasis of sepsis.

Acknowledgment

This chapter is a revised version of chapters that have appeared in prior editions of Harrison's in which Marshall M. Kaplan was a co-author together with Daniel Pratt.

CHAPTER 9

ABDOMINAL SWELLING AND ASCITES

Kathleen E. Corey ■ Lawrence S. Friedman

ABDOMINAL SWELLING

Abdominal swelling is a manifestation of numerous diseases. Patients may complain of bloating or abdominal fullness and may note increasing abdominal girth on the basis of increased clothing or belt size. Abdominal discomfort is often reported, but pain is less frequent. When abdominal pain does accompany swelling, it is frequently the result of an intraabdominal infection, peritonitis, or pancreatitis. Patients with abdominal distention from *ascites* (fluid in the abdomen) may report the new onset of an inguinal or umbilical hernia. Dyspnea may result from pressure against the diaphragm and the inability to expand the lungs fully.

CAUSES

The causes of abdominal swelling can be remembered conveniently as the *six Fs*: flatus, fat, fluid, fetus, feces, or a "fatal growth" (often a neoplasm).

Flatus

Abdominal swelling may be the result of increased intestinal gas. The normal small intestine contains approximately 200 mL of gas made up of nitrogen, oxygen, carbon dioxide, hydrogen, and methane. Nitrogen and oxygen are consumed (swallowed), whereas carbon dioxide, hydrogen, and methane are produced intraluminally by bacterial fermentation. Increased intestinal gas can occur in a number of conditions. *Aerophagia*, the swallowing of air, can result in increased amounts of oxygen and nitrogen in the small intestine and lead to abdominal swelling. Aerophagia typically results from gulping food; chewing gum; smoking; or as a response to anxiety, which can lead to repetitive belching. In some cases, increased intestinal gas is the consequence of bacterial metabolism of excess fermentable substances such as lactose and other oligosaccharides, which can lead to production of hydrogen, carbon dioxide, or methane. In many cases, the precise cause of abdominal distention cannot be determined. In some persons, particularly those with irritable bowel syndrome and bloating, the subjective sense of abdominal pressure is attributable to impaired intestinal transit of gas rather than increased gas volume. Abdominal distention—an objective increase in girth—is the result of a lack of coordination between diaphragmatic contraction and anterior abdominal wall relaxation, a response in some cases to an increase in intraabdominal volume loads. Occasionally, increased lumbar lordosis accounts for apparent abdominal distention.

Fat

Weight gain with an increase in abdominal fat can result in an increase in abdominal girth and can be perceived as abdominal swelling. Abdominal fat may be caused by an imbalance between caloric intake and energy expenditure associated with a poor diet and sedentary lifestyle; it also can be a manifestation of certain diseases, such as Cushing's syndrome. Excess abdominal fat has been associated with an increased risk of insulin resistance and cardiovascular disease.

Fluid

The accumulation of fluid within the abdominal cavity (ascites) often results in abdominal distention and is discussed in detail below.

Fetus

Pregnancy results in increased abdominal girth. Typically, an increase in abdominal size is first noted at 12–14 weeks of gestation, when the uterus moves from the pelvis into the abdomen. Abdominal distention may be seen before this point as a result of fluid retention and relaxation of the abdominal muscles.

Feces

In the setting of severe constipation or intestinal obstruction, increased stool in the colon leads to increased abdominal girth. These conditions are often accompanied by abdominal discomfort or pain, nausea, and vomiting and can be diagnosed by imaging studies.

Fatal growth

An abdominal mass can result in abdominal swelling. Enlargement of the intraabdominal organs, specifically the liver (hepatomegaly) or spleen (splenomegaly), or an abdominal aortic aneurysm can result in abdominal distention. Bladder distention also may result in abdominal swelling. In addition, malignancies, abscesses, or cysts can grow to sizes that lead to increased abdominal girth.

APPROACH TO THE PATIENT: Abdominal Swelling

HISTORY Determining the etiology of abdominal swelling begins with history-taking and a physical examination. Patients should be questioned regarding symptoms suggestive of malignancy, including weight loss, night sweats, and anorexia. Inability to pass stool or flatus together with nausea or vomiting suggests bowel obstruction, severe constipation, or an ileus (lack of peristalsis). Increased eructation and flatus may point toward aerophagia or increased intestinal production of gas. Patients should be questioned about risk factors for or symptoms of chronic liver disease, including excessive alcohol use and jaundice, which suggest ascites. Patients should also be asked about other symptoms of medical conditions, including heart failure and tuberculosis, which may cause ascites.

PHYSICAL EXAMINATION Physical examination should include an assessment for signs of systemic disease. The presence of lymphadenopathy, especially supraclavicular lymphadenopathy (*Virchow's node*), suggests metastatic abdominal malignancy. Care should be taken during the cardiac examination to evaluate for elevation of jugular venous pressure (JVP); *Kussmaul's sign* (elevation of the JVP during inspiration); a pericardial knock, which may be seen in heart failure or constrictive pericarditis; or a murmur of tricuspid regurgitation. Spider angiomas, palmar erythema, dilated superficial veins around the umbilicus (*caput medusae*), and gynecomastia suggest chronic liver disease.

The abdominal examination should begin with inspection for the presence of uneven distention or an obvious mass. Auscultation should follow. The absence of bowel sounds or the presence of high-pitched localized bowel sounds points toward an ileus or intestinal obstruction. An umbilical venous hum may suggest the presence of portal hypertension, and a harsh bruit over the liver is heard rarely in patients with hepatocellular carcinoma or alcoholic hepatitis. Abdominal swelling caused by intestinal gas can be differentiated from swelling caused by fluid or a solid mass by percussion; an abdomen filled with gas is tympanic, whereas an abdomen containing a mass or fluid is dull to percussion. The absence of abdominal dullness, however, does not exclude ascites, because a minimum of 1500 mL of ascitic fluid is required for detection on physical examination. Finally, the abdomen should be palpated to assess for tenderness, a mass, enlargement of the spleen or liver, or presence of a nodular liver suggesting cirrhosis or tumor. Light palpation of the liver may detect pulsations suggesting retrograde vascular flow from the heart in patients with right-sided heart failure, particularly tricuspid regurgitation.

IMAGING AND LABORATORY EVALUATION

Abdominal x-rays can be used to detect dilated loops of bowel suggesting intestinal obstruction or ileus. Abdominal ultrasonography can detect as little as 100 mL of ascitic fluid, hepatosplenomegaly, a nodular liver, or a mass. Ultrasonography is often inadequate to detect retroperitoneal lymphadenopathy or a pancreatic lesion because of overlying bowel gas. If malignancy or pancreatic disease is suspected, CT can be performed. CT may also detect changes associated with advanced cirrhosis and portal hypertension (Fig. 9-1).

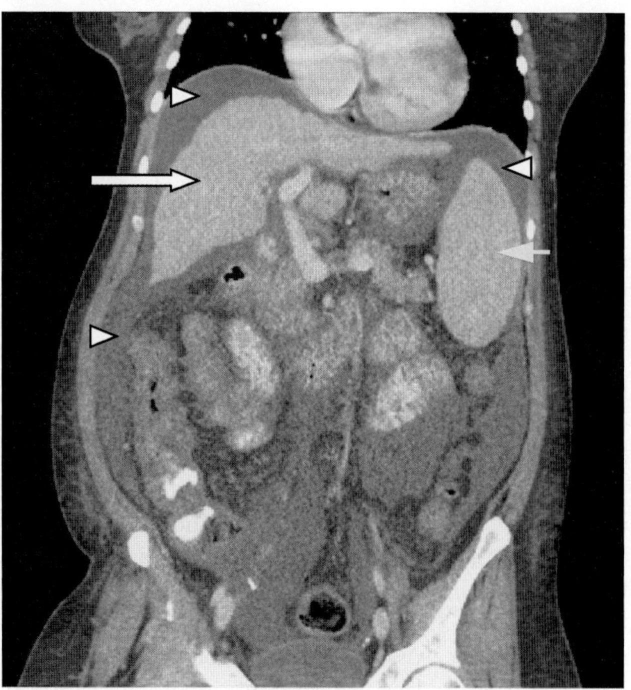

FIGURE 9-1
CT of a patient with a cirrhotic, nodular liver (white arrow), splenomegaly (yellow arrow), and ascites (arrowheads).

Laboratory evaluation should include liver biochemical testing, serum albumin level measurement, and prothrombin time determination (international normalized ratio) to assess hepatic function as well as a complete blood count to evaluate for the presence of cytopenias that may result from portal hypertension or of leukocytosis, anemia, and thrombocytosis that may result from systemic infection. Serum amylase and lipase levels should be checked to evaluate the patient for acute pancreatitis. Urinary protein quantitation is indicated when nephrotic syndrome, which may cause ascites, is suspected.

In selected cases, the hepatic venous pressure gradient (pressure across the liver between the portal and hepatic veins) can be measured via cannulation of the hepatic vein to confirm that ascites is caused by cirrhosis **(Chap. 44)**. In some cases, a liver biopsy may be necessary to confirm cirrhosis.

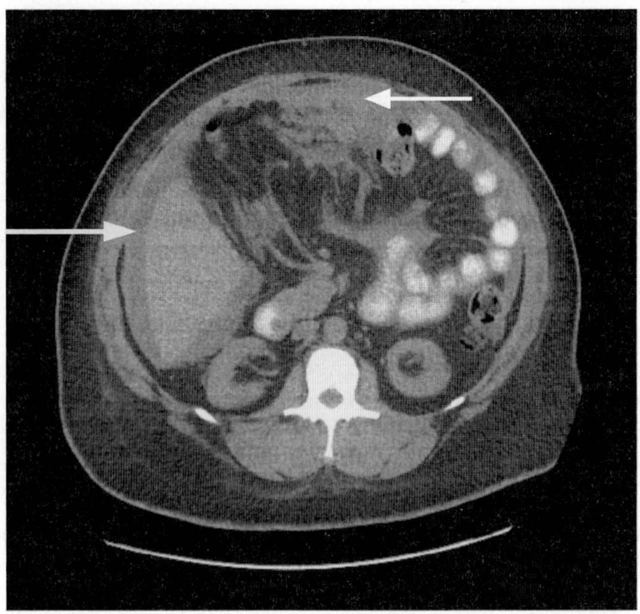

FIGURE 9-2
CT of a patient with peritoneal carcinomatosis *(white arrow)* and ascites *(yellow arrow)*.

ASCITES

PATHOGENESIS IN THE PRESENCE OF CIRRHOSIS

Ascites in patients with cirrhosis is the result of portal hypertension and renal salt and water retention. Similar mechanisms contribute to ascites formation in heart failure. Portal hypertension signifies elevation of the pressure within the portal vein. According to Ohm's law, pressure is the product of resistance and flow. Increased hepatic resistance occurs by several mechanisms. First, the development of hepatic fibrosis, which defines cirrhosis, disrupts the normal architecture of the hepatic sinusoids and impedes normal blood flow through the liver. Second, activation of hepatic stellate cells, which mediate fibrogenesis, leads to smooth-muscle contraction and fibrosis. Finally, cirrhosis is associated with a decrease in endothelial nitric oxide synthetase (eNOS) production, which results in decreased nitric oxide production and increased intrahepatic vasoconstriction.

The development of cirrhosis is also associated with increased systemic circulating levels of nitric oxide (contrary to the decrease seen intrahepatically) as well as increased levels of vascular endothelial growth factor and tumor necrosis factor that result in splanchnic arterial vasodilation. Vasodilation of the splanchnic circulation results in pooling of blood and a decrease in the effective circulating volume, which is perceived by the kidneys as hypovolemia. Compensatory vasoconstriction via release of antidiuretic hormone ensues; the consequences are free water retention and activation of the sympathetic nervous system and the renin angiotensin aldosterone system, which lead in turn to renal sodium and water retention.

PATHOGENESIS IN THE ABSENCE OF CIRRHOSIS

Ascites in the absence of cirrhosis generally results from peritoneal carcinomatosis, peritoneal infection, or pancreatic disease. Peritoneal carcinomatosis can result from primary peritoneal malignancies such as mesothelioma or sarcoma, abdominal malignancies such as gastric or colonic adenocarcinoma, or metastatic disease from breast or lung carcinoma or melanoma (Fig. 9-2). The tumor cells lining the peritoneum produce a protein-rich fluid that contributes to the development of ascites. Fluid from the extracellular space is drawn into the peritoneum, further contributing to the development of ascites. Tuberculous peritonitis causes ascites via a similar mechanism; tubercles deposited on the peritoneum exude a proteinaceous fluid. Pancreatic ascites results from leakage of pancreatic enzymes into the peritoneum.

CAUSES

Cirrhosis accounts for 84% of cases of ascites. Cardiac ascites, peritoneal carcinomatosis, and "mixed" ascites resulting from cirrhosis and a second disease account for 10–15% of cases. Less common causes of ascites include massive hepatic metastasis, infection (tuberculosis, *Chlamydia* infection), pancreatitis, and renal disease (nephrotic syndrome). Rare causes of ascites include hypothyroidism and familial Mediterranean fever.

EVALUATION

Once the presence of ascites has been confirmed, the etiology of the ascites is best determined by *paracentesis*, a bedside procedure in which a needle or small catheter is passed transcutaneously to extract ascitic fluid from the peritoneum. The lower quadrants are the most frequent sites for paracentesis. The left lower quadrant is preferred because of the greater depth of ascites and the thinner abdominal wall. Paracentesis is a safe procedure even in patients with coagulopathy; complications, including abdominal wall hematomas, hypotension, hepatorenal syndrome, and infection, are infrequent.

Once ascitic fluid has been extracted, its gross appearance should be examined. Turbid fluid can result from the presence of infection or tumor cells. White, milky fluid indicates a triglyceride level >200 mg/dL (and often >1000 mg/dL), which is the hallmark of *chylous ascites*. Chylous ascites results from lymphatic disruption that may occur with trauma, cirrhosis, tumor, tuberculosis, or certain congenital abnormalities. Dark brown fluid can reflect a high bilirubin concentration and indicates biliary tract perforation. Black fluid may indicate the presence of pancreatic necrosis or metastatic melanoma.

The ascitic fluid should be sent for measurement of albumin and total protein levels, cell and differential counts, and, if infection is suspected, Gram's stain and culture, with inoculation into blood culture bottles at the patient's bedside to maximize the yield. A serum albumin level should be measured simultaneously to permit calculation of the *serum-ascites albumin gradient* (SAAG).

The SAAG is useful for distinguishing ascites caused by portal hypertension from nonportal hypertensive ascites (Fig. 9-3). The SAAG reflects the pressure within the hepatic sinusoids and correlates with the hepatic venous pressure gradient. The SAAG is calculated by subtracting the ascitic albumin concentration from the serum albumin level and does not change with diuresis. A SAAG ≥1.1 g/dL reflects the presence of portal hypertension and indicates that the ascites is due to increased pressure in the hepatic sinusoids. According to Starling's law, a high SAAG reflects the oncotic pressure that counterbalances the portal pressure. Possible causes include cirrhosis, cardiac ascites, hepatic vein thrombosis (Budd-Chiari syndrome), sinusoidal obstruction syndrome (veno-occlusive disease), or massive liver metastases. A SAAG <1.1 g/dL indicates that the ascites is not related to portal hypertension, as in tuberculous peritonitis, peritoneal carcinomatosis, or pancreatic ascites.

For high-SAAG (≥1.1) ascites, the ascitic protein level can provide further clues to the etiology (Fig. 9-3). An ascitic protein level of ≥2.5 g/dL indicates that the hepatic sinusoids are normal and are allowing passage of protein into the ascites, as occurs in cardiac ascites, early Budd-Chiari syndrome, or sinusoidal obstruction syndrome. An ascitic protein level <2.5 g/dL indicates that the hepatic sinusoids have been damaged and scarred and no longer allow passage of protein, as occurs with cirrhosis, late Budd-Chiari syndrome, or massive liver metastases. Pro-brain-type natriuretic peptide (BNP) is a natriuretic hormone released by the heart as a result of increased volume and ventricular wall stretch. High levels of BNP in serum occur in heart failure and may be useful in identifying heart failure as the cause of high-SAAG ascites.

Further tests are indicated only in specific clinical circumstances. When secondary peritonitis resulting from a perforated hollow viscus is suspected, ascitic glucose and lactate dehydrogenase (LDH) levels can be measured. In contrast to "spontaneous" bacterial peritonitis, which may complicate cirrhotic ascites (see "Complications," below), secondary peritonitis is suggested by an ascitic glucose level <50 mg/dL, an ascitic LDH level higher than the serum LDH level, and the detection of multiple pathogens on ascitic fluid culture. When pancreatic ascites is suspected, the ascitic amylase level should be measured and is typically >1000 mg/dL.

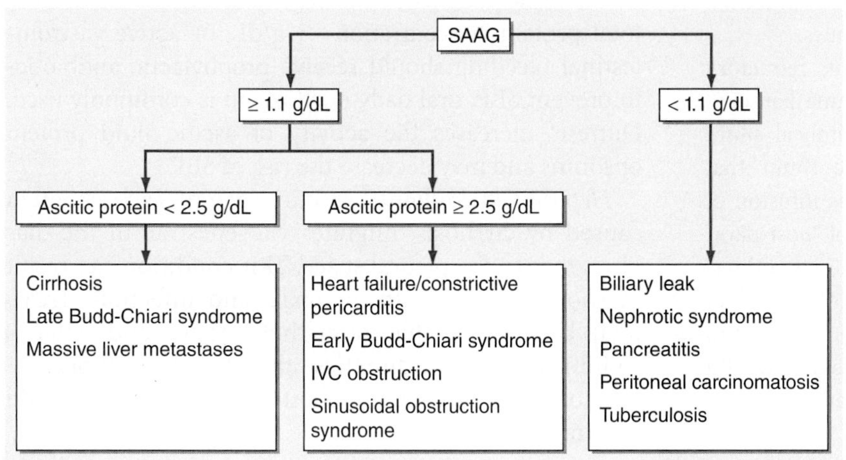

FIGURE 9-3
Algorithm for the diagnosis of ascites according to the serum-ascites albumin gradient (SAAG). IVC, inferior vena cava.

Cytology can be useful in the diagnosis of peritoneal carcinomatosis. At least 50 mL of fluid should be obtained and sent for immediate processing. Tuberculous peritonitis is typically associated with ascitic fluid lymphocytosis but can be difficult to diagnose by paracentesis. A smear for acid-fast bacilli has a diagnostic sensitivity of only 0 to 3%; a culture increases the sensitivity to 35–50%. In patients without cirrhosis, an elevated ascitic adenosine deaminase level has a sensitivity of >90% when a cut-off value of 30–45 U/L is used. When the cause of ascites remains uncertain, laparotomy or laparoscopy with peritoneal biopsies for histology and culture remains the gold standard.

TREATMENT Ascites

The initial treatment for cirrhotic ascites is restriction of sodium intake to 2 g/d. When sodium restriction alone is inadequate to control ascites, oral diuretics—typically the combination of spironolactone and furosemide—are used. Spironolactone is an aldosterone antagonist that inhibits sodium resorption in the distal convoluted tubule of the kidney. Use of spironolactone may be limited by hyponatremia, hyperkalemia, and painful gynecomastia. If the gynecomastia is distressing, amiloride (5–40 mg/d) may be substituted for spironolactone. Furosemide is a loop diuretic that is generally combined with spironolactone in a ratio of 40:100; maximal daily doses of spironolactone and furosemide are 400 mg and 160 mg, respectively.

Refractory cirrhotic ascites is defined by the persistence of ascites despite sodium restriction and maximal (or maximally tolerated) diuretic use. Pharmacologic therapy for refractory ascites includes the addition of midodrine, an α_1-adrenergic antagonist, or clonidine, an α_2-adrenergic antagonist, to diuretic therapy. These agents act as vasoconstrictors, counteracting splanchnic vasodilation. Midodrine alone or in combination with clonidine improves systemic hemodynamics and control of ascites over that obtained with diuretics alone. Although β-adrenergic blocking agents (beta blockers) are often prescribed to prevent variceal hemorrhage in patients with cirrhosis, the use of beta blockers in patients with refractory ascites is associated with decreased survival rates.

When medical therapy alone is insufficient, refractory ascites can be managed by repeated large-volume paracentesis (LVP) or a transjugular intrahepatic peritoneal shunt (TIPS)—a radiologically placed portosystemic shunt that decompresses the hepatic sinusoids. Intravenous infusion of albumin accompanying LVP decreases the risk of "post-paracentesis circulatory dysfunction" and death. Patients undergoing LVP should receive IV albumin infusions of 6–8 g/L of ascitic fluid removed. TIPS placement is superior to LVP in reducing the reaccumulation of ascites but is associated with an increased frequency of hepatic encephalopathy, with no difference in mortality rates.

Malignant ascites does not respond to sodium restriction or diuretics. Patients must undergo serial LVPs, transcutaneous drainage catheter placement, or, rarely, creation of a peritoneovenous shunt (a shunt from the abdominal cavity to the vena cava).

Ascites caused by tuberculous peritonitis is treated with standard antituberculosis therapy. Noncirrhotic ascites of other causes is treated by correction of the precipitating condition.

COMPLICATIONS

Spontaneous bacterial peritonitis (SBP; **Chap. 26**) is a common and potentially lethal complication of cirrhotic ascites. Occasionally, SBP also complicates ascites caused by nephrotic syndrome, heart failure, acute hepatitis, and acute liver failure but is rare in malignant ascites. Patients with SBP generally note an increase in abdominal girth; however, abdominal tenderness is found in only 40% of patients, and rebound tenderness is uncommon. Patients may present with fever, nausea, vomiting, or the new onset of or exacerbation of preexisting hepatic encephalopathy.

SBP is defined by a polymorphonuclear neutrophil (PMN) count of ≥250/μL in the ascitic fluid. Cultures of ascitic fluid typically reveal one bacterial pathogen. The presence of multiple pathogens in the setting of an elevated ascitic PMN count suggests *secondary peritonitis* from a ruptured viscus or abscess **(Chap. 26)**. The presence of multiple pathogens without an elevated PMN count suggests bowel perforation from the paracentesis needle. SBP is generally the result of enteric bacteria that have translocated across an edematous bowel wall. The most common pathogens are gram-negative rods, including *Escherichia coli* and *Klebsiella*, as well as streptococci and enterococci.

Treatment of SBP with an antibiotic such as IV cefotaxime is effective against gram-negative and gram-positive aerobes. A 5-day course of treatment is sufficient if the patient improves clinically. Nosocomial or health care–acquired SBP is frequently caused by multidrug-resistant bacteria, and initial antibiotic therapy should be guided by the local bacterial epidemiology.

Cirrhotic patients with a history of SBP, an ascitic fluid total protein concentration <1 g/dL, or active gastrointestinal bleeding should receive prophylactic antibiotics to prevent SBP; oral daily norfloxacin is commonly used. Diuresis increases the activity of ascitic fluid protein opsonins and may decrease the risk of SBP.

Hepatic hydrothorax occurs when ascites, often caused by cirrhosis, migrates via fenestrae in the diaphragm into the pleural space. This condition can result in shortness of breath, hypoxia, and infection. Treatment is similar to that for cirrhotic ascites and includes sodium restriction, diuretics, and, if needed, thoracentesis or TIPS placement. Chest tube placement should be avoided.

CHAPTER 10

INVOLUNTARY WEIGHT LOSS

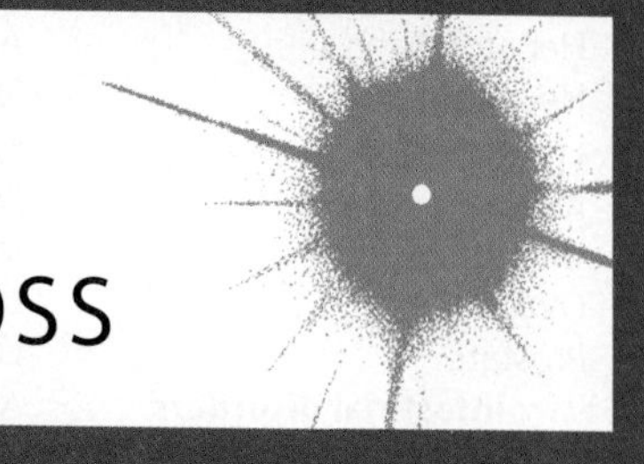

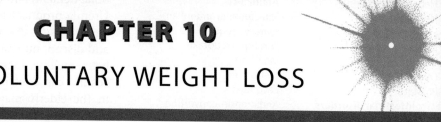

Russell G. Robertson ■ J. Larry Jameson

Involuntary weight loss (IWL) is frequently insidious and can have important implications, often serving as a harbinger of serious underlying disease. Clinically important weight loss is defined as the loss of 10 pounds (4.5 kg) or >5% of one's body weight over a period of 6–12 months. IWL is encountered in up to 8% of all adult outpatients and 27% of frail persons age 65 years and older. There is no identifiable cause in up to one-quarter of patients despite extensive investigation. Conversely, up to half of people who claim to have lost weight have no documented evidence of weight loss. People with no known cause of weight loss generally have a better prognosis than do those with known causes, particularly when the source is neoplastic. Weight loss in older persons is associated with a variety of deleterious effects, including hip fracture, pressure ulcers, impaired immune function, and decreased functional status. Not surprisingly, significant weight loss is associated with increased mortality, which can range from 9% to as high as 38% within 1 to 2.5 years in the absence of clinical awareness and attention.

PHYSIOLOGY OF WEIGHT REGULATION WITH AGING

(See also Chap. 60) Among healthy aging people, total body weight peaks in the sixth decade of life and generally remains stable until the ninth decade, after which it gradually falls. In contrast, lean body mass (fat-free mass) begins to decline at a rate of 0.3 kg per year in the third decade, and the rate of decline increases further beginning at age 60 in men and age 65 in women. These changes in lean body mass largely reflect the age-dependent decline in growth hormone secretion and, consequently, circulating levels of insulin-like growth factor type I (IGF-I) that occur with normal aging. Loss of sex steroids, at menopause in women and more gradually with aging in men, also contributes to these changes in body composition. In the healthy elderly, an increase in fat tissue balances the loss in lean body mass until very old age, when loss of both fat and skeletal muscle occurs. Age-dependent changes also occur at the cellular level. Telomeres shorten, and body cell mass—the fat-free portion of cells—declines steadily with aging.

Between ages 20 and 80, mean energy intake is reduced by up to 1200 kcal/d in men and 800 kcal/d in women. Decreased hunger is a reflection of reduced physical activity and loss of lean body mass, producing lower demand for calories and food intake. Several important age-associated physiologic changes also predispose elderly persons to weight loss, such as declining chemosensory function (smell and taste), reduced efficiency of chewing, slowed gastric emptying, and alterations in the neuroendocrine axis, including changes in levels of leptin, cholecystokinin, neuropeptide Y, and other hormones and peptides. These changes are associated with early satiety and a decline in both appetite and the hedonistic appreciation of food. Collectively, they contribute to the "anorexia of aging."

CAUSES OF INVOLUNTARY WEIGHT LOSS

Most causes of IWL belong to one of four categories: (1) malignant neoplasms, (2) chronic inflammatory or infectious diseases, (3) metabolic disorders (e.g., hyperthyroidism and diabetes), or (4) psychiatric disorders (Table 10-1). Not infrequently, more than one of these causes can be responsible for IWL. In most series, IWL is caused by malignant disease in a quarter of patients and by organic disease in one-third, with the remainder due to psychiatric disease, medications, or uncertain causes.

The most common malignant causes of IWL are gastrointestinal, hepatobiliary, hematologic, lung, breast, genitourinary, ovarian, and prostate. Half of all patients with cancer lose some body weight; one-third lose more than 5% of their original body weight, and up to 20% of all cancer deaths are caused directly by cachexia

TABLE 10-1

CAUSES OF INVOLUNTARY WEIGHT LOSS

Cancer	**Medications**
Colon	Sedatives
Hepatobiliary	Antibiotics
Hematologic	Nonsteroidal anti-inflammatory drugs
Lung	
Breast	Serotonin reuptake inhibitors
Genitourinary	
Ovarian	Metformin
Prostate	Levodopa
Gastrointestinal disorders	Angiotensin-converting enzyme inhibitors
Malabsorption	
Peptic ulcer	Other drugs
Inflammatory bowel disease	**Disorders of the mouth and teeth**
Pancreatitis	Caries
Obstruction/constipation	Dysgeusia
Pernicious anemia	**Age-related factors**
Endocrine and metabolic	Physiologic changes
Hyperthyroidism	Visual impairment
Diabetes mellitus	Decreased taste and smell
Pheochromocytoma	Functional disabilities
Adrenal insufficiency	**Neurologic**
Cardiac disorders	Stroke
Chronic ischemia	Parkinson's disease
Chronic congestive heart failure	Neuromuscular disorders
	Dementia
Respiratory disorders	**Social**
Emphysema	Isolation
Chronic obstructive pulmonary disease	Economic hardship
	Psychiatric and behavioral
Renal insufficiency	Depression
Rheumatologic disease	Anxiety
Infections	Paranoia
HIV	Bereavement
Tuberculosis	Alcoholism
Parasitic infection	Eating disorders
Subacute bacterial endocarditis	Increased activity or exercise
	Idiopathic

(through immobility and/or cardiac/respiratory failure). The greatest incidence of weight loss is seen among patients with solid tumors. Malignancy that reveals itself through significant weight loss usually has a very poor prognosis.

In addition to malignancies, gastrointestinal causes are among the most prominent causes of IWL. Peptic ulcer disease, inflammatory bowel disease, dysmotility syndromes, chronic pancreatitis, celiac disease, constipation, and atrophic gastritis are some of the more common entities. Oral and dental problems are easily overlooked and may manifest with halitosis, poor oral hygiene, xerostomia, inability to chew, reduced masticatory force, nonocclusion, temporomandibular joint syndrome, edentulousness, and pain due to caries or abscesses.

Tuberculosis, fungal diseases, parasites, subacute bacterial endocarditis, and HIV are well-documented causes of IWL. Cardiovascular and pulmonary diseases cause unintentional weight loss through increased metabolic demand and decreased appetite and caloric intake. Uremia produces nausea, anorexia, and vomiting. Connective tissue diseases may increase metabolic demand and disrupt nutritional balance. As the incidence of diabetes mellitus increases with aging, the associated glucosuria can contribute to weight loss. Hyperthyroidism in the elderly may have less prominent sympathomimetic features and may present as "apathetic hyperthyroidism" or T_3 toxicosis.

Neurologic injuries such as stroke, quadriplegia, and multiple sclerosis may lead to visceral and autonomic dysfunction that can impair caloric intake. Dysphagia from these neurologic insults is a common mechanism. Functional disability that compromises activities of daily living (ADLs) is a common cause of undernutrition in the elderly. Visual impairment from ophthalmic or central nervous system disorders such as a tremor can limit the ability of people to prepare and eat meals. IWL may be one of the earliest manifestations of Alzheimer's dementia.

Isolation and depression are significant causes of IWL that may manifest as an inability to care for oneself, including nutritional needs. A cytokine-mediated inflammatory metabolic cascade can be both a cause of and a manifestation of depression. Bereavement can be a cause of IWL and, when present, is more pronounced in men. More intense forms of mental illness such as paranoid disorders may lead to delusions about food and cause weight loss. Alcoholism can be a significant source of weight loss and malnutrition.

Elderly persons living in poverty may have to choose whether to purchase food or use the money for other expenses, including medications. Institutionalization is an independent risk factor, as up to 30–50% of nursing home patients have inadequate food intake.

Medications can cause anorexia, nausea, vomiting, gastrointestinal distress, diarrhea, dry mouth, and changes in taste. This is particularly an issue in the elderly, many of whom take five or more medications.

ASSESSMENT

The four major manifestations of IWL are (1) anorexia (loss of appetite), (2) sarcopenia (loss of muscle mass), (3) cachexia (a syndrome that combines weight loss, loss of muscle and adipose tissue, anorexia, and weakness), and (4) dehydration. The current obesity epidemic adds complexity, as excess adipose tissue can mask the development of sarcopenia and delay awareness of the development of cachexia. If it is not possible to measure weight directly, a change in clothing size, corroboration of weight loss by a relative or friend, and a numeric estimate of weight loss provided by the patient are suggestive of true weight loss.

Initial assessment includes a comprehensive history and physical, a complete blood count, tests of liver enzyme levels, C-reactive protein, erythrocyte sedimentation rate, renal function studies, thyroid function tests, chest radiography, and an abdominal ultrasound (Table 10-2). Age, sex, and risk factor–specific cancer screening tests, such as mammography and colonoscopy, should be performed. Patients at risk should have HIV testing. All elderly patients with weight loss should undergo screening for dementia and depression by using instruments such as the Mini-Mental State Examination and the Geriatric Depression Scale, respectively. The Mini Nutritional Assessment (*www.mna-elderly.com*) and the Nutrition Screening Initiative (*http://www.ncbi.nlm.nih.gov/pmc/articles/PMC1694757/*) are also available for the nutritional assessment of elderly patients. Almost all patients with a malignancy and >90% of those with other organic diseases have at least one laboratory abnormality. In patients presenting with substantial IWL, major organic and malignant diseases are unlikely when a baseline evaluation is completely normal. Careful follow-up rather than undirected testing is advised since the prognosis of weight loss of undetermined cause is generally favorable.

TABLE 10-2

ASSESSMENT AND TESTING FOR INVOLUNTARY WEIGHT LOSS

INDICATIONS	LABORATORY
5% weight loss in 30 d 10% weight loss in 180 d	Complete blood count Comprehensive electrolyte and metabolic panel, including liver and renal function tests
Body mass index <21 25% of food left uneaten after 7 d Change in fit of clothing Change in appetite, smell, or taste	Thyroid function tests Erythrocyte sedimentation rate C-reactive protein Ferritin
Abdominal pain, nausea, vomiting, diarrhea, constipation, dysphagia	HIV testing, if indicated
Assessment	**Radiology**
Complete physical exam, including dental evaluation Medication review Recommended cancer screening Mini-Mental State Examination[a] Mini-Nutritional Assessment[a] Nutrition Screening Initiative[a] Simplified Nutritional Assessment Questionnaire[a] Observation of eating[a] Activities of daily living[a] Instrumental activities of daily living[a]	Chest x-ray Abdominal ultrasound

[a]May be more specific to assess weight loss in the elderly.

TREATMENT Unintentional Weight Loss

The first priority in managing weight loss is to identify and treat the underlying causes systematically. Treatment of underlying metabolic, psychiatric, infectious, or other systemic disorders may be sufficient to restore weight and functional status gradually. Medications that cause nausea or anorexia should be withdrawn or changed, if possible. For those with unexplained IWL, oral nutritional supplements such as high-energy drinks sometimes reverse weight loss. Advising patients to consume supplements between meals rather than with a meal may help minimize appetite suppression and facilitate increased overall intake. Orexigenic, anabolic, and anticytokine agents are under investigation. In selected patients, the antidepressant mirtazapine results in a significant increase in body weight, body fat mass, and leptin concentration. Patients with wasting conditions who can comply with an appropriate exercise program gain muscle protein mass, strength, and endurance and may be more capable of performing ADLs.

SECTION II

EVALUATION OF THE PATIENT WITH ALIMENTARY TRACT SYNDROMES

CHAPTER 11

APPROACH TO THE PATIENT WITH GASTROINTESTINAL DISEASE

William L. Hasler ■ Chung Owyang

ANATOMIC CONSIDERATIONS

The gastrointestinal (GI) tract extends from the mouth to the anus and is composed of several organs with distinct functions. Specialized independently controlled thickened sphincters that assist in gut compartmentalization separate the organs. The gut wall is organized into well-defined layers that contribute to functional activities in each region. The mucosa is a barrier to luminal contents or a site for transfer of fluids or nutrients. Gut smooth muscle in association with the enteric nervous system mediates propulsion from one region to the next. Many GI organs possess a serosal layer that provides a supportive foundation but that also permits external input.

Interactions with other organ systems serve the needs both of the gut and the body. Pancreaticobiliary conduits deliver bile and enzymes into the duodenum. A rich vascular supply is modulated by GI tract activity. Lymphatic channels assist in gut immune activities. Intrinsic gut wall nerves provide the basic controls for propulsion and fluid regulation. Extrinsic neural input provides volitional or involuntary control to degrees that are specific for each gut region.

FUNCTIONS OF THE GASTROINTESTINAL TRACT

The GI tract serves two main functions—assimilating nutrients and eliminating waste. The gut anatomy is organized to serve these functions. In the mouth, food is processed, mixed with salivary amylase, and delivered to the gut lumen. The esophagus propels the bolus into the stomach; the lower esophageal sphincter prevents oral reflux of gastric contents. The esophageal mucosa has a protective squamous histology, which does not permit significant diffusion or absorption. Propulsive esophageal activities are exclusively aboral and coordinate with relaxation of the upper and lower esophageal sphincters on swallowing.

The stomach furthers food preparation by triturating and mixing the bolus with pepsin and acid. Gastric acid also sterilizes the upper gut. The proximal stomach serves a storage function by relaxing to accommodate the meal. The distal stomach exhibits phasic contractions that propel solid food residue against the pylorus, where it is repeatedly propelled proximally for further mixing before it is emptied into the duodenum. Finally, the stomach secretes intrinsic factor for vitamin B_{12} absorption.

The small intestine serves most of the nutrient absorptive function of the gut. The intestinal mucosa exhibits villus architecture to provide maximal surface area for absorption and is endowed with specialized enzymes and transporters. Triturated food from the stomach mixes with pancreatic juice and bile in the duodenum to facilitate digestion. Pancreatic juice contains the main enzymes for carbohydrate, protein, and fat digestion as well as bicarbonate to optimize the pH for activation of these enzymes. Bile secreted by the liver and stored in the gallbladder is essential for intestinal lipid digestion. The proximal intestine is optimized for rapid absorption of nutrient breakdown products and most minerals, whereas the ileum is better suited for absorption of vitamin B_{12} and bile acids. The small intestine also aids in waste elimination. Bile contains by-products of erythrocyte degradation, toxins, metabolized and unmetabolized medications, and cholesterol. Motor function of the small intestine delivers indigestible food residue and sloughed enterocytes into the colon for further processing. The small intestine terminates in the ileocecal junction, a sphincteric structure that prevents coloileal reflux and maintains small-intestinal sterility.

The colon prepares the waste material for controlled evacuation. The colonic mucosa dehydrates the stool, decreasing daily fecal volumes from 1000–1500 mL delivered from the ileum to 100–200 mL expelled from the rectum. The colonic lumen possesses a dense bacterial colonization that ferments undigested carbohydrates and short-chain fatty acids. Whereas transit times in the esophagus are on the order of seconds and times in the stomach and small intestine range from minutes to a few hours, propagation through the colon takes more than 1 day in most individuals. Colonic motor patterns exhibit a to-and-fro character that facilitates slow fecal desiccation. The proximal colon serves to mix and absorb fluid, while the distal colon exhibits peristaltic contractions and mass actions that function to expel the stool. The colon terminates in the anus, a structure with volitional and involuntary controls to permit retention of the fecal bolus until it can be released in a socially convenient setting.

EXTRINSIC MODULATION OF GUT FUNCTION

GI function is modified by influences outside of the gut. Unlike other organ systems, the gut is in continuity with the outside environment. Thus, protective mechanisms are vigilant against deleterious effects of foods, medications, toxins, and infectious organisms. Mucosal immune mechanisms include chronic lymphocyte and plasma cell populations in the epithelial layer and lamina propria backed up by lymph node chains to prevent noxious agents from entering the circulation. Antimicrobial peptides secreted by Paneth cells in the intestine further contribute to the defense mechanisms against pathogens in the lumen. All substances absorbed into the bloodstream are filtered through the liver via the portal venous circulation. In the liver, many drugs and toxins are detoxified by a variety of mechanisms. Although intrinsic nerves control most basic gut activities, extrinsic neural input modulates many functions. Two activities under voluntary control are swallowing and defecation. Many normal GI reflexes involve extrinsic vagus or splanchnic nerve pathways. The brain-gut axis further alters function in regions not under volitional regulation. As an example, stress has potent effects on gut motor, secretory, and sensory functions.

OVERVIEW OF GASTROINTESTINAL DISEASES

GI diseases develop as a result of abnormalities within or outside of the gut and range in severity from those that produce mild symptoms and no long-term morbidity to those with intractable symptoms or adverse outcomes. Diseases may be localized to one organ or exhibit diffuse involvement at many sites.

CLASSIFICATION OF GI DISEASES

GI diseases are manifestations of alterations in nutrient assimilation or waste evacuation or in the activities supporting these main functions.

Impaired digestion and absorption

Diseases of the stomach, intestine, biliary tree, and pancreas can disrupt digestion and absorption. The most common intestinal maldigestion syndrome, lactase deficiency, produces gas and diarrhea after ingestion of dairy products and has no adverse outcomes. Other intestinal enzyme deficiencies produce similar symptoms after ingestion of other simple sugars. Conversely, celiac disease, bacterial overgrowth, infectious enteritis, Crohn's ileitis, and radiation damage, which affect digestion and/or absorption more diffusely, produce anemia, dehydration, electrolyte disorders, or malnutrition. Gastric hypersecretory conditions such as Zollinger-Ellison syndrome damage the intestinal mucosa, impair pancreatic enzyme activation, and accelerate transit due to excess gastric acid. Biliary obstruction from stricture or neoplasm impairs fat digestion. Impaired pancreatic enzyme release in chronic pancreatitis or pancreatic cancer decreases intraluminal digestion and can lead to malnutrition.

Altered secretion

Selected GI diseases result from dysregulation of gut secretion. Gastric acid hypersecretion occurs in Zollinger-Ellison syndrome, G cell hyperplasia, retained antrum syndrome, and some individuals with duodenal ulcers. Conversely, patients with atrophic gastritis or pernicious anemia release little or no gastric acid. Inflammatory and infectious small-intestinal and colonic diseases produce fluid loss through impaired absorption or enhanced secretion. Common intestinal and colonic hypersecretory conditions cause diarrhea and include acute bacterial or viral infection, chronic *Giardia* or cryptosporidia infections, small-intestinal bacterial overgrowth, bile salt diarrhea, microscopic colitis, diabetic diarrhea, and abuse of certain laxatives. Less common causes include large colonic villus adenomas and endocrine neoplasias with tumor overproduction of secretagogue transmitters like vasoactive intestinal polypeptide.

Altered gut transit

Impaired gut transit may be secondary to mechanical obstruction. Esophageal occlusion often results from acid-induced stricture or neoplasm. Gastric outlet obstruction develops from peptic ulcer disease or gastric cancer. Small-intestinal obstruction most commonly results from adhesions but may also occur with Crohn's disease, radiation- or drug-induced strictures, and less likely malignancy. The most common cause of colonic obstruction is colon cancer, although inflammatory strictures develop in patients with inflammatory bowel disease, after certain infections such as diverticulitis, or with some drugs.

Retardation of propulsion also develops from disordered motor function. Achalasia is characterized by impaired esophageal body peristalsis and incomplete lower esophageal sphincter relaxation. Gastroparesis is the symptomatic delay in gastric emptying of meals due to impaired gastric motility. Intestinal pseudoobstruction causes marked delays in small-bowel transit due to enteric nerve or intestinal smooth-muscle injury. Slow-transit constipation is produced by diffusely impaired colonic propulsion. Constipation also is produced by outlet abnormalities such as rectal prolapse, intussusception, or dyssynergia—a failure of anal or puborectalis relaxation upon attempted defecation.

Disorders of rapid propulsion are less common than those with delayed transit. Rapid gastric emptying occurs in postvagotomy dumping syndrome, with gastric hypersecretion, and in some cases of functional dyspepsia and cyclic vomiting syndrome. Exaggerated intestinal or colonic motor patterns may be responsible for diarrhea in irritable bowel syndrome. Accelerated transit with hyperdefecation is noted in hyperthyroidism.

Immune dysregulation

Many inflammatory GI conditions are consequences of altered gut immune function. The mucosal inflammation of celiac disease results from dietary ingestion of gluten-containing grains. Some patients with food allergy also exhibit altered immune populations. Eosinophilic esophagitis and eosinophilic gastroenteritis are inflammatory disorders with prominent mucosal eosinophils. Ulcerative colitis and Crohn's disease are disorders of uncertain etiology that produce mucosal injury primarily in the lower gut. The microscopic colitides, lymphocytic and collagenous colitis, exhibit colonic subepithelial infiltrates without visible mucosal damage. Bacterial, viral, and protozoal organisms may produce ileitis or colitis in selected patient populations.

Impaired gut blood flow

Different GI regions are at variable risk for ischemic damage from impaired blood flow. Rare cases of gastroparesis result from blockage of the celiac and superior mesenteric arteries. More commonly encountered are intestinal and colonic ischemia that are consequences of arterial embolus, arterial thrombosis, venous thrombosis, or hypoperfusion from dehydration, sepsis, hemorrhage, or reduced cardiac output. These may produce mucosal injury, hemorrhage, or even perforation. Chronic ischemia may result in intestinal stricture. Some cases of radiation enterocolitis exhibit reduced mucosal blood flow.

Neoplastic degeneration

All GI regions are susceptible to malignant degeneration to varying degrees. In the United States, colorectal cancer is most common and usually presents after age 50 years. Worldwide, gastric cancer is prevalent especially in certain Asian regions. Esophageal cancer develops with chronic acid reflux or after an extensive alcohol or tobacco use history. Small-intestinal neoplasms are rare and occur with underlying inflammatory disease. Anal cancers arise after prior anal infection or inflammation. Pancreatic and biliary cancers elicit severe pain, weight loss, and jaundice and have poor prognoses. Hepatocellular carcinoma usually arises in the setting of chronic viral hepatitis or cirrhosis secondary to other causes. Most GI cancers exhibit carcinomatous histology; however, lymphomas and other cell types also are observed.

Disorders without obvious organic abnormalities

The most common GI disorders show no abnormalities on biochemical or structural testing and include irritable bowel syndrome, functional dyspepsia, functional chest pain, and functional heartburn. These disorders exhibit altered gut motor function; however, the pathogenic relevance of these abnormalities is uncertain. Exaggerated visceral sensory responses to noxious stimulation may cause discomfort in these disorders. Symptoms in other patients result from altered processing of visceral pain sensations in the central nervous system. Functional bowel patients with severe symptoms may exhibit significant emotional disturbances on psychometric testing. Subtle immunologic defects may contribute to functional symptoms as well.

Genetic influences

Although many GI diseases result from environmental factors, others exhibit hereditary components. Family members of inflammatory bowel disease patients show a genetic predisposition to disease development themselves. Colonic and esophageal malignancies arise in certain inherited disorders. Rare genetic dysmotility syndromes are described. Familial clustering is even observed in the functional bowel disorders, although

TABLE 11-1

COMMON CAUSES OF COMMON GASTROINTESTINAL (GI) SYMPTOMS

ABDOMINAL PAIN	NAUSEA AND VOMITING	DIARRHEA	GI BLEEDING	OBSTRUCTIVE JAUNDICE
Appendicitis	Medications	Infection	Ulcer disease	Bile duct stones
Gallstone disease	GI obstruction	Poorly absorbed sugars	Esophagitis	Cholangiocarcinoma
Pancreatitis	Motor disorders	Inflammatory bowel disease	Varices	Cholangitis
Diverticulitis	Functional bowel disorder	Microscopic colitis	Vascular lesions	Sclerosing cholangitis
Ulcer disease	Enteric infection	Functional bowel disorder	Neoplasm	Ampullary stenosis
Esophagitis	Pregnancy	Celiac disease	Diverticula	Ampullary carcinoma
GI obstruction	Endocrine disease	Pancreatic insufficiency	Hemorrhoids	Pancreatitis
Inflammatory bowel disease	Motion sickness	Hyperthyroidism	Fissures	Pancreatic tumor
Functional bowel disorder	Central nervous system disease	Ischemia	Inflammatory bowel disease	
Vascular disease		Endocrine tumor	Infectious colitis	
Gynecologic causes				
Renal stone				

this may be secondary learned familial illness behavior rather than a true hereditary factor.

SYMPTOMS OF GASTROINTESTINAL DISEASE

The most common GI symptoms are abdominal pain, heartburn, nausea and vomiting, altered bowel habits, GI bleeding, and jaundice (Table 11-1). Others are dysphagia, anorexia, weight loss, fatigue, and extraintestinal symptoms.

Abdominal pain

Abdominal pain results from GI disease and extraintestinal conditions involving the genitourinary tract, abdominal wall, thorax, or spine. Visceral pain generally is midline in location and vague in character, whereas parietal pain is localized and precisely described. Common inflammatory diseases with pain include peptic ulcer, appendicitis, diverticulitis, inflammatory bowel disease, and infectious enterocolitis. Other intraabdominal causes of pain include gallstone disease and pancreatitis. Noninflammatory visceral sources include mesenteric ischemia and neoplasia. The most common causes of abdominal pain are irritable bowel syndrome and functional dyspepsia.

Heartburn

Heartburn, a burning substernal sensation, is reported intermittently by at least 40% of the population. Classically, heartburn is felt to result from excess gastroesophageal reflux of acid. However, some cases exhibit normal esophageal acid exposure and may result from reflux of nonacidic material or heightened sensitivity of esophageal mucosal nerves.

Nausea and vomiting

Nausea and vomiting are caused by GI diseases, medications, toxins, acute and chronic infection, endocrine disorders, labyrinthine conditions, and central nervous system disease. The best-characterized GI etiologies relate to mechanical obstruction of the upper gut; however, disorders of propulsion including gastroparesis and intestinal pseudoobstruction also elicit prominent symptoms. Nausea and vomiting also are commonly reported by patients with irritable bowel syndrome and functional disorders of the upper gut (including chronic idiopathic nausea and functional vomiting).

Altered bowel habits

Altered bowel habits are common complaints of patients with GI disease. Constipation is reported as infrequent defecation, straining with defecation, passage of hard stools, or a sense of incomplete fecal evacuation. Causes of constipation include obstruction, motor disorders of the colon, medications, and endocrine diseases such as hypothyroidism and hyperparathyroidism. Diarrhea is reported as frequent defecation, passage of loose or watery stools, fecal urgency, or a similar sense of incomplete evacuation. The differential diagnosis of diarrhea is broad and includes infections, inflammatory causes, malabsorption, and medications. Irritable bowel syndrome produces constipation, diarrhea, or an alternating bowel pattern. Fecal mucus is common in irritable bowel syndrome, whereas pus characterizes inflammatory disease. Steatorrhea develops with malabsorption.

GI bleeding

Hemorrhage may develop from any gut organ. Most commonly, upper GI bleeding presents with melena or hematemesis, whereas lower GI bleeding produces passage of bright red or maroon stools. However, briskly bleeding upper sites can elicit voluminous red rectal bleeding, whereas slowly bleeding ascending colon sites may produce melena. Chronic slow GI bleeding may present with iron deficiency anemia. The most common upper GI causes of bleeding are ulcer disease, gastroduodenitis, and esophagitis. Other etiologies include portal hypertensive causes, malignancy, tears across the gastroesophageal junction, and vascular lesions. The most prevalent lower GI sources of hemorrhage include hemorrhoids, anal fissures, diverticula, ischemic colitis, and arteriovenous malformations. Other causes include neoplasm, inflammatory bowel disease, infectious colitis, drug-induced colitis, and other vascular lesions.

Jaundice

Jaundice results from prehepatic, intrahepatic, or posthepatic disease. Posthepatic causes of jaundice include biliary diseases, such as choledocholithiasis, acute cholangitis, primary sclerosing cholangitis, other strictures, and neoplasm, and pancreatic disorders, such as acute and chronic pancreatitis, stricture, and malignancy.

Other symptoms

Other symptoms are manifestations of GI disease. Dysphagia, odynophagia, and unexplained chest pain suggest esophageal disease. A globus sensation is reported with esophagopharyngeal conditions, but also occurs with functional GI disorders. Weight loss, anorexia, and fatigue are nonspecific symptoms of neoplastic, inflammatory, gut motility, pancreatic, small-bowel mucosal, and psychiatric conditions. Fever is reported with inflammatory illness, but malignancies also evoke febrile responses. GI disorders also produce extraintestinal symptoms. Inflammatory bowel disease is associated with hepatobiliary dysfunction, skin and eye lesions, and arthritis. Celiac disease may present with dermatitis herpetiformis. Jaundice can produce pruritus. Conversely, systemic diseases can have GI consequences. Systemic lupus may cause gut ischemia, presenting with pain or bleeding. Overwhelming stress or severe burns may lead to gastric ulcer formation.

EVALUATION OF THE PATIENT WITH GASTROINTESTINAL DISEASE

Evaluation of the patient with GI disease begins with a careful history and examination. Subsequent investigation with a variety of tools designed to test gut structure or function are indicated in selected cases. Some patients exhibit normal findings on diagnostic testing. In these individuals, validated symptom profiles are used to confidently diagnose a functional bowel disorder.

HISTORY

The history of the patient with suspected GI disease has several components. Symptom timing suggests specific etiologies. Symptoms of short duration commonly result from acute infection, toxin exposure, or abrupt inflammation or ischemia. Long-standing symptoms point to underlying chronic inflammatory or neoplastic conditions or functional bowel disorders. Symptoms from mechanical obstruction, ischemia, inflammatory bowel disease, and functional bowel disorders are worsened by meals. Conversely, ulcer symptoms may be relieved by eating or antacids. Symptom patterns and duration may suggest underlying etiologies. Ulcer pain occurs at intermittent intervals lasting weeks to months, whereas biliary colic has a sudden onset and lasts up to several hours. Pain from acute inflammation as with acute pancreatitis is severe and persists for days to weeks. Meals elicit diarrhea in some cases of inflammatory bowel disease and irritable bowel syndrome. Defecation relieves discomfort in inflammatory bowel disease and irritable bowel syndrome. Functional bowel disorders are exacerbated by stress. Sudden awakening from sound sleep suggests organic rather than functional disease. Diarrhea from malabsorption usually improves with fasting, whereas secretory diarrhea persists without oral intake.

Symptom relation to other factors narrows the list of diagnostic possibilities. Obstructive symptoms with prior abdominal surgery raise concern for adhesions, whereas loose stools after gastrectomy or gallbladder excision suggest dumping syndrome or postcholecystectomy diarrhea. Symptom onset after travel prompts a search for enteric infection. Medications may produce pain, altered bowel habits, or GI bleeding. Lower GI bleeding likely results from neoplasms, diverticula, or vascular lesions in an older person and from anorectal abnormalities or inflammatory bowel disease in a younger individual. Celiac disease is prevalent in people of northern European descent, whereas inflammatory bowel disease is more common in certain Jewish populations. A sexual history may raise concern for sexually transmitted diseases or immunodeficiency.

For more than two decades, working groups have been convened to devise symptom criteria to improve the confident diagnosis of functional bowel disorders and to minimize the numbers of unnecessary diagnostic tests performed. The most widely accepted symptom-based criteria are the Rome criteria. When tested against findings of structural investigations, the Rome criteria exhibit diagnostic specificities exceeding 90% for many of the functional bowel disorders.

PHYSICAL EXAMINATION

The physical exam complements information from the history. Abnormal vital signs provide diagnostic clues and determine the need for acute intervention. Fever suggests inflammation or neoplasm. Orthostasis is found with significant blood loss, dehydration, sepsis, or autonomic neuropathy. Skin, eye, or joint findings may point to specific diagnoses. Neck exam with swallowing assessment evaluates dysphagia. Cardiopulmonary disease may present with abdominal pain or nausea; thus lung and cardiac exams are important. Pelvic examination tests for a gynecologic source of abdominal pain. Rectal exam may detect blood, indicating gut mucosal injury or neoplasm or a palpable inflammatory mass in appendicitis. Metabolic conditions and gut motor disorders have associated peripheral neuropathy.

Inspection of the abdomen may reveal distention from obstruction, tumor, or ascites or vascular abnormalities with liver disease. Ecchymoses develop with severe pancreatitis. Auscultation can detect bruits or friction rubs from vascular disease or hepatic tumors. Loss of bowel sounds signifies ileus, whereas high-pitched, hyperactive sounds characterize intestinal obstruction. Percussion assesses liver size and can detect shifting dullness from ascites. Palpation assesses for hepatosplenomegaly as well as neoplastic or inflammatory masses. Abdominal exam is helpful in evaluating unexplained pain. Intestinal ischemia elicits severe pain but little tenderness. Patients with visceral pain may exhibit generalized discomfort, whereas those with parietal pain or peritonitis have directed pain, often with involuntary guarding, rigidity, or rebound. Patients with musculoskeletal abdominal wall pain may note tenderness exacerbated by Valsalva or straight-leg lift maneuvers.

TOOLS FOR PATIENT EVALUATION

Laboratory, radiographic, and functional tests can assist in diagnosis of suspected GI disease. The GI tract also is amenable to internal evaluation with upper and lower endoscopy and to examination of luminal contents. Histopathologic exams of GI tissues complement these tests.

Laboratory

Selected laboratory tests facilitate the diagnosis of GI disease. Iron-deficiency anemia suggests mucosal blood loss, whereas vitamin B_{12} deficiency results from small-intestinal, gastric, or pancreatic disease. Either also can result from inadequate oral intake. Leukocytosis and increased sedimentation rates and C-reactive protein levels are found in inflammatory conditions, whereas leukopenia is seen in viremic illness. Severe vomiting or diarrhea elicits electrolyte disturbances, acid-base abnormalities, and elevated blood urea nitrogen. Pancreaticobiliary or liver disease is suggested by elevated pancreatic or liver chemistries. Thyroid chemistries, cortisol, and calcium levels are obtained to exclude endocrinologic causes of GI symptoms. Pregnancy testing is considered for women with unexplained nausea. Serologic tests can screen for celiac disease, inflammatory bowel disease, rheumatologic diseases like lupus or scleroderma, and paraneoplastic dysmotility syndromes. Hormone levels are obtained for suspected endocrine neoplasia. Intraabdominal malignancies produce other tumor markers including the carcinoembryonic antigen CA 19-9 and α-fetoprotein. Blood testing also monitors medication therapy in some diseases, as with thiopurine metabolite levels in inflammatory bowel disease. Other body fluids are sampled under certain circumstances. Ascitic fluid is analyzed for infection, malignancy, or findings of portal hypertension. Cerebrospinal fluid is obtained for suspected central nervous system causes of vomiting. Urine samples screen for carcinoid, porphyria, and heavy metal intoxication.

Luminal contents

Luminal contents can be examined for diagnostic clues. Stool samples are cultured for bacterial pathogens, examined for leukocytes and parasites, or tested for *Giardia* antigen. Duodenal aspirates can be examined for parasites or cultured for bacterial overgrowth. Fecal fat is quantified in possible malabsorption. Stool electrolytes can be measured in diarrheal conditions. Laxative screens are done when laxative abuse is suspected. Gastric acid is quantified to rule out Zollinger-Ellison syndrome. Esophageal pH testing is done for refractory symptoms of acid reflux, whereas impedance techniques assess for nonacidic reflux. Pancreatic juice is analyzed for enzyme or bicarbonate content to exclude pancreatic exocrine insufficiency.

Endoscopy

The gut is accessible with endoscopy, which can provide the diagnosis of the causes of bleeding, pain, nausea and vomiting, weight loss, altered bowel function, and fever. Table 11-2 lists the most common indications for the major endoscopic procedures. Upper endoscopy evaluates the esophagus, stomach, and duodenum, whereas colonoscopy assesses the colon and distal ileum. Upper endoscopy is advocated as the initial structural test performed in patients with suspected ulcer disease, esophagitis, neoplasm, malabsorption, and Barrett's metaplasia because of its ability to directly visualize as well as biopsy the abnormality. Colonoscopy is the

TABLE 11-2

COMMON INDICATIONS FOR ENDOSCOPY

UPPER ENDOSCOPY	COLONOSCOPY	ENDOSCOPIC RETROGRADE CHOLANGIOPANCREATOGRAPHY	ENDOSCOPIC ULTRASOUND	CAPSULE ENDOSCOPY	DOUBLE-BALLOON ENDOSCOPY
Dyspepsia despite treatment Dyspepsia with signs of organic disease Refractory vomiting Dysphagia Upper GI bleeding Anemia Weight loss Malabsorption Biopsy radiologic abnormality Polypectomy Place gastrostomy Barrett's surveillance Palliate neoplasm Sample duodenal tissue/fluid Remove foreign body Endoscopic mucosal resection or ablation of dysplastic Barrett's mucosa Place stent across stenosis	Cancer screening Lower GI bleeding Anemia Diarrhea Polypectomy Obstruction Biopsy radiologic abnormality Cancer surveillance: family history prior polyp/cancer, colitis Palliate neoplasm Remove foreign body Place stent across stenosis	Jaundice Postbiliary surgery complaints Cholangitis Gallstone pancreatitis Pancreatic/biliary/ampullary tumor Unexplained pancreatitis Pancreatitis with unrelenting pain Fistulas Biopsy radiologic abnormality Pancreaticobiliary drainage Sample bile Sphincter of Oddi manometry	Staging of malignancy Characterize and biopsy submucosal mass Bile duct stones Chronic pancreatitis Drain pseudocyst Anal continuity	Obscure gastrointestinal (GI) bleeding Suspected Crohn's disease of the small intestine	Ablation of small-intestinal bleeding sources Biopsy of suspicious small-intestinal masses/ulcers

procedure of choice for colon cancer screening and surveillance as well as diagnosis of colitis secondary to infection, ischemia, radiation, and inflammatory bowel disease. Sigmoidoscopy examines the colon up to the splenic flexure and is currently used to exclude distal colonic inflammation or obstruction in young patients not at significant risk for colon cancer. For elusive GI bleeding secondary to arteriovenous malformations or superficial ulcers, small-intestinal examination is performed with push enteroscopy, capsule endoscopy, or double-balloon enteroscopy. Capsule endoscopy also can visualize small-intestinal Crohn's disease in individuals with negative barium radiography. Endoscopic retrograde cholangiopancreaticography (ERCP) provides diagnoses of pancreatic and biliary disease. Endoscopic ultrasound is useful for evaluating extent of disease in GI malignancy as well as exclusion of choledocholithiasis, evaluation of pancreatitis, drainage of pancreatic pseudocysts, and assessment of anal continuity.

Radiography/nuclear medicine

Radiographic tests evaluate diseases of the gut and extraluminal structures. Oral or rectal contrast agents like barium provide mucosal definition from the esophagus to the rectum. Contrast radiography also assesses gut transit and pelvic floor dysfunction. Barium swallow is the initial procedure for evaluation of dysphagia to exclude subtle rings or strictures and assess for achalasia, whereas small-bowel contrast radiology reliably diagnoses intestinal tumors and Crohn's ileitis. Contrast enemas are performed when colonoscopy is unsuccessful or contraindicated. Ultrasound and computed tomography (CT) evaluate regions not accessible by endoscopy or contrast studies, including the liver, pancreas, gallbladder, kidneys, and retroperitoneum. These tests are useful for diagnosis of mass lesions, fluid collections, organ enlargement, and, in the case of ultrasound, gallstones. CT and magnetic resonance (MR) colonography are being evaluated as alternatives to colonoscopy for colon cancer screening. MR imaging assesses the pancreaticobiliary ducts to exclude neoplasm, stones, and sclerosing cholangitis, and the liver to characterize benign and malignant tumors. Specialized CT or MR enterography can assess intensity of inflammatory bowel disease. Angiography excludes mesenteric ischemia and determines spread of malignancy. Angiographic techniques also access the biliary tree in obstructive jaundice. CT and MR techniques can be used to screen for mesenteric occlusion, thereby limiting exposure to angiographic dyes. Positron emission tomography can facilitate distinguishing malignant from benign disease in several organ systems.

Scintigraphy both evaluates structural abnormalities and quantifies luminal transit. Radionuclide bleeding scans localize bleeding sites in patients with brisk hemorrhage so that therapy with endoscopy, angiography, or surgery may be directed. Radiolabeled leukocyte scans can search for intraabdominal abscesses not visualized on CT. Biliary scintigraphy is complementary to ultrasound in the assessment of cholecystitis. Scintigraphy to quantify esophageal and gastric emptying is well established, whereas techniques to measure small-intestinal or colonic transit are less widely used.

Histopathology

Gut mucosal biopsies obtained at endoscopy evaluate for inflammatory, infectious, and neoplastic disease. Deep rectal biopsies assist with diagnosis of Hirschsprung's disease or amyloid. Liver biopsy is indicated in cases with abnormal liver chemistries, in unexplained jaundice, following liver transplant to exclude rejection, and to characterize the degree of inflammation in patients with chronic viral hepatitis prior to initiating antiviral therapy. Biopsies obtained during CT or ultrasound can evaluate for other intraabdominal conditions not accessible by endoscopy.

Functional testing

Tests of gut function provide important data when structural testing is nondiagnostic. In addition to gastric acid and pancreatic function testing, functional testing of motor activity is provided by manometric techniques. Esophageal manometry is useful for suspected achalasia, whereas small-intestinal manometry tests for pseudoobstruction. A wireless motility capsule is now available to measure transit and contractile activity in the stomach, small intestine, and colon in a single test. Anorectal manometry with balloon expulsion testing is used for unexplained incontinence or constipation from outlet dysfunction. Anorectal manometry and electromyography also assess anal function in fecal incontinence. Biliary manometry tests for sphincter of Oddi dysfunction with unexplained biliary pain. Measurement of breath hydrogen while fasting and after oral mono- or oligosaccharide challenge can screen for carbohydrate intolerance and small-intestinal bacterial overgrowth.

TREATMENT Gastrointestinal Disease

Management options for the patient with GI disease depend on the cause of symptoms. Available treatments include modifications in dietary intake, medications, interventional endoscopy or radiology techniques, surgery, and therapies directed to external influences.

NUTRITIONAL MANIPULATION Dietary modifications for GI disease include treatments that only reduce symptoms, therapies that correct pathologic defects, and measures that replace normal food intake with enteral or parenteral formulations. Changes that improve symptoms but do not reverse an organic abnormality include lactose restriction for lactase deficiency, liquid meals in gastroparesis, carbohydrate restrictions with dumping syndrome, and low-FODMAP (fermentable oligo-di-mono-saccharides and polyols) diets in irritable bowel syndrome. The gluten-free diet for celiac disease exemplifies a modification that serves as primary therapy to reduce mucosal inflammation. Enteral medium-chain triglycerides replace normal fats in short-gut syndrome or severe ileal disease. Perfusion of liquid meals through a gastrostomy is performed in those who cannot swallow safely. Enteral feeding through a jejunostomy is considered for gastric dysmotility syndromes that preclude feeding into the stomach. Intravenous hyperalimentation is used for individuals with generalized gut malfunction who cannot tolerate or who cannot be sustained with enteral nutrition.

PHARMACOTHERAPY Several medications are available to treat GI diseases. Considerable health care resources are expended on over-the-counter remedies. Many prescription drug classes are offered as short-term or continuous therapy of GI illness. A plethora of alternative treatments have gained popularity in GI conditions for which traditional therapies provide incomplete relief.

Over-the-counter agents Over-the-counter agents are reserved for mild GI symptoms. Antacids and histamine H_2 antagonists decrease symptoms in gastroesophageal reflux and dyspepsia, whereas antiflatulents and adsorbents reduce gaseous symptoms. More potent acid inhibitors such as proton pump inhibitors are now available over the counter for treatment of chronic gastroesophageal reflux disease (GERD). Fiber supplements, stool softeners, enemas, and laxatives are used for constipation. Laxatives are categorized as stimulants, osmotic agents (including isotonic preparations containing polyethylene glycol), and poorly absorbed sugars. Nonprescription antidiarrheal agents include bismuth subsalicylate, kaolin-pectin combinations, and loperamide. Supplemental enzymes include lactase pills for lactose intolerance and bacterial α-galactosidase to treat excess gas. In general, use of a nonprescription preparation for more than a short time for chronic persistent symptoms should be supervised by a health care provider.

Prescription drugs Prescription drugs for GI diseases are a major focus of attention from pharmaceutical companies. Potent acid suppressants, including drugs that inhibit the proton pump, are advocated for acid reflux when over-the-counter preparations are inadequate. Cytoprotective agents rarely are used for upper gut ulcers. Prokinetic drugs stimulate GI propulsion in gastroparesis and pseudoobstruction. Prosecretory drugs are prescribed for constipation refractory to other agents. Prescription antidiarrheals include opiate drugs, anticholinergic antispasmodics, tricyclics, bile acid binders, and serotonin antagonists. Antispasmodics and antidepressants also are useful for functional abdominal pain, whereas narcotics are used for pain control in organic conditions such as disseminated malignancy and chronic pancreatitis. Antiemetics in several classes reduce nausea and vomiting. Potent pancreatic enzymes decrease malabsorption and pain from pancreatic disease. Antisecretory drugs such as the somatostatin analogue octreotide treat hypersecretory states. Antibiotics treat ulcer disease secondary to *Helicobacter pylori*, infectious diarrhea, diverticulitis, intestinal bacterial overgrowth, and Crohn's disease. Some cases of irritable bowel syndrome (especially those with diarrhea) respond to nonabsorbable antibiotic therapy. Anti-inflammatory and immunosuppressive drugs are used in ulcerative colitis, Crohn's disease, microscopic colitis, refractory celiac disease, and gut vasculitis. Chemotherapy with or without radiotherapy is offered for GI malignancies. Most GI carcinomas respond poorly to such therapy, whereas lymphomas may be cured with such intervention.

Alternative therapies Alternative treatments are marketed to treat selected GI symptoms. Ginger, acupressure, and acustimulation have been advocated for nausea, whereas pyridoxine has been investigated for nausea of first-trimester pregnancy. Probiotics containing active bacterial cultures are used as adjuncts in some cases of infectious diarrhea and irritable bowel syndrome. Probiotics that selectively nourish benign commensal bacteria may ultimately show benefit in functional disorders as well. Low-potency pancreatic enzyme preparations are sold as general digestive aids but have little evidence to support their efficacy.

ENTERIC THERAPIES/INTERVENTIONAL ENDOSCOPY AND RADIOLOGY Simple luminal interventions are commonly performed for GI diseases. Nasogastric tube suction decompresses the upper gut in ileus or mechanical obstruction. Nasogastric lavage of saline or water in the patient with upper GI hemorrhage determines the rate of bleeding and helps evacuate blood prior to endoscopy. Enteral feedings can be initiated through a nasogastric or nasoenteric tube. Enemas relieve fecal impaction or assist in gas evacuation in acute colonic pseudoobstruction. A rectal tube can be left in place to vent the distal colon in colonic pseudoobstruction and other colonic distention disorders.

In addition to its diagnostic role, endoscopy has therapeutic capabilities in certain settings. Cautery techniques can stop hemorrhage from ulcers, vascular malformations, and tumors. Injection with vasoconstrictor substances or sclerosants is used for bleeding ulcers, vascular malformations, varices, and hemorrhoids. Endoscopic encirclement of varices and hemorrhoids with constricting bands stops hemorrhage from these sites, whereas endoscopically placed clips can occlude arterial bleeding sites. Endoscopy can remove polyps or debulk lumen-narrowing malignancies. Endoscopic mucosal resection and radiofrequency techniques can remove or ablate some cases of Barrett's esophagus with dysplasia. Endoscopic sphincterotomy of the ampulla of Vater relieves symptoms of choledocholithiasis. Obstructions of the gut lumen and pancreaticobiliary tree are relieved by endoscopic dilatation or placement of plastic or expandable metal stents. In cases of acute colonic pseudoobstruction, colonoscopy is used to withdraw luminal gas. Finally, endoscopy is commonly used to insert feeding tubes.

Radiologic measures also are useful in GI disease. Angiographic embolization or vasoconstriction decreases bleeding from sites not amenable to endoscopic intervention. Dilatation or stenting with fluoroscopic guidance relieves luminal strictures. Contrast enemas can reduce volvulus and evacuate air in acute colonic pseudoobstruction. CT and ultrasound help drain abdominal fluid collections, in many cases obviating the need for surgery. Percutaneous transhepatic cholangiography relieves biliary obstruction when ERCP is contraindicated. Lithotripsy can fragment gallstones in patients who are not candidates for surgery. In some instances, radiologic approaches offer advantages over endoscopy for gastroenterostomy placement. Finally, central venous catheters for parenteral nutrition may be placed using radiographic techniques.

SURGERY Surgery is performed to cure disease, control symptoms without cure, maintain nutrition, or palliate unresectable neoplasm. Medication-unresponsive ulcerative colitis, diverticulitis, cholecystitis, appendicitis, and intraabdominal abscess are curable with surgery, whereas only symptom control without cure is possible with Crohn's disease. Surgery is mandated for ulcer complications such as bleeding, obstruction, or perforation and intestinal obstructions that persist after conservative care. Fundoplication of the gastroesophageal junction is performed for severe ulcerative esophagitis and drug-refractory symptomatic acid reflux. Achalasia responds to operations to relieve lower esophageal sphincter pressure. Operations for motor disorders have been introduced including implanted electrical stimulators for gastroparesis and electrical devices and artificial sphincters for fecal incontinence. Surgery may be needed to place a jejunostomy for long-term enteral feedings. The threshold for performing surgery depends on the clinical setting. In all cases, the benefits of operation must be weighed against the potential for postoperative complications.

THERAPY DIRECTED TO EXTERNAL INFLUENCES In some conditions, GI symptoms respond to treatments directed outside the gut. Psychological therapies including psychotherapy, behavior modification, hypnosis, and biofeedback have shown efficacy in functional bowel disorders. Patients with significant psychological dysfunction and those with little response to treatments targeting the gut are likely to benefit from this form of therapy.

CHAPTER 12
GASTROINTESTINAL ENDOSCOPY

Louis Michel Wong Kee Song ■ Mark Topazian

Gastrointestinal endoscopy has been attempted for over 200 years, but the introduction of semirigid gastroscopes in the middle of the twentieth century marked the dawn of the modern endoscopic era. Since then, rapid advances in endoscopic technology have led to dramatic changes in the diagnosis and treatment of many digestive diseases. Innovative endoscopic devices and new endoscopic treatment modalities continue to expand the use of endoscopy in patient care.

Current flexible endoscopes provide an electronic video image generated by a charge-coupled device in the tip of the endoscope. Operator controls permit deflection of the endoscope tip; fiberoptic bundles or light-emitting diodes bring light to the tip of the endoscope; and working channels allow washing, suctioning, and the passage of instruments. Progressive changes in the diameter and stiffness of endoscopes have improved the ease and patient tolerance of endoscopy.

ENDOSCOPIC PROCEDURES

UPPER ENDOSCOPY

Upper endoscopy, also referred to as esophagogastroduodenoscopy (EGD), is performed by passing a flexible endoscope through the mouth into the esophagus, stomach, and duodenum. The procedure is the best method for examining the upper gastrointestinal mucosa. While the upper gastrointestinal radiographic series has similar accuracy for diagnosis of duodenal ulcer (Fig. 12-1), EGD is superior for detection of gastric ulcers (Fig. 12-2) and flat mucosal lesions such as Barrett's esophagus (Fig. 12-3), and it permits directed biopsy and endoscopic therapy. Intravenous conscious sedation is given to most patients in the United States to ease the anxiety and discomfort of the procedure, although in many countries EGD is routinely performed with topical pharyngeal anesthesia only. Patient tolerance of unsedated EGD is improved by the use of an ultrathin, 5-mm diameter endoscope that can be passed transorally or transnasally.

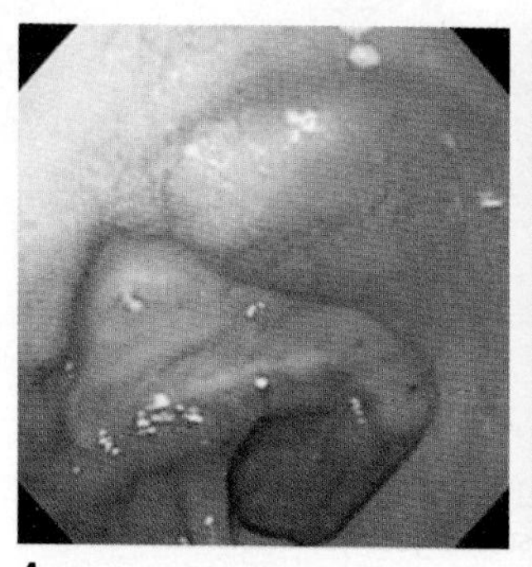

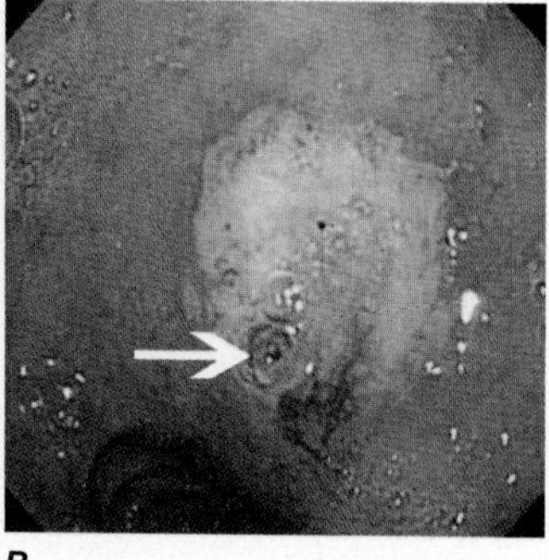

A B

FIGURE 12-1
Duodenal ulcers. *A.* Ulcer with a clean base. ***B.*** Ulcer with a visible vessel (*arrow*) in a patient with recent hemorrhage.

COLONOSCOPY

Colonoscopy is performed by passing a flexible colonoscope through the anal canal into the rectum and colon. The cecum is reached in >95% of cases, and the terminal ileum can often be examined. Colonoscopy is the gold

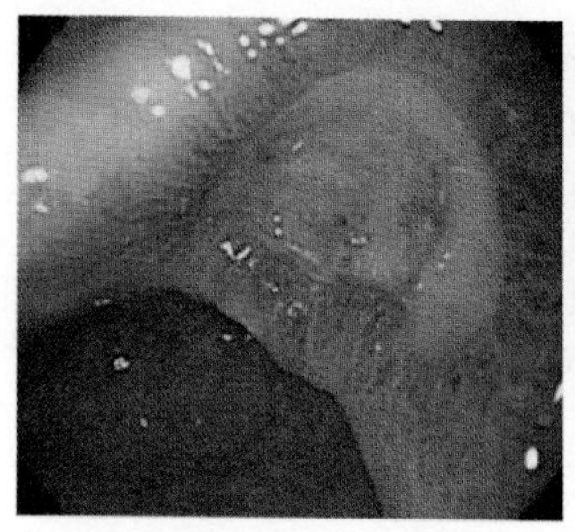

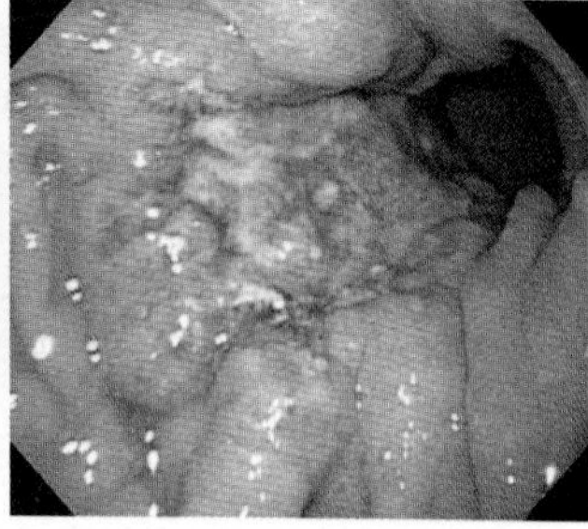

A B

FIGURE 12-2
Gastric ulcers. *A.* Benign gastric ulcer. ***B.*** Malignant gastric ulcer involving greater curvature of stomach.

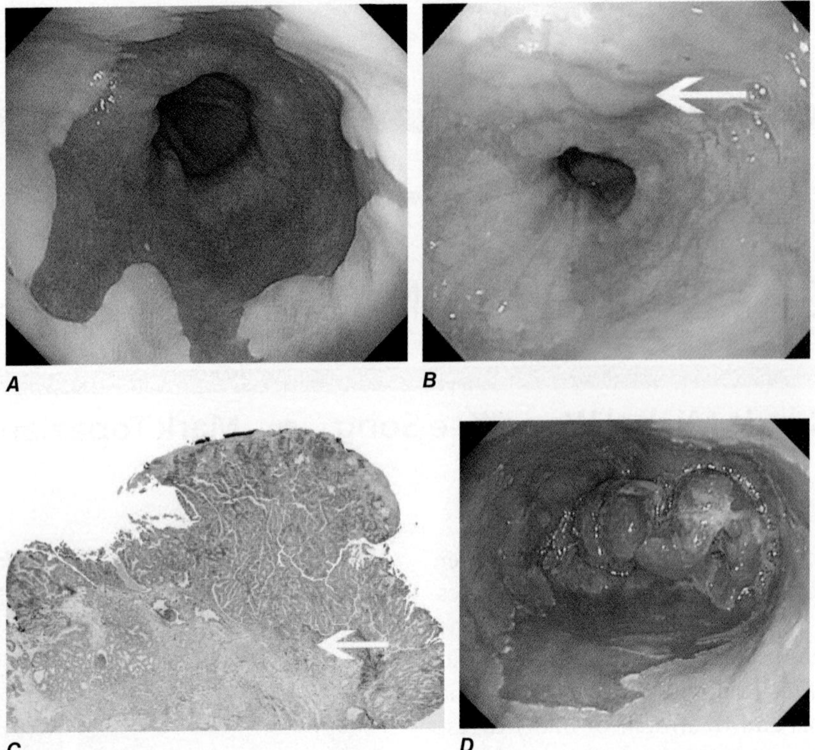

FIGURE 12-3
Barrett's esophagus. *A.* Pink tongues of Barrett's mucosa extending proximally from the gastroesophageal junction. ***B.*** Barrett's esophagus with a suspicious nodule (*arrow*) identified during endoscopic surveillance. ***C.*** Histologic finding of intramucosal adenocarcinoma in the endoscopically resected nodule. Tumor extends into the esophageal submucosa (*arrow*). ***D.*** Barrett's esophagus with locally advanced adenocarcinoma.

standard for imaging the colonic mucosa. Colonoscopy has greater sensitivity than barium enema for colitis (Fig. 12-4), polyps (Fig. 12-5), and cancer (Fig. 12-6). Computed tomography (CT) colonography is an emerging technology that rivals the accuracy of colonoscopy for detection of some polyps and cancer, although it may not be sensitive for the detection of flat lesions, such as serrated polyps (Fig. 12-7). Conscious sedation is usually given before colonoscopy in the United States, although a willing patient and a skilled examiner can complete the procedure without sedation in many cases.

FLEXIBLE SIGMOIDOSCOPY

Flexible sigmoidoscopy is similar to colonoscopy, but visualizes only the rectum and a variable portion of the left colon, typically to 60 cm from the anal verge. This procedure causes abdominal cramping, but it is brief and is usually performed without sedation. Flexible sigmoidoscopy is primarily used for evaluation of diarrhea and rectal outlet bleeding.

SMALL-BOWEL ENDOSCOPY

Three endoscopic techniques are currently used to evaluate the small intestine, most often in patients presenting with presumed small-bowel bleeding. For *capsule*

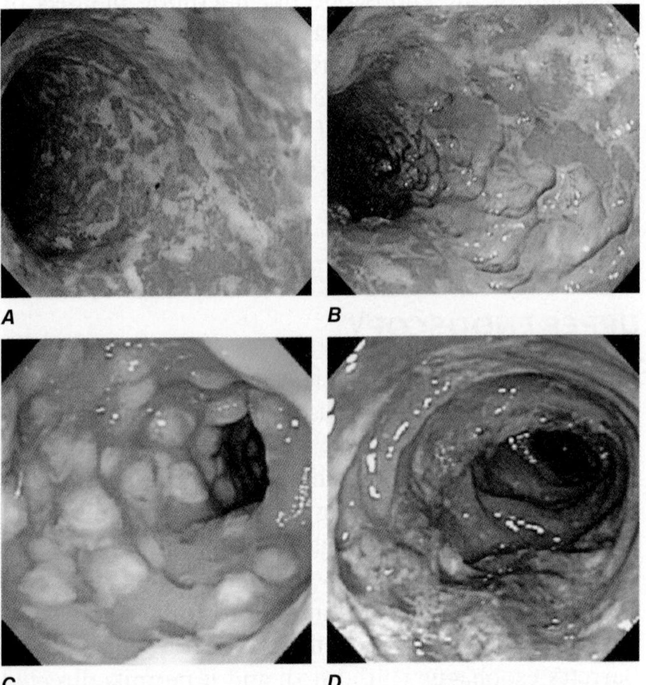

FIGURE 12-4
Causes of colitis. *A.* Chronic ulcerative colitis with diffuse ulcerations and exudates. ***B.*** Severe Crohn's colitis with deep ulcers. ***C.*** Pseudomembranous colitis with yellow, adherent pseudomembranes. ***D.*** Ischemic colitis with patchy mucosal edema, subepithelial hemorrhage, and cyanosis.

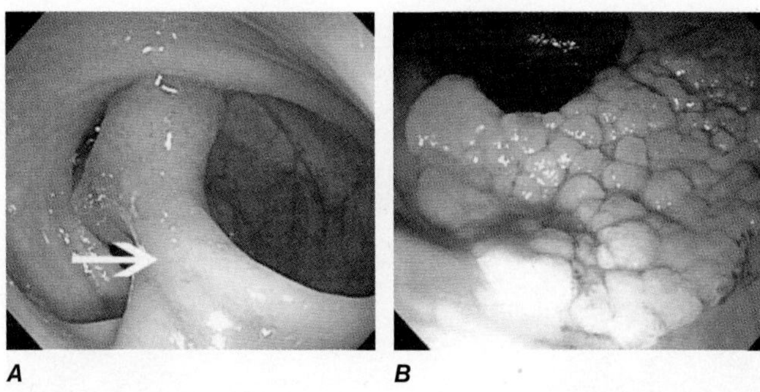

A *B*

FIGURE 12-5
Colonic polyps. *A.* Pedunculated colon polyp on a thick stalk covered with normal mucosa (*arrow*). ***B.*** Sessile rectal polyp.

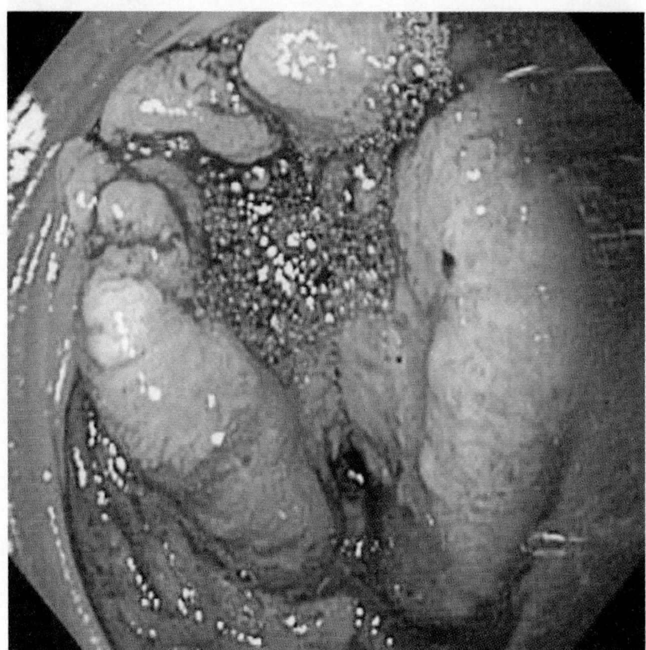

FIGURE 12-6
Colon adenocarcinoma growing into the lumen.

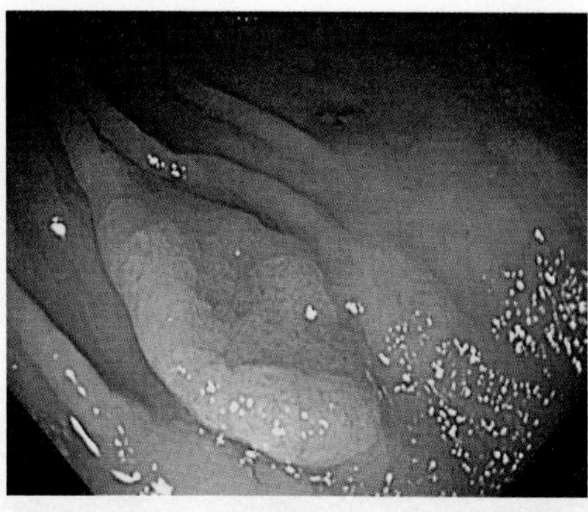

A

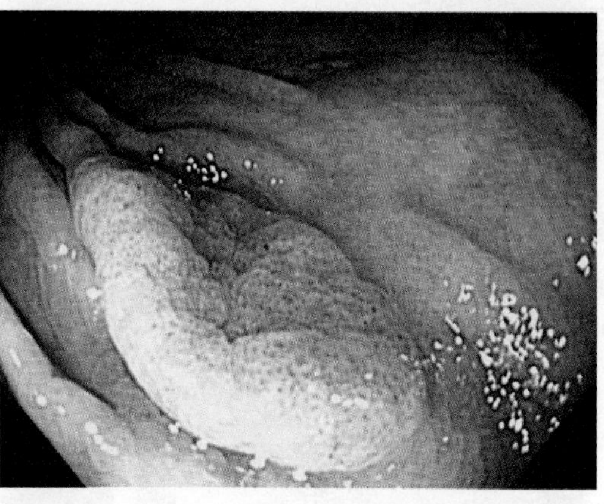

B

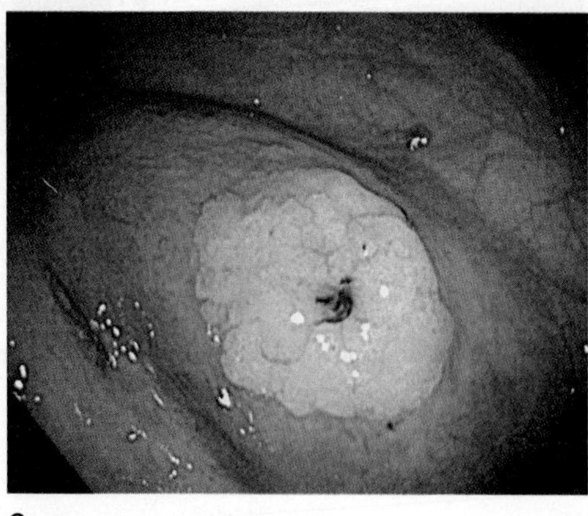

C

FIGURE 12-7
Flat serrated polyp in the cecum. *A.* Appearance of the lesion under conventional white-light imaging. ***B.*** Mucosal patterns and boundary of the lesion enhanced with narrow band imaging. ***C.*** Submucosal lifting of the lesion with dye (methylene blue) injection prior to resection.

endoscopy, the patient swallows a disposable capsule that contains a complementary metal oxide silicon (CMOS) chip camera. Color still images (Fig. 12-8) are transmitted wirelessly to an external receiver at several frames per second until the capsule's battery is exhausted or it is passed into the toilet. Capsule endoscopy enables visualization of the small-bowel mucosa beyond the reach of a conventional endoscope and, at present, is solely a diagnostic procedure.

Push enteroscopy is performed with a long endoscope similar in design to an upper endoscope. The enteroscope is pushed down the small bowel, sometimes with the help of a stiffening overtube that extends from the mouth to the small intestine. The proximal to mid-jejunum is usually reached, and the instrument channel of the endoscope allows for biopsy or endoscopic therapy.

Deeper insertion into the small bowel can be accomplished by *single-* or *double-balloon enteroscopy* or *spiral enteroscopy* (Fig. 12-9). These instruments enable pleating of the small intestine onto an overtube **(see Video 13-1)**. With balloon-assisted enteroscopy, the entire intestinal tract can be visualized in some patients when both the oral and anal routes of insertion are used. Biopsies and endoscopic therapy can be performed throughout the visualized small bowel (Fig. 12-10).

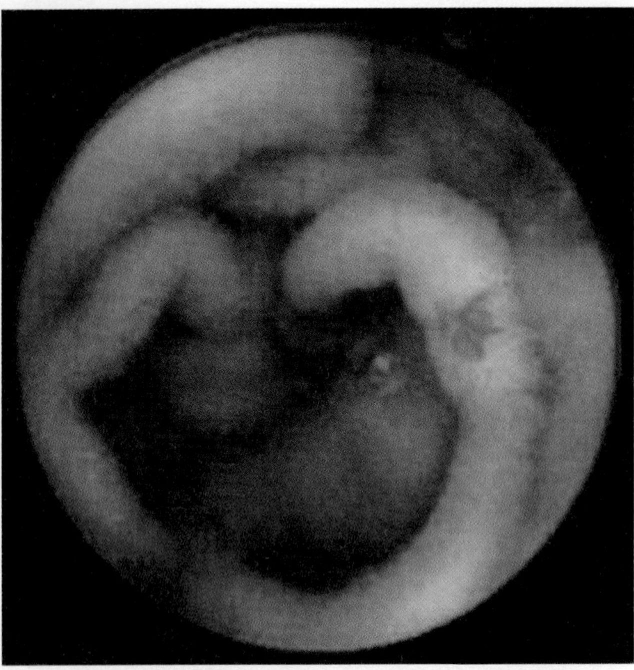

FIGURE 12-8
Capsule endoscopy image of jejunal vascular ectasia.

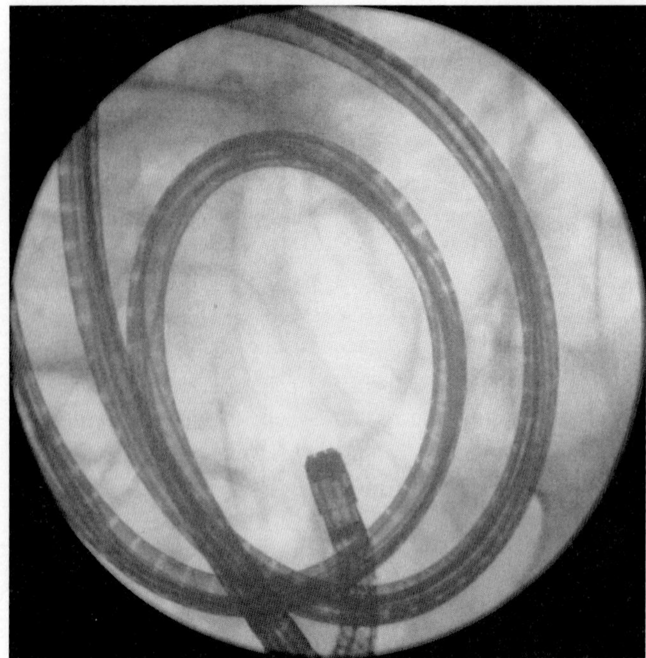

FIGURE 12-9
Radiograph of a double-balloon enteroscope in the small intestine.

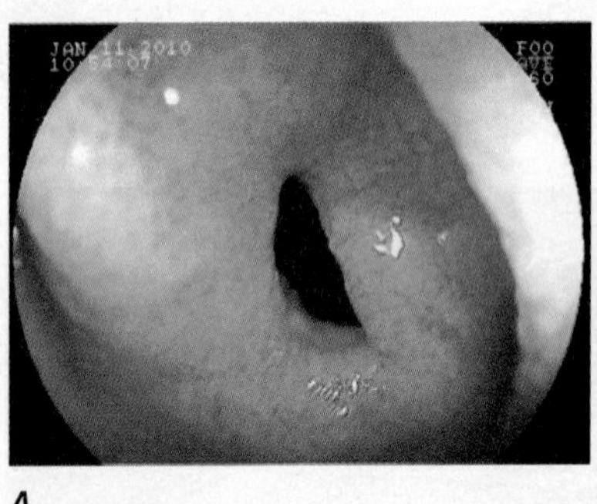
A

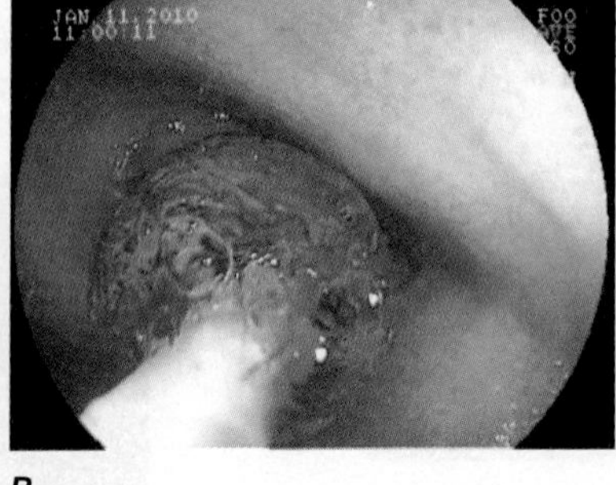
B

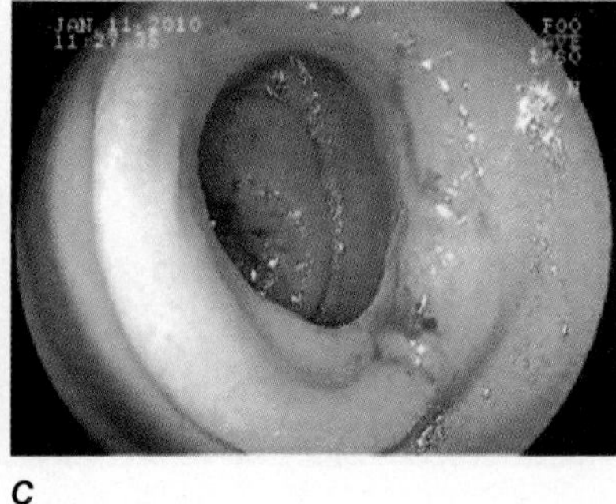
C

FIGURE 12-10
Nonsteroidal anti-inflammatory drug (NSAID)–induced proximal ileal stricture diagnosed by double-balloon endoscopy. *A.* Ileal stricture causing obstructive symptoms. ***B.*** Balloon dilatation of the ileal stricture. ***C.*** Appearance of stricture after dilatation.

ENDOSCOPIC RETROGRADE CHOLANGIOPANCREATOGRAPHY (ERCP)

During ERCP a side-viewing endoscope is passed through the mouth to the duodenum, the ampulla of Vater is identified and cannulated with a thin plastic catheter, and radiographic contrast material is injected into the bile duct and pancreatic duct under fluoroscopic guidance (Fig. 12-11). When indicated, the sphincter of Oddi can be opened using the technique of endoscopic sphincterotomy (Fig. 12-12). Stones can be retrieved from the ducts (see **Video 13-15**), biopsies can be performed, strictures can be dilated and/or stented (Fig. 12-13), and ductal leaks can be stented (Fig. 12-14). ERCP is often performed for therapy but remains important in diagnosis, especially for sphincter of Oddi dysfunction and for tissue sampling of ductal strictures.

ENDOSCOPIC ULTRASOUND (EUS)

EUS utilizes high-frequency ultrasound transducers incorporated into the tip of a flexible endoscope. Ultrasound images are obtained of the gut wall and adjacent organs, vessels, and lymph nodes. By sacrificing depth of ultrasound penetration and bringing the ultrasound transducer close to the area of interest via endoscopy, high-resolution images are obtained. EUS provides the most accurate preoperative local staging of esophageal,

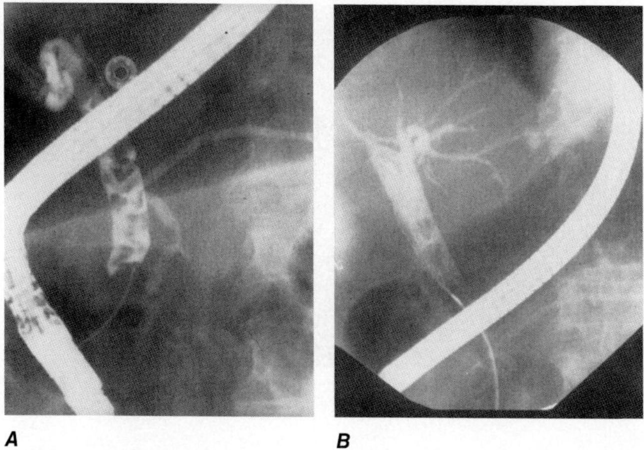

FIGURE 12-11

Endoscopic retrograde cholangiopancreatography (ERCP) for bile duct stones with cholangitis. *A.* Faceted bile duct stones are demonstrated in the common bile duct. ***B.*** After endoscopic sphincterotomy, the stones are extracted with a Dormia basket. A small abscess communicates with the left hepatic duct.

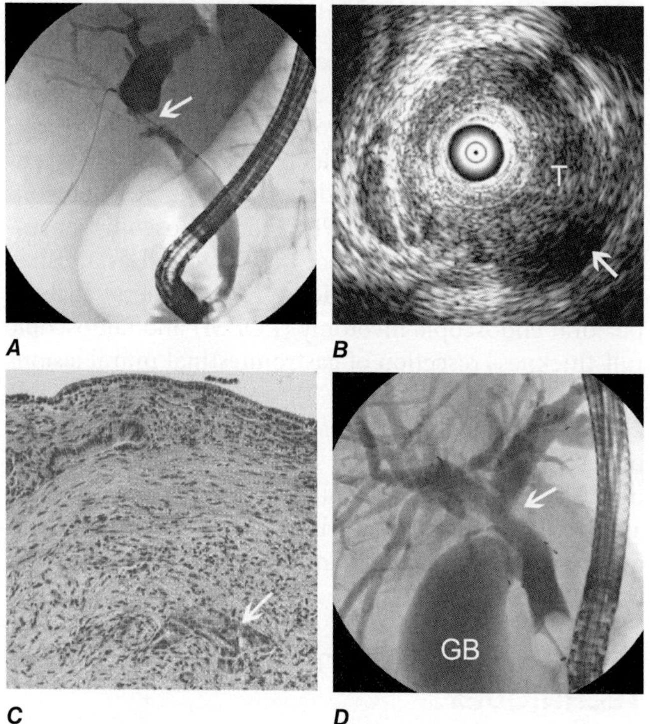

FIGURE 12-13

Endoscopic diagnosis, staging, and palliation of hilar cholangiocarcinoma. *A.* Endoscopic retrograde cholangiopancreatography (ERCP) in a patient with obstructive jaundice demonstrates a malignant-appearing stricture of the biliary confluence extending into the left and right intrahepatic ducts. ***B.*** Intraductal ultrasound of the biliary stricture demonstrates marked bile duct wall thickening due to tumor (T) with partial encasement of the hepatic artery (*arrow*). ***C.*** Intraductal biopsy obtained during ERCP demonstrates malignant cells infiltrating the submucosa of the bile duct wall (*arrow*). ***D.*** Endoscopic placement of bilateral self-expanding metal stents (*arrow*) relieves the biliary obstruction. GB, gallbladder. (*Image C courtesy of Dr. Thomas Smyrk; with permission.*)

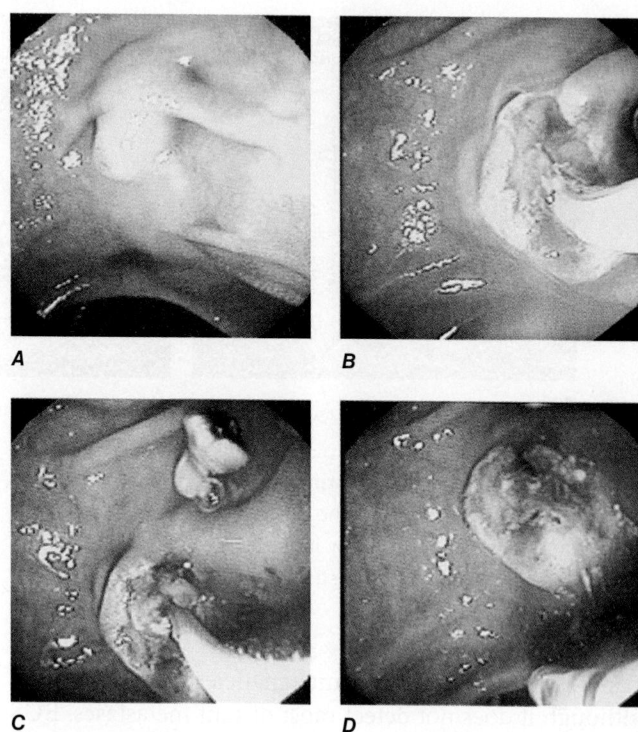

FIGURE 12-12

Endoscopic sphincterotomy. *A.* A normal-appearing ampulla of Vater. ***B.*** Sphincterotomy is performed with electrocautery. ***C.*** Bile duct stones are extracted with a balloon catheter. ***D.*** Final appearance of the sphincterotomy.

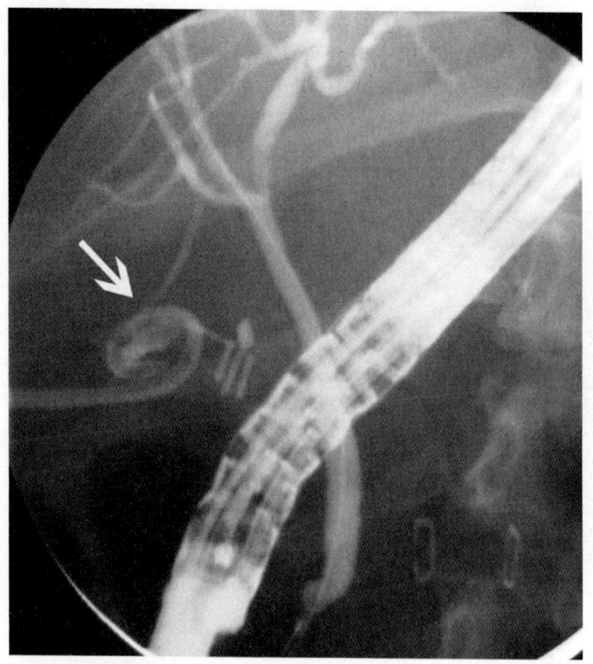

FIGURE 12-14

Bile leak (*arrow*) from a duct of Luschka after laparoscopic cholecystectomy. Contrast leaks from a small right intrahepatic duct into the gallbladder fossa and then flows into the pigtail of a percutaneous drainage catheter.

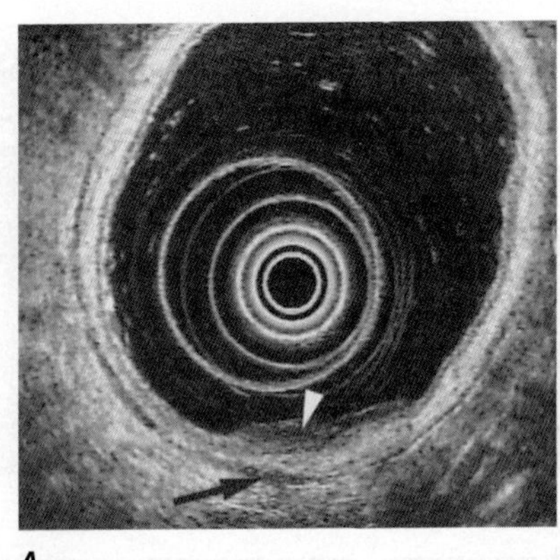

A

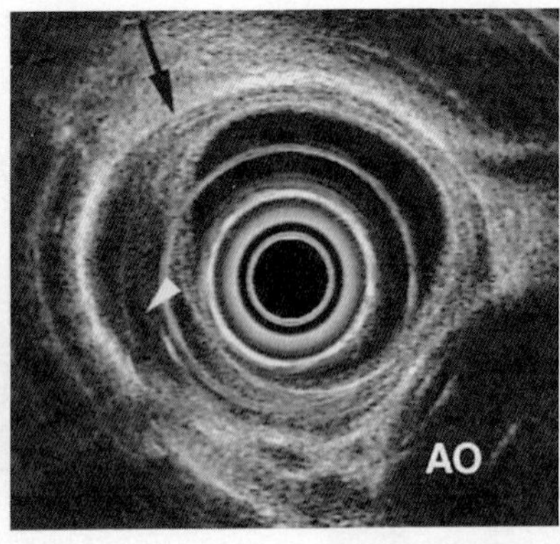

B

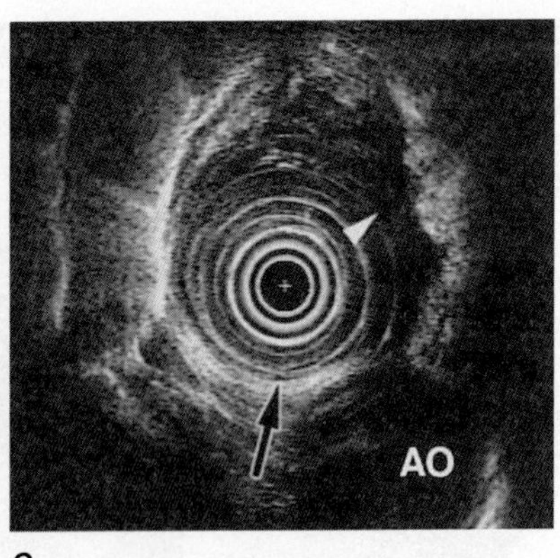

C

FIGURE 12-15

Local staging of gastrointestinal cancers with endoscopic ultrasound. In each example, the *white arrowhead* marks the primary tumor and the *black arrow* indicates the muscularis propria of the intestinal wall. ***A.*** T1 gastric cancer. The tumor does not invade the mp. ***B.*** T2 esophageal cancer. The tumor invades the muscularis propria. ***C.*** T3 esophageal cancer. The tumor extends through the muscularis propria into the surrounding tissue and focally abuts the aorta. AO, aorta.

pancreatic, and rectal malignancies (Fig. 12-15), although it does not detect most distant metastases. EUS is also useful for diagnosis of bile duct stones, gallbladder disease, submucosal gastrointestinal lesions, and chronic pancreatitis. Fine-needle aspirates and core biopsies of masses and lymph nodes in the posterior mediastinum, abdomen, pancreas, retroperitoneum, and pelvis can be obtained under EUS guidance (Fig. 12-16). EUS-guided therapeutic procedures are increasingly performed, including drainage of abscesses, pseudocysts, and pancreatic necrosis into the gut lumen **(see Video 13-2)**, celiac plexus neurolysis for treatment of pancreatic pain, ethanol ablation of pancreatic neuroendocrine tumors, treatment of gastrointestinal hemorrhage, and drainage of obstructed biliary and pancreatic ducts.

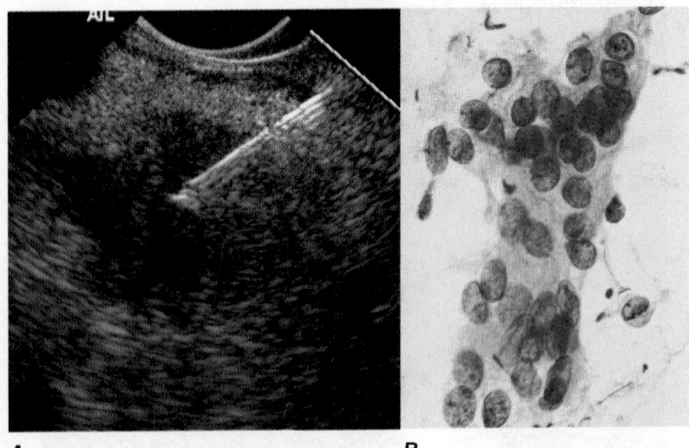

A B

FIGURE 12-16

Endoscopic ultrasound (EUS)–guided fine-needle aspiration (FNA). ***A.*** Ultrasound image of a 22-gauge needle passed through the duodenal wall and positioned in a hypoechoic pancreatic head mass. ***B.*** Micrograph of aspirated malignant cells. *(Image B courtesy of Dr. Michael R. Henry; with permission.)*

NATURAL ORIFICE TRANSLUMINAL ENDOSCOPIC SURGERY (NOTES)

NOTES is an evolving collection of endoscopic methods that entail passage of an endoscope or its accessories into or through the wall of the gastrointestinal tract to perform diagnostic or therapeutic interventions. Some NOTES procedures, such as percutaneous endoscopic gastrostomy (PEG) or endoscopic necrosectomy of pancreatic necrosis, are well-established clinical procedures **(see Video 13-2)**; others, such as per-oral endoscopic myotomy (POEM) and endoscopic full-thickness resection of gastrointestinal mural lesions (Fig. 12-17, **see Video 13-3**), are emerging as viable clinical therapeutic options; and still others, such as endoscopic appendectomy, cholecystectomy, and tubal ligation, are in development, and their ultimate clinical application is presently unclear. NOTES is currently an area of intense innovation and endoscopic research.

ENDOSCOPIC RESECTION AND CLOSURE TECHNIQUES

Endoscopic mucosal resection (EMR) **(see Video 13-4)** and endoscopic submucosal dissection (ESD) (Fig. 12-18, **see Video 13-5**) are two commonly used techniques for the resection of benign and early-stage malignant gastrointestinal neoplasms. In addition to providing larger specimens for more accurate histopathologic assessment and diagnosis, these techniques can be potentially curative for certain dysplastic lesions and focal intramucosal carcinomas involving the esophagus, stomach, and colon. Several devices are also available for closure of EMR and ESD defects, as well as gastrointestinal fistulas and perforations. Endoscopic clips deployed through the working channel of an endoscope

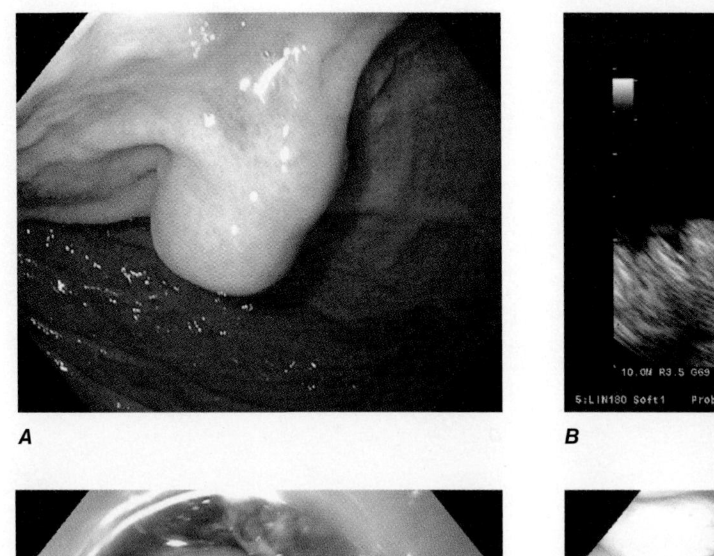

A *B*

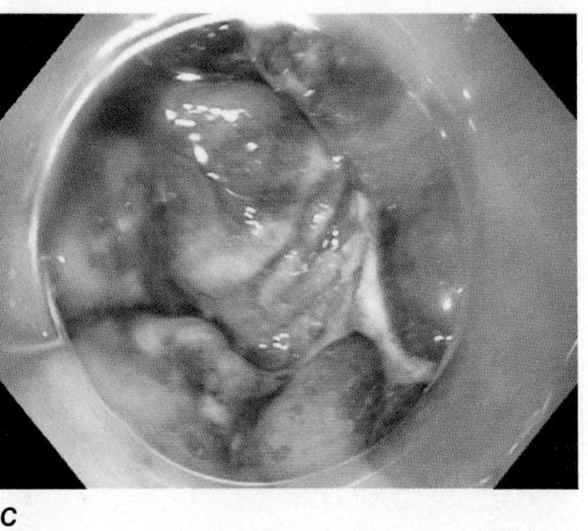

C D

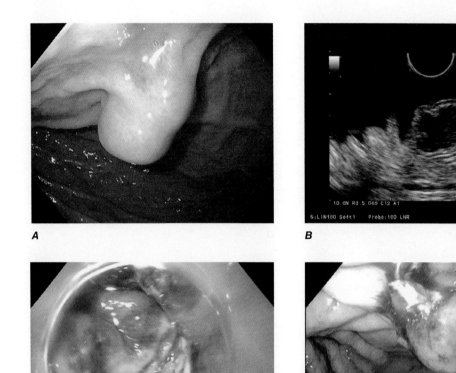

FIGURE 12-17

Endoscopic full-thickness resection of a gastrointestinal stromal tumor. *A.* Subepithelial lesion in the proximal stomach. ***B.*** Hypoechoic lesion arising from the fourth layer (muscularis propria) at endoscopic ultrasound. ***C.*** Full-thickness resection defect. ***D.*** Closure of defect using an over-the-scope clip.

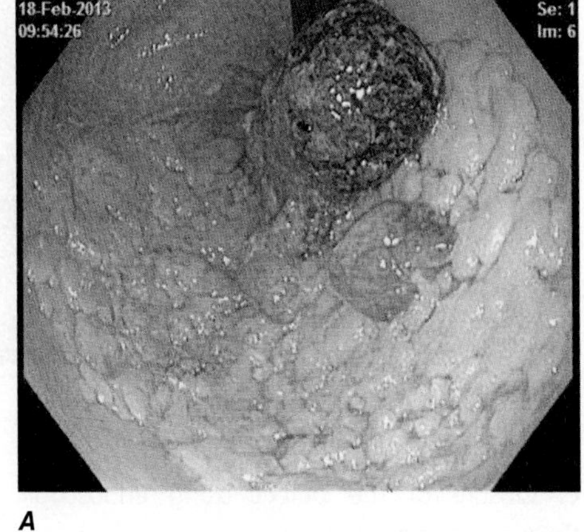

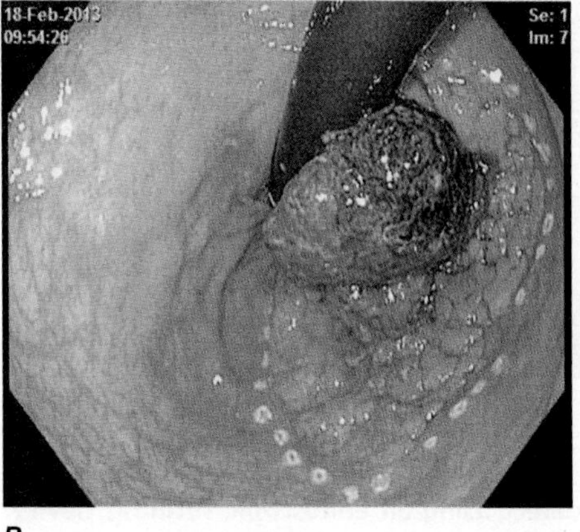

A *B*

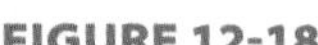

FIGURE 12-18

Endoscopic submucosal dissection. *A.* Large flat distal rectal adenoma with central lobulation. ***B.*** Marking the periphery of the lesion with coagulation dots. ***C.*** Rectal defect following endoscopic submucosal dissection. ***D.*** Specimen resected en bloc.

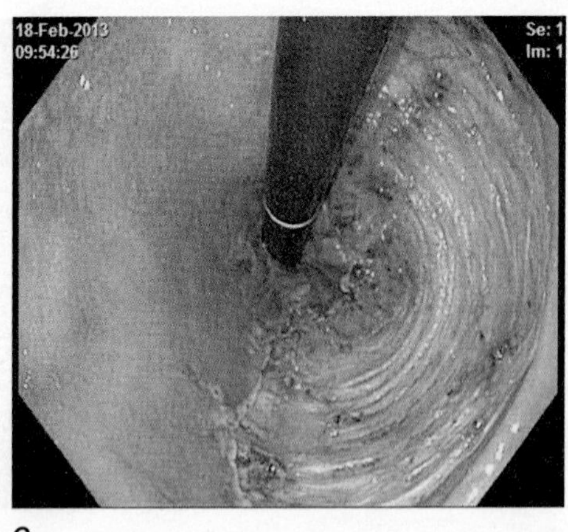

C

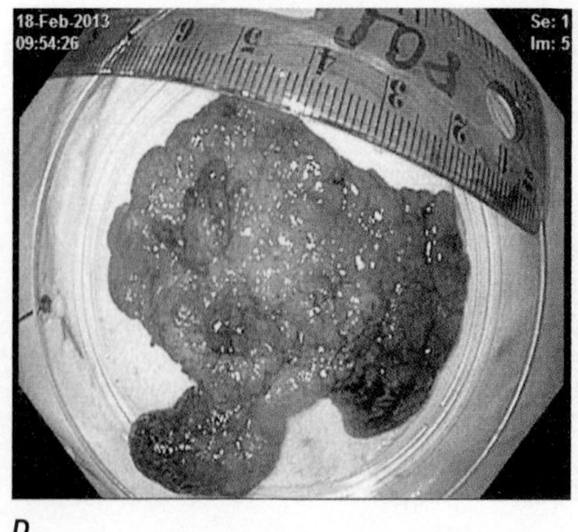

D

FIGURE 12-18
(*continued*)

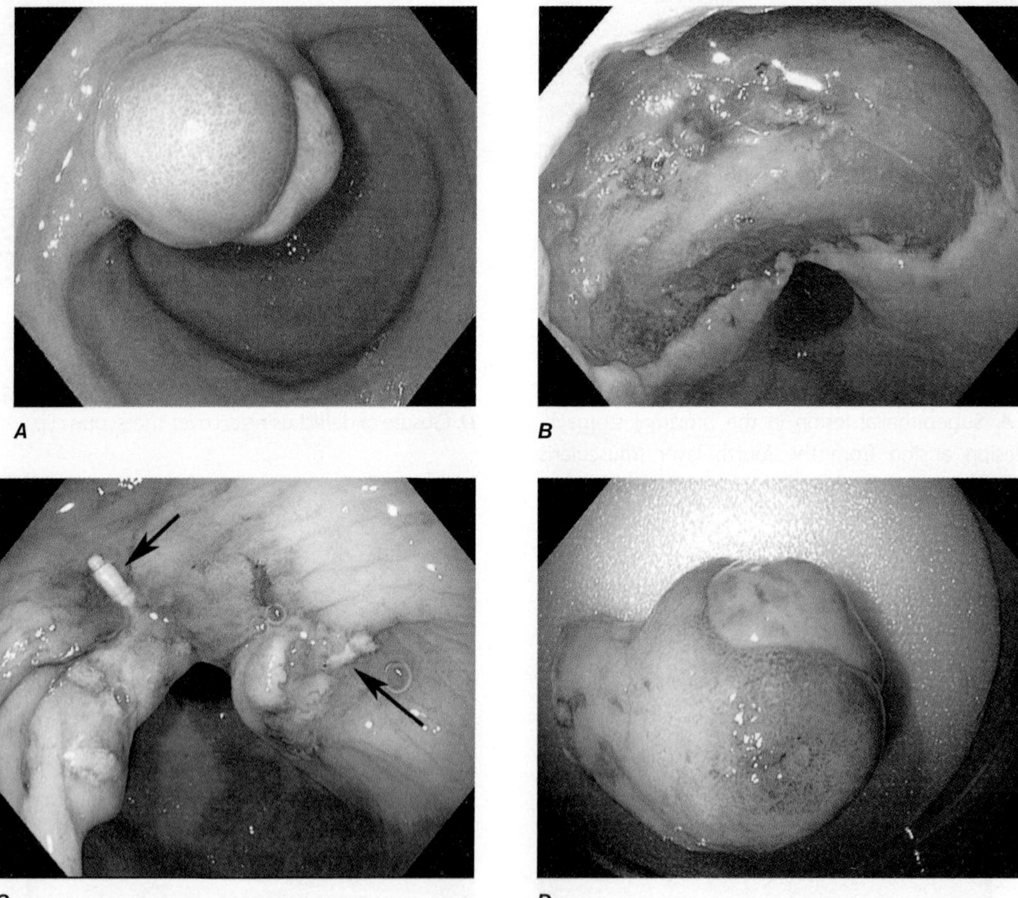

FIGURE 12-19
Closure of large defect using an endoscopic suturing device. ***A.*** Ulcerated inflammatory fibroid polyp in the antrum. ***B.*** Large defect following endoscopic submucosal dissection of the lesion. ***C.*** Closure of the defect using endoscopic sutures (*arrows*). ***D.*** Resected specimen.

have been used for many years to treat bleeding lesions, but the development of more robust over-the-scope clips has facilitated endoscopic closure of gastrointestinal fistulas and perforations not previously amenable to endoscopic therapy **(see Video 13-6)**. Endoscopic suturing is also feasible, and the technique can be used to close perforations and large defects (Fig. 12-19, **see Video 13-7**), anastomotic leaks, and fistulas. Other

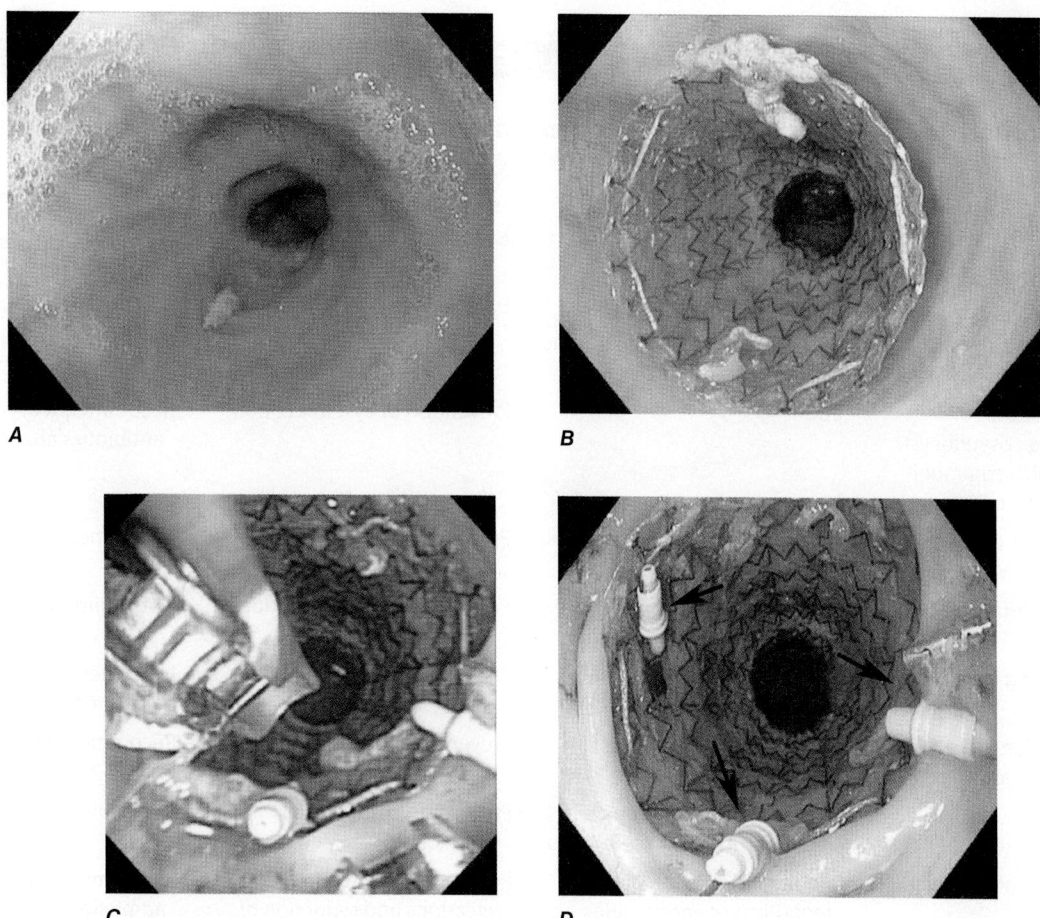

FIGURE 12-20
Prevention of stent migration using endoscopic sutures. ***A.*** Esophagogastric anastomotic stricture refractory to balloon dilation. ***B.*** Temporary placement of covered esophageal stent. ***C.*** Endoscopic suturing device to anchor stent to esophageal wall. ***D.*** Stent fixation with endoscopic sutures (*arrows*).

potential indications for endoscopic suturing include stent fixation to prevent its migration (Fig. 12-20), and endoscopic bariatric procedures. These technologies are likely to have an expanding role in patient care.

RISKS OF ENDOSCOPY

Medications used during conscious sedation may cause respiratory depression or allergic reactions. All endoscopic procedures carry some risk of bleeding and gastrointestinal perforation. The risk is small with diagnostic upper endoscopy and colonoscopy (<1:1000 procedures), but ranges from 0.5 to 5% when therapeutic procedures, such as EMR and ESD, control of hemorrhage, or stricture dilatation, are performed. Bleeding and perforation are rare adverse events with flexible sigmoidoscopy. The risk of adverse events for diagnostic EUS (without needle aspiration) is similar to that for diagnostic upper endoscopy.

Infectious complications are uncommon with most endoscopic procedures. Some procedures carry a higher incidence of postprocedure bacteremia, and prophylactic antibiotics may be indicated (Table 12-1). Management of antithrombotic agents prior to endoscopic procedures should take into account the procedural risk of hemorrhage, the agent, and the patient condition, as summarized in Table 12-2.

ERCP carries additional risks. Pancreatitis occurs in about 5% of patients undergoing the procedure and in up to 30% of patients with sphincter of Oddi dysfunction. Young anicteric patients with normal ducts are at increased risk. Post-ERCP pancreatitis is usually mild and self-limited, but may result in prolonged hospitalization, surgery, diabetes, or death when severe. Bleeding occurs in 1% of endoscopic sphincterotomies. Ascending cholangitis, pseudocyst infection, retroperitoneal perforation, and abscess formation may occur as a result of ERCP.

Percutaneous gastrostomy tube placement during EGD is associated with a 10–15% incidence of adverse events, most often wound infections. Fasciitis, pneumonia, bleeding, buried bumper syndrome, and colonic injury may result from gastrostomy tube placement.

TABLE 12-1

ANTIBIOTIC PROPHYLAXIS FOR ENDOSCOPIC PROCEDURES

PATIENT CONDITION	PROCEDURE CONTEMPLATED	GOAL OF PROPHYLAXIS	PERIPROCEDURAL ANTIBIOTIC PROPHYLAXIS
All cardiac conditions	Any endoscopic procedure	Prevention of infective endocarditis	Not indicated
Bile duct obstruction in the absence of cholangitis	ERCP with complete drainage	Prevention of cholangitis	Not recommended
Bile duct obstruction in absence of cholangitis	ERCP with anticipated incomplete drainage (e.g., sclerosing cholangitis, hilar strictures)	Prevention of cholangitis	Recommended; continue antibiotics after the procedure
Sterile pancreatic fluid collection (e.g., pseudocyst, necrosis), which communicates with pancreatic duct	ERCP	Prevention of cyst infection	Recommended; continue antibiotics after the procedure
Sterile pancreatic fluid collection	Transmural drainage	Prevention of cyst infection	Recommended
Solid lesion along upper GI tract	EUS-FNA	Prevention of local infection	Not recommended[a]
Solid lesion along lower GI tract	EUS-FNA	Prevention of local infection	Insufficient data to make firm recommendation[b]
Cystic lesions along GI tract (including mediastinum)	EUS-FNA	Prevention of cyst infection	Recommended
All patients	Percutaneous endoscopic feeding tube placement	Prevention of peristomal infection	Recommended
Cirrhosis with acute GI bleeding	Required for all such patients, regardless of endoscopic procedures	Prevention of infectious complications and reduction of mortality	Recommended, upon admission[c]
Synthetic vascular graft and other nonvalvular cardiovascular devices	Any endoscopic procedure	Prevention of graft and device infection	Not recommended[d]
Prosthetic joints	Any endoscopic procedure	Prevention of septic arthritis	Not recommended[e]

[a]Low rates of bacteremia and local infection.
[b]Endoscopists may choose on a case-by-case basis.
[c]Risk for bacterial infection associated with cirrhosis and GI bleeding is well established.
[d]No reported cases of infection associated with endoscopy.
[e]Very low risk of infection.
Abbreviations: ERCP, endoscopic retrograde cholangiopancreatography; EUS-FNA, endoscopic ultrasound–fine-needle aspiration; GI, gastrointestinal.
Source: Adapted from S Banerjee et al: *Gastrointest Endosc* 67:719, 2008; with permission from Elsevier.

TABLE 12-2

MANAGEMENT OF ANTITHROMBOTIC DRUGS BEFORE ENDOSCOPIC PROCEDURES

DRUG	BLEEDING RISK OF PROCEDURE	MANAGEMENT	INTERVAL BETWEEN LAST DOSE AND PROCEDURE	COMMENTS
Warfarin	Low[a]	Continue	N/A	Ensure that INR is not supratherapeutic
	High[b]	Discontinue	3–7 days (usually 5), INR should be ≤1.5 for procedure	Consider bridging therapy with heparin[c]
New oral anticoagulants (dabigatran, rivaroxaban, apixaban)	Low[a]	Continue	N/A	

(*continued*)

TABLE 12-2

MANAGEMENT OF ANTITHROMBOTIC DRUGS BEFORE ENDOSCOPIC PROCEDURES (*CONTINUED*)

DRUG	BLEEDING RISK OF PROCEDURE	MANAGEMENT	INTERVAL BETWEEN LAST DOSE AND PROCEDURE	COMMENTS
	High[b]	Discontinue	Varies from 1 to 5 days, depending on the drug and the patient's renal function	Bridging therapy generally unnecessary
Heparin	Low[a]	Continue	N/A	
	High[b]	Discontinue	4-6 h for unfractionated heparin	Skip one dose if using low-molecular-weight heparin
Aspirin	Any	Continue	N/A	Low-dose aspirin does not substantially increase the risk of endoscopic procedures
Aspirin with dipyridamole	Low[a]	Continue	N/A	
	High[b]	Discontinue	2–7 days	Consider continuing aspirin monotherapy
Thienopyridines	Low[a]	Continue	N/A	
	High[b]	Discontinue	5 days (clopidogrel or ticagrelor), 7 days (prasugrel), 10–14 days (ticlopidine)	Consider bridging therapy with aspirin

[a]Low-risk endoscopic procedures include esophagogastroduodenoscopy (EGD) or colonoscopy with or without biopsy, endoscopic ultrasound (EUS) without fine-needle aspiration (FNA), and endoscopic retrograde cholangiopancreatography (ERCP) with stent exchange.

[b]High-risk endoscopic procedures include EGD or colonoscopy with dilation, polypectomy, or thermal ablation; percutaneous endoscopic gastrostomy; EUS with FNA; and ERCP with sphincterotomy or pseudocyst drainage.

[c]Bridging therapy with heparin may be considered for patients discontinuing warfarin who are at high risk for thromboembolism, including those with mitral valve replacement or aortic valve replacement with other risk factors; those with nonvalvular atrial fibrillation with a history of stroke, embolic event, cardiac thrombus, or $CHADS_2$ score ≥4; and those with venous thromboembolism within the past 3 months or severe underlying thrombophilia.

Source: TH Baron et al: *N Engl J Med* 368:2113, 2013; MA Anderson et al: *Gastrointest Endosc* 70:1060, 2009; MJ Zuckerman et al: *Gastrointest Endosc* 61:189, 2005.

URGENT ENDOSCOPY

ACUTE GASTROINTESTINAL HEMORRHAGE

Endoscopy is an important diagnostic and therapeutic technique for patients with acute gastrointestinal hemorrhage. Although gastrointestinal bleeding stops spontaneously in most cases, some patients will have persistent or recurrent hemorrhage that may be life-threatening. Clinical predictors of rebleeding help identify patients most likely to benefit from urgent endoscopy and endoscopic, angiographic, or surgical hemostasis.

Initial evaluation

The initial evaluation of the bleeding patient focuses on the severity of hemorrhage as reflected by the postural vital signs, the frequency of hematemesis or melena, and (in some cases) findings on nasogastric lavage. Decreases in hematocrit and hemoglobin lag behind the clinical course and are not reliable gauges of the magnitude of acute bleeding. This initial evaluation, completed well before the bleeding source is confidently identified, guides immediate supportive care of the patient, triage to the ward or intensive care unit, and timing of endoscopy. The severity of the initial hemorrhage is the most important indication for urgent endoscopy, since a large initial bleed increases the likelihood of ongoing or recurrent bleeding. Patients with resting hypotension or orthostatic change in vital signs, repeated hematemesis, or bloody nasogastric aspirate that does not clear with large-volume lavage, or those requiring blood transfusions, should be considered for urgent endoscopy. In addition, patients with cirrhosis, coagulopathy, or respiratory or renal failure and those over 70 years of age are more likely to have significant rebleeding.

Bedside evaluation also suggests an upper or lower gastrointestinal source of bleeding in most patients. Over 90% of patients with melena are bleeding proximal to the ligament of Treitz, and about 85% of patients with hematochezia are bleeding from the colon. Melena can result from bleeding in the small bowel or right colon, especially in older patients with slow colonic transit. Conversely, some patients with massive hematochezia may be bleeding from an upper gastrointestinal source, such as a gastric Dieulafoy lesion or duodenal ulcer, with rapid intestinal transit. Early upper endoscopy should be considered in such patients.

Endoscopy should be performed after the patient has been resuscitated with intravenous fluids and transfusions, as necessary. Marked coagulopathy or thrombocytopenia is usually treated before endoscopy, since correction of these abnormalities may lead to resolution of bleeding, and techniques for endoscopic hemostasis are limited in such patients. Metabolic derangements should also be addressed. Tracheal intubation for airway protection should be considered before upper endoscopy in patients with repeated recent hematemesis, encephalopathy, and suspected variceal hemorrhage.

Most patients with significant hematochezia can undergo colonoscopy after a rapid colonic purge with a polyethylene glycol solution; the preparation fluid may be administered via a nasogastric tube. Colonoscopy has a higher diagnostic yield than radionuclide bleeding scans or angiography in lower gastrointestinal bleeding, and endoscopic therapy can be applied in some cases. In a minority of cases, endoscopic assessment is hindered by poor visualization due to persistent vigorous bleeding with recurrent hemodynamic instability, and other techniques (such as angiography or emergent subtotal colectomy) must be employed. In such patients, massive bleeding originating from an upper gastrointestinal source should also be considered and excluded by upper endoscopy. The anal and rectal mucosa should be visualized endoscopically early in the course of massive rectal bleeding, because bleeding lesions in or close to the anal canal may be identified that are amenable to endoscopic or surgical transanal hemostatic techniques.

Peptic ulcer

The endoscopic appearance of peptic ulcers provides useful prognostic information and guides the need for endoscopic therapy in patients with acute hemorrhage (Fig. 12-21). A clean-based ulcer is associated with a low risk (3–5%) of rebleeding; patients with melena and a clean-based ulcer are often discharged home from the

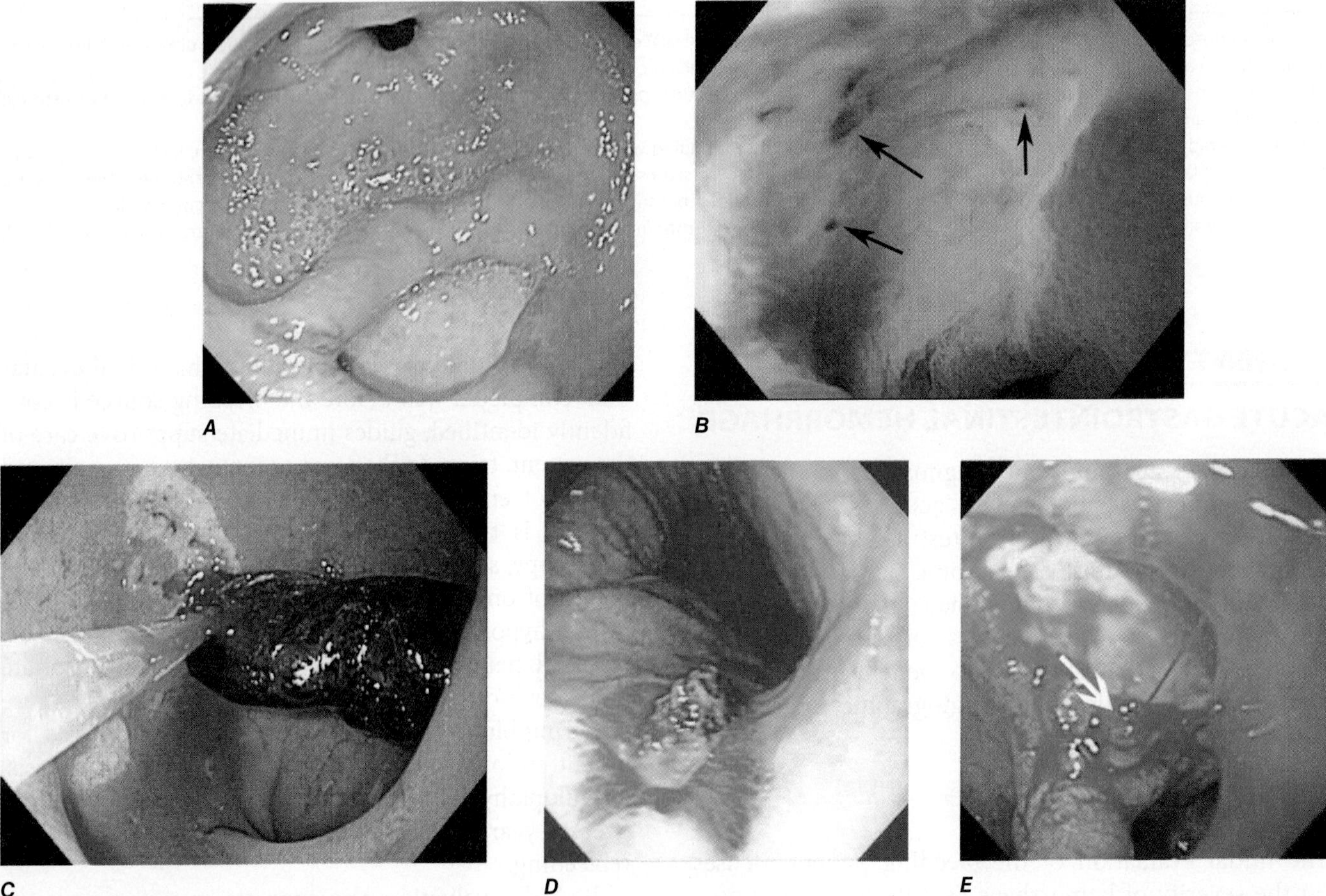

FIGURE 12-21

Stigmata of hemorrhage in peptic ulcers. ***A.*** Gastric antral ulcer with a clean base. ***B.*** Duodenal ulcer with flat pigmented spots (*arrows*). ***C.*** Duodenal ulcer with a dense adherent clot. ***D.*** Gastric ulcer with a pigmented protuberance/visible vessel. ***E.*** Duodenal ulcer with active spurting (*arrow*).

emergency room or endoscopy suite if they are young, reliable, and otherwise healthy. Flat pigmented spots and adherent clots covering the ulcer base have a 10% and 20% risk of rebleeding, respectively. Endoscopic therapy is often considered for an ulcer with an adherent clot. When a fibrin plug is seen protruding from a vessel wall in the base of an ulcer (so-called sentinel clot or visible vessel), the risk of rebleeding from the ulcer is 40%. This finding generally leads to endoscopic therapy to decrease the rebleeding rate. Occasionally, active spurting from an ulcer is seen, with >90% risk of ongoing bleeding without therapy.

Endoscopic therapy of ulcers with high-risk stigmata typically lowers the rebleeding rate to 5–10%. Several hemostatic techniques are available, including injection of epinephrine or a sclerosant into and around the vessel, "coaptive coagulation" of the vessel in the base of the ulcer using a thermal probe that is pressed against the site of bleeding, placement of hemoclips (Fig. 12-22), or a combination of these modalities **(see Video 13-8)**. In conjunction with endoscopic therapy, the administration of a proton pump inhibitor decreases the risk of rebleeding and improves patient outcome.

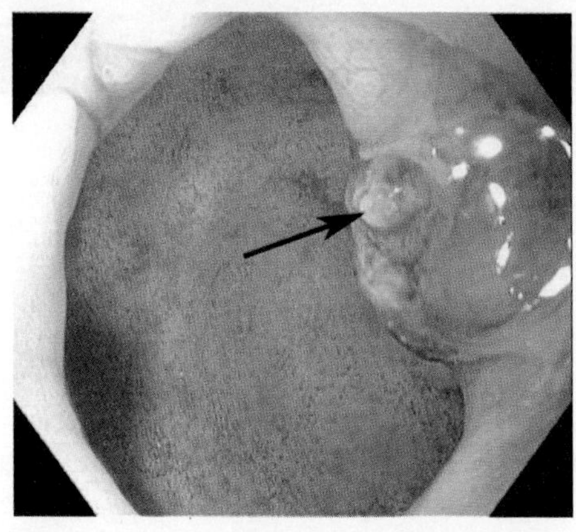

A

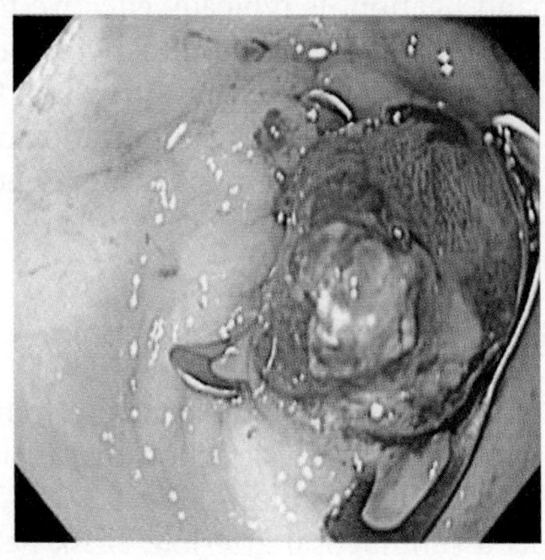

B

FIGURE 12-22

Endoscopic hemostasis of ulcer bleeding. ***A.*** Pyloric channel ulcer with visible vessel (*arrow*). ***B.*** Ulcer hemostasis with placement of an over-the-scope clip.

Varices

Two complementary strategies guide therapy of bleeding varices: local treatment of the bleeding varices and treatment of the underlying portal hypertension. Local therapies, including endoscopic variceal band ligation, endoscopic variceal sclerotherapy, and balloon tamponade with a Sengstaken-Blakemore tube, effectively control acute hemorrhage in most patients, although therapies that decrease portal pressure (pharmacologic treatment, surgical shunts, or radiologically placed intrahepatic portosystemic shunts) also play an important role.

Endoscopic variceal ligation (EVL) is indicated for the prevention of a first bleed (primary prophylaxis) from large esophageal varices, particularly in patients in whom beta blockers are contraindicated or not tolerated. EVL is also the preferred endoscopic therapy for control of active esophageal variceal bleeding and for subsequent eradication of esophageal varices (secondary prophylaxis). During EVL, a varix is suctioned into a cap fitted on the end of the endoscope, and a rubber band is released from the cap, ligating the varix (Fig. 12-24, **see Video 13-9**). EVL controls acute hemorrhage in up to 90% of patients. Complications of EVL, such as postbanding ulcer bleeding and esophageal stenosis, are uncommon. Endoscopic variceal sclerotherapy (EVS) involves the injection of a sclerosing, thrombogenic solution into or next to esophageal varices. EVS also controls acute hemorrhage in most patients, but it is generally used as salvage therapy when band ligation fails because of its higher complication rate compared to EVL. These techniques are used when varices are actively bleeding during endoscopy or (more commonly) when varices are the only identifiable cause of acute hemorrhage. Bleeding from large gastric fundic

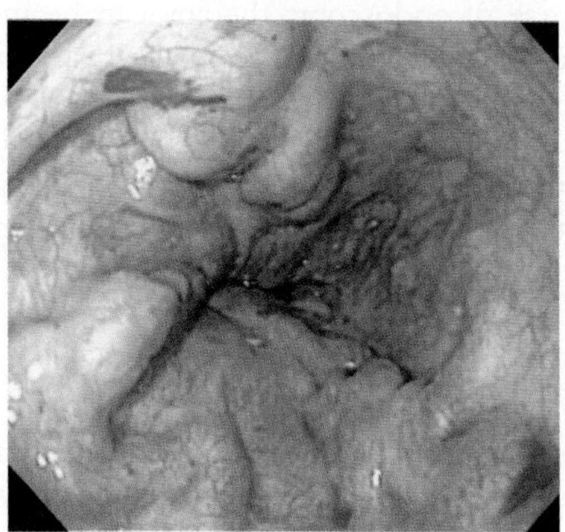

FIGURE 12-23

Esophageal varices.

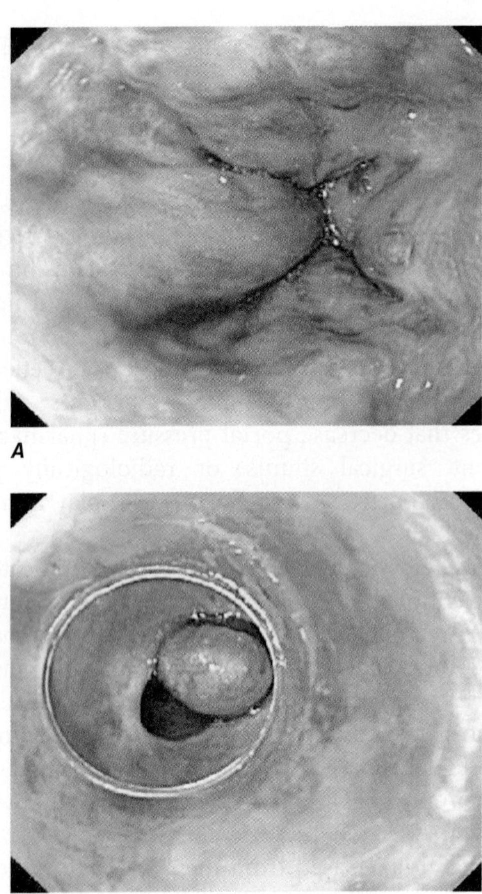

FIGURE 12-24
Endoscopic band ligation of esophageal varices. *A.* Large esophageal varices with stigmata of recent bleeding. ***B.*** Band ligation of varices.

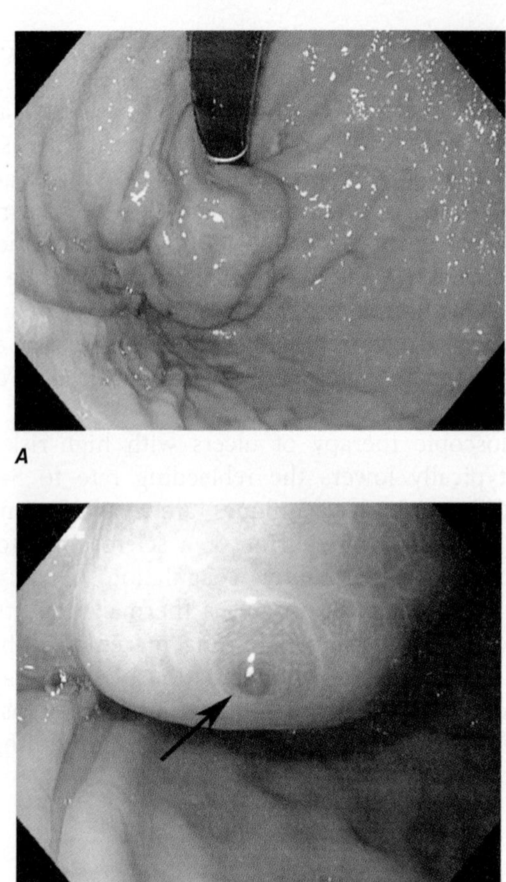

FIGURE 12-25
Gastric varices. *A.* Large gastric fundal varices. ***B.*** Stigmata of recent bleeding from the same gastric varices (*arrow*).

varices (Fig. 12-25) is best treated with endoscopic cyanoacrylate ("glue") injection **(see Video 13-10)**, because EVL or EVS of these varices is associated with a high rebleeding rate. Complications of cyanoacrylate injection include infection and glue embolization to other organs, such as the lungs, brain, and spleen.

After treatment of the acute hemorrhage, an elective course of endoscopic therapy can be undertaken with the goal of eradicating esophageal varices and preventing rebleeding months to years later. However, this chronic therapy is less successful, preventing long-term rebleeding in ~50% of patients. Pharmacologic therapies that decrease portal pressure have similar efficacy, and the two modalities may be combined.

Dieulafoy's lesion

This lesion, also called *persistent caliber artery*, is a large-caliber arteriole that runs immediately beneath the gastrointestinal mucosa and bleeds through a pinpoint mucosal erosion (Fig. 12-26). Dieulafoy's lesion is seen most commonly on the lesser curvature of the proximal stomach, causes impressive arterial hemorrhage, and may be difficult to diagnose; it is often recognized only after repeated endoscopy for recurrent bleeding. Endoscopic therapy, such as thermal coagulation or band ligation, is typically effective for control of bleeding and ablation of the underlying vessel once the lesion has been identified **(see Video 13-11)**. Rescue therapies, such as angiographic embolization or surgical oversewing, are considered in situations where endoscopic therapy has failed.

Mallory-Weiss tear

A Mallory-Weiss tear is a linear mucosal rent near or across the gastroesophageal junction that is often associated with retching or vomiting (Fig. 12-27). When the tear disrupts a submucosal arteriole, brisk hemorrhage may result. Endoscopy is the best method of diagnosis, and an actively bleeding tear can be treated endoscopically with epinephrine injection, coaptive coagulation, band ligation, or hemoclips **(see Video 13-12)**. Unlike peptic ulcer, a Mallory-Weiss tear with a nonbleeding

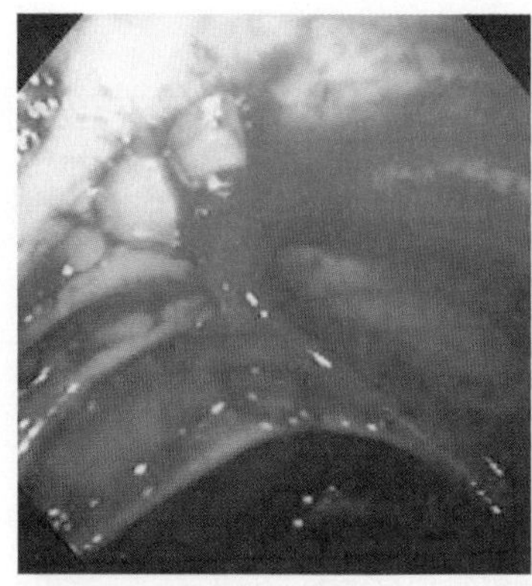

A

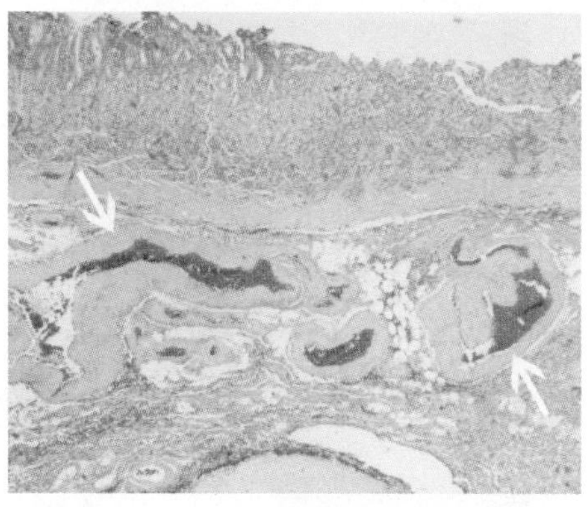

B

FIGURE 12-26
Dieulafoy's lesion. *A.* Actively spurting jejunal Dieulafoy's lesion. There is no underlying mucosal lesion. ***B.*** Histology of a gastric Dieulafoy's lesion. A persistent caliber artery (*arrows*) is present in the gastric submucosa, immediately beneath the mucosa.

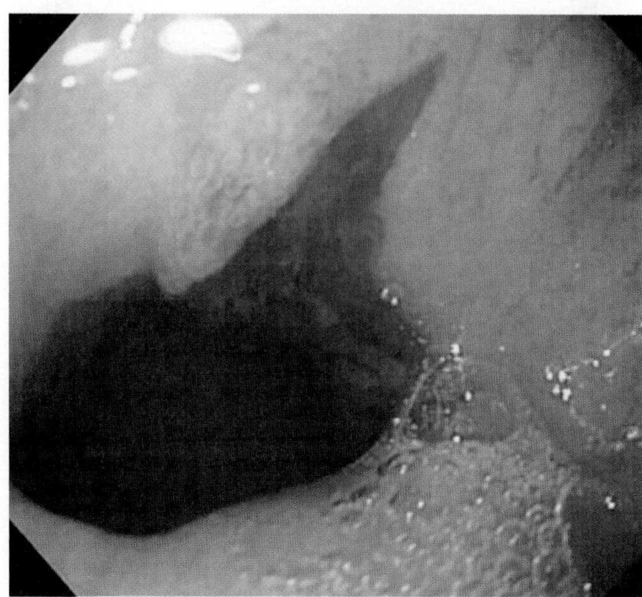

FIGURE 12-27
Mallory-Weiss tear at the gastroesophageal junction.

sentinel clot in its base rarely rebleeds and thus does not necessitate endoscopic therapy.

Vascular ectasias

Vascular ectasias are flat mucosal vascular anomalies that are best diagnosed by endoscopy. They usually cause slow intestinal blood loss and occur either in a sporadic fashion or in a well-defined pattern of distribution (e.g., gastric antral vascular ectasia [GAVE] or "watermelon stomach") (Fig. 12-28). Cecal vascular ectasias, GAVE, and radiation-induced rectal ectasias are often responsive to local endoscopic ablative therapy, such as argon plasma coagulation **(see Video 13-13)**. Patients with diffuse small-bowel vascular ectasias (associated with chronic renal failure and with hereditary hemorrhagic telangiectasia) may continue to bleed despite endoscopic treatment of easily accessible lesions by conventional endoscopy. These patients may benefit from deep enteroscopy with endoscopic therapy, pharmacologic treatment with octreotide or estrogen/progesterone therapy, or intraoperative enteroscopy.

Colonic diverticula

Diverticula form where nutrient arteries penetrate the muscular wall of the colon en route to the colonic

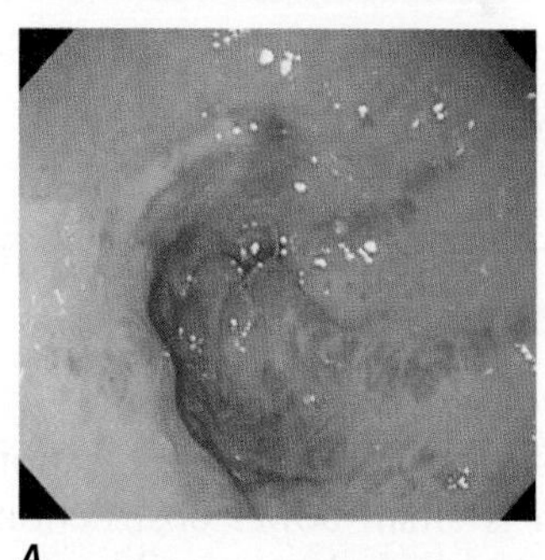

A

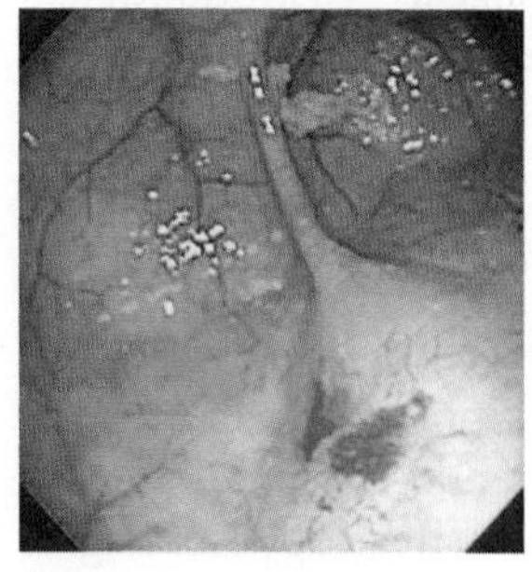

B

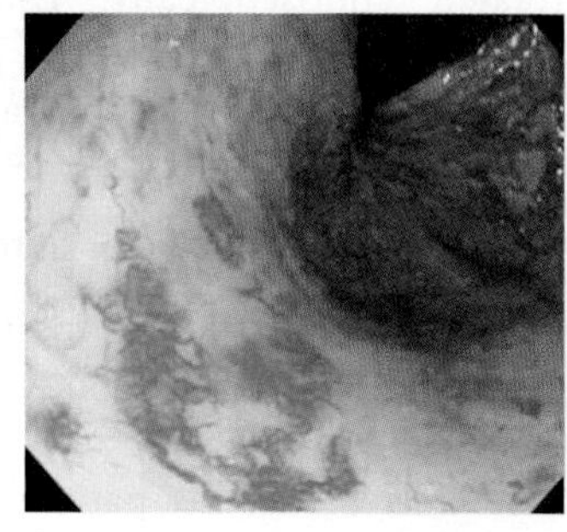

C

FIGURE 12-28
Gastrointestinal vascular ectasias. *A.* Gastric antral vascular ectasia ("watermelon stomach") characterized by stripes of prominent flat or raised vascular ectasias. ***B.*** Cecal vascular ectasias. ***C.*** Radiation-induced vascular ectasias of the rectum in a patient previously treated for prostate cancer.

mucosa (Fig. 12-29). The artery found in the base of a diverticulum may bleed, causing painless and impressive hematochezia. Colonoscopy is indicated in patients with hematochezia and suspected diverticular hemorrhage, because other causes of bleeding (such as vascular ectasias, colitis, and colon cancer) must be excluded. In addition, an actively bleeding diverticulum may be seen and treated during colonoscopy (Fig. 12-30, **see Video 13-14**).

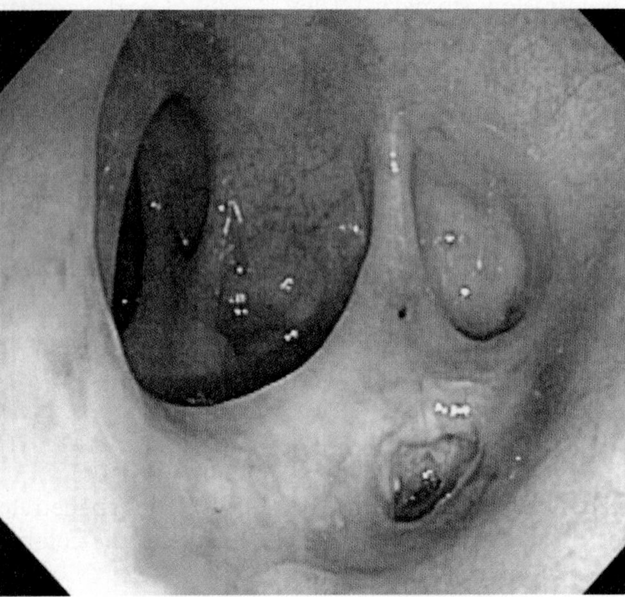

FIGURE 12-29
Colonic diverticula.

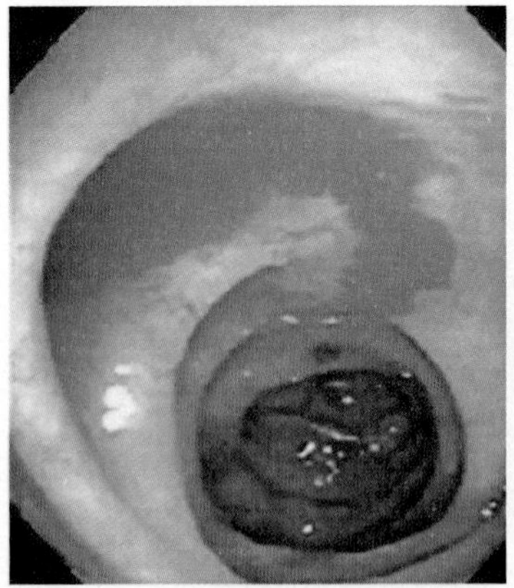

A

B

FIGURE 12-30
Diverticular hemorrhage. ***A.*** Actively bleeding sigmoid diverticulum. ***B.*** Hemostasis achieved using endoscopic clips.

GASTROINTESTINAL OBSTRUCTION AND PSEUDOOBSTRUCTION

Endoscopy is useful for evaluation and treatment of some forms of gastrointestinal obstruction. An important exception is small-bowel obstruction due to surgical adhesions, which is generally not diagnosed or treated endoscopically. Esophageal, gastroduodenal, and colonic obstruction or pseudoobstruction can all be diagnosed and often managed endoscopically.

Acute esophageal obstruction

Esophageal obstruction by impacted food (Fig. 12-31) or an ingested foreign body is a potentially life-threatening event and represents an endoscopic emergency. Left untreated, the patient may develop esophageal ulceration, ischemia, and perforation. Patients with persistent esophageal obstruction often have hypersalivation and are usually unable to swallow water; endoscopy is generally the best initial test in such patients, because endoscopic removal of the obstructing material is usually possible, and the presence of an underlying esophageal pathology can often be determined.

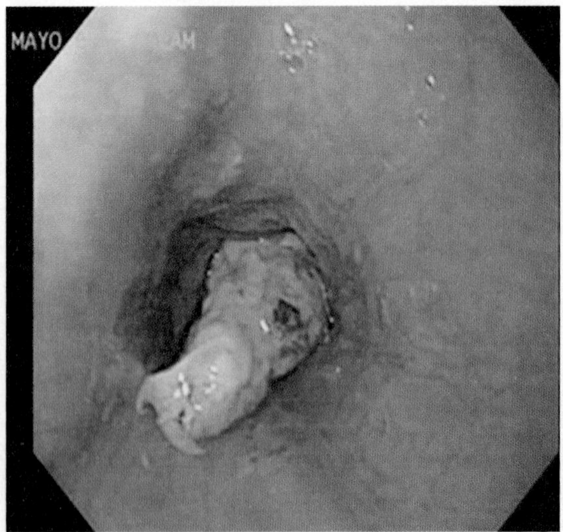

FIGURE 12-31
Esophageal food (meat) impaction.

Radiographs of the chest and neck should be considered before endoscopy in patients with fever, obstruction for ≥24 h, or ingestion of a sharp object, such as a fishbone. Radiographic contrast studies interfere with subsequent endoscopy and are not advisable in most patients with a clinical picture of esophageal obstruction. Sips of a carbonated beverage, sublingual nifedipine or nitrates, or intravenous glucagon may resolve an esophageal food impaction, but in most patients, an underlying web, ring, or stricture is present and endoscopic removal of the obstructing food bolus is necessary.

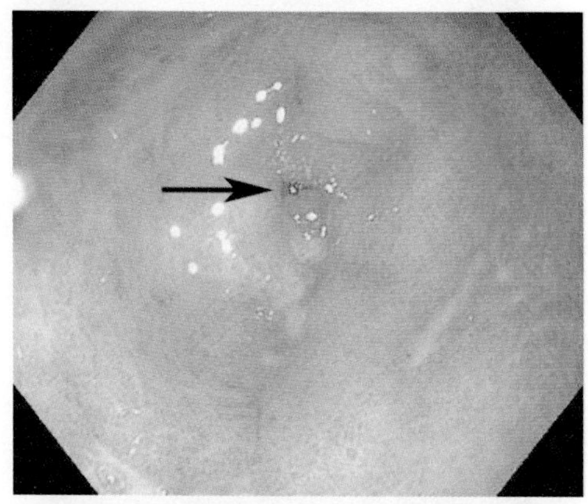

A

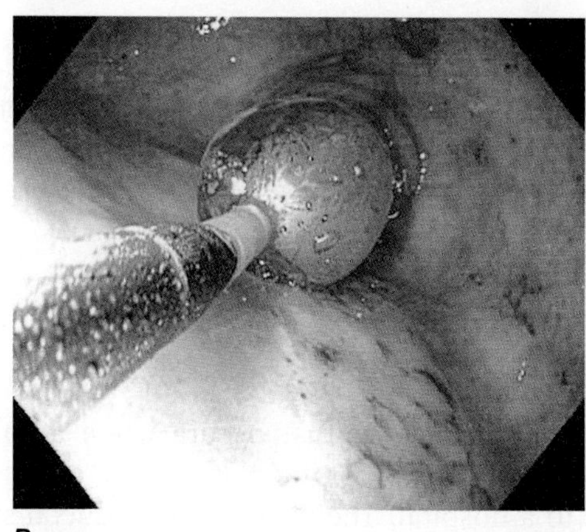

B

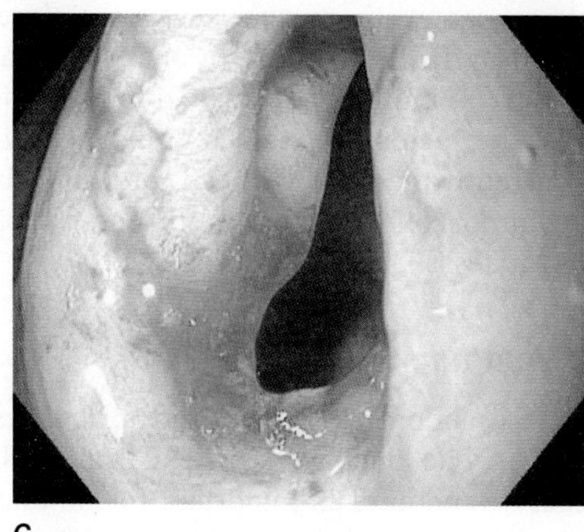

C

FIGURE 12-32

Gastric outlet obstruction due to pyloric stenosis. *A.* Sequela of nonsteroidal anti-inflammatory drug (NSAID)–induced ulcer disease with severe stenosis of the pylorus (*arrow*). ***B.*** Balloon dilation of the stenosis. ***C.*** Appearance of pyloric ring after dilation.

Gastric outlet obstruction

Obstruction of the gastric outlet is commonly caused by gastric, duodenal, or pancreatic malignancy or chronic peptic ulceration with stenosis of the pylorus (Fig. 12-32). Patients vomit partially digested food many hours after eating. Gastric decompression with a nasogastric tube and subsequent lavage for removal of retained material is the first step in treatment. The diagnosis can then be confirmed with a saline load test, if desired. Endoscopy is useful for diagnosis and treatment. Patients with benign pyloric stenosis may be treated with endoscopic balloon dilatation of the pylorus, and a course of endoscopic dilatation results in long-term relief of symptoms in about 50% of patients. Malignant gastric outlet obstruction can be relieved with endoscopically placed expandable stents in patients with inoperable malignancy (Fig. 12-33).

Colonic obstruction and pseudoobstruction

These both present with abdominal distention and discomfort; tympany; and a dilated, air-filled colon on plain abdominal radiography. The radiographic appearance can be characteristic of a particular condition, such as

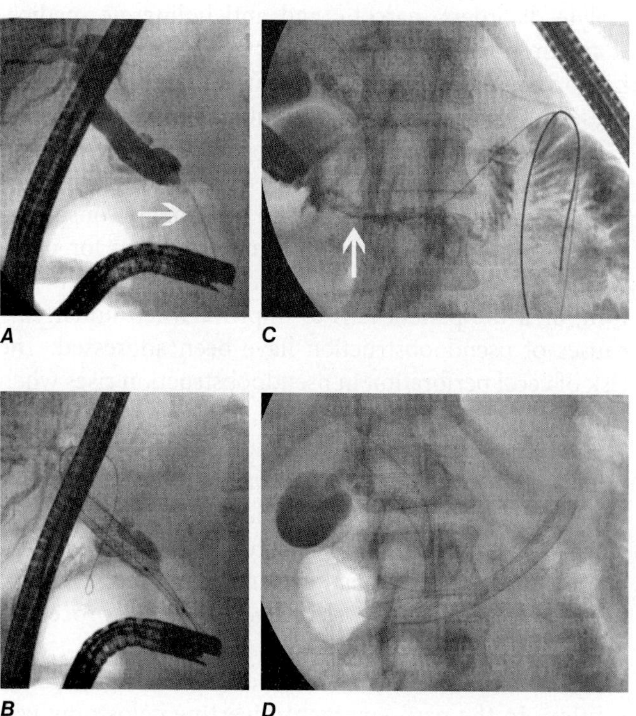

FIGURE 12-33

Biliary and duodenal self-expanding metal stents (SEMS) for obstruction caused by pancreatic cancer. *A.* Endoscopic retrograde cholangiopancreatography (ERCP) demonstrates a distal-bile duct stricture (*arrow*). ***B.*** A biliary SEMS is placed. ***C.*** Contrast injection demonstrates a duodenal stricture (*arrow*). ***D.*** Biliary and duodenal SEMS in place.

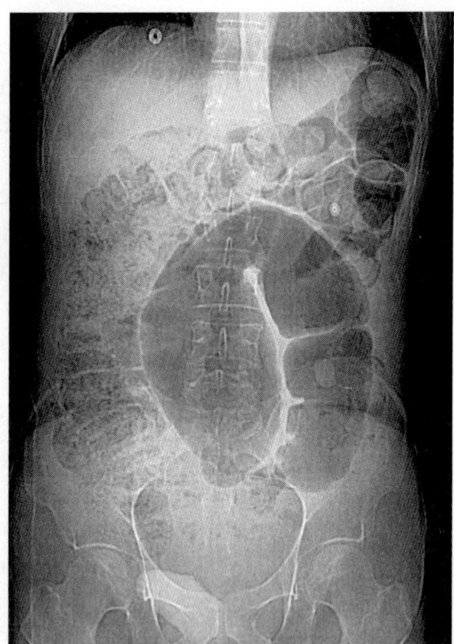

FIGURE 12-34
Sigmoid volvulus with the characteristic radiologic appearance of a "bent inner tube."

sigmoid volvulus (Fig. 12-34). Both structural obstruction and pseudoobstruction may lead to colonic perforation if left untreated. Acute colonic pseudoobstruction is a form of colonic ileus that is usually attributable to electrolyte disorders, narcotic and anticholinergic medications, immobility (as after surgery), and retroperitoneal hemorrhage or mass. Multiple causative factors are often present. Colonoscopy, water-soluble contrast enema, or CT may be used to assess for an obstructing lesion and differentiate obstruction from pseudoobstruction. One of these diagnostic studies should be strongly considered if the patient does not have clear risk factors for pseudoobstruction, if radiographs do not show air in the rectum, or if the patient fails to improve when underlying causes of pseudoobstruction have been addressed. The risk of cecal perforation in pseudoobstruction rises when the cecal diameter exceeds 12 cm, and decompression of the colon may be achieved using intravenous neostigmine or via colonoscopic decompression (Fig. 12-35). Most patients should receive a trial of conservative therapy (with correction of electrolyte disorders, removal of offending medications, and increased mobilization) before undergoing an invasive decompressive procedure for colonic pseudoobstruction.

Colonic obstruction is an indication for urgent intervention. In the past, emergent diverting colostomy was usually performed with a subsequent second operation after bowel preparation to treat the underlying cause of obstruction. Colonoscopic placement of an expandable stent is now a widely used alternative that can relieve malignant colonic obstruction without emergency surgery and permit bowel preparation for an elective one-stage operation (Fig. 12-36, **see Video 13-15**).

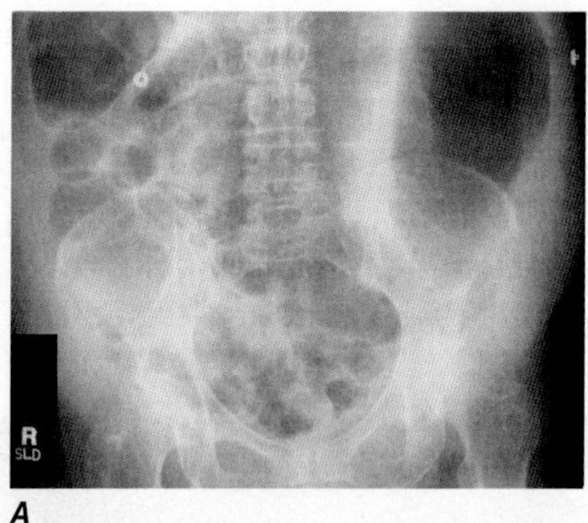

A

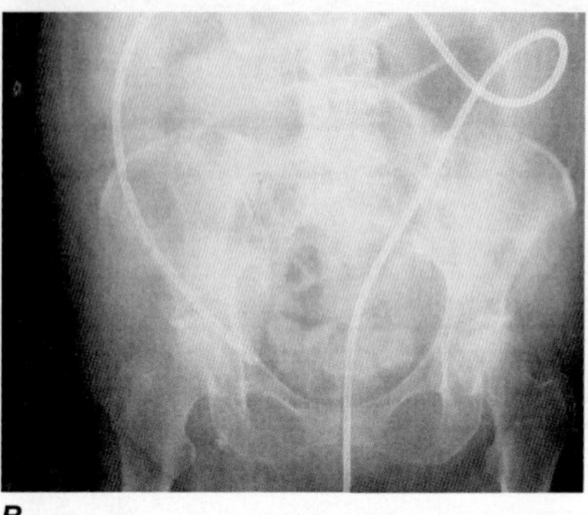

B

FIGURE 12-35
Acute colonic pseudoobstruction. ***A.*** Acute colonic dilatation occurring in a patient soon after knee surgery. ***B.*** Colonoscopic placement of decompression tube with marked improvement in colonic dilatation.

ACUTE BILIARY OBSTRUCTION

The steady, severe pain that occurs when a gallstone acutely obstructs the common bile duct often brings patients to a hospital. The diagnosis of a ductal stone is suspected when the patient is jaundiced or when serum liver tests or pancreatic enzyme levels are elevated; it is confirmed by EUS, magnetic resonance cholangiography (MRCP), or direct cholangiography (performed endoscopically, percutaneously, or during surgery). ERCP is currently the primary means of diagnosing and treating common bile duct stones in most hospitals in the United States (Figs. 345-11 and 345-12).

Bile duct imaging

Whereas transabdominal ultrasound diagnoses only a minority of bile duct stones, MRCP and EUS are >90% accurate and have an important role in diagnosis. Examples of these modalities are shown in Fig. 12-37.

If the suspicion for a bile duct stone is high and urgent treatment is required (as in a patient with obstructive jaundice and biliary sepsis), ERCP is the procedure of choice, because it remains the gold standard for diagnosis and allows for immediate treatment (**see Video 13-16**). If a persistent bile duct stone is

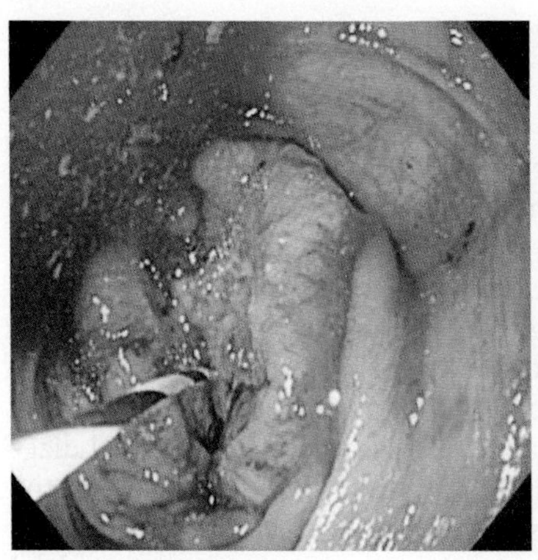

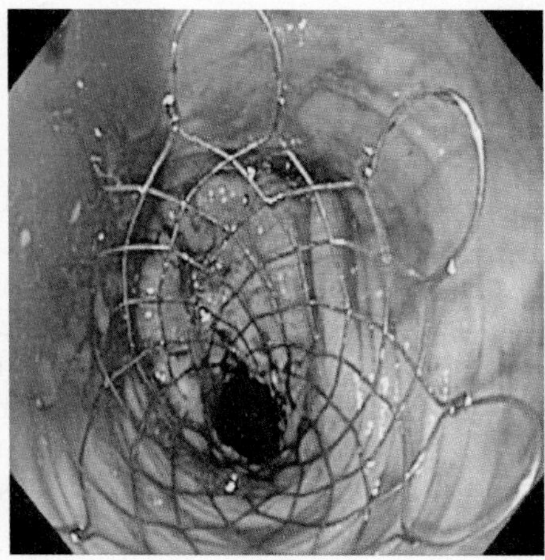

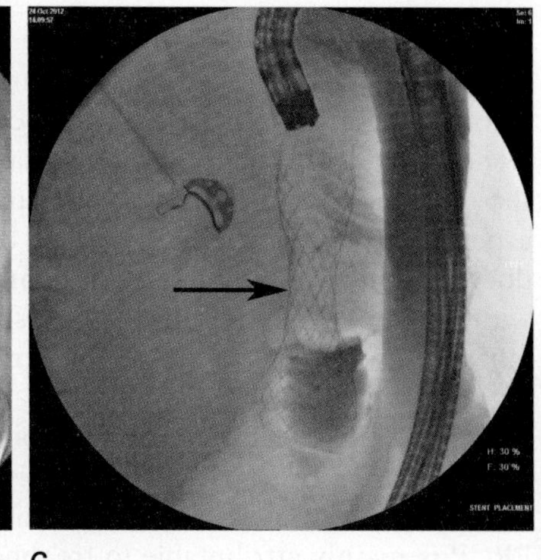

A B C

FIGURE 12-36

Obstructing colonic carcinoma. *A.* Colonic adenocarcinoma causing marked luminal narrowing of the distal transverse colon. ***B.*** Endoscopic placement of a self-expandable metal stent. ***C.*** Radiograph of expanded stent across the obstructing tumor with a residual waist (*arrow*).

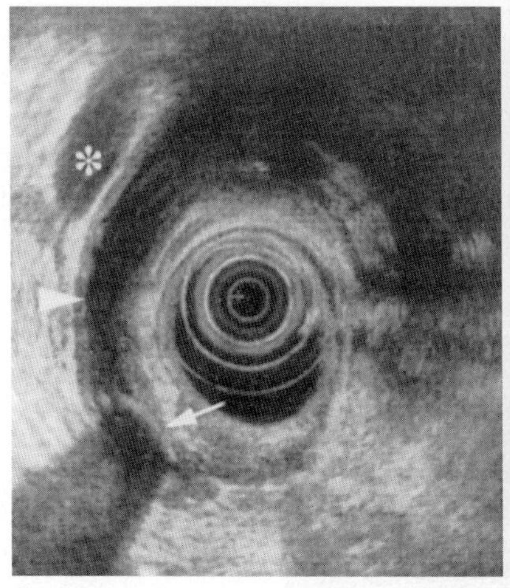

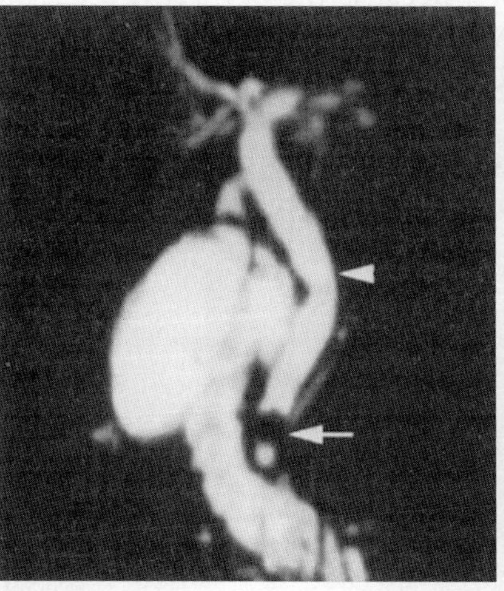

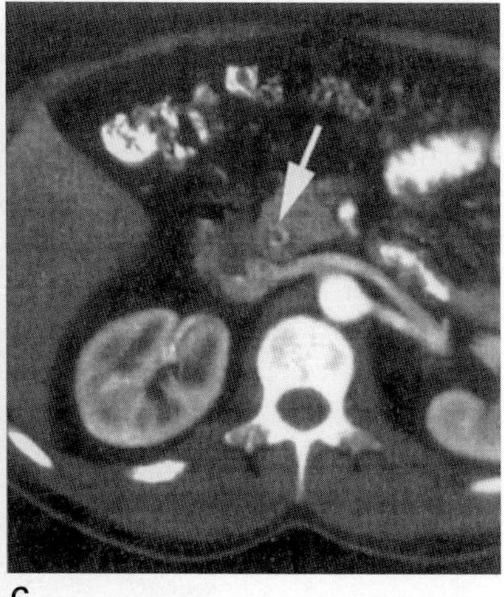

A B C

FIGURE 12-37

Methods of bile duct imaging. *Arrows* mark bile duct stones. *Arrowheads* indicate the common bile duct, and the *asterisk* marks the portal vein. ***A.*** Endoscopic ultrasound (EUS). ***B.*** Magnetic resonance cholangiopancreatography (MRCP). ***C.*** Helical computed tomography (CT).

relatively unlikely (as in a patient with gallstone pancreatitis), ERCP may be supplanted by less invasive imaging techniques, such as EUS, MRCP, or intraoperative cholangiography performed during cholecystectomy, sparing patients the risk and discomfort of ERCP.

Ascending cholangitis

Charcot's triad of jaundice, abdominal pain, and fever is present in about 70% of patients with ascending cholangitis and biliary sepsis. These patients are managed initially with fluid resuscitation and intravenous antibiotics. Abdominal ultrasound is often performed to assess for gallbladder stones and bile duct dilation. However, the bile duct may not be dilated early in the course of acute biliary obstruction. Medical management usually improves the patient's clinical status, providing a window of approximately 24 h during which biliary drainage should be established, typically by ERCP. Undue delay can result in recrudescence of overt sepsis and increased morbidity and mortality rates. In addition to Charcot's triad, the additional presence of shock and confusion (Reynolds's pentad) is associated with high mortality rate and should prompt urgent intervention to restore biliary drainage.

Gallstone pancreatitis

Gallstones may cause acute pancreatitis as they pass through the ampulla of Vater. The occurrence of gallstone pancreatitis usually implies passage of a stone into the duodenum, and only about 20% of patients harbor a persistent stone in the ampulla or the common bile duct. Retained stones are more common in patients with jaundice, rising serum liver tests following hospitalization, severe pancreatitis, or superimposed ascending cholangitis.

Urgent ERCP decreases the morbidity rate of gallstone pancreatitis in a subset of patients with retained bile duct stones. It is unclear whether the benefit of ERCP is mainly attributable to treatment and prevention of ascending cholangitis or to relief of pancreatic ductal obstruction. ERCP is warranted early in the course of gallstone pancreatitis if ascending cholangitis is suspected, especially in a jaundiced patient. Urgent ERCP may also benefit patients predicted to have severe pancreatitis using a clinical index of severity, such as the Glasgow or Ranson score. Because the benefit of ERCP is limited to patients with a retained bile duct stone, a strategy of initial MRCP or EUS for diagnosis decreases the utilization of ERCP in gallstone pancreatitis and improves clinical outcomes by limiting the occurrence of ERCP-related adverse events.

ELECTIVE ENDOSCOPY

DYSPEPSIA

Dyspepsia is a chronic or recurrent burning discomfort or pain in the upper abdomen that may be caused by diverse processes such as gastroesophageal reflux, peptic ulcer disease, and "nonulcer dyspepsia," a heterogeneous category that includes disorders of motility, sensation, and somatization. Gastric and esophageal malignancies are less common causes of dyspepsia. Careful history-taking allows accurate differential diagnosis of dyspepsia in only about half of patients. In the remainder, endoscopy can be a useful diagnostic tool, especially in patients whose symptoms are not resolved by an empirical trial of symptomatic treatment. Endoscopy should be performed at the outset in patients with dyspepsia and alarm features, such as weight loss or iron-deficiency anemia.

GASTROESOPHAGEAL REFLUX DISEASE (GERD)

When classic symptoms of gastroesophageal reflux are present, such as water brash and substernal heartburn, presumptive diagnosis and empirical treatment are often sufficient. Endoscopy is a sensitive test for diagnosis of esophagitis (Fig. 12-38), but will

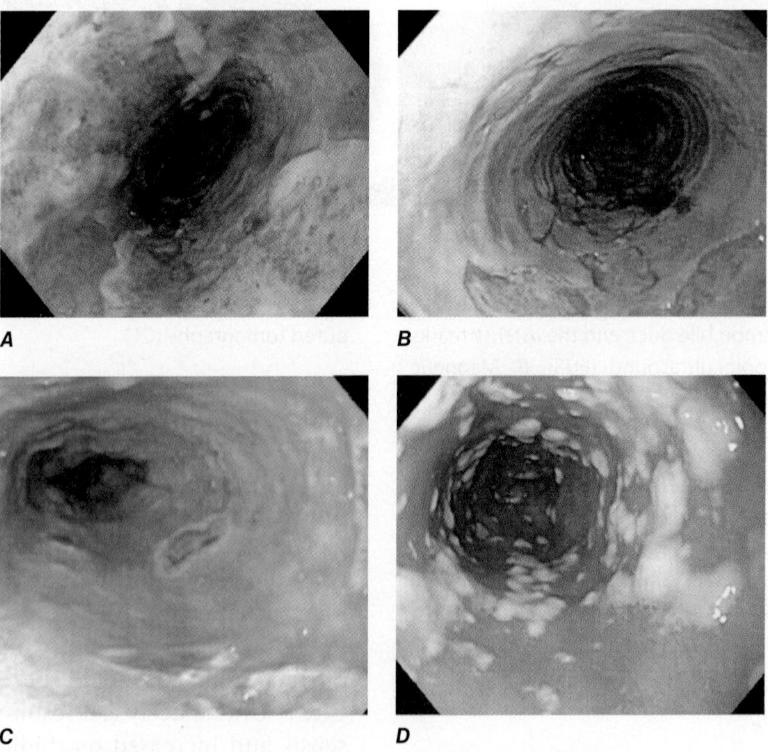

FIGURE 12-38
Causes of esophagitis. ***A.*** Severe reflux esophagitis with mucosal ulceration and friability. ***B.*** Cytomegalovirus esophagitis. ***C.*** Herpes simplex virus esophagitis with target-type shallow ulcerations. ***D.*** *Candida* esophagitis with white plaques adherent to the esophageal mucosa.

miss nonerosive reflux disease (NERD) because some patients have symptomatic reflux without esophagitis. The most sensitive test for diagnosis of GERD is 24-h ambulatory pH monitoring. Endoscopy is indicated in patients with reflux symptoms refractory to antisecretory therapy; in those with alarm symptoms, such as dysphagia, weight loss, or gastrointestinal bleeding; and in those with recurrent dyspepsia after treatment that is not clearly due to reflux on clinical grounds alone. Endoscopy should be considered in patients with long-standing (≥10 years) GERD, because they have a sixfold increased risk of harboring Barrett's esophagus compared to a patient with <1 year of reflux symptoms. Patients with Barrett's esophagus (Fig. 12-3) generally undergo a surveillance program of periodic endoscopy with biopsies to detect dysplasia or early carcinoma.

Barrett's esophagus

Barrett's esophagus is specialized columnar metaplasia that replaces the normal squamous mucosa of the distal esophagus in some persons with GERD. Barrett's epithelium is a major risk factor for adenocarcinoma of the esophagus and is readily detected endoscopically, due to proximal displacement of the squamocolumnar junction (Fig. 12-3). A screening EGD for Barrett's esophagus should be considered in patients with a chronic (≥10 year) history of GERD symptoms. Endoscopic biopsy is the gold standard for confirmation of Barrett's esophagus and for dysplasia or cancer arising in Barrett's mucosa.

PEPTIC ULCER

Peptic ulcer classically causes epigastric gnawing or burning, often occurring nocturnally and promptly relieved by food or antacids. Although endoscopy is the most sensitive diagnostic test for peptic ulcer, it is not a cost-effective strategy in young patients with ulcer-like dyspeptic symptoms unless endoscopy is available at low cost. Patients with suspected peptic ulcer should be evaluated for *Helicobacter pylori* infection. Serology (past or present infection), urea breath testing (current infection), and stool tests are noninvasive and less costly than endoscopy with biopsy. Patients with alarm symptoms and those with persistent symptoms despite treatment should undergo endoscopy to exclude gastric malignancy and other etiologies.

NONULCER DYSPEPSIA

Nonulcer dyspepsia may be associated with bloating and, unlike peptic ulcer, tends not to remit and recur. Most patients describe marginal relief on acid-reducing, prokinetic, or anti-*Helicobacter* therapy, and are referred for endoscopy to exclude a refractory ulcer and assess for other causes. Although endoscopy is useful for excluding other diagnoses, its impact on the treatment of patients with nonulcer dyspepsia is limited.

DYSPHAGIA

About 50% of patients presenting with difficulty swallowing have a mechanical obstruction; the remainder has a motility disorder, such as achalasia or diffuse esophageal spasm. Careful history-taking often points to a presumptive diagnosis and leads to the appropriate use of diagnostic tests. Esophageal strictures (Fig. 12-39) typically cause progressive dysphagia, first for solids, then for liquids; motility disorders often cause intermittent dysphagia for both solids and liquids. Some underlying disorders have characteristic historic features: Schatzki's ring (Fig. 12-40) causes episodic dysphagia for solids, typically at the beginning of a meal; oropharyngeal motor disorders typically present with difficulty initiating deglutition (*transfer dysphagia*) and nasal reflux or coughing with swallowing; and achalasia may cause nocturnal regurgitation of undigested food.

When mechanical obstruction is suspected, endoscopy is a useful initial diagnostic test, because it permits immediate biopsy and/or dilatation of strictures, masses, or rings. The presence of linear furrows and multiple corrugated rings throughout a narrowed esophagus (*feline esophagus*) should raise suspicion for eosinophilic esophagitis, an increasingly recognized cause for recurrent dysphagia and food impaction

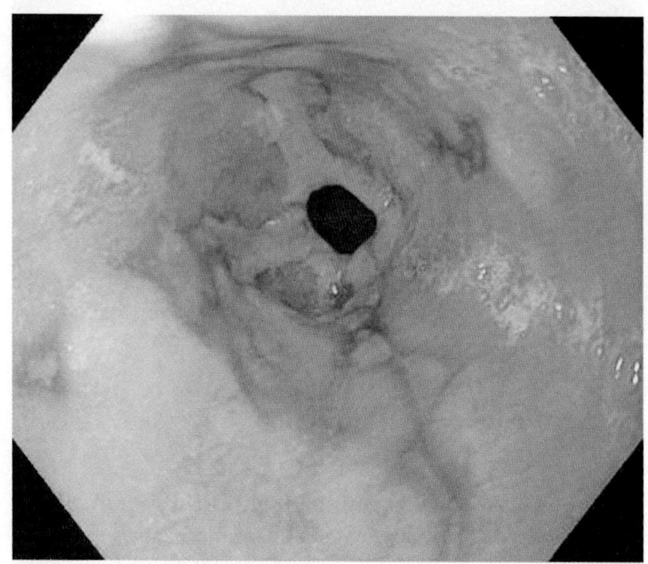

FIGURE 12-39
Peptic esophageal stricture associated with esophagitis.

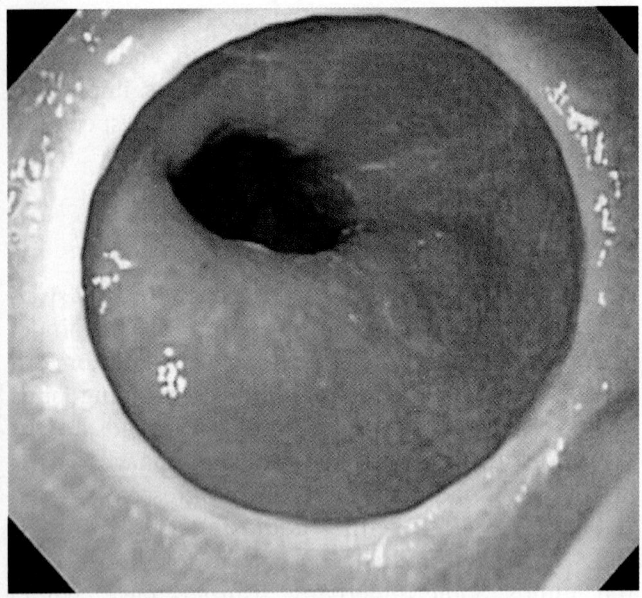

FIGURE 12-40
Schatzki's ring at the gastroesophageal junction.

(Fig. 12-41). Blind or forceful passage of an endoscope may lead to perforation in a patient with stenosis of the cervical esophagus or a Zenker's diverticulum, but gentle passage of an endoscope under direct visual guidance is reasonably safe. Endoscopy can miss a subtle stricture or ring in some patients.

When transfer dysphagia is evident or an esophageal motility disorder is suspected, esophageal radiography and/or a video-swallow study are the best initial diagnostic tests. The oropharyngeal swallowing mechanism, esophageal peristalsis, and the lower esophageal sphincter can all be assessed. In some disorders, subsequent esophageal manometry may also be important for diagnosis.

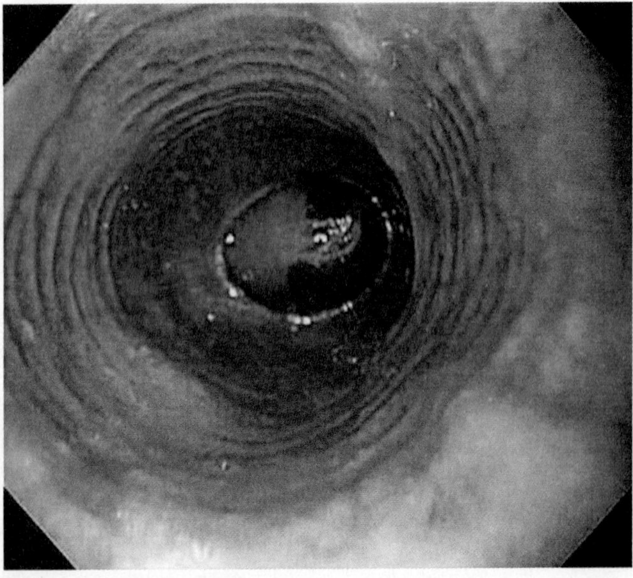

FIGURE 12-41
Eosinophilic esophagitis with multiple circular rings of the esophagus creating a corrugated appearance, and an impacted grape at the narrowed esophagogastric junction. The diagnosis requires biopsy with histologic finding of > 15–20 eosinophils per high-power field.

TREATMENT OF MALIGNANCIES

Endoscopy plays an important role in the treatment of gastrointestinal malignancies. Early-stage malignancies limited to the superficial layers of the gastrointestinal mucosa may be resected using the techniques of endoscopic mucosal resection (EMR) **(see Video 13-4)** or endoscopic submucosal dissection (ESD) **(see Video 13-5)**. Photodynamic therapy (PDT) and radiofrequency ablation (RFA) are effective modalities for ablative treatment of high-grade dysplasia and intramucosal cancer in Barrett's esophagus. Gastrointestinal stromal tumors can be removed en bloc by endoscopic full-thickness resection **(see Video 13-3)**. In general, endoscopic techniques offer the advantage of a minimally invasive approach to treatment, but rely on other imaging techniques (such as CT, magnetic resonance imaging [MRI], positron emission tomography [PET], and EUS) to exclude distant metastases or locally advanced disease better treated by surgery or other modalities. The decision to treat an early-stage gastrointestinal malignancy endoscopically is often made in collaboration with a surgeon and/or oncologist.

Endoscopic palliation of gastrointestinal malignancies relieves symptoms and in many cases prolongs survival. Malignant obstruction can be relieved by endoscopic stent placement **(see Video 13-15)**, and malignant gastrointestinal bleeding can often be palliated endoscopically as well. EUS-guided celiac plexus neurolysis may relieve pancreatic cancer pain.

ANEMIA AND OCCULT BLOOD IN THE STOOL

Iron-deficiency anemia may be attributed to poor iron absorption (as in celiac sprue) or, more commonly, chronic blood loss. Intestinal bleeding should be strongly suspected in men and postmenopausal women with iron-deficiency anemia, and colonoscopy is indicated in such patients, even in the absence of detectable occult blood in the stool. Approximately 30% will have large colonic polyps, 10% will have colorectal cancer, and a few additional patients will have colonic vascular lesions. When a convincing source of blood loss is not found in the colon, upper gastrointestinal endoscopy should be considered; if no lesion is found, duodenal biopsies should be obtained to exclude sprue

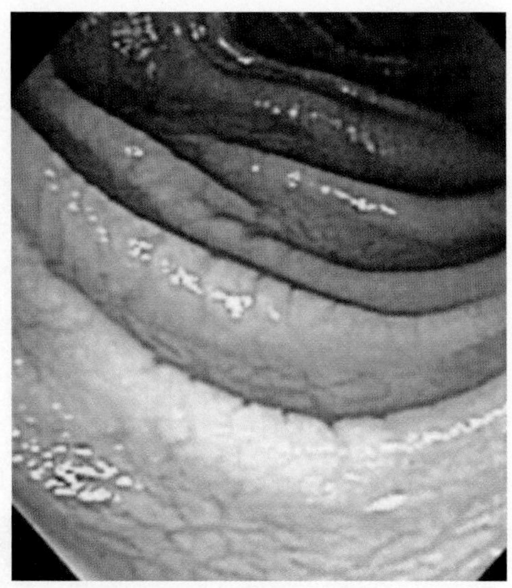

FIGURE 12-42
Scalloped duodenal folds in a patient with celiac sprue.

(Fig. 12-42). Small-bowel evaluation with capsule endoscopy (Fig. 12-43), CT or magnetic resonance (MR) enterography, or balloon-assisted enteroscopy may be appropriate if both EGD and colonoscopy are unrevealing.

Tests for occult blood in the stool detect hemoglobin or the heme moiety and are most sensitive for colonic blood loss, although they will also detect larger amounts of upper gastrointestinal bleeding. Patients over age 50 with occult blood in normal-appearing stool should undergo colonoscopy to diagnose or exclude colorectal neoplasia. The diagnostic yield is lower than in iron-deficiency anemia. Whether upper endoscopy is also indicated depends on the patient's symptoms.

The small intestine may be the source of chronic intestinal bleeding, especially if colonoscopy and upper endoscopy are not diagnostic. The utility of small-bowel evaluation varies with the clinical setting and is most important in patients in whom bleeding causes chronic or recurrent anemia. In contrast to the low diagnostic yield of small-bowel radiography, positive findings on capsule endoscopy are seen in 50–70% of patients with suspected small intestinal bleeding. The most common finding is mucosal vascular ectasias. CT or MR enterography accurately detects small-bowel masses and inflammation and is also useful for initial small-bowel evaluation. Deep enteroscopy may follow capsule endoscopy for biopsy of lesions or to provide specific therapy, such as argon plasma coagulation of vascular ectasias (Fig. 12-44).

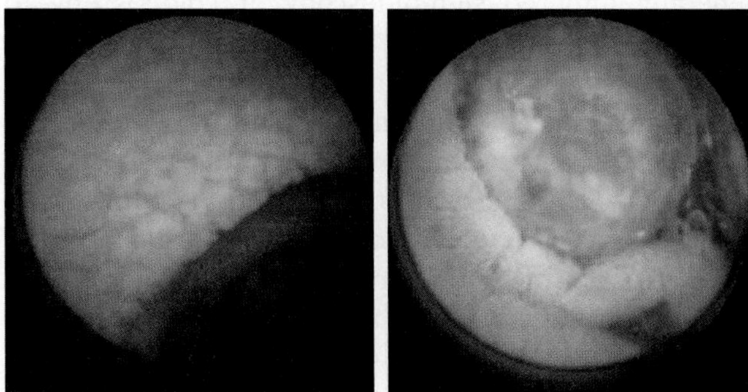

FIGURE 12-43
Capsule endoscopy images of a mildly scalloped jejunal fold (*left*) and an ileal tumor (*right*) in a patient with celiac sprue. *(Images courtesy of Dr. Elizabeth Rajan; with permission.)*

COLORECTAL CANCER SCREENING

The majority of colon cancers develop from preexisting colonic adenomas, and colorectal cancer can be largely prevented by the detection and removal of adenomatous polyps **(see Video 13-17)**. The choice of screening strategy for an asymptomatic person depends on personal and family history. Individuals with inflammatory bowel disease, a history of colorectal polyps or cancer, family members with adenomatous polyps or cancer, or certain familial cancer syndromes (Fig. 12-45) are at increased risk for colorectal cancer. An individual without these factors is generally considered at average risk.

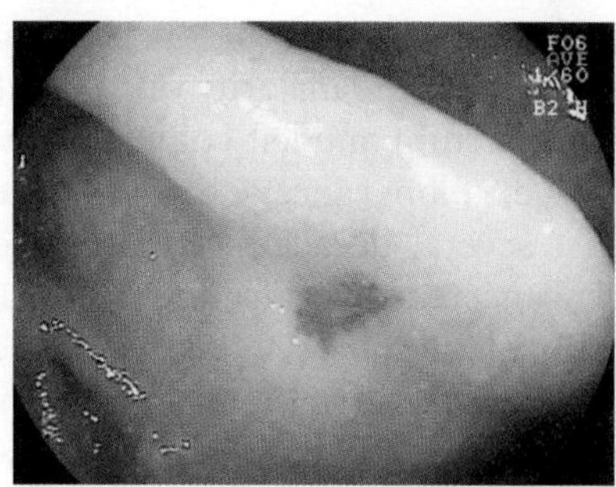

A

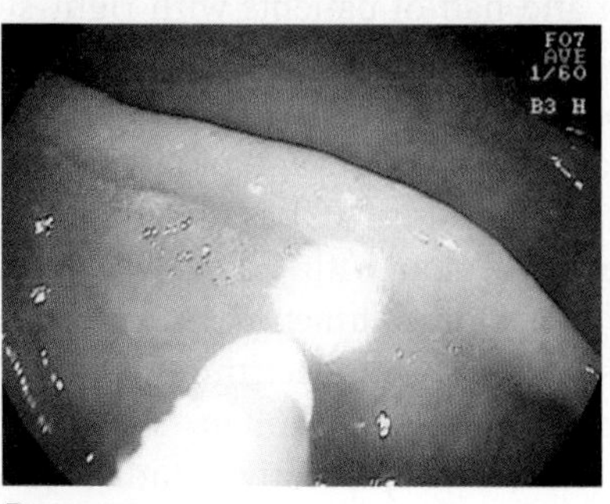

B

FIGURE 12-44
A. Mid-jejunal vascular ectasia identified by double-balloon endoscopy. ***B.*** Ablation of vascular ectasia with argon plasma coagulation.

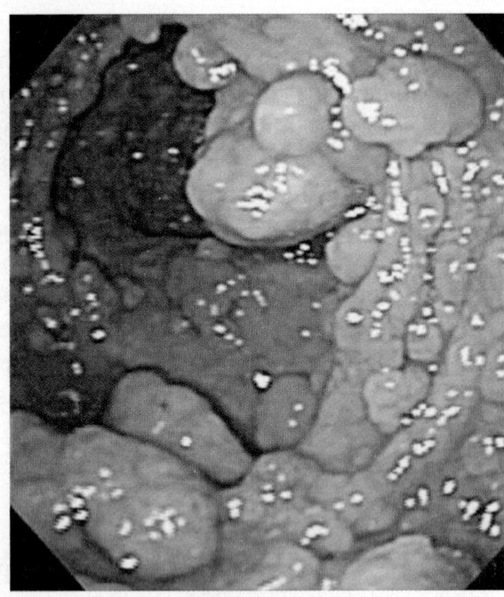

FIGURE 12-45
Innumerable colon polyps of various sizes in a patient with familial adenomatous polyposis syndrome.

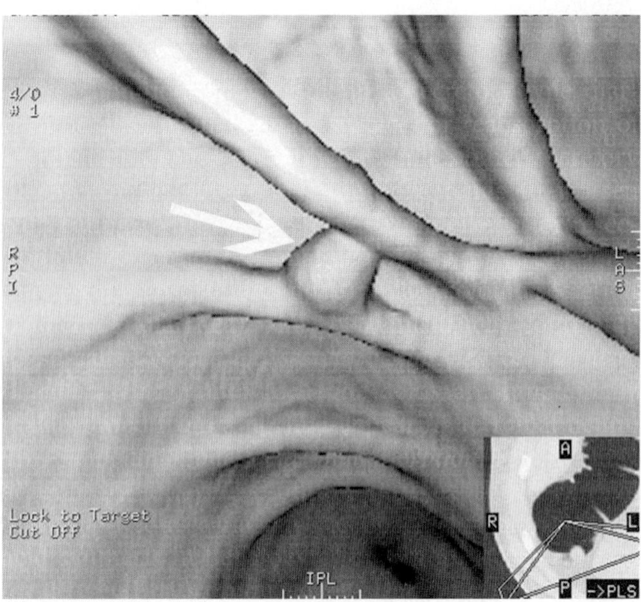

FIGURE 12-46
Virtual colonoscopy image of a colon polyp *(arrow). (Image courtesy of Dr. Jeff Fidler; with permission.)*

Screening strategies are summarized in Table 12-3. Although stool tests for occult blood have been shown to decrease mortality rate from colorectal cancer, they do not detect some cancers and many polyps, and direct visualization of the colon is a more effective screening strategy. Either sigmoidoscopy or colonoscopy may be used for cancer screening in asymptomatic average-risk individuals. The use of sigmoidoscopy was based on the historical finding that the majority of colorectal cancers occurred in the rectum and left colon and that patients with right-sided colon cancers had left-sided polyps. Over the past several decades, however, the distribution of colon cancers has changed in the United States, with proportionally fewer rectal and left-sided cancers than in the past. Large American studies of colonoscopy for screening of average-risk individuals show that cancers are roughly equally distributed between left and right colon and half of patients with right-sided lesions have no polyps in the left colon. Visualization of the entire colon thus appears to be the optimal strategy for colorectal cancer screening and prevention.

Virtual colonoscopy (VC) is a radiologic technique that images the colon with CT following rectal insufflation of the colonic lumen. Computer rendering of CT images generates an electronic display of a virtual "flight" along the colonic lumen, simulating colonoscopy (Fig. 12-46). Comparative studies of virtual and routine colonoscopy have shown conflicting results, but technical refinements have improved the performance characteristics of VC. The use of VC for colorectal cancer screening may become more widespread in the future, particularly at institutions with demonstrated skill with this technique. Findings detected during virtual colonoscopy often require subsequent conventional colonoscopy for confirmation and treatment.

DIARRHEA

Most cases of diarrhea are acute, self-limited, and due to infections or medication. Chronic diarrhea (lasting >6 weeks) is more often due to a primary inflammatory, malabsorptive, or motility disorder; is less likely to resolve spontaneously; and generally requires diagnostic evaluation. Patients with chronic diarrhea or severe, unexplained acute diarrhea often undergo endoscopy if stool tests for pathogens are unrevealing. The choice of endoscopic testing depends on the clinical setting.

Patients with colonic symptoms and findings such as bloody diarrhea, tenesmus, fever, or leukocytes in stool generally undergo sigmoidoscopy or colonoscopy to assess for colitis (Fig. 12-4). Sigmoidoscopy is an appropriate initial test in most patients. Conversely, patients with symptoms and findings suggesting small-bowel disease, such as large-volume watery stools, substantial weight loss, and malabsorption of iron, calcium, or fat, may undergo upper endoscopy with duodenal aspirates for assessment of bacterial overgrowth and biopsies for assessment of mucosal diseases, such as celiac sprue.

Many patients with chronic diarrhea do not fit either of these patterns. In the setting of a long-standing history of alternating constipation and diarrhea dating to early adulthood, without findings such as blood in the stool or anemia, a diagnosis of irritable bowel syndrome may be made without direct visualization of the bowel.

TABLE 12-3

COLORECTAL CANCER SCREENING STRATEGIES

	CHOICES/RECOMMENDATIONS	COMMENTS
Average-Risk Patients		
Asymptomatic individuals ≥50 years of age (≥45 years of age for African Americans)	Colonoscopy every 10 years[a]	Preferred cancer prevention strategy
	Annual fecal immunochemical test (FIT) or fecal occult blood test (FOBT), multiple take-home specimen cards	Cancer detection strategy; fails to detect most polyps; colonoscopy if results are positive
	Computed tomography (CT) colonography every 5 years	Colonoscopy if results are positive
	Flexible sigmoidoscopy every 5 years	Fails to detect proximal colon polyps and cancers
	Double-contrast barium enema every 5 years	Less sensitive than colonoscopy or CT colonography; misses some cancers and polyps
Personal History of Polyps or Colorectal Cancer		
1 or 2 small (<1 cm) adenomas with low-grade dysplasia	Repeat colonoscopy in 5–10 years	Assuming complete polyp resection; interval may vary based on prior history, family history
3 to 9 adenomas, or any high-risk adenoma[b]	Repeat colonoscopy in 3 years; subsequent colonoscopy based on findings	Assuming complete polyp resection
≥10 adenomas	Repeat colonoscopy in <3 years based on clinical judgment	Consider evaluation for FAP or HNPCC; see recommendations below
Piecemeal removal of a sessile polyp	Exam in 2–6 months to verify complete removal	
Small (<1 cm) hyperplastic polyps of sigmoid and rectum	Repeat colonoscopy in 10 years	Those with hyperplastic polyposis syndrome merit more frequent follow-up
Sessile serrated adenoma/polyp <10 mm, without dysplasia	Repeat colonoscopy in 5 years	
Sessile serrated adenoma/polyp ≥10 mm or with dysplasia, or ≥2 serrated polyps	Repeat colonoscopy in 3 years	Serrated polyposis syndrome merits more frequent follow-up
Incompletely removed serrated polyp ≥1 cm	Exam in 2–6 months to verify complete removal	
Colon cancer	Evaluate entire colon around the time of resection, then repeat colonoscopy in 1 year	Subsequent colonoscopy in 3 years if the 1-year exam is normal
Inflammatory Bowel Disease		
Long-standing (>8 years) ulcerative pancolitis or Crohn's colitis, or left-sided ulcerative colitis of >15 years in duration	Colonoscopy with biopsies every 1–3 years	
Family History of Polyps or Colorectal Cancer		
First-degree relatives with only small tubular adenomas	Same as average risk	
Single first-degree relative with CRC or advanced adenoma at age ≥60 years	Colonoscopy every 10 years starting at age 40	
Single first-degree relative with CRC or advanced adenoma at age <60 years, OR two first-degree relatives with CRC or advanced adenomas at any age	Colonoscopy every 5 years beginning at age 40 years or 10 years younger than age at diagnosis of the youngest affected relative, whichever is earlier	
FAP	Sigmoidoscopy or colonoscopy annually, beginning at age 10–12 years	Consider genetic counseling and testing
HNPCC	Colonoscopy every 2 years beginning at age 20–25 years (or 10 years younger than the youngest affected first-degree relative) until age 40, then annually thereafter	Consider histologic evaluation for microsatellite instability in tumor specimens of patients who meet Bethesda criteria; consider genetic counseling and testing

[a]Assumes good colonic preparation and complete exam to cecum.

[b]High-risk adenoma: any adenoma ≥1 cm in size or containing high-grade dysplasia or villous features.

Abbreviations: CRC, colorectal cancer; FAP, familial adenomatous polyposis; HNPCC, hereditary nonpolyposis colorectal cancer.

Source: Adapted from DA Lieberman et al: *Gastroenterology* 143:844, 2012; B Levin et al: *CA Cancer J Clin* 58:130, 2008; American Cancer Society Guidelines *(http://www.cancer.org/cancer/colonandrectumcancer/moreinformation/colonandrectumcancerearlydetection/colorectal-cancer-early-detection-acs-recommendations)*, accessed November 15, 2013.

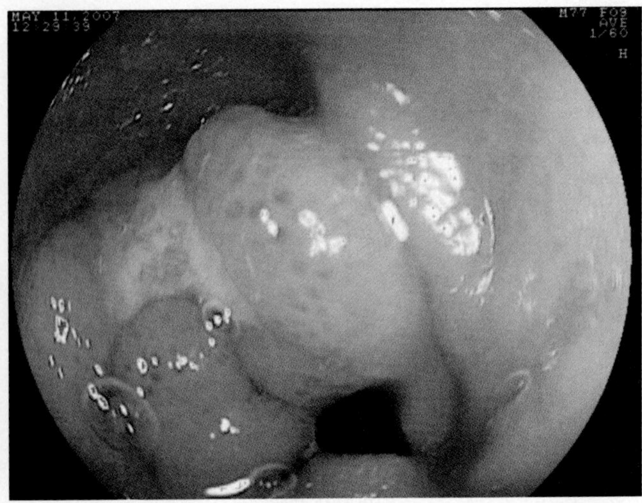

FIGURE 12-47
Ulcerated ileal carcinoid tumor.

Steatorrhea and upper abdominal pain may prompt evaluation of the pancreas rather than the gut. Patients whose chronic diarrhea is not easily categorized often undergo initial colonoscopy to examine the entire colon and terminal ileum for inflammatory or neoplastic disease (Fig. 12-47).

MINOR HEMATOCHEZIA

Bright red blood passed with or on formed brown stool usually has a rectal, anal, or distal sigmoid source (Fig. 12-48). Patients with even trivial amounts of hematochezia should be investigated with flexible sigmoidoscopy and anoscopy to exclude polyps or cancers in the distal colon. Patients reporting red blood on the toilet tissue only, without blood in the toilet or on the stool, are generally bleeding from a lesion in the anal canal. Careful external inspection, digital examination, and proctoscopy with anoscopy are sufficient for diagnosis in most cases.

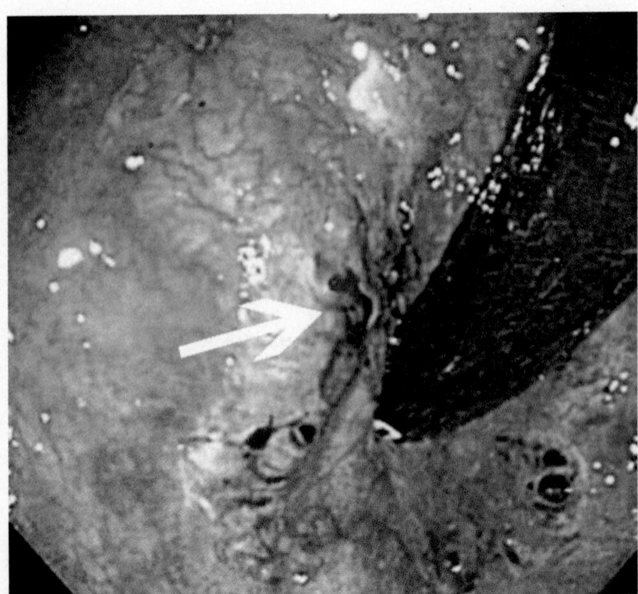

FIGURE 12-48
Internal hemorrhoids with bleeding (*arrow*) as seen on a retroflexed view of the rectum.

PANCREATITIS

About 20% of patients with pancreatitis have no identified cause after routine clinical investigation (including a review of medication and alcohol use, measurement of serum triglyceride and calcium levels, abdominal ultrasonography, and CT). Endoscopic assessment leads to a specific diagnosis in the majority of such patients, often altering clinical management. Endoscopic investigation is particularly appropriate if the patient has had more than one episode of pancreatitis.

Microlithiasis, or the presence of microscopic crystals in bile, is a leading cause of previously unexplained acute pancreatitis and is sometimes seen during abdominal ultrasonography as layering sludge or flecks of floating, echogenic material in the gallbladder. Gallbladder bile can be obtained for microscopic analysis by administering a cholecystokinin analogue during endoscopy, causing contraction of the gallbladder. Bile is suctioned from the duodenum as it drains from the papilla, and the darkest fraction is examined for cholesterol crystals or bilirubinate granules. The combination of EUS of the gallbladder and bile microscopy is probably the most sensitive means of diagnosing microlithiasis.

Previously undetected chronic pancreatitis, pancreatic malignancy, or pancreas divisum may be diagnosed by either ERCP or EUS. Sphincter of Oddi dysfunction or stenosis is a potential cause for pancreatitis and can be diagnosed by manometric studies performed during ERCP. Autoimmune pancreatitis may require EUS-guided pancreatic biopsy for histologic diagnosis.

Severe pancreatitis often results in pancreatic fluid collections. Both pseudocysts and areas of walled-off pancreatic necrosis can be drained into the stomach or duodenum endoscopically, using transpapillary and transmural endoscopic techniques. Pancreatic necrosis can be treated by direct endoscopic necrosectomy **(see Video 13-2)**.

CANCER STAGING

Local staging of esophageal, gastric, pancreatic, bile duct, and rectal cancers can be obtained with EUS (Fig. 12-15). EUS with fine-needle aspiration (Fig. 12-16) currently provides the most accurate preoperative assessment of local tumor and nodal staging, but it does not detect most distant metastases. Details of the local tumor stage can guide treatment decisions including resectability and need for neoadjuvant therapy. EUS with transesophageal needle biopsy may also be used to assess the presence of non-small-cell lung cancer in mediastinal nodes.

OPEN-ACCESS ENDOSCOPY

Direct scheduling of endoscopic procedures by primary care physicians without preceding gastroenterology consultation, or *open-access endoscopy*, is common. When the indications for endoscopy are clear-cut and appropriate, the procedural risks are low, and the patient understands what to expect, open-access endoscopy streamlines patient care and decreases costs.

Patients referred for open-access endoscopy should have a recent history, physical examination, and medication review. A copy of such an evaluation should be available when the patient comes to the endoscopy suite. Patients with unstable cardiovascular or respiratory conditions should not be referred directly for open-access endoscopy. Patients with particular conditions and undergoing certain procedures should be prescribed prophylactic antibiotics prior to endoscopy (Table 12-1). In addition, patients taking anticoagulants and/or antiplatelet drugs may require adjustment of these agents before endoscopy based on the procedure risk for bleeding and condition risk for a thromboembolic event (Table 12-2).

Common indications for open-access EGD include dyspepsia resistant to a trial of appropriate therapy; dysphagia; gastrointestinal bleeding; and persistent anorexia or early satiety. Open-access colonoscopy is often requested in men or postmenopausal women with iron-deficiency anemia, in patients over age 50 with occult blood in the stool, in patients with a previous history of colorectal adenomatous polyps or cancer, and for colorectal cancer screening. Flexible sigmoidoscopy is commonly performed as an open-access procedure.

When patients are referred for open-access colonoscopy, the primary care provider may need to choose a colonic preparation. Commonly used oral preparations include polyethylene glycol lavage solution, with or without citric acid. A "split-dose" regimen improves the quality of colonic preparation. Sodium phosphate purgatives may cause fluid and electrolyte abnormalities and renal toxicity, especially in patients with renal failure or congestive heart failure and those over 70 years of age.

CHAPTER 13

VIDEO ATLAS OF GASTROINTESTINAL ENDOSCOPY

Louis Michel Wong Kee Song ■ Mark Topazian

Videos can be accessed via the following link: https://www.mhprofessional.com/mediacenter/

(Animations courtesy of Dr. Mark Stark and Dr. Jonathan Leighton; with permission.)

Gastrointestinal endoscopy is an increasingly important method for diagnosis and treatment of disease. This atlas demonstrates endoscopic findings in a variety of gastrointestinal infectious, inflammatory, vascular, and neoplastic conditions. Cancer screening and prevention are common indications for gastrointestinal endoscopy, and the premalignant conditions of Barrett's esophagus and colonic polyps are illustrated. Endoscopic treatment modalities for gastrointestinal bleeding, polyps, and biliary stones are demonstrated in video clips. The images shown in this atlas are also found in **Chap. 12** of the book.

Video 13–1 Methods of deep enteroscopy.

Video 13–2 Pancreatic necrosis treated by transduodenal endoscopic drainage and necrosectomy.

Video 13–3 Endoscopic full-thickness resection of a gastric subepithelial lesion.

Video 13–4 Endoscopic submucosal dissection of a large rectal adenoma.

Video 13–5 Over-the-scope clip closure of a spontaneous esophageal perforation.

Video 13–6 Endoscopic suturing for stent fixation.

Video 13–7 Actively bleeding duodenal ulcer treated with dilute epinephrine injection, thermal probe application, and hemoclips.
(Video courtesy of Dr. Navtej Buttar; with permission.)

Video 13–8 Actively bleeding esophageal varices treated with endoscopic band ligation.

Video 13–9 Large, bleeding gastric varix treated with endoscopic cyanoacrylate injection.

Video 13–10 Dieulafoy's lesion treated endoscopically.

Video 13–11 Bleeding Mallory-Weiss tear treated with hemoclip placement.

Video 13–12 Radiation proctopathy treated with argon plasma coagulation.

Video 13–13 Actively bleeding colonic diverticulum treated with dilute epinephrine injection and band ligation.

Video 13–14 Stent placement for palliation of malignant colonic obstruction.

Video 13–15 Bile duct stones removed after endoscopic sphincterotomy.

Video 13–16 Barrett's esophagus with high-grade dysplasia treated with endoscopic mucosal resection.

Video 13–17 Pedunculated and sessile colonic polyps removed with snare cautery during colonoscopy.

SECTION III

DISORDERS OF THE ALIMENTARY TRACT

CHAPTER 14

DISEASES OF THE ESOPHAGUS

Peter J. Kahrilas ■ Ikuo Hirano

ESOPHAGEAL STRUCTURE AND FUNCTION

The esophagus is a hollow, muscular tube coursing through the posterior mediastinum joining the hypopharynx to the stomach with a sphincter at each end. It functions to transport food and fluid between these ends, otherwise remaining empty. The physiology of swallowing, esophageal motility, and oral and pharyngeal dysphagia are described in **Chap. 4**. Esophageal diseases can be manifested by impaired function or pain. Key functional impairments are swallowing disorders and excessive gastroesophageal reflux. Pain, sometimes indistinguishable from cardiac chest pain, can result from inflammation, infection, dysmotility, or neoplasm.

SYMPTOMS OF ESOPHAGEAL DISEASE

The clinical history remains central to the evaluation of esophageal symptoms. A thoughtfully obtained history will often expedite management. Important details include weight gain or loss, gastrointestinal bleeding, dietary habits including the timing of meals, smoking, and alcohol consumption. The major esophageal symptoms are heartburn, regurgitation, chest pain, dysphagia, odynophagia, and globus sensation.

Heartburn (pyrosis), the most common esophageal symptom, is characterized by a discomfort or burning sensation behind the sternum that arises from the epigastrium and may radiate toward the neck. Heartburn is an intermittent symptom, most commonly experienced after eating, during exercise, and while lying recumbent. The discomfort is relieved with drinking water or antacid but can occur frequently interfering with normal activities including sleep. The association between heartburn and gastroesophageal reflux disease (GERD) is so strong that empirical therapy for GERD has become accepted management. However, the term "heartburn" is often misused and/or referred to with other terms such as "indigestion" or "repeating," making it important to clarify the intended meaning.

Regurgitation is the effortless return of food or fluid into the pharynx without nausea or retching. Patients report a sour or burning fluid in the throat or mouth that may also contain undigested food particles. Bending, belching, or maneuvers that increase intraabdominal pressure can provoke regurgitation. A clinician needs to discriminate among regurgitation, vomiting, and rumination. *Vomiting* is preceded by nausea and accompanied by retching. *Rumination* is a behavior in which recently swallowed food is regurgitated and then reswallowed repetitively for up to an hour. Although there is some linkage between rumination and mental deficiency, the behavior is also exhibited by unimpaired individuals who sometimes even find it pleasurable.

Chest pain is a common esophageal symptom with characteristics similar to cardiac pain, sometimes making this distinction difficult. Esophageal pain is usually experienced as a pressure type sensation in the mid chest, radiating to the mid back, arms, or jaws. The similarity to cardiac pain is likely because the two organs share a nerve plexus and the nerve endings in the esophageal wall have poor discriminative ability among stimuli. Esophageal distention or even chemostimulation (e.g., with acid) will often be perceived as chest pain. Gastroesophageal reflux is the most common cause of esophageal chest pain.

Esophageal *dysphagia* (**Chap. 4**) is often described as a feeling of food "sticking" or even lodging in the chest. Important distinctions are between uniquely solid food dysphagia as opposed to liquid and solid, episodic versus constant dysphagia, and progressive versus static dysphagia. If the dysphagia is for liquids as well as solid food, it suggests a motility disorder such as achalasia. Conversely, uniquely solid food dysphagia is suggestive of a stricture, ring, or tumor. Of note, a patient's localization of food hang-up in the esophagus is notoriously imprecise. Approximately 30% of distal esophageal obstructions are perceived as cervical dysphagia. In such instances, the absence of concomitant symptoms generally associated with oropharyngeal dysphagia such as aspiration, nasopharyngeal regurgitation, cough, drooling, or obvious neuromuscular compromise should suggest an esophageal etiology.

Odynophagia is pain either caused by or exacerbated by swallowing. Although typically considered distinct from dysphagia, odynophagia may manifest concurrently with dysphagia. Odynophagia is more common with pill or infectious esophagitis than with reflux esophagitis and should prompt a search for these entities. When odynophagia does occur in GERD, it is likely related to an esophageal ulcer or deep erosion.

Globus sensation, alternatively labeled "globus hystericus," is the perception of a lump or fullness in the throat that is felt irrespective of swallowing. Although such patients are frequently referred for an evaluation of dysphagia, globus sensation is often relieved by the act of swallowing. As implied by its alternative name (globus hystericus), globus sensation often occurs in the setting of anxiety or obsessive-compulsive disorders. Clinical experience teaches that it is often attributable to GERD.

Water brash is excessive salivation resulting from a vagal reflex triggered by acidification of the esophageal mucosa. This is not a common symptom. Afflicted individuals will describe the unpleasant sensation of the mouth rapidly filling with salty thin fluid, often in the setting of concomitant heartburn.

DIAGNOSTIC STUDIES

ENDOSCOPY

Endoscopy, also known as esophagogastroduodenoscopy (EGD), is the most useful test for the evaluation of the proximal gastrointestinal tract. Modern instruments produce high-quality, color images of the esophageal, gastric, and duodenal lumen. Endoscopes also have an instrumentation channel through which biopsy forceps, injection catheters for local delivery of therapeutic agents, balloon dilators, or hemostatic devices can be used. The key advantages of endoscopy over barium radiography are: (1) increased sensitivity for the detection of mucosal lesions, (2) vastly increased sensitivity for the detection of abnormalities mainly identifiable by color such as Barrett's metaplasia or vascular lesions, (3) the ability to obtain biopsy specimens for histologic examination of suspected abnormalities, and (4) the ability to dilate strictures during the examination. The main disadvantages of endoscopy are cost and the utilization of sedatives or anesthetics.

RADIOGRAPHY

Contrast radiography of the esophagus, stomach, and duodenum can demonstrate reflux of the contrast media, hiatal hernia, mucosal granularity, erosions, ulcerations, and strictures. The sensitivity of radiography compared with endoscopy for detecting reflux esophagitis reportedly ranges from 22–95%, with higher grades of esophagitis (i.e., ulceration or stricture) exhibiting greater detection rates. Conversely, the sensitivity of barium radiography for detecting esophageal strictures is greater than that of endoscopy, especially when the study is done in conjunction with barium-soaked bread or a 13-mm barium tablet. Barium studies also provide an assessment of esophageal function and morphology that may be undetected on endoscopy. Tracheoesophageal fistula, altered postsurgical anatomy, and extrinsic esophageal compression are conditions where radiographic imaging complements endoscopic assessment. Hypopharyngeal pathology and disorders of the cricopharyngeus muscle are better appreciated on radiographic examination than with endoscopy, particularly with rapid sequence or video fluoroscopic recording. The major shortcoming of barium radiography is that it rarely obviates the need for endoscopy. Either a positive or a negative study is usually followed by an endoscopic evaluation either to obtain biopsies, provide therapy, or clarify findings in the case of a positive examination or to add a level of certainty in the case of a negative one.

ENDOSCOPIC ULTRASOUND

Endoscopic ultrasound (EUS) instruments combine an endoscope with an ultrasound transducer to create a transmural image of the tissue surrounding the endoscope tip. The key advantage of EUS over alternative radiologic imaging techniques is much greater resolution attributable to the proximity of the ultrasound transducer to the area being examined. Available devices can provide either radial imaging (360-degree, cross-sectional) or a curved linear image that can guide fine-needle aspiration of imaged structures such as lymph nodes or tumors. Major esophageal applications of EUS are to stage esophageal cancer, to evaluate dysplasia in Barrett's esophagus, and to assess submucosal lesions.

ESOPHAGEAL MANOMETRY

Esophageal manometry, or motility testing, entails positioning a pressure-sensing catheter within the esophagus and then observing the contractility following test swallows. The upper and lower esophageal sphincters appear as zones of high pressure that relax on swallowing, while the intersphincteric esophagus exhibits peristaltic contractions. Manometry is used to

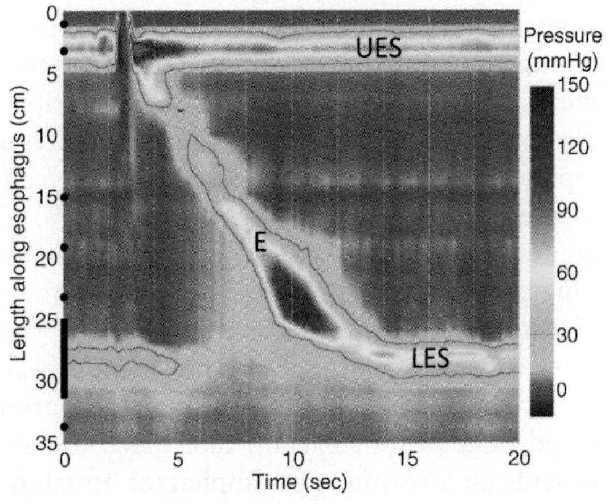

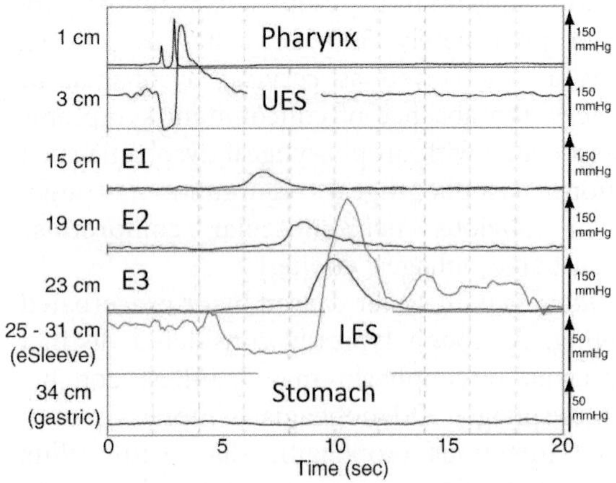

FIGURE 14-1

High-resolution esophageal pressure topography (*right*) and conventional manometry (*left*) of a normal swallow. E, esophageal body; LES, lower esophageal sphincter; UES, upper esophageal sphincter.

diagnose motility disorders (achalasia, diffuse esophageal spasm) and to assess peristaltic integrity prior to the surgery for reflux disease. Technologic advances have enhanced esophageal manometry as high-resolution esophageal pressure topography (Fig. 14-1). Manometry can also be combined with intraluminal impedance monitoring. Impedance recordings use a catheter with a series of paired electrodes. Esophageal luminal contents in contact with the electrodes decrease (liquid) or increase (air) the impedance signal, allowing detection of anterograde or retrograde esophageal bolus transit.

REFLUX TESTING

GERD is often diagnosed in the absence of endoscopic esophagitis, which would otherwise define the disease. This occurs in the settings of partially treated disease, an abnormally sensitive esophageal mucosa, or without obvious explanation. In such instances, reflux testing can demonstrate excessive esophageal exposure to refluxed gastric juice, the physiologic abnormality of GERD. This can be done by ambulatory 24- to 48-h esophageal pH recording using either a wireless pH-sensitive transmitter that is anchored to the esophageal mucosa or a transnasally positioned wire electrode with the tip stationed in the distal esophagus. Either way, the outcome is expressed as the percentage of the day that the pH was less than 4 (indicative of recent acid reflux), with values exceeding 5% indicative of GERD. Reflux testing is useful with atypical symptoms or an inexplicably poor response to therapy. Intraluminal impedance monitoring can be added to pH monitoring to detect reflux events irrespective of whether or not they are acidic, potentially increasing the sensitivity of the study.

STRUCTURAL DISORDERS

HIATAL HERNIA

Hiatus hernia is a herniation of viscera, most commonly the stomach, into the mediastinum through the esophageal hiatus of the diaphragm. Four types of hiatus hernia are distinguished with type I, or sliding hiatal hernia, comprising at least 95% of the overall total. A sliding hiatal hernia is one in which the gastroesophageal junction and gastric cardia translocate cephalad as a result of weakening of the phrenoesophageal ligament attaching the gastroesophageal junction to the diaphragm at the hiatus and dilatation of the diaphragmatic hiatus. The incidence of sliding hernia increases with age. True to its name, sliding hernias enlarge with increased intraabdominal pressure, swallowing, and respiration. Conceptually, sliding hernias are the result of wear and tear: increased intraabdominal pressure from abdominal obesity, pregnancy, etc., along with hereditary factors predisposing to the condition. The main significance of sliding hernias is the propensity of affected individuals to have GERD.

Types II, III, and IV hiatal hernias are all subtypes of paraesophageal hernia in which the herniation into the mediastinum includes a visceral structure other than the gastric cardia. With type II and III paraesophageal hernias, the gastric fundus also herniates with the distinction being that in type II, the gastroesophageal junction remains fixed at the hiatus, whereas type III is a combined sliding and paraesophageal hernia. With type IV hiatal hernias, viscera other than the stomach herniate into the mediastinum, most commonly the colon. With type II and III paraesophageal hernias, the stomach inverts as it herniates and large paraesophageal hernias can lead to an upside down stomach, gastric volvulus, and even strangulation of the stomach.

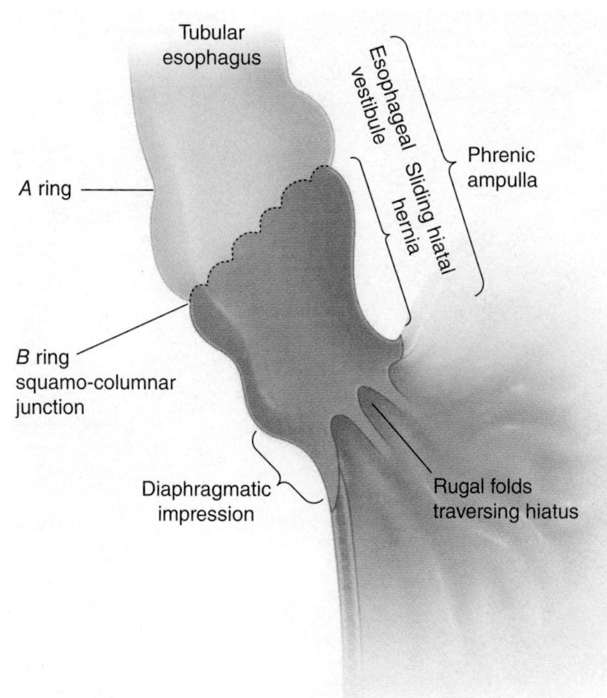

FIGURE 14-2
Radiographic anatomy of the gastroesophageal junction.

Because of this risk, surgical repair is often advocated for large paraesophageal hernias.

RINGS AND WEBS

A lower esophageal mucosal ring, also called a *B ring*, is a thin membranous narrowing at the squamocolumnar mucosal junction (Fig. 14-2). Its origin is unknown, but B rings are demonstrable in about 10–15% of the general population and are usually asymptomatic. When the lumen diameter is less than 13 mm, distal rings are usually associated with episodic solid food dysphagia and are called *Schatzki rings*. Patients typically present older than 40 years, consistent with an acquired rather than congenital origin. Schatzki ring is one of the most common causes of intermittent food impaction, also known as "steakhouse syndrome" because meat is a typical instigator. Symptomatic rings are easily treated by dilation.

Web-like constrictions higher in the esophagus can be of congenital or inflammatory origin. Asymptomatic cervical esophageal webs are demonstrated in about 10% of people and typically originate along the anterior aspect of the esophagus. When circumferential, they can cause intermittent dysphagia to solids similar to Schatzki rings and are similarly treated with dilatation. The combination of symptomatic proximal esophageal webs and iron-deficiency anemia in middle-aged women constitutes Plummer-Vinson syndrome.

DIVERTICULA

Esophageal diverticula are categorized by location with the most common being epiphrenic, hypopharyngeal (Zenker's), and midesophageal. Epiphrenic and Zenker's diverticula are false diverticula involving herniation of the mucosa and submucosa through the muscular layer of the esophagus. These lesions result from increased intraluminal pressure associated with distal obstruction. In the case of Zenker's, the obstruction is a stenotic cricopharyngeus muscle (upper esophageal sphincter), and the hypopharyngeal herniation most commonly occurs in an area of natural weakness proximal to the cricopharyngeus known as *Killian's triangle* (Fig. 14-3). Small Zenker's diverticula are usually

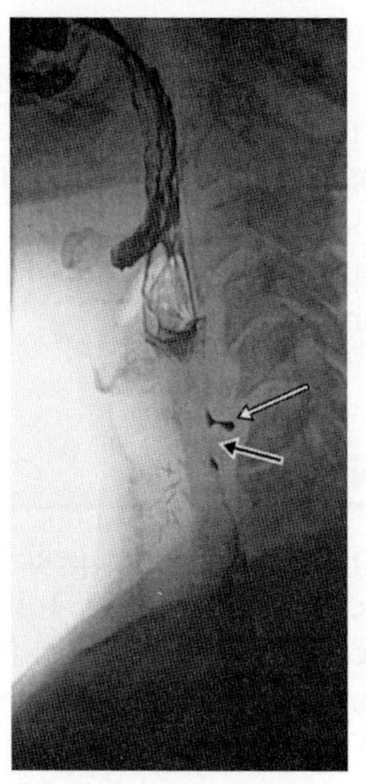

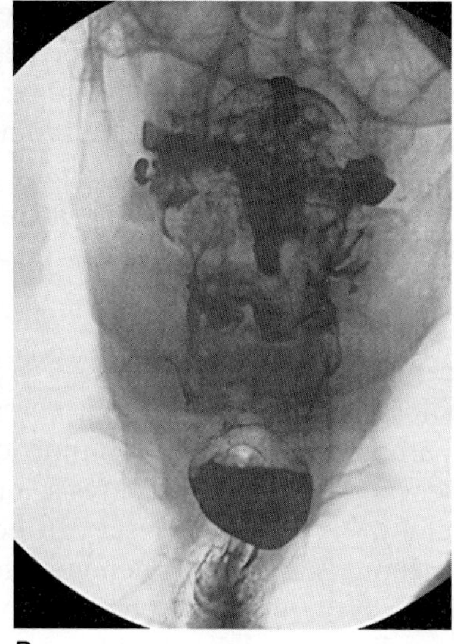

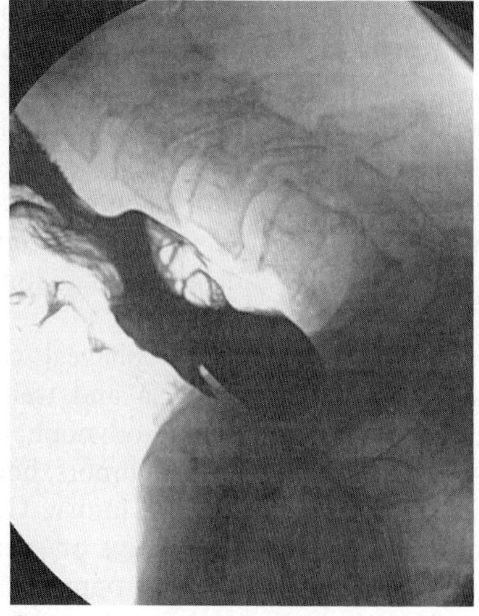

FIGURE 14-3
Examples of small (*A*) and large (*B, C*) Zenker's diverticula arising from Killian's triangle in the distal hypopharynx. Smaller diverticula are evident only during the swallow, whereas larger ones retain food and fluid.

asymptomatic, but when they enlarge sufficiently to retain food and saliva they can be associated with dysphagia, halitosis, and aspiration. Treatment is by surgical diverticulectomy and cricopharyngeal myotomy or a marsupialization procedure in which an endoscopic stapling device is used to divide the cricopharyngeus.

Epiphrenic diverticula are usually associated with achalasia or a distal esophageal stricture. Midesophageal diverticula may be caused by traction from adjacent inflammation (classically tuberculosis) in which case they are true diverticula involving all layers of the esophageal wall, or by pulsion associated with esophageal motor disorders. Midesophageal and epiphrenic diverticula are usually asymptomatic until they enlarge sufficiently to retain food and cause dysphagia and regurgitation. Symptoms attributable to the diverticula tend to correlate more with the underlying esophageal disorder than the size of the diverticula. Large diverticula can be removed surgically, usually in conjunction with a myotomy if the underlying cause is achalasia. Diffuse intramural esophageal diverticulosis is a rare entity that results from dilatation of the excretory ducts of submucosal esophageal glands (Fig. 14-4). Esophageal candidiasis and proximal esophageal strictures are commonly found in association with this disorder.

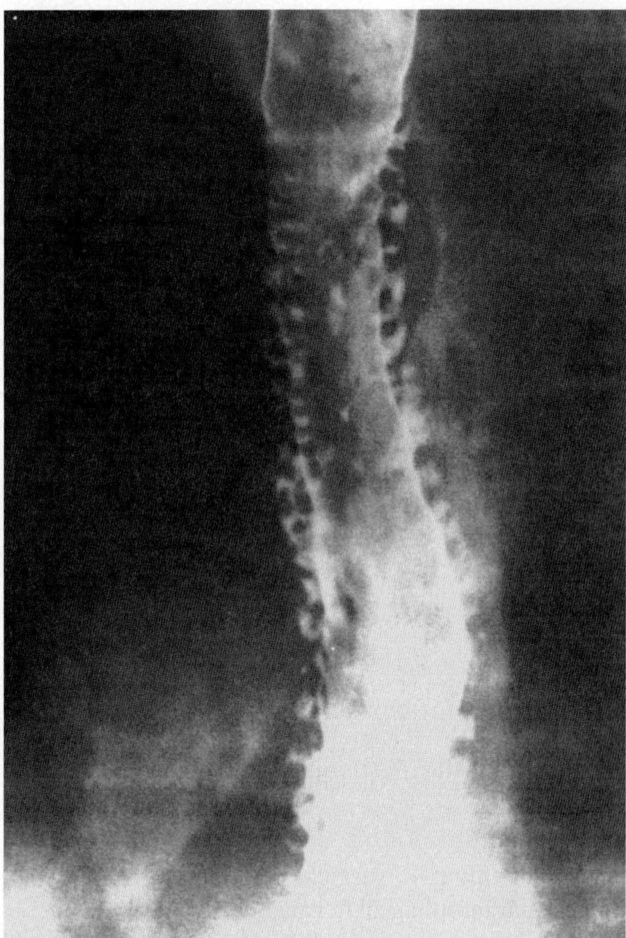

FIGURE 14-4
Intramural esophageal pseudodiverticulosis associated with chronic obstruction. Invaginations of contrast into the esophageal wall outline deep esophageal glands.

TUMORS

Esophageal cancer occurs in about 4.5:100,000 people in the United States with the associated mortality being only slightly less at 4.4:100,000. It is about 10 times less common than colorectal cancer but kills about one-quarter as many patients. These statistics emphasize both the rarity and lethality of esophageal cancer. One notable trend is the shift of dominant esophageal cancer type from squamous cell to adenocarcinoma, strongly linked to reflux disease and Barrett's metaplasia. Other distinctions between cell types are the predilection for adenocarcinoma to affect the distal esophagus in white males and squamous cell to affect the more proximal esophagus in black males with the added risk factors of smoking, alcohol consumption, caustic injury, and human papilloma virus infection **(Chap. 51)**.

The typical presentation of esophageal cancer is of progressive solid food dysphagia and weight loss. Associated symptoms may include odynophagia, iron deficiency, and, with midesophageal tumors, hoarseness from left recurrent laryngeal nerve injury. Generally, these are indications of locally invasive or even metastatic disease manifest by tracheoesophageal fistulas and vocal cord paralysis. Even when detected as a small lesion, esophageal cancer has poor survival because of the abundant esophageal lymphatics leading to regional lymph node metastases.

Benign esophageal tumors are uncommon and usually discovered incidentally. In decreasing frequency of occurrence, cell types include leiomyoma, fibrovascular polyps, squamous papilloma, granular cell tumors, lipomas, neurofibromas, and inflammatory fibroid polyps. These generally become symptomatic only when they are associated with dysphagia and merit removal only under the same circumstances.

CONGENITAL ANOMALIES

The most common congenital esophageal anomaly is esophageal atresia, occurring in about 1 in 5000 live births. Atresia can occur in several permutations, the common denominator being developmental failure of fusion between the proximal and distal esophagus associated with a tracheoesophageal fistula, most commonly with the distal segment excluded. Alternatively, there can be an H-type configuration in which esophageal fusion has occurred, but with a tracheoesophageal fistula. Esophageal atresia is usually recognized and corrected surgically within the first few days of life. Later life complications include dysphagia from anastomotic strictures or absent peristalsis and reflux, which can be severe. Less common developmental anomalies include congenital esophageal stenosis, webs, and duplications.

Dysphagia can also result from congenital abnormalities that cause extrinsic compression of the esophagus. In dysphagia lusoria, the esophagus is compressed by an aberrant right subclavian artery arising from the descending aorta and passing behind the esophagus. Alternatively vascular rings may surround and constrict the esophagus.

Heterotopic gastric mucosa, also known as an esophageal inlet patch, is a focus of gastric type epithelium in the proximal cervical esophagus; the estimated prevalence is 4.5%. The inlet patch is thought to result from incomplete replacement of embryonic columnar epithelium with squamous epithelium. The majority of inlet patches are asymptomatic, but acid production can occur as most contain fundic type gastric epithelium with parietal cells.

ESOPHAGEAL MOTILITY DISORDERS

Esophageal motility disorders are diseases attributable to esophageal neuromuscular dysfunction commonly associated with dysphagia, chest pain, or heartburn. The major entities are achalasia, diffuse esophageal spasm (DES), and GERD. Motility disorders can also be secondary to broader disease processes as is the case with pseudoachalasia, Chagas' disease, and scleroderma. Not included in this discussion are diseases affecting the pharynx and proximal esophagus, the impairment of which is almost always part of a more global neuromuscular disease process.

ACHALASIA

Achalasia is a rare disease caused by loss of ganglion cells within the esophageal myenteric plexus with a population incidence of about 1:100,000 and usually presenting between age 25 and 60. With longstanding disease, aganglionosis is noted. The disease involves both excitatory (cholinergic) and inhibitory (nitric oxide) ganglionic neurons. Functionally, inhibitory neurons mediate deglutitive lower esophageal sphincter (LES) relaxation and the sequential propagation of peristalsis. Their absence leads to impaired deglutitive LES relaxation and absent peristalsis. Increasing evidence suggests that the ultimate cause of ganglion cell degeneration in achalasia is an autoimmune process attributable to a latent infection with human herpes simplex virus 1 combined with genetic susceptibility.

Long-standing achalasia is characterized by progressive dilatation and sigmoid deformity of the esophagus with hypertrophy of the LES. Clinical manifestations may include dysphagia, regurgitation, chest pain, and weight loss. Most patients report solid and liquid food dysphagia. Regurgitation occurs when food, fluid, and secretions are retained in the dilated esophagus. Patients with advanced achalasia are at risk for bronchitis, pneumonia, or lung abscess from chronic regurgitation and aspiration. Chest pain is frequent early in the course of achalasia, thought to result from esophageal spasm. Patients describe a squeezing, pressure-like retrosternal pain, sometimes radiating to the neck, arms, jaw, and back. Paradoxically, some patients complain of heartburn that may be a chest pain equivalent. Treatment of achalasia is less effective in relieving chest pain than it is in relieving dysphagia or regurgitation.

The differential diagnosis of achalasia includes DES, Chagas' disease, and pseudoachalasia. Chagas' disease is endemic in areas of central Brazil, Venezuela, and northern Argentina and spread by the bite of the reduviid (kissing) bug that transmits the protozoan, *Trypanosoma cruzi.* The chronic phase of the disease develops years after infection and results from destruction of autonomic ganglion cells throughout the body, including the heart, gut, urinary tract, and respiratory tract. Tumor infiltration, most commonly seen with carcinoma in the gastric fundus or distal esophagus, can mimic idiopathic achalasia. The resultant "pseudoachalasia" accounts for up to 5% of suspected cases and is more likely with advanced age, abrupt onset of symptoms (<1 year), and weight loss. Hence, endoscopy is a necessary part of the evaluation of achalasia. When the clinical suspicion for pseudoachalasia is high and endoscopy nondiagnostic, computed tomography (CT) scanning or EUS may be of value. Rarely, pseudoachalasia can result from a paraneoplastic syndrome with circulating antineuronal antibodies.

Achalasia is diagnosed by barium swallow x-ray and/or esophageal manometry; endoscopy has a relatively minor role other than to exclude pseudoachalasia. The barium swallow x-ray appearance is of a dilated esophagus with poor emptying, an air-fluid level, and tapering at the LES giving it a beak-like appearance (Fig. 14-5). Occasionally, an epiphrenic diverticulum is observed. In long-standing achalasia, the esophagus may assume a sigmoid configuration. The diagnostic criteria for achalasia with esophageal manometry are impaired LES relaxation and absent peristalsis. High-resolution manometry has somewhat advanced this diagnosis; three subtypes of achalasia are differentiated based on the pattern of pressurization in the nonperistaltic esophagus (Fig. 14-6). Because manometry identifies early disease before esophageal dilatation and food retention, it is the most sensitive diagnostic test.

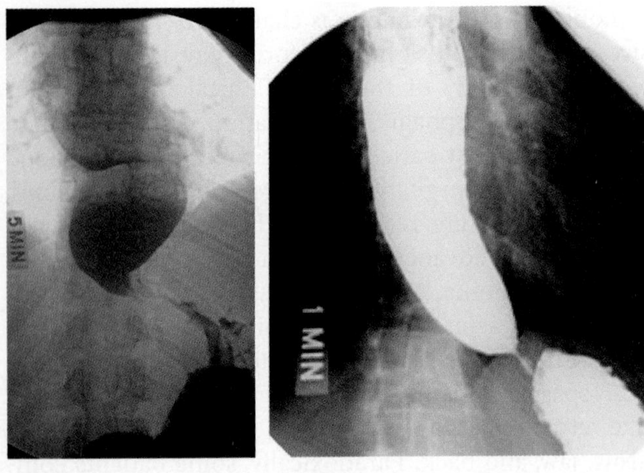

FIGURE 14-5

Achalasia with esophageal dilatation, tapering at the gastroesophageal junction, and an air-fluid level within the esophagus. The example on the *left* shows sigmoid deformity with very advanced disease.

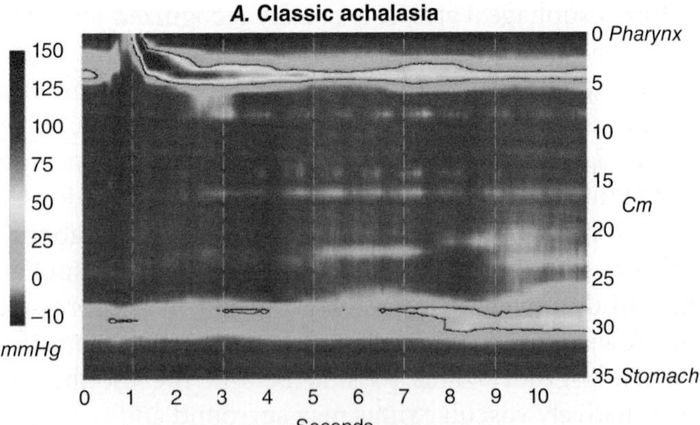

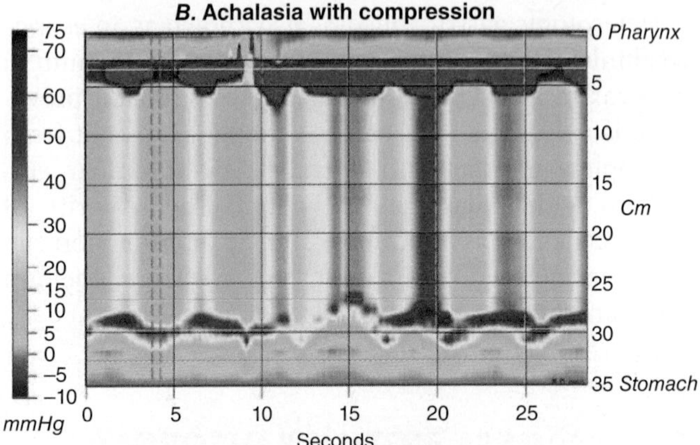

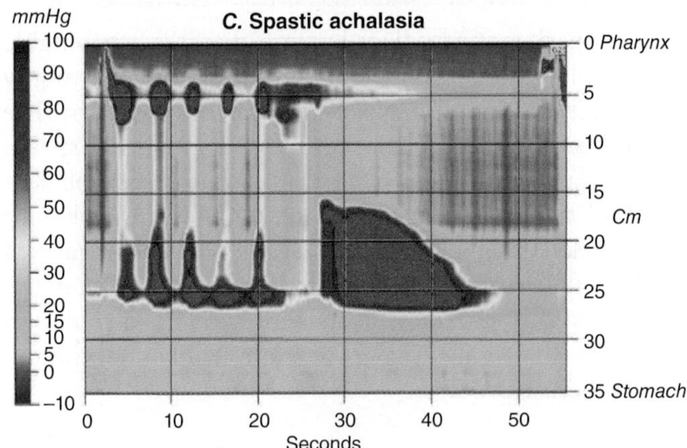

FIGURE 14-6

Three subtypes of achalasia: classic (*A*), with esophageal compression (*B*), and spastic achalasia (*C*) imaged with pressure topography. All are characterized by impaired lower esophageal sphincter (LES) relaxation and absent peristalsis. However, classic achalasia has minimal pressurization of the esophageal body, whereas substantial fluid pressurization is observed in achalasia with esophageal compression, and spastic esophageal contractions are observed with spastic achalasia.

There is no known way of preventing or reversing achalasia. Therapy is directed at reducing LES pressure so that gravity and esophageal pressurization promote esophageal emptying. Peristalsis rarely, if ever, recovers. However, in many instances, remnants of peristalsis masked by esophageal pressurization and dilatation prior to therapy are demonstrable following effective treatment. LES pressure can be reduced by pharmacologic therapy, pneumatic balloon dilatation, or surgical myotomy. No large, controlled trials of the therapeutic alternatives exist, and the optimal approach is debated. Pharmacologic therapies are relatively ineffective but are often used as temporizing therapies. Nitrates or calcium channel blockers are administered before eating, advising caution because of their effects on blood pressure. Botulinum toxin, injected into the LES under endoscopic guidance, inhibits acetylcholine release from nerve endings and improves dysphagia in about 66% of cases for at least 6 months. Sildenafil and alternative phosphodiesterase inhibitors effectively decrease LES pressure, but practicalities limit their clinical use in achalasia.

The only durable therapies for achalasia are pneumatic dilatation and Heller myotomy. Pneumatic dilatation, with a reported efficacy ranging from 32–98%, is an endoscopic technique using a noncompliant, cylindrical balloon dilator positioned across the LES and inflated to a diameter of 3–4 cm. The major complication is perforation with a reported incidence of 0.5–5%. The most common surgical procedure for achalasia is laparoscopic Heller myotomy, usually performed in conjunction with an antireflux procedure (partial fundoplication); good to excellent results are reported in 62–100% of cases. A European randomized controlled trial demonstrated an equivalent response rate of approximately 90% for both pneumatic dilation and laparoscopic Heller myotomy at 2-year follow-up. Occasionally, patients with advanced disease fail to respond to pneumatic dilatation or Heller myotomy. In such refractory cases, esophageal resection with gastric pull-up or interposition of a segment of transverse colon may be the only option other than gastrostomy feeding.

An endoscopic approach to LES myotomy has been introduced, referred to as per oral esophageal myotomy. This technique involves the creation of a tunnel within the esophageal wall through which the circular muscle of the LES and distal esophagus are transected with electrocautery. Short-term studies of efficacy have been favorable. Potential advantages over the conventional laparoscopic approach include avoidance of surgical disruption of the diaphragmatic hiatus and more rapid recovery.

In untreated or inadequately treated achalasia, esophageal dilatation predisposes to stasis esophagitis. Prolonged stasis esophagitis is the likely explanation for the association between achalasia and esophageal squamous cell cancer. Tumors develop after years of achalasia, usually in the setting of a greatly dilated esophagus with the overall squamous cell cancer risk increased 17-fold compared to controls.

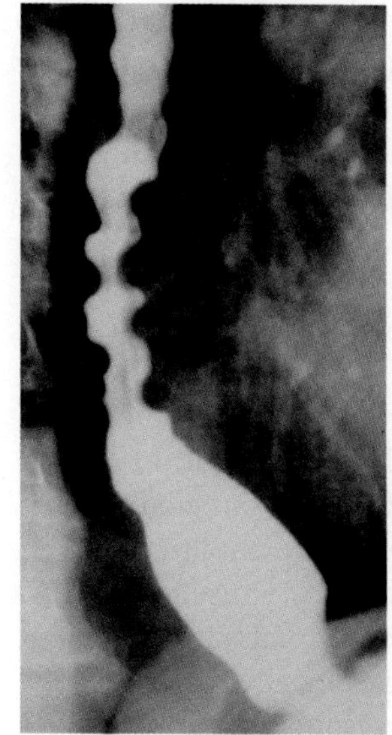
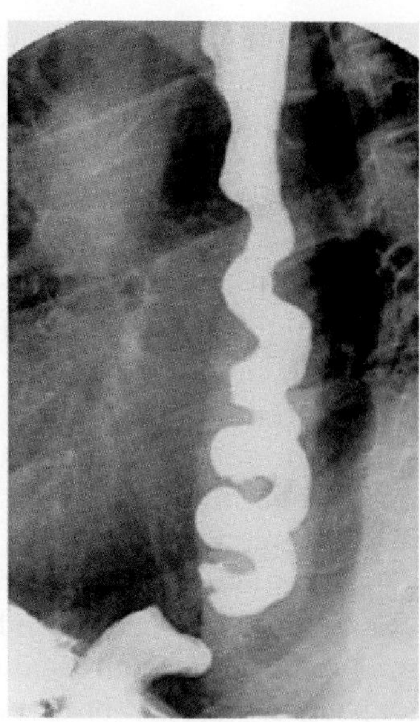

FIGURE 14-7

Diffuse esophageal spasm. The characteristic "corkscrew" esophagus results from spastic contraction of the circular muscle in the esophageal wall; more precisely, this is actually a helical array of muscle. These findings are also seen with spastic achalasia.

DIFFUSE ESOPHAGEAL SPASM (DES)

DES is manifested by episodes of dysphagia and chest pain attributable to abnormal esophageal contractions with normal deglutitive LES relaxation. Beyond that, there is little consensus. The pathophysiology and natural history of DES are ill defined. Radiographically, DES has been characterized by tertiary contractions or a "corkscrew esophagus" (Fig. 14-7), but in many instances, these abnormalities are actually indicative of achalasia. Manometrically, a variety of defining features have been proposed including uncoordinated ("spastic") activity in the distal esophagus, spontaneous and repetitive contractions, or high-amplitude and prolonged contractions. The current consensus, derived from high-resolution manometry studies, is to define spasm by the occurrence of contractions in the distal esophagus with short latency relative to the time of the pharyngeal contraction, a dysfunction indicative of impairment of inhibitory myenteric plexus neurons. When defined in this restrictive fashion (Fig. 14-8), DES is actually much less common than achalasia.

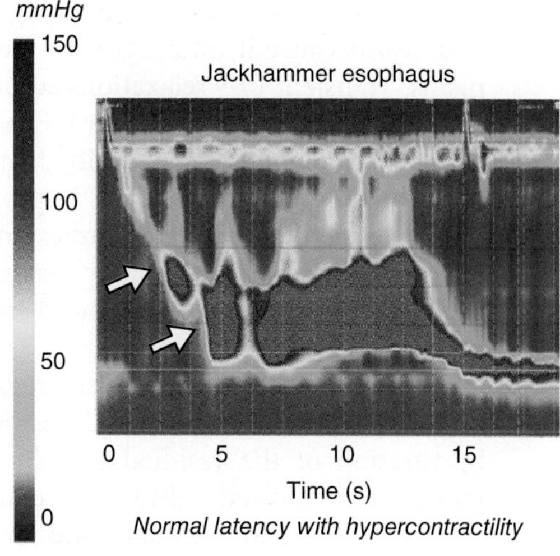

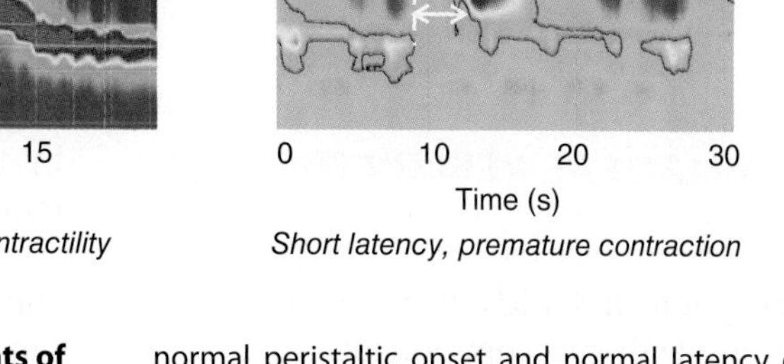

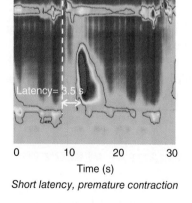

FIGURE 14-8

Esophageal pressure topography of the two major variants of esophageal spasm: jackhammer esophagus (*left*) and diffuse esophageal spasm (*right*). Jackhammer esophagus is defined by the extraordinarily vigorous and repetitive contractions with normal peristaltic onset and normal latency of the contraction. Diffuse esophageal spasm is similar but primarily defined by a short latency (premature) contraction.

Esophageal chest pain closely mimics angina pectoris. Features suggesting esophageal pain include pain that is nonexertional, prolonged, interrupts sleep, meal-related, relieved with antacids, and accompanied by heartburn, dysphagia, or regurgitation. However, all of these features exhibit overlap with cardiac pain, which still must be the primary consideration. Furthermore, even within the spectrum of esophageal diseases, both chest pain and dysphagia are also characteristic of peptic or infectious esophagitis. Only after these more common entities have been excluded by evaluation and/or treatment should a diagnosis of DES be pursued.

Although the defining criteria are in flux, DES is diagnosed by manometry. Endoscopy is useful to identify alternative structural and inflammatory lesions that may cause chest pain. Radiographically, a "corkscrew esophagus," "rosary bead esophagus," pseudodiverticula, or curling can be indicative of DES, but these are also found with spastic achalasia. Given these vagaries of defining DES, and the resultant heterogeneity of patients identified for inclusion in therapeutic trials, it is not surprising that trial results have been disappointing. Only small, uncontrolled trials exist, reporting response to nitrates, calcium channel blockers, hydralazine, botulinum toxin, and anxiolytics. The only controlled trial showing efficacy was with an anxiolytic. Surgical therapy (long myotomy or even esophagectomy) should be considered only with severe weight loss or unbearable pain. These indications are extremely rare.

NONSPECIFIC MANOMETRIC FINDINGS

Manometric studies done to evaluate chest pain and/or dysphagia often report minor abnormalities (e.g., hypertensive or hypotensive peristalsis, hypertensive LES) that are insufficient to diagnose either achalasia or DES. These findings are of unclear significance. Reflux and psychiatric diagnoses, particularly anxiety and depression, are common among such individuals. A lower visceral pain threshold and symptoms of irritable bowel syndrome are noted in more than half of such patients. Consequently, therapy for these individuals should either target the most common esophageal disorder, GERD, or more global conditions such as depression or somatization neurosis that are found to be coexistent.

GASTROESOPHAGEAL REFLUX DISEASE (GERD)

The current conception of GERD is to encompass a family of conditions with the commonality that they are caused by gastroesophageal reflux resulting in either troublesome symptoms or an array of potential esophageal and extraesophageal manifestations. It is estimated that 15% of adults in the United States are affected by GERD, although such estimates are based only on population studies of self-reported chronic heartburn. With respect to the esophagus, the spectrum of injury includes esophagitis, stricture, Barrett's esophagus, and adenocarcinoma (Fig. 14-9). Of particular concern is the rising incidence of esophageal adenocarcinoma, an epidemiologic trend that parallels the increasing incidence of GERD. There were about 8000 incident cases of esophageal adenocarcinoma in the United States in 2013 (half of all esophageal cancers); it is estimated that this disease burden has increased two- to sixfold in the last 20 years.

PATHOPHYSIOLOGY

The best-defined subset of GERD patients, albeit a minority overall, have esophagitis. Esophagitis occurs when refluxed gastric acid and pepsin cause necrosis of the esophageal mucosa causing erosions and ulcers. Note that some degree of gastroesophageal reflux is normal, physiologically intertwined with the mechanism of belching (transient LES relaxation), but esophagitis results from excessive reflux, often accompanied by impaired clearance of the refluxed gastric juice. Restricting reflux to that which is physiologically intended depends on the anatomic and physiologic integrity of the esophagogastric junction, a complex sphincter comprised of both the LES and the surrounding crural diaphragm. Three dominant mechanisms of esophagogastric junction incompetence are recognized: (1) transient LES relaxations (a vagovagal reflex in which LES relaxation is elicited by gastric distention), (2) LES hypotension, or (3) anatomic distortion of the esophagogastric junction inclusive of hiatus hernia. Of note, the third factor, esophagogastric junction anatomic disruption, is both significant unto itself and also because it interacts with the first two mechanisms. Transient LES relaxations account for about 90% of reflux in normal subjects or GERD patients without hiatus hernia, but patients with hiatus hernia have a more heterogeneous mechanistic profile. Factors tending to exacerbate reflux regardless of mechanism are abdominal obesity, pregnancy, gastric hypersecretory states, delayed gastric emptying, disruption of esophageal peristalsis, and gluttony.

After acid reflux, peristalsis returns the refluxed fluid to the stomach and acid clearance is completed by titration of the residual acid by bicarbonate contained in swallowed saliva. Consequently, two causes of prolonged acid clearance are impaired peristalsis and reduced salivation. Impaired peristaltic emptying can be attributable to disrupted peristalsis or superimposed reflux associated with a hiatal hernia. With superimposed reflux, fluid retained within a sliding hiatal hernia refluxes back into the esophagus during

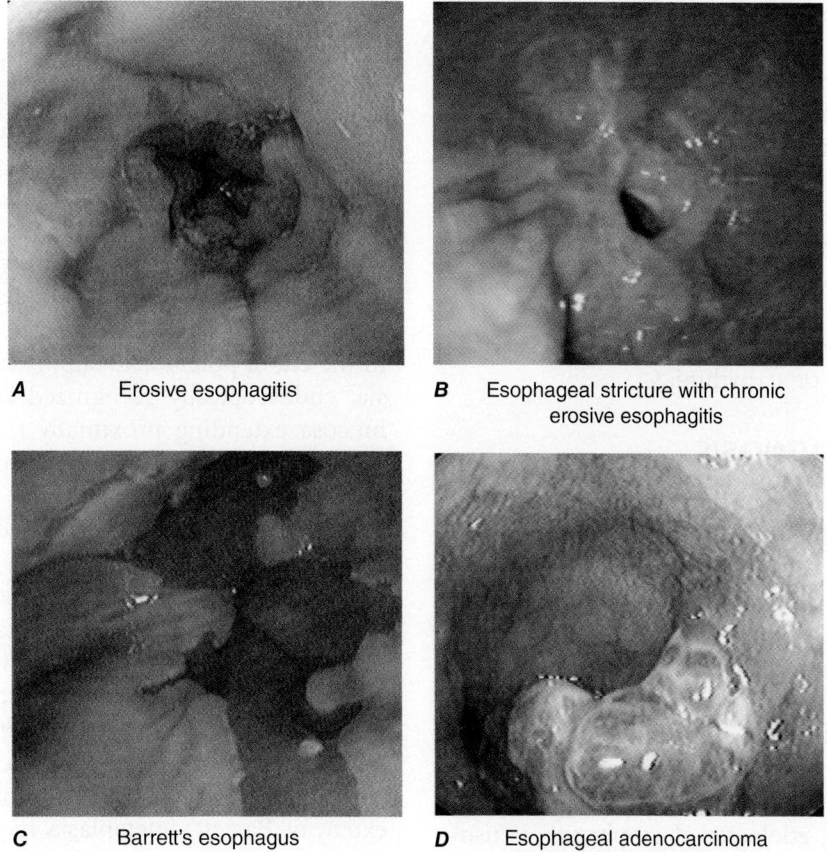

FIGURE 14-9

Endoscopic appearance of (*A*) peptic esophagitis, (***B***) a peptic stricture, (***C***) Barrett's metaplasia, and (***D***) adenocarcinoma developing within an area of Barrett's esophagus.

swallow-related LES relaxation, a phenomenon that does not normally occur.

Inherent in the pathophysiologic model of GERD is that gastric juice is harmful to the esophageal epithelium. However, gastric acid hypersecretion is usually not a dominant factor in the development of esophagitis. An obvious exception is with Zollinger-Ellison syndrome, which is associated with severe esophagitis in about 50% of patients. Another caveat is with chronic *Helicobacter pylori* gastritis, which may have a protective effect by inducing atrophic gastritis with concomitant hypoacidity. Pepsin, bile, and pancreatic enzymes within gastric secretions can also injure the esophageal epithelium, but their noxious properties are either lessened without an acidic environment or dependent on acidity for activation. Bile warrants attention because it persists in refluxate despite acid-suppressing medications. Bile can transverse the cell membrane, imparting severe cellular injury in a weakly acidic environment, and has also been invoked as a cofactor in the pathogenesis of Barrett's metaplasia and adenocarcinoma. Hence, the causticity of gastric refluxate extends beyond hydrochloric acid.

SYMPTOMS

Heartburn and regurgitation are the typical symptoms of GERD. Somewhat less common are dysphagia and chest pain. In each case, multiple potential mechanisms for symptom genesis operate that extend beyond the basic concepts of mucosal erosion and activation of afferent sensory nerves. Specifically, hypersensitivity and functional pain are increasingly recognized as cofactors. Nonetheless, the dominant clinical strategy is empirical treatment with acid inhibitors, reserving further evaluation for those who fail to respond. Important exceptions to this are patients with chest pain or persistent dysphagia, each of which may be indicative of more morbid conditions. With chest pain, cardiac disease must be carefully considered. In the case of persistent dysphagia, chronic reflux can lead to the development of a peptic stricture or adenocarcinoma, each of which benefits from early detection and/or specific therapy.

Extraesophageal syndromes with an established association to GERD include chronic cough, laryngitis, asthma, and dental erosions. A multitude of other conditions including pharyngitis, chronic bronchitis, pulmonary fibrosis, chronic sinusitis, cardiac arrhythmias, sleep apnea, and recurrent aspiration pneumonia have proposed associations with GERD. However, in both cases, it is important to emphasize the word *association* as opposed to *causation*. In many instances, the disorders likely coexist because of shared pathogenetic mechanisms rather than strict causality. Potential mechanisms for extraesophageal GERD manifestations are either regurgitation with direct contact between the refluxate and supraesophageal structures or via a vagovagal reflex wherein reflux activation of esophageal afferent nerves triggers efferent vagal reflexes such as bronchospasm, cough, or arrhythmias.

DIFFERENTIAL DIAGNOSIS

Although generally quite characteristic, symptoms from GERD need to be distinguished from symptoms related to infectious, pill, or eosinophilic esophagitis, peptic ulcer disease, dyspepsia, biliary colic, coronary artery disease, and esophageal motility disorders. It is especially important that coronary artery disease be given early consideration because of its potentially lethal implications. The remaining elements of the differential diagnosis can be addressed by endoscopy, upper gastrointestinal series, or biliary tract ultrasonography as appropriate. The distinction among etiologies of esophagitis is usually easily made by endoscopy with mucosal biopsies, which are necessary to evaluate for infection or eosinophilic inflammation. In terms of endoscopic appearance, infectious esophagitis is diffuse and tends to involve the proximal esophagus far more frequently than does reflux esophagitis. The ulcerations seen in peptic esophagitis are usually solitary and distal, whereas infectious ulcerations are punctate and diffuse. Eosinophilic esophagitis characteristically exhibits multiple esophageal rings, linear furrows, or white punctate exudate. Esophageal ulcerations from pill esophagitis are usually singular and deep at points of luminal narrowing, especially near the carina, with sparing of the distal esophagus.

COMPLICATIONS

The complications of GERD are related to chronic esophagitis (bleeding and stricture) and the relationship between GERD and esophageal adenocarcinoma. However, both esophagitis and peptic strictures have become increasingly rare in the era of potent antisecretory medications. Conversely, the most severe histologic consequence of GERD is Barrett's metaplasia with the associated risk of esophageal adenocarcinoma, and the incidence of these lesions has increased, not decreased, in the era of potent acid suppression. Barrett's metaplasia, endoscopically recognized by tongues of reddish mucosa extending proximally from the gastroesophageal junction (Fig. 14-9) or histopathologically by the finding of specialized columnar metaplasia, is associated with a substantially increased risk for development of esophageal adenocarcinoma.

Barrett's metaplasia can progress to adenocarcinoma through the intermediate stages of low- and high-grade dysplasia (Fig. 14-10). Owing to this risk, areas of Barrett's and especially any included areas of mucosal irregularity should be extensively biopsied. The rate of cancer development is estimated at 0.1–0.3% per year, but vagaries in definitional criteria and of the extent of Barrett's metaplasia requisite to establish the diagnosis have contributed to variability and inconsistency in this risk assessment. The group at greatest risk is obese white males in their sixth decade of life. However, despite common practice, the utility of endoscopic screening and surveillance programs intended to control the adenocarcinoma risk has not been established. Also of note, no high-level evidence confirms that aggressive antisecretory therapy or antireflux surgery causes regression of Barrett's esophagus or prevents adenocarcinoma.

Although the management of Barrett's esophagus remains controversial, the finding of dysplasia in Barrett's, particularly high-grade dysplasia, mandates

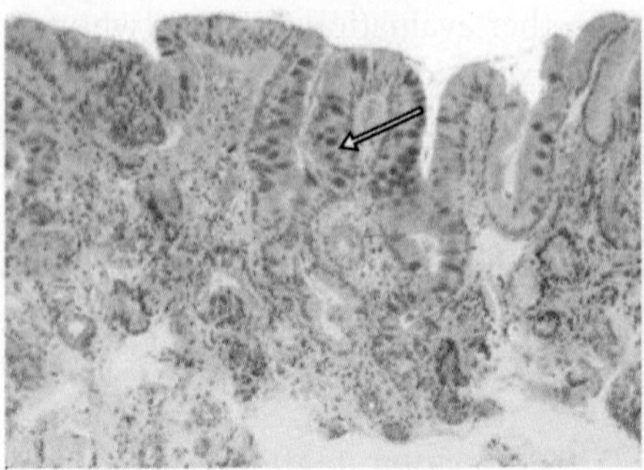

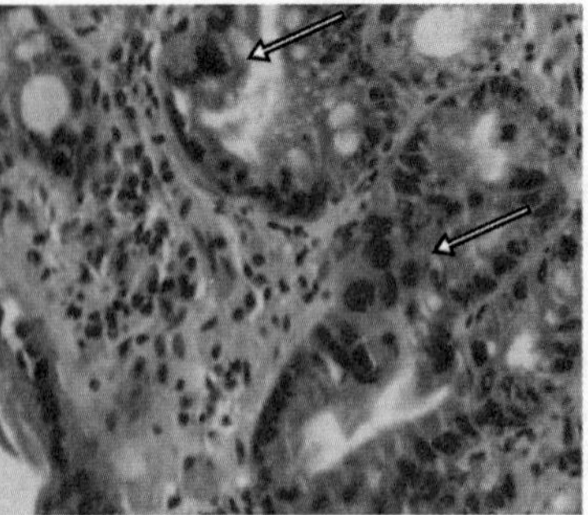

FIGURE 14-10
Histopathology of Barrett's metaplasia and Barrett's with high-grade dysplasia. H&E, hematoxylin and eosin.

further intervention. In addition to the high rate of progression to adenocarcinoma, there is also a high prevalence of unrecognized coexisting cancer with high-grade dysplasia. Nonetheless, treatment remains controversial. Esophagectomy, intensive endoscopic surveillance, and mucosal ablation have all been advocated. Currently, esophagectomy is the gold standard treatment for high-grade dysplasia in an otherwise healthy patient with minimal surgical risk. However, esophagectomy has a mortality ranging from 3–10%, along with substantial morbidity. That, along with increasing evidence of the effectiveness of endoscopic therapy with purpose-built radiofrequency ablation devices, has led many to favor this therapy as a preferable management strategy.

TREATMENT Gastroesophageal Reflux Disease (GERD)

Lifestyle modifications are routinely advocated as GERD therapy. Broadly speaking, these fall into three categories: (1) avoidance of foods that reduce LES pressure, making them "refluxogenic" (these commonly include fatty foods, alcohol, spearmint, peppermint, tomato-based foods, and possibly coffee and tea); (2) avoidance of acidic foods that are inherently irritating; and (3) adoption of behaviors to minimize reflux and/or heartburn. In general, minimal evidence supports the efficacy of these measures. However, clinical experience dictates that subsets of patients are benefitted by specific recommendations, based on their unique history and symptom profile. A patient with sleep disturbance from nighttime heartburn is likely to benefit from elevation of the head of the bed and avoidance of eating before retiring, but those recommendations are superfluous for a patient without nighttime symptoms. The most broadly applicable recommendation is for weight reduction. Even though the benefit with respect to reflux cannot be assured, the strong epidemiologic relationship between body mass index and GERD and the secondary health gains of weight reduction are beyond dispute.

The dominant pharmacologic approach to GERD management is with inhibitors of gastric acid secretion, and abundant data support the effectiveness of this approach. Pharmacologically reducing the acidity of gastric juice does not prevent reflux, but it ameliorates reflux symptoms and allows esophagitis to heal. The hierarchy of effectiveness among pharmaceuticals parallels their antisecretory potency. Proton pump inhibitors (PPIs) are more efficacious than histamine$_2$ receptor antagonists (H_2RAs), and both are superior to placebo. No major differences exist among PPIs, and only modest gain is achieved by increased dosage.

Paradoxically, the perceived frequency and severity of heartburn correlate poorly with the presence or severity of esophagitis. When GERD treatments are assessed in terms of resolving heartburn, both efficacy and differences among pharmaceuticals are less clear-cut than with the objective of healing esophagitis. Although the same overall hierarchy of effectiveness exists, observed efficacy rates are lower and vary widely, likely reflecting patient heterogeneity.

Reflux symptoms tend to be chronic, irrespective of esophagitis. Thus, a common management strategy is indefinite treatment with PPIs or H_2RAs as necessary for symptom control. The side effects of PPI therapy are generally minimal. Vitamin B_{12} and iron absorption may be compromised and susceptibility to enteric infections, particularly *Clostridium difficile* colitis, increased with treatment. Population studies have also suggested a slight increased risk of bone fracture with chronic PPI use suggesting an impairment of calcium absorption, but prospective studies have failed to corroborate this. Nonetheless, as with any medication, PPI dosage should be minimized to that necessary for the clinical indication.

Laparoscopic Nissen fundoplication, wherein the proximal stomach is wrapped around the distal esophagus to create an antireflux barrier, is a surgical alternative to the management of chronic GERD. Just as with PPI therapy, evidence on the utility of fundoplication is strongest for treating esophagitis, and controlled trials suggest similar efficacy to PPI therapy. However, the benefits of fundoplication must be weighed against potential deleterious effects, including surgical morbidity and mortality, postoperative dysphagia, failure or breakdown requiring reoperation, an inability to belch, and increased bloating, flatulence, and bowel symptoms after surgery.

EOSINOPHILIC ESOPHAGITIS

Eosinophilic esophagitis (EoE) is increasingly recognized in adults and children around the world. Current prevalence estimates identified 4–6 cases per 10,000 with a predilection for white males. The increasing prevalence of EoE is attributable to a combination of an increasing incidence and a growing recognition of the condition. There is also an incompletely understood, but important, overlap between EoE and GERD that confuses diagnosis of the disease.

EoE is diagnosed based on the combination of typical esophageal symptoms and esophageal mucosal biopsies demonstrating squamous epithelial eosinophil-predominant inflammation. Alternative etiologies of esophageal eosinophilia include GERD, drug hypersensitivity, connective tissue disorders, hypereosinophilic syndrome, and infection. Current evidence indicates that EoE is an immunologic disorder induced by antigen sensitization in susceptible individuals. Dietary factors play an important role in both the pathogenesis and treatment of EoE. Aeroallergens may also contribute, but the evidence is weaker. The natural history of EoE is unclear, but an increased risk of esophageal stricture development paralleling the duration of untreated disease has been noted.

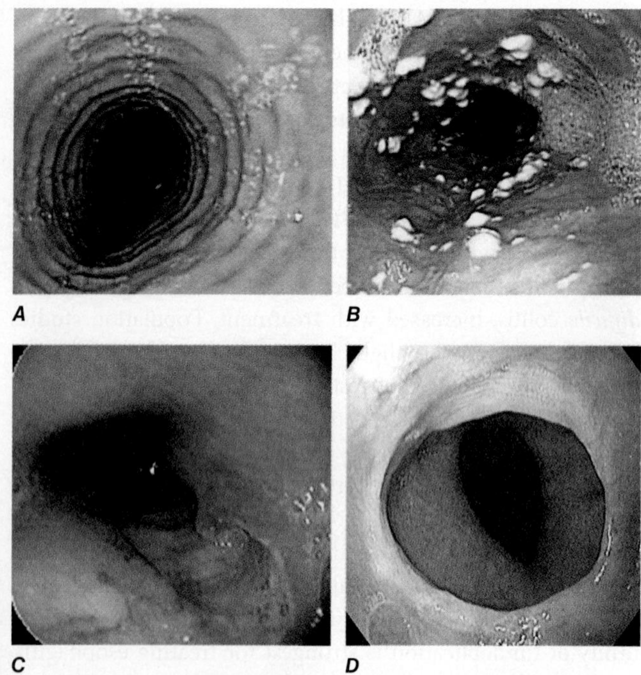

FIGURE 14-11
Endoscopic features of (*A*) eosinophilic esophagitis (EoE), (***B***) *Candida* esophagitis, (***C***) giant ulcer associated with HIV, and (***D***) a Schatzki ring.

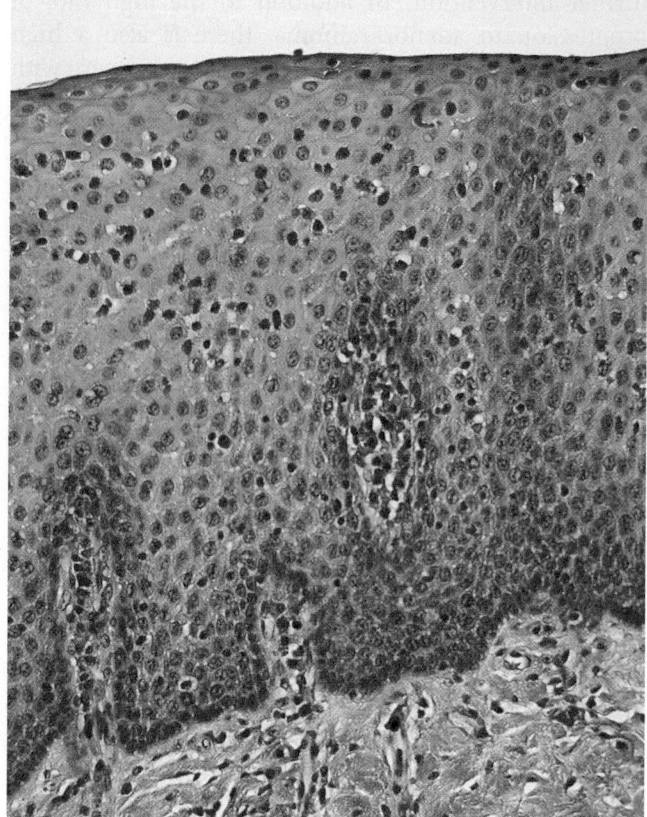

FIGURE 14-12
Histopathology of eosinophilic esophagitis (EoE) showing infiltration of the esophageal squamous epithelium with eosinophils. Additional features of basal cell hyperplasia and lamina propria fibrosis are present. Eosinophilic inflammation can also be seen with gastroesophageal reflux disease.

EoE should be strongly considered in children and adults with dysphagia and esophageal food impactions. In preadolescent children, symptom presentations of EoE include chest or abdominal pain, nausea, vomiting, and food aversion. Other symptoms in adults may include atypical chest pain and heartburn, particularly heartburn that is refractory to PPI therapy. An atopic history of food allergy, asthma, eczema, or allergic rhinitis is present in the majority of patients. Peripheral blood eosinophilia is demonstrable in up to 50% of patients, but the specificity of this finding is problematic in the setting of concomitant atopy. The characteristic endoscopic esophageal findings are loss of vascular markings (edema), multiple esophageal rings, longitudinally oriented furrows, and punctate exudate (Fig. 14-11). Histologic confirmation is made with the demonstration of esophageal mucosal eosinophilia (greatest density ±15 eosinophils per high-power field) (Fig. 14-12). Complications of EoE include esophageal stricture, narrow-caliber esophagus, food impaction, and esophageal perforation.

The goals of EoE management are symptom control and the prevention of complications. Once esophageal eosinophilia is demonstrated, patients typically undergo a trial of PPI therapy as a practical means of excluding a contribution of GERD to the esophageal mucosal inflammation. PPI-responsive esophageal eosinophilia, characterized by elimination of mucosal eosinophilia, occurs in 30–50% of cases of suspected EoE. Patients with persistent symptoms and eosinophilic inflammation following PPI therapy are subsequently considered for EoE treatments such as elimination diets or swallowed topical glucocorticoids. Elemental formula diets are a highly effective therapy that have primarily been studied in children but are limited by palatability. Notably, allergy testing by means of either serum IgE or skin prick testing has demonstrated poor sensitivity and specificity in the identification of foods that incite the esophageal inflammatory response. Allergy testing combining skin prick and atopy patch testing has been effective in children with EoE, but additional validation is needed. Empiric elimination of common food allergies (milk, wheat, egg, soy, nuts, and seafood) followed by systematic reintroduction has been an effective diet therapy in both children and adults with EoE. The intent of the elimination diet approach is the identification of a single food trigger or a small number of food triggers. Swallowed, topical glucocorticoids (fluticasone propionate or budesonide) are highly effective, but recurrence of disease is common following the cessation of therapy. Systemic glucocorticoids are reserved for severely afflicted patients refractory to less morbid treatments. Esophageal dilation is very effective at relieving dysphagia in patients with fibrostenosis. Dilation should be approached conservatively because of the risk of deep, esophageal mural laceration or perforation in the stiff-walled esophagus that is characteristic of the disease.

INFECTIOUS ESOPHAGITIS

With the increased use of immunosuppression for organ transplantation as well as chronic inflammatory diseases and chemotherapy along with the AIDS epidemic, infections with *Candida* species, herpesvirus, and cytomegalovirus (CMV) have become relatively common. Although rare, infectious esophagitis also occurs among the nonimmunocompromised, with herpes simplex and *Candida albicans* being the most common pathogens. Among AIDS patients, infectious esophagitis becomes more common as the CD4 count declines; cases are rare with a CD4 count >200 and common when <100. HIV itself may also be associated with a self-limited syndrome of acute esophageal ulceration with oral ulcers and a maculopapular skin rash at the time of seroconversion. Additionally, some patients with advanced disease have deep, persistent esophageal ulcers treated with oral glucocorticoids or thalidomide. However, with the widespread use of protease inhibitors, a reduction in these HIV complications has been noted.

Regardless of the infectious agent, odynophagia is a characteristic symptom of infectious esophagitis; dysphagia, chest pain, and hemorrhage are also common. Odynophagia is uncommon with reflux esophagitis, so its presence should always raise suspicion of an alternative etiology.

CANDIDA ESOPHAGITIS

Candida is normally found in the throat, but can become pathogenic and produce esophagitis in a compromised host; *C. albicans* is most common. *Candida* esophagitis also occurs with esophageal stasis secondary to esophageal motor disorders and diverticula. Patients complain of odynophagia and dysphagia. If oral thrush is present, empirical therapy is appropriate, but co-infection is common, and persistent symptoms should lead to prompt endoscopy with biopsy, which is the most useful diagnostic evaluation. *Candida* esophagitis has a characteristic appearance of white plaques with friability. Rarely, *Candida* esophagitis is complicated by bleeding, perforation, stricture, or systemic invasion. Oral fluconazole (200–400 mg on the first day, followed by 100–200 mg daily) for 14–21 days is the preferred treatment. Patients refractory to fluconazole may respond to itraconazole, voriconazole, or posaconazole. Alternatively, poorly responsive patients or those who cannot swallow medications can be treated with an intravenous echinocandin (caspofungin 50 mg daily for 7–21 days).

HERPETIC ESOPHAGITIS

Herpes simplex virus type 1 or 2 may cause esophagitis. Vesicles on the nose and lips may coexist and are suggestive of a herpetic etiology. Varicella-zoster virus can also cause esophagitis in children with chickenpox or adults with zoster. The characteristic endoscopic findings are vesicles and small, punched-out ulcerations. Because herpes simplex infections are limited to squamous epithelium, biopsies from the ulcer margins are most likely to reveal the characteristic ground-glass nuclei, eosinophilic Cowdry's type A inclusion bodies, and giant cells. Culture or polymerase chain reaction (PCR) assays are helpful to identify acyclovir-resistant strains. Acyclovir (200 mg orally five times a day for 7–10 days) can be used for immunocompetent hosts, although the disease is typically self-limited after a 1- to 2-week period in such patients. Immunocompromised patients are treated with acyclovir (400 mg orally five times a day for 14–21 days), famciclovir (500 mg orally three times a day), or valacyclovir (1 g orally three times a day). In patients with severe odynophagia, intravenous acyclovir, 5 mg/kg every 8 h for 7–14 days, reduces this morbidity.

CYTOMEGALOVIRUS

CMV esophagitis occurs primarily in immunocompromised patients, particularly organ transplant recipients. CMV is usually activated from a latent stage. Endoscopically, CMV lesions appear as serpiginous ulcers in an otherwise normal mucosa, particularly in the distal esophagus. Biopsies from the ulcer bases have the greatest diagnostic yield for finding the pathognomonic large nuclear or cytoplasmic inclusion bodies. Immunohistology with monoclonal antibodies to CMV and in situ hybridization tests are useful for early diagnosis. Data on therapy for CMV esophagitis are limited. Treatment studies of CMV gastrointestinal disease have demonstrated effectiveness of both ganciclovir (5 mg/kg every 12 h intravenously) and foscarnet (90 mg/kg every 12 h intravenously). Valganciclovir (900 mg two times a day), an oral formulation of ganciclovir, can also be used. Therapy is continued until healing, which may take 3–6 weeks. Maintenance therapy may be needed for patients with relapsing disease.

MECHANICAL TRAUMA AND IATROGENIC INJURY

ESOPHAGEAL PERFORATION

Most cases of esophageal perforation are from instrumentation of the esophagus or trauma. Alternatively, forceful vomiting or retching can lead to spontaneous rupture at the gastroesophageal junction (Boerhaave's syndrome). More rarely, corrosive esophagitis or neoplasms lead to perforation. Instrument perforation from endoscopy or nasogastric tube placement typically occurs in the hypopharynx or at the gastroesophageal junction. Perforation may also occur at the site of a stricture in the setting of endoscopic food disimpaction or esophageal dilation. Esophageal perforation causes pleuritic retrosternal pain that can be associated with pneumomediastinum and subcutaneous emphysema. Mediastinitis is a major complication of esophageal perforation, and prompt recognition is key to optimizing outcome. CT of the chest is most sensitive in detecting mediastinal air. Esophageal perforation is confirmed by a contrast swallow, usually Gastrografin followed by thin barium. Treatment includes nasogastric suction and parenteral broad-spectrum antibiotics with prompt surgical drainage and repair in noncontained leaks. Conservative therapy with NPO status and antibiotics without surgery may be appropriate in cases of contained perforation that are detected early. Endoscopic clipping or stent placement may be indicated in nonoperated iatrogenic perforations or nonoperable cases such as perforated tumors.

MALLORY-WEISS TEAR

Vomiting, retching, or vigorous coughing can cause a nontransmural tear at the gastroesophageal junction that is a common cause of upper gastrointestinal bleeding. Most patients present with hematemesis. Antecedent vomiting is anticipated but not always evident. Bleeding usually abates spontaneously, but protracted bleeding may respond to local epinephrine or cauterization therapy, endoscopic clipping, or angiographic embolization. Surgery is rarely needed.

RADIATION ESOPHAGITIS

Radiation esophagitis can complicate treatment for thoracic cancers, especially breast and lung, with the risk proportional to radiation dosage. Radiosensitizing drugs such as doxorubicin, bleomycin, cyclophosphamide, and cisplatin also increase the risk. Dysphagia and odynophagia may last weeks to months after therapy. The esophageal mucosa becomes erythematous, edematous, and friable. Submucosal fibrosis and degenerative tissue changes and stricturing may occur years after the radiation exposure. Radiation exposure in excess of 5000 cGy has been associated with increased risk of esophageal stricture. Treatment for acute radiation esophagitis is supportive. Chronic strictures are managed with esophageal dilation.

CORROSIVE ESOPHAGITIS

Caustic esophageal injury from ingestion of alkali or, less commonly, acid can be accidental or from attempted suicide. Absence of oral injury does not exclude possible esophageal involvement. Thus, early endoscopic evaluation is recommended to assess and grade the injury to the esophageal mucosa. Severe corrosive injury may lead to esophageal perforation, bleeding, stricture, and death. Glucocorticoids have not been shown to improve the clinical outcome of acute corrosive esophagitis and are not recommended. Healing of more severe grades of caustic injury is commonly associated with severe stricture formation and often requires repeated dilatation.

PILL ESOPHAGITIS

Pill-induced esophagitis occurs when a swallowed pill fails to traverse the entire esophagus and lodges within the lumen. Generally, this is attributed to poor "pill taking habits": inadequate liquid with the pill or lying down immediately after taking a pill. The most common location for the pill to lodge is in the mid-esophagus near the crossing of the aorta or carina. Extrinsic compression from these structures halts the movement of the pill or capsule. Since initially reported in 1970, more than 1000 cases of pill esophagitis have been reported, suggesting that this is not an unusual occurrence. A wide variety of medications are implicated with the most common being doxycycline, tetracycline, quinidine, phenytoin, potassium chloride, ferrous sulfate, nonsteroidal anti-inflammatory drugs (NSAIDs), and bisphosphonates. However, virtually any pill can result in pill esophagitis if taken carelessly.

Typical symptoms of pill esophagitis are the sudden onset of chest pain and odynophagia. Characteristically, the pain will develop over a period of hours or will awaken the individual from sleep. A classic history in the setting of ingestion of recognized pill offenders obviates the need for diagnostic testing in most patients. When endoscopy is performed, localized ulceration or inflammation is evident. Histologically, acute inflammation is typical. Chest CT imaging will sometimes reveal esophageal thickening consistent with transmural inflammation. Although the condition usually resolves within days to weeks, symptoms may persist for months and stricture can develop in severe cases. No specific therapy is known to hasten the healing process, but antisecretory medications are frequently prescribed to remove concomitant reflux as an aggravating factor. When healing results in stricture formation, dilation is indicated.

FOREIGN BODIES AND FOOD IMPACTION

Food or foreign bodies may lodge in the esophagus causing complete obstruction, which in turn can cause an inability to handle secretions (foaming at the mouth) and severe chest pain. Food impaction may occur due to stricture, carcinoma, Schatzki ring, eosinophilic esophagitis, or simply inattentive eating. If it does not spontaneously resolve, impacted food can be dislodged endoscopically. Use of meat tenderizer enzymes to facilitate passage of a meat bolus is discouraged because of potential esophageal injury. Glucagon (1 mg IV) is sometimes tried before endoscopic dislodgement. After emergent treatment, patients should be evaluated for potential causes of the impaction with treatment rendered as indicated.

ESOPHAGEAL MANIFESTATIONS OF SYSTEMIC DISEASE

SCLERODERMA AND COLLAGEN VASCULAR DISEASES

Scleroderma esophagus (hypotensive LES and absent esophageal peristalsis) was initially described as a manifestation of scleroderma or other collagen vascular diseases and thought to be specific for these disorders. However, this nomenclature subsequently proved unfortunate and has been discarded because an estimated half of qualifying patients do not have an identifiable systemic disease, and reflux disease is often the only identifiable association. When scleroderma esophagus occurs as a manifestation of a collagen vascular disease, the histopathologic findings are of infiltration and destruction of the esophageal muscularis propria with collagen deposition and fibrosis. The pathogenesis of absent peristalsis and LES hypotension in the absence of a collagen vascular disease is unknown. Regardless of the underlying cause, the manometric abnormalities predispose patients to severe GERD due to inadequate LES barrier function combined with poor esophageal clearance of refluxed acid. Dysphagia may also be manifest but is generally mild and alleviated by eating in an upright position and using liquids to facilitate solid emptying.

DERMATOLOGIC DISEASES

A host of dermatologic disorders (pemphigus vulgaris, bullous pemphigoid, cicatricial pemphigoid, Behçet's syndrome, and epidermolysis bullosa) can affect the oropharynx and esophagus, particularly the proximal esophagus with blisters, bullae, webs, and strictures. Glucocorticoid treatment is usually effective. Erosive lichen planus, Stevens-Johnson syndrome, and graft-versus-host disease can also involve the esophagus. Esophageal dilatation may be necessary to treat strictures.

CHAPTER 15

PEPTIC ULCER DISEASE AND RELATED DISORDERS

John Del Valle

PEPTIC ULCER DISEASE

Burning epigastric pain exacerbated by fasting and improved with meals is a symptom complex associated with peptic ulcer disease (PUD). An *ulcer* is defined as disruption of the mucosal integrity of the stomach and/or duodenum leading to a local defect or excavation due to active inflammation. Ulcers occur within the stomach and/or duodenum and are often chronic in nature. Acid peptic disorders are very common in the United States, with 4 million individuals (new cases and recurrences) affected per year. Lifetime prevalence of PUD in the United States is ~12% in men and 10% in women. PUD significantly affects quality of life by impairing overall patient well-being and contributing substantially to work absenteeism. Moreover, an estimated 15,000 deaths per year occur as a consequence of complicated PUD. The financial impact of these common disorders has been substantial, with an estimated burden on direct and indirect health care costs of ~$6 billion per year in the United States, with $3 billion spent on hospitalizations, $2 billion on physician office visits, and $1 billion in decreased productivity and days lost from work.

GASTRIC PHYSIOLOGY

Despite the constant attack on the gastroduodenal mucosa by a host of noxious agents (acid, pepsin, bile acids, pancreatic enzymes, drugs, and bacteria), integrity is maintained by an intricate system that provides mucosal defense and repair.

Gastric anatomy

The gastric epithelial lining consists of rugae that contain microscopic gastric pits, each branching into four or five gastric glands made up of highly specialized epithelial cells. The makeup of gastric glands varies with their anatomic location. Glands within the gastric cardia comprise <5% of the gastric gland area and contain mucous and endocrine cells. The 75% of gastric glands are found within the oxyntic mucosa and contain mucous neck, parietal, chief, endocrine, enterochromaffin, and enterochromaffin-like (ECL) cells (Fig. 15-1). Pyloric glands contain mucous and endocrine cells (including gastrin cells) and are found in the antrum.

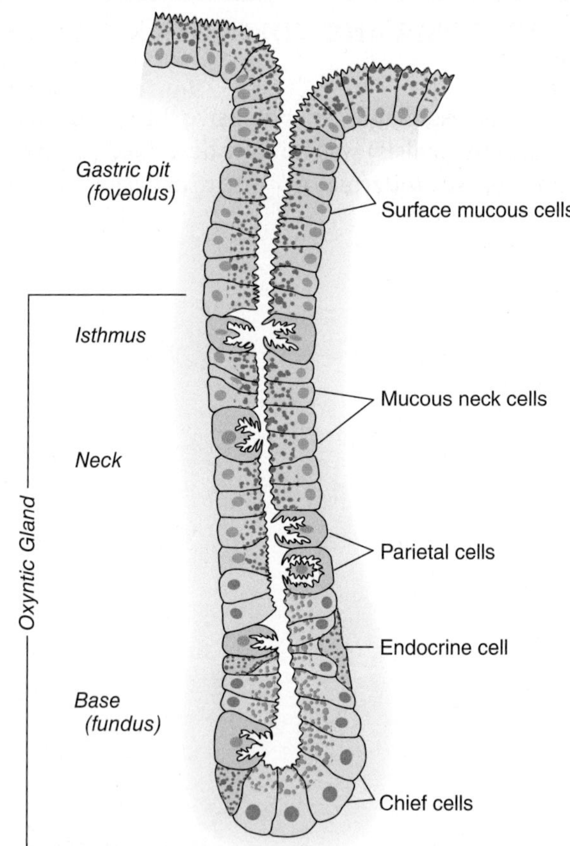

FIGURE 15-1

Diagrammatic representation of the oxyntic gastric gland. *(Adapted from S Ito, RJ Winchester: J Cell Biol 16:541, 1963. doi:10.1083/jcb.16.3.541. © 1963 Ito and Winchester.)*

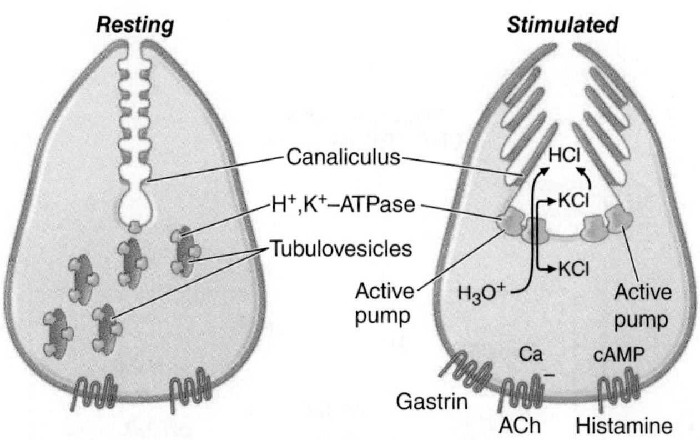

FIGURE 15-2
Gastric parietal cell undergoing transformation after secretagogue-mediated stimulation. cAMP, cyclic adenosine monophosphate. *(Adapted from SJ Hersey, G Sachs: Physiol Rev 75:155, 1995.)*

The parietal cell, also known as the oxyntic cell, is usually found in the neck, or isthmus, or in the oxyntic gland. The resting, or unstimulated, parietal cell has prominent cytoplasmic tubulovesicles and intracellular canaliculi containing short microvilli along its apical surface (Fig. 15-2). H^+,K^+-adenosine triphosphatase (ATPase) is expressed in the tubulovesicle membrane; upon cell stimulation, this membrane, along with apical membranes, transforms into a dense network of apical intracellular canaliculi containing long microvilli. Acid secretion, a process requiring high energy, occurs at the apical canalicular surface. Numerous mitochondria (30–40% of total cell volume) generate the energy required for secretion.

Gastroduodenal mucosal defense

The gastric epithelium is under constant assault by a series of endogenous noxious factors, including hydrochloric acid (HCl), pepsinogen/pepsin, and bile salts. In addition, a steady flow of exogenous substances such as medications, alcohol, and bacteria encounter the gastric mucosa. A highly intricate biologic system is in place to provide defense from mucosal injury and to repair any injury that may occur.

The mucosal defense system can be envisioned as a three-level barrier, composed of preepithelial, epithelial, and subepithelial elements (Fig. 15-3). The first line of defense is a mucus-bicarbonate-phospholipid layer, which serves as a physicochemical barrier to multiple molecules, including hydrogen ions. Mucus is secreted in a regulated fashion by gastroduodenal surface epithelial cells. It consists primarily of water (95%) and a mixture of phospholipids and glycoproteins (mucin). The mucous gel functions as a nonstirred water layer impeding diffusion of ions and molecules such as pepsin. Bicarbonate, secreted in a regulated manner by surface epithelial cells of the gastroduodenal mucosa into the mucous gel, forms a pH gradient ranging from 1 to 2 at the gastric luminal surface and reaching 6 to 7 along the epithelial cell surface.

Surface epithelial cells provide the next line of defense through several factors, including mucus production, epithelial cell ionic transporters that maintain intracellular pH and bicarbonate production, and intracellular tight junctions. Surface epithelial cells generate heat shock proteins that prevent protein denaturation and protect cells from certain factors such as increased temperature, cytotoxic agents, or oxidative stress. Epithelial cells also generate trefoil factor family peptides and cathelicidins, which also play a role in surface cell protection and regeneration. If the preepithelial barrier were breached, gastric epithelial cells bordering a site of injury can migrate to restore a damaged region (*restitution*). This process occurs independent of cell division and requires uninterrupted blood flow and an alkaline pH in the surrounding environment. Several growth factors, including epidermal growth factor (EGF), transforming growth factor (TGF) α, and basic fibroblast growth factor (FGF), modulate the process of restitution. Larger defects that are not effectively repaired by restitution require cell proliferation. Epithelial cell regeneration is regulated by prostaglandins and growth factors such as EGF and TGF-α. In tandem with epithelial cell renewal, formation of new vessels (*angiogenesis*) within the injured microvascular bed occurs. Both FGF and vascular endothelial growth factor (VEGF) are important in regulating angiogenesis in the gastric mucosa.

An elaborate microvascular system within the gastric submucosal layer is the key component of the subepithelial defense/repair system, providing HCO_3^-, which neutralizes the acid generated by the parietal cell. Moreover, this microcirculatory bed provides an adequate supply of micronutrients and oxygen while removing toxic metabolic by-products.

Prostaglandins play a central role in gastric epithelial defense/repair (Fig. 15-4). The gastric mucosa contains abundant levels of prostaglandins that regulate the release of mucosal bicarbonate and mucus, inhibit parietal cell secretion, and are important in maintaining mucosal blood flow and epithelial cell restitution. Prostaglandins are derived from esterified arachidonic acid, which is formed from phospholipids (cell membrane) by the action of phospholipase A_2. A key enzyme that controls the rate-limiting step in prostaglandin synthesis is cyclooxygenase (COX), which is present in two isoforms (COX-1, COX-2), each having distinct characteristics regarding structure, tissue distribution, and expression. COX-1 is expressed in a host of tissues, including the stomach, platelets, kidneys, and endothelial cells. This isoform is expressed in a constitutive manner and plays an important role in maintaining the integrity of renal function, platelet aggregation,

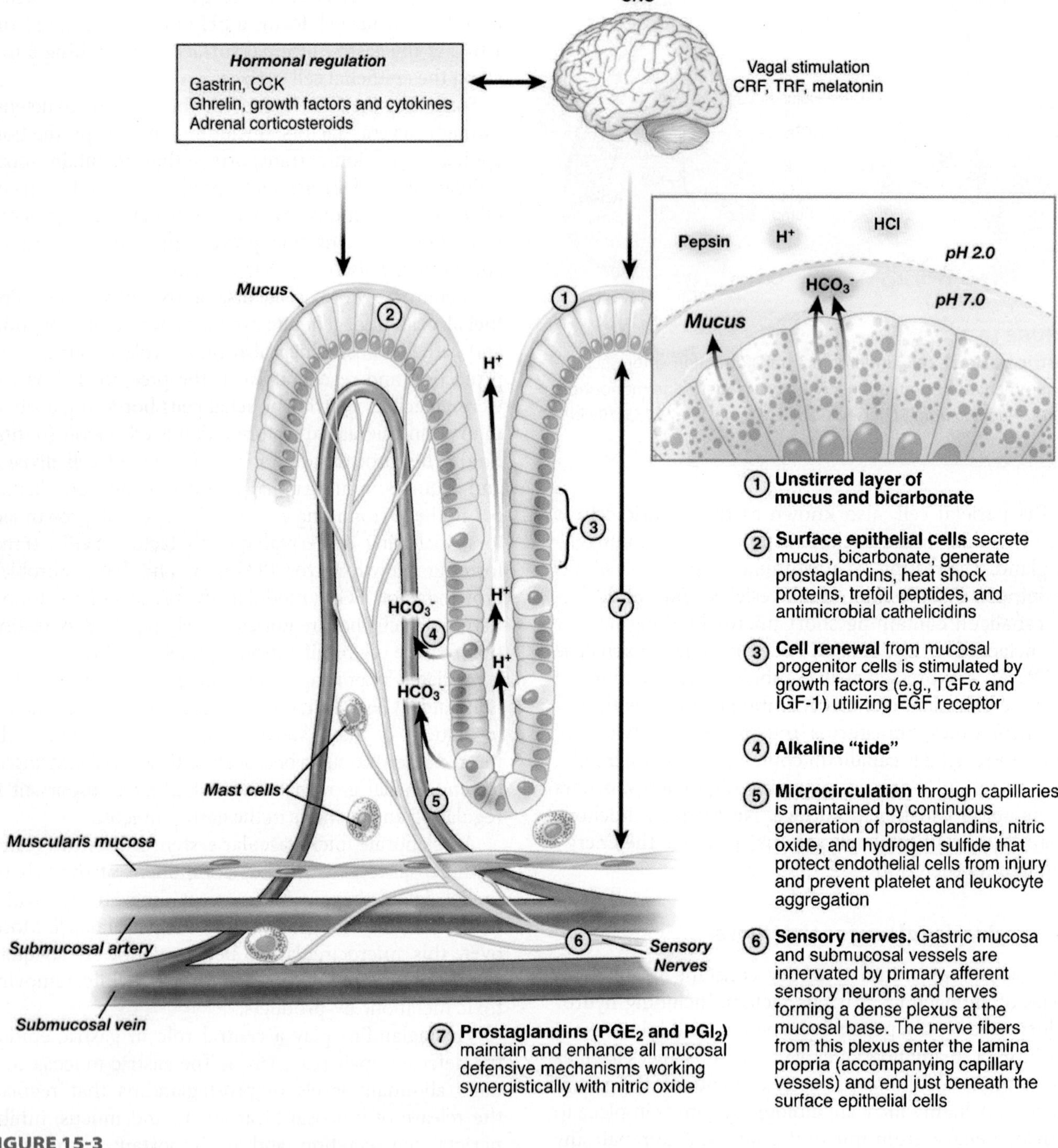

CNS
Hormonal regulation
Gastrin, CCK
Ghrelin, growth factors and cytokines
Adrenal corticosteroids
Vagal stimulation
CRF, TRF, melatonin
Pepsin
H+
HCl
pH 2.0
HCO3-
pH 7.0
Mucus
Mucus
H+
H+
H+
HCO3-
HCO3-
Mast cells
Muscularis mucosa
Submucosal artery
Submucosal vein
Sensory Nerves
1 Unstirred layer of mucus and bicarbonate
2 Surface epithelial cells secrete mucus, bicarbonate, generate prostaglandins, heat shock proteins, trefoil peptides, and antimicrobial cathelicidins
3 Cell renewal from mucosal progenitor cells is stimulated by growth factors (e.g., TGFα and IGF-1) utilizing EGF receptor
4 Alkaline "tide"
5 Microcirculation through capillaries is maintained by continuous generation of prostaglandins, nitric oxide, and hydrogen sulfide that protect endothelial cells from injury and prevent platelet and leukocyte aggregation
6 Sensory nerves. Gastric mucosa and submucosal vessels are innervated by primary afferent sensory neurons and nerves forming a dense plexus at the mucosal base. The nerve fibers from this plexus enter the lamina propria (accompanying capillary vessels) and end just beneath the surface epithelial cells
7 Prostaglandins (PGE2 and PGI2) maintain and enhance all mucosal defensive mechanisms working synergistically with nitric oxide

FIGURE 15-3

Components involved in providing gastroduodenal mucosal defense and repair. CCK, cholecystokinin; CRF, corticotropin-releasing factor; EGF, epidermal growth factor; HCl, hydrochloride; IGF, insulin-like growth factor; TGFα, transforming growth factor α; TRF, thyrotropin releasing factor. *(Modified and updated from Tarnawski A. Cellular and molecular mechanisms of mucosal defense and repair. In: Yoshikawa T, Arakawa T. Bioregulation and Its Disorders in the Gastrointestinal Tract. Tokyo, Japan: Blackwell Science, 1998:3–17.)*

and gastrointestinal (GI) mucosal integrity. In contrast, the expression of COX-2 is inducible by inflammatory stimuli, and it is expressed in macrophages, leukocytes, fibroblasts, and synovial cells. The beneficial effects of nonsteroidal anti-inflammatory drugs (NSAIDs) on tissue inflammation are due to inhibition of COX-2; the toxicity of these drugs (e.g., GI mucosal ulceration and renal dysfunction) is related to inhibition of the COX-1 isoform. The highly COX-2–selective NSAIDs have the potential to provide the beneficial effect of

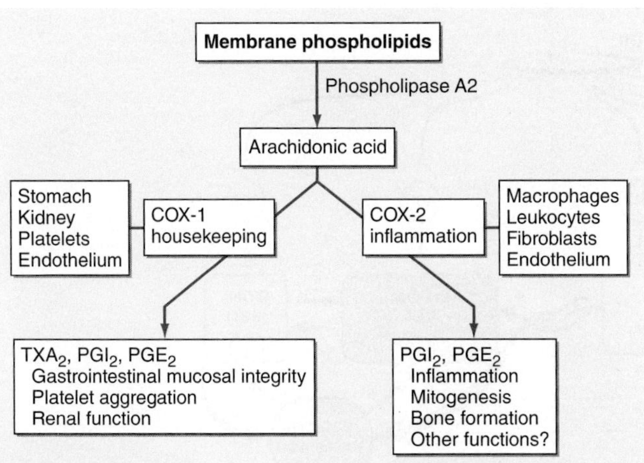

FIGURE 15-4

Schematic representation of the steps involved in synthesis of prostaglandin E_2 (PGE$_2$) and prostacyclin (PGI$_2$). Characteristics and distribution of the cyclooxygenase (COX) enzymes 1 and 2 are also shown. TXA$_2$, thromboxane A_2.

decreasing tissue inflammation while minimizing toxicity in the GI tract. Selective COX-2 inhibitors have had adverse effects on the cardiovascular system, leading to increased risk of myocardial infarction. Therefore, the U.S. Food and Drug Administration (FDA) has removed two of these agents (valdecoxib and rofecoxib) from the market (see below).

Nitric oxide (NO) is important in the maintenance of gastric mucosal integrity. The key enzyme NO synthase is constitutively expressed in the mucosa and contributes to cytoprotection by stimulating gastric mucus, increasing mucosal blood flow, and maintaining epithelial cell barrier function. The central nervous system (CNS) and hormonal factors also play a role in regulating mucosal defense through multiple pathways (Fig. 15-3).

Physiology of gastric secretion

Hydrochloric acid and pepsinogen are the two principal gastric secretory products capable of inducing mucosal injury. Gastric acid and pepsinogen play a physiologic role in protein digestion; absorption of iron, calcium, magnesium, and vitamin B_{12}; and killing ingested bacteria. Acid secretion should be viewed as occurring under basal and stimulated conditions. Basal acid production occurs in a circadian pattern, with highest levels occurring during the night and lowest levels during the morning hours. Cholinergic input via the vagus nerve and histaminergic input from local gastric sources are the principal contributors to basal acid secretion. Stimulated gastric acid secretion occurs primarily in three phases based on the site where the signal originates (cephalic, gastric, and intestinal). Sight, smell, and taste of food are the components of the cephalic phase, which stimulates gastric secretion via the vagus nerve. The gastric phase is activated once food enters the stomach. This component of secretion is driven by nutrients (amino acids and amines) that directly stimulate the G cell to release gastrin, which in turn activates the parietal cell via direct and indirect mechanisms. Distention of the stomach wall also leads to gastrin release and acid production. The last phase of gastric acid secretion is initiated as food enters the intestine and is mediated by luminal distention and nutrient assimilation. A series of pathways that inhibit gastric acid production are also set into motion during these phases. The GI hormone somatostatin is released from endocrine cells found in the gastric mucosa (D cells) in response to HCl. Somatostatin can inhibit acid production by both direct (parietal cell) and indirect mechanisms (decreased histamine release from ECL cells and gastrin release from G cells). Additional neural (central and peripheral) and humoral (amylin, atrial natriuretic peptide [ANP], cholecystokinin, ghrelin, interleukin 11 [IL-11], obestatin, secretin, and serotonin) factors play a role in counterbalancing acid secretion. Under physiologic circumstances, these phases occur simultaneously. Ghrelin, the appetite-regulating hormone expressed in Gr cells in the stomach, may increase gastric acid secretion through stimulation of histamine release from ECL cells, but this remains to be confirmed.

The acid-secreting parietal cell is located in the oxyntic gland, adjacent to other cellular elements (ECL cell, D cell) important in the gastric secretory process (Fig. 15-5). This unique cell also secretes intrinsic factor (IF) and IL-11. The parietal cell expresses receptors for several stimulants of acid secretion, including histamine (H_2), gastrin (cholecystokinin B/gastrin receptor), and acetylcholine (muscarinic, M_3). Binding of histamine to the H_2 receptor leads to activation of adenylate cyclase and an increase in cyclic adenosine monophosphate (AMP). Activation of the gastrin and muscarinic receptors results in activation of the protein kinase C/phosphoinositide signaling pathway. Each of these signaling pathways in turn regulates a series of downstream kinase cascades that control the acid-secreting pump, H^+,K^+-ATPase. The discovery that different ligands and their corresponding receptors lead to activation of different signaling pathways explains the potentiation of acid secretion that occurs when histamine and gastrin or acetylcholine are combined. More importantly, this observation explains why blocking one receptor type (H_2) decreases acid secretion stimulated by agents that activate a different pathway (gastrin, acetylcholine). Parietal cells also express receptors for ligands that inhibit acid production (prostaglandins, somatostatin, and EGF). Histamine also stimulates gastric acid secretion indirectly by activating the histamine H_3 receptor on D-cells, which inhibits somatostatin release.

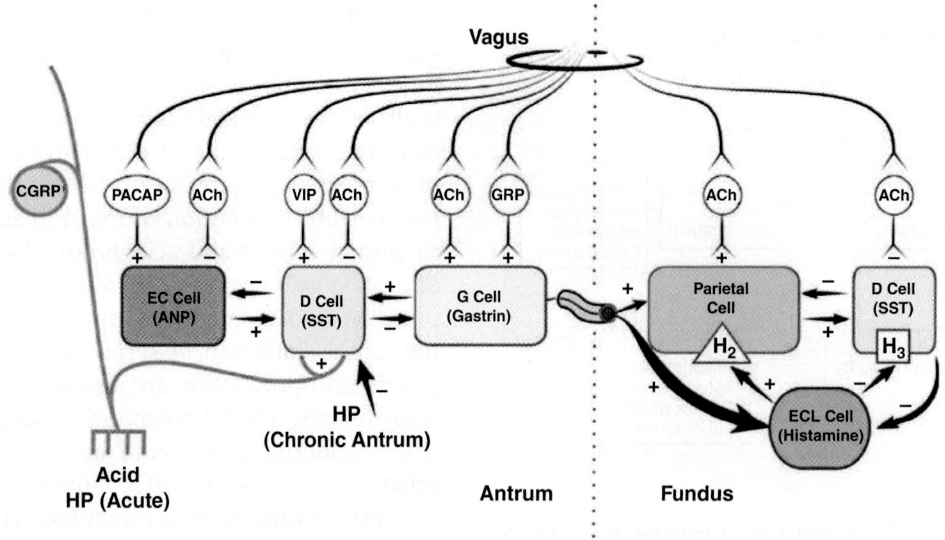

FIGURE 15-5

Regulation of gastric acid secretion at the cellular level. ACh, acetylcholine; ANP, atrial natriuretic peptide; CGRP, calcitonin gene-related peptide; EC, enterochromaffin; ECL, enterochromaffin-like; GRP, gastrin-releasing peptide; PACAP, pituitary adenylate-cyclase activating peptide; SST, somatostatin; VIP, vasoactive intestinal peptide.

The enzyme H^+,K^+-ATPase is responsible for generating the large concentration of H^+. It is a membrane-bound protein that consists of two subunits, α and β. The active catalytic site is found within the α subunit; the function of the β subunit is unclear. This enzyme uses the chemical energy of adenosine triphosphate (ATP) to transfer H^+ ions from parietal cell cytoplasm to the secretory canaliculi in exchange for K^+. The H^+,K^+-ATPase is located within the secretory canaliculus and in nonsecretory cytoplasmic tubulovesicles. The tubulovesicles are impermeable to K^+, which leads to an inactive pump in this location. The distribution of pumps between the nonsecretory vesicles and the secretory canaliculus varies according to parietal cell activity (Fig. 15-2). Proton pumps are recycled back to the inactive state in cytoplasmic vesicles once parietal cell activation ceases. Small G proteins of the Rab family and secretory carrier membrane proteins (SCAMPS) are postulated to participate in parietal cell membrane translocation. In addition, acid secretion requires a number of apical and basolateral parietal cell membrane chloride and potassium channels.

The chief cell, found primarily in the gastric fundus, synthesizes and secretes pepsinogen, the inactive precursor of the proteolytic enzyme pepsin. The acid environment within the stomach leads to cleavage of the inactive precursor to pepsin and provides the low pH (<2) required for pepsin activity. Pepsin activity is significantly diminished at a pH of 4 and irreversibly inactivated and denatured at a pH of ≥7. Many of the secretagogues that stimulate acid secretion also stimulate pepsinogen release. The precise role of pepsin in the pathogenesis of PUD remains to be established.

PATHOPHYSIOLOGIC BASIS OF PEPTIC ULCER DISEASE

PUD encompasses both gastric and duodenal ulcers. *Ulcers* are defined as breaks in the mucosal surface >5 mm in size, with depth to the submucosa. Duodenal ulcers (DUs) and gastric ulcers (GUs) share many common features in terms of pathogenesis, diagnosis, and treatment, but several factors distinguish them from one another. *Helicobacter pylori* and NSAIDs are the most common risk factors for PUD, with estimated odds ratios in the United States of 3.7 and 3.3, respectively. Additional risk factors (odds ratio) include chronic obstructive lung disease (2.34), chronic renal insufficiency (2.29), current tobacco use (1.99), former tobacco use (1.55), older age (1.67), three or more doctor visits in a year (1.49), coronary heart disease (1.46), former alcohol use (1.29), African-American race (1.20), obesity (1.18), and diabetes (1.13). The mechanisms by which some of these risk factors lead to ulcer disease are highlighted below.

Epidemiology

Duodenal ulcers

DUs are estimated to occur in 6–15% of the Western population. The incidence of DUs declined steadily from 1960 to 1980 and has remained stable since then. The death rates, need for surgery, and physician visits have decreased by >50% over the past 30 years. The reason for the reduction in the frequency of DUs is likely related to the decreasing frequency of *H. pylori*. Before the discovery of *H. pylori*, the natural history of DUs was typified by frequent recurrences after initial therapy. Eradication of *H. pylori* has greatly reduced these recurrence rates.

Gastric ulcers

GUs tend to occur later in life than duodenal lesions, with a peak incidence reported in the sixth decade. More than one-half of GUs occur in males and are less common than DUs, perhaps due to the higher likelihood of GUs being silent and presenting only after a complication develops. Autopsy studies suggest a similar incidence of DUs and GUs.

Pathology

Duodenal ulcers

DUs occur most often in the first portion of the duodenum (>95%), with ~90% located within 3 cm of the pylorus. They are usually ≤1 cm in diameter but can occasionally reach 3–6 cm (giant ulcer). Ulcers are sharply demarcated, with depth at times reaching the muscularis propria. The base of the ulcer often consists of a zone of eosinophilic necrosis with surrounding fibrosis. Malignant DUs are extremely rare.

Gastric ulcers

In contrast to DUs, GUs can represent a malignancy and should be biopsied upon discovery. Benign GUs are most often found distal to the junction between the antrum and the acid secretory mucosa. Benign GUs are quite rare in the gastric fundus and are histologically similar to DUs. Benign GUs associated with *H. pylori* are also associated with antral gastritis. In contrast, NSAID-related GUs are not accompanied by chronic active gastritis but may instead have evidence of a chemical gastropathy, typified by foveolar hyperplasia, edema of the lamina propria, and epithelial regeneration in the absence of *H. pylori.* Extension of smooth-muscle fibers into the upper portions of the mucosa, where they are not typically found, may also occur.

Pathophysiology

Duodenal ulcers

H. pylori and NSAID-induced injury account for the majority of DUs. Many acid secretory abnormalities have been described in DU patients. Of these, average basal and nocturnal gastric acid secretion appears to be increased in DU patients as compared to controls; however, the level of overlap between DU patients and control subjects is substantial. The reason for this altered secretory process is unclear, but *H. pylori* infection may contribute. Bicarbonate secretion is significantly decreased in the duodenal bulb of patients with an active DU as compared to control subjects. *H. pylori* infection may also play a role in this process (see below).

Gastric ulcers

As in DUs, the majority of GUs can be attributed to either *H. pylori* or NSAID-induced mucosal damage. GUs that occur in the prepyloric area or those in the body associated with a DU or a duodenal scar are similar in pathogenesis to DUs. Gastric acid output (basal and stimulated) tends to be normal or decreased in GU patients. When GUs develop in the presence of minimal acid levels, impairment of mucosal defense factors may be present. GUs have been classified based on their location: Type I occur in the gastric body and tend to be associated with low gastric acid production; type II occur in the antrum and gastric acid can vary from low to normal; type III occur within 3 cm of the pylorus and are commonly accompanied by DUs and normal or high gastric acid production; and type IV are found in the cardia and are associated with low gastric acid production.

H. Pylori and acid peptic disorders

Gastric infection with the bacterium *H. pylori* accounts for the majority of PUD **(Chap. 27)**. This organism also plays a role in the development of gastric mucosa-associated lymphoid tissue (MALT) lymphoma and gastric adenocarcinoma. Although the entire genome of *H. pylori* has been sequenced, it is still not clear how this organism, which resides in the stomach, causes ulceration in the duodenum, or whether its eradication will lead to a decrease in gastric cancer.

The bacterium

The bacterium, initially named *Campylobacter pyloridis,* is a gram-negative microaerophilic rod found most commonly in the deeper portions of the mucous gel coating the gastric mucosa or between the mucous layer and the gastric epithelium. It may attach to gastric epithelium but under normal circumstances does not appear to invade cells. It is strategically designed to live within the aggressive environment of the stomach. It is S-shaped (~0.5–3 μm in size) and contains multiple sheathed flagella. Initially, *H. pylori* resides in the antrum but, over time, migrates toward the more proximal segments of the stomach. The organism is capable of transforming into a coccoid form, which represents a dormant state that may facilitate survival in adverse conditions. The genome of *H. pylori* (1.65 million base pairs) encodes ~1500 proteins. Among this multitude of proteins there are factors that are essential determinants of *H. pylori*–mediated pathogenesis and colonization such as the outer membrane protein (Hop proteins), urease, and the vacuolating cytotoxin (Vac A). Moreover, the majority of *H. pylori* strains contain a genomic fragment that encodes the cag pathogenicity island (cag-PAI). Several of the genes that make up cag-PAI encode components of a type IV secretion island that translocates Cag A into host cells. Once in the cell, Cag A activates a series of cellular events important in cell growth and cytokine production. *H. pylori* also has extensive genetic diversity that in turn enhances its ability to promote disease. The first step in infection by *H. pylori* is dependent on the bacteria's motility and its ability to produce urease. Urease produces ammonia from urea, an essential step in alkalinizing the surrounding pH. Additional bacterial factors include catalase, lipase, adhesins, platelet-activating factor, and pic B (induces cytokines). Multiple strains of *H. pylori* exist and are characterized by their ability to express several of these factors (Cag A, Vac A, etc.). It is possible that the different diseases related to *H. pylori* infection can be attributed to different strains of the organism with distinct pathogenic features.

Epidemiology

The prevalence of *H. pylori* varies throughout the world and depends largely on the overall standard of living in the region. In developing parts of the world, 80% of the population may be infected by the age of 20, whereas the prevalence is 20–50% in industrialized countries. In contrast, in the United States this organism is rare in childhood. The overall prevalence of *H. pylori* in the United States is ~30%, with individuals born before 1950 having a higher rate of infection than those born later. About 10% of Americans <30 years of age are colonized with the bacteria. The rate of infection with *H. pylori* in industrialized countries has decreased substantially in recent decades. The steady increase in the prevalence of *H. pylori* noted with increasing age is due primarily to a cohort effect, reflecting higher transmission during a period in which the earlier cohorts were children. It has been calculated through mathematical models that improved sanitation during the latter half of the nineteenth century dramatically decreased transmission of *H. pylori*. Moreover, with the present rate of intervention, the organism will be ultimately eliminated from the United States. Two factors that predispose to higher colonization rates include poor socioeconomic status and less education. These factors, not race, are responsible for the rate of *H. pylori* infection in blacks and Hispanic Americans being double the rate seen in whites of comparable age. Other risk factors for *H. pylori* infection are (1) birth or residence in a developing country, (2) domestic crowding, (3) unsanitary living conditions, (4) unclean food or water, and (5) exposure to gastric contents of an infected individual.

Transmission of *H. pylori* occurs from person to person, following an oral-oral or fecal-oral route. The risk of *H. pylori* infection is declining in developing countries. The rate of infection in the United States has fallen by >50% when compared to 30 years ago.

Pathophysiology

H. pylori infection is virtually always associated with a chronic active gastritis, but only 10–15% of infected individuals develop frank peptic ulceration. The basis for this difference is unknown, but is likely due to a combination of host and bacterial factors some of which are outlined below. Initial studies suggested that >90% of all DUs were associated with *H. pylori*, but *H. pylori* is present in only 30–60% of individuals with GUs and 50–70% of patients with DUs. The pathophysiology of ulcers not associated with *H. pylori* or NSAID ingestion (or the rare Zollinger-Ellison syndrome [ZES]) is becoming more relevant as the incidence of *H. pylori* is dropping, particularly in the Western world (see below).

The particular end result of *H. pylori* infection (gastritis, PUD, gastric MALT lymphoma, gastric cancer) is determined by a complex interplay between bacterial and host factors (Fig. 15-6).

1. *Bacterial factors: H. pylori* is able to facilitate gastric residence, induce mucosal injury, and avoid host defense. Different strains of *H. pylori* produce different virulence factors. A specific region of the bacterial genome, the pathogenicity island (cag-PAI), encodes the virulence factors Cag A and pic B. Vac A also contributes to pathogenicity, although it is not encoded within the pathogenicity island. These virulence factors, in conjunction with additional bacterial constituents, can cause mucosal damage, in part through their ability to target the host immune cells. For example, Vac A targets human CD4 T cells, inhibiting their proliferation and in addition can disrupt normal function of B cells, CD8 T cells, macrophages, and mast cells. Multiple studies have demonstrated that *H. pylori* strains that are cag-PAI positive are associated with a higher risk of PUD, premalignant gastric lesions, and gastric cancer than are strains that lack the cag-PAI. In addition, *H. pylori* may directly inhibit

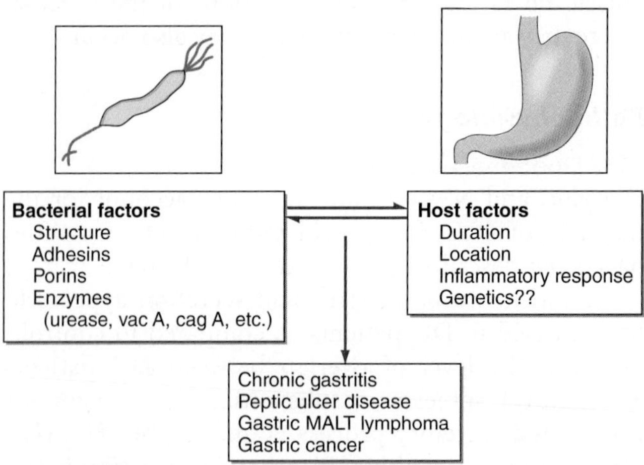

FIGURE 15-6
Outline of the bacterial and host factors important in determining *H. pylori*–induced gastrointestinal disease. MALT, mucosal-associated lymphoid tissue.

parietal cell H^+,K^+-ATPase activity through a Cag A–dependent mechanism, leading in part to the low acid production observed after acute infection with the organism. Urease, which allows the bacteria to reside in the acidic stomach, generates NH_3, which can damage epithelial cells. The bacteria produce surface factors that are chemotactic for neutrophils and monocytes, which in turn contribute to epithelial cell injury (see below). *H. pylori* makes proteases and phospholipases that break down the glycoprotein lipid complex of the mucous gel, thus reducing the efficacy of this first line of mucosal defense. *H. pylori* expresses adhesins (OMPs like BabA), which facilitate attachment of the bacteria to gastric epithelial cells. Although lipopolysaccharide (LPS) of gram-negative bacteria often plays an important role in the infection, *H. pylori* LPS has low immunologic activity compared to that of other organisms. It may promote a smoldering chronic inflammation.

2. *Host factors:* Studies in twins suggest that there may be genetic predisposition to acquire *H. pylori.* The inflammatory response to *H. pylori* includes recruitment of neutrophils, lymphocytes (T and B), macrophages, and plasma cells. The pathogen leads to local injury by binding to class II major histocompatibility complex (MHC) molecules expressed on gastric epithelial cells, leading to cell death (*apoptosis*). Moreover, bacterial strains that encode cag-PAI can introduce Cag A into the host cells, leading to further cell injury and activation of cellular pathways involved in cytokine production and repression of tumor-suppressor genes. Elevated concentrations of multiple cytokines are found in the gastric epithelium of *H. pylori*–infected individuals, including interleukin (IL) 1α/β, IL-2, IL-6, IL-8, tumor necrosis factor (TNF) α, and interferon (IFN) γ. *H. pylori* infection also leads to both a mucosal and a systemic humoral response, which does not lead to eradication of the bacteria but further compounds epithelial cell injury. Additional mechanisms by which *H. pylori* may cause epithelial cell injury include (1) activated neutrophil-mediated production of reactive oxygen or nitrogen species and enhanced epithelial cell turnover and (2) apoptosis related to interaction with T cells (T helper 1, or T_H1, cells) and IFN-γ. Finally, the human stomach can be colonized by a host of commensal organisms that may affect the likelihood of *H. pylori*–mediated mucosal injury.

The reason for *H. pylori*–mediated duodenal ulceration remains unclear. Studies suggest that *H. pylori* associated with duodenal ulceration may be more virulent. In addition, certain specific bacterial factors such as the DU-promoting gene A (*dupA*), may be associated with the development of DUs. Another potential contributing factor is that gastric metaplasia in the duodenum of DU patients, which may be due to high acid exposure (see below), permits *H. pylori* to bind to it and produce local injury secondary to the host response. Another hypothesis is that *H. pylori* antral infection could lead to increased acid production, increased duodenal acid, and mucosal injury. Basal and stimulated (meal, gastrin-releasing peptide [GRP]) gastrin release are increased in *H. pylori*–infected individuals, and somatostatin-secreting D cells may be decreased. *H. pylori* infection might induce increased acid secretion through both direct and indirect actions of *H. pylori* and proinflammatory cytokines (IL-8, TNF, and IL-1) on G, D, and parietal cells (Fig. 15-7). GUs, in contrast, are associated with *H. pylori*–induced pangastritis and normal or low gastric acid secretion. *H. pylori* infection has also been associated with decreased duodenal mucosal bicarbonate production. Data supporting and contradicting each of these interesting theories have been demonstrated. Thus, the mechanism by which *H. pylori* infection of the stomach leads to duodenal ulceration remains to be established.

In summary, the final effect of *H. pylori* on the GI tract is variable and determined by microbial and host factors. The type and distribution of gastritis correlate with the ultimate gastric and duodenal pathology observed. Specifically, the presence of antral-predominant gastritis is associated with DU formation; gastritis involving primarily the corpus predisposes to the

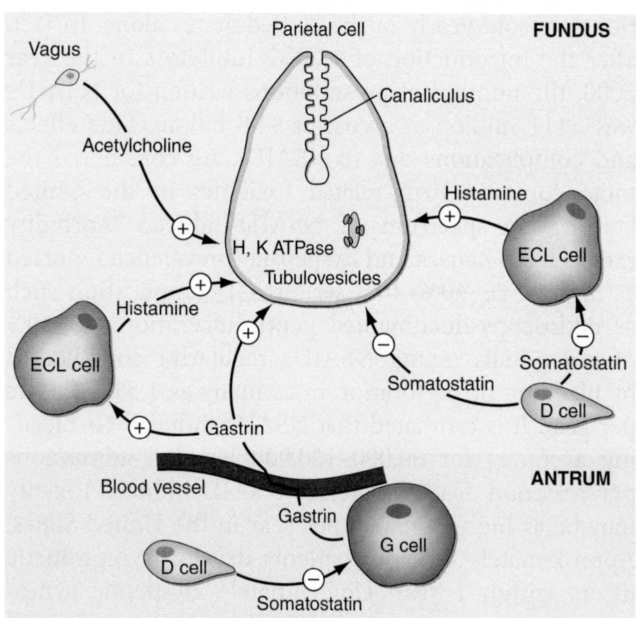

FIGURE 15-7
Summary of potential mechanisms by which *H. pylori* may lead to gastric secretory abnormalities. D, somatostatin cell; ECL, enterochromaffin-like cell; G, G cell. *(Adapted from J Calam et al: Gastroenterology 113:543, 1997.)*

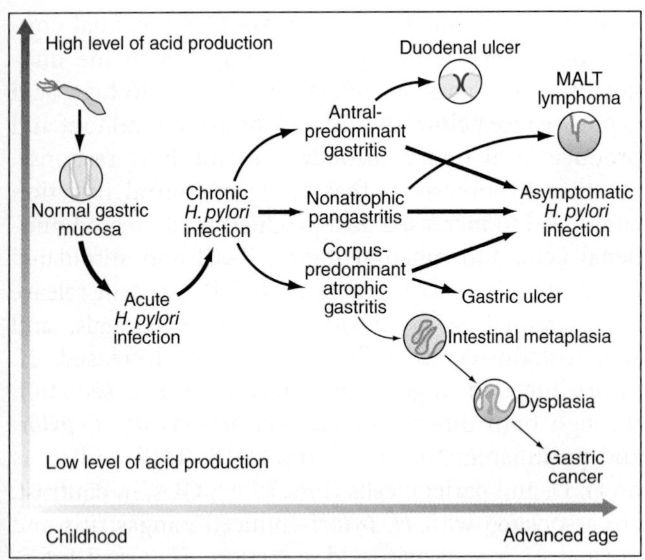

FIGURE 15-8

Natural history of *H. pylori* infection. MALT, mucosal-associated lymphoid tissue. *(Used with permission from S Suerbaum, P Michetti: N Engl J Med 347:1175, 2002.)*

development of GUs, gastric atrophy, and ultimately gastric carcinoma (Fig. 15-8).

NSAID-induced disease

Epidemiology

NSAIDs represent a group of the most commonly used medications in the United States. More than 30 billion over-the-counter tablets and over 100 million prescriptions are sold yearly in the United States alone. In fact, after the introduction of COX-2 inhibitors in the year 2000, the number of prescriptions written for NSAIDs was >111 million at a cost of $4.8 billion. Side effects and complications due to NSAIDs are considered the most common drug-related toxicities in the United States. The spectrum of NSAID-induced morbidity ranges from nausea and dyspepsia (prevalence reported as high as 50–60%) to a serious GI complication such as endoscopy-documented peptic ulceration (15–30% of individuals taking NSAIDs regularly) complicated by bleeding or perforation in as many as 1.5% of users per year. It is estimated that NSAID-induced GI bleeding accounts for 60,000–120,000 hospital admissions per year, and deaths related to NSAID-induced toxicity may be as high as 16,000 per year in the United States. Approximately 4–5% of patients develop symptomatic ulcers within 1 year. Unfortunately, dyspeptic symptoms do not correlate with NSAID-induced pathology. Over 80% of patients with serious NSAID-related complications did not have preceding dyspepsia. In view of the lack of warning signs, it is important to identify patients who are at increased risk for morbidity and mortality related to NSAID usage. Even 75 mg/d of aspirin may lead to serious GI ulceration; thus, no dose of NSAID is completely safe. In fact, the incidence of mucosal injury (ulcers and erosions) in patients taking low-dose aspirin (75–325 mg) has been estimated to range from as low as 8% to as high as 60%. It appears that *H. pylori* infection increases the risk of PUD-associated GI bleeding in chronic users of low-dose aspirin. Established risk factors include advanced age, history of ulcer, concomitant use of glucocorticoids, high-dose NSAIDs, multiple NSAIDs, concomitant use of anticoagulants, clopidogrel, and serious or multisystem disease. Possible risk factors include concomitant infection with *H. pylori*, cigarette smoking, and alcohol consumption.

Pathophysiology

Prostaglandins play a critical role in maintaining gastroduodenal mucosal integrity and repair. It therefore follows that interruption of prostaglandin synthesis can impair mucosal defense and repair, thus facilitating mucosal injury via a systemic mechanism. Animal studies have demonstrated that neutrophil adherence to the gastric microcirculation plays an essential role in the initiation of NSAID-induced mucosal injury. A summary of the pathogenetic pathways by which systemically administered NSAIDs may lead to mucosal injury is shown in Fig. 15-9. Single nucleotide polymorphisms (SNPs) have been found in several genes, including those encoding certain subtypes of cytochrome P450 (see below), interleukin-1β (*IL-1β*), angiotensinogen (*AGT*), and an organic ion transporting polypeptide (*SLCO1B1*), but these findings need confirmation in larger scale studies.

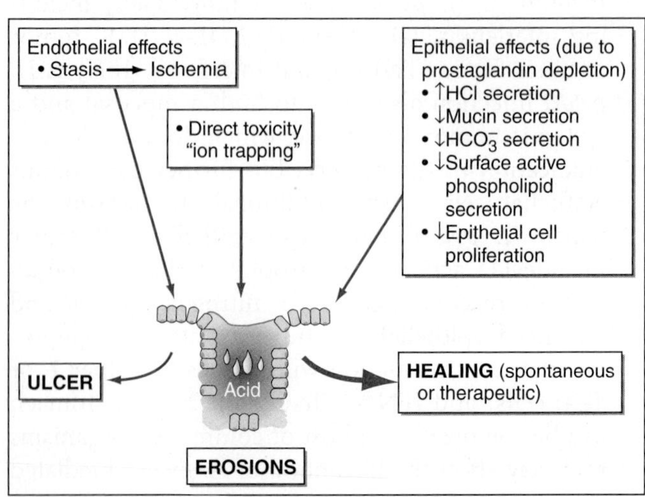

FIGURE 15-9

Mechanisms by which nonsteroidal anti-inflammatory drugs may induce mucosal injury. *(Adapted from J Scheiman et al: J Clin Outcomes Management 3:23, 1996. Copyright 2003 Turner White Communications, Inc., www.turner-white.com. Used with permission.)*

Injury to the mucosa also occurs as a result of the topical encounter with NSAIDs. Aspirin and many NSAIDs are weak acids that remain in a nonionized lipophilic form when found within the acid environment of the stomach. Under these conditions, NSAIDs migrate across lipid membranes of epithelial cells, leading to cell injury once trapped intracellularly in an ionized form. Topical NSAIDs can also alter the surface mucous layer, permitting back diffusion of H^+ and pepsin, leading to further epithelial cell damage. Moreover, enteric-coated or buffered preparations are also associated with risk of peptic ulceration.

The interplay between *H. pylori* and NSAIDs in the pathogenesis of PUD is complex. Meta-analysis supports the conclusion that each of these aggressive factors is independent and synergistic risk factors for PUD and its complications such as GI bleeding. For example, eradication of *H. pylori* reduces the likelihood of GI complications in high-risk individuals to levels observed in individuals with average risk of NSAID-induced complications.

Pathogenetic factors unrelated to *H. pylori* and NSAIDs in acid peptic disease

Cigarette smoking has been implicated in the pathogenesis of PUD. Not only have smokers been found to have ulcers more frequently than do nonsmokers, but smoking appears to decrease healing rates, impair response to therapy, and increase ulcer-related complications such as perforation. The mechanism responsible for increased ulcer diathesis in smokers is unknown. Theories have included altered gastric emptying, decreased proximal duodenal bicarbonate production, increased risk for *H. pylori* infection, and cigarette-induced generation of noxious mucosal free radicals. Genetic predisposition may play a role in ulcer development. First-degree relatives of DU patients are three times as likely to develop an ulcer; however, the potential role of *H. pylori* infection in contacts is a major consideration. Increased frequencies of blood group O and of the nonsecretor status have also been implicated as genetic risk factors for peptic diathesis. However, *H. pylori* preferentially binds to group O antigens. Additional genetic factors have been postulated to predispose certain individuals to developing PUD and/or upper GI bleeding. Specifically, genes encoding the NSAID-metabolizing enzymes cytochrome P450 2C9 and 2C8 (CYP2C9 and CYP2C8) are potential susceptibility genes for NSAID-induced PUD, but unfortunately, the studies have not been consistent in demonstrating this association. In a United Kingdom study, the *CYP2C19*17* gain-of-function polymorphism was associated with PUD in a Caucasian cohort, irrespective of ulcer etiology. These findings need to be confirmed in broader studies. Psychological stress has been thought to contribute to PUD, but studies examining the role of psychological factors in its pathogenesis have generated conflicting results. Although PUD is associated with certain personality traits (neuroticism), these same traits are also present in individuals with nonulcer dyspepsia (NUD) and other functional and organic disorders.

Diet has also been thought to play a role in peptic diseases. Certain foods and beverages can cause dyspepsia, but no convincing studies indicate an association between ulcer formation and a specific diet. Specific chronic disorders have been shown to have a strong association with PUD: (1) advanced age, (2) chronic pulmonary disease, (3) chronic renal failure, (4) cirrhosis, (5) nephrolithiasis, (6) α_1-antitrypsin deficiency, and (7) systemic mastocytosis. Disorders with a possible association are (1) hyperparathyroidism, (2) coronary artery disease, (3) polycythemia vera, (4) chronic pancreatitis, (5) former alcohol use, (6) obesity, (7) African-American race, and (8) three or more doctor visits in a year.

Multiple factors play a role in the pathogenesis of PUD. The two predominant causes are *H. pylori* infection and NSAID ingestion. PUD not related to *H. pylori* or NSAIDs is increasing. Other less common causes of PUD are shown in Table 15-1. These etiologic agents should be considered as the incidence of *H. pylori* is decreasing. Independent of the inciting or injurious agent, peptic

TABLE 15-1

CAUSES OF ULCERS NOT CAUSED BY *HELICOBACTER PYLORI* AND NSAIDS

Pathogenesis of Non-Hp and Non-NSAID Ulcer Disease
Infection
Cytomegalovirus
Herpes simplex virus
Helicobacter heilmannii
Drug/Toxin
Bisphosphonates
Chemotherapy
Clopidogrel
Crack cocaine
Glucocorticoids (when combined with NSAIDs)
Mycophenolate mofetil
Potassium chloride
Miscellaneous
Basophilia in myeloproliferative disease
Duodenal obstruction (e.g., annular pancreas)
Infiltrating disease
Ischemia
Radiation therapy
Eosinophilic infiltration
Sarcoidosis
Crohn's disease
Idiopathic hypersecretory state

Abbreviations: Hp, *H. pylori*; NSAIDs, nonsteroidal anti-inflammatory drugs.

ulcers develop as a result of an imbalance between mucosal protection/repair and aggressive factors. Gastric acid plays an important role in mucosal injury.

CLINICAL FEATURES

History

Abdominal pain is common to many GI disorders, including DU and GU, but has a poor predictive value for the presence of either DU or GU. Up to 10% of patients with NSAID-induced mucosal disease can present with a complication (bleeding, perforation, and obstruction) without antecedent symptoms. Despite this poor correlation, a careful history and physical examination are essential components of the approach to a patient suspected of having peptic ulcers.

Epigastric pain described as a burning or gnawing discomfort can be present in both DU and GU. The discomfort is also described as an ill-defined, aching sensation or as hunger pain. The typical pain pattern in DU occurs 90 minutes to 3 hours after a meal and is frequently relieved by antacids or food. Pain that awakes the patient from sleep (between midnight and 3 A.M.) is the most discriminating symptom, with two-thirds of DU patients describing this complaint. Unfortunately, this symptom is also present in one-third of patients with NUD (see below). Elderly patients are less likely to have abdominal pain as a manifestation of PUD and may instead present with a complication such as ulcer bleeding or perforation. The pain pattern in GU patients may be different from that in DU patients, where discomfort may actually be precipitated by food. Nausea and weight loss occur more commonly in GU patients. Endoscopy detects ulcers in <30% of patients who have dyspepsia.

The mechanism for development of abdominal pain in ulcer patients is unknown. Several possible explanations include acid-induced activation of chemical receptors in the duodenum, enhanced duodenal sensitivity to bile acids and pepsin, or altered gastroduodenal motility.

Variation in the intensity or distribution of the abdominal pain, as well as the onset of associated symptoms such as nausea and/or vomiting, may be indicative of an ulcer complication. Dyspepsia that becomes constant, is no longer relieved by food or antacids, or radiates to the back may indicate a penetrating ulcer (pancreas). Sudden onset of severe, generalized abdominal pain may indicate perforation. Pain worsening with meals, nausea, and vomiting of undigested food suggest gastric outlet obstruction. Tarry stools or coffee-ground emesis indicate bleeding.

Physical examination

Epigastric tenderness is the most frequent finding in patients with GU or DU. Pain may be found to the right of the midline in 20% of patients. Unfortunately, the predictive value of this finding is rather low. Physical examination is critically important for discovering evidence of ulcer complication. Tachycardia and orthostasis suggest dehydration secondary to vomiting or active GI blood loss. A severely tender, board-like abdomen suggests a perforation. Presence of a succussion splash indicates retained fluid in the stomach, suggesting gastric outlet obstruction.

PUD-related complications

Gastrointestinal bleeding

GI bleeding is the most common complication observed in PUD. Bleeding is estimated to occur in 19.4–57 per 100,000 individuals in a general population or in approximately 15% of patients. Bleeding and complications of ulcer disease occur more often in individuals >60 years of age. The 30-day mortality rate is as high as 5–10%. The higher incidence in the elderly is likely due to the increased use of NSAIDs in this group. In addition, up to 80% of the mortality in PUD-related bleeding is due to nonbleeding causes such as multiorgan failure (24%), pulmonary complications (24%), and malignancy (34%).

Up to 20% of patients with ulcer-related hemorrhage bleed without any preceding warning signs or symptoms.

Perforation

The second most common ulcer-related complication is perforation, being reported in as many as 6–7% of PUD patients with an estimated 30-day mortality of over 20%. As in the case of bleeding, the incidence of perforation in the elderly appears to be increasing secondary to increased use of NSAIDs. *Penetration* is a form of perforation in which the ulcer bed tunnels into an adjacent organ. DUs tend to penetrate posteriorly into the pancreas, leading to pancreatitis, whereas GUs tend to penetrate into the left hepatic lobe. Gastrocolic fistulas associated with GUs have also been described.

Gastric outlet obstruction

Gastric outlet obstruction is the least common ulcer-related complication, occurring in 1–2% of patients. A patient may have relative obstruction secondary to ulcer-related inflammation and edema in the peripyloric region. This process often resolves with ulcer healing. A fixed, mechanical obstruction secondary to scar formation in the peripyloric areas is also possible. The latter requires endoscopic (balloon dilation) or surgical intervention. Signs and symptoms relative to mechanical obstruction may develop insidiously. New onset of early satiety, nausea, vomiting, increase of postprandial abdominal pain, and weight loss should make gastric outlet obstruction a possible diagnosis.

Differential diagnosis

The list of GI and non-GI disorders that can mimic ulceration of the stomach or duodenum is quite extensive. The most commonly encountered diagnosis among patients seen for upper abdominal discomfort is NUD. NUD, also known as *functional dyspepsia* or *essential dyspepsia,* refers to a group of heterogeneous disorders typified by upper abdominal pain without the presence of an ulcer. Dyspepsia has been reported to occur in up to 30% of the U.S. population. Up to 60% of patients seeking medical care for dyspepsia have a negative diagnostic evaluation. The etiology of NUD is not established, and the potential role of *H. pylori* in NUD remains controversial.

Several additional disease processes that may present with "ulcer-like" symptoms include proximal GI tumors, gastroesophageal reflux, vascular disease, pancreaticobiliary disease (biliary colic, chronic pancreatitis), and gastroduodenal Crohn's disease.

Diagnostic evaluation

In view of the poor predictive value of abdominal pain for the presence of a gastroduodenal ulcer and the multiple disease processes that can mimic this disease, the clinician is often confronted with having to establish the presence of an ulcer. Documentation of an ulcer requires either a radiographic (barium study) or an endoscopic procedure. However, a large percentage of patients with symptoms suggestive of an ulcer have NUD; testing for *H. pylori* and antibiotic therapy (see below) is appropriate for individuals who are otherwise healthy and <45 years of age, before embarking on a diagnostic evaluation **(Chap. 5)**.

Barium studies of the proximal GI tract are still occasionally used as a first test for documenting an ulcer. The sensitivity of older single-contrast barium meals for detecting a DU is as high as 80%, with a double-contrast study providing detection rates as high as 90%. Sensitivity for detection is decreased in small ulcers (<0.5 cm), with presence of previous scarring, or in postoperative patients. A DU appears as a well-demarcated crater, most often seen in the bulb (Fig. 15-10*A*). A GU may represent benign or malignant disease. Typically, a benign GU also appears as a discrete crater with radiating mucosal folds originating from the ulcer margin (Fig. 15-10*B*). Ulcers >3 cm in size or those associated with a mass are more often malignant. Unfortunately, up to 8% of GUs that appear to be benign by radiographic appearance are malignant by endoscopy or surgery. Radiographic studies that show a GU must be followed by endoscopy and biopsy.

Endoscopy provides the most sensitive and specific approach for examining the upper GI tract (Fig. 15-11). In addition to permitting direct visualization of the mucosa, endoscopy facilitates photographic documentation of a mucosal defect and tissue biopsy to rule out malignancy (GU) or *H. pylori.* Endoscopic examination is particularly helpful in identifying lesions too small to detect by radiographic examination, for evaluation of atypical radiographic abnormalities, or to determine if an ulcer is a source of blood loss.

Although the methods for diagnosing *H. pylori* are outlined in Chap. 27, a brief summary will be included here (Table 15-2). Several biopsy urease tests have been developed (PyloriTek, CLOtest, Hpfast, Pronto Dry) that have a sensitivity and specificity of >90–95%. Several noninvasive methods for detecting this organism

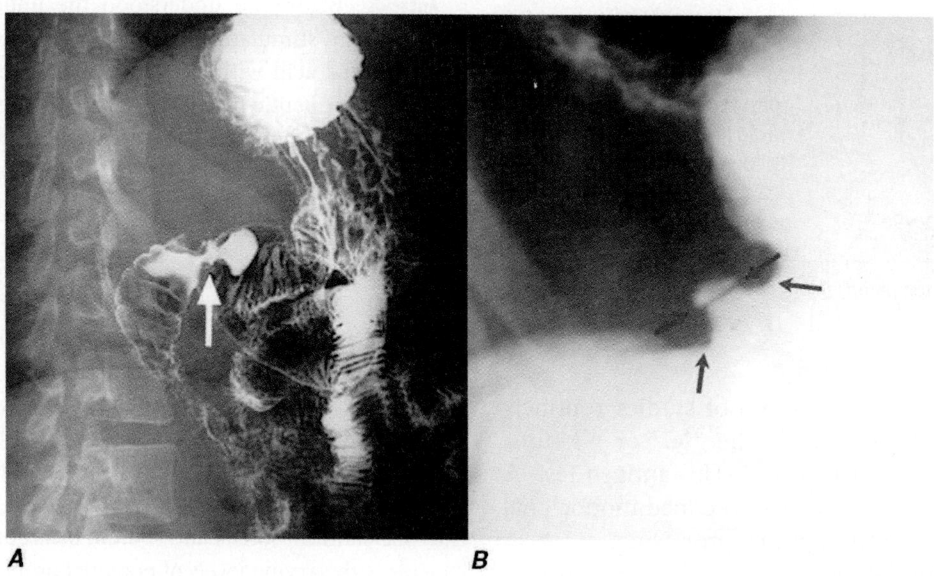

FIGURE 15-10
Barium study demonstrating (*A*) a benign duodenal ulcer and (***B***) a benign gastric ulcer.

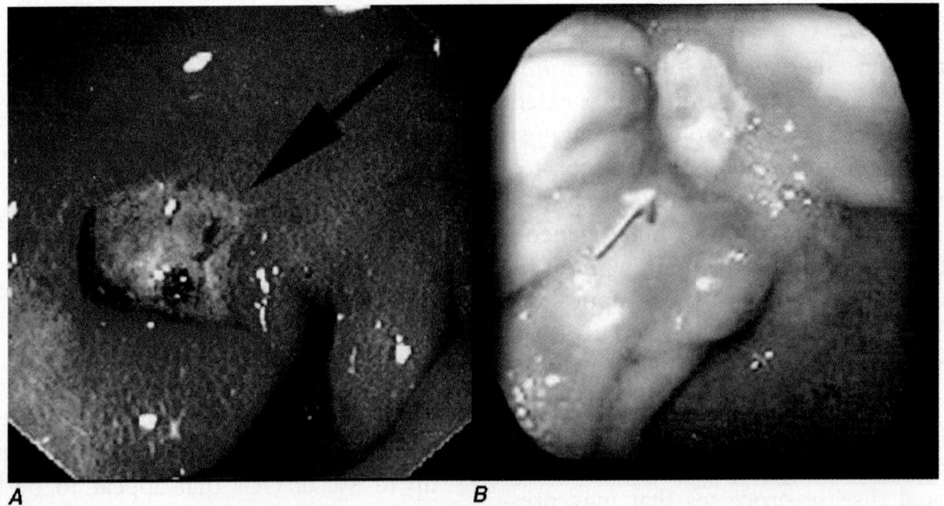

FIGURE 15-11
Endoscopy demonstrating (*A*) a benign duodenal ulcer and (*B*) a benign gastric ulcer.

TABLE 15-2

TESTS FOR DETECTION OF *H. PYLORI*

TEST	SENSITIVITY/ SPECIFICITY, %	COMMENTS
Invasive (Endoscopy/Biopsy Required)		
Rapid urease	80–95/95–100	Simple, false negative with recent use of PPIs, antibiotics, or bismuth compounds
Histology	80–90/>95	Requires pathology processing and staining; provides histologic information
Culture	—/—	Time-consuming, expensive, dependent on experience; allows determination of antibiotic susceptibility
Noninvasive		
Serology	>80/>90	Inexpensive, convenient; not useful for early follow-up
Urea breath test	>90/>90	Simple, rapid; useful for early follow-up; false negatives with recent therapy (see rapid urease test); exposure to low-dose radiation with ^{14}C test
Stool antigen	>90/>90	Inexpensive, convenient

Abbreviation: PPIs, proton pump inhibitors.

have been developed. Three types of studies routinely used include serologic testing, the ^{13}C- or ^{14}C-urea breath test, and the fecal *H. pylori* (Hp) antigen test. A urinary Hp antigen test, as well as a refined monoclonal antibody stool antigen test, appears promising.

Occasionally, specialized testing such as serum gastrin and gastric acid analysis or sham feeding may be needed in individuals with complicated or refractory PUD (see "Zollinger-Ellison Syndrome [ZES]," below). Screening for aspirin or NSAIDs (blood or urine) may also be necessary in refractory *H. pylori*–negative PUD patients.

TREATMENT Peptic Ulcer Disease

Before the discovery of *H. pylori,* the therapy of PUD was centered on the old dictum by Schwartz of "no acid, no ulcer." Although acid secretion is still important in the pathogenesis of PUD, eradication of *H. pylori* and therapy/prevention of NSAID-induced disease is the mainstay of treatment. A summary of commonly used drugs for treatment of acid peptic disorders is shown in Table 15-3.

ACID-NEUTRALIZING/INHIBITORY DRUGS

Antacids Before we understood the important role of histamine in stimulating parietal cell activity, neutralization of secreted acid with antacids constituted the main form of therapy for peptic ulcers. They are now rarely, if ever, used as the primary therapeutic agent but instead are often used by patients for symptomatic relief of dyspepsia. The most commonly used agents are mixtures of aluminum hydroxide and magnesium hydroxide. Aluminum hydroxide can produce constipation and phosphate depletion; magnesium hydroxide may cause loose stools. Many of the commonly used antacids (e.g., Maalox, Mylanta) have a combination of both aluminum and magnesium hydroxide in order to avoid these side effects. The magnesium-containing preparation should not be used in chronic renal failure patients because of possible hypermagnesemia, and aluminum may cause chronic neurotoxicity in these patients.

Calcium carbonate and sodium bicarbonate are potent antacids with varying levels of potential problems. The long-term use of calcium carbonate (converts to calcium chloride in the stomach) can lead to milk-alkali syndrome (hypercalcemia,

TABLE 15-3

DRUGS USED IN THE TREATMENT OF PEPTIC ULCER DISEASE

DRUG TYPE/ MECHANISM	EXAMPLES	DOSE
Acid-suppressing drugs		
Antacids	Mylanta, Maalox, Tums, Gaviscon	100–140 meq/L 1 and 3 h after meals and hs
H_2 receptor antagonists	Cimetidine	400 mg bid
	Ranitidine	300 mg hs
	Famotidine	40 mg hs
	Nizatidine	300 mg hs
Proton pump inhibitors	Omeprazole	20 mg/d
	Lansoprazole	30 mg/d
	Rabeprazole	20 mg/d
	Pantoprazole	40 mg/d
	Esomeprazole	20 mg/d
	Dexlansoprazole	30 mg/d
Mucosal protective agents		
Sucralfate	Sucralfate	1 g qid
Prostaglandin analogue	Misoprostol	200 μg qid
Bismuth-containing compounds	Bismuth subsalicylate (BSS)	See anti-*H. pylori* regimens (Table 15-4)

Abbreviation: hs, at bedtime (*hora somni*).

hyperphosphatemia with possible renal calcinosis and progression to renal insufficiency). Sodium bicarbonate may induce systemic alkalosis.

H_2 receptor antagonists Four of these agents are presently available (cimetidine, ranitidine, famotidine, and nizatidine), and their structures share homology with histamine. Although each has different potency, all will significantly inhibit basal and stimulated acid secretion to comparable levels when used at therapeutic doses. Moreover, similar ulcer-healing rates are achieved with each drug when used at the correct dosage. Presently, this class of drug is often used for treatment of active ulcers (4–6 weeks) in combination with antibiotics directed at eradicating *H. pylori* (see below).

Cimetidine was the first H_2 receptor antagonist used for the treatment of acid peptic disorders. The initial recommended dosing profile for cimetidine was 300 mg qid. Subsequent studies have documented the efficacy of using 800 mg at bedtime for treatment of active ulcer, with healing rates approaching 80% at 4 weeks. Cimetidine may have weak antiandrogenic side effects resulting in reversible gynecomastia and impotence, primarily in patients receiving high doses for prolonged periods of time (months to years, as in ZES). In view of cimetidine's ability to inhibit cytochrome P450, careful monitoring of drugs such as warfarin, phenytoin, and theophylline is indicated with long-term usage. Other rare reversible adverse effects reported with cimetidine include confusion and elevated levels of serum aminotransferases, creatinine, and serum prolactin. Ranitidine, famotidine, and nizatidine are more potent H_2 receptor antagonists than cimetidine. Each can be used once a day at bedtime for ulcer prevention, which was commonly done before the discovery of *H. pylori* and the development of proton pump inhibitors (PPIs). Patients may develop tolerance to H_2 blockers, a rare event with PPIs (see below). Comparable nighttime dosing regimens are ranitidine 300 mg, famotidine 40 mg, and nizatidine 300 mg.

Additional rare, reversible systemic toxicities reported with H_2 receptor antagonists include pancytopenia, neutropenia, anemia, and thrombocytopenia, with a prevalence rate varying from 0.01–0.2%. Cimetidine and ranitidine (to a lesser extent) can bind to hepatic cytochrome P450; famotidine and nizatidine do not.

Proton pump (H^+,K^+-ATPase) inhibitors Omeprazole, esomeprazole, lansoprazole, rabeprazole, and pantoprazole are substituted benzimidazole derivatives that covalently bind and irreversibly inhibit H^+,K^+-ATPase. Esomeprazole, one of the newest members of this drug class, is the S-enantiomer of omeprazole, which is a racemic mixture of both S- and R-optical isomers. The R-isomer of lansoprazole, dexlansoprazole, is the most recent PPI approved for clinical use. Its reported advantage is a dual delayed-release system, aimed at improving treatment of gastroesophageal reflux disease (GERD). These are the most potent acid inhibitory agents available. Omeprazole and lansoprazole are the PPIs that have been used for the longest time. Both are acid-labile and are administered as enteric-coated granules in a sustained-release capsule that dissolves within the small intestine at a pH of 6. Lansoprazole is available in an orally disintegrating tablet that can be taken with or without water, an advantage for individuals who have significant dysphagia. Absorption kinetics are similar to the capsule. In addition, a lansoprazole-naproxen combination preparation that has been made available is targeted at decreasing NSAID-related GI injury (see below). Omeprazole is available as nonenteric-coated granules mixed with sodium bicarbonate in a powder form that can be administered orally or via gastric tube. The sodium bicarbonate has two purposes: to protect the omeprazole from acid degradation and to promote rapid gastric alkalinization and subsequent proton pump activation, which facilitates rapid action of the PPI. Pantoprazole and rabeprazole are available as enteric-coated tablets. Pantoprazole is also available as a parenteral formulation for intravenous use. These agents are lipophilic compounds; upon entering the parietal cell, they are protonated and trapped within the acid environment of the tubulovesicular and canalicular system. These agents potently inhibit all phases of gastric acid secretion. Onset of action is rapid, with a maximum acid inhibitory effect between 2 and 6 h after administration and duration of inhibition lasting up to 72–96 h. With repeated daily dosing, progressive acid inhibitory effects are observed, with basal and secretagogue-stimulated acid production being inhibited by >95% after 1 week of therapy. The half-life of PPIs is ~18 h; thus, it can take between 2 and 5 days for gastric acid secretion to return to normal levels once these drugs have been discontinued. Because the pumps need to be activated for these agents to be effective, their efficacy is maximized if they are administered before a meal (except for the immediate-release formulation of omeprazole) (e.g., in the morning before breakfast). Mild to moderate hypergastrinemia has been observed in patients taking these drugs. Carcinoid tumors developed in some animals given the drugs preclinically; however, extensive experience has failed to demonstrate gastric carcinoid tumor development in humans. Serum gastrin levels return to normal levels within 1–2 weeks after drug cessation. Rebound gastric acid hypersecretion has been described in *H. pylori*–negative individuals after discontinuation of PPIs. It occurs even after relatively short-term usage (2 months) and may last for up to 2 months after the PPI has been discontinued. The mechanism involves gastrin-induced hyperplasia and hypertrophy of histamine-secreting ECL cells. The clinical relevance of this observation is that individuals may have worsening symptoms of GERD or dyspepsia upon stopping the PPI. Gradual tapering of the PPI and switching to an H_2 receptor antagonist may prevent this from occurring. *H. pylori*–induced inflammation and concomitant decrease in acid production may explain why this does not occur in *H. pylori*–positive patients. IF production is also inhibited, but vitamin B_{12}-deficiency anemia is uncommon, probably because of the large stores of the vitamin. As with any agent that leads to significant hypochlorhydria, PPIs may interfere with absorption of drugs such as ketoconazole, ampicillin, iron, and digoxin. Hepatic cytochrome P450 can be inhibited by the earlier PPIs (omeprazole, lansoprazole). Rabeprazole, pantoprazole, and esomeprazole do not appear to interact significantly with drugs metabolized by the cytochrome P450 system. The overall clinical significance of this observation is not definitely established. Caution should be taken when using theophylline, warfarin, diazepam, atazanavir, and phenytoin concomitantly with PPIs. Long-term acid suppression, especially with PPIs, has been associated with a higher incidence of community-acquired pneumonia as well as community and hospital acquired *Clostridium difficile*–associated disease. These observations require confirmation but should alert the practitioner to take caution when recommending these agents for long-term use, especially in elderly patients at risk for developing pneumonia or *C. difficile* infection. A population-based study revealed that long-term use of PPIs was associated with the development of hip fractures in older women. The absolute risk of fracture remained low despite an observed increase associated with the dose and duration of acid suppression. The mechanism for this observation is not clear, and this finding must be confirmed before making broad recommendations regarding the discontinuation of these agents in patients who benefit from them. Long-term use of PPIs has also been implicated in the development of iron and magnesium deficiency, but here again, the studies are limited and inconclusive. PPIs may exert a negative effect on the antiplatelet effect of clopidogrel. Although the evidence is mixed and inconclusive, a small increase in mortality and readmission rate for coronary events was seen in patients receiving a PPI while on clopidogrel in earlier studies. Subsequently, three meta-analyses reported an inverse correlation between clopidogrel and PPI use; therefore, the influence of this drug interaction on mortality is not clearly established. The mechanism involves the competition of the PPI and clopidogrel with the same cytochrome P450 (CYP2C19). Whether this is a class effect of PPIs is unclear; there appears to be at least a theoretical advantage of pantoprazole over the other PPIs, but this has not been confirmed. This drug interaction is particularly relevant in light of the common use of aspirin and clopidogrel for prevention of coronary events and the efficacy of PPIs in preventing GI bleeding in these patients. The FDA has made several recommendations while awaiting further evidence to clarify the impact of PPI therapy on clopidogrel use. Health care providers should continue to prescribe clopidogrel to patients who require it and should reevaluate the need for starting or continuing treatment with a PPI. From a practical standpoint, additional recommendations to consider include the following: Patients taking clopidogrel with aspirin, especially with other GI risk factors for bleeding, should receive GI protective therapy. Although high-dose H_2 blockers have been considered an option, these do not appear to be as effective as PPIs. If PPIs are to be given, some have recommended that there be a 12-h separation between administration of the PPI and clopidogrel to minimize competition of the two agents with the involved cytochrome P450. One option is to give the PPI 30 min before breakfast and the clopidogrel at bedtime. Insufficient data are available to firmly recommend one PPI over another. Patients 65 years of age or older have a higher risk for some of the long-term side effects of PPIs highlighted above, in part due to the higher prevalence of concomitant chronic diseases. It is therefore important to carefully select individuals, especially among the elderly, who need long-term PPI therapy and discontinue it in those individuals who do not need it.

Two new formulations of acid inhibitory agents are being developed. Tenatoprazole is a PPI containing an imidazopyridine ring instead of a benzimidazole ring, which promotes irreversible proton pump inhibition. This agent has a longer half-life than the other PPIs and may be beneficial for inhibiting nocturnal acid secretion, which has significant relevance in GERD. A second new class of agents is the potassium-competitive acid pump antagonists (P-CABs). These compounds inhibit gastric acid secretion via potassium competitive binding of the H^+,K^+-ATPase.

CYTOPROTECTIVE AGENTS

Sucralfate Sucralfate is a complex sucrose salt in which the hydroxyl groups have been substituted by aluminum hydroxide and sulfate. This compound is insoluble in water and becomes a viscous paste within the stomach and duodenum, binding primarily to sites of active ulceration. Sucralfate may act by several mechanisms: serving as a physicochemical barrier, promoting a trophic action by binding growth factors such as EGF, enhancing prostaglandin synthesis, stimulating mucus and bicarbonate secretion, and enhancing mucosal defense and repair. Toxicity from this drug is rare, with constipation being most common (2–3%). It should be avoided in patients with chronic renal insufficiency to prevent aluminum-induced neurotoxicity. Hypophosphatemia and gastric bezoar formation have also been reported rarely. Standard dosing of sucralfate is 1 g qid.

Bismuth-containing preparations Sir William Osler considered bismuth-containing compounds the drug of choice for treating PUD. The resurgence in the use of these agents is due to their effect against *H. pylori.* Colloidal bismuth subcitrate (CBS) and bismuth subsalicylate (BSS, Pepto-Bismol) are the most widely used preparations. The mechanism by which these agents induce ulcer healing is unclear. Adverse effects with short-term use include black stools, constipation, and darkening of the tongue. Long-term use with high doses, especially with the avidly absorbed CBS, may lead to neurotoxicity. These compounds are commonly used as one of the agents in an anti-*H. pylori* regimen (see below).

Prostaglandin analogues In view of their central role in maintaining mucosal integrity and repair, stable prostaglandin analogues were developed for the treatment of PUD. The mechanism by which this rapidly absorbed drug provides its therapeutic effect is through enhancement of mucosal defense and repair. The most common toxicity noted with this drug is diarrhea (10–30% incidence). Other major toxicities include uterine bleeding and contractions; misoprostol is contraindicated in women who may be pregnant, and women of childbearing age must be made clearly aware of this potential drug toxicity. The standard therapeutic dose is 200 μg qid.

Miscellaneous drugs A number of drugs including anticholinergic agents and tricyclic antidepressants were used for treating acid peptic disorders, but in light of their toxicity and the development of potent antisecretory agents, these are rarely, if ever, used today.

THERAPY OF *H. PYLORI*

The physician's goal in treating PUD is to provide relief of symptoms (pain or dyspepsia), promote ulcer healing, and ultimately prevent ulcer recurrence and complications. The greatest influence of understanding the role of *H. pylori* in peptic disease has been the ability to prevent recurrence. Documented eradication of *H. pylori* in patients with PUD is associated with a dramatic decrease in ulcer recurrence to <10–20% as compared to 59% in GU patients and 67% in DU patients when the organism is not eliminated. Eradication of the organism may lead to diminished recurrent ulcer bleeding. The effect of its eradication on ulcer perforation is unclear.

Extensive effort has been made in determining who of the many individuals with *H. pylori* infection should be treated. The common conclusion arrived at by multiple consensus conferences around the world is that *H. pylori* should be eradicated in patients with documented PUD. This holds true independent of time of presentation (first episode or not), severity of symptoms, presence of confounding factors such as ingestion of NSAIDs, or whether the ulcer is in remission. Some have advocated treating patients with a history of documented PUD who are found to be *H. pylori*–positive by serology or breath testing. Over one-half of patients with gastric MALT lymphoma experience complete remission of the tumor in response to *H. pylori* eradication. The Maastricht IV/Florence Consensus Report recommends a test-and-treat approach for patients with uninvestigated dyspepsia if the local incidence of *H. pylori* is greater than 20%. In addition, recommendations from this consensus report include testing and eradicating *H. pylori* in patients who will be using NSAIDs (including low-dose aspirin) on a long-term basis, especially if there is a prior history of PUD. These individuals will require continued PPI treatment as well as eradication treatment, because eradication of the organism alone does not eliminate the risk of gastroduodenal ulcers in patients already receiving long-term NSAIDs. Treating patients with NUD to prevent gastric cancer or patients with GERD requiring long-term acid suppression remains controversial. Guidelines from the American College of Gastroenterology suggest eradication of *H. pylori* in patients who have undergone resection of early gastric cancer. The Maastricht IV/Florence Consensus Report also evaluated *H. pylori* treatment in gastric cancer prevention and recommends that eradication should be considered in the following situations: first-degree relatives of family members with gastric cancer; patients with previous gastric neoplasm treated by endoscopic or subtotal resection; individuals with a risk of gastritis (severe pangastritis or body-predominant gastritis) or severe atrophy; patients with gastric acid inhibition for more than 1 year; individuals with strong environmental risk factors for gastric cancer (heavy smoking; high exposure to dust, coal, quartz, or cement; and/or work in quarries); and *H. pylori*–positive patients with a fear of gastric cancer.

Multiple drugs have been evaluated in the therapy of *H. pylori.* No single agent is effective in eradicating the organism. Combination therapy for 14 days provides the greatest efficacy, although regimens based on sequential administration of antibiotics also appear promising (see below). A shorter administration course (7–10 days), although attractive, has not proved as successful as the 14-day regimens. The agents used with the greatest frequency include amoxicillin, metronidazole, tetracycline, clarithromycin, and bismuth compounds.

Suggested treatment regimens for *H. pylori* are outlined in Table 15-4. Choice of a particular regimen will be influenced by several factors, including efficacy, patient tolerance, existing antibiotic resistance, and cost of the drugs. The aim for initial eradication rates should be 85–90%. Dual therapy (PPI plus amoxicillin, PPI plus clarithromycin, ranitidine bismuth citrate [Tritec] plus clarithromycin) is not recommended in view of studies demonstrating eradication rates of <80–85%. The combination of bismuth, metronidazole,

TABLE 15-4

REGIMENS RECOMMENDED FOR ERADICATION OF *H. PYLORI* INFECTION

DRUG	DOSE
Triple Therapy	
1. Bismuth subsalicylate *plus*	2 tablets qid
Metronidazole *plus*	250 mg qid
Tetracycline[a]	500 mg qid
2. Ranitidine bismuth citrate *plus*	400 mg bid
Tetracycline *plus*	500 mg bid
Clarithromycin or metronidazole	500 mg bid
3. Omeprazole (lansoprazole) *plus*	20 mg bid (30 mg bid)
Clarithromycin *plus*	250 or 500 mg bid
Metronidazole[b] *or*	500 mg bid
Amoxicillin[c]	1 g bid
Quadruple Therapy	
Omeprazole (lansoprazole)	20 mg (30 mg) daily
Bismuth subsalicylate	2 tablets qid
Metronidazole	250 mg qid
Tetracycline	500 mg qid

[a]Alternative: use prepacked Helidac (see text).
[b]Alternative: use prepacked Prevpac (see text).
[c]Use either metronidazole or amoxicillin, not both.

and tetracycline was the first triple regimen found effective against *H. pylori.* The combination of two antibiotics plus either a PPI, H_2 blocker, or bismuth compound has comparable success rates. Addition of acid suppression assists in providing early symptom relief and enhances bacterial eradication.

Triple therapy, although effective, has several drawbacks, including the potential for poor patient compliance and drug-induced side effects. Compliance is being addressed by simplifying the regimens so that patients can take the medications twice a day. Simpler (dual therapy) and shorter regimens (7 and 10 days) are not as effective as triple therapy for 14 days. Two anti-*H. pylori* regimens are available in prepackaged formulation: Prevpac (lansoprazole, clarithromycin, and amoxicillin) and Helidac (BSS, tetracycline, and metronidazole). The contents of the Prevpac are to be taken twice per day for 14 days, whereas Helidac constituents are taken four times per day with an antisecretory agent (PPI or H_2 blocker), also for at least 14 days. Clarithromycin-based triple therapy should be avoided in settings where *H. pylori* resistance to this agent exceeds 15–20%.

Side effects have been reported in up to 20–30% of patients on triple therapy. Bismuth may cause black stools, constipation, or darkening of the tongue. The most feared complication with amoxicillin is pseudomembranous colitis, but this occurs in <1–2% of patients. Amoxicillin can also lead to antibiotic-associated diarrhea, nausea, vomiting, skin rash, and allergic reaction. Concomitant use of probiotics may ameliorate some of the antibiotic side effects (see below). Tetracycline has been reported to cause rashes and, very rarely, hepatotoxicity and anaphylaxis.

One important concern with treating patients who may not need therapy is the potential for development of antibiotic-resistant strains. The incidence and type of antibiotic-resistant *H. pylori* strains vary worldwide. Strains resistant to metronidazole, clarithromycin, amoxicillin, and tetracycline have been described, with the latter two being uncommon. Antibiotic-resistant strains are the most common cause for treatment failure in compliant patients. Unfortunately, in vitro resistance does not predict outcome in patients. Culture and sensitivity testing of *H. pylori* is not performed routinely. Although resistance to metronidazole has been found in as many as 30% of isolates in North America and 80% in developing countries, triple therapy is effective in eradicating the organism in >50% of patients infected with a resistant strain. Clarithromycin resistance is seen in 13% of individuals in the United States, with resistance to amoxicillin being <1% and resistance to both metronidazole and clarithromycin in the 5% range.

Failure of *H. pylori* eradication with triple therapy in a compliant patient is usually due to infection with a resistant organism. Quadruple therapy (Table 15-4), where clarithromycin is substituted for metronidazole (or vice versa), should be the next step. The combination of pantoprazole, amoxicillin, and rifabutin for 10 days has also been used successfully (86% cure rate) in patients infected with resistant strains. Additional regimens considered for second-line therapy include levofloxacin-based triple therapy (levofloxacin, amoxicillin, PPI) for 10 days and furazolidone-based triple therapy (furazolidone, amoxicillin, PPI) for 14 days. Unfortunately, there is no universally accepted treatment regimen recommended for patients who have failed two courses of antibiotics. If eradication is still not achieved in a compliant patient, then culture and sensitivity of the organism should be considered. Additional factors that may lower eradication rates include the patient's country of origin (higher in Northeast Asia than other parts of Asia or Europe) and cigarette smoking. In addition, meta-analysis suggests that even the most effective regimens (quadruple therapy including PPI, bismuth, tetracycline, and metronidazole and triple therapy including PPI, clarithromycin, and amoxicillin) may have suboptimal eradication rates (<80%), thus demonstrating the need for the development of more efficacious treatments.

In view of the observation that 15–25% of patients treated with first-line therapy may still remain infected with the organism, new approaches to treatment have been explored. One promising approach is sequential therapy. Regimens examined consist of 5 days of amoxicillin and a PPI, followed by an additional 5 days of PPI plus tinidazole and clarithromycin or levofloxacin. One promising regimen that has the benefit of being shorter in duration, easier to take, and less expensive is 5 days of concomitant therapy

(PPI twice daily, amoxicillin 1 g twice daily, levofloxacin 500 mg twice daily, and tinidazole 500 mg twice daily). Initial studies have demonstrated eradication rates of >90% with good patient tolerance. Confirmation of these findings and applicability of this approach in the United States are needed, although some experts are recommending abandoning clarithromycin-based triple therapy in the United States for the concomitant therapy or the alternative sequential therapies highlighted above.

Innovative non–antibiotic-mediated approaches have been explored in an effort to improve eradication rates of *H. pylori*. Pretreatment of patients with *N*-acetylcysteine as a mucolytic agent to destroy the *H. pylori* biofilm and therefore impair antibiotic resistance has been examined, but more studies are needed to confirm the applicability of this approach. In vitro studies suggest that certain probiotics like *Lactobacillus* or its metabolites can inhibit *H. pylori*. Administration of probiotics has been attempted in several clinical studies in an effort to maximize antibiotic-mediated eradication with varying results. Overall, it appears that the use of certain probiotics, such as *Lactobacillus* spp., *Saccharomyces* spp., *Bifidobacterium* spp., and *Bacillus clausii*, did not alter eradication rates but importantly decreased antibiotic-associated side effects including nausea, dysgeusia, diarrhea, and abdominal discomfort/pain, resulting in enhanced tolerability of *H. pylori* therapies. Additional studies are needed to confirm the potential benefits of probiotics in this setting.

Reinfection after successful eradication of *H. pylori* is rare in the United States (<1% per year). If recurrent infection occurs within the first 6 months after completing therapy, the most likely explanation is recrudescence as opposed to reinfection.

THERAPY OF NSAID-RELATED GASTRIC OR DUODENAL INJURY

Medical intervention for NSAID-related mucosal injury includes treatment of an active ulcer and primary prevention of future injury. Recommendations for the treatment and primary prevention of NSAID-related mucosal injury are listed in Table 15-5. Ideally, the injurious agent should be stopped as the first step in the therapy of an active NSAID-induced ulcer. If that is possible, then treatment with one of the acid inhibitory agents (H_2 blockers, PPIs) is indicated. Cessation of NSAIDs is not always possible because of the patient's severe underlying disease. Only PPIs can heal GUs or DUs, independent of whether NSAIDs are discontinued.

The approach to primary prevention has included avoiding the agent, using the lowest possible dose of the agent, using NSAIDs that are theoretically less injurious, using newer topical NSAID preparations, and/or using concomitant medical therapy to prevent NSAID-induced injury. Several nonselective NSAIDs that are associated with a lower likelihood of GI toxicity include diclofenac, aceclofenac, and ibuprofen, although the beneficial effect may be eliminated if higher dosages of the agents are used. Primary prevention of NSAID-induced ulceration can be accomplished by misoprostol (200 μg qid) or a PPI. High-dose H_2 blockers (famotidine, 40 mg bid) have also shown some promise in preventing endoscopically documented ulcers, although PPIs are superior. The highly selective COX-2 inhibitors, celecoxib and rofecoxib, are 100 times more selective inhibitors of COX-2 than standard NSAIDs, leading to gastric or duodenal mucosal injury that is comparable to placebo; their utilization led to an increase in cardiovascular events and withdrawal from the market. Additional caution was engendered when the CLASS study demonstrated that the advantage of celecoxib in preventing GI complications was offset when low-dose aspirin was used simultaneously. Therefore, gastric protection therapy is required in individuals taking COX-2 inhibitors and aspirin prophylaxis. Finally, much of the work demonstrating the benefit of COX-2 inhibitors and PPIs on GI injury has been performed in individuals of average risk; it is unclear if the same level of benefit will be achieved in high-risk patients. For example, concomitant use of warfarin and a COX-2 inhibitor was associated with rates of GI bleeding similar to those observed in patients taking nonselective NSAIDs. A combination of factors, including withdrawal of the majority of COX-2 inhibitors from the market, the observation that low-dose aspirin appears to diminish the beneficial effect of COX-2 selective inhibitors, and the growing use of aspirin for prophylaxis of cardiovascular events, have significantly altered the approach to gastric protective therapy during the use of NSAIDs. A set of guidelines for the approach to the use of NSAIDs was published by the American College of Gastroenterology and is shown in Table 15-6. Individuals who are not at risk for cardiovascular events, do not use aspirin, and are without risk for GI complications can receive nonselective NSAIDs without gastric protection. In those without cardiovascular risk factors but with a high potential risk (prior GI bleeding or multiple GI risk factors) for NSAID-induced GI toxicity, cautious use of a selective COX-2 inhibitor and co-therapy with misoprostol or high-dose PPI are recommended. Individuals at moderate GI risk without cardiac risk factors can be treated with a COX-2 inhibitor alone or with a nonselective NSAID with misoprostol or a PPI. Individuals with cardiovascular risk

TABLE 15-5

RECOMMENDATIONS FOR TREATMENT OF NSAID-RELATED MUCOSAL INJURY

CLINICAL SETTING	RECOMMENDATION
Active ulcer	
NSAID discontinued	H_2 receptor antagonist or PPI
NSAID continued	PPI
Prophylactic therapy	Misoprostol
	PPI
	Selective COX-2 inhibitor
H. pylori infection	Eradication if active ulcer present or there is a past history of peptic ulcer disease

Abbreviations: COX-2, isoenzyme of cyclooxygenase; NSAID, nonsteroidal anti-inflammatory drug; PPI, proton pump inhibitor.

TABLE 15-6

GUIDE TO NSAID THERAPY

	NO/LOW NSAID GI RISK	NSAID GI RISK
No CV risk (no aspirin)	Traditional NSAID	Coxib *or* Traditional NSAID + PPI *or* misoprostol Consider non-NSAID therapy
CV risk (consider aspirin)	Traditional NSAID + PPI *or* misoprostol if GI risk warrants gastroprotection Consider non-NSAID therapy	A gastroprotective agent must be added if a traditional NSAID is prescribed Consider non-NSAID therapy

Abbreviations: CV, cardiovascular; GI, gastrointestinal; NSAID, nonsteroidal anti-inflammatory drug; PPI, proton pump inhibitor.
Source: Adapted from AM Fendrick: *Am J Manag Care* 10:740, 2004. Reproduced with permission of Intellisphere, LLC via Copyright Clearance Center.

factors, who require low-dose aspirin and have low potential for NSAID-induced toxicity, should be considered for a non-NSAID agent or use of a traditional NSAID in combination with gastric protection, if warranted. Finally, individuals with cardiovascular and GI risks who require aspirin must be considered for non-NSAID therapy, but if that is not an option, then gastric protection with any type of NSAID must be considered. Any patient, regardless of risk status, who is being considered for long-term traditional NSAID therapy, should also be considered for *H. pylori* testing and treatment if positive. Assuring the use of GI protective agents with NSAIDs is difficult, even in high-risk patients. This is in part due to underprescribing of the appropriate protective agent; other times the difficulty is related to patient compliance. The latter may be due to patients forgetting to take multiple pills or preferring not to take the extra pill, especially if they have no GI symptoms. Several NSAID gastroprotective-containing combination pills are now commercially available, including double-dose famotidine with ibuprofen, diclofenac with misoprostol, and naproxen with esomeprazole. Although initial studies suggested improved compliance and a cost advantage when taking these combination drugs, their clinical benefit over the use of separate pills has not been established. Efforts continue toward developing safer NSAIDs, including NO-releasing NSAIDs, hydrogen sulfide–releasing NSAIDs, dual COX/5-LOX inhibitors, NSAID prodrugs, or agents that can effectively sequester unbound NSAIDs without interfering with their efficacy.

APPROACH AND THERAPY: SUMMARY

Controversy continues regarding the best approach to the patient who presents with dyspepsia (**Chap. 5**). The discovery of *H. pylori* and its role in pathogenesis of ulcers has added a new variable to the equation. Previously, if a patient <50 years of age presented with dyspepsia and without alarming signs or symptoms suggestive of an ulcer complication or malignancy, an empirical therapeutic trial with acid suppression was commonly recommended. Although this approach is practiced by some today, an approach presently gaining approval for the treatment of patients with dyspepsia is outlined in Fig. 15-12. The referral to a gastroenterologist is for the potential need of endoscopy and subsequent evaluation and treatment if the endoscopy is negative.

Once an ulcer (GU or DU) is documented, the main issue at stake is whether *H. pylori* or an NSAID is involved. With *H. pylori* present, independent of the NSAID status, triple therapy is recommended for 14 days, followed by continued acid-suppressing drugs (H_2 receptor antagonist or PPIs) for a total of 4–6 weeks. Selection of patients for documentation of *H. pylori* eradication (organisms gone at least 4 weeks after completing antibiotics) is an area of some debate. The test of choice for documenting eradication is the laboratory-based validated monoclonal stool antigen test or a urea breath test (UBT). The patient must be off antisecretory agents when being tested for eradication of *H. pylori* with UBT or stool antigen. Serologic testing is not useful for the purpose of documenting eradication because antibody titers fall slowly and often do not become undetectable. Two approaches toward documentation of eradication exist: (1) Test for eradication only in individuals with a complicated course or in individuals who are frail or with multisystem

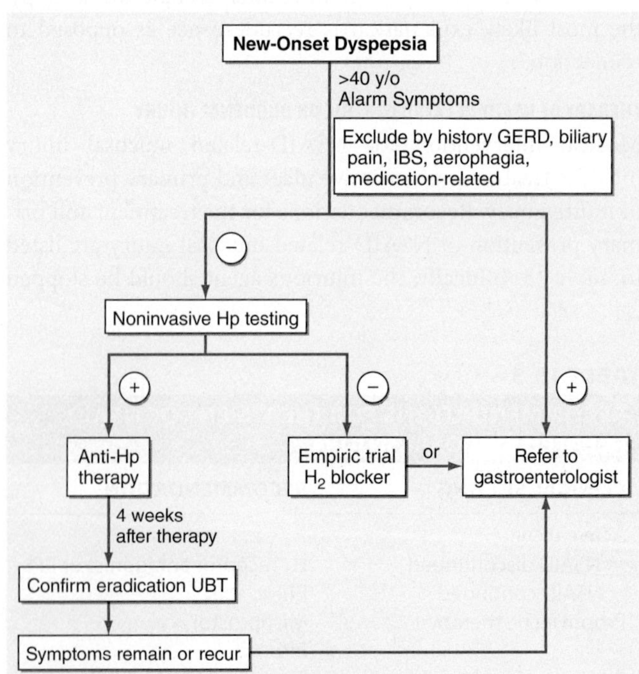

FIGURE 15-12

Overview of new-onset dyspepsia. GERD, gastroesophageal reflux disease; Hp, *Helicobacter pylori*; IBS, irritable bowel syndrome; UBT, urea breath test. *(Adapted from BS Anand and DY Graham: Endoscopy 31:215, 1999.)*

disease who would do poorly with an ulcer recurrence, and (2) test all patients for successful eradication. Some recommend that patients with complicated ulcer disease, or who are frail, should be treated with long-term acid suppression, thus making documentation of *H. pylori* eradication a moot point. In view of this discrepancy in practice, it would be best to discuss with the patient the different options available.

Several issues differentiate the approach to a GU versus a DU. GUs, especially of the body and fundus, have the potential of being malignant. Multiple biopsies of a GU should be taken initially; even if these are negative for neoplasm, repeat endoscopy to document healing at 8–12 weeks should be performed, with biopsy if the ulcer is still present. About 70% of GUs eventually found to be malignant undergo significant (usually incomplete) healing. Repeat endoscopy is warranted in patients with DU if symptoms persist despite medical therapy or a complication is suspected.

The majority (>90%) of GUs and DUs heal with the conventional therapy outlined above. A GU that fails to heal after 12 weeks and a DU that does not heal after 8 weeks of therapy should be considered refractory. Once poor compliance and persistent *H. pylori* infection have been excluded, NSAID use, either inadvertent or surreptitious, must be excluded. In addition, cigarette smoking must be eliminated. For a GU, malignancy must be meticulously excluded. Next, consideration should be given to a gastric acid hypersecretory state such as ZES (see "Zollinger-Ellison Syndrome," below) or the idiopathic form, which can be excluded with gastric acid analysis. Although a subset of patients have gastric acid hypersecretion of unclear etiology as a contributing factor to refractory ulcers, ZES should be excluded with a fasting gastrin or secretin stimulation test (see below). More than 90% of refractory ulcers (either DUs or GUs) heal after 8 weeks of treatment with higher doses of PPI (omeprazole, 40 mg/d; lansoprazole 30–60 mg/d). This higher dose is also effective in maintaining remission. Surgical intervention may be a consideration at this point; however, other rare causes of refractory ulcers must be excluded before recommending surgery. Rare etiologies of refractory ulcers that may be diagnosed by gastric or duodenal biopsies include ischemia, Crohn's disease, amyloidosis, sarcoidosis, lymphoma, eosinophilic gastroenteritis, or infection (cytomegalovirus [CMV], tuberculosis, or syphilis).

SURGICAL THERAPY

Surgical intervention in PUD can be viewed as being either elective, for treatment of medically refractory disease, or as urgent/emergent, for the treatment of an ulcer-related complication. The development of pharmacologic and endoscopic approaches for the treatment of peptic disease and its complications has led to a substantial decrease in the number of operations needed for this disorder with a drop of over 90% for elective ulcer surgery over the last four decades. Refractory ulcers are an exceedingly rare occurrence. Surgery is more often required for treatment of an ulcer-related complication.

Hemorrhage is the most common ulcer-related complication, occurring in ~15–25% of patients. Bleeding may occur in any age group but is most often seen in older patients (sixth decade or beyond). The majority of patients stop bleeding spontaneously, but endoscopic therapy **(Chap. 12)** is necessary in some. Parenterally and orally administered PPIs also decrease ulcer rebleeding in patients who have undergone endoscopic therapy. Patients unresponsive or refractory to endoscopic intervention will require surgery (~5% of transfusion-requiring patients).

Free peritoneal perforation occurs in ~2–3% of DU patients. As in the case of bleeding, up to 10% of these patients will not have antecedent ulcer symptoms. Concomitant bleeding may occur in up to 10% of patients with perforation, with mortality being increased substantially. Peptic ulcer can also penetrate into adjacent organs, especially with a posterior DU, which can penetrate into the pancreas, colon, liver, or biliary tree.

Pyloric channel ulcers or DUs can lead to gastric outlet obstruction in ~2–3% of patients. This can result from chronic scarring or from impaired motility due to inflammation and/or edema with pylorospasm. Patients may present with early satiety, nausea, vomiting of undigested food, and weight loss. Conservative management with nasogastric suction, intravenous hydration/nutrition, and antisecretory agents is indicated for 7–10 days with the hope that a functional obstruction will reverse. If a mechanical obstruction persists, endoscopic intervention with balloon dilation may be effective. Surgery should be considered if all else fails.

SPECIFIC OPERATIONS FOR DUODENAL ULCERS

Surgical treatment was originally designed to decrease gastric acid secretion. Operations most commonly performed include (1) vagotomy and drainage (by pyloroplasty, gastroduodenostomy, or gastrojejunostomy), (2) highly selective vagotomy (which does not require a drainage procedure), and (3) vagotomy with antrectomy. The specific procedure performed is dictated by the underlying circumstances: elective versus emergency, the degree and extent of duodenal ulceration, the etiology of the ulcer (*H. pylori*, NSAIDs, malignancy), and the expertise of the surgeon. Moreover, the trend has been toward a dramatic decrease in the need for surgery for treatment of refractory PUD, and when needed, minimally invasive and anatomy-preserving operations are preferred.

Vagotomy is a component of each of these procedures and is aimed at decreasing acid secretion through ablating cholinergic input to the stomach. Unfortunately, both truncal and selective vagotomy (preserves the celiac and hepatic branches) result in gastric atony despite successful reduction of both basal acid output (BAO; decreased by 85%) and maximal acid output (MAO; decreased by 50%). Drainage through pyloroplasty or gastroduodenostomy is required in an effort to compensate for the vagotomy-induced gastric motility disorder. This procedure has an intermediate complication rate and a 10% ulcer recurrence rate. To minimize gastric dysmotility, highly selective vagotomy (also known as parietal cell, super-selective, or proximal vagotomy) was developed. Only the vagal fibers innervating the portion of the stomach that contains parietal cells is transected, thus leaving fibers important for regulating gastric motility intact. Although this procedure leads to an immediate decrease in both BAO and stimulated acid output, acid secretion recovers over time. By the end of the first postoperative year, basal and stimulated acid output are ~30 and 50%, respectively, of preoperative levels. Ulcer recurrence rates are higher with highly selective vagotomy (≥10%), although the overall complication rates are the lowest of the three procedures.

The procedure that provides the lowest rates of ulcer recurrence (1%) but has the highest complication rate is vagotomy (truncal or selective) in combination with antrectomy. Antrectomy is aimed at eliminating an additional stimulant of gastric acid secretion, gastrin. Two principal types of reanastomoses are used after antrectomy: gastroduodenostomy (Billroth I) or gastrojejunostomy (Billroth II) (Fig. 15-13). Although Billroth I is often preferred over II, severe duodenal inflammation or scarring may preclude its performance. Prospective, randomized studies confirm that partial gastrectomy followed by Roux-en-Y reconstruction leads to a significantly better clinical, endoscopic, and histologic outcome than Billroth II reconstruction.

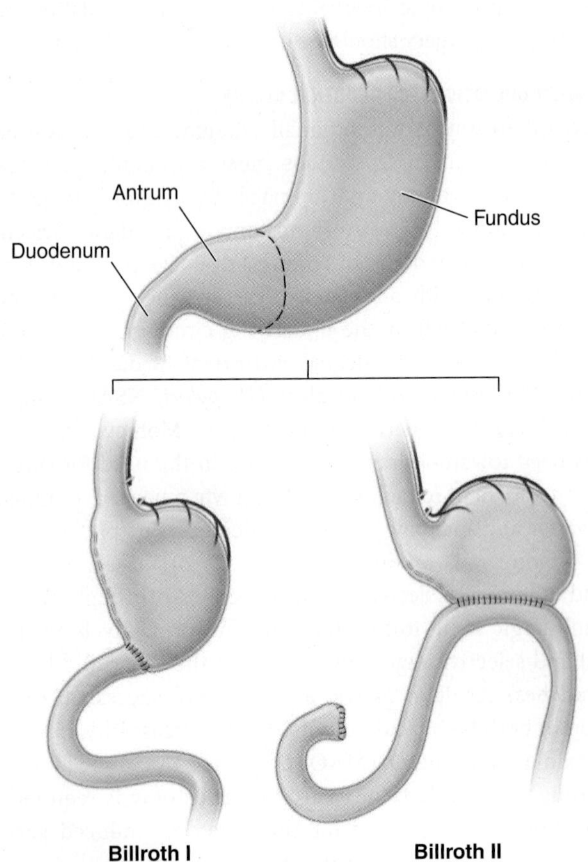

FIGURE 15-13
Schematic representation of Billroth I and II procedures.

Of these procedures, highly selective vagotomy may be the one of choice in the elective setting, except in situations where ulcer recurrence rates are high (prepyloric ulcers and those refractory to medical therapy). Selection of vagotomy and antrectomy may be more appropriate in these circumstances.

These procedures have been traditionally performed by standard laparotomy. The advent of laparoscopic surgery has led several surgical teams to successfully perform highly selective vagotomy, truncal vagotomy/pyloroplasty, and truncal vagotomy/antrectomy through this approach. An increase in the number of laparoscopic procedures for treatment of PUD has occurred. Laparoscopic repair of perforated peptic ulcers is safe, feasible for the experienced surgeon and is associated with decreased postoperative pain, although it does take longer than an open approach. Moreover, no difference between the two approaches is noted in postoperative complications or length of hospital stay.

Specific operations for gastric ulcers The location and the presence of a concomitant DU dictate the operative procedure performed for a GU. Antrectomy (including the ulcer) with a Billroth I anastomosis is the treatment of choice for an antral ulcer. Vagotomy is performed only if a DU is present. Although ulcer excision with vagotomy and drainage procedure has been proposed, the higher incidence of ulcer recurrence makes this a less desirable approach. Ulcers located near the esophagogastric junction may require a more radical approach, a subtotal gastrectomy with a Roux-en-Y esophagogastrojejunostomy (Csendes' procedure). A less aggressive approach, including antrectomy, intraoperative ulcer biopsy, and vagotomy (Kelling-Madlener procedure), may be indicated in fragile patients with a high GU. Ulcer recurrence approaches 30% with this procedure.

Surgery-related complications Complications seen after surgery for PUD are related primarily to the extent of the anatomic modification performed. Minimal alteration (highly selective vagotomy) is associated with higher rates of ulcer recurrence and less GI disturbance. More aggressive surgical procedures have a lower rate of ulcer recurrence but a greater incidence of GI dysfunction. Overall, morbidity and mortality related to these procedures are quite low. Morbidity associated with vagotomy and antrectomy or pyloroplasty is ≤5%, with mortality ~1%. Highly selective vagotomy has lower morbidity and mortality rates of 1 and 0.3%, respectively.

In addition to the potential early consequences of any intraabdominal procedure (bleeding, infection, thromboembolism), gastroparesis, duodenal stump leak, and efferent loop obstruction can be observed.

Recurrent ulceration The risk of ulcer recurrence is directly related to the procedure performed. Ulcers that recur after partial gastric resection tend to develop at the anastomosis (stomal or marginal ulcer). Epigastric abdominal pain is the most frequent presenting complaint (>90%). Severity and duration of pain tend to be more progressive than observed with DUs before surgery.

Ulcers may recur for several reasons, including incomplete vagotomy, inadequate drainage, retained antrum, and, less likely, persistent or recurrent *H. pylori* infection. ZES should have been excluded preoperatively. Surreptitious use of NSAIDs is an important reason for recurrent ulcers after surgery, especially if the initial procedure was done for an NSAID-induced ulcer. Once *H. pylori* and NSAIDs have been excluded as etiologic factors, the question of incomplete vagotomy or retained gastric antrum should be explored. For the latter, fasting plasma gastrin levels should be determined. If elevated, retained antrum or ZES (see below) should be considered. Incomplete vagotomy can be ruled out by gastric acid analysis coupled with sham feeding. In this test, gastric acid output is measured while the patient sees, smells, and chews a meal (without swallowing). The cephalic phase of gastric secretion, which is mediated by the vagus, is being assessed with this study. An increase in gastric acid output in response to sham feeding is evidence that the vagus nerve is intact. A rise in serum pancreatic polypeptide >50% within 30 min of sham feeding is also suggestive of an intact vagus nerve.

Medical therapy with H_2 blockers will heal postoperative ulceration in 70–90% of patients. The efficacy of PPIs has not been fully assessed in this group, but one may anticipate greater rates of ulcer healing compared to those obtained with H_2 blockers. Repeat operation (complete vagotomy, partial gastrectomy) may be required in a small subgroup of patients who have not responded to aggressive medical management.

Afferent loop syndromes Although rarely seen today as a result of the decrease in the performance of Billroth II anastomosis, two types of afferent loop syndrome can occur in patients who have undergone this type of partial gastric resection. The more common of the two is bacterial overgrowth in the afferent limb secondary to stasis. Patients may experience postprandial abdominal pain, bloating, and diarrhea with concomitant malabsorption of fats and vitamin B_{12}. Cases refractory to antibiotics may require surgical revision of the loop. The less common afferent loop syndrome can present with severe abdominal pain and bloating that occur 20–60 min after meals. Pain is often followed by nausea and vomiting of bile-containing material. The pain and bloating may improve after emesis. The cause of this clinical picture is theorized to be incomplete drainage of bile and pancreatic secretions from an afferent loop that is partially obstructed. Cases refractory to dietary measures may need surgical revision or conversion of the Billroth II anastomosis to a Roux-en-Y gastrojejunostomy.

Dumping syndrome Dumping syndrome consists of a series of vasomotor and GI signs and symptoms and occurs in patients who have undergone vagotomy and drainage (especially Billroth procedures). Two phases of dumping, early and late, can occur. Early dumping takes place 15–30 min after meals and consists of crampy abdominal discomfort, nausea, diarrhea, belching, tachycardia, palpitations, diaphoresis, light-headedness, and, rarely, syncope. These signs and symptoms arise from the rapid emptying of hyperosmolar gastric contents into the small intestine, resulting in a fluid shift into the gut lumen with plasma volume contraction and acute intestinal distention. Release of vasoactive GI hormones (vasoactive intestinal polypeptide, neurotensin, motilin) is also theorized to play a role in early dumping.

The late phase of dumping typically occurs 90 min to 3 h after meals. Vasomotor symptoms (light-headedness, diaphoresis, palpitations, tachycardia, and syncope) predominate during this phase. This component of dumping is thought to be secondary to hypoglycemia from excessive insulin release.

Dumping syndrome is most noticeable after meals rich in simple carbohydrates (especially sucrose) and high osmolarity. Ingestion of large amounts of fluids may also contribute. Up to 50% of postvagotomy and drainage patients will experience dumping syndrome to some degree early on. Signs and symptoms often improve with time, but a severe protracted picture can occur in up to 1% of patients.

Dietary modification is the cornerstone of therapy for patients with dumping syndrome. Small, multiple (six) meals devoid of simple carbohydrates coupled with elimination of liquids during meals is important. Antidiarrheals and anticholinergic agents are complementary to diet. Guar and pectin, which increase the viscosity of intraluminal contents, may be beneficial in more symptomatic individuals. Acarbose, an α-glucosidase inhibitor that delays digestion of ingested carbohydrates, has also been shown to be beneficial in the treatment of the late phases of dumping. The somatostatin analogue octreotide has been successful in diet-refractory cases. This drug is administered subcutaneously (50 μg tid), titrated according to clinical response. A long-acting depot formulation of octreotide can be administered once every 28 days and provides symptom relief comparable to the short-acting agent. In addition, patient weight gain and quality of life appear to be superior with the long-acting form.

Postvagotomy diarrhea Up to 10% of patients may seek medical attention for the treatment of postvagotomy diarrhea. This complication is most commonly observed after truncal vagotomy, which is rarely performed today. Patients may complain of intermittent diarrhea that occurs typically 1–2 h after meals. Occasionally the symptoms may be severe and relentless. This is due to a motility disorder from interruption of the vagal fibers supplying the luminal gut. Other contributing factors may include decreased absorption of nutrients (see below), increased excretion of bile acids, and release of luminal factors that promote secretion. Diphenoxylate or loperamide is often useful in symptom control. The bile salt–bindingagent cholestyramine may be helpful in severe cases. Surgical reversal of a 10-cm segment of jejunum may yield a substantial improvement in bowel frequency in a subset of patients.

Bile reflux gastropathy A subset of post–partial gastrectomy patients who present with abdominal pain, early satiety, nausea, and vomiting will have mucosal erythema of the gastric remnant as the only finding. Histologic examination of the gastric mucosa reveals minimal inflammation but the presence of epithelial cell injury. This clinical picture is categorized as bile or alkaline reflux gastropathy/gastritis. Although reflux of bile is implicated as the reason for this disorder, the mechanism is unknown. Prokinetic agents, cholestyramine, and sucralfate have been somewhat effective treatments. Severe refractory symptoms may require using either nuclear scanning with ^{99m}Tc-HIDA to document reflux or an alkaline challenge test, where 0.1 *N* NaOH is infused into the stomach in an effort to reproduce the patient's symptoms. Surgical diversion of pancreaticobiliary secretions away from the gastric remnant with a Roux-en-Y gastrojejunostomy consisting of a long (50–60 cm) Roux limb has been used in severe cases. Bilious vomiting improves, but early satiety and bloating may persist in up to 50% of patients.

Maldigestion and malabsorption Weight loss can be observed in up to 60% of patients after partial gastric resection. Patients can experience a 10% loss of body weight, which stabilizes 3 months postoperatively. A significant component of this weight reduction is due to decreased oral intake. However, mild steatorrhea can also develop. Reasons for maldigestion/malabsorption include decreased gastric acid production, rapid gastric emptying, decreased food dispersion in the stomach, reduced luminal bile concentration, reduced pancreatic secretory response to feeding, and rapid intestinal transit.

Decreased serum vitamin B_{12} levels can be observed after partial gastrectomy. This is usually not due to deficiency of IF, since a minimal amount of parietal cells (source of IF) are removed during antrectomy. Reduced vitamin B_{12} may be due to competition for the vitamin by bacterial overgrowth or inability to split the vitamin from its protein-bound source due to hypochlorhydria.

Iron-deficiency anemia may be a consequence of impaired absorption of dietary iron in patients with a Billroth II gastrojejunostomy. Absorption of iron salts is normal in these individuals; thus, a favorable response to oral iron supplementation can be anticipated. Folate deficiency with concomitant anemia can also develop in these patients. This deficiency may be secondary to decreased absorption or diminished oral intake.

Malabsorption of vitamin D and calcium resulting in osteoporosis and osteomalacia is common after partial gastrectomy and gastrojejunostomy (Billroth II). Osteomalacia can occur as a late complication in up to 25% of post–partial gastrectomy patients. Bone fractures occur twice as commonly in men after gastric surgery as in a control population. It may take years before x-ray findings demonstrate diminished bone density. Elevated alkaline phosphatase, reduced serum calcium, bone pain, and pathologic fractures may be seen in patients with osteomalacia. The high incidence of these abnormalities in this subgroup of patients justifies treating them with vitamin D and calcium supplementation indefinitely. Therapy is especially important in females. Copper deficiency has also been reported in patients undergoing surgeries that bypass the duodenum, where copper is primarily absorbed. Patients may present with a rare syndrome that includes ataxia, myelopathy, and peripheral neuropathy.

Gastric adenocarcinoma The incidence of adenocarcinoma in the gastric stump is increased 15 years after resection. Some have reported a four- to fivefold increase in gastric cancer 20–25 years after resection. The pathogenesis is unclear but may involve alkaline reflux, bacterial proliferation, or hypochlorhydria. The role of endoscopic screening is not clear, and most guidelines do not support its use.

Additional complications Reflux esophagitis and a higher incidence of gallstones and cholecystitis have been reported to patients undergoing subtotal gastrectomy. The latter is thought to be due to decreased gallbladder contractility associated with vagotomy and bypass of the duodenum, leading to decreased postprandial release of cholecystokinin.

RELATED CONDITIONS

ZOLLINGER–ELLISON SYNDROME

Severe peptic ulcer diathesis secondary to gastric acid hypersecretion due to unregulated gastrin release from a non-β cell endocrine tumor (gastrinoma) defines the components of ZES. Initially, ZES was typified by aggressive and refractory ulceration in which total gastrectomy provided the only chance for enhancing survival. Today it can be cured by surgical resection in up to 40% of patients.

Epidemiology

The incidence of ZES varies from 0.1–1% of individuals presenting with PUD. Males are more commonly affected than females, and the majority of patients are diagnosed between ages 30 and 50. Gastrinomas are classified into sporadic tumors (more common) and those associated with multiple endocrine neoplasia (MEN) type 1 (see below). The widespread availability and use of PPIs has led to a decreased patient referral for gastrinoma evaluation, delay in diagnosis, and an increase in false-positive diagnoses of ZES. In fact, diagnosis may be delayed for 6 or more years after symptoms consistent with ZES are displayed.

Pathophysiology

Hypergastrinemia originating from an autonomous neoplasm is the driving force responsible for the clinical manifestations in ZES. Gastrin stimulates acid secretion through gastrin receptors on parietal cells and by inducing histamine release from ECL cells. Gastrin also has a trophic action on gastric epithelial cells. Longstanding hypergastrinemia leads to markedly increased gastric acid secretion through both parietal cell stimulation and increased parietal cell mass. The increased gastric acid output leads to peptic ulcer diathesis, erosive esophagitis, and diarrhea.

Tumor distribution

Although early studies suggested that the vast majority of gastrinomas occurred within the pancreas, a significant number of these lesions are extrapancreatic. Over 80% of these tumors are found within the hypothetical gastrinoma triangle (confluence of the cystic and common bile ducts superiorly, junction of the second and third portions of the duodenum inferiorly, and junction of the neck and body of the pancreas medially). Duodenal tumors constitute the most common nonpancreatic lesion; between 50 and 75% of gastrinomas are found here. Duodenal tumors are smaller, slower growing, and less likely to metastasize than pancreatic lesions. Less common extrapancreatic sites include stomach, bones, ovaries, heart, liver, and lymph nodes. More than 60% of tumors are considered malignant, with up to 30–50% of patients having multiple lesions or metastatic disease at presentation. Histologically, gastrin-producing cells appear well-differentiated, expressing markers typically found in endocrine neoplasms (chromogranin, neuron-specific enolase).

Clinical manifestations

Gastric acid hypersecretion is responsible for the signs and symptoms observed in patients with ZES. Peptic ulcer is the most common clinical manifestation, occurring in >90% of gastrinoma patients. Initial presentation and ulcer location (duodenal bulb) may be indistinguishable from common PUD. Clinical situations that should create suspicion of gastrinoma are ulcers in unusual locations (second part of the duodenum and beyond), ulcers refractory to standard medical therapy, ulcer recurrence after acid-reducing surgery, ulcers presenting with frank complications (bleeding, obstruction, and perforation), or ulcers in the absence of *H. pylori* or NSAID ingestion. Symptoms of esophageal origin are present in up to two-thirds of patients with ZES, with a spectrum ranging from mild esophagitis to frank ulceration with stricture and Barrett's mucosa.

Diarrhea, the next most common clinical manifestation, is found in up to 50% of patients. Although diarrhea often occurs concomitantly with acid peptic disease, it may also occur independent of an ulcer. Etiology of the diarrhea is multifactorial, resulting from marked volume overload to the small bowel, pancreatic enzyme inactivation by acid, and damage of the intestinal epithelial surface by acid. The epithelial damage can lead to a mild degree of maldigestion and malabsorption of nutrients. The diarrhea may also have a secretory component due to the direct stimulatory effect of gastrin on enterocytes or the co-secretion of additional hormones from the tumor such as vasoactive intestinal peptide.

Gastrinomas can develop in the presence of MEN 1 syndrome **(Chap. 55)** in ~25% of patients. This autosomal dominant disorder involves primarily three organ sites: the parathyroid glands (80–90%), pancreas (40–80%), and pituitary gland (30–60%). The syndrome is caused by inactivating mutations of the *MEN1* tumor suppressor gene found on the long arm of chromosome 11q13. The gene encodes for Menin, which has an important role in DNA replication and transcriptional regulation. A genetic diagnosis is obtained by sequencing of the *MEN1* gene, which can reveal mutations in 70–90% of typical MEN 1 cases. A family may have an unknown mutation, making a genetic diagnosis impossible, and therefore certain individuals will require a clinical diagnosis, which is determined by whether a patient has tumors in two of the three endocrine organs (parathyroid, pancreas/duodenum, or pituitary) or has a family history of MEN 1 and one of the endocrine organ tumors. In view of the stimulatory effect of calcium on gastric secretion, the hyperparathyroidism and hypercalcemia seen in MEN 1 patients may have a direct effect on ulcer disease. Resolution of hypercalcemia by parathyroidectomy reduces gastrin and gastric acid output in gastrinoma patients. An additional distinguishing feature in ZES patients with MEN 1 is the higher incidence of gastric carcinoid tumor development (as compared to patients with sporadic gastrinomas). ZES presents and is diagnosed earlier in MEN 1 patients, and they have a more indolent course as compared to patients with sporadic gastrinoma. Gastrinomas tend to be smaller, multiple, and located in the duodenal wall more often than is seen in patients with sporadic ZES. Establishing the diagnosis of MEN 1 is critical in order to provide genetic counseling to the patient and his or her family and also to determine the recommended surgical approach.

Diagnosis

Biochemical measurements of gastrin and acid secretion in patients suspected of ZES play an important role is establishing this rare diagnosis. Often, patients suspected of having ZES will be treated with a PPI in an effort to ameliorate symptoms and decrease the likelihood of possible acid-related complications. The presence of the PPI, which will lower acid secretion and potentially elevate fasting gastrin levels in normal individuals, will make the diagnostic approach in these individuals somewhat difficult. Significant morbidity related to peptic diathesis has been described when stopping PPIs in gastrinoma patients; therefore,

TABLE 15-7

WHEN TO OBTAIN A FASTING SERUM GASTRIN LEVEL
Multiple ulcers
Ulcers in unusual locations; associated with severe esophagitis; resistant to therapy with frequent recurrences; in the absence of nonsteroidal anti-inflammatory drug ingestion or *H. pylori* infection
Ulcer patients awaiting surgery
Extensive family history for peptic ulcer disease
Postoperative ulcer recurrence
Basal hyperchlorhydria
Unexplained diarrhea or steatorrhea
Hypercalcemia
Family history of pancreatic islet, pituitary, or parathyroid tumor
Prominent gastric or duodenal folds

a systematic approach in stopping these agents is warranted (see below). The first step in the evaluation of a patient suspected of having ZES is to obtain a fasting gastrin level. A list of clinical scenarios that should arouse suspicion regarding this diagnosis is shown in Table 15-7. Fasting gastrin levels obtained using a dependable assay are usually <150 pg/mL. A normal fasting gastrin, on two separate occasions, especially if the patient is on a PPI, virtually excludes this diagnosis. Virtually all gastrinoma patients will have a gastrin level >150–200 pg/mL. Measurement of fasting gastrin should be repeated to confirm the clinical suspicion. Some of the commercial biochemical assays used for measuring serum gastrin may be inaccurate. Variable specificity of the antibodies used have led to both false-positive and false-negative fasting gastrin levels, placing in jeopardy the ability to make an accurate diagnosis of ZES.

Multiple processes can lead to an elevated fasting gastrin level, the most frequent of which are gastric hypochlorhydria and achlorhydria, with or without pernicious anemia. Gastric acid induces feedback inhibition of gastrin release. A decrease in acid production will subsequently lead to failure of the feedback inhibitory pathway, resulting in net hypergastrinemia. Gastrin levels will thus be high in patients using antisecretory agents for the treatment of acid peptic disorders and dyspepsia. *H. pylori* infection can also cause hypergastrinemia. Additional causes of elevated gastrin include retained gastric antrum; G cell hyperplasia; gastric outlet obstruction; renal insufficiency; massive small-bowel obstruction; and conditions such as rheumatoid arthritis, vitiligo, diabetes mellitus, and pheochromocytoma. Although a fasting gastrin >10 times normal is highly suggestive of ZES, two-thirds of patients will have fasting gastrin levels that overlap with levels found in the more common disorders outlined above, especially if a PPI is being taken by the patient. The effect of the PPI on gastrin levels and acid secretion will linger several days after stopping the PPI; therefore, it should be stopped for a minimum of 7 days before testing. During this period, the patient should be placed on a histamine H_2 antagonist, such as famotidine, twice to three times per day. Although this type of agent has a short-term effect on gastrin and acid secretion, it needs to be stopped 24 h before repeating fasting gastrin levels or performing some the tests highlighted below. The patient may take antacids for the final day, stopping them approximately 12 h before testing is performed. Heightened awareness of complications related to gastric acid hypersecretion during the period of PPI cessation is critical.

The next step in establishing a biochemical diagnosis of gastrinoma is to assess acid secretion. Nothing further needs to be done if decreased acid output in the absence of a PPI is observed. A pH can be measured on gastric fluid obtained either during endoscopy or through nasogastric aspiration; a pH <3 is suggestive of a gastrinoma, but a pH >3 is not helpful in excluding the diagnosis. In those situations where the pH is >3, formal gastric acid analysis should be performed if available. Normal BAO in nongastric surgery patients is typically <5 meq/h. A BAO >15 meq/h in the presence of hypergastrinemia is considered pathognomonic of ZES, but up to 12% of patients with common PUD may have elevated BAO to a lesser degree that can overlap with levels seen in ZES patients. In an effort to improve the sensitivity and specificity of gastric secretory studies, a BAO/MAO ratio was established using pentagastrin infusion as a way to maximally stimulate acid production, with a BAO/MAO ratio >0.6 being highly suggestive of ZES. Pentagastrin is no longer available in the United States, making measurement of MAO virtually impossible. An endoscopic method for measuring gastric acid output has been developed but requires further validation.

Gastrin provocative tests have been developed in an effort to differentiate between the causes of hypergastrinemia and are especially helpful in patients with indeterminate acid secretory studies. The tests are the secretin stimulation test and the calcium infusion study. The most sensitive and specific gastrin provocative test for the diagnosis of gastrinoma is the secretin study. An increase in gastrin of ≥120 pg within 15 min of secretin injection has a sensitivity and specificity of >90% for ZES. PPI-induced hypochlorhydria or achlorhydria may lead to a false-positive secretin test; thus, this agent must be stopped for 1 week before testing.

The calcium infusion study is less sensitive and specific than the secretin test, which, coupled with it being a more cumbersome study with greater potential for adverse effects, relegates it to rare utilization in the cases where the patient's clinical characteristics are highly suggestive of ZES but the secretin stimulation is inconclusive.

TABLE 15-8

SENSITIVITY OF IMAGING STUDIES IN ZOLLINGER-ELLISON SYNDROME

STUDY	SENSITIVITY, % PRIMARY GASTRINOMA	SENSITIVITY, % METASTATIC GASTRINOMA
Ultrasound	21–28	14
CT scan	55–70	>85
Selective angiography	35–68	33–86
Portal venous sampling	70–90	N/A
SASI	55–78	41
MRI	55–70	>85
OctreoScan	67–86	80–100
EUS	80–100	N/A

Abbreviations: CT, computed tomography; EUS, endoscopic ultrasonography; MRI, magnetic resonance imaging; N/A, not applicable; OctreoScan, imaging with ^{111}In-pentreotide; SASI, selective arterial secretin injection.

Tumor localization

Once the biochemical diagnosis of gastrinoma has been confirmed, the tumor must be located. Multiple imaging studies have been used in an effort to enhance tumor localization (Table 15-8). The broad range of sensitivity is due to the variable success rates achieved by the different investigative groups. Endoscopic ultrasound (EUS) permits imaging of the pancreas with a high degree of resolution (<5 mm). This modality is particularly helpful in excluding small neoplasms within the pancreas and in assessing the presence of surrounding lymph nodes and vascular involvement, but it is not very sensitive for finding duodenal lesions. Several types of endocrine tumors express cell-surface receptors for somatostatin. This permits the localization of gastrinomas by measuring the uptake of the stable somatostatin analogue ^{111}In-pentreotide (OctreoScan) with sensitivity and specificity rates of >85%.

Up to 50% of patients have metastatic disease at diagnosis. Success in controlling gastric acid hypersecretion has shifted the emphasis of therapy toward providing a surgical cure. Detecting the primary tumor and excluding metastatic disease are critical in view of this paradigm shift. Once a biochemical diagnosis has been confirmed, the patient should first undergo an abdominal computed tomography (CT) scan, magnetic resonance imaging (MRI), or OctreoScan (depending on availability) to exclude metastatic disease. In addition, the positron emitter ^{68}Ga has been used to label somatostatin analogues for positron emission tomography (PET) with some success. In addition, hybrid scanners combining CT scan with PET scan are also available in certain specialized centers. Once metastatic disease has been excluded, an experienced endocrine surgeon may opt for exploratory laparotomy with intraoperative ultrasound or transillumination. In other centers, careful examination of the peripancreatic area with EUS, accompanied by endoscopic exploration of the duodenum for primary tumors, will be performed before surgery. Selective arterial secretin injection may be a useful adjuvant for localizing tumors in a subset of patients. The extent of the diagnostic and surgical approach must be carefully balanced with the patient's overall physiologic condition and the natural history of a slow-growing gastrinoma.

TREATMENT Zollinger-Ellison Syndrome

Treatment of functional endocrine tumors is directed at ameliorating the signs and symptoms related to hormone overproduction, curative resection of the neoplasm, and attempts to control tumor growth in metastatic disease.

PPIs are the treatment of choice and have decreased the need for total gastrectomy. Initial PPI doses tend to be higher than those used for treatment of GERD or PUD. The initial dose of omeprazole, lansoprazole, rabeprazole, or esomeprazole should be in the range of 60 mg in divided doses in a 24-h period. Dosing can be adjusted to achieve a BAO <10 meq/h (at the drug trough) in surgery-naive patients and to <5 meq/h in individuals who have previously undergone an acid-reducing operation. Although the somatostatin analogue has inhibitory effects on gastrin release from receptor-bearing tumors and inhibits gastric acid secretion to some extent, PPIs have the advantage of reducing parietal cell activity to a greater degree. Despite this, octreotide may be considered as adjunctive therapy to the PPI in patients with tumors that express somatostatin receptors and have peptic symptoms that are difficult to control with high-dose PPI.

The ultimate goal of surgery would be to provide a definitive cure. Improved understanding of tumor distribution has led to immediate cure rates as high as 60% with 10-year disease-free intervals as high as 34% in sporadic gastrinoma patients undergoing surgery. A positive outcome is highly dependent on the experience of the surgical team treating these rare tumors. Surgical therapy of gastrinoma patients with MEN 1 remains controversial because of the difficulty in rendering these patients disease-free with surgery. In contrast to the encouraging postoperative results observed in patients with sporadic disease, only 6% of MEN 1 patients are disease free 5 years after an operation. Moreover, in contrast to patients with sporadic ZES, the clinical course of MEN 1 patients is benign and rarely leads to disease-related mortality, recommending that early surgery be deferred. Some groups suggest surgery only if a clearly identifiable, nonmetastatic lesion is documented by structural studies. Others advocate a more aggressive approach, where all patients free of hepatic metastasis are explored and all detected tumors in the duodenum are resected; this is followed by enucleation of lesions in the pancreatic head, with a distal pancreatectomy to follow.

The outcome of the two approaches has not been clearly defined. Laparoscopic surgical interventions may provide attractive approaches in the future but currently seem to be of some limited benefit in patients with gastrinoma because a significant percentage of the tumors may be extrapancreatic and difficult to localize with a laparoscopic approach. Finally, patients selected for surgery should be individuals whose health status would lead them to tolerate a more aggressive operation and obtain the long-term benefits from such aggressive surgery, which are often witnessed after 10 years.

Therapy of metastatic endocrine tumors in general remains suboptimal; gastrinomas are no exception. In light of the observation that in many instances tumor growth is indolent and that many individuals with metastatic disease remain relatively stable for significant periods of time, many advocate not instituting systemic tumor-targeted therapy until evidence of tumor progression or refractory symptoms not controlled with PPIs are noted. Medical approaches, including biological therapy (IFN-α, long-acting somatostatin analogues, peptide receptor radionuclides), systemic chemotherapy (streptozotocin, 5-fluorouracil, and doxorubicin), and hepatic artery embolization, may lead to significant toxicity without a substantial improvement in overall survival. ^{111}In-pentetreotide has been used in the therapy of metastatic neuroendocrine tumors; further studies are needed. Several novel therapies are being explored, including radiofrequency ablation or cryoablation of liver lesions and use of agents that block the vascular endothelial growth receptor pathway (bevacizumab, sunitinib) or the mammalian target of rapamycin **(Chap. 55)**.

Surgical approaches, including debulking surgery and liver transplantation for hepatic metastasis, have also produced limited benefit.

The overall 5- and 10-year survival rates for gastrinoma patients are 62–75% and 47–53%, respectively. Individuals with the entire tumor resected or those with a negative laparotomy have 5- and 10-year survival rates >90%. Patients with incompletely resected tumors have 5- and 10-year survival rates of 43% and 25%, respectively. Patients with hepatic metastasis have <20% survival at 5 years. Favorable prognostic indicators include primary duodenal wall tumors, isolated lymph node tumor, the presence of MEN 1, and undetectable tumor upon surgical exploration. Poor outcome is seen in patients with shorter disease duration; higher gastrin levels (>10,000 pg/mL); large pancreatic primary tumors (>3 cm); metastatic disease to lymph nodes, liver, and bone; and Cushing's syndrome. Rapid growth of hepatic metastases is also predictive of poor outcome.

STRESS-RELATED MUCOSAL INJURY

Patients suffering from shock, sepsis, massive burns, severe trauma, or head injury can develop acute erosive gastric mucosal changes or frank ulceration with bleeding. Classified as stress-induced gastritis or ulcers, injury is most commonly observed in the acid-producing (fundus and body) portions of the stomach. The most common presentation is GI bleeding, which is usually minimal but can occasionally be life threatening. Respiratory failure requiring mechanical ventilation and underlying coagulopathy are risk factors for bleeding, which tends to occur 48–72 h after the acute injury or insult.

Histologically, stress injury does not contain inflammation or *H. pylori*; thus, "gastritis" is a misnomer. Although elevated gastric acid secretion may be noted in patients with stress ulceration after head trauma (Cushing's ulcer) and severe burns (Curling's ulcer), mucosal ischemia, breakdown of the normal protective barriers of the stomach, systemic release of cytokines, poor GI motility, and oxidative stress also play an important role in the pathogenesis. Acid must contribute to injury in view of the significant drop in bleeding noted when acid inhibitors are used as prophylaxis for stress gastritis.

Improvement in the general management of intensive care unit patients has led to a significant decrease in the incidence of GI bleeding due to stress ulceration. The estimated decrease in bleeding is from 20–30% to <5%. This improvement has led to some debate regarding the need for prophylactic therapy. The high mortality associated with stress-induced clinically important GI bleeding (>40%) and the limited benefit of medical (endoscopic, angiographic) and surgical therapy in a patient with hemodynamically compromising bleeding associated with stress ulcer/gastritis support the use of preventive measures in high-risk patients (mechanically ventilated, coagulopathy, multiorgan failure, or severe burns). Maintenance of gastric pH >3.5 with continuous infusion of H_2 blockers or liquid antacids administered every 2–3 h are viable options. Tolerance to the H_2 blocker is likely to develop; thus, careful monitoring of the gastric pH and dose adjustment are important if H_2 blockers are used. Sucralfate slurry (1 g every 4–6 h) has also been somewhat successful but requires a gastric tube and may lead to constipation and aluminum toxicity. Sucralfate use in endotracheal intubated patients has also been associated with aspiration pneumonia. Meta-analysis comparing H_2 blockers with PPIs for the prevention of stress-associated clinically important and overt GI bleeding demonstrates superiority of the latter without increasing the risk of nosocomial infections, increasing mortality, or prolonging intensive care unit length of stay. Therefore, PPIs are the treatment of choice for stress prophylaxis. Oral PPI is the best option if the patient can tolerate enteral administration. Pantoprazole is available as an intravenous formulation for individuals in whom enteral administration is not possible. If bleeding occurs despite these measures, endoscopy, intraarterial vasopressin, and embolization are options. If all else fails, then surgery should be considered. Although vagotomy and antrectomy may be used, the better approach would be a total gastrectomy, which has an exceedingly high mortality rate in this setting.

GASTRITIS

The term *gastritis* should be reserved for histologically documented inflammation of the gastric mucosa. Gastritis is not the mucosal erythema seen during endoscopy and is not interchangeable with "dyspepsia." The etiologic factors leading to gastritis are broad and heterogeneous. Gastritis has been classified based on time course (acute vs chronic), histologic features, and anatomic distribution or proposed pathogenic mechanism (Table 15-9).

The correlation between the histologic findings of gastritis, the clinical picture of abdominal pain or dyspepsia, and endoscopic findings noted on gross inspection of the gastric mucosa is poor. Therefore, there is no typical clinical manifestation of gastritis.

Acute gastritis

The most common causes of acute gastritis are infectious. Acute infection with *H. pylori* induces gastritis. However, *H. pylori* acute gastritis has not been extensively studied. It is reported as presenting with sudden onset of epigastric pain, nausea, and vomiting, and limited mucosal histologic studies demonstrate a marked infiltrate of neutrophils with edema and hyperemia. If not treated, this picture will evolve into one of chronic gastritis. Hypochlorhydria lasting for up to 1 year may follow acute *H. pylori* infection.

TABLE 15-9

CLASSIFICATION OF GASTRITIS

- I. Acute gastritis
  - A. Acute *H. pylori* infection
  - B. Other acute Infectious gastritides
    1. Bacterial (other than *H. pylori)*
    2. *H. heilmannii*
    3. Phlegmonous
    4. Mycobacterial
    5. Syphilitic
    6. Viral
    7. Parasitic
    8. Fungal
- II. Chronic atrophic gastritis
  - A. Type A: Autoimmune, body-predominant
  - B. Type B: *H. pylori*–related, antral-predominant
  - C. Indeterminate
- III. Uncommon forms of gastritis
  - A. Lymphocytic
  - B. Eosinophilic
  - C. Crohn's disease
  - D. Sarcoidosis
  - E. Isolated granulomatous gastritis
  - F. Russell body gastritis

Bacterial infection of the stomach or phlegmonous gastritis is a rare, potentially life-threatening disorder characterized by marked and diffuse acute inflammatory infiltrates of the entire gastric wall, at times accompanied by necrosis. Elderly individuals, alcoholics, and AIDS patients may be affected. Potential iatrogenic causes include polypectomy and mucosal injection with India ink. Organisms associated with this entity include streptococci, staphylococci, *Escherichia coli, Proteus,* and *Haemophilus* species. Failure of supportive measures and antibiotics may result in gastrectomy.

Other types of infectious gastritis may occur in immunocompromised individuals such as AIDS patients. Examples include herpetic (herpes simplex) or CMV gastritis. The histologic finding of intranuclear inclusions would be observed in the latter.

Chronic gastritis

Chronic gastritis is identified histologically by an inflammatory cell infiltrate consisting primarily of lymphocytes and plasma cells, with very scant neutrophil involvement. Distribution of the inflammation may be patchy, initially involving superficial and glandular portions of the gastric mucosa. This picture may progress to more severe glandular destruction, with atrophy and metaplasia. Chronic gastritis has been classified according to histologic characteristics. These include superficial atrophic changes and gastric atrophy. The association of atrophic gastritis with the development of gastric cancer has led to the development of endoscopic and serologic markers of severity. Some of these include gross inspection and classification of mucosal abnormalities during standard endoscopy, magnification endoscopy, endoscopy with narrow band imaging and/or autofluorescence imaging, and measurement of several serum biomarkers including pepsinogen I and II levels, gastrin-17, and anti-*H. pylori* serologies. The clinical utility of these tools is currently being explored.

The early phase of chronic gastritis is *superficial gastritis.* The inflammatory changes are limited to the lamina propria of the surface mucosa, with edema and cellular infiltrates separating intact gastric glands. The next stage is *atrophic gastritis.* The inflammatory infiltrate extends deeper into the mucosa, with progressive distortion and destruction of the glands. The final stage of chronic gastritis is *gastric atrophy.* Glandular structures are lost, and there is a paucity of inflammatory infiltrates. Endoscopically, the mucosa may be substantially thin, permitting clear visualization of the underlying blood vessels.

Gastric glands may undergo morphologic transformation in chronic gastritis. Intestinal metaplasia denotes the conversion of gastric glands to a small intestinal phenotype with small-bowel mucosal glands containing goblet cells. The metaplastic changes may vary in distribution from patchy to fairly extensive gastric involvement. Intestinal metaplasia is an important predisposing factor for gastric cancer **(Chap. 51)**.

Chronic gastritis is also classified according to the predominant site of involvement. Type A refers to the body-predominant form (autoimmune), and type B is the antral-predominant form (*H. pylori*–related). This classification is artificial in view of the difficulty in distinguishing between these two entities. The term *AB gastritis* has been used to refer to a mixed antral/body picture.

Type A gastritis

The less common of the two forms involves primarily the fundus and body, with antral sparing. Traditionally, this form of gastritis has been associated with pernicious anemia in the presence of circulating antibodies against parietal cells and IF; thus, it is also called *autoimmune gastritis. H. pylori* infection can lead to a similar distribution of gastritis. The characteristics of an autoimmune picture are not always present.

Antibodies to parietal cells have been detected in >90% of patients with pernicious anemia and in up to 50% of patients with type A gastritis. The parietal cell antibody is directed against H^+,K^+-ATPase. T cells are also implicated in the injury pattern of this form of gastritis. A subset of patients infected with *H. pylori* develop antibodies against H^+,K^+-ATPase, potentially leading to the atrophic gastritis pattern seen in some patients infected with this organism. The mechanism is thought to involve molecular mimicry between *H. pylori* LPS and H^+,K^+-ATPase.

Parietal cell antibodies and atrophic gastritis are observed in family members of patients with pernicious anemia. These antibodies are observed in up to 20% of individuals over age 60 and in ~20% of patients with vitiligo and Addison's disease. About one-half of patients with pernicious anemia have antibodies to thyroid antigens, and about 30% of patients with thyroid disease have circulating antiparietal cell antibodies. Anti-IF antibodies are more specific than parietal cell antibodies for type A gastritis, being present in ~40% of patients with pernicious anemia. Another parameter consistent with this form of gastritis being autoimmune in origin is the higher incidence of specific familial histocompatibility haplotypes such as HLA-B8 and HLA-DR3.

The parietal cell–containing gastric gland is preferentially targeted in this form of gastritis, and achlorhydria results. Parietal cells are the source of IF, the lack of which will lead to vitamin B_{12} deficiency and its sequelae (megaloblastic anemia, neurologic dysfunction).

Gastric acid plays an important role in feedback inhibition of gastrin release from G cells. Achlorhydria, coupled with relative sparing of the antral mucosa (site of G cells), leads to hypergastrinemia. Gastrin levels can be markedly elevated (>500 pg/mL) in patients with pernicious anemia. ECL cell hyperplasia with frank development of gastric carcinoid tumors may result from gastrin trophic effects. Hypergastrinemia and achlorhydria may also be seen in nonpernicious anemia–associated type A gastritis.

Type B gastritis

Type B, or antral-predominant, gastritis is the more common form of chronic gastritis. *H. pylori* infection is the cause of this entity. Although described as "antral-predominant," this is likely a misnomer in view of studies documenting the progression of the inflammatory process toward the body and fundus of infected individuals. The conversion to a pangastritis is time-dependent and estimated to require 15–20 years. This form of gastritis increases with age, being present in up to 100% of persons over age 70. Histology improves after *H. pylori* eradication. The number of *H. pylori* organisms decreases dramatically with progression to gastric atrophy, and the degree of inflammation correlates with the level of these organisms. Early on, with antral-predominant findings, the quantity of *H. pylori* is highest and a dense chronic inflammatory infiltrate of the lamina propria is noted, accompanied by epithelial cell infiltration with polymorphonuclear leukocytes (Fig. 15-14).

Multifocal atrophic gastritis, gastric atrophy with subsequent metaplasia, has been observed in chronic *H. pylori*–induced gastritis. This may ultimately lead to development of gastric adenocarcinoma (Fig. 15-8; **Chap. 51**). *H. pylori* infection is now considered an

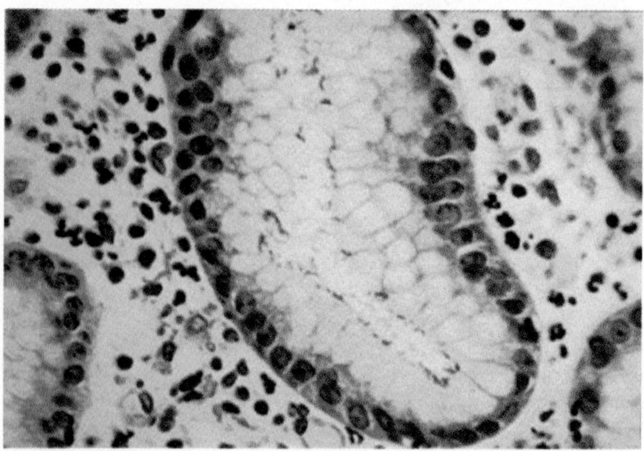

FIGURE 15-14

Chronic gastritis and *H. pylori* organisms. Steiner silver stain of superficial gastric mucosa showing abundant darkly stained microorganisms layered over the apical portion of the surface epithelium. Note that there is no tissue invasion.

independent risk factor for gastric cancer. Worldwide epidemiologic studies have documented a higher incidence of *H. pylori* infection in patients with adenocarcinoma of the stomach as compared to control subjects. Seropositivity for *H. pylori* is associated with a three- to sixfold increased risk of gastric cancer. This risk may be as high as ninefold after adjusting for the inaccuracy of serologic testing in the elderly. The mechanism by which *H. pylori* infection leads to cancer is unknown, but it appears to be related to the chronic inflammation induced by the organism. Eradication of *H. pylori* as a general preventative measure for gastric cancer is being evaluated but is not yet recommended.

Infection with *H. pylori* is also associated with development of a low-grade B cell lymphoma, gastric MALT lymphoma. The chronic T cell stimulation caused by the infection leads to production of cytokines that promote the B cell tumor. The tumor should be initially staged with a CT scan of the abdomen and EUS. Tumor growth remains dependent on the presence of *H. pylori,* and its eradication is often associated with complete regression of the tumor. The tumor may take more than a year to regress after treating the infection. Such patients should be followed by EUS every 2–3 months. If the tumor is stable or decreasing in size, no other therapy is necessary. If the tumor grows, it may have become a high-grade B cell lymphoma. When the tumor becomes a high-grade aggressive lymphoma histologically, it loses responsiveness to *H. pylori* eradication.

TREATMENT CHRONIC GASTRITIS

Treatment in chronic gastritis is aimed at the sequelae and not the underlying inflammation. Patients with pernicious anemia will require parenteral vitamin B_{12} supplementation on a long-term basis. Eradication of *H. pylori* is often recommended even if PUD or a low-grade MALT lymphoma is not present.

Miscellaneous forms of gastritis

Lymphocytic gastritis is characterized histologically by intense infiltration of the surface epithelium with lymphocytes. The infiltrative process is primarily in the body of the stomach and consists of mature T cells and plasmacytes. The etiology of this form of chronic gastritis is unknown. It has been described in patients with celiac sprue, but whether there is a common factor associating these two entities is unknown. No specific symptoms suggest lymphocytic gastritis. A subgroup of patients have thickened folds noted on endoscopy. These folds are often capped by small nodules that contain a central depression or erosion; this form of the disease is called *varioliform gastritis. H. pylori* probably plays no significant role in lymphocytic gastritis. Therapy with glucocorticoids or sodium cromoglycate has obtained unclear results.

Marked eosinophilic infiltration involving any layer of the stomach (mucosa, muscularis propria, and serosa) is characteristic of *eosinophilic gastritis.* Affected individuals will often have circulating eosinophilia with clinical manifestation of systemic allergy. Involvement may range from isolated gastric disease to diffuse eosinophilic gastroenteritis. Antral involvement predominates, with prominent edematous folds being observed on endoscopy. These prominent antral folds can lead to outlet obstruction. Patients can present with epigastric discomfort, nausea, and vomiting. Treatment with glucocorticoids has been successful.

Several systemic disorders may be associated with *granulomatous gastritis.* Gastric involvement has been observed in Crohn's disease. Involvement may range from granulomatous infiltrates noted only on gastric biopsies to frank ulceration and stricture formation. Gastric Crohn's disease usually occurs in the presence of small-intestinal disease. Several rare infectious processes can lead to granulomatous gastritis, including histoplasmosis, candidiasis, syphilis, and tuberculosis. Other unusual causes of this form of gastritis include sarcoidosis, idiopathic granulomatous gastritis, and eosinophilic granulomas involving the stomach. Establishing the specific etiologic agent in this form of gastritis can be difficult, at times requiring repeat endoscopy with biopsy and cytology. Occasionally, a surgically obtained full-thickness biopsy of the stomach may be required to exclude malignancy.

Russell body gastritis (RBG) is a mucosal lesion of unknown etiology that has a pseudotumoral endoscopic appearance. Histologically, it is defined by the presence of numerous plasma cells containing Russell bodies (RBs) that express kappa and lambda light chains. Only 10 cases have been reported, and 7 of these have been associated with ***H. pylori*** infection. The lesion can be confused with a neoplastic process, but it is benign in nature, and the natural history of the lesion is not known. There have been cases of resolution of the lesion when *H. pylori* was eradicated.

MÉNÉTRIER'S DISEASE

Ménétrier's disease (MD) is a very rare gastropathy characterized by large, tortuous mucosal folds. MD has an average age of onset of 40–60 years with a male predominance. The differential diagnosis of large gastric folds includes ZES, malignancy (lymphoma, infiltrating carcinoma), infectious etiologies (CMV, histoplasmosis, syphilis, tuberculosis), gastritis polyposa profunda, and infiltrative disorders such as sarcoidosis. MD is most commonly confused with large or multiple gastric polyps (prolonged PPI use) or familial polyposis syndromes. The mucosal folds in MD are often most prominent in the body and fundus, sparing the antrum. Histologically, massive foveolar hyperplasia (hyperplasia of surface and glandular mucous cells) and a marked reduction in oxyntic glands and parietal cells and chief cells are noted. This hyperplasia produces the prominent folds observed. The pits of the gastric glands elongate and may become extremely dilated and tortuous. Although the lamina propria may contain a mild chronic inflammatory infiltrate including eosinophils and plasma cells, MD is not considered a form of gastritis. The etiology of this unusual clinical picture in children is often CMV, but the etiology in adults is unknown. Overexpression of the growth factor TGF-α has been demonstrated in patients with MD. The overexpression of TGF-α in turn results in overstimulation of the epidermal growth factor receptor (EGFR) pathway and increased proliferation of mucus cells, resulting in the observed foveolar hyperplasia.

The clinical presentation in adults is usually insidious and progressive. Epigastric pain, nausea, vomiting, anorexia, peripheral edema, and weight loss are signs and symptoms in patients with MD. Occult GI bleeding may occur, but overt bleeding is unusual and, when present, is due to superficial mucosal erosions. In fact, bleeding is more often seen in one of the common mimics of MD, gastric polyposis. Twenty to 100% of patients (depending on time of presentation) develop a protein-losing gastropathy due to hypersecretion of gastric mucus accompanied by hypoalbuminemia and edema. Gastric acid secretion is usually reduced or absent because of the decreased parietal cells. Large gastric folds are readily detectable by either radiographic (barium meal) or endoscopic methods. Endoscopy with deep mucosal biopsy, preferably full thickness with a snare technique, is required to establish the diagnosis and exclude other entities that may present similarly. A nondiagnostic biopsy may lead to a surgically obtained full-thickness biopsy to exclude malignancy. Although MD is considered premalignant by some, the risk of neoplastic progression is not defined. Complete blood count, serum gastrin, serum albumin, CMV and *H. pylori* serology, and pH testing of gastric aspirate during endoscopy should be included as part of the initial evaluation of patients with large gastric folds.

TREATMENT MÉNÉTRIER'S DISEASE

Medical therapy with anticholinergic agents, prostaglandins, PPIs, prednisone, somatostatin analogues (octreotide) and H_2 receptor antagonists yields varying results. Ulcers should be treated with a standard approach. The discovery that MD is associated with overstimulation of the EGFR pathway has led to the successful use of the EGF inhibitory antibody, cetuximab, in these patients. Specifically, four of seven patients who completed a 1-month trial with this agent demonstrated near complete histologic remission and improvement in symptoms. Cetuximab is now considered the first-line treatment for MD, leaving total gastrectomy for severe disease with persistent and substantial protein loss despite therapy with this agent.

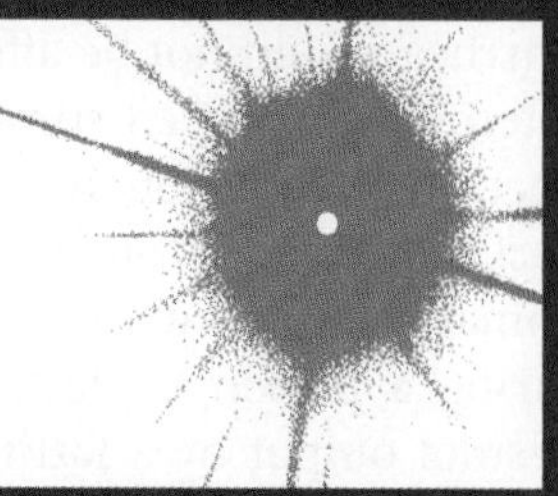

CHAPTER 16

DISORDERS OF ABSORPTION

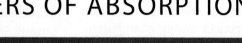

Henry J. Binder

Disorders of absorption constitute a broad spectrum of conditions with multiple etiologies and varied clinical manifestations. Almost all of these clinical problems are associated with *diminished* intestinal absorption of one or more dietary nutrients and are often referred to as the *malabsorption syndrome.* This term is not ideal as it represents a pathophysiologic state, does *not* provide an etiologic explanation for the underlying problem, and should not be considered an adequate final diagnosis. The only clinical conditions in which absorption is *increased* are hemochromatosis and Wilson's disease, in which absorption of iron and copper, respectively, is elevated.

Most malabsorption syndromes are associated with *steatorrhea*, an increase in stool fat excretion to >6% of dietary fat intake. Some malabsorption disorders are not associated with steatorrhea: primary lactase deficiency, a congenital absence of the small-intestinal brush border disaccharidase enzyme lactase, is associated with lactose "malabsorption," and pernicious anemia is associated with a marked decrease in intestinal absorption of cobalamin (vitamin B_{12}) due to an absence of gastric parietal-cell intrinsic factor, which is required for cobalamin absorption.

Disorders of absorption must be included in the differential diagnosis of diarrhea **(Chap. 6)**. First, diarrhea is frequently associated with and/or is a consequence of the diminished absorption of one or more dietary nutrients. The diarrhea may be secondary either to the intestinal process that is responsible for the steatorrhea or to steatorrhea per se. Thus, celiac disease (see below) is associated with both extensive morphologic changes in the small-intestinal mucosa and reduced absorption of several dietary nutrients; in contrast, the diarrhea of steatorrhea is the result of the effect of nonabsorbed dietary fatty acids on intestinal (usually colonic) ion transport. For example, oleic acid and ricinoleic acid (a bacterially hydroxylated fatty acid that is also the active ingredient in castor oil, a widely used laxative) induce active colonic Cl ion secretion, most likely secondary to increasing intracellular Ca. In addition, diarrhea per se may result in mild steatorrhea (<11 g of fat excretion while on a 100-g fat diet). Second, most patients will indicate that they have diarrhea, not that they have fat malabsorption. Third, many intestinal disorders that have diarrhea as a prominent symptom (e.g., ulcerative colitis, traveler's diarrhea secondary to an enterotoxin produced by *Escherichia coli*) do not necessarily have diminished absorption of any dietary nutrient.

Diarrhea as a *symptom* (i.e., when the term is used by patients to describe their bowel movement pattern) may reflect a decrease in stool consistency, an increase in stool volume, an increase in number of bowel movements, or any combination of these three changes. In contrast, diarrhea as a *sign* is a quantitative increase in stool water or weight of >200–225 mL or g per 24 h when a Western-type diet is consumed. Individuals consuming a diet with higher fiber content may normally have a stool weight of up to 400 g/24 h. Thus, the clinician must clarify what an individual patient means by diarrhea. Some 10% of patients referred to gastroenterologists for further evaluation of unexplained diarrhea do not have an increase in stool water when this variable is determined quantitatively. Such patients may have small, frequent, somewhat loose bowel movements with stool urgency that is indicative of proctitis but do not have an increase in stool weight or volume.

It is also critical to establish whether a patient's diarrhea is secondary to diminished absorption of one or more dietary nutrients rather than being due to small- and/or large-intestinal fluid and electrolyte secretion. The former has often been termed *osmotic diarrhea*, while the latter has been referred to as *secretory diarrhea.* Unfortunately, both secretory and osmotic elements can be present simultaneously in the same disorder; thus, this distinction is not always precise. Nonetheless, two studies—determination of stool electrolytes and observation of the effect of a fast on stool output—can help make this distinction.

The demonstration of the effect of prolonged (>24 h) fasting on stool output can suggest that a *dietary nutrient* is responsible for the individual's diarrhea. Secretory diarrhea associated with enterotoxin-induced traveler's diarrhea would not be affected by prolonged fasting, as enterotoxin-induced stimulation of intestinal fluid and electrolyte secretion is not altered by eating. In contrast, diarrhea secondary to lactose malabsorption in primary lactase deficiency would undoubtedly cease during a prolonged fast. Thus, a substantial decrease in stool output by a fasting patient during quantitative stool collection lasting at least 24 h is presumptive evidence that the diarrhea is related to malabsorption of a dietary nutrient. The persistence of stool output during fasting indicates that the diarrhea is likely secretory and that its cause is *not* a dietary nutrient. Either a luminal (e.g., *E. coli* enterotoxin) or a circulating (e.g., vasoactive intestinal peptide) secretagogue could be responsible for unaltered persistence of a patient's diarrhea during a prolonged fast. The observed effects of fasting can be compared and correlated with stool electrolyte and osmolality determinations.

Measurement of stool electrolytes and osmolality requires comparison of Na^+ and K^+ concentrations in liquid stool with the osmolality of the stool in order to determine the presence or absence of a so-called stool osmotic gap. The following formula is used:

$$2 \times (\text{stool } [Na^+] + \text{stool } [K^+]) \leq \text{stool osmolality}$$

The cation concentrations are doubled to estimate stool anion concentrations. The presence of a significant osmotic gap suggests the presence in stool water of a substance (or substances) other than Na/K/anions that is presumably responsible for the patient's diarrhea. Originally, stool osmolality was measured, but it is almost invariably greater than the required 290–300 mosmol/kg H_2O, reflecting bacterial degradation of nonabsorbed carbohydrate either immediately before defecation or in the stool jar while specimen awaits chemical analysis, even when the stool is refrigerated. As a result, the stool osmolality should be assumed to be 300 mosmol/kg H_2O. A low stool osmolality (<290 mosmol/kg H_2O) reflects the addition of either dilute urine or water, indicating either collection of urine and stool together or so-called factitious diarrhea, a form of Münchausen's syndrome. When the calculated difference in the formula above is >50, an osmotic gap exists; its presence suggests that the diarrhea is due to a nonabsorbed dietary nutrient—e.g., a fatty acid and/or a carbohydrate. When this difference is <25, it is presumed that a dietary nutrient is not responsible for the diarrhea. Since elements of both osmotic diarrhea (i.e., due to malabsorption of a dietary nutrient) and secretory diarrhea may be present, this distinction at times is less clear-cut at the bedside than when used as a teaching example. Ideally, the presence of an osmotic gap will be associated with a marked decrease in stool output during a prolonged fast, while an osmotic gap will likely be absent in an individual whose stool output is not reduced substantially during a period of fasting.

NUTRIENT DIGESTION AND ABSORPTION

The lengths of the small intestine and the colon are ~300 cm and ~80 cm, respectively. However, the effective functional surface area is ~600-fold greater than that of a hollow tube as a result of folds, villi (in the small intestine), and microvilli. The functional surface area of the small intestine is somewhat greater than that of a doubles tennis court. In addition to nutrient digestion and absorption, the intestinal epithelia have several other functions:

1. *Barrier and immune defense.* The intestine is exposed to a large number of potential antigens and enteric and invasive microorganisms, and it is extremely effective at preventing the entry of almost all of these agents. The intestinal mucosa also synthesizes and secretes secretory IgA.
2. *Fluid and electrolyte absorption and secretion.* The intestine absorbs ~7–8 L of fluid daily, a volume comprising dietary fluid intake (1–2 L/d) and salivary, gastric, pancreatic, biliary, and intestinal fluid (6–7 L/d). Several stimuli, especially bacteria and bacterial enterotoxins, induce fluid and electrolyte secretion that may lead to diarrhea **(Chap. 24)**.
3. *Synthesis and secretion of several proteins.* The intestinal mucosa is a major site for the production of proteins, including apolipoproteins.
4. *Production of several bioactive amines and peptides.* The intestine is one of the largest endocrine organs in the body and produces several amines (e.g., 5-hydroxytryptophan) and peptides that serve as paracrine and hormonal mediators of intestinal function.

The small and large intestines are distinct anatomically (villi are present in the small intestine but are absent in the colon) and functionally (nutrient digestion and absorption take place in the small intestine but not in the colon). No precise anatomic characteristics separate duodenum, jejunum, and ileum, although certain nutrients are absorbed exclusively in specific areas of the small intestine. However, villous cells in the small intestine (surface epithelial cells in the colon) and crypt cells have distinct anatomic and functional characteristics. Intestinal epithelial cells are continuously renewed; new proliferating epithelial cells at the base of the crypt migrate over 48–72 h to the tip of the villus (or surface of the colon), where they exist as well-developed epithelial cells with digestive and absorptive function. This high rate of cell turnover explains the relatively rapid resolution of diarrhea and other digestive-tract side effects during chemotherapy as new cells not exposed to these toxic agents are produced. Equally important is the paradigm of separation of villous/surface cell and crypt cell functions. Digestive hydrolytic enzymes are present primarily in the brush border of villous epithelial cells. Absorptive and secretory functions are also separate: villous/surface cells are primarily, but not exclusively, the site for absorptive function, while secretory function is located in crypts of both the small and large intestines.

Nutrients, minerals, and vitamins are absorbed by one or more active-transport mechanisms. These mechanisms are energy dependent and are mediated by membrane transport proteins. These processes will result in the *net* movement of a substance against or in the absence of an electrochemical concentration gradient. Intestinal absorption of amino acids and monosaccharides (e.g., glucose) is also a specialized form of active transport—*secondary active transport.* The movement of actively transported nutrients against a concentration gradient is Na^+ dependent and is due to a Na^+ gradient across the apical membrane. The Na^+ gradient is maintained by Na^+,K^+-adenosine triphosphatase (ATPase), the so-called Na^+ pump located on the basolateral membrane, which extrudes Na^+ and maintains low intracellular [Na] as well as the Na^+ gradient across the apical membrane. As a result, active glucose absorption and glucose-stimulated Na^+ absorption require both the apical membrane transport protein SGLT1 and the basolateral Na^+,K^+-ATPase. In addition to exhibiting Na^+ for its absorption, glucose stimulates Na^+ and fluid absorption; this effect is the physiologic basis of oral rehydration therapy for the treatment of diarrhea **(Chap. 6). The mechanisms of intestinal fluid and electrolyte absorption and secretion are discussed in Chap. 6.**

Although the intestinal epithelial cells are crucial mediators of absorption and of ion and water flow, the several cell types in the lamina propria (e.g., mast cells, macrophages, myofibroblasts) and the enteric nervous system interact with the epithelium to regulate mucosal cell function. Intestinal function results from the integrated responses and interactions of intestinal epithelial cells and intestinal muscle.

ENTEROHEPATIC CIRCULATION OF BILE ACIDS

Bile acids are not present in the diet but are synthesized in the liver by a series of enzymatic steps that also represent cholesterol catabolism. Indeed, interruption of the enterohepatic circulation of bile acids can reduce serum cholesterol levels by 10% before a new steady state is established. Bile acids are either primary or secondary. Primary bile acids are synthesized in the liver from cholesterol, and secondary bile acids are synthesized from primary bile acids in the intestine by colonic bacterial enzymes. The two primary bile acids in humans are cholic acid and chenodeoxycholic acid; the two most abundant secondary bile acids are deoxycholic acid and lithocholic acid. The liver synthesizes ~500 mg of bile acids daily; the bile acids are conjugated to either taurine or glycine (to form tauroconjugated and glycoconjugated bile acids, respectively) and are secreted into the duodenum in bile. The primary functions of bile acids are (1) to promote bile flow, (2) to solubilize cholesterol and phospholipid in the gallbladder by mixed micelle formation, and (3) to enhance dietary lipid digestion and absorption by forming mixed micelles in the proximal small intestine.

Bile acids are primarily absorbed by an active, Na^+-dependent process that takes place exclusively in the ileum; to a lesser extent, they are absorbed by non-carrier-mediated transport processes in the jejunum, ileum, and colon. Conjugated bile acids that enter the colon are deconjugated by colonic bacterial enzymes. The unconjugated bile acids are rapidly absorbed by nonionic diffusion. Colonic bacterial enzymes also dehydroxylate bile acids to secondary bile acids.

Bile acids absorbed from the intestine return to the liver via the portal vein and are then re-secreted (Fig. 16-1). Bile acid synthesis is largely autoregulated by 7α-hydroxylase, the initial enzyme in cholesterol

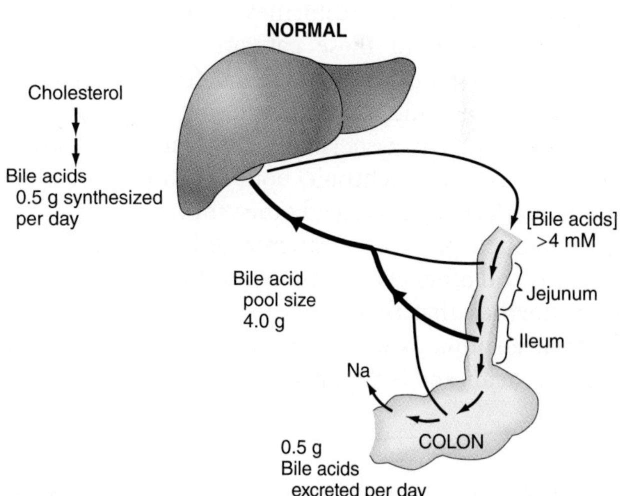

FIGURE 16-1

Schematic representation of the enterohepatic circulation of bile acids. Bile acid synthesis is cholesterol catabolism and occurs in the liver. Bile acids are secreted in bile and are stored in the gallbladder between meals and at night. Food in the duodenum induces the release of cholecystokinin, a potent stimulus for gallbladder contraction resulting in bile acid entry into the duodenum. Bile acids are primarily absorbed via an Na-dependent transport process that is located only in the ileum. A relatively small quantity of bile acids (~500 mg) is not absorbed in a 24-h period and is lost in stool. Fecal bile acid losses are matched by bile acid synthesis. The bile acid pool (the total amount of bile acids in the body) is ~4 g and is circulated twice during each meal or six to eight times in a 24-h period.

degradation. A decrease in the volume of bile acids returning to the liver from the intestine is associated with an increase in bile acid synthesis/cholesterol catabolism, which helps keep the bile-acid pool size relatively constant. However, the capacity to increase bile acid synthesis is limited to ~2- to 2.5-fold (see below). The bile-acid pool size is ~4 g. The pool is circulated via the enterohepatic circulation about twice during each meal, or six to eight times during a 24-h period. A relatively small quantity of bile acids is not absorbed and is excreted in stool daily; this fecal loss is matched by hepatic bile-acid synthesis.

Defects in any of the steps in enterohepatic circulation of bile acids can result in a decrease in the duodenal concentration of conjugated bile acids and consequently in the development of steatorrhea. Thus, steatorrhea can be caused by abnormalities in bile acid synthesis and excretion, their physical state in the intestinal lumen, and reabsorption (Table 16-1).

Synthesis

Decreased bile acid synthesis and steatorrhea have been demonstrated in chronic liver disease, but steatorrhea often is not a major component of illness in these patients.

Secretion

Although bile acid secretion may be reduced or absent in biliary obstruction, steatorrhea is rarely a significant medical problem in these patients. In contrast, primary biliary cirrhosis represents a defect in canalicular excretion of organic anions, including bile acids, and not infrequently is associated with steatorrhea and its consequences (e.g., chronic bone disease). Thus, the osteopenia/osteomalacia and other chronic bone abnormalities often present in patients with primary biliary cirrhosis and other cholestatic syndromes are secondary to steatorrhea that then leads to calcium and vitamin D malabsorption as well as to the effects of cholestasis (e.g., bile acids and inflammatory cytokines).

Maintenance of conjugated bile acids

In bacterial overgrowth syndromes associated with diarrhea, steatorrhea, and macrocytic anemia, a colonic type of bacterial flora is increased in the small intestine. Steatorrhea is primarily a result of the decrease in conjugated bile acids secondary to their deconjugation by colonic-type bacteria. Two complementary explanations account for the resulting impairment of micelle formation: (1) Unconjugated bile acids are rapidly absorbed in the jejunum by nonionic diffusion, and the result is a reduced concentration of duodenal bile acids. (2) The critical micellar concentration (CMC) of unconjugated bile acids is higher than that of conjugated bile acids; therefore, unconjugated bile acids are less effective than conjugated bile acids in micelle formation.

Reabsorption

Ileal dysfunction caused by either Crohn's disease or surgical resection results in a decrease in bile acid reabsorption in the ileum and an *increase* in the delivery of bile acids to the large intestine. The resulting clinical consequences—diarrhea with or without steatorrhea—are determined by the *degree* of ileal dysfunction and the *response* of the enterohepatic circulation to bile acid losses (Table 16-2). Patients with limited ileal disease or resection often have diarrhea but not steatorrhea. The diarrhea, a result of stimulation of active Cl secretion by bile acids in the colon, has been called *bile acid diarrhea* or *choleretic enteropathy* and responds promptly to cholestyramine, an anion-binding resin. Steatorrhea does not develop because hepatic synthesis of bile acids increases to compensate for the rate of fecal bile-acid losses, resulting in maintenance of both the bile-acid pool size and the intraduodenal concentrations of bile acids. In contrast, patients with greater degrees of ileal disease and/or resection often have diarrhea

TABLE 16-1

DEFECTS IN ENTEROHEPATIC CIRCULATION OF BILE ACIDS

PROCESS	PATHOPHYSIOLOGIC DEFECT	DISEASE EXAMPLE
Synthesis	Decreased hepatic function	Cirrhosis
Biliary secretion	Altered canalicular function	Primary biliary cirrhosis
Maintenance of conjugated bile acids	Bacterial overgrowth	Jejunal diverticulosis
Reabsorption	Abnormal ileal function	Crohn's disease

TABLE 16-2

COMPARISON OF BILE ACID AND FATTY ACID DIARRHEA

	BILE ACID DIARRHEA	FATTY ACID DIARRHEA
Extent of ileal disease	Limited	Extensive
Ileal bile-acid absorption	Reduced	Reduced
Fecal bile-acid excretion	Increased	Increased
Fecal bile-acid loss compensated by hepatic synthesis	Yes	No
Bile-acid pool size	Normal	Reduced
Intraduodenal (bile acid)	Normal	Reduced
Steatorrhea	None or mild	>20 g
Response to cholestyramine	Yes	No
Response to low-fat diet	No	Yes

TABLE 16-3

COMPARISON OF DIFFERENT TYPES OF FATTY ACIDS

	LONG-CHAIN	MEDIUM-CHAIN	SHORT-CHAIN
Carbon chain length	>12	8–12	<8
Present in diet	In large amounts	In small amounts	No
Origin	In diet as triglycerides	Only in small amounts in diet as triglycerides	Bacterial degradation in colon of non-absorbed carbohydrate to fatty acids
Primary site of absorption	Small intestine	Small intestine	Colon
Requires pancreatic lipolysis	Yes	No	No
Requires micelle formation	Yes	No	No
Present in stool	Minimal	No	Substantial

and steatorrhea that do not respond to cholestyramine. In this situation, ileal disease is also associated with increased volumes of bile acids entering the colon; however, hepatic synthesis can no longer increase sufficiently to maintain the bile-acid pool size. As a consequence, the intraduodenal concentration of bile acids is reduced to less than the CMC, and the result is impaired micelle formation and steatorrhea. This second situation is often called *fatty acid diarrhea*. Cholestyramine may not be effective (and may even exacerbate the diarrhea by further depleting the intraduodenal bile-acid concentration); however, a low-fat diet to reduce fatty acid entry into the colon can be effective. Two clinical features—the length of the ileal section removed and the degree of steatorrhea—can predict whether an individual patient will respond to cholestyramine. Unfortunately, these predictors are imperfect, and a therapeutic trial of cholestyramine is often necessary to establish whether an individual patient will benefit from cholestyramine. Table 16-2 contrasts the characteristics of bile acid diarrhea (small ileal dysfunction) and fatty acid diarrhea (large ileal dysfunction).

Bile acid diarrhea can also occur in the absence of ileal inflammation and/or resection and is characterized by an abnormal ^{75}SeHCAT retention study and reduced ileal release of fibroblast growth factor 19, a negative regulator of bile acid synthesis, with a consequent increase in bile acid synthesis and secretion that exceeds ileal bile-acid absorption. The diarrhea in these patients also responds to cholestyramine.

LIPIDS

Steatorrhea is caused by one or more defects in the digestion and absorption of dietary fat. The average intake of dietary fat in the United States is ~120–150 g/d, and fat absorption is linear to dietary fat intake. The total load of fat presented to the small intestine is considerably greater, as substantial amounts of lipid are secreted in bile each day (see "Enterohepatic Circulation of Bile Acids," above). Three types of fatty acids compose fats: long-chain fatty acids (LCFAs), medium-chain fatty acids (MCFAs), and short-chain fatty acids (SCFAs) (Table 16-3). Dietary fat is exclusively composed of long-chain triglycerides (LCTs)—i.e., glycerol that is bound via ester linkages to three LCFAs. While the majority of dietary LCFAs have carbon chain lengths of 16 or 18, all fatty acids of carbon chain length >12 are metabolized in the same manner; saturated and unsaturated fatty acids are handled identically.

Assimilation of dietary lipid requires three integrated processes: (1) an intraluminal, or digestive, phase; (2) a mucosal, or absorptive, phase; and (3) a delivery, or postabsorptive, phase. An abnormality at any site involved in these processes can cause steatorrhea (Table 16-4).

TABLE 16-4

DEFECTS IN LIPID DIGESTION AND ABSORPTION IN STEATORRHEA

PHASE, PROCESS	PATHOPHYSIOLOGIC DEFECT	DISEASE EXAMPLE
Digestive		
Lipolysis formation	Decreased lipase secretion	Chronic pancreatitis
Micelle formation	Decreased intraduodenal bile acids	See Table 16-1
Absorptive		
Mucosal uptake and re-esterification	Mucosal dysfunction	Celiac disease
Postabsorptive		
Chylomicron formation	Absent betalipoproteins	Abetalipoproteinemia
Delivery from intestine	Abnormal lymphatics	Intestinal lymphangiectasia

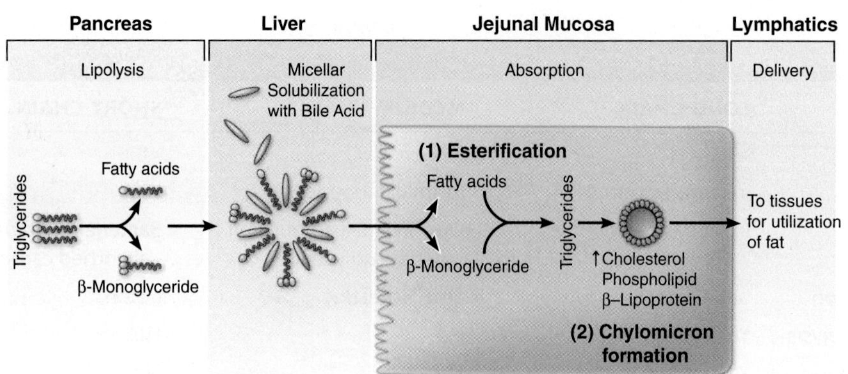

FIGURE 16-2

Schematic representation of lipid digestion and absorption. Dietary lipid is in the form of long-chain triglycerides. The overall process can be divided into (1) a digestive phase that includes both lipolysis and micelle formation requiring pancreatic lipase and conjugated bile acids, respectively, in the duodenum; (2) an absorptive phase for mucosal uptake and re-esterification; and (3) a postabsorptive phase that includes chylomicron formation and exit from the intestinal epithelial cell via lymphatics. *(Courtesy of John M. Dietschy, MD; with permission.)*

Therefore, it is essential that any patient with steatorrhea be evaluated to identify the specific physiologic defect in overall lipid digestion/absorption, as therapy will be determined by the specific etiology.

The digestive phase has two components, *lipolysis* and *micelle formation.* Although dietary lipid is in the form of LCTs, the intestinal mucosa does not absorb triglycerides; they must first be hydrolyzed (Fig. 16-2). The initial step in lipid digestion is the formation of emulsions of finely dispersed lipid, which is accomplished by mastication and gastric contractions. Lipolysis, the hydrolysis of triglycerides to free fatty acids, monoglycerides, and glycerol by lipase, is initiated in the stomach by lingual and gastric lipases that have a pH optimum of 4.5–6.0. About 20–30% of total lipolysis occurs in the stomach. Lipolysis is completed in the duodenum and jejunum by pancreatic lipase, which is inactivated by a pH <7.0. Pancreatic lipolysis is greatly enhanced by the presence of a second pancreatic enzyme, colipase, which facilitates the movement of lipase to the triglyceride.

Impaired lipolysis can lead to steatorrhea and can occur in the presence of pancreatic insufficiency due to chronic pancreatitis in adults or cystic fibrosis in children and adolescents. Normal lipolysis can be maintained by ~5% of maximal pancreatic lipase secretion; thus, steatorrhea is a late manifestation of these disorders. A reduction in intraduodenal pH can also result in altered lipolysis, as pancreatic lipase is inactivated at pH <7. Thus, ~15% of patients who have gastrinoma **(Chap. 15)**, with substantial increases in gastric acid secretion from ectopic production of gastrin (usually from an islet cell adenoma), have diarrhea, and some have steatorrhea believed to be secondary to acid inactivation of pancreatic lipase. Similarly, patients who have chronic pancreatitis (with reduced lipase secretion) often have a decrease in pancreatic bicarbonate secretion, which will also result in a lowering of intraduodenal pH and inactivation of endogenous pancreatic lipase or of therapeutically administered lipase.

Overlying the microvillus membrane of the small intestine is the so-called unstirred water layer, a relatively stagnant aqueous phase that must be traversed by the products of lipolysis that are primarily water insoluble. Water-soluble mixed micelles provide a mechanism by which the water-insoluble products of lipolysis can reach the luminal plasma membrane of villous epithelial cells—the site for lipid absorption. Mixed micelles are molecular aggregates composed of fatty acids, monoglycerides, phospholipids, cholesterol, and conjugated bile acids. These mixed micelles are formed when the concentration of conjugated bile acids is greater than its CMC, which differs among the several bile acids present in the small-intestinal lumen. Conjugated bile acids, synthesized in the liver and excreted into the duodenum in bile, are regulated by the enterohepatic circulation (see above). Steatorrhea can result from impaired movement of fatty acids across the unstirred aqueous fluid layer in two situations: (1) an increase in the relative thickness of the unstirred water layer that occurs in bacterial overgrowth syndromes (see below) secondary to functional stasis (e.g., scleroderma); and (2) a decrease in the *duodenal* concentration of conjugated bile acids below the CMC, resulting in impaired micelle formation. Thus, steatorrhea can be caused by one or more defects in the enterohepatic circulation of bile acids.

Uptake and re-esterification constitute the *absorptive phase* of lipid digestion/absorption. Although passive diffusion has been thought to be responsible, a carrier-mediated process may mediate fatty acid and monoglyceride uptake. Regardless of the uptake process, fatty acids and monoglycerides are re-esterified by a series of enzymatic steps in the endoplasmic reticulum to form triglycerides, in which lipid exits from the intestinal epithelial cell. Impaired lipid absorption as a result of mucosal inflammation (e.g., celiac disease) and/or intestinal resection can also lead to steatorrhea.

The re-esterified triglycerides require the formation of *chylomicrons* to permit their exit from the small-intestinal epithelial cell and their delivery to the liver via the lymphatics. Chylomicrons are composed of β-lipoprotein and contain triglycerides, cholesterol, cholesterol esters, and phospholipids and enter the lymphatics, not the portal vein. Defects in the *postabsorptive phase* of lipid digestion/absorption can also result in steatorrhea, but these disorders are uncommon. Abetalipoproteinemia, or acanthocytosis, is a rare disorder of impaired synthesis of β-lipoprotein associated with abnormal erythrocytes (acanthocytes), neurologic problems, and steatorrhea. Lipolysis, micelle formation, and lipid uptake are all normal in patients with abetalipoproteinemia, but the re-esterified triglyceride cannot exit the epithelial cell because of the failure to produce chylomicrons. Small-intestinal biopsy samples obtained from these rare patients in the postprandial state reveal lipid-laden small-intestinal epithelial cells that become perfectly normal in appearance after a 72- to 96-h fast. Similarly, abnormalities of intestinal lymphatics (e.g., intestinal lymphangiectasia) may also be associated with steatorrhea as well as protein loss (see below). Steatorrhea can result from defects at any of the several steps in lipid digestion/absorption.

The mechanism of lipid digestion/absorption outlined above is limited to *dietary* lipid, which is almost exclusively in the form of LCTs (Table 16-3). Medium-chain triglycerides (MCTs), composed of fatty acids with carbon chain lengths of 8–12, are present in large amounts in coconut oil and are used as a nutritional supplement. MCTs can be digested and absorbed by a pathway different from that involved in LCT digestion and absorption; at one time, MCTs held promise as an important treatment for steatorrhea of almost all etiologies. Unfortunately, they have been less therapeutically effective than expected because, for reasons that are not completely understood, their use often is not associated with an increase in body weight.

In contrast to LCTs, MCTs do not require pancreatic lipolysis as they can be absorbed intact by the intestinal epithelial cell. Further, micelle formation is not necessary for the absorption of MCTs (or MCFAs, if hydrolyzed by pancreatic lipase). MCTs are absorbed more efficiently than LCTs for the following reasons: (1) The rate of absorption is greater for MCTs than for LCFAs. (2) After absorption, MCFAs are not re-esterified. (3) After absorption, MCTs are hydrolyzed to MCFAs. (4) MCTs do not require chylomicron formation to exit intestinal epithelial cells. (5) The route of MCT exit is via the portal vein and not via lymphatics. Thus, the absorption of MCTs is greater than that of LCTs in pancreatic insufficiency, conditions with reduced intraduodenal bile acid concentrations, small-intestinal mucosal disease, abetalipoproteinemia, and intestinal lymphangiectasia.

SCFAs are not dietary lipids but are synthesized by colonic bacterial enzymes from nonabsorbed carbohydrate and are the anions present at the highest concentration in stool (80–130 m*M*). The SCFAs in stool are primarily acetate, propionate, and butyrate, whose carbon chain lengths are 2, 3, and 4, respectively. Butyrate is the primary nutrient for colonic epithelial cells, and its deficiency can be associated with one or more colitides. SCFAs conserve calories and carbohydrate: carbohydrates that are not completely absorbed in the small intestine will not be absorbed in the large intestine because of the absence of both disaccharidases and SGLT1, the transport protein that mediates monosaccharide absorption. In contrast, SCFAs are rapidly absorbed and stimulate colonic NaCl and fluid absorption. Most antibiotic-associated diarrhea not caused by *Clostridium difficile* is due to antibiotic suppression of the colonic microbiota, with a resulting decrease in SCFA production. As *C. difficile* accounts for only ~15–20% of all antibiotic-associated diarrhea, a relative decrease in colonic production of SCFA is likely the cause of most antibiotic-associated diarrhea.

The clinical manifestations of steatorrhea are a consequence both of the underlying disorder responsible for its development and of steatorrhea per se. Depending on the degree of steatorrhea and the level of dietary intake, significant fat malabsorption may lead to weight loss. Steatorrhea per se can be responsible for diarrhea; if the primary cause of the steatorrhea has not been identified, a low-fat diet can often ameliorate the diarrhea by decreasing fecal fat excretion. Steatorrhea is commonly associated with fat-soluble vitamin deficiency, which requires replacement with water-soluble preparations of these vitamins.

Disorders of absorption may also be associated with malabsorption of other dietary nutrients — most often carbohydrates—with or without a decrease in dietary lipid digestion and absorption. Therefore, knowledge of the mechanisms of digestion and absorption of carbohydrates, proteins, and other minerals and vitamins is useful in the evaluation of patients with altered intestinal nutrient absorption.

CARBOHYDRATES

Carbohydrates in the diet are present in the form of starch, disaccharides (sucrose and lactose), and glucose. Carbohydrates are absorbed only in the small intestine and only in the form of monosaccharides. Therefore, before their absorption, starch and disaccharides must first be digested by pancreatic amylase and intestinal brush border disaccharidases to monosaccharides. Monosaccharide absorption occurs by a Na-dependent process mediated by the brush border transport protein SGLT1.

Lactose malabsorption is the only clinically important disorder of carbohydrate absorption. Lactose, the disaccharide present in milk, requires digestion by brush border lactase to its two constituent monosaccharides, glucose and galactose. Lactase is present in almost all species in the postnatal period but then disappears throughout the animal kingdom, except in humans. Lactase activity persists in many individuals throughout life. Two different types of lactase deficiency exist—primary and secondary. In *primary lactase deficiency*, a genetically determined decrease or absence of lactase is noted, while all other aspects of both intestinal absorption and brush border enzymes are normal. In a number of nonwhite groups, primary lactase deficiency is common in adulthood. In fact, Northern European and North American whites are the only groups to maintain small-intestinal lactase activity throughout adult life. Table 16-5 presents the incidence of primary lactase deficiency in several ethnic groups. Lactase persistence in adults is an abnormality due to a defect in the regulation of its maturation. In contrast, *secondary lactase deficiency* occurs in association with small-intestinal mucosal disease, with abnormalities in both structure and function of other brush border enzymes and transport processes. Secondary lactase deficiency is often seen in celiac disease.

As lactose digestion is rate-limiting compared to glucose/galactose absorption, lactase deficiency is associated with significant lactose malabsorption. Some individuals with lactose malabsorption develop symptoms such as diarrhea, abdominal pain, cramps, and/or flatus. Most individuals with primary lactase deficiency do not have symptoms. Since lactose intolerance may be associated with symptoms suggestive of irritable bowel syndrome, persistence of such symptoms in an individual who exhibits lactose intolerance while on a strict lactose-free diet suggests that the person's symptoms were related to irritable bowel syndrome.

The development of symptoms of lactose intolerance is related to several factors:

1. *Amount of lactose in the diet.*
2. *Rate of gastric emptying.* Symptoms are more likely when gastric emptying is rapid than when it is slower. Therefore, skim milk is more likely to be associated with symptoms of lactose intolerance than whole milk, as the rate of gastric emptying after skim milk intake is more rapid. Similarly, diarrhea following subtotal gastrectomy is often a result of lactose intolerance, as gastric emptying is accelerated in patients with a gastrojejunostomy.
3. *Small-intestinal transit time.* Although the small and large intestines both contribute to the development of symptoms, many symptoms of lactase deficiency are related to the interaction of colonic bacteria and nonabsorbed lactose. More rapid small-intestinal transit makes symptoms more likely.
4. *Colonic compensation by production of SCFAs from nonabsorbed lactose.* Reduced levels of colonic microflora, which can follow antibiotic use, are associated with increased symptoms after lactose ingestion, especially in a lactase-deficient individual.

Glucose-galactose or monosaccharide malabsorption may also be associated with diarrhea and is due to a congenital absence of SGLT1. Diarrhea develops when individuals with this disorder ingest carbohydrates that contain actively transported monosaccharides (e.g., glucose, galactose) but not when they ingest monosaccharides that are not actively transported (e.g., fructose). Fructose is absorbed by the brush border transport protein GLUT 5, a facilitated diffusion process that is not Na-dependent and is distinct from SGLT1. In contrast, some individuals develop diarrhea as a result of the consumption of large quantities of sorbitol, a sugar used in diabetic candy; sorbitol is only minimally absorbed because of the absence of an intestinal absorptive transport mechanism for this sugar.

TABLE 16-5

PRIMARY LACTASE DEFICIENCY IN ADULT ETHNIC GROUPS

ETHNIC GROUP	PREVALENCE OF LACTASE DEFICIENCY, %
Northern European	5–15
Mediterranean	60–85
African black	85–100
American black	45–80
American white	10–25
Native American	50–95
Mexican American	40–75
Asian	90–100

Source: From FJ Simoons: *Am J Dig Dis* 23:963, 1978.

PROTEINS

Protein is present in food almost exclusively as polypeptides and requires extensive hydrolysis to di- and tripeptides and amino acids before absorption. Proteolysis occurs in both the stomach and the small intestine; it is mediated by pepsin, which is secreted as pepsinogen by gastric chief cells, and by trypsinogen and other peptidases from pancreatic acinar cells. The proenzymes pepsinogen and trypsinogen must be activated to pepsin (by pepsin at a pH <5) and to trypsin (by the intestinal brush border enzyme enterokinase and subsequently by trypsin), respectively. Proteins are absorbed by separate transport systems for di- and tripeptides and for different types of amino acids—e.g., neutral and dibasic. Alterations in either protein or amino acid digestion and absorption are rarely observed clinically, even in the presence of extensive small-intestinal mucosal inflammation. However, three rare genetic disorders involve protein digestion/absorption: (1) *Enterokinase deficiency* is due to an absence of the brush border enzyme that converts the proenzyme trypsinogen to trypsin and is associated with diarrhea, growth retardation, and hypoproteinemia. (2) *Hartnup's syndrome*, a defect in neutral amino acid transport, is characterized by a pellagra-like rash and neuropsychiatric symptoms. (3) *Cystinuria*, a defect in dibasic amino acid transport, is associated with renal calculi and chronic pancreatitis.

APPROACH TO THE PATIENT: Malabsorption

The clues provided by the history, symptoms, and initial preliminary observations will serve to limit extensive, ill-focused, and expensive laboratory and imaging studies. For example, a clinician evaluating a patient who has symptoms suggestive of malabsorption and who has recently undergone extensive small-intestinal resection for mesenteric ischemia should direct the initial assessment almost exclusively to defining whether a short-bowel syndrome might explain the entire clinical picture. Similarly, the development of a pattern of bowel movements suggestive of steatorrhea in a patient with long-standing alcohol abuse and chronic pancreatitis should prompt an assessment of pancreatic exocrine function.

The classic picture of malabsorption is rarely seen today in most parts of the United States. As a consequence, diseases with malabsorption must be suspected in individuals who have less severe symptoms and signs and subtle evidence of the altered absorption of only a *single* nutrient rather than obvious evidence of the malabsorption of multiple nutrients.

Although diarrhea can be caused by changes in fluid and electrolyte movement in either the small or the large intestine, dietary nutrients are absorbed almost exclusively in the small intestine.

Therefore, the demonstration of diminished absorption of a dietary nutrient provides unequivocal evidence for small-intestinal disease, although colonic dysfunction may also be present (e.g., Crohn's disease may involve both the small and large intestines). Dietary nutrient absorption may be segmental or diffuse along the small intestine and is site specific. Thus, for example, calcium, iron, and folic acid are exclusively absorbed by active-transport processes in the proximal small intestine, especially the duodenum; in contrast, the active-transport mechanisms for both cobalamin and bile acids are operative only in the ileum. Therefore, in an individual who years previously has had an intestinal resection, the details of which are not presently available, a presentation with evidence of calcium, folic acid, and/or iron malabsorption but without cobalamin deficiency makes it likely that the duodenum and proximal jejunum, but not the ileum, were resected.

Some nutrients—e.g., glucose, amino acids, and lipids—are absorbed throughout the small intestine, although their rate of absorption is greater in the proximal than in the distal segments. However, after segmental resection of the small intestine, the remaining segments undergo both morphologic and functional "adaptation" to enhance absorption. Such adaptation is secondary to the presence of luminal nutrients and hormonal stimuli and may not be complete in humans for several months after resection. Adaptation is critical for the survival of individuals who have undergone massive resection of the small intestine and/or colon.

Establishing the diagnosis of steatorrhea and identifying its specific cause are often quite difficult. The "gold standard" remains a timed, quantitative stool-fat determination. From a practical standpoint, stool collections are invariably difficult and often incomplete, as nobody wants to handle stool. A qualitative test—Sudan III staining—has long been available to document an increase in stool fat. This test is rapid and inexpensive but, as a qualitative test, does not establish the degree of fat malabsorption and is best used as a preliminary screening study. Many of the blood, breath, and isotopic tests that have been developed (1) do not directly measure fat absorption; (2) exhibit excellent sensitivity when steatorrhea is obvious and severe but poor sensitivity when steatorrhea is mild (e.g., assays for stool chymotrypsin and elastase, which can potentially distinguish pancreatic from nonpancreatic etiologies of steatorrhea); or (3) have not survived the transition from the research laboratory to commercial application.

Nevertheless, routine laboratory studies (i.e., complete blood count, prothrombin time, serum protein determination, alkaline phosphatase) may suggest dietary nutrient depletion, especially deficiencies of iron, folate, cobalamin, and vitamins D and K. Additional studies include measurement of serum carotene, cholesterol, albumin, iron, folate, and cobalamin levels. The serum carotene level can also be reduced if the patient's dietary intake of leafy vegetables is poor.

If steatorrhea and/or altered absorption of other nutrients is suspected, then history, clinical observations, and laboratory testing can help detect deficiency of a nutrient, especially of a fat-soluble vitamin (A, D, E, or K). Thus, evidence of metabolic bone disease with elevated alkaline phosphatase concentrations and/or reduced serum calcium levels suggests vitamin D malabsorption. A deficiency of vitamin K is suggested by an elevated prothrombin time in an individual without liver disease who is not taking anticoagulants. Macrocytic anemia leads to an evaluation for possible cobalamin or folic acid malabsorption. Iron-deficiency anemia in the absence of occult bleeding from the gastrointestinal tract in either a male patient or a nonmenstruating female patient requires an evaluation for iron malabsorption and the exclusion of celiac disease, as iron is absorbed exclusively in the proximal small intestine.

At times, however, a timed (72-h) quantitative stool collection, preferably while the patient is on a defined diet, must be undertaken in order to determine stool fat content and establish the diagnosis of steatorrhea. The presence of steatorrhea then requires further assessment to identify the pathophysiologic process(es) responsible for the defect in dietary lipid digestion/absorption (Table 16-4). Other studies include the Schilling test **(Chap. 17)**, the D-xylose test, duodenal mucosal biopsy, small-intestinal radiologic examination, and tests of pancreatic exocrine function.

THE SCHILLING TEST This test (**Chap. 17**) is performed to determine the cause of cobalamin malabsorption. An understanding of the physiology and pathophysiology of cobalamin absorption is very valuable, enhancing comprehension of aspects of gastric, pancreatic, and ileal function. Unfortunately, the Schilling test has not been available commercially in the United States for the past few years.

URINARY D-XYLOSE TEST The urinary D-xylose test for carbohydrate absorption provides an assessment of proximal small-intestinal mucosal function. D-Xylose, a pentose, is absorbed almost exclusively in the proximal small intestine. The D-xylose test is usually performed by administering 25 g of D-xylose and collecting urine for 5 h. An abnormal test (excretion of <4.5 g) primarily reflects duodenal/jejunal mucosal disease. The D-xylose test can also be abnormal in patients with blind loop syndrome (as a consequence primarily of an abnormal intestinal mucosa) and, as a false-positive study, in patients with large collections of fluid in a third space (i.e., ascites, pleural fluid). The ease of obtaining a mucosal biopsy of the small intestine by endoscopy and the false-negative rate of the D-xylose test have led to its diminished use. When small-intestinal mucosal disease is suspected, a small-intestinal mucosal biopsy should be performed.

RADIOLOGIC EXAMINATION Radiologic examination of the small intestine using barium contrast (small-bowel series or study) can provide important information in the evaluation of the patient with presumed or suspected malabsorption. This study is most often performed in conjunction with an examination of the esophagus, stomach, and duodenal bulb. Because insufficient barium is given to the patient to permit an adequate examination of the small-intestinal mucosa, especially in the ileum, many gastrointestinal radiologists alter the procedure by performing either a small-bowel series in which a large amount of barium is given by mouth, without concurrent examination of the esophagus and stomach, or an enteroclysis study in which a large amount of barium is introduced into the duodenum via a fluoroscopically placed tube. In addition, many of the diagnostic features initially described by radiologists to denote the presence of small-intestinal disease (e.g., flocculation, segmentation) are rarely seen with current barium suspensions. Nonetheless, in skilled hands, barium contrast examination of the small intestine can yield important information. For example, with extensive mucosal disease, intestinal dilation can be seen as a dilution of barium from increased intestinal fluid secretion (Fig. 16-3). A normal barium contrast study does *not* exclude the possibility of small-intestinal disease. However, a small-bowel series remains useful in the search for anatomic abnormalities, such as strictures and fistulas (as in Crohn's disease) or blind loop syndrome (e.g., multiple jejunal diverticula) and to define the extent of a previous surgical resection. Other imaging studies that assess the integrity of small-intestinal morphology are CT enterography and magnetic resonance enterography. Capsule endoscopy and double-balloon enteroscopy are other useful aids in the diagnostic assessment of small-intestinal pathology.

BIOPSY OF SMALL-INTESTINAL MUCOSA A small-intestinal mucosal biopsy is essential in the evaluation of a patient with documented steatorrhea or chronic diarrhea (i.e., that lasting >3 weeks) (**Chap. 6**). The ready availability of endoscopic equipment to examine the stomach and duodenum has led to its almost uniform use as the preferred method of obtaining histologic material from the proximal small-intestinal mucosa. The primary indications for a small-intestinal biopsy are evaluation of a patient (1) either with documented or suspected steatorrhea or with chronic diarrhea, and (2) with diffuse or focal abnormalities of the small intestine defined on a small-intestinal series. Lesions seen on small-bowel biopsy can be classified into three categories (Table 16-6):

1. *Diffuse, specific lesions.* Relatively few diseases associated with altered nutrient absorption have specific histopathologic abnormalities on small-intestinal mucosal biopsy, and these diseases are uncommon. *Whipple's disease* is characterized by the presence of periodic acid–Schiff (PAS)–positive macrophages in the lamina propria; the bacilli that are also present may require electron microscopic examination for identification (Fig. 16-4). *Abetalipoproteinemia* is characterized by a normal mucosal appearance except for the presence of mucosal absorptive cells that contain lipid postprandially and disappear after a prolonged period of either fat-free intake or fasting. *Immune globulin deficiency* is associated with a variety of histopathologic findings on small-intestinal mucosal biopsy. The characteristic feature is the absence of or substantial reduction in the number of plasma cells in the lamina propria; the mucosal architecture may be

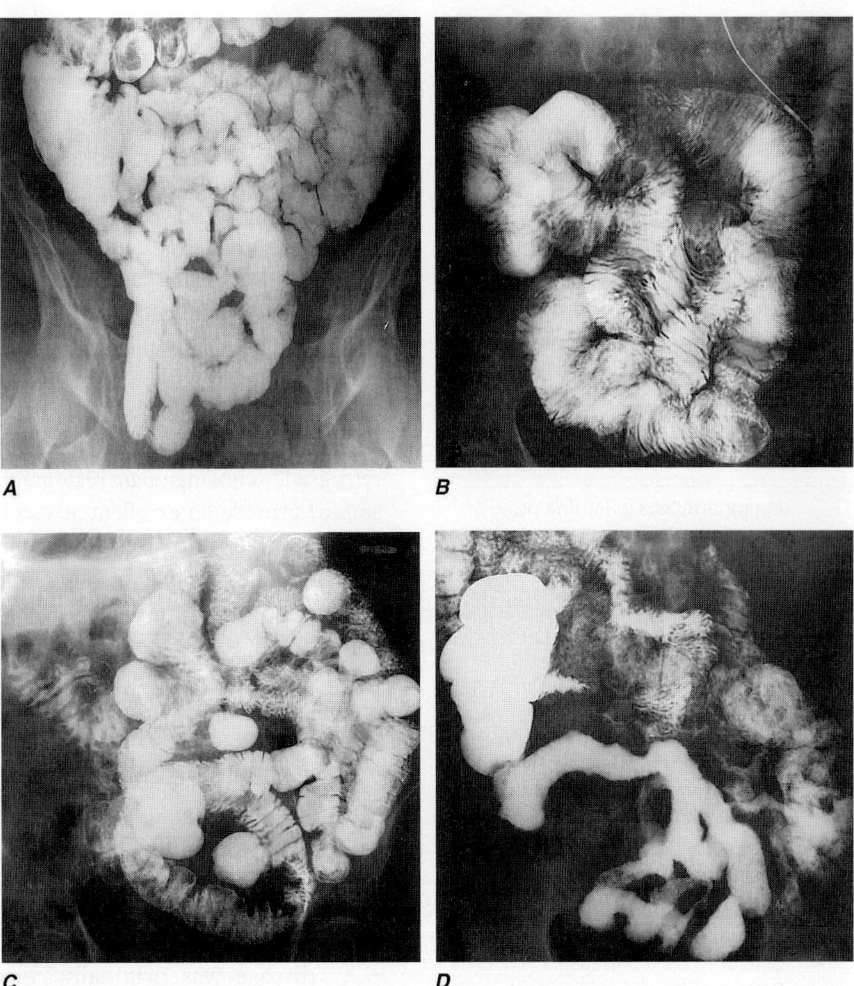

FIGURE 16-3

Barium contrast small-intestinal radiologic examinations. ***A.*** Normal individual. ***B.*** Celiac sprue. ***C.*** Jejunal diverticulosis. ***D.*** Crohn's disease. *(Courtesy of Morton Burrell, MD, Yale University; with permission.)*

either perfectly normal or flat (i.e., villous atrophy). As patients with immune globulin deficiency are often infected with *Giardia lamblia, Giardia* trophozoites may also be seen in the biopsy.

2. *Patchy, specific lesions.* Several diseases feature an abnormal small-intestinal mucosa with a patchy distribution. As a result, biopsy samples obtained randomly or in the absence of endoscopically visualized abnormalities may not reveal diagnostic features. Intestinal *lymphoma* can at times be diagnosed on mucosal biopsy by the identification of malignant lymphoma cells in the lamina propria and submucosa. Dilated lymphatics in the submucosa and sometimes in the lamina propria indicate *lymphangiectasia* associated with hypoproteinemia secondary to protein loss into the intestine. *Eosinophilic gastroenteritis* comprises a heterogeneous group of disorders with a spectrum of presentations and symptoms, with an eosinophilic infiltrate of the lamina propria, and with or without peripheral eosinophilia. The patchy nature of the infiltrate and its presence in the submucosa often lead to an absence of histopathologic findings on mucosal biopsy. As the involvement of the duodenum in *Crohn's disease* is also submucosal and not necessarily continuous, mucosal biopsies are not the most direct approach to the diagnosis of duodenal Crohn's disease **(Chap. 18)**. Amyloid deposition can be identified by Congo Red staining in some patients with *amyloidosis* involving the duodenum.

3. *Diffuse, nonspecific lesions. Celiac disease* presents with a characteristic mucosal appearance on duodenal/proximal jejunal mucosal biopsy that is *not* diagnostic of the disease. The diagnosis of celiac disease is established by clinical, histologic, and immunologic responses to a gluten-free diet. *Tropical sprue* (see below) is associated with histologic findings similar to those of celiac disease after a tropical or subtropical exposure but does not respond to gluten restriction; most often symptoms improve with antibiotics and folate administration.

TABLE 16-6

DISEASES THAT CAN BE DIAGNOSED BY SMALL-INTESTINAL MUCOSAL BIOPSIES

LESIONS	PATHOLOGIC FINDINGS
Diffuse, Specific	
Whipple's disease	Lamina propria includes macrophages containing material positive on periodic acid–Schiff staining
Agammaglobulinemia	No plasma cells; either normal or absent villi ("flat mucosa")
Abetalipoproteinemia	Normal villi; epithelial cells vacuolated with fat postprandially
Patchy, Specific	
Intestinal lymphoma	Malignant cells in lamina propria and submucosa
Intestinal lymphangiectasia	Dilated lymphatics; clubbed villi
Eosinophilic gastroenteritis	Eosinophil infiltration of lamina propria and mucosa
Amyloidosis	Amyloid deposits
Crohn's disease	Noncaseating granulomas
Infection by one or more microorganisms (see text)	Specific organisms
Mastocytosis	Mast cell infiltration of lamina propria
Diffuse, Nonspecific	
Celiac disease	Short or absent villi; mononuclear infiltrate; epithelial cell damage; hypertrophy of crypts
Tropical sprue	Similar to celiac disease
Bacterial overgrowth	Patchy damage to villi; lymphocyte infiltration
Folate deficiency	Short villi; decreased mitosis in crypts; megalocytosis
Vitamin B12 deficiency	Similar to folate deficiency
Radiation enteritis	Similar to folate deficiency
Zollinger-Ellison syndrome	Mucosal ulceration and erosion from acid
Protein-calorie malnutrition	Villous atrophy; secondary bacterial overgrowth
Drug-induced enteritis	Variable histology

Several microorganisms can be identified in small-intestinal biopsy samples, establishing a correct diagnosis. At times, the biopsy is performed specifically to diagnose infection (e.g., Whipple's disease or giardiasis). In most other instances, the infection is detected incidentally during the workup for diarrhea or other abdominal symptoms. Many of these infections occur in immunocompromised patients with diarrhea; the etiologic agents include *Cryptosporidium, Isospora belli,* microsporidia, *Cyclospora, Toxoplasma*, cytomegalovirus, adenovirus, *Mycobacterium avium-intracellulare*, and *G. lamblia*. In immunocompromised patients, when *Candida, Aspergillus, Cryptococcus*, or *Histoplasma* organisms are seen on duodenal biopsy, their presence generally reflects systemic infection. Apart from Whipple's disease and infections in the immunocompromised host, small-bowel biopsy is seldom used as the primary mode of diagnosis of infection. Even giardiasis is more easily diagnosed by stool antigen studies and/or duodenal aspiration than by duodenal biopsy.

Patients with steatorrhea require assessment of *pancreatic exocrine function*, which is often abnormal in chronic pancreatitis. The secretin test that collects pancreatic secretions by duodenal intubation following intravenous administration of secretin is the only test that directly measures pancreatic exocrine function but is available only at a few specialized centers. Endoscopic approaches (endoscopic retrograde cholangiopancreatography, endoscopic ultrasound) provide an excellent assessment of pancreatic duct anatomy but do *not* assess exocrine function **(Chap. 49)**.

Table 16-7 summarizes the results of the D-xylose test, the Schilling test, and small-intestinal mucosal biopsy in patients with steatorrhea of various etiologies.

SPECIFIC DISEASE ENTITIES

CELIAC DISEASE

Celiac disease is a common cause of malabsorption of one or more nutrients. Although celiac disease was originally considered largely a disease of white individuals, especially persons of European descent, recent observations have established that it is a common disease with protean manifestations, a worldwide distribution, and an estimated incidence in the United States that is as high as 1 in 113 people. Its incidence has increased over the past 50 years. Celiac disease has had several other names, including nontropical sprue, celiac sprue, adult celiac disease, and gluten-sensitive enteropathy. The etiology of celiac disease is not known, but environmental, immunologic, and genetic factors are important. Celiac disease is considered an "iceberg" disease. A small number of individuals have classical symptoms and manifestations related to nutrient malabsorption along with a varied natural history; the onset of symptoms can occur at all points from the first year of life through the eighth decade. A much larger number of individuals have "atypical celiac disease", with manifestations that are not obviously related to intestinal malabsorption (e.g., anemia, osteopenia, infertility, and neurologic symptoms). Finally, an even larger number of persons have "silent celiac disease"; they are essentially asymptomatic despite abnormal small-intestinal histopathology and serologies (see below).

The hallmark of celiac disease is an abnormal small-intestinal biopsy (Fig. 16-4) and the response of the

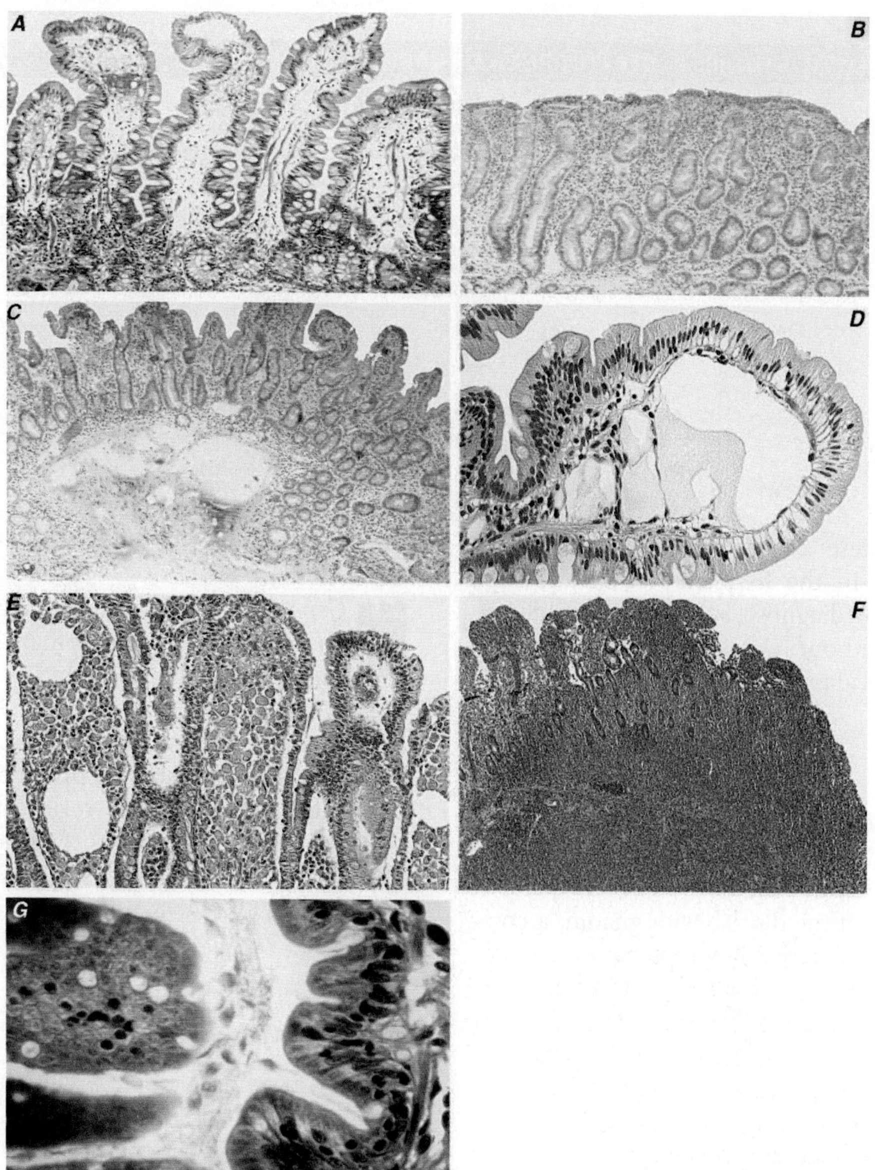

FIGURE 16-4

Small-intestinal mucosal biopsies. ***A.*** Normal individual. ***B.*** Untreated celiac sprue. ***C.*** Treated celiac sprue. **D.** Intestinal lymphangiectasia. ***E.*** Whipple's disease. ***F.*** Lymphoma. ***G.*** Giardiasis. *(Courtesy of Marie Robert, MD, Yale University; with permission.)*

condition (including symptoms and histologic changes on small-intestinal biopsy) to the elimination of gluten from the diet. The histologic changes have a proximal-to-distal intestinal distribution of severity, which probably reflects the exposure of the intestinal mucosa to varied amounts of dietary gluten. The symptoms do not necessarily correlate with histologic changes, especially as many newly diagnosed patients with celiac disease may be asymptomatic or only minimally symptomatic (often with no gastrointestinal symptoms).

The symptoms of celiac disease may appear with the introduction of cereals into an infant's diet, although spontaneous remissions often occur during the second decade of life that may be either permanent or followed by the reappearance of symptoms over several years. Alternatively, the symptoms of celiac disease may first become evident at almost any age throughout adulthood. In many patients, frequent spontaneous remissions and exacerbations occur. The symptoms range from significant malabsorption of multiple nutrients, with diarrhea, steatorrhea, weight loss, and the consequences of nutrient depletion (i.e., anemia and metabolic bone disease), to the absence of gastrointestinal symptoms despite evidence of the depletion of a single nutrient (e.g., iron or folate deficiency, osteomalacia, edema from protein loss). Asymptomatic relatives of patients with celiac disease have been identified as having this disease either by small-intestinal biopsy or by serologic studies (e.g., antiendomysial antibodies, tissue transglutaminase [tTG], deamidated gliadin peptide).

TABLE 16-7

RESULTS OF DIAGNOSTIC STUDIES IN STEATORRHEA OF VARIOUS ETIOLOGIES

	D-XYLOSE TEST	SCHILLING TEST	DUODENAL MUCOSAL BIOPSY
Chronic pancreatitis	Normal	50% abnormal; if abnormal, normal with pancreatic enzyme treatment	Normal
Bacterial overgrowth syndromes	Normal or only modestly abnormal	Often abnormal; if abnormal, normal after antibiotic treatment	Usually normal
Ileal disease	Normal	Abnormal	Normal
Celiac disease	Decreased	Normal	Abnormal: probably "flat"
Intestinal lymphangiectasiaia	Normal	Normal	Abnormal: "dilated lymphatics"

The availability of these "celiac serologies" has led to a substantial increase in the frequency of diagnosis of celiac disease, and the diagnosis is now being made primarily in patients without "classic" symptoms but with atypical and subclinical presentations.

Etiology

The etiology of celiac disease is not known, but environmental, immunologic, and genetic factors all appear to contribute to the disease. One *environmental* factor is the clear association of the disease with gliadin, a component of gluten that is present in wheat, barley, and rye. In addition to the role of gluten restriction in treatment, the instillation of gluten into both the normal-appearing rectum and the distal ileum of patients with celiac disease results in morphologic changes within hours.

An *immunologic* component in the pathogenesis of celiac disease is critical and involves both adaptive and innate immune responses. Serum antibodies—IgA antigliadin, antiendomysial, and anti-tTG antibodies—are present, but it is not known whether such antibodies are primary or secondary to the tissue damage. The presence of antiendomysial antibody is 90–95% sensitive and 90–95% specific; the antigen recognized by antiendomysial antibody is tTG, which deaminates gliadin, which is presented to HLA-DQ2 or HLA-DQ8 (see below). Antibody studies are frequently used to identify patients with celiac disease; patients with these antibodies should undergo duodenal biopsy. This autoantibody has not been linked to a pathogenetic mechanism (or mechanisms) responsible for celiac disease. Nonetheless, this antibody is useful in establishing the true prevalence of celiac disease in the general population. A 4-week course of treatment with prednisolone induces a remission in a patient with celiac disease who continues to eat gluten and converts the "flat" abnormal duodenal biopsy to a more normal-appearing one. In addition, gliadin peptides interact with gliadin-specific T cells that mediate tissue injury and induce the release of one or more cytokines (e.g., interferon γ) that cause tissue injury.

Genetic factor(s) are also involved in celiac disease. The incidence of symptomatic celiac disease varies widely in different population groups (high among whites, low among blacks and Asians) and is 10% among first-degree relatives of celiac disease patients. However, serologic studies provide clear evidence that celiac disease is present worldwide. Furthermore, all patients with celiac disease express the HLA-DQ2 or HLA-DQ8 allele, although only a minority of people expressing DQ2/DQ8 have celiac disease. Absence of DQ2/DQ8 excludes the diagnosis of celiac disease.

Diagnosis

A small-intestinal biopsy is required to establish a diagnosis of celiac disease (Fig. 16-4). A biopsy should be performed when patients have symptoms and laboratory findings suggestive of nutrient malabsorption and/or deficiency as well as a positive tTG antibody test. Since the presentation of celiac disease is often subtle, without overt evidence of malabsorption or nutrient deficiency, a relatively low threshold for biopsy performance is important. It is more prudent to perform a biopsy than another test of intestinal absorption that can never completely exclude or establish this diagnosis.

The diagnosis of celiac disease requires the detection of characteristic histologic changes on small-intestinal biopsy together with a prompt clinical and histologic response after the institution of a gluten-free diet. If IgA antiendomysial or tTG antibodies have been detected in serologic studies, they too should disappear after a gluten-free diet is started. With the increase in the number of patients diagnosed with celiac disease (mostly by serologic studies), the spectrum of histologic changes seen on duodenal biopsy has increased and includes findings that are not as severe as the classic changes shown in Fig. 16-4. The classic changes seen on duodenal/jejunal biopsy are restricted to the mucosa and include (1) an increase in the number of intraepithelial lymphocytes; (2) absence or a reduced height of villi, which causes a flat appearance with increased crypt cell proliferation resulting in crypt hyperplasia and loss of villous structure, with consequent villous, but not mucosal, atrophy; (3) a cuboidal appearance and nuclei that are no longer oriented basally in surface epithelial cells; and (4) increased numbers of lymphocytes and plasma cells in the lamina propria (Fig. 16-4*B*). Although these features are characteristic of celiac disease, they are *not* diagnostic because a similar appearance can develop in tropical sprue, eosinophilic enteritis, and milk-protein intolerance in children and occasionally in lymphoma, bacterial overgrowth, Crohn's disease, and gastrinoma with acid hypersecretion. However, a characteristic histologic appearance that reverts toward normal after the initiation of a gluten-free diet establishes the diagnosis of celiac disease (Fig. 16-4*C*). Readministration of gluten, with or without an additional small-intestinal biopsy, is not necessary.

A number of patients exhibit *gluten sensitivity*; i.e., they have gastrointestinal symptoms that respond to gluten restriction but do not have celiac disease. The basis for such gluten sensitivity is not known.

Failure to respond to gluten restriction

The most common cause of persistent symptoms in a patient who fulfills all the criteria for the diagnosis of celiac disease is *continued intake of gluten*. Gluten is ubiquitous, and a significant effort must be made to exclude all gluten from the diet. Use of rice flour in place of wheat flour is very helpful, and several support groups provide important aid to patients with celiac disease and to their families. More than 90% of patients who have the characteristic findings of celiac disease respond to complete dietary gluten restriction. The remainder constitute a heterogeneous group (whose condition is often called *refractory celiac disease* or *refractory sprue*) that includes some patients who (1) respond to restriction of other dietary protein (e.g., soy); (2) respond to glucocorticoid treatment; (3) are "temporary" (i.e., whose clinical and morphologic findings disappear after several months or years); or (4) fail to respond to all measures and have a fatal outcome, with or without documented complications of celiac disease, such as the development of intestinal T cell lymphoma or autoimmune enteropathy.

Therapeutic approaches that do not include a gluten-free diet are being developed and include the use of peptidases to inactivate toxic gliadin peptides and of small molecules to block toxic peptide uptake across intestinal tight junctions.

Mechanism of diarrhea

The diarrhea in celiac disease has several pathogenetic mechanisms. Diarrhea may be secondary to (1) steatorrhea, which is primarily a result of changes in jejunal mucosal function; (2) secondary lactase deficiency, a consequence of changes in jejunal brush border enzymatic function; (3) bile acid malabsorption resulting in bile acid–induced fluid secretion in the colon (in cases with more extensive disease involving the ileum); and (4) endogenous fluid secretion resulting from crypt hyperplasia. Celiac disease patients with more severe involvement may improve temporarily with *dietary lactose and fat restriction* while awaiting the full effects of total gluten restriction, which constitutes primary therapy.

Associated diseases

Celiac disease is associated with dermatitis herpetiformis (DH), but this association has not been explained. Patients with DH have characteristic papulovesicular lesions that respond to dapsone. Almost all patients with DH have histologic changes in the small intestine consistent with celiac disease, although usually much milder and less diffuse in distribution. Most patients with DH have mild or no gastrointestinal symptoms. In contrast, relatively few patients with celiac disease have DH.

Celiac disease is also associated with diabetes mellitus type 1, IgA deficiency, Down syndrome, and Turner's syndrome. The clinical importance of the association with diabetes is that, although severe watery diarrhea without evidence of malabsorption is most often diagnosed as "diabetic diarrhea", assay of antiendomysial antibodies and/or a small-intestinal biopsy must be considered to exclude celiac disease.

Complications

The most important complication of celiac disease is the development of cancer. The incidences of both gastrointestinal and nongastrointestinal neoplasms as well as intestinal lymphoma are elevated among patients with celiac disease. For unexplained reasons, the frequency of lymphoma in patients with celiac disease is higher in Ireland and the United Kingdom than in the United States. The possibility of lymphoma must be considered whenever a patient with celiac disease who has previously done well on a gluten-free diet is no longer responsive to gluten restriction or a patient who presents with clinical and histologic features consistent with celiac disease does not respond to a gluten-free diet. Other complications of celiac disease include the development of intestinal ulceration independent of lymphoma and so-called refractory sprue (see above) and collagenous sprue. In *collagenous sprue*, a layer of collagen-like material is present beneath the basement membrane; patients with collagenous sprue generally do not respond to a gluten-free diet and often have a poor prognosis.

TROPICAL SPRUE

Tropical sprue is a poorly understood syndrome that affects both expatriates and natives in certain but not all tropical areas and is manifested by chronic diarrhea, steatorrhea, weight loss, and nutritional deficiencies, including those of both folate and cobalamin. This disease affects 5–10% of the population in some tropical areas.

Chronic diarrhea in a tropical environment is most often caused by infectious agents, including *G. lamblia, Yersinia enterocolitica, C. difficile, Cryptosporidium parvum*, and *Cyclospora cayetanensis*. Tropical sprue should not be entertained as a possible diagnosis until the presence of cysts and trophozoites has been excluded in three stool samples. **Chronic infections of the gastrointestinal tract and diarrhea in patients with or without AIDS are discussed in Chaps. 24 and 25.**

The small-intestinal mucosa of individuals living in tropical areas is not identical to that of individuals who reside in temperate climates. In residents of tropical areas, biopsies reveal a mild alteration of villous architecture with a modest increase in mononuclear cells in the lamina propria, which on occasion can be as severe as that seen in celiac disease. These changes are observed both in native residents and in expatriates living in tropical regions and are usually associated with mild decreases in absorptive function, but they revert to "normal" when an individual moves or returns to a temperate area. Some have suggested that the changes seen in tropical enteropathy and in tropical sprue represent different ends of the spectrum of a single entity, but convincing evidence to support this concept is lacking.

Etiology

Because tropical sprue responds to antibiotics, the consensus is that it may be caused by one or more infectious agents. Nonetheless, the etiology and pathogenesis of tropical sprue are uncertain. First, its occurrence is not evenly distributed in all tropical areas; rather, it is found in specific locations, including southern India, the Philippines, and several Caribbean islands (e.g., Puerto Rico, Haiti), but is rarely observed in Africa, Jamaica, or Southeast Asia. Second, an occasional individual does not develop symptoms of tropical sprue until long after having left an endemic area. For this reason, celiac disease (often referred to as celiac sprue) was originally called *nontropical sprue* to distinguish it from tropical sprue. Third, multiple microorganisms have been identified in jejunal aspirates, with relatively little consistency among studies. *Klebsiella pneumoniae, Enterobacter cloacae*, and *E. coli* have been implicated in some studies of tropical sprue, while other studies have favored a role for a toxin produced by one or more of these bacteria. Fourth, the incidence of tropical sprue appears to have decreased substantially during the past two or three decades, perhaps in relation to improved sanitation in many tropical countries during this time. Some have speculated that the reduced occurrence is attributable to the wider use of antibiotics in acute diarrhea, especially in travelers to tropical areas from temperate countries. Fifth, the role of folic acid deficiency in the pathogenesis of tropical sprue requires clarification. Folic acid is absorbed exclusively in the duodenum and proximal jejunum, and most patients with tropical sprue have evidence of folate malabsorption and depletion. Although folate deficiency can cause changes in small-intestinal mucosa that are corrected by folate replacement, several earlier studies reporting that tropical sprue could be cured by folic acid did not provide an explanation for the "insult" that was initially responsible for folate malabsorption.

The clinical pattern of tropical sprue varies in different areas of the world (e.g., India vs. Puerto Rico). Not infrequently, individuals in southern India initially report the occurrence of acute enteritis before the development of steatorrhea and malabsorption. In contrast, in Puerto Rico, a more insidious onset of symptoms and a more dramatic response to antibiotics are seen than in some other locations. Tropical sprue in different areas of the world may not be the same disease, and similar clinical entities may have different etiologies.

Diagnosis

The diagnosis of tropical sprue is best based on an abnormal small-intestinal mucosal biopsy in an individual with chronic diarrhea and evidence of malabsorption who is either residing or has recently lived in a tropical country. The small-intestinal biopsy in tropical sprue does not reveal pathognomonic features but resembles, and can often be indistinguishable from, that seen in celiac disease (Fig. 16-4). The biopsy sample in tropical sprue has less villous architectural alteration and more mononuclear cell infiltrate in the lamina propria. In contrast to those of celiac disease, the histologic features of tropical sprue manifest with a similar degree of severity throughout the small intestine, and a gluten-free diet does not result in either clinical or histologic improvement in tropical sprue.

TREATMENT Tropical Sprue

Broad-spectrum antibiotics and folic acid are most often curative, especially if the patient leaves the tropical area and does not return. Tetracycline should be used for up to 6 months and may be associated with improvement within 1–2 weeks. Folic acid alone induces hematologic remission as well as improvement in appetite, weight gain, and some morphologic changes in small-intestinal biopsy. Because of marked folate deficiency, folic acid is most often given together with antibiotics.

SHORT-BOWEL SYNDROME

Short-bowel syndrome is a descriptive term for the myriad clinical problems that follow resection of various lengths of small intestine or, on rare occasions, are congenital (e.g., microvillous inclusion disease). The factors that determine both the type and degree of symptoms include (1) the specific segment (jejunum vs. ileum) resected, (2) the length of the resected segment, (3) the integrity of the ileocecal valve, (4) whether any large intestine has also been removed, (5) residual disease in the remaining small and/or large intestine (e.g., Crohn's disease, mesenteric artery disease), and (6) the degree of adaptation in the remaining intestine. Short-bowel syndrome can occur in persons of any age, from neonates to the elderly.

Three different situations in adults mandate intestinal resection: (1) mesenteric vascular disease, including atherosclerosis, thrombotic phenomena, and vasculitides; (2) primary mucosal and submucosal disease (e.g., Crohn's disease); and (3) operations without preexisting small-intestinal disease (e.g., after trauma).

After resection of the small intestine, the residual intestine undergoes adaptation of both structure and function that may last for up to 6–12 months. Continued intake of dietary nutrients and calories is required to stimulate adaptation via direct contact with the intestinal mucosa, the release of one or more intestinal hormones, and pancreatic and biliary secretions. Thus, enteral nutrition with calorie administration must be maintained, especially in the early postoperative period, even if an extensive intestinal resection requiring parenteral nutrition (PN) has been performed. The subsequent ability of such patients to absorb nutrients will not be known for several months, until adaptation is complete.

Multiple factors besides the absence of intestinal mucosa (required for lipid, fluid, and electrolyte absorption) contribute to diarrhea and steatorrhea in these patients. Removal of the ileum, and especially the ileocecal valve, is often associated with more severe diarrhea than jejunal resection. Without part or all of the ileum, diarrhea can be caused by an increase in bile acids entering the colon; these acids stimulate colonic fluid and electrolyte secretion. Absence of the ileocecal valve is also associated with a decrease in intestinal transit time and bacterial overgrowth from the colon. The presence of the colon (or a major portion) is associated with substantially less diarrhea and a lower likelihood of *intestinal failure* (an inability to maintain nutrition without parenteral support) as a result of fermentation of nonabsorbed carbohydrates to SCFAs. The latter are absorbed in the colon and stimulate Na and water absorption, improving overall fluid balance. Lactose intolerance as a result of the removal of lactase-containing mucosa as well as gastric hypersecretion may also contribute to the diarrhea.

In addition to diarrhea and/or steatorrhea, a range of nonintestinal symptoms is observed in some patients. The frequency of renal calcium oxalate calculi increases significantly in patients with a small-intestinal resection and an intact colon; this greater frequency is due to an increase in oxalate absorption by the large intestine, with subsequent *enteric hyperoxaluria*. Two possible mechanisms for the increase in oxalate absorption in the colon have been suggested: (1) increased bile acids and fatty acids that augment colonic mucosal permeability, resulting in enhanced oxalate absorption; and (2) increased fatty acids that bind calcium, resulting in an enhanced amount of soluble oxalate that is then absorbed. Since oxalate is high in relatively few foods (e.g., spinach, rhubarb, tea), dietary restrictions alone do not constitute adequate treatment. Cholestyramine (an anion-binding resin) and calcium have proved useful in reducing hyperoxaluria. Similarly, an increase in cholesterol gallstones is related to a decrease in the bile-acid pool size, which results in the generation of cholesterol supersaturation in gallbladder bile. Gastric hypersecretion of acid occurs in many patients after large resections of the small intestine. The etiology is unclear but may be related to either reduced hormonal inhibition of acid secretion or increased gastrin levels due to reduced small-intestinal catabolism of circulating gastrin. The resulting gastric acid secretion may be an important factor contributing to diarrhea and steatorrhea. A reduced pH in the duodenum can inactivate pancreatic lipase and/or precipitate duodenal bile acids, thereby increasing steatorrhea, and an increase in gastric secretion can create a volume overload relative to the reduced small-intestinal absorptive capacity. Inhibition of gastric acid secretion with proton pump inhibitors can help reduce diarrhea and steatorrhea, but only for the first 6 months.

TREATMENT Short-Bowel Syndrome

Treatment of short-bowel syndrome depends on the severity of symptoms and on whether the individual is able to maintain caloric and electrolyte balance with oral intake alone. Initial treatment includes judicious use of opiates (including codeine) to reduce stool output and to establish an effective diet. If the colon is in situ, the initial diet should be low in fat and high in carbohydrate in order to minimize diarrhea from fatty acid stimulation of colonic fluid secretion. MCTs (see Table 16-3), a low-lactose diet, and various soluble fiber–containing diets should also be tried. In the absence of an ileocecal valve, possible bacterial overgrowth must be considered and treated. If gastric acid hypersecretion is contributing to diarrhea and steatorrhea, a proton pump inhibitor may be helpful. Usually none of these therapeutic approaches provides an instant solution, but each can contribute to the reduction of disabling diarrhea.

The patient's vitamin and mineral status must also be monitored; replacement therapy should be initiated if indicated. Fat-soluble vitamins, folate, cobalamin, calcium, iron, magnesium, and zinc are the most critical factors to monitor on a regular basis. If these approaches are not successful, home PN is an established therapy that can be maintained for many years. Small-intestinal transplantation is becoming established as a possible approach for individuals with extensive intestinal resection who cannot be maintained without PN—i.e., those with intestinal failure. A recombinant analogue of glucagon-like peptide 2 (GLP-2; teduglutide) is approved for use in patients with PN-dependent short-bowel syndrome on the basis of its ability to increase intestinal growth and improve absorption.

BACTERIAL OVERGROWTH SYNDROMES

Bacterial overgrowth syndromes comprise a group of disorders with diarrhea, steatorrhea, and macrocytic anemia whose common feature is the proliferation of colonic-type bacteria within the small intestine. This bacterial proliferation is due to stasis caused by impaired peristalsis (*functional stasis*), changes in intestinal anatomy (*anatomic stasis*), or direct communication between the small and large intestine. These conditions have also been referred to as *stagnant bowel syndrome* or *blind loop syndrome*.

Pathogenesis

The manifestations of bacterial overgrowth syndromes are a direct consequence of the presence of increased amounts of a colonic-type bacterial flora, such as *E. coli* or *Bacteroides*, in the small intestine. *Macrocytic anemia* is due to cobalamin—not folate—deficiency. Most bacteria require cobalamin for growth, and increasing concentrations of bacteria use up the relatively small amounts of dietary cobalamin. *Steatorrhea* is due to impaired micelle formation as a consequence of a reduced intraduodenal concentration of conjugated bile acids and the presence of unconjugated bile acids. Certain bacteria, including *Bacteroides*, deconjugate conjugated bile acids to unconjugated bile acids. Unconjugated bile acids are absorbed more rapidly than conjugated bile acids; as a result, the intraduodenal concentration of bile acids is reduced. In addition, the CMC of unconjugated bile acids is higher than that of conjugated bile acids, and the result is a decrease in micelle formation. *Diarrhea* is due, at least in part, to steatorrhea, when it is present. However, some patients manifest diarrhea *without* steatorrhea, and it is assumed that the colonic-type bacteria in these patients are producing one or more bacterial enterotoxins that are responsible for fluid secretion and diarrhea.

Etiology

The etiology of these different disorders is bacterial proliferation in the small-intestinal lumen secondary to anatomic or functional stasis or to a communication between the relatively sterile small intestine and the colon, with its high levels of aerobic and anaerobic bacteria. Several examples of *anatomic* stasis have been identified: (1) one or more diverticula (both duodenal and jejunal) (Fig. 16-3*C*); (2) fistulas and strictures related to Crohn's disease (Fig. 16-3*D*); (3) a proximal duodenal afferent loop following subtotal gastrectomy and gastrojejunostomy; (4) a bypass of the intestine (e.g., a jejunoileal bypass for obesity); and (5) dilation at the site of a previous intestinal anastomosis. These anatomic derangements are often associated with the presence of a segment (or segments) of intestine out of continuity of propagated peristalsis, with consequent stasis and bacterial proliferation. Bacterial overgrowth syndromes can also occur in the *absence* of an anatomic blind loop when *functional* stasis is present. Impaired peristalsis and bacterial overgrowth in the absence of a blind loop occur in scleroderma, where motility abnormalities exist in both the esophagus and the small intestine. Functional stasis and bacterial overgrowth can also develop in association with diabetes mellitus and in the small intestine when a direct connection exists between the small and large intestines, including an ileocolonic resection, or occasionally after an enterocolic anastomosis that permits entry of bacteria into the small intestine as a result of bypassing the ileocecal valve.

Diagnosis

The diagnosis may be suspected from the combination of a low serum cobalamin level and an elevated serum folate level, as enteric bacteria frequently produce folate compounds that are absorbed in the duodenum. Ideally, the bacterial overgrowth syndromes are diagnosed by the demonstration of increased levels of aerobic and/or anaerobic colonic-type bacteria in a jejunal aspirate obtained by intubation. However, this specialized test is rarely available. Breath hydrogen testing with administration of lactulose (a nondigestible disaccharide) has also been used to detect bacterial overgrowth. The Schilling test can diagnose bacterial overgrowth (see **Chap. 17**) but is not available routinely. Often the diagnosis is suspected clinically and confirmed by the response to treatment.

TREATMENT Bacterial Overgrowth Syndromes

Primary treatment should be directed, if at all possible, to the surgical correction of an anatomic blind loop. In the absence of functional stasis, it is important to define the anatomic relationships responsible for stasis and bacterial overgrowth.

For example, bacterial overgrowth secondary to strictures, one or more diverticula, or a proximal afferent loop can potentially be cured by surgical correction of the anatomic state. In contrast, the functional stasis of scleroderma or certain anatomic stasis states (e.g., multiple jejunal diverticula) cannot be corrected surgically, and these conditions should be treated with broad-spectrum antibiotics. Tetracycline used to be the initial drug of choice; because of increasing resistance, however, other antibiotics, such as metronidazole, amoxicillin/clavulanic acid, rifaximin and cephalosporins, have been employed. The antibiotic should be given for ~3 weeks or until symptoms remit. Although the natural history of these conditions is chronic, antibiotics should not be given continuously. Symptoms usually remit within 2–3 weeks of initial antibiotic therapy. Treatment need not be repeated until symptoms recur. For frequent recurrences, several treatment strategies exist, but the use of antibiotics for 1 week per month, whether or not symptoms are present, is often most effective.

Unfortunately, therapy for bacterial overgrowth syndromes is largely empirical, with an absence of clinical trials on which to base rational decisions regarding antibiotic choice, treatment duration, and/or the best approach to therapy for recurrences. Bacterial overgrowth may also occur as a component of another chronic disease, such as Crohn's disease, radiation enteritis, or short-bowel syndrome. Treatment of the bacterial overgrowth in these settings will not cure the underlying problem but may be very important in ameliorating a subset of clinical problems that are related to bacterial overgrowth.

WHIPPLE'S DISEASE

Whipple's disease is a chronic multisystemic disease associated with diarrhea, steatorrhea, weight loss, arthralgia, and central nervous system (CNS) and cardiac problems; it is caused by the bacterium *Tropheryma whipplei*. Until the identification of *T. whipplei* by polymerase chain reaction, the hallmark of Whipple's disease had been the presence of PAS-positive macrophages in the small intestine (Fig. 16-4*E*) and other organs with evidence of disease.

Etiology

T. whipplei, a small (50–500 nm) gram-positive bacillus in the group Actinobacteria, has low virulence but high infectivity. Symptoms of Whipple's disease are relatively minimal compared to the bacterial burden in multiple tissues.

Clinical presentation

The onset of Whipple's disease is insidious and is characterized by diarrhea, steatorrhea, abdominal pain, weight loss, migratory large-joint arthropathy, and fever as well as ophthalmologic and CNS symptoms. Dementia is a relatively late symptom and an extremely poor prognostic sign, especially in patients who experience relapse after the induction of a remission with antibiotics. For unexplained reasons, the disease occurs primarily in middle-aged white men. The steatorrhea in these patients is generally believed to be secondary to both small-intestinal mucosal injury and lymphatic obstruction due to the increased number of PAS-positive macrophages in the lamina propria of the small intestine.

Diagnosis

The diagnosis of Whipple's disease is suggested by a multisystemic disease in a patient with diarrhea and steatorrhea. Tissue biopsy of the small intestine and/or other organs that may be involved (e.g., liver, lymph nodes, heart, eyes, CNS, or synovial membranes), given the patient's symptoms, is the primary approach. The presence of PAS-positive macrophages containing the characteristic small bacilli is suggestive of this diagnosis. However, *T. whipplei*–containing macrophages can be confused with PAS-positive macrophages containing *M. avium* complex, which may be a cause of diarrhea in AIDS. The presence of the *T. whipplei* bacillus outside of macrophages is a more important indicator of active disease than is their presence within the macrophages. *T. whipplei* has now been successfully grown in culture.

TREATMENT Whipple's Disease

The treatment for Whipple's disease is prolonged use of antibiotics. The current regimen of choice is ceftriaxone or meropenem for 2 weeks followed by oral TMP-SMX (160/800 mg) twice a day for 1 year. PAS-positive macrophages can persist after successful treatment, and the presence of bacilli outside of macrophages is indicative of persistent infection or an early sign of recurrence. Recurrence of disease activity, especially with dementia, is an extremely poor prognostic sign and requires an antibiotic that crosses the blood-brain barrier. If trimethoprim-sulfamethoxazole is not tolerated, chloramphenicol is an appropriate second choice.

PROTEIN-LOSING ENTEROPATHY

Protein-losing enteropathy is not a specific disease but rather a group of gastrointestinal and nongastrointestinal disorders with hypoproteinemia and edema in the absence of either proteinuria or defects in protein synthesis (e.g., chronic liver disease). These diseases are characterized by excess protein loss into the gastrointestinal tract. Normally, ~10% of total protein catabolism occurs via the gastrointestinal tract. Evidence of

TABLE 16-8

CLASSIFICATION OF MALABSORPTION SYNDROMES

Inadequate digestion
- Postgastrectomy[a]
- Deficiency or inactivation of pancreatic lipase
  - Exocrine pancreatic insufficiency
    - Chronic pancreatitis
    - Pancreatic carcinoma
    - Cystic fibrosis
    - Pancreatic insufficiency—congenital or acquired
- Gastrinoma—acid inactivation of lipasea
- Drugs—orlistat

Reduced intraduodenal bile acid concentration/impaired micelle formation
- Liver disease
  - Parenchymal liver disease
  - Cholestatic liver disease
- Bacterial overgrowth in small intestine:
  - Anatomic stasis
    - Afferent loop
    - Stasis/blind
    - Loop/strictures/fistulae
  - Functional stasis
    - Diabetes[a]
    - Scleroderma[a]
    - Intestinal pseudo-obstruction
- Interrupted enterohepatic circulation of bile salts
  - Ileal resection
  - Crohn's diseasea
- Drugs (binding or precipitating bile salts)—neomycin, cholestyramine, calcium carbonate

Impaired mucosal absorption/mucosal loss or defect
- Intestinal resection or bypass[a]
- Inflammation, infiltration, or infection:
  - Crohn's disease[a]
  - Amyloidosis
  - Scleroderma[a]
  - Lymphoma[a]
  - Eosinophilic enteritis
  - Mastocytosis
  - Tropical sprue
  - Celiac disease
  - Collagenous sprue
  - Whipple's disease[a]
  - Radiation enteritis[a]
  - Folate and vitamin B12 deficiency
  - Infections—giardiasis
  - Graft versus host disease
- Genetic disorders
  - Disaccharidase deficiency
  - Agammaglobulinemia
  - Abetalipoproteinemia
  - Hartnup's disease
  - Cystinuria

Impaired nutrient delivery to and/or from intestine:
- Lymphatic obstruction
  - Lymphomaa
  - Lymphangiectasia
- Circulatory disorders
  - Congestive heart failure
  - Constrictive pericarditis
  - Mesenteric artery atherosclerosis
  - Vasculitis

Endocrine and metabolic disorders
- Diabetes[a]
- Hypoparathyroidism
- Adrenal insufficiency
- Hyperthyroidism
- Carcinoid syndrome

[a]Malabsorption caused by more than one mechanism.

TABLE 16-9

PATHOPHYSIOLOGY OF CLINICAL MANIFESTATIONS OF MALABSORPTION DISORDERS

SYMPTOM OR SIGN	MECHANISM
Weight loss/ malnutrition	Anorexia, malabsorption of nutrients
Diarrhea	Impaired absorption or secretion of water and electrolytes; colonic fluid secretion secondary to unabsorbed dihydroxy bile acids and fatty acids
Flatus	Bacterial fermentation of unabsorbed carbohydrate
Glossitis, cheilosis, stomatitis	Deficiency of iron, vitamin B_{12}, folate, and vitamin A
Abdominal pain	Bowel distention or inflammation, pancreatitis
Bone pain	Calcium, vitamin D malabsorption, protein deficiency, osteoporosis
Tetany, paresthesia	Calcium and magnesium malabsorption
Weakness	Anemia, electrolyte depletion (particularly K^+)
Azotemia, hypotension	Fluid and electrolyte depletion
Amenorrhea, decreased libido	Protein depletion, decreased calories, secondary hypopituitarism
Anemia	Impaired absorption of iron, folate, vitamin B_{12}
Bleeding	Vitamin K malabsorption, hypoprothrombinemia
Night blindness/ xerophthalmia	Vitamin A malabsorption
Peripheral neuropathy	Vitamin B_{12} and thiamine deficiency
Dermatitis	Deficiency of vitamin A, zinc, and essential fatty acid

increased protein loss into the gastrointestinal tract is found in more than 65 different diseases, which can be classified into three groups: (1) mucosal ulceration, such that the protein loss primarily represents exudation across damaged mucosa (e.g., ulcerative colitis, gastrointestinal carcinomas, and peptic ulcer); (2) nonulcerated mucosa, but with evidence of mucosal damage so that the protein loss represents loss across epithelia with altered permeability (e.g., celiac disease and Ménétrier's disease in the small intestine and stomach, respectively); and (3) lymphatic dysfunction, representing either primary lymphatic disease or lymphatic disease secondary to partial lymphatic obstruction that may occur as a result of enlarged lymph nodes or cardiac disease.

Diagnosis

The diagnosis of protein-losing enteropathy is suggested by peripheral edema and low serum albumin and globulin levels in the absence of renal and hepatic disease. An individual with protein-losing enteropathy only rarely has selective loss of *only* albumin or *only* globulins. Therefore, marked reduction of serum albumin with normal serum globulins should not initiate an evaluation for protein-losing enteropathy but should suggest renal and/or hepatic disease. Likewise, reduced serum globulins with normal serum albumin levels are more likely a result of reduced globulin synthesis rather than enhanced globulin loss into the intestine. An increase in protein loss into the gastrointestinal tract has been documented by the administration of one of several radiolabeled proteins and its quantitation in stool during a 24- or 48-h period. Unfortunately, none of these radiolabeled proteins is available for routine clinical use. α_1-Antitrypsin, a protein that accounts for ~4% of total serum proteins and is resistant to proteolysis, can be used to detect enhanced rates of serum protein loss into the intestinal tract but cannot be used to assess gastric protein loss because of its degradation in an acid milieu. α_1-Antitrypsin clearance is measured by determining stool volume as well as both stool and plasma α_1-antitrypsin concentrations. In addition to the loss of protein via abnormal and distended lymphatics, peripheral lymphocytes may be lost via lymphatics, with consequent relative lymphopenia. Thus, lymphopenia in a patient with hypoproteinemia indicates increased loss of protein into the gastrointestinal tract.

Patients with increased protein loss into the gastrointestinal tract from lymphatic obstruction often have steatorrhea and diarrhea. The steatorrhea is a result of altered lymphatic flow as lipid-containing chylomicrons exit from intestinal epithelial cells via intestinal lymphatics (Table 16-4; Fig. 16-4). In the absence of mechanical or anatomic lymphatic obstruction, intrinsic intestinal lymphatic dysfunction—with or without lymphatic dysfunction in the peripheral extremities—has been designated *intestinal lymphangiectasia.* Similarly, ~50% of individuals with intrinsic peripheral lymphatic disease (Milroy's disease) also have intestinal lymphangiectasia and hypoproteinemia. Other than steatorrhea and enhanced protein loss into the gastrointestinal tract, all other aspects of intestinal absorptive function are normal in intestinal lymphangiectasia.

Other causes

Patients who appear to have idiopathic protein-losing enteropathy without evidence of gastrointestinal disease should be examined for cardiac disease—especially right-sided valvular disease and chronic pericarditis. On occasion, hypoproteinemia can be the only presenting manifestation in these two types of heart disease. Ménétrier's disease (also called *hypertrophic gastropathy*) is an uncommon entity that involves the body and fundus of the stomach and is characterized by large gastric folds, reduced gastric acid secretion, and, at times, enhanced protein loss into the stomach.

TREATMENT Protein-Losing Enteropathy

As excess protein loss into the gastrointestinal tract is most often secondary to a specific disease, treatment should be directed primarily to the underlying disease process and not to the hypoproteinemia. For example, if significant hypoproteinemia with resulting peripheral edema is secondary to celiac disease or ulcerative colitis, a gluten-free diet and mesalamine, respectively, would be the initial therapy. When enhanced protein loss is secondary to lymphatic obstruction, it is critical to establish the nature of this obstruction. Identification of mesenteric nodes or lymphoma may be possible by imaging studies. Similarly, it is important to exclude cardiac disease as a cause of protein-losing enteropathy, either by echosonography or, on occasion, by a right-heart catheterization.

The increased protein loss that occurs in intestinal lymphangiectasia is a result of distended lymphatics associated with lipid malabsorption. The hypoproteinemia is treated with a low-fat diet and the administration of MCTs (Table 16-3), which do not exit from the intestinal epithelial cells via lymphatics but are delivered to the body via the portal vein.

SUMMARY

The many conditions that can produce malabsorption are classified by their pathophysiology in Table 16-8. The pathophysiology of the various clinical manifestations of malabsorption is summarized in Table 16-9.

CHAPTER 17
THE SCHILLING TEST

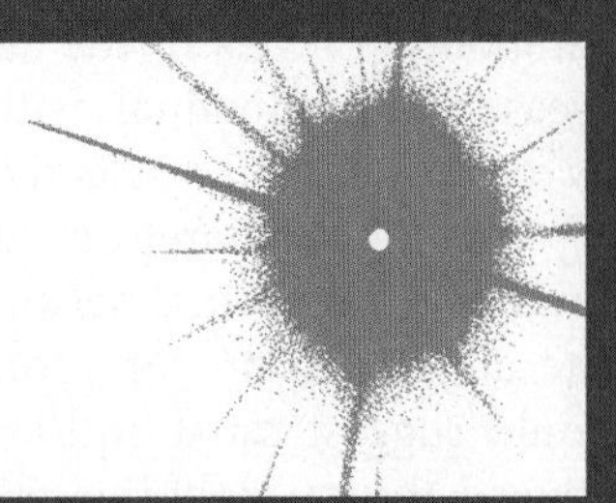

Henry J. Binder

The Schilling test is performed to determine the cause of cobalamin malabsorption. Unfortunately, this test has not been available commercially in the United States for the last few years. Since an understanding of the physiology and pathophysiology of cobalamin absorption is very valuable in enhancing one's understanding of aspects of gastric, pancreatic, and ileal function, discussion of the Schilling test is provided as supplemental information to **Chap. 16**. Because cobalamin absorption requires multiple steps, including gastric, pancreatic, and ileal processes, the Schilling test also can be used to assess the integrity of the organs involved in those processes.

Cobalamin is present primarily in meat. Except in strict vegans, *dietary* cobalamin deficiency is exceedingly uncommon. Dietary cobalamin is bound in the stomach to a glycoprotein called *R-binder protein*, which is synthesized in both the stomach and the salivary glands. This cobalamin–R binder complex is formed in the acid milieu of the stomach. Cobalamin absorption has an absolute requirement for *intrinsic factor*, another glycoprotein synthesized and released by gastric parietal cells, to promote its uptake by specific cobalamin receptors on the brush border of ileal enterocytes. Pancreatic protease enzymes split the cobalamin–R binder complex to release cobalamin in the proximal small intestine, where cobalamin then is bound by intrinsic factor.

As a consequence, cobalamin absorption may be abnormal in the following conditions:

1. *Pernicious anemia*. In this disease, immunologically mediated atrophy of gastric parietal cells leads to an absence of both gastric acid and intrinsic factor secretion.
2. *Chronic pancreatitis* can result from a deficiency of pancreatic proteases to split the cobalamin–R binder complex. Although 50% of patients with chronic pancreatitis reportedly have an abnormal Schilling test that is corrected by pancreatic enzyme replacement, cobalamin-responsive macrocytic anemia in chronic pancreatitis is extremely rare. Although this probably reflects a difference in the digestion/absorption of cobalamin in food versus that in a crystalline form, the Schilling test still can be used to assess pancreatic exocrine function.
3. *Achlorhydria* is the absence of hydrochloric acid; intrinsic factor is also secreted with acid which is responsible for splitting cobalamin away from the proteins in food to which it is bound. Up to one-third of individuals >60 years of age have marginal vitamin B_{12} absorption because of an inability to release cobalamin from food; these people have no defects in the absorption of crystalline vitamin B_{12}.
4. *Bacterial overgrowth syndromes*, which are most often secondary to stasis in the small intestine, lead to bacterial utilization of cobalamin (often referred to as *stagnant bowel syndrome*; see below).
5. *Ileal dysfunction* (as a result of either inflammation or prior intestinal resection) is due to impaired function of the mechanism of cobalamin–intrinsic factor uptake by ileal intestinal epithelial cells.

In the Schilling test, ^{58}Co-labeled cobalamin is administered orally, and urine is collected for 24 h. The test is dependent on normal renal and bladder function. Urinary excretion of cobalamin reflects cobalamin absorption, provided that intrahepatic binding sites for cobalamin are fully occupied. To ensure saturation of these binding sites so that all absorbed radiolabeled cobalamin will be excreted in urine, 1 mg of cobalamin is administered intramuscularly 1 h after ingestion of the radiolabeled cobalamin. The Schilling test may yield an abnormal result (usually defined as <10% excretion in 24 h) in pernicious anemia, chronic pancreatitis, blind loop syndrome, and ileal disease (Table 17-1). Therefore, whenever an abnormal Schilling result is obtained, ^{58}Co-labeled cobalamin should be administered on another occasion, this time bound to intrinsic factor, with pancreatic enzymes, or after a 5-day

TABLE 17-1

DIFFERENTIAL RESULTS OF THE SCHILLING TEST IN SEVERAL DISEASES ASSOCIATED WITH COBALAMIN MALABSORPTION

	^{58}CO-LABELED COBALAMIN	WITH INTRINSIC FACTOR	WITH PANCREATIC ENZYMES	AFTER 5 DAYS OF ANTIBIOTICS
Pernicious anemia	Reduced	Normal	Reduced	Reduced
Chronic pancreatitis	Reduced	Reduced	Normal	Reduced
Bacterial overgrowth	Reduced	Reduced	Reduced	Normal
Ileal disease	Reduced	Reduced	Reduced	Reduced

course of antibiotic treatment (often with tetracycline). A variation of the Schilling test can detect failure to split cobalamin from food proteins. The labeled cobalamin is cooked together with a scrambled egg and administered orally. People with achlorydria excrete <10% of the labeled cobalamin in the urine. In addition to establishing the etiology for cobalamin deficiency, the Schilling test can help delineate the pathologic process responsible for steatorrhea by assessing ileal, pancreatic, and small-intestinal luminal function. Unfortunately, the Schilling test is performed infrequently because of the unavailability of human intrinsic factor.

CHAPTER 18

INFLAMMATORY BOWEL DISEASE

Sonia Friedman ■ Richard S. Blumberg

Inflammatory bowel disease (IBD) is an immune-mediated chronic intestinal condition. Ulcerative colitis (UC) and Crohn's disease (CD) are the two major types of IBD.

GLOBAL CONSIDERATIONS: EPIDEMIOLOGY

The incidence and prevalence of IBD are highest in Westernized nations, with UC incidence estimates ranging from 0.6 to 24.3 per 100,000 in Europe, 0 to 19.2 per 100,000 in North America, and 0.1 to 6.3 per 100,000 in the Middle East and Asia and CD estimates ranging from 0.3 to 12.7 per 100,000 in Europe, 0 to 20.2 per 100,000 in North America, and 0.04 to 5.0 per 100,000 in the Middle East and Asia (Table 18-1). For prevalence rates, the UC estimates range from 4.9 to 505 per 100,000 in Europe, 37.5 to 248.6 per 100,000 in North America, and 4.9 to 168.3 per 100,000 in the Middle East and Asia, and the CD estimates range from 0.6 to 322 per 100,000 in Europe, 16.7 to 318.5 per 100,000 in North America, and 0.88 to 67.9 per 100,000 in Asia and the Middle East. The highest reported incidence rates are in Canada (19.2 per 100,000 for UC and 20.2 per 100,000 for CD), with approximately 0.6% of the Canadian population having IBD. Countries in the Pacific, including New Zealand and Australia, which share many possible environmental risk factors and similar genetic background as northwest Europe and North America, have high incidence rates of IBD.

In countries that are becoming more Westernized, including China, South Korea, India, Lebanon, Iran, Thailand, and countries in the French West Indies and North Africa, IBD appears to be emerging, emphasizing the importance of environmental factors in disease pathogenesis. In Japan, the prevalence of CD has risen rapidly from 2.9 cases per 100,000 in 1986 to 13.5 per 100,000 in 1998, whereas in South Korea, the prevalence of UC has quadrupled from 7.6 per 100,000 in 1997 to 30.9 per 100,000 in 2005. In Hong Kong, the prevalence of UC almost tripled from 2.3 in 1997 to 6.3 per 100,000 over a 9-year period. In Singapore, the prevalence of CD increased from 1.3 in 1990 to 7.2 per 100,000 in 2004. In China the number of cases of UC has increased by fourfold between 1981–1990 and 1991–2000.

TABLE 18-1

EPIDEMIOLOGY OF IBD

	ULCERATIVE COLITIS	CROHN'S DISEASE
Incidence (North America) per person-years	0–19.2 per 100,000	0–20.2 per 100,000
Age of onset	Second to fourth decades and seventh to ninth decades	Second to fourth decades and seventh to ninth decades
Ethnicity	Jewish > non-Jewish white > African American > Hispanic > Asian	
Female/male ratio	0.51–1.58	0.34–1.65
Smoking	May prevent disease (odds ratio 0.58)	May cause disease (odds ratio 1.76)
Oral contraceptives	No increased risk	Odds ratio 1.4
Appendectomy	Protective (risk reduction of 13–26%)	Not protective
Monozygotic twins	6–18% concordance	38–58% concordance
Dizygotic twins	0–2% concordance	4% concordance
Antibiotic use in the first year of life	2.9× the risk of developing childhood IBD	

***Abbreviation*:** IBD, inflammatory bowel disease.

Increasing immigration to Western societies also has an impact on the incidence and prevalence of IBD. The prevalence of UC among southern Asians who immigrated to the United Kingdom (UK) was higher in comparison to the European UK population (17 cases per 100,000 persons vs 7 per 100,000). Spanish patients who emigrated within Europe, but not those who immigrated to Latin America, developed IBD more frequently than controls. Individuals who have immigrated to Westernized countries and then returned to their country of birth also continue to demonstrate an increased risk of developing IBD.

Peak incidence of UC and CD is in the second to fourth decades, with 78% of CD studies and 51% of UC studies reporting the highest incidence among those age 20–29 years old. A second modest rise in incidence occurs between the seventh and ninth decades of life. The female-to-male ratio ranges from 0.51 to 1.58 for UC studies and 0.34 to 1.65 for CD studies, suggesting that the diagnosis of IBD is not gender specific. The greatest incidence of IBD is among white and Jewish people, but the incidence of IBD in Hispanic and Asian people is increasing, as noted above. Urban areas have a higher prevalence of IBD than rural areas, and high socioeconomic classes have a higher prevalence than lower socioeconomic classes.

Epidemiologic studies have identified a number of potential environmental factors that are associated with disease risk (Fig. 18-1). In Caucasian populations, smoking is an important risk factor in IBD with opposite effects on UC (odds ratio [OR] 0.58) and CD (OR 1.76), whereas in other ethnic groups with different genetic susceptibility, smoking may play a lesser role. There is a protective effect of previous appendectomy with confirmed appendicitis (reduction of 13–26%), particularly at a young age, on the development of UC across different geographical regions and populations. There is a modest association with the development of

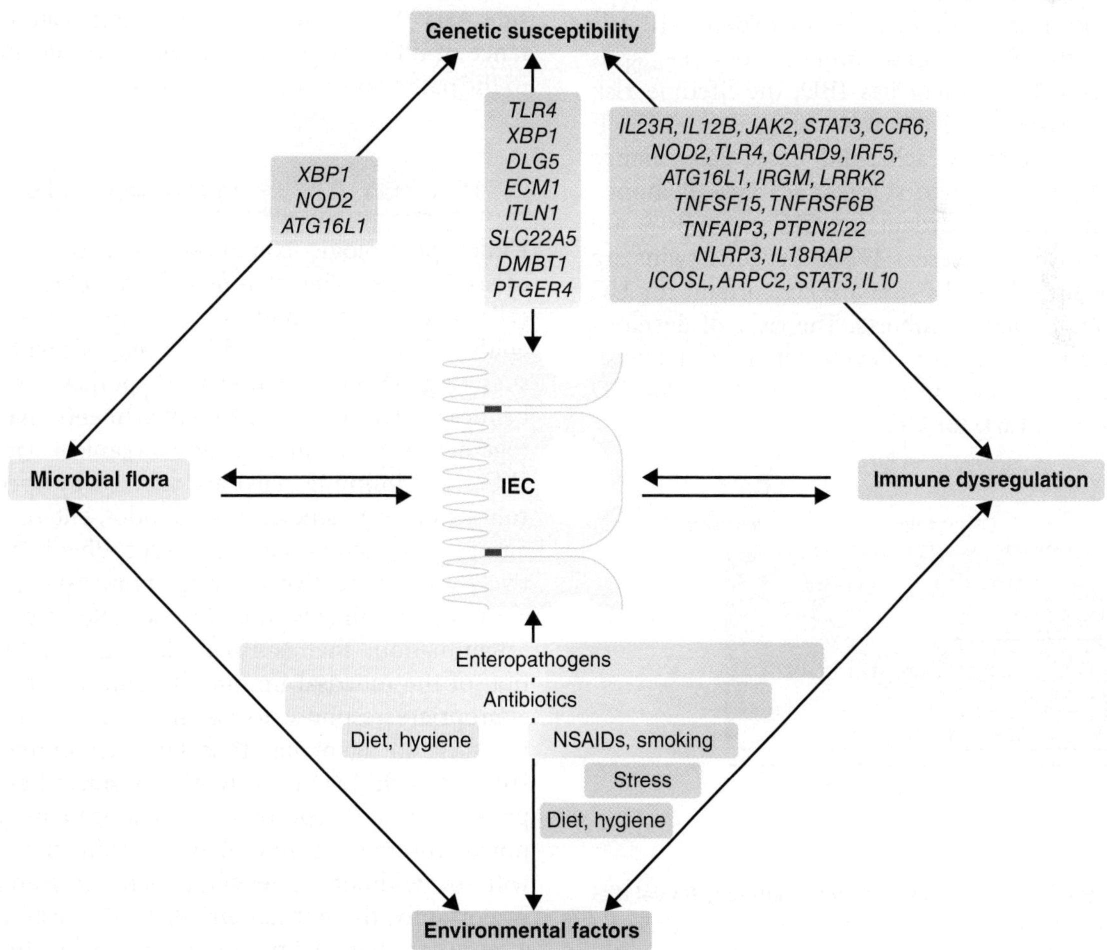

FIGURE 18-1

Pathogenesis of inflammatory bowel disease (IBD). In IBD, the tridirectional relationship between the commensal flora (microbiota), intestinal epithelial cells (IEC), and mucosal immune system is dysregulated, leading to chronic inflammation. Each of these three factors is affected by genetic and environmental factors that determine risk for the disease. NSAIDs, nonsteroidal anti-inflammatory drugs. *(Adapted from A Kaser et al: Annu Rev Immunol 28:573, 2010.)*

CD. Oral contraceptive use is associated with the risk of CD (OR 1.4). The association between oral contraceptive use and UC is limited to women with a history of smoking. There is an association between antibiotic use and the development of childhood IBD with children who received one or more dispensations of antibiotics during the first year of life having a 2.9-fold increase in the risk of developing IBD during childhood. Breast-feeding may also protect against the development of IBD. These factors are consistent with the rapid increase in IBD incidence recently noted during the first decade of life. Infectious gastroenteritis with pathogens (e.g., *Salmonella, Shigella, Campylobacter* spp., *Clostridium difficile*) increases IBD risk by two- to threefold. Diets high in animal protein, sugars, sweets, oils, fish and shellfish, and dietary fat, especially ω-6 fatty acids, and low in ω-3 fatty acids have been implicated in increasing the risk of IBD.

IBD is a familial disease in 5–10% of patients (Fig. 18-2). Some of these patients may exhibit early-onset disease during the first decade of life and, in CD, a concordance of anatomic site and clinical type within families. In the remainder of patients, IBD is observed in the absence of a family history (i.e., sporadic disease). If a patient has IBD, the lifetime risk that a first-degree relative will be affected is ~10%. If two parents have IBD, each child has a 36% chance of being affected. In twin studies, 38–58% of monozygotic twins are concordant for CD and 6–18% are concordant for UC, whereas 4% of dizygotic twins are concordant for CD and 0–2% are concordant for UC in Swedish and Danish cohorts. The risks of developing IBD are higher in first-degree relatives of Jewish versus non-Jewish patients: 7.8% versus 5.2% for CD and 4.5% versus 1.6% for UC.

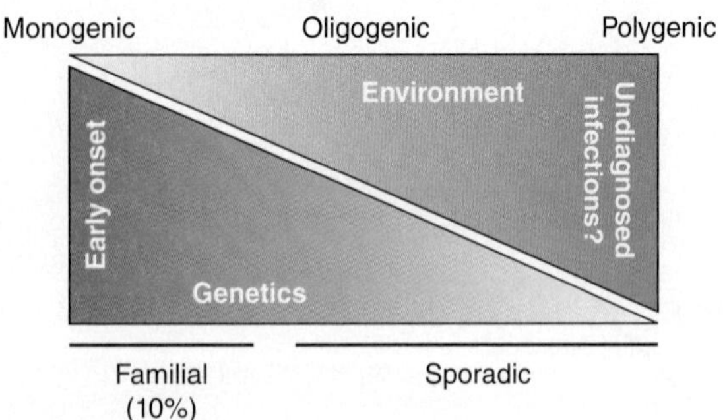

FIGURE 18-2

A model for the syndromic nature of inflammatory bowel disease. Genetic and environmental factors variably influence the development and phenotypic manifestations of IBD. At the one extreme, IBD is a exemplified as a simple Mendelian disorder as observed in "early-onset IBD" due to single gene defects such as *IL10, IL10RA*, and *IL10RB*; and at the other extreme, it may be exemplified by as yet to be described emerging infectious diseases. *(Adapted from A Kaser et al: Dig Dis 28:395, 2010.)*

GLOBAL CONSIDERATIONS: IBD PHENOTYPES

There are racial differences in IBD location and behavior that may reflect underlying genetic variations and have important implications for diagnosis and management of disease. For example, African-American patients are more likely than non-Hispanic whites to develop esophagogastroduodenal CD, colorectal disease, and perianal disease and are less likely to have ileal involvement. They are also at higher risk for uveitis and sacroiliitis. Hispanics have a higher prevalence of perianal CD and erythema nodosum and a more proximal extent of disease. Fistulizing CD has been reported in nearly one-third of Hispanic patients, up to one-quarter of African-American patients, and up to one-half of Asian patients. Both African-American and Hispanic CD patients, but not UC patients, had a lower prevalence of family history of IBD than their white counterparts. There are few data on all aspects of disease in Hispanics, in the incidence and prevalence of IBD in African Americans, and in Asians with IBD outside Asia. These ethnic variations implicate the importance of different genetic and/or environmental factors in the pathogenesis of this disorder.

ETIOLOGY AND PATHOGENESIS

Under physiologic conditions, homeostasis normally exists between the commensal microbiota, epithelial cells that line the interior of the intestines (intestinal epithelial cells [IECs]) and immune cells within the tissues (Fig. 18-1). A consensus hypothesis is that each of these three major host compartments that function together as an integrated "supraorganism" (microbiota, IECs, and immune cells) are affected by specific environmental (e.g., smoking, antibiotics, enteropathogens) and genetic factors that, in a susceptible host, cumulatively and interactively disrupt homeostasis, which in so doing culminates in a chronic state of dysregulated inflammation; that is IBD. Although chronic activation of the mucosal immune system may represent an appropriate response to an infectious agent, a search for such an agent has thus far been unrewarding in IBD. As such, IBD is currently considered an inappropriate immune response to the endogenous (autocthonous) commensal microbiota within the intestines, with or without some component of autoimmunity. Importantly, the normal, uninflamed intestines contain a large number of immune cells that are in a unique state of activation, in which the gut is restrained from full immunologic responses to the commensal microbiota and dietary antigens by very powerful regulatory pathways that function within the immune system (e.g., T regulatory cells that express the FoxP3 transcription factor and suppress inflammation). During the course of infections or other environmental stimuli in the normal host, full activation of the gut-associated lymphoid tissues occurs but is rapidly superseded by dampening of the immune response and tissue repair. In IBD such processes may not be regulated normally.

GENETIC CONSIDERATIONS

The genetic underpinning of IBD is known from its occurrence in the context of several genetic syndromes and the development of severe, refractory IBD in early life in the setting of single gene defects that affect the immune system (Table 18-2). In addition, IBD has a familial origin in at least 10% of afflicted individuals (Fig. 18-2). In the majority of patients, IBD is considered to be a polygenic disorder that gives rise to multiple clinical subgroups within UC and CD. A variety of genetic approaches including candidate gene studies, linkage analysis, and genome-wide association studies (GWASs) that focus on the identification of disease-associated, single-nucleotide polymorphisms (SNPs) within the human genome and, more recently, whole-genome sequencing have elucidated many of the genetic factors that affect risk for these diseases. GWASs have, to date, identified 163 genetic loci with 100 of these loci observed to be associated with both disease phenotypes (Table 18-3). The remainder are specific for either CD (30 loci) or UC (20 loci). These genetic similarities account for the overlapping immunopathogenesis and consequently epidemiologic observations of both diseases in the same families and similarities in response to therapies. Because the specific causal variants for each identified gene or locus are largely unknown, it is not clear whether the similarities in the genetic risk factors associated with CD and UC that are observed are shared at structural or functional levels. The risk conferred by each identified gene or locus is unequal and generally small, such that only ~20% of the genetic variance is considered to be explained by the current genetic information. Further, many of the genetic risk factors identified are also observed to be associated with risk for other immune-mediated diseases, suggesting that related immunogenetic pathways are involved in the pathogenesis of multiple different disorders accounting for the common responsiveness to similar types of biologic therapies (e.g., anti–tumor necrosis factor therapies) and possibly the simultaneous occurrence of these disorders. The diseases and the genetic risk factors that are shared with IBD include rheumatoid arthritis (*TNFAIP3*), psoriasis (*IL23R*, *IL12B*), ankylosing spondylitis (*IL23R*), type 1 diabetes mellitus (*IL10*, *PTPN2*), asthma (*ORMDL3*), and systemic lupus erythematosus (*TNFAIP3*, *IL10*) among others.

The genetic factors defined to date that are recognized to mediate risk for IBD have highlighted the importance of several common mechanisms of disease (Table 18-3). These include the following: those genes that are associated with fundamental cell biologic processes such as endoplasmic reticulum (ER) and metabolic stress (e.g., *XBP1*, *ORMDL3*, *OCTN*), which serve to regulate the secretory activity of cells involved in responses to the commensal microbiota such as Paneth and goblet cells and the manner in which intestinal cells respond to the metabolic products of bacteria; those associated with innate immunity and autophagy (e.g., *NOD2*, *ATG16L1*, *IRGM*, *JAK2*, *STAT3*) that function in innate immune cells (both parenchymal and hematopoietic) to respond to and effectively clear bacteria, mycobacteria, and viruses; those that are associated

TABLE 18-2

PRIMARY GENETIC DISORDERS ASSOCIATED WITH IBD

NAME	GENETIC ASSOCIATION	PHENOTYPE
Turner's syndrome	Loss of part or all of X chromosome	Associated with UC and colonic CD
Hermansky-Pudlak	Autosomal recessive chromosome 10q23	Granulomatous colitis, oculocutaneous albinism, platelet dysfunction, pulmonary fibrosis
Wiskott-Aldrich syndrome (WAS)	X-linked recessive disorder, loss of WAS protein function	Colitis, immunodeficiency, severely dysfunctional platelets, and thrombocytopenia
Glycogen storage disease	Deficiency of the glucose-6-phosphate transport protein type B1	Granulomatous colitis, presents in infancy with hypoglycemia, growth failure, hepatomegaly, and neutropenia
Immune dysregulation polyendocrinopathy, enteropathy X-linked (IPEX)	Loss of FoxP3 transcription factor and T regulatory cell function	UC-like autoimmune enteropathy, with endocrinopathy (neonatal type 1 diabetes or thyroiditis), dermatitis
Early-onset IBD	Deficient IL-10 and IL-10 receptor function	Severe, refractory IBD in early life

Abbreviations: CD, Crohn's disease; IBD, inflammatory bowel disease; IL, interleukin; UC, ulcerative colitis.

TABLE 18-3

EXAMPLES OF GENETIC LOCI ASSOCIATED WITH CD AND/OR UC

CHROMOSOME	PUTATIVE GENE	GENE NAME	PROTEIN FUNCTION	CD	UC
ER Stress and Metabolism					
5q31	*SLC22A5*	Solute carrier family 22, member 5	β carnitine transporter	+	
7p21	*AGR2*	Anterior gradient 2	ER stress	+	+
17q21	*ORMDL3*	Orosomucoid related member 1-like 3	ER stress and lipid synthesis	+	+
22q12	*XBP1*	X-box binding protein 1	ER stress	+	+
1q23	*ITLN1*	Intelectin 1	Bacterial binding	+	
2q37	*ATG16L1*	ATG16 autophagy related 16-like 1	Autophagy	+	
5q33	*IRGM*	Immunity-related GTPase family, M	Autophagy	+	
9p24	*JAK2*	Janus kinase 2	IL-6R and IL-23R signaling	+	+
12q12	*LRRK2*	Leucine-rich repeat kinase 2	Autophagy?	+	
16q12	*NOD2*	Nucleotide-binding oligomerization domain containing 2	Bacterial sensing and autophagy activation	+	
17q21	*STAT3*	Signal transducer and activator of transcription 3	IL-6R, IL-23R, and IL-10R signaling	+	+
Adaptive Immunity					
1p31	*IL23R*	Interleukin 23 receptor	Th17 cell stimulation	+	+
1q32	*IL10*	Interleukin 10	Treg-associated cytokine	+	+
5q33	*IL12B*	Interleukin 12B	IL-12 p40 chain of IL-12/IL-23	+	+
18p11	*PTPN2*	Protein tyrosine phosphatase, nonreceptor type 2	T cell regulation	+	
Inflammation					
3p21	*MST1*	Macrophage stimulating 1	Macrophage activation	+	+
5p13	*PTGER4*	Prostaglandin E receptor 4	PGE_2 receptor	+	+
6q23	*TNFAIP3*	Tumor necrosis factor, alpha-induced protein 3 (A20)	Toll-like receptor regulation	+	
6q27	*CCR6*	Chemokine (C-C motif) receptor 6	Dendritic cell migration	+	

Abbreviations: CD, Crohn's disease; ER, endoplasmic reticulum; GTPase, guanosine triphosphatase; IL, interleukin; PGE_2, prostaglandin E_2; UC, ulcerative colitis.

Source: Adapted from A Kaser et al: *Ann Rev Immunol* 28:573, 2010; B Khor et al: *Nature* 474:307, 2011; and L Jostins et al: *Nature* 491:119, 2012.

with the regulation of adaptive immunity (e.g., *IL23R, IL12B, IL10, PTPN2*), which regulate the balance between inflammatory and anti-inflammatory (regulatory) cytokines; and, finally, those that are involved in the development and resolution of inflammation (e.g., *MST1, CCR6, TNFAIP3, PTGER4*) and ultimately leukocyte recruitment and inflammatory mediator production. Some of these loci are associated with specific subtypes of disease such as the association between *NOD2* polymorphisms and fibrostenosing CD or *ATG16L1* and fistulizing disease, especially within the ileum. However, the clinical utility of these genetic risk factors for the diagnosis or determination of prognosis and therapeutic responses remains to be defined.

COMMENSAL MICROBIOTA AND IBD

The endogenous commensal microbiota within the intestines plays a central role in the pathogenesis of IBD. Humans are born sterile and acquire their commensal microbiota initially from the mother during egress through the birth canal and subsequently from environmental sources. A stable configuration of up to 1000 species of bacteria that achieves a biomass of approximately 10^{12} colony-forming units per gram of feces is achieved by 3 years of age, which likely persists into adult life, with each individual human possessing a unique combination of species. In addition, the intestines contain other microbial life forms including archae, viruses, and protists. The microbiota is thus considered as a critical and sustaining component of the organism. The establishment and maintenance of the intestinal microbiota composition and function is under the control of host (e.g., immune and epithelial responses), environmental (e.g., diet and antibiotics), and likely genetic (e.g., *NOD2*) factors (Fig. 18-1). In turn, the microbiota, through its structural components and metabolic activity, has major influences on the epithelial and immune function of the host, which, through epigenetic effects, may have durable consequences. During early life when the commensal microbiota is being established, these microbial effects on the host may be particularly important in determining later life risk for IBD. Specific components of the microbiota can promote or protect from disease. The commensal microbiota in patients with both UC and CD is demonstrably different from nonafflicted individuals, a state of dysbiosis, suggesting the presence of microorganisms that drive disease (e.g., Proteobacteria such as enteroinvasive and adherent *Escherichia coli*) and to which the immune response is directed and/or the loss of microorganisms that hinder inflammation (e.g., Firmicutes such as *Faecalibacterium prausnitzii*). Many of the changes in the commensal microbiota occur as a consequence of the inflammation. In addition, agents that alter the intestinal microbiota such as metronidazole, ciprofloxacin, and elemental diets, may improve CD. CD may also respond to fecal diversion, demonstrating the ability of luminal contents to exacerbate disease.

DEFECTIVE IMMUNE REGULATION IN IBD

The mucosal immune system is normally unreactive to luminal contents due to oral (mucosal) tolerance. When soluble antigens are administered orally rather than subcutaneously or intramuscularly, antigen-specific nonresponsiveness is induced. Multiple mechanisms are involved in the induction of oral tolerance and include deletion or anergy of antigen-reactive T cells or induction of CD4+ T cells that suppress gut inflammation (e.g., T regulatory cells expressing the FoxP3 transcription factor) that secrete anti-inflammatory cytokines such as interleukin (IL) 10, IL-35, and transforming growth factor β (TGF-β). Oral tolerance may be responsible for the lack of immune responsiveness to dietary antigens and the commensal microbiota in the intestinal lumen. In IBD this suppression of inflammation is altered, leading to uncontrolled inflammation. The mechanisms of this regulated immune suppression are incompletely known.

Gene knockout ($^{-/-}$) or transgenic (Tg) mouse models of IBD, which include those that are directed at genes demonstrated to be associated with risk for the human disease, have revealed that deleting specific cytokines (e.g., IL-2, IL-10, TGF-β) or their receptors, deleting molecules associated with T cell antigen recognition (e.g., T cell antigen receptors), or interfering with IEC barrier function and the regulation of responses to commensal bacteria (e.g., XBP1, N-cadherin, mucus glycoprotein, or nuclear factor-κB [NF-κB]) leads to spontaneous colitis or enteritis. In the majority of circumstances, intestinal inflammation in these animal models requires the presence of the commensal microbiota. Thus, a variety of specific alterations can lead to immune activation by commensal microbiota and inflammation directed at the intestines in mice. How these relate to human IBD remains to be defined, but they are consistent with inappropriate responses of the genetically susceptible host to the commensal microbiota.

In both UC and CD, an inflammatory pathway thus likely emerges from the genetic predisposition that is associated with inappropriate innate immune and epithelial sensing and reactivity to commensal bacteria that secrete inflammatory mediators together with inadequate regulatory pathways that lead to activated CD4+ and $CD8^+$ T cells within the epithelium and lamina propria that altogether secrete excessive quantities of inflammatory cytokines relative to anti-inflammatory cytokines. Some cytokines activate other inflammatory cells (macrophages and B cells), and others act indirectly to recruit other lymphocytes, inflammatory leukocytes, and mononuclear cells from the bloodstream into the gut through interactions between homing receptors on leukocytes (e.g., α4β7 integrin) and addressins on vascular endothelium (e.g., MadCAM1). Consistent with this, neutralization of tumor necrosis factor (TNF) or α4β7 integrin demonstrate therapeutic efficacy in IBD. CD4+ T helper (T_H) cells that promote inflammation are of three major types, all of which may be associated with colitis in animal models and perhaps humans: T_H1 cells (secrete interferon [IFN] γ), T_H2 cells (secrete IL-4, IL-5, IL-13), and T_H17 cells (secrete IL-17, IL-21). T_H1 cells induce transmural granulomatous inflammation that resembles CD; T_H2 cells, and related natural killer T cells that secrete IL-13, induce superficial mucosal inflammation resembling UC in animal models; and T_H17 cells may be responsible for neutrophilic recruitment. However, neutralization of the cytokines produced by these cells, such as IFN-γ or IL-17, has yet to show efficacy in therapeutic trials. Each of these T cell subsets cross-regulate each other. The T_H1 cytokine pathway is initiated by IL-12, a key cytokine in the pathogenesis of experimental models of mucosal inflammation. IL-4 and IL-23, together with IL-6 and TGF-β, induce T_H2 and T_H17 cells, respectively, and IL-23 inhibits the suppressive function of regulatory T cells. Activated macrophages secrete TNF and IL-6. These characteristics of the immune response in IBD explain the beneficial therapeutic effects of antibodies to block proinflammatory cytokines or the signaling by their receptors (e.g., anti-TNF, anti-IL-12, anti-IL-23, anti-IL-6, or Janus kinase [JAK] inhibitors) or molecules associated with leukocyte recruitment (e.g., anti-α4β7), or the use of cytokines that inhibit inflammation and promote regulatory T cells (e.g., IL-10) or promote intestinal barrier function and may be beneficial to humans with intestinal inflammation.

THE INFLAMMATORY CASCADE IN IBD

Once initiated in IBD by abnormal innate immune sensing of bacteria by parenchymal cells (e.g., IECs) and hematopoietic cells (e.g., dendritic cells), the immune inflammatory response is perpetuated by T cell activation. A sequential cascade of inflammatory mediators extends the response; each step is a potential target for therapy. Inflammatory cytokines such as IL-1, IL-6, and TNF have diverse effects on tissues. They promote fibrogenesis, collagen production, activation of tissue metalloproteinases, and the production of other inflammatory mediators; they also activate the coagulation cascade in local blood vessels (e.g., increased production of von Willebrand's factor). These cytokines are normally produced in response to infection but are usually turned off or inhibited at the appropriate time to limit tissue damage. In IBD their activity is not regulated, resulting in an imbalance between the proinflammatory and anti-inflammatory mediators. Therapies such as the 5-aminosalicylic acid (5-ASA) compounds and glucocorticoids are potent inhibitors of these inflammatory mediators through inhibition of transcription factors such as NF-κB that regulate their expression.

PATHOLOGY

ULCERATIVE COLITIS: MACROSCOPIC FEATURES

UC is a mucosal disease that usually involves the rectum and extends proximally to involve all or part of the colon. About 40–50% of patients have disease limited to the rectum and rectosigmoid, 30–40% have disease extending beyond the sigmoid but not involving the whole colon, and 20% have a total colitis. Proximal spread occurs in continuity without areas of uninvolved mucosa. When the whole colon is involved, the inflammation extends 2–3 cm into the terminal ileum in 10–20% of patients. The endoscopic changes of *backwash ileitis* are superficial and mild and are of little clinical significance. Although variations in macroscopic activity may suggest skip areas, biopsies from normal-appearing mucosa are usually abnormal. Thus, it is important to obtain multiple biopsies from apparently uninvolved mucosa, whether proximal or distal, during endoscopy. One caveat is that effective medical therapy can change the appearance of the mucosa such that either skip areas or the entire colon can be microscopically normal.

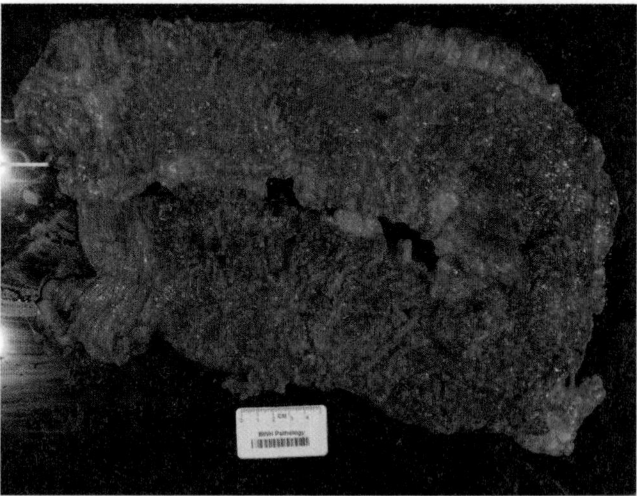

FIGURE 18-3
Ulcerative colitis. Diffuse (nonsegmental) mucosal disease, with broad areas of ulceration. The bowel wall is not thickened, and there is no cobblestoning. *(Courtesy of Dr. R. Odze, Division of Gastrointestinal Pathology, Department of Pathology, Brigham and Women's Hospital, Boston, Massachusetts; with permission.)*

With mild inflammation, the mucosa is erythematous and has a fine granular surface that resembles sandpaper. In more severe disease, the mucosa is hemorrhagic, edematous, and ulcerated (Fig. 18-3). In longstanding disease, inflammatory polyps (pseudopolyps) may be present as a result of epithelial regeneration. The mucosa may appear normal in remission, but in patients with many years of disease it appears atrophic and featureless, and the entire colon becomes narrowed and shortened. Patients with fulminant disease can develop a toxic colitis or megacolon where the bowel wall thins and the mucosa is severely ulcerated; this may lead to perforation.

ULCERATIVE COLITIS: MICROSCOPIC FEATURES

Histologic findings correlate well with the endoscopic appearance and clinical course of UC. The process is limited to the mucosa and superficial submucosa, with deeper layers unaffected except in fulminant disease. In UC, two major histologic features suggest chronicity and help distinguish it from infectious or acute self-limited colitis. First, the crypt architecture of the colon is distorted; crypts may be bifid and reduced in number, often with a gap between the crypt bases and the

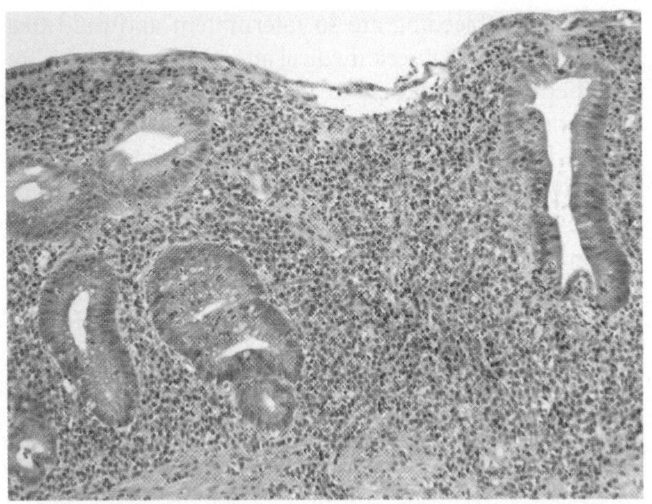

FIGURE 18-4
Medium-power view of colonic mucosa in ulcerative colitis showing diffuse mixed inflammation, basal lymphoplasmacytosis, crypt atrophy and irregularity, and superficial erosion. These features are typical of chronic active ulcerative colitis. *(Courtesy of Dr. R. Odze, Division of Gastrointestinal Pathology, Department of Pathology, Brigham and Women's Hospital, Boston, Massachusetts; with permission.)*

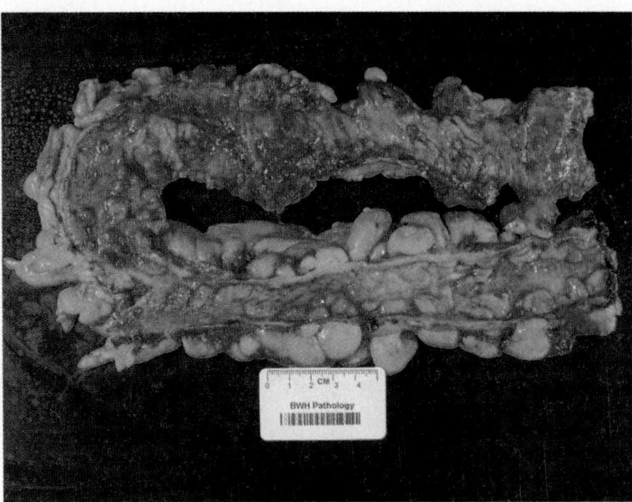

FIGURE 18-5
Crohn's disease of the colon showing thickening of the wall, with stenosis, linear serpiginous ulcers and cobblestoning of the mucosa. *(Courtesy of Dr. R Odze, Division of Gastrointestinal Pathology, Department of Pathology, Brigham and Women's Hospital, Boston, Massachusetts; with permission.)*

muscularis mucosae. Second, some patients have basal plasma cells and multiple basal lymphoid aggregates. Mucosal vascular congestion, with edema and focal hemorrhage, and an inflammatory cell infiltrate of neutrophils, lymphocytes, plasma cells, and macrophages may be present. The neutrophils invade the epithelium, usually in the crypts, giving rise to cryptitis and, ultimately, to crypt abscesses (Fig. 18-4). Ileal changes in patients with backwash ileitis include villous atrophy and crypt regeneration with increased inflammation, increased neutrophil and mononuclear inflammation in the lamina propria, and patchy cryptitis and crypt abscesses.

CROHN'S DISEASE: MACROSCOPIC FEATURES

CD can affect any part of the gastrointestinal (GI) tract from the mouth to the anus. Some 30–40% of patients have small bowel disease alone, 40–55% have disease involving both the small and large intestines, and 15–25% have colitis alone. In the 75% of patients with small intestinal disease, the terminal ileum is involved in 90%. Unlike UC, which almost always involves the rectum, the rectum is often spared in CD. CD is segmental with skip areas in the midst of diseased intestine (Fig. 18-5). Perirectal fistulas, fissures, abscesses, and anal stenosis are present in one-third of patients with CD, particularly those with colonic involvement. Rarely, CD may also involve the liver and the pancreas.

Unlike UC, CD is a transmural process. Endoscopically, aphthous or small superficial ulcerations characterize mild disease; in more active disease, stellate ulcerations fuse longitudinally and transversely to demarcate islands of mucosa that frequently are histologically normal. This "cobblestone" appearance is characteristic of CD, both endoscopically and by barium radiography. As in UC, pseudopolyps can form in CD.

Active CD is characterized by focal inflammation and formation of fistula tracts, which resolve by fibrosis and stricturing of the bowel. The bowel wall thickens and becomes narrowed and fibrotic, leading to chronic, recurrent bowel obstructions. Projections of thickened mesentery encase the bowel ("creeping fat"), and serosal and mesenteric inflammation promotes adhesions and fistula formation.

CROHN'S DISEASE: MICROSCOPIC FEATURES

The earliest lesions are aphthoid ulcerations and focal crypt abscesses with loose aggregations of macrophages, which form noncaseating granulomas in all layers of the bowel wall (Fig. 18-6). Granulomas can be seen in lymph nodes, mesentery, peritoneum, liver, and pancreas. Although granulomas are a pathognomonic feature of CD, they are rarely found on mucosal biopsies. Surgical resection reveals granulomas in about one-half of cases. Other histologic features of CD include submucosal or subserosal lymphoid aggregates, particularly away from areas of ulceration, gross and microscopic skip areas, and transmural inflammation that is

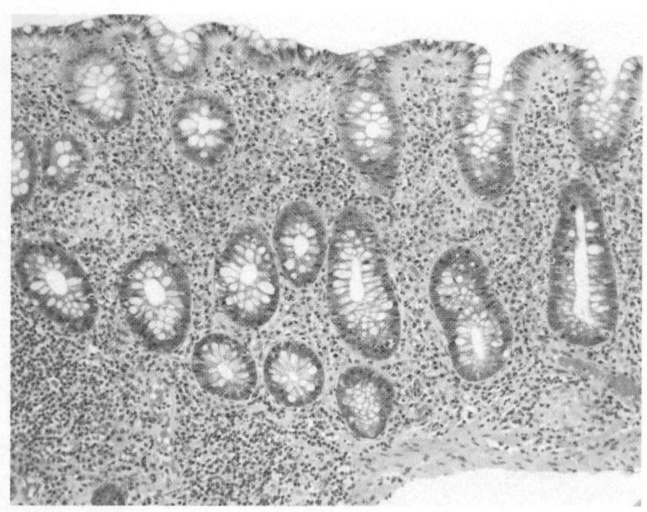

FIGURE 18-6
Medium-power view of Crohn's colitis showing mixed acute and chronic inflammation, crypt atrophy, and multiple small epithelioid granulomas in the mucosa. *(Courtesy of Dr. R Odze, Division of Gastrointestinal Pathology, Department of Pathology, Brigham and Women's Hospital, Boston, Massachusetts; with permission.)*

accompanied by fissures that penetrate deeply into the bowel wall and sometimes form fistulous tracts or local abscesses.

CLINICAL PRESENTATION

ULCERATIVE COLITIS

Signs and symptoms

The major symptoms of UC are diarrhea, rectal bleeding, tenesmus, passage of mucus, and crampy abdominal pain. The severity of symptoms correlates with the extent of disease. Although UC can present acutely, symptoms usually have been present for weeks to months. Occasionally, diarrhea and bleeding are so intermittent and mild that the patient does not seek medical attention.

Patients with proctitis usually pass fresh blood or blood-stained mucus, either mixed with stool or streaked onto the surface of a normal or hard stool. They also have tenesmus, or urgency with a feeling of incomplete evacuation, but rarely have abdominal pain. With proctitis or proctosigmoiditis, proximal transit slows, which may account for the constipation commonly seen in patients with distal disease.

When the disease extends beyond the rectum, blood is usually mixed with stool or grossly bloody diarrhea may be noted. Colonic motility is altered by inflammation with rapid transit through the inflamed intestine. When the disease is severe, patients pass a liquid stool containing blood, pus, and fecal matter. Diarrhea is often nocturnal and/or postprandial. Although severe pain is not a prominent symptom, some patients with active disease may experience vague lower abdominal discomfort or mild central abdominal cramping. Severe cramping and abdominal pain can occur with severe attacks of the disease. Other symptoms in moderate to severe disease include anorexia, nausea, vomiting, fever, and weight loss.

Physical signs of proctitis include a tender anal canal and blood on rectal examination. With more extensive disease, patients have tenderness to palpation directly over the colon. Patients with a toxic colitis have severe pain and bleeding, and those with megacolon have hepatic tympany. Both may have signs of peritonitis if a perforation has occurred. The classification of disease activity is shown in Table 18-4.

Laboratory, endoscopic, and radiographic features

Active disease can be associated with a rise in acute-phase reactants (C-reactive protein [CRP]), platelet count, and erythrocyte sedimentation rate (ESR), and

TABLE 18-4
ULCERATIVE COLITIS: DISEASE PRESENTATION

	MILD	MODERATE	SEVERE
Bowel movements	<4 per day	4–6 per day	>6 per day
Blood in stool	Small	Moderate	Severe
Fever	None	<37.5°C mean (<99.5°F)	>37.5°C mean (>99.5°F)
Tachycardia	None	<90 mean pulse	>90 mean pulse
Anemia	Mild	>75%	≤75%
Sedimentation rate	<30 mm		>30 mm
Endoscopic appearance	Erythema, decreased vascular pattern, fine granularity	Marked erythema, coarse granularity, absent vascular markings, contact bleeding, no ulcerations	Spontaneous bleeding, ulcerations

a decrease in hemoglobin. Fecal lactoferrin is a highly sensitive and specific marker for detecting intestinal inflammation. Fecal calprotectin levels correlate well with histologic inflammation, predict relapses, and detect pouchitis. Both fecal lactoferrin and calprotectin are becoming an integral part of IBD management and are used frequently to rule out active inflammation versus symptoms of irritable bowel or bacterial overgrowth. In severely ill patients, the serum albumin level will fall rather quickly. Leukocytosis may be present but is not a specific indicator of disease activity. Proctitis or proctosigmoiditis rarely causes a rise in CRP. Diagnosis relies on the patient's history; clinical symptoms; negative stool examination for bacteria, *C. difficile* toxin, and ova and parasites; sigmoidoscopic appearance **(see Fig. 12-4*A*)**; and histology of rectal or colonic biopsy specimens.

Sigmoidoscopy is used to assess disease activity and is usually performed before treatment. If the patient is not having an acute flare, colonoscopy is used to assess disease extent and activity (Fig. 18-7). Endoscopically mild disease is characterized by erythema, decreased vascular pattern, and mild friability. Moderate disease is characterized by marked erythema, absent vascular pattern, friability and erosions, and severe disease by spontaneous bleeding and ulcerations. Histologic features change more slowly than clinical features but can also be used to grade disease activity.

The earliest radiologic change of UC seen on single-contrast barium enema is a fine mucosal granularity. With increasing severity, the mucosa becomes thickened, and superficial ulcers are seen. Deep ulcerations can appear as "collar-button" ulcers, which indicate that the ulceration has penetrated the mucosa. Haustral folds may be normal in mild disease, but as activity progresses they become edematous and thickened. Loss of haustration can occur, especially in patients with long-standing disease. In addition, the colon becomes shortened and narrowed. Polyps in the colon may be postinflammatory polyps or pseudopolyps, adenomatous polyps, or carcinoma.

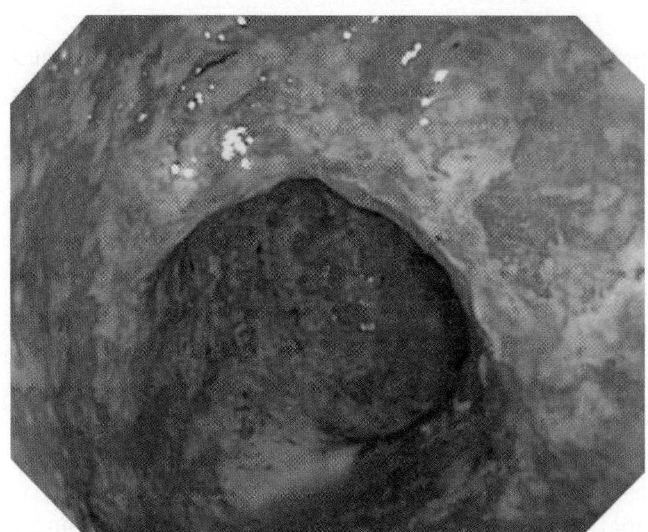

FIGURE 18-7
Colonoscopy with acute ulcerative colitis: severe colon inflammation with erythema, friability, and exudates. *(Courtesy of Dr. M. Hamilton, Gastroenterology Division, Department of Medicine, Brigham and Women's Hospital, Boston, Massachusetts; with permission.)*

Computed tomography (CT) scanning or magnetic resonance imaging (MRI) is not as helpful as endoscopy in making the diagnosis of UC, but typical findings include mild mural thickening (<1.5 cm), inhomogeneous wall density, absence of small bowel thickening, increased perirectal and presacral fat, target appearance of the rectum, and adenopathy.

Complications

Only 15% of patients with UC present initially with catastrophic illness. Massive hemorrhage occurs with severe attacks of disease in 1% of patients, and treatment for the disease usually stops the bleeding. However, if a patient requires 6–8 units of blood within 24–48 h, colectomy is indicated. *Toxic megacolon* is defined as a transverse or right colon with a diameter of >6 cm, with loss of haustration in patients with severe attacks of UC. It occurs in about 5% of attacks and can be triggered by electrolyte abnormalities and narcotics. About 50% of acute dilations will resolve with medical therapy alone, but urgent colectomy is required for those that do not improve. Perforation is the most dangerous of the local complications, and the physical signs of peritonitis may not be obvious, especially if the patient is receiving glucocorticoids. Although perforation is rare, the mortality rate for perforation complicating a toxic megacolon is about 15%. In addition, patients can develop a toxic colitis and such severe ulcerations that the bowel may perforate without first dilating.

Strictures occur in 5–10% of patients and are always a concern in UC because of the possibility of underlying neoplasia. Although benign strictures can form from the inflammation and fibrosis of UC, strictures that are impassable with the colonoscope should be presumed malignant until proven otherwise. A stricture that prevents passage of the colonoscope is an indication for surgery. UC patients occasionally develop anal fissures, perianal abscesses, or hemorrhoids, but the occurrence of extensive perianal lesions should suggest CD.

CROHN'S DISEASE

Signs and symptoms

Although CD usually presents as acute or chronic bowel inflammation, the inflammatory process evolves toward one of two patterns of disease: a fibrostenotic obstructing pattern or a penetrating fistulous pattern, each with different treatments and prognoses. The site of disease influences the clinical manifestations.

Ileocolitis

Because the most common site of inflammation is the terminal ileum, the usual presentation of ileocolitis is a chronic history of recurrent episodes of right lower quadrant pain and diarrhea. Sometimes the initial presentation mimics acute appendicitis with pronounced right lower quadrant pain, a palpable mass, fever, and leukocytosis. Pain is usually colicky; it precedes and is relieved by defecation. A low-grade fever is usually noted. High-spiking fever suggests intraabdominal abscess formation. Weight loss is common—typically 10–20% of body weight—and develops as a consequence of diarrhea, anorexia, and fear of eating.

An inflammatory mass may be palpated in the right lower quadrant of the abdomen. The mass is composed of inflamed bowel, adherent and indurated mesentery, and enlarged abdominal lymph nodes. Extension of the mass can cause obstruction of the right ureter or bladder inflammation, manifested by dysuria and fever. Edema, bowel wall thickening, and fibrosis of the bowel wall within the mass account for the radiographic "string sign" of a narrowed intestinal lumen.

Bowel obstruction may take several forms. In the early stages of disease, bowel wall edema and spasm produce intermittent obstructive manifestations and increasing symptoms of postprandial pain. Over several years, persistent inflammation gradually progresses to fibrostenotic narrowing and stricture. Diarrhea will decrease and be replaced by chronic bowel obstruction. Acute episodes of obstruction occur as well, precipitated by bowel inflammation and spasm or sometimes by impaction of undigested food or medication. These episodes usually resolve with intravenous fluids and gastric decompression.

Severe inflammation of the ileocecal region may lead to localized wall thinning, with microperforation and fistula formation to the adjacent bowel, the skin, or the urinary bladder, or to an abscess cavity in the mesentery. Enterovesical fistulas typically present as dysuria or recurrent bladder infections or, less commonly, as pneumaturia or fecaluria. Enterocutaneous fistulas follow tissue planes of least resistance, usually draining through abdominal surgical scars. Enterovaginal fistulas are rare and present as dyspareunia or as a feculent or foul-smelling, often painful vaginal discharge. They are unlikely to develop without a prior hysterectomy.

Jejunoileitis

Extensive inflammatory disease is associated with a loss of digestive and absorptive surface, resulting in malabsorption and steatorrhea. Nutritional deficiencies can also result from poor intake and enteric losses of protein and other nutrients. Intestinal malabsorption can cause anemia, hypoalbuminemia, hypocalcemia, hypomagnesemia, coagulopathy, and hyperoxaluria with nephrolithiasis in patients with an intact colon. Many patients need to take oral and often intravenous iron. Vertebral fractures are caused by a combination of vitamin D deficiency, hypocalcemia, and prolonged glucocorticoid use. Pellagra from niacin deficiency can occur in extensive small-bowel disease, and malabsorption of vitamin B_{12} can lead to megaloblastic anemia and neurologic symptoms. Other important nutrients to measure and replete if low are folate and vitamins A, E, and K. Levels of minerals such as zinc, selenium, copper, and magnesium are often low in patients with extensive small-bowel inflammation or resections, and these should be repleted as well. Most patients should take a daily multivitamin, calcium, and vitamin D supplements.

Diarrhea is characteristic of active disease; its causes include (1) bacterial overgrowth in obstructive stasis or fistulization, (2) bile-acid malabsorption due to a diseased or resected terminal ileum, and (3) intestinal inflammation with decreased water absorption and increased secretion of electrolytes.

Colitis and perianal disease

Patients with colitis present with low-grade fevers, malaise, diarrhea, crampy abdominal pain, and sometimes hematochezia. Gross bleeding is not as common as in UC and appears in about one-half of patients with exclusively colonic disease. Only 1–2% bleed massively. Pain is caused by passage of fecal material through narrowed and inflamed segments of the large bowel. Decreased rectal compliance is another cause for diarrhea in Crohn's colitis patients. Toxic megacolon is rare but may be seen with severe inflammation and short duration disease.

Stricturing can occur in the colon in 4–16% of patients and produce symptoms of bowel obstruction. If the endoscopist is unable to traverse a stricture in Crohn's colitis, surgical resection should be considered, especially if the patient has symptoms of chronic obstruction. Colonic disease may fistulize into the stomach or duodenum, causing feculent vomiting, or to the proximal or mid-small bowel, causing malabsorption by "short circuiting" and bacterial overgrowth. Ten percent of women with Crohn's colitis will develop a rectovaginal fistula.

Perianal disease affects about one-third of patients with Crohn's colitis and is manifested by incontinence, large hemorrhoidal tags, anal strictures, anorectal fistulae, and perirectal abscesses. Not all patients with perianal fistula will have endoscopic evidence of colonic inflammation.

Gastroduodenal disease

Symptoms and signs of upper GI tract disease include nausea, vomiting, and epigastric pain. Patients usually have an *Helicobacter pylori*–negative gastritis. The second portion of the duodenum is more commonly involved than the bulb. Fistulas involving the stomach or duodenum arise from the small or large bowel and do not necessarily signify the presence of upper GI tract involvement. Patients with advanced gastroduodenal CD may develop a chronic gastric outlet obstruction.

Laboratory, endoscopic, and radiographic features

Laboratory abnormalities include elevated ESR and CRP. In more severe disease, findings include hypoalbuminemia, anemia, and leukocytosis.

Endoscopic features of CD include rectal sparing, aphthous ulcerations, fistulas, and skip lesions. Colonoscopy allows examination and biopsy of mass lesions or strictures and biopsy of the terminal ileum. Upper endoscopy is useful in diagnosing gastroduodenal involvement in patients with upper tract symptoms. Ileal or colonic strictures may be dilated with balloons introduced through the colonoscope. Strictures ≤4 cm and those at anastomotic sites respond better to endoscopic dilation. The perforation rate is as high as 10%. Most endoscopists dilate only fibrotic strictures and not those associated with active inflammation. Wireless capsule endoscopy (WCE) allows direct visualization of the entire small-bowel mucosa (Fig. 18-8). The diagnostic yield of detecting lesions suggestive of active CD is higher with WCE than CT or magnetic resonance (MR) enterography or small-bowel series. WCE cannot be used in the setting of a small-bowel stricture. Capsule retention occurs in <1% of patients with suspected CD, but retention rates of 4–6% are seen in patients with established CD. It is helpful to give the patient with CD a patency capsule, which is made of barium and starts to dissolve 30 h after ingestion. An abdominal x-ray can be taken at around 30 h after ingestion to see if the capsule is still present in the small bowel, which would indicate a stricture.

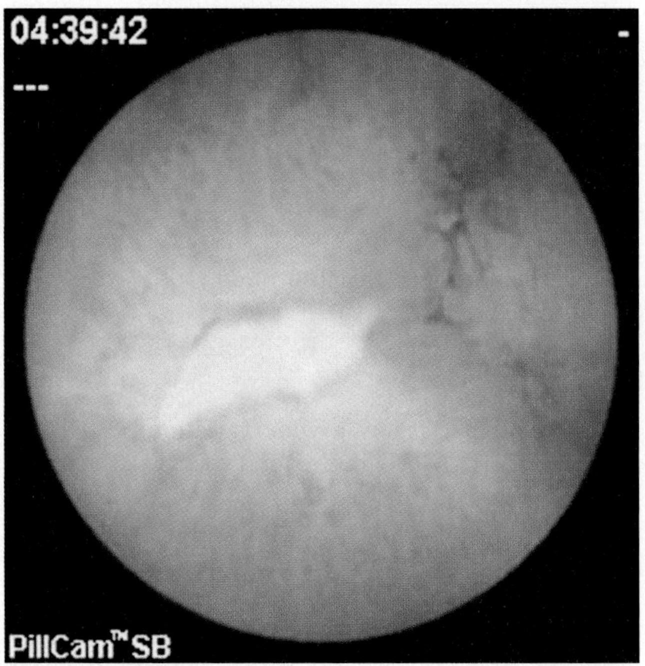

FIGURE 18-8

Wireless capsule endoscopy image in a patient with Crohn's disease of the ileum shows ulcerations and narrowing of the intestinal lumen. *(Courtesy of Dr. S. Reddy, Gastroenterology Division, Department of Medicine, Brigham and Women's Hospital, Boston, Massachusetts; with permission.)*

In CD, early radiographic findings in the small bowel include thickened folds and aphthous ulcerations. "Cobblestoning" from longitudinal and transverse ulcerations most frequently involves the small bowel. In more advanced disease, strictures, fistulas, inflammatory masses, and abscesses may be detected. The earliest macroscopic findings of colonic CD are aphthous ulcers. These small ulcers are often multiple and separated by normal intervening mucosa. As the disease progresses, aphthous ulcers become enlarged, deeper, and occasionally connected to one another, forming longitudinal stellate, serpiginous, and linear ulcers **(see Fig. 12-4*B*)**.

The transmural inflammation of CD leads to decreased luminal diameter and limited distensibility. As ulcers progress deeper, they can lead to fistula formation. The radiographic "string sign" represents long areas of circumferential inflammation and fibrosis, resulting in long segments of luminal narrowing. The segmental nature of CD results in wide gaps of normal or dilated bowel between involved segments.

Both CT and MRI of the small bowel can be performed by enterography (CTE or MRE), using oral and IV contrast, as well as enteroclysis. Although institutional preference guides technique selection, CTE and MRE tend to be preferred over enteroclysis due to ease and patient preference. Although CTE, MRE, and small-bowel follow-through (SBFT) have been shown to be equally accurate in the identification of active small-bowel inflammation, CTE and MRE have been shown to be superior to SBFT in the detection of extraluminal complications, including fistulas, sinus tracts, and abscesses. Currently, the use of CT scans is more common than MRI due to institutional availability and expertise. However, MRI is thought to offer superior soft tissue contrast and has the added advantage of avoiding radiation exposure changes. The lack of ionizing radiation is particularly appealing in younger patients and when monitoring response to therapy where serial images will be obtained. Either CTE or MRE is the first-line test for the evaluation of suspected CD and its complications. Pelvic MRI is superior to CT for demonstrating pelvic lesions such as ischiorectal abscesses and perianal fistulae (Fig. 18-11).

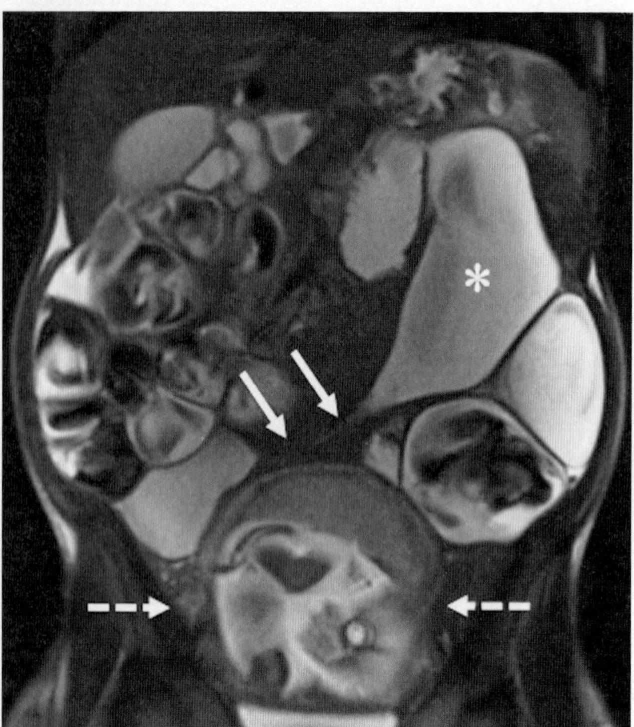

FIGURE 18-9

A coronal magnetic resonance image was obtained using a half Fourier single-shot T2-weighted acquisition with fat saturation in a 27-year-old pregnant (23 weeks' gestation) woman. The patient had Crohn's disease and was maintained on 6-mercaptopurine and prednisone. She presented with abdominal pain, distension, vomiting, and small-bowel obstruction. The image reveals a 7- to 10-cm long stricture at the terminal ileum (*white arrows*) causing obstruction and significant dilatation of the proximal small bowel (*white asterisk*). A fetus is seen in the uterus (*dashed white arrows*). *(Courtesy of Drs. J. F. B. Chick and P. B. Shyn, Abdominal Imaging and Intervention, Department of Radiology, Brigham and Women's Hospital, Harvard Medical School, Boston, Massachusetts; with permission.)*

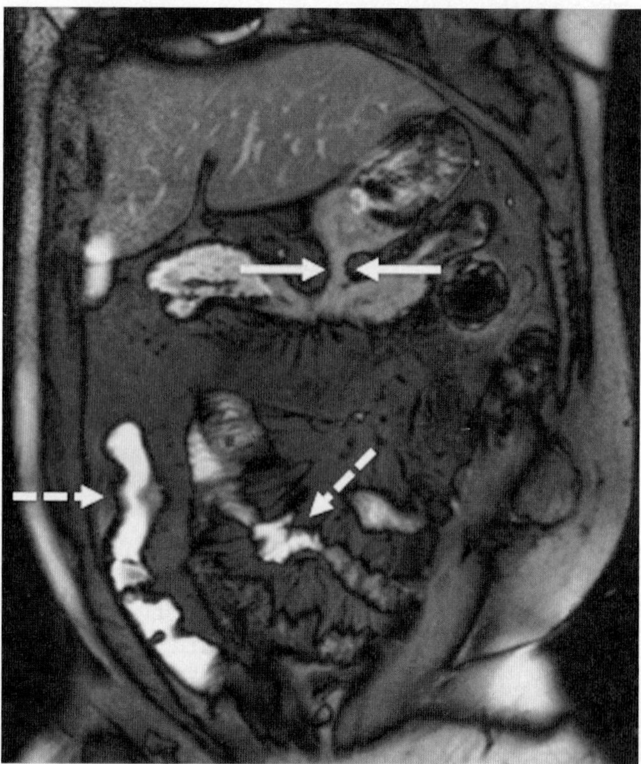

FIGURE 18-10

A coronal balanced, steady-state, free precession, T2-weighted image with fat saturation was obtained in a 32-year-old man with Crohn's disease and prior episodes of bowel obstruction, fistulas, and abscesses. He was being treated with 6-mercaptopurine and presented with abdominal distention and diarrhea. The image demonstrates a new gastrocolic fistula (*solid white arrows*). Multifocal involvement of the small bowel and terminal ileum is also present (*dashed white arrows*). *(Courtesy of Drs. J. F. B. Chick and P. B. Shyn, Abdominal Imaging and Intervention, Department of Radiology, Brigham and Women's Hospital, Harvard Medical School, Boston, Massachusetts; with permission.)*

Complications

Because CD is a transmural process, serosal adhesions develop that provide direct pathways for fistula formation and reduce the incidence of free perforation. Perforation occurs in 1–2% of patients, usually in the ileum but occasionally in the jejunum or as a complication of toxic megacolon. The peritonitis of free perforation, especially colonic, may be fatal. Intraabdominal and pelvic abscesses occur in 10–30% of patients with CD at some time in the course of their illness. CT-guided percutaneous drainage of the abscess is standard therapy. Despite adequate drainage, most patients need resection of the offending bowel segment. Percutaneous drainage has an especially high failure rate in abdominal wall abscesses. Systemic glucocorticoid therapy increases the risk of intraabdominal and pelvic abscesses in CD patients who have never had an operation. Other complications include intestinal obstruction in 40%, massive hemorrhage, malabsorption, and severe perianal disease.

Serologic markers

Patients with CD show a wide variation in the way they present and progress over time. Some patients present with mild disease activity and do well with generally safe and mild medications, but many others exhibit more severe disease and can develop serious complications that will require surgery. Current and developing biologic therapies can help halt progression of disease and give patients with moderate to severe CD a better quality of life. There are potential risks of biologic therapies such as infection and malignancy, and it would be optimal to determine at the time of diagnosis which patients will require more aggressive medical therapy. This same argument holds true for UC patients as well.

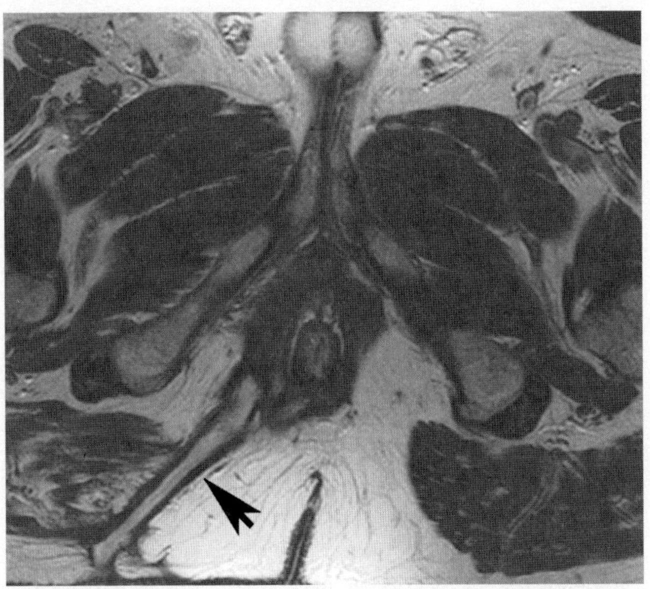

FIGURE 18-11

Axial T2-weighted magnetic resonance image obtained in a 37-year-old man with Crohn's disease shows a linear fluid-filled perianal fistula (*arrow*) in the right ischioanal fossa. *(Courtesy of Dr. K. Mortele, Gastrointestinal Radiology, Department of Radiology, Brigham and Women's Hospital, Boston, Massachusetts; with permission.)*

Subsets of patients with differing immune responses to microbial antigens have been described, and serology is often tested for perinuclear antineutrophil cytoplasmic antibodies (pANCAs) and anti-*Saccharomyces cerevisiae* antibodies (ASCAs). Unfortunately, these serologic markers are only marginally useful in helping to make the diagnosis of UC or CD and in predicting the course of disease. For success in diagnosing IBD and in differentiating between CD and UC, the efficacy of these serologic tests depends on the prevalence of IBD in a specific population. pANCA positivity is found in about 60–70% of UC patients and 5–10% of CD patients; 5–15% of first-degree relatives of UC patients are pANCA positive, whereas only 2–3% of the general population is pANCA positive. Sixty to 70% of CD patients, 10–15% of UC patients, and up to 5% of non-IBD controls are ASCA positive. In a patient population with a combined prevalence of UC and CD of 62%, pANCA/ASCA serology showed a sensitivity of 64% and a specificity of 94%. Positive and negative predictive values (PPVs and NPVs) for pANCA/ASCA also vary based on the prevalence of IBD in a given population. For the patient population with a prevalence of IBD of 62%, the PPV is 94%, and the NPV is 63%.

Other serologic tests include antibodies to *Escherichia coli* outer membrane porin protein C (OmpC), which is found in 55% of CD patients; antibodies to I_2, a homologue of the bacterial transcription factor families from a *Pseudomonas fluorescens*–associated sequence that is found in 50–54% of CD patients; and anti-flagellin (anti-CBir1) antibodies, which have been identified in approximately 50% of CD patients.

Children with CD positive for all four immune responses (ASCA+, OmpC+, I_2+, and anti-Cbir1+) may have more aggressive disease and a shorter time to progression to internal perforating and/or stricturing disease. However, larger prospective studies in both children and adults have not yet been performed and compared to CRP or other markers.

Clinical factors described at diagnosis are more helpful than serologies at predicting the natural history of CD. The initial requirements for glucocorticoid use, an age at diagnosis below 40 years and the presence of perianal disease at diagnosis, have been shown to be independently associated with subsequent disabling CD after 5 years. Except in special circumstances (such as before consideration of an ileoanal pouch anastomosis [IPAA] in a patient with indeterminate colitis), serologic markers have only minimal clinical utility.

DIFFERENTIAL DIAGNOSIS OF UC AND CD

UC and CD have similar features to many other diseases. In the absence of a key diagnostic test, a combination of features is used (Table 18-5). Once a diagnosis of IBD is made, distinguishing between UC and CD is impossible initially in up to 15% of cases. These are termed *indeterminate colitis.* Fortunately, in most cases, the true nature of the underlying colitis becomes evident later in the course of the patient's disease. Approximately 5% (range 1–20%) of colon resection specimens are difficult to classify as either UC or CD because they exhibit overlapping histologic features.

INFECTIOUS DISEASES

Infections of the small intestines and colon can mimic CD or UC. They may be bacterial, fungal, viral, or protozoal in origin (Table 18-6). *Campylobacter* colitis can mimic the endoscopic appearance of severe UC and can cause a relapse of established UC. *Salmonella* can cause watery or bloody diarrhea, nausea, and vomiting. Shigellosis causes watery diarrhea, abdominal pain, and fever followed by rectal tenesmus and by the passage of blood and mucus per rectum. All three are usually self-limited, but 1% of patients infected with *Salmonella* become asymptomatic carriers. *Yersinia enterocolitica* infection occurs mainly in the terminal ileum and causes mucosal ulceration, neutrophil invasion, and thickening of the ileal wall. Other bacterial infections that may mimic IBD include *C. difficile,* which presents with watery diarrhea, tenesmus, nausea, and vomiting;

TABLE 18-5

DIFFERENT CLINICAL, ENDOSCOPIC, AND RADIOGRAPHIC FEATURES

	ULCERATIVE COLITIS	CROHN'S DISEASE
Clinical		
Gross blood in stool	Yes	Occasionally
Mucus	Yes	Occasionally
Systemic symptoms	Occasionally	Frequently
Pain	Occasionally	Frequently
Abdominal mass	Rarely	Yes
Significant perineal disease	No	Frequently
Fistulas	No	Yes
Small intestinal obstruction	No	Frequently
Colonic obstruction	Rarely	Frequently
Response to antibiotics	No	Yes
Recurrence after surgery	No	Yes
Endoscopic		
Rectal sparing	Rarely	Frequently
Continuous disease	Yes	Occasionally
"Cobblestoning"	No	Yes
Granuloma on biopsy	No	Occasionally
Radiographic		
Small bowel significantly abnormal	No	Yes
Abnormal terminal ileum	No	Yes
Segmental colitis	No	Yes
Asymmetric colitis	No	Yes
Stricture	Occasionally	Frequently

TABLE 18-6

DISEASES THAT MIMIC IBD

Infectious Etiologies		
Bacterial	**Mycobacterial**	**Viral**
Salmonella	Tuberculosis	Cytomegalovirus
Shigella	*Mycobacterium avium*	Herpes simplex
Toxigenic *Escherichia coli*		HIV
Campylobacter	**Parasitic**	**Fungal**
Yersinia	Amebiasis	Histoplasmosis
Clostridium difficile	*Isospora*	*Candida*
Gonorrhea	*Trichuris trichiura*	*Aspergillus*
Chlamydia trachomatis	Hookworm	
	Strongyloides	
Noninfectious Etiologies		
Inflammatory	**Neoplastic**	**Drugs and Chemicals**
Appendicitis	Lymphoma	NSAIDs
Diverticulitis	Metastatic	Phosphosoda
Diversion colitis	Carcinoma	Cathartic colon
Collagenous/lymphocytic colitis	Carcinoma of the ileum	Gold
Ischemic colitis	Carcinoid	Oral contraceptives
Radiation colitis/enteritis	Familial polyposis	Cocaine
Solitary rectal ulcer syndrome		Ipilimumab
Eosinophilic gastroenteritis		Mycophenolate mofetil
Neutropenic colitis		
Behçet's syndrome		
Graft-versus-host disease		

Abbreviation: IBD, inflammatory bowel disease; NSAIDs, nonsteroidal anti-inflammatory drugs.

and *E. coli,* three categories of which can cause colitis. These are enterohemorrhagic, enteroinvasive, and enteroadherent *E. coli,* all of which can cause bloody diarrhea and abdominal tenderness. Diagnosis of bacterial colitis is made by sending stool specimens for bacterial culture and *C. difficile* toxin analysis. Gonorrhea, *Chlamydia*, and syphilis can also cause proctitis.

GI involvement with mycobacterial infection occurs primarily in the immunosuppressed patient but may occur in patients with normal immunity. Distal ileal and cecal involvement predominates, and patients present with symptoms of small-bowel obstruction and a tender abdominal mass. The diagnosis is made most directly by colonoscopy with biopsy and culture. *Mycobacterium avium-intracellulare* complex infection occurs in advanced stages of HIV infection and in other immunocompromised states; it usually manifests as a systemic infection with diarrhea, abdominal pain, weight loss, fever, and malabsorption. Diagnosis is established by acid-fast smear and culture of mucosal biopsies.

Although most of the patients with viral colitis are immunosuppressed, cytomegalovirus (CMV) and herpes simplex proctitis may occur in immunocompetent individuals. CMV occurs most commonly in the esophagus, colon, and rectum but may also involve the small intestine. Symptoms include abdominal pain, bloody diarrhea, fever, and weight loss. With severe disease, necrosis and perforation can occur. Diagnosis is made by identification of characteristic intranuclear inclusions in mucosal cells on biopsy. Herpes simplex infection of the GI tract is limited to the oropharynx, anorectum, and perianal areas. Symptoms include anorectal pain, tenesmus, constipation, inguinal adenopathy, difficulty with urinary voiding, and sacral paresthesias. Diagnosis is made by rectal biopsy with identification of characteristic cellular inclusions and viral culture. HIV itself can cause diarrhea, nausea, vomiting, and anorexia. Small intestinal biopsies show partial villous atrophy; small bowel bacterial overgrowth and fat malabsorption may also be noted.

Protozoan parasites include *Isospora belli,* which can cause a self-limited infection in healthy hosts but causes a chronic profuse, watery diarrhea, and weight loss in AIDS patients. *Entamoeba histolytica* or related species infect about 10% of the world's population; symptoms include abdominal pain, tenesmus, frequent loose stools containing blood and mucus, and abdominal tenderness. Colonoscopy reveals focal punctate ulcers with normal intervening mucosa; diagnosis is made by biopsy or serum amebic antibodies. Fulminant amebic colitis is rare but has a mortality rate of >50%.

Other parasitic infections that may mimic IBD include hookworm (*Necator americanus*), whipworm (*Trichuris trichiura*), and *Strongyloides stercoralis.* In severely immunocompromised patients, *Candida* or *Aspergillus* can be identified in the submucosa. Disseminated histoplasmosis can involve the ileocecal area.

NONINFECTIOUS DISEASES

Diverticulitis can be confused with CD clinically and radiographically. Both diseases cause fever, abdominal pain, tender abdominal mass, leukocytosis, elevated ESR, partial obstruction, and fistulas. Perianal disease or ileitis on small-bowel series favors the diagnosis of CD. Significant endoscopic mucosal abnormalities are more likely in CD than in diverticulitis. Endoscopic or clinical recurrence following segmental resection favors CD. Diverticular-associated colitis is similar to CD, but mucosal abnormalities are limited to the sigmoid and descending colon.

Ischemic colitis is commonly confused with IBD. The ischemic process can be chronic and diffuse, as in UC, or segmental, as in CD. Colonic inflammation due to ischemia may resolve quickly or may persist and result in transmural scarring and stricture formation. Ischemic bowel disease should be considered in the elderly following abdominal aortic aneurysm repair or when a patient has a hypercoagulable state or a severe cardiac or peripheral vascular disorder. Patients usually present with sudden onset of left lower quadrant pain, urgency to defecate, and the passage of bright red blood per rectum. Endoscopic examination often demonstrates a normal-appearing rectum and a sharp transition to an area of inflammation in the descending colon and splenic flexure.

The effects of radiotherapy on the GI tract can be difficult to distinguish from IBD. Acute symptoms can occur within 1–2 weeks of starting radiotherapy. When the rectum and sigmoid are irradiated, patients develop bloody, mucoid diarrhea and tenesmus, as in distal UC. With small-bowel involvement, diarrhea is common. Late symptoms include malabsorption and weight loss. Stricturing with obstruction and bacterial overgrowth may occur. Fistulas can penetrate the bladder, vagina, or abdominal wall. Flexible sigmoidoscopy reveals mucosal granularity, friability, numerous telangiectasias, and occasionally discrete ulcerations. Biopsy can be diagnostic.

Solitary rectal ulcer syndrome is uncommon and can be confused with IBD. It occurs in persons of all ages and may be caused by impaired evacuation and failure of relaxation of the puborectalis muscle. Single or multiple ulcerations may arise from anal sphincter overactivity, higher intrarectal pressures during defecation, and digital removal of stool. Patients complain of constipation with straining and pass blood and mucus per rectum. Other symptoms include abdominal pain, diarrhea, tenesmus, and perineal pain. Ulceration as large as 5 cm in diameter is usually seen anteriorly or anterior-laterally 3–15 cm from the anal verge. Biopsies can be diagnostic.

Several types of colitis are associated with nonsteroidal anti-inflammatory drugs (NSAIDs), including de novo colitis, reactivation of IBD, and proctitis caused by use of suppositories. Most patients with NSAID-related colitis present with diarrhea and abdominal pain, and complications include stricture, bleeding, obstruction, perforation, and fistulization. Withdrawal of these agents is crucial, and in cases of reactivated IBD, standard therapies are indicated.

There are complications of two drugs used in a hospital setting that mimic IBD. The first is ipilimumab, a drug that targets cytotoxic T lymphocyte antigen 4 (CTLA-4) and reverses T cell inhibition and is used to treat metastatic melanoma; ipilimumab has an incidence of IBD in 0.0017 cases per 100 person-years. Ipilimumab-induced colitis is typically treated with glucocorticoids or infliximab. The second is mycophenolate mofetil (MMF), an immunosuppressive agent commonly used to prevent posttransplant rejection. The colitis associated with MMF is common and can occur in more than one-third of patients taking the drug. Treatment is dose reduction or cessation of the drug.

THE ATYPICAL COLITIDES

Two atypical colitides—collagenous colitis and lymphocytic colitis—have completely normal endoscopic appearances. Collagenous colitis has two main histologic components: increased subepithelial collagen deposition and colitis with increased intraepithelial lymphocytes. The female to male ratio is 9:1, and most patients present in the sixth or seventh decades of life. The main symptom is chronic watery diarrhea. Treatments range from sulfasalazine or mesalamine and diphenoxylate/atropine (Lomotil) to bismuth to budesonide to prednisone or azathioprine/6-mercaptopurine for refractory disease. Risk factors include smoking; use of NSAIDs, proton pump inhibitors, or beta blockers; and a history of autoimmune disease.

Lymphocytic colitis has features similar to collagenous colitis, including age at onset and clinical presentation, but it has almost equal incidence in men and women and no subepithelial collagen deposition on pathologic section. However, intraepithelial lymphocytes are increased. Use of sertraline (but not beta blockers) is an additional risk factor. The frequency of celiac disease is increased in lymphocytic colitis and ranges from 9 to 27%. Celiac disease should be excluded in all patients with lymphocytic colitis, particularly if diarrhea does not respond to conventional therapy. Treatment is similar to that of collagenous colitis with the exception of a gluten-free diet for those who have celiac disease.

Diversion colitis is an inflammatory process that arises in segments of the large intestine that are excluded from the fecal stream. It usually occurs in patients with ileostomy or colostomy when a mucus fistula or a Hartmann's pouch has been created. Clinically, patients have mucus or bloody discharge from the rectum. Erythema, granularity, friability, and, in more severe cases, ulceration can be seen on endoscopy. Histopathology shows areas of active inflammation with foci of cryptitis and crypt abscesses. Crypt architecture is normal, which differentiates it from UC. It may be impossible to distinguish from CD. Short-chain fatty acid enemas may help in diversion colitis, but the definitive therapy is surgical reanastomosis.

EXTRAINTESTINAL MANIFESTATIONS

Up to one-third of IBD patients have at least one extraintestinal disease manifestation.

DERMATOLOGIC

Erythema nodosum (EN) occurs in up to 15% of CD patients and 10% of UC patients. Attacks usually correlate with bowel activity; skin lesions develop after the onset of bowel symptoms, and patients frequently have concomitant active peripheral arthritis. The lesions of EN are hot, red, tender nodules measuring 1–5 cm in diameter and are found on the anterior surface of the lower legs, ankles, calves, thighs, and arms. Therapy is directed toward the underlying bowel disease.

Pyoderma gangrenosum (PG) is seen in 1–12% of UC patients and less commonly in Crohn's colitis. Although it usually presents after the diagnosis of IBD, PG may occur years before the onset of bowel symptoms, run a course independent of the bowel disease, respond poorly to colectomy, and even develop years after proctocolectomy. It is usually associated with severe disease. Lesions are commonly found on the dorsal surface of the feet and legs but may occur on the arms, chest, stoma, and even the face. PG usually begins as a pustule and then spreads concentrically to rapidly undermine healthy skin. Lesions then ulcerate, with violaceous edges surrounded by a margin of erythema. Centrally, they contain necrotic tissue with blood and exudates. Lesions may be single or multiple and grow as large as 30 cm. They are sometimes very difficult to treat and often require IV antibiotics, IV glucocorticoids, dapsone, azathioprine, thalidomide, IV cyclosporine, or infliximab.

Other dermatologic manifestations include pyoderma vegetans, which occurs in intertriginous areas; pyostomatitis vegetans, which involves the mucous membranes; Sweet syndrome, a neutrophilic dermatosis; and metastatic CD, a rare disorder defined by cutaneous granuloma formation. Psoriasis affects 5–10% of patients with IBD and is unrelated to bowel activity consistent with the potential shared immunogenetic basis of these diseases. Perianal skin tags are found in 75–80% of patients with CD, especially those with colon involvement. Oral mucosal lesions, seen often in CD and rarely in UC, include aphthous stomatitis and "cobblestone" lesions of the buccal mucosa.

RHEUMATOLOGIC

Peripheral arthritis develops in 15–20% of IBD patients, is more common in CD, and worsens with exacerbations of bowel activity. It is asymmetric, polyarticular, and migratory and most often affects large joints of the upper and lower extremities. Treatment is directed at reducing bowel inflammation. In severe UC, colectomy frequently cures the arthritis.

Ankylosing spondylitis (AS) occurs in about 10% of IBD patients and is more common in CD than UC. About two-thirds of IBD patients with AS express the HLA-B27 antigen. The AS activity is not related to bowel activity and does not remit with glucocorticoids or colectomy. It most often affects the spine and pelvis, producing symptoms of diffuse low-back pain, buttock pain, and morning stiffness. The course is continuous and progressive, leading to permanent skeletal damage and deformity. Anti-TNF therapy reduces spinal inflammation and improves functional status and quality of life.

Sacroiliitis is symmetric, occurs equally in UC and CD, is often asymptomatic, does not correlate with bowel activity, and does not always progress to AS. Other rheumatic manifestations include hypertrophic osteoarthropathy, pelvic/femoral osteomyelitis, and relapsing polychondritis.

OCULAR

The incidence of ocular complications in IBD patients is 1–10%. The most common are conjunctivitis, anterior uveitis/iritis, and episcleritis. Uveitis is associated with both UC and Crohn's colitis, may be found during periods of remission, and may develop in patients following bowel resection. Symptoms include ocular pain, photophobia, blurred vision, and headache. Prompt intervention, sometimes with systemic glucocorticoids, is required to prevent scarring and visual impairment. Episcleritis is a benign disorder that presents with symptoms of mild ocular burning. It occurs in 3–4% of IBD patients, more commonly in Crohn's colitis, and is treated with topical glucocorticoids.

HEPATOBILIARY

Hepatic steatosis is detectable in about one-half of the abnormal liver biopsies from patients with CD and UC; patients usually present with hepatomegaly. Fatty liver usually results from a combination of chronic debilitating illness, malnutrition, and glucocorticoid therapy. Cholelithiasis occurs in 10–35% of CD patients with ileitis or ileal resection. Gallstone formation is caused by malabsorption of bile acids, resulting in depletion of the bile salt pool and the secretion of lithogenic bile.

Primary sclerosing cholangitis (PSC) is a disorder characterized by both intrahepatic and extrahepatic bile duct inflammation and fibrosis, frequently leading to biliary cirrhosis and hepatic failure; approximately 5% of patients with UC have PSC, but 50–75% of patients with PSC have IBD. PSC occurs less often in patients with CD. Although it can be recognized after the diagnosis of IBD, PSC can be detected earlier or even years after proctocolectomy. Consistent with this, the immunogenetic basis for PSC appears to be overlapping but distinct from UC based on GWAS, although both IBD and PSC are commonly pANCA positive. Most patients have no symptoms at the time of diagnosis; when symptoms are present, they consist of fatigue, jaundice, abdominal pain, fever, anorexia, and malaise. The traditional gold standard diagnostic test is endoscopic retrograde cholangiopancreatography (ERCP), but magnetic resonance cholangiopancreatography (MRCP) is also sensitive and specific. MRCP is reasonable as an initial diagnostic test in children and can visualize irregularities, multifocal strictures, and dilatations of all levels of the biliary tree. In patients with PSC, both ERCP and MRCP demonstrate multiple bile duct strictures alternating with relatively normal segments.

The bile acid ursodeoxycholic acid (ursodiol) may reduce alkaline phosphatase and serum aminotransferase levels, but histologic improvement has been marginal. High doses (25–30 mg/kg per day) may decrease the risk of colorectal dysplasia and cancer in patients with UC and PSC. Endoscopic stenting may be palliative for cholestasis secondary to bile duct obstruction. Patients with symptomatic disease develop cirrhosis and liver failure over 5–10 years and eventually require liver transplantation. PSC patients have a 10–15% lifetime risk of developing cholangiocarcinoma and then cannot be transplanted. Patients with IBD and PSC are at increased risk of colon cancer and should be surveyed yearly by colonoscopy and biopsy.

In addition, cholangiography is normal in a small percentage of patients who have a variant of PSC known as *small duct primary sclerosing cholangitis*. This variant (sometimes referred to as "pericholangitis") is probably a form of PSC involving small-caliber bile ducts. It has similar biochemical and histologic features to classic PSC. It appears to have a significantly better prognosis than classic PSC, although it may evolve into classic PSC. Granulomatous hepatitis and hepatic amyloidosis are much rarer extraintestinal manifestations of IBD.

UROLOGIC

The most frequent genitourinary complications are calculi, ureteral obstruction, and ileal bladder fistulas. The highest frequency of nephrolithiasis (10–20%) occurs in patients with CD following small bowel resection. Calcium oxalate stones develop secondary to hyperoxaluria, which results from increased absorption of dietary oxalate. Normally, dietary calcium combines with luminal oxalate to form insoluble calcium oxalate, which is eliminated in the stool. In patients with ileal dysfunction, however, nonabsorbed fatty acids bind calcium and leave oxalate unbound. The unbound oxalate is then delivered to the colon, where it is readily absorbed, especially in the presence of inflammation.

METABOLIC BONE DISORDERS

Low bone mass occurs in 3–30% of IBD patients. The risk is increased by glucocorticoids, cyclosporine, methotrexate, and total parenteral nutrition (TPN). Malabsorption and inflammation mediated by IL-1, IL-6, TNF, and other inflammatory mediators also contribute to low bone density. An increased incidence of hip, spine, wrist, and rib fractures has been noted: 36% in CD and 45% in UC. The absolute risk of an osteoporotic fracture is about 1% per person per year. Fracture rates, particularly in the spine and hip, are highest among the elderly (age >60). One study noted an OR of 1.72 for vertebral fracture and an OR of 1.59 for hip fracture. The disease severity predicted the risk of a fracture. Only 13% of IBD patients who had a fracture were on any kind of antifracture treatment. Up to 20% of bone mass can be lost per year with chronic glucocorticoid use. The effect is dosage-dependent. Budesonide may also suppress the pituitary-adrenal axis and thus carries a risk of causing osteoporosis.

Osteonecrosis is characterized by death of osteocytes and adipocytes and eventual bone collapse. The pain is aggravated by motion and swelling of the joints. It affects the hips more often than knees and shoulders, and in one series, 4.3% of patients developed osteonecrosis within 6 months of starting glucocorticoids. Diagnosis is made by bone scan or MRI, and treatment consists of pain control, cord decompression, osteotomy, and joint replacement.

THROMBOEMBOLIC DISORDERS

Patients with IBD have an increased risk of both venous and arterial thrombosis even if the disease is not active. Factors responsible for the hypercoagulable state have included abnormalities of the platelet-endothelial interaction, hyperhomocysteinemia, alterations in the coagulation cascade, impaired fibrinolysis, involvement of tissue factor-bearing microvesicles, disruption of the normal coagulation system by autoantibodies, and a genetic predisposition. A spectrum of vasculitides involving small, medium, and large vessels has also been observed.

OTHER DISORDERS

More common cardiopulmonary manifestations include endocarditis, myocarditis, pleuropericarditis, and interstitial lung disease. A secondary or reactive amyloidosis can occur in patients with long-standing IBD, especially in patients with CD. Amyloid material is deposited systemically and can cause diarrhea, constipation, and renal failure. The renal disease can be successfully treated with colchicine. Pancreatitis is a rare extraintestinal manifestation of IBD and results from duodenal fistulas; ampullary CD; gallstones; PSC; drugs such as 6-mercaptopurine, azathioprine, or, very rarely, 5-ASA agents; autoimmune pancreatitis; and primary CD of the pancreas.

TREATMENT Inflammatory Bowel Disease

5-ASA AGENTS The mainstay of therapy for mild to moderate UC is sulfasalazine and the other 5-ASA agents. These agents are effective at inducing and maintaining remission in UC. They may have a limited role in inducing remission in CD but no clear role in maintenance of CD. Newer sulfa-free aminosalicylate preparations deliver increased amounts of the pharmacologically active ingredient of sulfasalazine (5-ASA, mesalamine) to the site of active bowel disease while limiting systemic toxicity. Peroxisome proliferator activated receptor γ (PPAR-γ) may mediate 5-ASA therapeutic action by decreasing nuclear localization of NF-κB. Sulfa-free aminosalicylate formulations include alternative azo-bonded carriers, 5-ASA dimers, and delayed-release and controlled-release preparations. Each has the same efficacy as sulfasalazine when equimolar concentrations are used.

Sulfasalazine was originally developed to deliver both antibacterial (sulfapyridine) and anti-inflammatory (5-ASA) therapy into the connective tissues of joints and the colonic mucosa. The molecular structure provides a convenient delivery system to the colon by allowing the intact molecule to pass through the small intestine after only partial absorption and to be broken down in the colon by bacterial azo reductases that cleave the azo bond linking the sulfa and 5-ASA moieties. Sulfasalazine is effective treatment for mild to moderate UC and is occasionally used in Crohn's colitis, but its high rate of side effects limits its use. Although sulfasalazine is more effective at higher doses, at 6 or 8 g/d up to 30% of patients experience allergic reactions or intolerable side effects such as headache, anorexia, nausea, and vomiting that are attributable to the sulfapyridine moiety. Hypersensitivity reactions, independent of sulfapyridine levels, include rash, fever, hepatitis, agranulocytosis, hypersensitivity pneumonitis, pancreatitis, worsening of colitis, and reversible sperm abnormalities. Sulfasalazine can also impair folate absorption, and patients should be given folic acid supplements.

Balsalazide contains an azo bond binding mesalamine to the carrier molecule 4-aminobenzoyl-β-alanine; it is effective in the colon.

Olsalazine is composed of two 5-ASA radicals linked by an azo bond, which is split in the colon by bacterial reduction, and two 5-ASA molecules are released. Olsalazine is similar in effectiveness to sulfasalazine in treating UC, but up to 17% of patients experience nonbloody diarrhea caused by increased secretion of fluid in the small bowel.

Delzicol and *Asacol HD* (high dose) are enteric-coated forms of mesalamine with the 5-ASA being released at pH >7. They disintegrate with complete breakup of the tablet occurring in many different parts of the gut ranging from the small intestine to the splenic flexure; they have increased gastric residence when taken with a meal. Asacol has recently been discontinued and replaced with Delzicol, which lacks dibutyl phthalate (DBP), an inactive ingredient in Asacol's enteric coating. DBP has been associated with adverse effects on the male reproductive system in animals at very high doses. Asacol HD with the same chemical in its coating is still on the market, but the human doses of DBP are within acceptable limits of toxicity.

Lialda is a once-a-day formulation of mesalamine (Multi-Matrix System [MMX]) designed to release mesalamine in the colon. The MMX technology incorporates mesalamine into a lipophilic matrix within a hydrophilic matrix encapsulated in a polymer resistant to degradation at a low pH (<7) to delay release throughout the colon. The safety profile appears to be comparable to other 5-ASA formulations.

Apriso is a formulation containing encapsulated mesalamine granules that delivers mesalamine to the terminal ileum and colon via a proprietary extended-release mechanism (Intellicor). The outer coating (Eudragit L) dissolves at a pH >6. In addition, there is a polymer matrix core that aids in sustained release throughout the colon. Because Lialda and Apriso are given once daily, an anticipated benefit is improved compliance compared with two to four daily doses required for other mesalamine preparations.

Pentasa is another mesalamine formulation that uses an ethylcellulose coating to allow water absorption into small beads containing the mesalamine. Water dissolves the 5-ASA, which then diffuses out of the bead into the lumen. Disintegration of the capsule occurs in the stomach. The microspheres then disperse throughout the entire GI tract from the small intestine through the distal colon in both fasted and fed conditions.

Salofalk® Granu-Stix, an unencapsulated version of mesalamine, has been in use in Europe for induction and maintenance of remission for several years.

Appropriate doses of the 5-ASA compounds are shown in Table 18-7. Some 50–75% of patients with mild to moderate UC improve when treated with 5-ASA doses equivalent to 2 g/d of mesalamine; the dose response continues up to at least 4.8 g/d. As a general rule, 5-ASA agents act within 2–4 weeks. 5-ASA doses equivalent to 1.5–4 g/d of mesalamine maintain remission in 50–75% of patients with UC.

More common side effects of the 5-ASA medications include headaches, nausea, hair loss, and abdominal pain. Rare side effects of the 5-ASA medications include renal impairment, hematuria, pancreatitis, and paradoxical worsening of colitis. Renal function tests and urinalysis should be checked yearly.

Topical *Rowasa* enemas are composed of mesalamine and are effective in mild-to-moderate distal UC. Clinical response occurs in up to 80% of UC patients with colitis distal to the splenic flexure. Combination therapy with mesalamine in both oral and enema form is more effective than either treatment alone for both distal and extensive UC.

Canasa suppositories composed of mesalamine are effective in treating proctitis.

GLUCOCORTICOIDS The majority of patients with moderate to severe UC benefit from oral or parenteral glucocorticoids. Prednisone is usually started at doses of 40–60 mg/d for active UC that is unresponsive to 5-ASA therapy. Parenteral glucocorticoids may be administered as hydrocortisone, 300 mg/d, or methylprednisolone, 40–60 mg/d. A new glucocorticoid for UC, budesonide (Uceris), is released entirely in the colon and has minimal to no glucocorticoid side effects. The dose is 9 mg/d for 8 weeks, and no taper is required. Topically applied glucocorticoids are also beneficial for distal colitis and may serve as an adjunct in those who have rectal involvement plus more proximal disease. Hydrocortisone enemas or foam may control active disease, although they have no proven role as maintenance therapy. These glucocorticoids are significantly absorbed from the rectum and can lead to adrenal suppression with prolonged administration. Topical 5-ASA therapy is more effective than topical steroid therapy in the treatment of distal UC.

Glucocorticoids are also effective for treatment of moderate to severe CD and induce a 60–70% remission rate compared to a 30% placebo response. The systemic effects of standard glucocorticoid formulations have led to the development of more potent formulations that are less well-absorbed

TABLE 18-7

ORAL 5-ASA PREPARATIONS

PREPARATION	FORMULATION	DELIVERY	DOSING PER DAY
Azo-Bond			
Sulfasalazine (500 mg) (Azulfidine)	Sulfapyridine-5-ASA	Colon	3–6 g (acute) 2–4 g (maintenance)
Olsalazine (250 mg) (Dipentum)	5-ASA–5-ASA	Colon	1–3 g
Balsalazide (750 mg) (Colazal)	Aminobenzoyl-alanine–5-ASA	Colon	6.75–9 g
Delayed-Release			
Mesalamine (400, 800 mg) (Delzicol, Asacol HD)	Eudragit S (pH 7)	Distal ileum-colon	2.4–4.8 g (acute) 1.6–4.8 g (maintenance)
Mesalamine (1.2 g) (Lialda)	MMX mesalamine (SPD476)	Ileum-colon	2.4–4.8 g
Controlled-Release			
Mesalamine (250, 500, 1000 mg) (Pentasa)	Ethylcellulose microgranules	Stomach-colon	2–4 g (acute) 1.5–4 g (maintenance)
Delayed- and Extended-Release			
Mesalamine (0.375 g) (Apriso)	Intellicor extended-release mechanism	Ileum-colon	1.5 g (maintenance)

and have increased first-pass metabolism. Controlled ileal-release budesonide has been nearly equal to prednisone for ileocolonic CD with fewer glucocorticoid side effects. Budesonide is used for 2–3 months at a dose of 9 mg/d, and then tapered. Budesonide 6 mg/d is effective in reducing relapse rates at 3–6 months but not at 12 months in CD patients with a medically induced remission.

Glucocorticoids play no role in maintenance therapy in either UC or CD. Once clinical remission has been induced, they should be tapered according to the clinical activity, normally at a rate of no more than 5 mg/week. They can usually be tapered to 20 mg/d within 4–5 weeks but often take several months to be discontinued altogether. The side effects are numerous, including fluid retention, abdominal striae, fat redistribution, hyperglycemia, subcapsular cataracts, osteonecrosis, osteoporosis, myopathy, emotional disturbances, and withdrawal symptoms. Most of these side effects, aside from osteonecrosis, are related to the dose and duration of therapy.

ANTIBIOTICS Antibiotics have no role in the treatment of active or quiescent UC. However, pouchitis, which occurs in about a third of UC patients after colectomy and IPAA, usually responds to treatment with metronidazole and/or ciprofloxacin.

Metronidazole is effective in active inflammatory, fistulous, and perianal CD and may prevent recurrence after ileal resection. The most effective dose is 15–20 mg/kg per day in three divided doses; it is usually continued for several months. Common side effects include nausea, metallic taste, and disulfiram-like reaction. Peripheral neuropathy can occur with prolonged administration (several months) and on rare occasions is permanent despite discontinuation. *Ciprofloxacin* (500 mg bid) is also beneficial for inflammatory, perianal, and fistulous CD but has been associated with Achilles tendinitis and rupture. Both ciprofloxacin and metronidazole antibiotics can be used as first-line drugs for short periods of time in active inflammatory, fistulizing, and perianal CD.

AZATHIOPRINE AND 6-MERCAPTOPURINE Azathioprine and 6-mercaptopurine (6-MP) are purine analogues commonly employed in the management of glucocorticoid-dependent IBD. Azathioprine is rapidly absorbed and converted to 6-MP, which is then metabolized to the active end product, thioinosinic acid, an inhibitor of purine ribonucleotide synthesis and cell proliferation. These agents also inhibit the immune response. Efficacy can be seen as early as 3–4 weeks but can take up to 4–6 months. Adherence can be monitored by measuring the levels of 6-thioguanine and 6-methyl-mercaptopurine, end products of 6-MP metabolism. Azathioprine (2–3 mg/kg per day) and 6-MP (1–1.5 mg/kg per day) have been used successfully as glucocorticoid-sparing agents in up to two-thirds of UC and CD patients previously unable to be weaned from glucocorticoids. They are also used as maintenance therapy in UC and CD and for treating active perianal disease and fistulas in CD. In addition, 6-MP or azathioprine is effective for postoperative prophylaxis of CD.

Although azathioprine and 6-MP are usually well tolerated, pancreatitis occurs in 3–4% of patients, typically presents within the first few weeks of therapy, and is completely reversible when the drug is stopped. Other side effects include nausea, fever, rash, and hepatitis. Bone marrow suppression (particularly leukopenia) is dose-related and often delayed, necessitating regular monitoring of the complete blood cell count (CBC). Additionally, 1 in 300 individuals lacks thiopurine methyltransferase, the enzyme responsible for drug metabolism to inactive end-products (6-methylmercaptopurine); an additional 11% of the population are heterozygotes with intermediate enzyme activity. Both are at increased risk of toxicity because of increased accumulation of active 6-thioguanine metabolites. Although 6-thioguanine and 6-methylmercaptopurine levels can be followed to determine correct drug dosing and reduce toxicity, weight-based dosing is an acceptable alternative. CBCs and liver function tests should be monitored frequently regardless of dosing strategy. IBD patients treated with azathioprine/6-MP are at approximately a fourfold increased risk of developing a lymphoma. This increased risk could be a result of the medications, the underlying disease, or both.

METHOTREXATE Methotrexate (MTX) inhibits dihydrofolate reductase, resulting in impaired DNA synthesis. Additional anti-inflammatory properties may be related to decreased IL-1 production. Intramuscular (IM) or subcutaneous (SC) MTX (25 mg/week) is effective in inducing remission and reducing glucocorticoid dosage; 15 mg/week is effective in maintaining remission in active CD. Potential toxicities include leukopenia and hepatic fibrosis, necessitating periodic evaluation of CBCs and liver enzymes. The role of liver biopsy in patients on long-term MTX is uncertain but is probably limited to those with increased liver enzymes. Hypersensitivity pneumonitis is a rare but serious complication of therapy.

CYCLOSPORINE Cyclosporine (CSA) is a lipophilic peptide with inhibitory effects on both the cellular and humoral immune systems. CSA blocks the production of IL-2 by T helper lymphocytes. CSA binds to cyclophilin, and this complex inhibits calcineurin, a cytoplasmic phosphatase enzyme involved in the activation of T cells. CSA also indirectly inhibits B cell function by blocking helper T cells. CSA has a more rapid onset of action than 6-MP and azathioprine.

CSA is most effective when given at 2–4 mg/kg per day IV in severe UC that is refractory to IV glucocorticoids, with 82% of patients responding. CSA can be an alternative to colectomy. The long-term success of oral CSA is not as dramatic, but if patients are started on 6-MP or azathioprine at the time of hospital discharge, remission can be maintained. For the 2 mg/kg dose, levels as measured by monoclonal radioimmunoassay or by the high-performance liquid chromatography assay should be maintained between 150 and 350 ng/mL.

CSA may cause significant toxicity; renal function should be monitored frequently. Hypertension, gingival hyperplasia, hypertrichosis, paresthesias, tremors, headaches, and electrolyte abnormalities are common side effects. Creatinine elevation calls for dose reduction or discontinuation. Seizures may also complicate therapy, especially if the patient is hypomagnesemic or if serum cholesterol levels are <3.1 mmol/L (<120 mg/dL). Opportunistic infections, most notably *Pneumocystis carinii* pneumonia, may occur with combination immunosuppressive treatment; prophylaxis should be given. Major adverse events occurred in 15% of patients in one large study, including nephrotoxicity not responding to dose adjustment, serious infections, seizures, anaphylaxis, and death of two patients. This high incidence suggests that vigorous monitoring by experienced clinicians at tertiary care centers may be required. To compare IV cyclosporine versus infliximab, a large trial was conducted in Europe by the GETAID group. The results indicated identical 7-day response rates between cyclosporine 2 mg/kg (with doses adjusted for levels of 150–250 ng/mL) and infliximab 5 mg/kg, with both groups achieving response rates of 85%. Serious infections occurred in 5 of 55 cyclosporine patients and 4 of 56 infliximab patients. Response rates were similar in the two groups at day 98 among patients treated with oral cyclosporine versus infliximab at the usual induction dose and maintenance dose regimen (40% and 46%, respectively). In light of data showing equal efficacy of CSA and infliximab in severe UC, more physicians are relying on infliximab rather than CSA in these patients.

TACROLIMUS Tacrolimus is a macrolide antibiotic with immunomodulatory properties similar to CSA. It is 100 times as potent as CSA and is not dependent on bile or mucosal integrity for absorption. These pharmacologic properties enable tacrolimus to have good oral absorption despite proximal small bowel Crohn's involvement. It has shown efficacy in children with refractory IBD and in adults with extensive involvement of the small bowel. It is also effective in adults with glucocorticoid-dependent or refractory UC and CD as well as refractory fistulizing CD.

BIOLOGIC THERAPIES Biologic therapy was traditionally reserved for moderately to severely ill patients with CD who had failed other therapies. However, it is now commonly given as an initial therapy for patients with moderate to severe CD in order to prevent future disease complications. Patients who respond to biologic therapies enjoy an improvement in clinical symptoms; a better quality of life; less disability, fatigue, and depression; and fewer surgeries and hospitalizations.

Anti-TNF therapies The first biologic therapy approved for CD was *infliximab*, a chimeric IgG1 antibody against TNF-α, which is now also approved for treatment of moderately to severely active UC. Of active CD patients refractory to glucocorticoids, 6-MP, or 5-ASA, 65% will respond to IV infliximab (5 mg/kg); one-third will enter complete remission. The ACCENT I (A Crohn's Disease Clinical Trial Evaluating Infliximab in a New Long-Term Treatment Regimen) study showed that of the patients who experience an initial response, 40% will maintain remission for at least 1 year with repeated infusions of infliximab every 8 weeks.

Infliximab is also effective in CD patients with refractory perianal and enterocutaneous fistulas, with the ACCENT II trial showing a 68% response rate (50% reduction in fistula drainage) and a 50% complete remission rate. Reinfusion, typically every 8 weeks, is necessary to continue therapeutic benefits in many patients.

The SONIC (Study of Biologic and Immunomodulator-Naive Patients with Crohn's Disease) trial compared infliximab plus azathioprine, infliximab alone, and azathioprine alone in immunomodulator- and biologic-naive patients with moderate to severe CD. At 1 year, the infliximab plus azathioprine group had a glucocorticoid-free remission rate of 46% compared with 35% for infliximab alone and 24% for azathioprine alone. There was also complete mucosal healing at week 26 with the combined approach relative to either infliximab or azathioprine alone (44% vs 30% vs 17%). The adverse events were equal between groups.

Two large trials of infliximab in moderate to severe UC also showed efficacy with a response rate of 37–49%, with about one-fifth of patients maintaining remission after 54 weeks. Dosing for UC and CD are identical, with induction dosing at 0, 2, and 6 weeks and every 8 weeks thereafter. There is a similar study to SONIC in patients with moderate to severe UC. After 16 weeks of therapy, UC patients taking azathioprine plus infliximab had a glucocorticoid-free remission rate of 40% compared to 24% (article now published) and 22% of those on azathioprine and infliximab alone, respectively. This is even further evidence for "top-down" or more aggressive therapy for both moderate to severe CD and UC.

Adalimumab is a recombinant human monoclonal IgG1 antibody containing only human peptide sequences and is injected subcutaneously. Adalimumab binds TNF and neutralizes its function by blocking the interaction between TNF and its cell-surface receptor. Therefore, it seems to have a similar mechanism of action to infliximab but with less immunogenicity. Adalimumab has been approved for treatment of moderate to severe CD. CHARM (Crohn's Trial of the Fully Human Adalimumab for Remission Maintenance) is an adalimumab maintenance study in patients who responded to adalimumab induction therapy. About 50% of the patients in this trial were previously treated with infliximab. Remission rates ranged from 42–48% of infliximab-naïve patients at 1 year compared with remission rates of 31–34% in patients who had previously received infliximab. Another trial showed a remission rate of 21% at 4 weeks in patients who had initially responded to and then failed infliximab. In clinical practice, the remission rate in patients taking adalimumab increases with a dose increase to 40 mg weekly instead of every other week. Adalimumab is now also approved for the treatment of moderately to severely active UC.

Certolizumab pegol is a pegylated form of an anti-TNF Fab portion of an antibody administered SC once monthly. SC certolizumab pegol was effective for induction of clinical response in patients with active inflammatory CD. In the PRECISE II (Pegylated Antibody Fragment Evaluation in Crohn's Disease) trial of maintenance therapy with certolizumab in patients who responded to certolizumab induction, the results were similar to the CHARM trial. At week 26, the subgroup of patients who were infliximab naïve had a response of 69% as compared to 44% in patients who had previously received infliximab.

Golimumab is another fully human IgG1 antibody against TNF-α and is currently approved for the treatment of moderately to severely active UC. All of the patients in the golimumab trial were infliximab-naive. Like adalimumab and certolizumab, golimumab is injected SC.

Side effects of anti-TNF therapies

Development of antibodies The development of antibodies to infliximab (ATIs) is associated with an increased risk of infusion reactions and a decreased response to treatment. Current practice does not include giving on-demand or episodic infusions in contrast to periodic (every 8 week) infusions because patients are most likely to develop ATIs. ATIs are generally present when the quality of response or the response duration to infliximab infusion decreases. Decreasing the dosing intervals or increasing the dosage to 10 mg/kg may restore the efficacy. There are commercial assays for both infliximab and adalimumab antibodies and trough levels to determine optimal dosing. If a patient has high ATIs and a low trough level of infliximab, it is best to switch to another anti-TNF therapy. Most acute infusion reactions and serum sickness can be managed with glucocorticoids and antihistamines. Some reactions can be serious and would necessitate a change in therapy, especially if a patient has ATIs.

Non-Hodgkin's lymphoma (NHL) The baseline risk of NHL in CD patients is 2:10,000, which is slightly higher than in the general population. Azathioprine and/or 6-MP therapy increases the risk to about 4:10,000. The highest risk for thiopurine-associated NHL is in patients over 65 years old, with a moderate risk in those between the ages of 50 and 65. Anti-TNF therapy increases the risk to approximately 6:10,000.

Hepatosplenic T cell lymphoma (HSTCL) HSTCL is a nearly universally fatal lymphoma in patients with or without CD. In patients with CD, events reported to the Food and Drug Administration Adverse Event Reporting System (FDA AERS) and search of PubMed and Embase published case reports demonstrate a total of 37 unique cases. Eighty-six percent of the patients were male, with a median age of 26 years. Patients had CD for a mean of 10 years before the diagnosis of HSTCL. Thirty-six cases had used either 6-MP or azathioprine, and 28 cases had used infliximab. Of these 28 cases, 27 had also used 6-MP or azathioprine. The other case had a history of both infliximab and adalimumab exposure.

Skin lesions New-onset psoriasiform skin lesions develop in nearly 5% of IBD patients treated with anti-TNF therapy. Most often, these can be treated topically, and rarely, anti-TNF therapy must be decreased, switched, or stopped. The risk of melanoma is increased almost twofold with anti-TNF and not thiopurine use. The risk of nonmelanoma skin cancer is increased with thiopurines and biologics, especially with 1 year of follow-up or greater. Patients on these medications should have a skin check at least once a year.

Infections All of the anti-TNF drugs are associated with an increased risk of infections, particularly reactivation of latent tuberculosis and opportunistic fungal infections including disseminated histoplasmosis and coccidioidomycosis. It is recommended that patients have a purified protein derivative (PPD) or a QuantiFERON-TB gold test as well as a chest x-ray before initiation of anti-TNF therapy. Patients over 65 have a higher rate of infections and death on infliximab or adalimumab than those younger than 65 years of age.

Other Acute liver injury due to reactivation of hepatitis B virus and to autoimmune effects and cholestasis has been reported. Rarely, infliximab and the other anti-TNF drugs have been associated with optic neuritis, seizures, new onset or exacerbation of clinical symptoms, and radiographic evidence of central nervous system demyelinating disorders, including multiple sclerosis. They may exacerbate symptoms in patients with New York Heart Association functional class III/IV heart failure.

Anti-integrins Integrins are expressed on the cell surface of leukocytes and serve as mediators of leukocyte adhesion to vascular endothelium. α4-Integrin along with its β1 or β7 subunit interact with endothelial ligands termed adhesion molecules. Interaction between α4β7 and mucosal addressin cellular adhesion molecule (MAdCAM-1) is important in lymphocyte trafficking to gut mucosa.

Natalizumab is a recombinant humanized IgG4 antibody against α4-integrin that has been shown to be effective in induction and maintenance of patients with CD. It has been approved since February 2008 for the treatment of patients with CD refractory or intolerant to anti-TNF therapy. The rates of response and remission at 3 months are about 60% and 40%, respectively, with a sustained remission rate of about 40% at 36 weeks.

One case of progressive multifocal leukoencephalopathy (PML) after eight infusions of natalizumab was observed among 1043 patients in the clinical trials for CD, and two patients developed PML in the multiple sclerosis (MS) trials after a median of 120 weeks. There were 410 postmarketing cases of PML, 408 in MS and 2 in CD. The most important risk factor for development of PML is exposure to the John Cunningham (JC) polyomavirus, seen in 50–55% of the adult population. The other two risk factors for development of PML are longer duration of treatment, especially beyond 2 years, and prior treatment with an immunosuppressant medication. Patients with all three risk factors have an estimated risk of 11:1000.

The FDA approved a commercial enzyme-linked immunosorbent assay (ELISA) kit to assay anti-JC viral antibodies (Stratify JCV Antibody ELISA; Focus Diagnostics, Cypress, CA) in early 2012. The test is 99% accurate in stratifying risk of PML. It is recommended that all patients be tested prior to initiating natalizumab therapy. JC virus serologies are then measured every 6 months because 1–2% of patients will seroconvert yearly. All patients taking natalizumab and their providers must be enrolled in the TOUCH (Tysabri Outreach Unified Commitment for Health) pharmacovigilance program. Natalizumab is administered IV, 300 mg every 4 weeks. Labeling requirements mandate that it not be used in combination with any immunosuppressant medications.

Vedolizumab, another leukocyte trafficking inhibitor, is indicated for patients who have had an inadequate response or lost response to, or were intolerant of a TNF blocker or immunomodulator; or had an inadequate response or were intolerant to, or demonstrated dependence on glucocorticoids. It is an option for patients who are JC antibody positive since it does not cross the blood-brain barrier. Vedolizumab is a monoclonal antibody directed against α4β7 integrin specifically and has the ability to convey gut-selective immunosuppression.

THERAPIES IN DEVELOPMENT *Ustekinumab*, a fully human IgG1 monoclonal antibody, blocks the biologic activity of IL-12 and IL-23 through their common p40 subunit by inhibiting the interaction of these cytokines with their receptors on T cells, natural killer cells, and antigen presenting cells. It shows efficacy in moderate to severe CD in clinical trials.

Tofacitinib is an oral inhibitor of Janus kinases 1, 3, and, to a lesser extent, 2. It is expected to block signaling involving common gamma chain–containing cytokines including IL-2, IL-4, IL-7, IL-9, IL-15, and IL-21. These cytokines are integral to lymphocyte activation, function, and proliferation. It is effective in moderate to severe UC in clinical trials.

NUTRITIONAL THERAPIES Dietary antigens may stimulate the mucosal immune response. Patients with active CD respond to bowel rest, along with TPN. Bowel rest and TPN are as effective as glucocorticoids at inducing remission of active CD but are not effective as maintenance therapy. Enteral nutrition in the form of elemental or peptide-based preparations is also as effective as glucocorticoids or TPN, but these diets are not palatable. Enteral diets may provide the small intestine with nutrients vital to cell growth and do not have the complications of TPN. In contrast to CD, dietary intervention does not reduce inflammation in UC. Standard medical management of UC and CD is shown in Fig. 18-12.

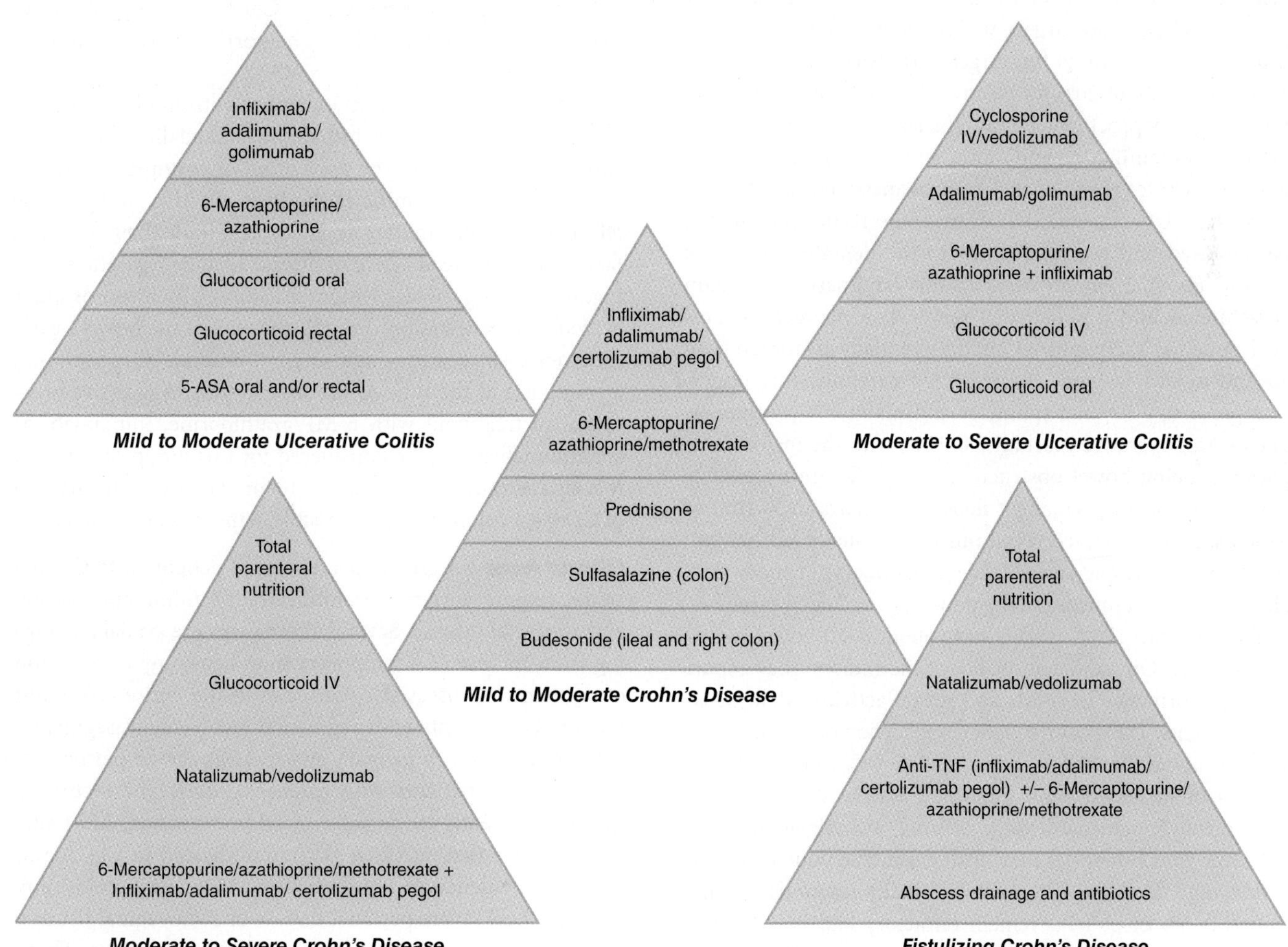

FIGURE 18-12
Medical management of inflammatory bowel disease. 5-ASA, 5-aminosalicylic acid; CD, Crohn's disease; UC, ulcerative colitis.

TABLE 18-8

INDICATIONS FOR SURGERY

ULCERATIVE COLITIS	CROHN'S DISEASE
Intractable disease	Small Intestine
Fulminant disease	Stricture and obstruction
Toxic megacolon	unresponsive to medical therapy
Colonic perforation	Massive hemorrhage
Massive colonic hemorrhage	Refractory fistula
Extracolonic disease	Abscess
Colonic obstruction	Colon and rectum
Colon cancer prophylaxis	Intractable disease
Colon dysplasia or cancer	Fulminant disease
	Perianal disease unresponsive to medical therapy
	Refractory fistula
	Colonic obstruction
	Cancer prophylaxis
	Colon dysplasia or cancer

SURGICAL THERAPY

Ulcerative colitis Nearly one-half of patients with extensive chronic UC undergo surgery within the first 10 years of their illness. The indications for surgery are listed in Table 18-8. Morbidity is about 20% for elective, 30% for urgent, and 40% for emergency proctocolectomy. The risks are primarily hemorrhage, contamination and sepsis, and neural injury. The operation of choice is an ileoanal J pouch anastomosis (IPAA).

Because UC is a mucosal disease, the rectal mucosa can be dissected and removed down to the dentate line of the anus or about 2 cm proximal to this landmark. The ileum is fashioned into a pouch that serves as a neorectum. This ileal pouch is then sutured circumferentially to the anus in an end-to-end fashion. If performed carefully, this operation preserves the anal sphincter and maintains continence. The overall operative morbidity is 10%, with the major complication being bowel obstruction. Pouch failure necessitating conversion to permanent ileostomy occurs in 5–10% of patients. Some inflamed rectal mucosa is usually left behind, and thus endoscopic surveillance is necessary. Primary dysplasia of the ileal mucosa of the pouch has occurred rarely.

Patients with IPAA usually have about 6–10 bowel movements a day. On validated quality-of-life indices, they report better performance in sports and sexual activities than ileostomy patients. The most frequent complication of IPAA is pouchitis in about 30–50% of patients with UC. This syndrome consists of increased stool frequency, watery stools, cramping, urgency, nocturnal leakage of stool, arthralgias, malaise, and fever. Pouch biopsies may distinguish true pouchitis from underlying CD. Although pouchitis usually responds to antibiotics, 3–5% of patients remain refractory and may require glucocorticoids, immunomodulators, anti-TNF therapy, or even pouch removal. A highly concentrated probiotic preparation with four strains of *Lactobacillus,* three strains of *Bifidobacterium,* and one strain of *Streptococcus salivarius* can prevent the recurrence of pouchitis when taken daily.

Crohn's disease Most patients with CD require at least one operation in their lifetime. The need for surgery is related to duration of disease and the site of involvement. Patients with small-bowel disease have an 80% chance of requiring surgery. Those with colitis alone have a 50% chance. Surgery is an option only when medical treatment has failed or complications dictate its necessity. The indications for surgery are shown in Table 18-8.

Small intestinal disease Because CD is chronic and recurrent, with no clear surgical cure, as little intestine as possible is resected. Current surgical alternatives for treatment of obstructing CD include resection of the diseased segment and strictureplasty. Surgical resection of the diseased segment is the most frequently performed operation, and in most cases, primary anastomosis can be done to restore continuity. If much of the small bowel has already been resected and the strictures are short, with intervening areas of normal mucosa, strictureplasties should be done to avoid a functionally insufficient length of bowel. The strictured area of intestine is incised longitudinally and the incision sutured transversely, thus widening the narrowed area. Complications of strictureplasty include prolonged ileus, hemorrhage, fistula, abscess, leak, and restricture.

There is evidence that mesalamine, nitroimidazole antibiotics, 6-MP/azathioprine, infliximab, and adalimumab are all superior to placebo for the prevention of postoperative recurrence of CD. Mesalamine is the least effective, and the side effects of the nitroimidazole antibiotics limit their use. Risk factors for early recurrence of disease include cigarette smoking, penetrating disease (internal fistulas, abscesses, or other evidence of penetration through the wall of the bowel), early recurrence since a previous surgery, multiple surgeries, and a young age at the time of the first surgery. Aggressive postoperative treatment with 6-MP/azathioprine, infliximab, or adalimumab should be considered for this group of patients. It is also recommended to evaluate for endoscopic recurrence of CD via a colonoscopy, if possible, 6 months after surgery.

Colorectal disease A greater percentage of patients with Crohn's colitis require surgery for intractability, fulminant disease, and anorectal disease. Several alternatives are available, ranging from the use of a temporary loop ileostomy to resection of segments of diseased colon or even the entire colon and rectum. For patients with segmental involvement, segmental colon resection with primary anastomosis can be performed. In 20–25% of patients with extensive colitis, the rectum is spared sufficiently to consider rectal preservation. Most surgeons believe that an IPAA is contraindicated in CD due to the high incidence of pouch failure. A diverting colostomy may help heal severe perianal disease or rectovaginal fistulas, but disease almost always recurs with reanastomosis. These patients often require a total proctocolectomy and ileostomy.

INFLAMMATORY BOWEL DISEASE AND PREGNANCY

Patients with quiescent UC and CD have normal fertility rates; the fallopian tubes can be scarred by the inflammatory process of CD, especially on the right side because of the proximity of the terminal ileum. In addition, perirectal, perineal, and rectovaginal abscesses and fistulae can result in dyspareunia. Infertility in men can be caused by sulfasalazine but reverses when treatment is stopped. In women who have an ileoanal J pouch anastomosis, most studies show that the fertility rate is reduced to about 50–80% of normal. This is due to scarring or occlusion of the fallopian tubes secondary to pelvic inflammation.

In mild or quiescent UC and CD, fetal outcome is nearly normal. Spontaneous abortions, stillbirths, and developmental defects are increased with increased disease activity, not medications. The courses of CD and UC during pregnancy mostly correlate with disease activity at the time of conception. Patients should be in remission for 6 months before conceiving. Most CD patients can deliver vaginally, but cesarean delivery may be the preferred route of delivery for patients with anorectal and perirectal abscesses and fistulas to reduce the likelihood of fistulas developing or extending into the episiotomy scar. Unless they desire multiple children, UC patients with an IPAA should consider a cesarean delivery due to an increased risk of future fecal incontinence.

Sulfasalazine, Lialda, Apriso, Delzicol, and balsalazide are safe for use in pregnancy and nursing with the caveat that additional folate supplementation must be given with sulfasalazine. Asacol HD and olsalazine are considered by the FDA to be class C agents in pregnancy and thus not recommended. Topical 5-ASA agents are also safe during pregnancy and nursing. Glucocorticoids are generally safe for use during pregnancy and are indicated for patients with moderate to severe disease activity. The amount of glucocorticoids received by the nursing infant is minimal. The safest antibiotics to use for CD in pregnancy for short periods of time (weeks, not months) are ampicillin and cephalosporins. Metronidazole can be used in the second or third trimester. Ciprofloxacin causes cartilage lesions in immature animals and should be avoided because of the absence of data on its effects on growth and development in humans.

6-MP and azathioprine pose minimal or no risk during pregnancy, but experience is limited. If the patient cannot be weaned from the drug or has an exacerbation that requires 6-MP/azathioprine during pregnancy, she should continue the drug with informed consent. Breast milk has been shown to contain negligible levels of 6-MP/azathioprine when measured in a limited number of patients.

Little data exist on CSA in pregnancy. In a small number of patients with severe IBD treated with IV CSA during pregnancy, 80% of pregnancies were successfully completed without development of renal toxicity or congenital malformations. However, because of the lack of data, CSA should probably be avoided unless the patient would otherwise require surgery.

MTX is contraindicated in pregnancy and nursing. In a large prospective study, no increased risk of stillbirths, miscarriages, or spontaneous abortions was seen with infliximab, adalimumab, or certolizumab, which are all class B drugs. Infliximab and adalimumab are IgG1 antibodies and are actively transported across the placenta in the late second and third trimester. Infants can have serum levels of both infliximab and adalimumab up to 7 months of age, and live vaccines should be avoided during this time. Certolizumab crosses the placenta by passive diffusion, and infant serum and cord blood levels are minimal. The anti-TNF drugs are relatively safe in nursing. Miniscule levels of both infliximab and adalimumab, but not certolizumab, have been reported in breast milk. These levels are of no clinical significance. It is recommended that drugs not be switched during pregnancy unless necessitated by the medical condition of the IBD. Natalizumab is considered as a class C drug because there is limited data in pregnancy.

Surgery in UC should be performed only for emergency indications, including severe hemorrhage, perforation, and megacolon refractory to medical therapy. Total colectomy and ileostomy carry a 50% risk of postoperative spontaneous abortion. Fetal mortality is also high in CD requiring surgery. Patients with IPAAs have increased nighttime stool frequency during pregnancy that resolves postpartum. Transient small-bowel obstruction or ileus has been noted in up to 8% of patients with ileostomies.

CANCER IN INFLAMMATORY BOWEL DISEASE

ULCERATIVE COLITIS

Patients with long-standing UC are at increased risk for developing colonic epithelial dysplasia and carcinoma (Fig. 18-13).

The risk of neoplasia in chronic UC increases with duration and extent of disease. From one large meta-analysis, the risk of cancer in patients with UC is estimated at 2% after 10 years, 8% after 20 years, and 18% after 30 years of disease. Data from a 30-year surveillance program in the United Kingdom calculated the risk of colorectal cancer to be 7.7% at 20 years and 15.8% at 30 years of disease. The rates of colon cancer are higher than in the general population, and colonoscopic surveillance is the standard of care.

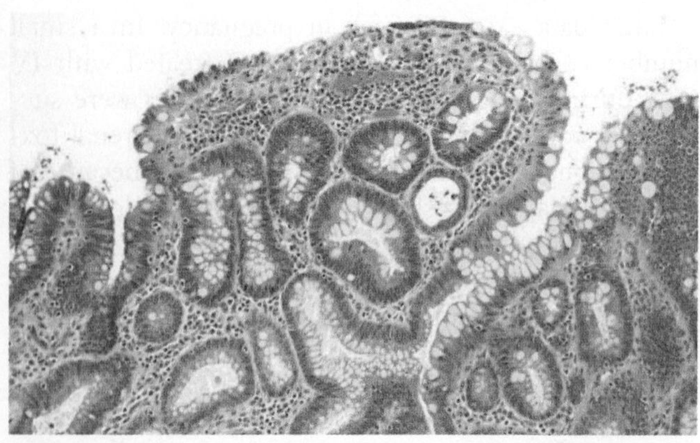

FIGURE 18-13

Medium-power view of low-grade dysplasia in a patient with chronic ulcerative colitis. Low-grade dysplastic crypts are interspersed among regenerating crypts. *(Courtesy of Dr. R. Odze, Division of Gastrointestinal Pathology, Department of Pathology, Brigham and Women's Hospital, Boston, Massachusetts; with permission.)*

Annual or biennial colonoscopy with multiple biopsies is recommended for patients with >8–10 years of extensive colitis (greater than one-third of the colon involved) or 12–15 years of proctosigmoiditis (less than one-third but more than just the rectum) and has been widely used to screen and survey for subsequent dysplasia and carcinoma. Risk factors for cancer in UC include long-duration disease, extensive disease, family history of colon cancer, PSC, a colon stricture, and the presence of postinflammatory pseudopolyps on colonoscopy.

CROHN'S DISEASE

Risk factors for developing cancer in Crohn's colitis are long-duration and extensive disease, bypassed colon segments, colon strictures, PSC, and family history of colon cancer. The cancer risks in CD and UC are probably equivalent for similar extent and duration of disease. In the CESAME study, a prospective observational cohort of IBD patients in France, the standardized incidence ratios of colorectal cancer were 2.2 for all IBD patients (95% confidence interval [CI], 1.5–3.0; $p < .001$) and 7.0 for patients with long-standing extensive colitis (both Crohn's and UC) (95% CI, 4.4–10.5; $p < .001$). Thus, the same endoscopic surveillance strategy used for UC is recommended for patients with chronic Crohn's colitis. A pediatric colonoscope can be used to pass narrow strictures in CD patients, but surgery should be considered in symptomatic patients with impassable strictures.

MANAGEMENT OF DYSPLASIA AND CANCER

Dysplasia can be flat or polypoid. If flat high-grade dysplasia is encountered on colonoscopic surveillance, the usual treatment is colectomy for UC and either colectomy or segmental resection for CD. If flat low-grade dysplasia is found (Fig. 18-13), most investigators recommend immediate colectomy. Adenomas may occur coincidently in UC and CD patients with chronic colitis and can be removed endoscopically provided that biopsies of the surrounding mucosa are free of dysplasia. High-definition and high-magnification colonoscopes and dye sprays have increased the rate of dysplasia detection.

IBD patients are also at greater risk for other malignancies. Patients with CD may have an increased risk of non-Hodgkin's lymphoma, leukemia, and myelodysplastic syndromes. Severe, chronic, complicated perianal disease in CD patients may be associated with an increased risk of cancer in the lower rectum and anal canal (squamous cell cancers). Although the absolute risk of small-bowel adenocarcinoma in CD is low (2.2% at 25 years in one study), patients with long-standing, extensive, small-bowel disease should consider screening.

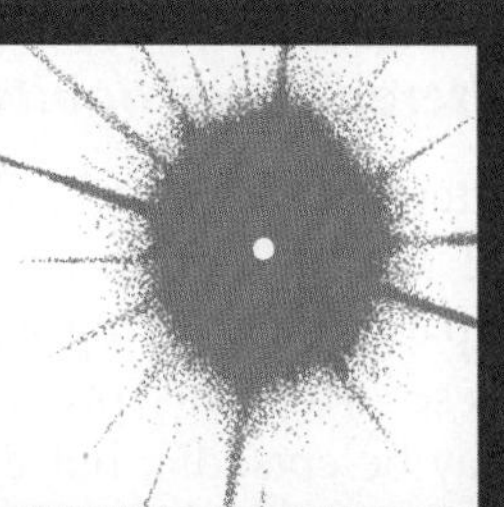

CHAPTER 19
IRRITABLE BOWEL SYNDROME

Chung Owyang

Irritable bowel syndrome (IBS) is a functional bowel disorder characterized by abdominal pain or discomfort and altered bowel habits in the absence of detectable structural abnormalities. No clear diagnostic markers exist for IBS; thus the diagnosis of the disorder is based on clinical presentation. In 2006, the Rome II criteria for the diagnosis of IBS were revised (Table 19-1). Throughout the world, about 10–20% of adults and adolescents have symptoms consistent with IBS, and most studies show a female predominance. IBS symptoms tend to come and go over time and often overlap with other functional disorders such as fibromyalgia, headache, backache, and genitourinary symptoms. Severity of symptoms varies and can significantly impair quality of life, resulting in high health care costs. Advances in basic, mechanistic, and clinical investigations have improved our understanding of this disorder and its physiologic and psychosocial determinants. Altered gastrointestinal (GI) motility, visceral hyperalgesia, disturbance of brain-gut interaction, abnormal central processing, autonomic and hormonal events, genetic and environmental factors, and psychosocial disturbances are variably involved, depending on the individual. This progress may result in improved methods of treatment.

TABLE 19-1

DIAGNOSTIC CRITERIA FOR IRRITABLE BOWEL SYNDROME[a]
Recurrent abdominal pain or discomfort[b] at least 3 days per month in the last 3 months associated with two or more of the following:
1. Improvement with defecation
2. Onset associated with a change in frequency of stool
3. Onset associated with a change in form (appearance) of stool

[a]Criteria fulfilled for the last 3 months with symptom onset at least 6 months prior to diagnosis.

[b]Discomfort means an uncomfortable sensation not described as pain. In pathophysiology research and clinical trials, a pain/discomfort frequency of at least 2 days a week during screening evaluation is required for subject eligibility.

Source: Adapted from GF Longstreth et al: *Gastroenterology* 130:1480, 2006.

CLINICAL FEATURES

IBS is a disorder that affects all ages, although most patients have their first symptoms before age 45. Older individuals have a lower reporting frequency. Women are diagnosed with IBS two to three times as often as men and make up 80% of the population with severe IBS. As indicated in Table 19-1, pain or abdominal discomfort is a key symptom for the diagnosis of IBS. These symptoms should be improved with defecation and/or have their onset associated with a change in frequency or form of stool. Painless diarrhea or constipation does not fulfill the diagnostic criteria to be classified as IBS. Supportive symptoms that are not part of the diagnostic criteria include defecation straining, urgency or a feeling of incomplete bowel movement, passing mucus, and bloating.

Abdominal pain

According to the current IBS diagnostic criteria, abdominal pain or discomfort is a prerequisite clinical feature of IBS. Abdominal pain in IBS is highly variable in intensity and location. It is frequently episodic and crampy, but it may be superimposed on a background of constant ache. Pain may be mild enough to be ignored or it may interfere with daily activities. Despite this, malnutrition due to inadequate caloric intake is exceedingly rare with IBS. Sleep deprivation is also unusual because abdominal pain is almost uniformly present only during waking hours. However, patients with severe IBS frequently wake repeatedly during the night; thus, nocturnal pain is a poor discriminating factor between organic and functional bowel disease. Pain is often exacerbated by eating or emotional stress and improved by passage of flatus or stools. In addition, female patients with IBS commonly report worsening symptoms during the premenstrual and menstrual phases.

Altered bowel habits

Alteration in bowel habits is the most consistent clinical feature in IBS. The most common pattern is constipation alternating with diarrhea, usually with one of these symptoms predominating. At first, constipation may be episodic, but eventually it becomes continuous and increasingly intractable to treatment with laxatives. Stools are usually hard with narrowed caliber, possibly reflecting excessive dehydration caused by prolonged colonic retention and spasm. Most patients also experience a sense of incomplete evacuation, thus leading to repeated attempts at defecation in a short time span. Patients whose predominant symptom is constipation may have weeks or months of constipation interrupted with brief periods of diarrhea. In other patients, diarrhea may be the predominant symptom. Diarrhea resulting from IBS usually consists of small volumes of loose stools. Most patients have stool volumes of <200 mL. Nocturnal diarrhea does not occur in IBS. Diarrhea may be aggravated by emotional stress or eating. Stool may be accompanied by passage of large amounts of mucus. Bleeding is not a feature of IBS unless hemorrhoids are present, and malabsorption or weight loss does not occur.

Bowel pattern subtypes are highly unstable. In a patient population with ~33% prevalence rates of IBS-diarrhea predominant (IBS-D), IBS-constipation predominant (IBS-C), and IBS-mixed (IBS-M) forms, 75% of patients change subtypes and 29% switch between IBS-C and IBS-D over 1 year. The heterogeneity and variable natural history of bowel habits in IBS increase the difficulty of conducting pathophysiology studies and clinical trials.

Gas and flatulence

Patients with IBS frequently complain of abdominal distention and increased belching or flatulence, all of which they attribute to increased gas. Although some patients with these symptoms actually may have a larger amount of gas, quantitative measurements reveal that most patients who complain of increased gas generate no more than a normal amount of intestinal gas. Most IBS patients have impaired transit and tolerance of intestinal gas loads. In addition, patients with IBS tend to reflux gas from the distal to the more proximal intestine, which may explain the belching.

Some patients with bloating may also experience visible distention with increase in abdominal girth. Both symptoms are more common among female patients and in those with higher overall Somatic Symptom Checklist scores. IBS patients who experienced bloating alone have been shown to have lower thresholds for pain and desire to defecate compared to those with concomitant distention irrespective of bowel habit. When patients were grouped according to sensory threshold, hyposensitive individuals had distention significantly more than those with hypersensitivity and this was observed more in the constipation subgroup. This suggests that the pathogenesis of bloating and distention may not be the same.

Upper gastrointestinal symptoms

Between 25 and 50% of patients with IBS complain of dyspepsia, heartburn, nausea, and vomiting. This suggests that other areas of the gut apart from the colon may be involved. Prolonged ambulant recordings of small-bowel motility in patients with IBS show a high incidence of abnormalities in the small bowel during the diurnal (waking) period; nocturnal motor patterns are not different from those of healthy controls. The overlap between dyspepsia and IBS is great. The prevalence of IBS is higher among patients with dyspepsia (31.7%) than among those who reported no symptoms of dyspepsia (7.9%). Conversely, among patients with IBS, 55.6% reported symptoms of dyspepsia. In addition, the functional abdominal symptoms can change over time. Those with predominant dyspepsia or IBS can flux between the two. Although the prevalence of functional gastrointestinal disorders is stable over time, the turnover in symptom status is high. Many episodes of symptom disappearance are due to subjects changing symptoms rather than total symptom resolution. Thus it is conceivable that functional dyspepsia and IBS are two manifestations of a single, more extensive digestive system disorder. Furthermore, IBS symptoms are prevalent in noncardiac chest pain patients, suggesting overlap with other functional gut disorders.

PATHOPHYSIOLOGY

The pathogenesis of IBS is poorly understood, although roles of abnormal gut motor and sensory activity, central neural dysfunction, psychological disturbances, mucosal inflammation, stress, and luminal factors have been proposed.

Gastrointestinal motor abnormalities

Studies of colonic myoelectrical and motor activity under unstimulated conditions have not shown consistent abnormalities in IBS. In contrast, colonic motor abnormalities are more prominent under stimulated conditions in IBS. IBS patients may exhibit increased rectosigmoid motor activity for up to 3 h after eating. Similarly, inflation of rectal balloons both in IBS-D and IBS-C patients leads to marked and prolonged distention-evoked contractile activity. Recordings from the transverse, descending, and sigmoid colon showed that the motility index and peak amplitude of high-amplitude propagating contractions (HAPCs) in diarrhea-prone IBS patients were greatly increased compared to those in healthy subjects and were associated with rapid colonic transit and accompanied by abdominal pain.

Visceral hypersensitivity

As with studies of motor activity, IBS patients frequently exhibit exaggerated sensory responses to visceral stimulation. The frequency of perceptions of food intolerance is at least twofold more common than in the general population. Postprandial pain has been temporally related to entry of the food bolus into the cecum in 74% of patients. On the other hand, prolonged fasting in IBS patients is often associated with significant improvement in symptoms. Rectal balloon inflation produces nonpainful and painful sensations at lower volumes in IBS patients than in healthy controls without altering rectal tension, suggestive of visceral afferent dysfunction in IBS. Similar studies show gastric and esophageal hypersensitivity in patients with nonulcer dyspepsia and noncardiac chest pain, raising the possibility that these conditions have a similar pathophysiologic basis. Lipids lower the thresholds for the first sensation of gas, discomfort, and pain in IBS patients. Hence, postprandial symptoms in IBS patients may be explained in part by a nutrient-dependent exaggerated sensory component of the gastrocolonic response. In contrast to enhanced gut sensitivity, IBS patients do not exhibit heightened sensitivity elsewhere in the body. Thus, the afferent pathway disturbances in IBS appear to be selective for visceral innervation with sparing of somatic pathways. The mechanisms responsible for visceral hypersensitivity are still under investigation. It has been proposed that these exaggerated responses may be due to (1) increased end-organ sensitivity with recruitment of "silent" nociceptors; (2) spinal hyperexcitability with activation of nitric oxide and possibly other neurotransmitters; (3) endogenous (cortical and brainstem) modulation of caudad nociceptive transmission; and (4) over time, the possible development of long-term hyperalgesia due to development of neuroplasticity, resulting in permanent or semipermanent changes in neural responses to chronic or recurrent visceral stimulation (Table 19-2).

TABLE 19-2

PROPOSED MECHANISMS FOR VISCERAL HYPERSENSITIVITY	
End-organ sensitivity	Long-term hyperalgesia
"Silent" nociceptors	Tonic cortical regulation
CNS modulation	Neuroplasticity
Cortex	
Brainstem	

Abbreviation: CNS, central nervous system.

Central neural dysregulation

The role of central nervous system (CNS) factors in the pathogenesis of IBS is strongly suggested by the clinical association of emotional disorders and stress with symptom exacerbation and the therapeutic response to therapies that act on cerebral cortical sites. Functional brain imaging studies such as magnetic resonance imaging (MRI) have shown that in response to distal colonic stimulation, the mid-cingulate cortex—a brain region concerned with attention processes and response selection—shows greater activation in IBS patients. Modulation of this region is associated with changes in the subjective unpleasantness of pain. In addition, IBS patients also show preferential activation of the prefrontal lobe, which contains a vigilance network within the brain that increases alertness. These may represent a form of cerebral dysfunction leading to the increased perception of visceral pain.

Abnormal psychological features

Abnormal psychiatric features are recorded in up to 80% of IBS patients, especially in referral centers; however, no single psychiatric diagnosis predominates. Most of these patients demonstrated exaggerated symptoms in response to visceral distention, and this abnormality persists even after exclusion of psychological factors.

Psychological factors influence pain thresholds in IBS patients, as stress alters sensory thresholds. An association between prior sexual or physical abuse and development of IBS has been reported. Abuse is associated with greater pain reporting, psychological distress, and poor health outcome. Brain functional MRI studies show greater activation of the posterior and middle dorsal cingulate cortex, which is implicated in affect processing in IBS patients with a past history of sexual abuse.

Thus, patients with IBS frequently demonstrate increased motor reactivity of the colon and small bowel to a variety of stimuli and altered visceral sensation associated with lowered sensation thresholds. These may result from CNS–enteric nervous system dysregulation (Fig. 19-1).

Postinfectious IBS

IBS may be induced by GI infection. In an investigation of 544 patients with confirmed bacterial gastroenteritis, one-quarter developed IBS subsequently. Conversely, about a third of IBS patients experienced an acute

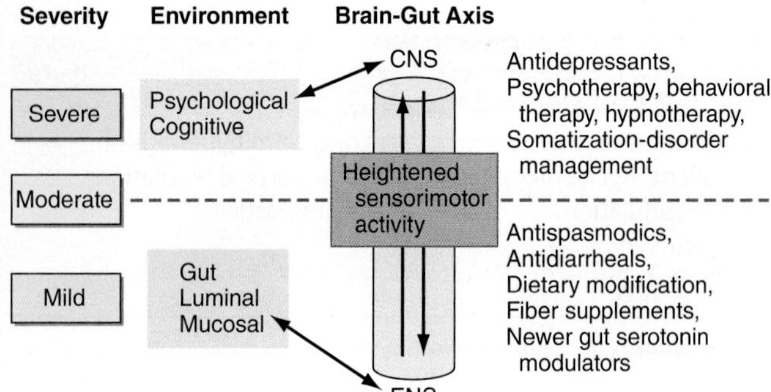

FIGURE 19-1

Therapeutic targets for irritable bowel syndrome. Patients with mild to moderate symptoms usually have intermittent symptoms that correlate with altered gut physiology. Treatments include gut-acting pharmacologic agents such as antispasmodics, antidiarrheals, fiber supplements, and gut serotonin modulators. Patients who have severe symptoms usually have constant pain and psychosocial difficulties. This group of patients is best managed with antidepressants and other psychosocial treatments. CNS, central nervous system; ENS, enteric nervous system.

"gastroenteritis-like" illness at the onset of their chronic IBS symptomatology. This group of "postinfective" IBS occurs more commonly in females and affects younger rather than older patients. Risk factors for developing postinfectious IBS include, in order of importance, prolonged duration of initial illness, toxicity of infecting bacterial strain, smoking, mucosal markers of inflammation, female gender, depression, hypochondriasis, and adverse life events in the preceding 3 months. Age older than 60 years might protect against postinfectious IBS, whereas treatment with antibiotics has been associated with increased risk. The microbes involved in the initial infection are *Campylobacter*, *Salmonella*, and *Shigella*. Those patients with *Campylobacter* infection who are toxin-positive are more likely to develop postinfective IBS. Increased rectal mucosal enteroendocrine cells, T lymphocytes, and increased gut permeability are acute changes following *Campylobacter* enteritis that could persist for more than a year and may contribute to postinfective IBS.

Immune activation and mucosal inflammation

Some patients with IBS display persistent signs of low-grade mucosal inflammation with activated lymphocytes, mast cells, and enhanced expression of proinflammatory cytokines. These abnormalities may contribute to abnormal epithelial secretion and visceral hypersensitivity. There is increasing evidence that some members of the superfamily of transient receptor potential (TRP) cation channels such as TRPV1 (vanilloid) channels are central to the initiation and persistence of visceral hypersensitivity. Mucosal inflammation can lead to increased expression of TRPV1 in the enteric nervous system. Enhanced expression of TRPV1 channels in the sensory neurons of the gut has been observed in IBS, and such expression appears to correlate with visceral hypersensitivity and abdominal pain. Interestingly, clinical studies have also shown increased intestinal permeability in patients with IBS-D. Psychological stress and anxiety can increase the release of proinflammatory cytokine, and this in turn may alter intestinal permeability. This provides a functional link between psychological stress, immune activation, and symptom generation in patients with IBS.

Altered gut flora

A high prevalence of small intestinal bacterial overgrowth in IBS patients has been noted based on positive lactulose hydrogen breath test. This finding, however, has been challenged by a number of other studies that found no increased incidence of bacterial overgrowth based on jejunal aspirate culture. Abnormal H_2 breath test can occur because of small-bowel rapid transit and may lead to erroneous interpretation. Hence, the role of testing for small intestinal bacterial overgrowth in IBS patients remains unclear.

Studies using culture-independent approaches such as 16S rRNA gene-based analysis found significant differences between the molecular profile of the fecal microbiota of IBS patients and that of healthy subjects. IBS patients had decreased proportions of the genera *Bifidobacterium* and *Lactobacillus* and increased ratios of Firmicutes:Bacteroidetes. It has been speculated that these changes may be related to stress and diet. A temporary reduction in lactobacilli has been reported in animal models of early-life stress. On the other hand, Firmicutes is the dominant phylum in adults consuming a diet high in animal fat and protein. However, it is still unclear whether such changes in fecal microbiota are causal, consequential, or merely the result of constipation and diarrhea. In addition, the stability of the change in the microbiota needs to be determined.

Abnormal serotonin pathways

The serotonin (5-HT)-containing enterochromaffin cells in the colon are increased in a subset of IBS-D patients compared to healthy individuals or patients with ulcerative colitis. Furthermore, postprandial plasma 5-HT levels were significantly higher in this group of patients compared to healthy controls. Because serotonin plays an important role in the regulation of GI motility and visceral perception, the increased release of serotonin may contribute to the postprandial symptoms of these patients and provides a rationale for the use of serotonin antagonists in the treatment of this disorder.

APPROACH TO THE PATIENT: Irritable Bowel Syndrome

Because IBS is a disorder for which no pathognomonic abnormalities have been identified, its diagnosis relies on recognition of positive clinical features and elimination of other organic diseases. Symptom-based criteria have been developed for the purpose of differentiating patients with IBS from those with organic diseases. These include the Manning, Rome I, Rome II, and Rome III criteria (Table 19-1). The diagnostic values of these criteria are shown in Table 19-3. In a validation study, Rome III performed less well than either the Rome I and II criteria and all criteria studied to date showed positive predictive values of <50%, which underscores the need for developing diagnostic strategies for IBS that are more cost-effective than the current approaches. A careful history and physical examination are frequently helpful in establishing the diagnosis. Clinical features suggestive of IBS include the following: recurrence of lower abdominal pain with altered bowel habits over a period of time without progressive deterioration, onset of symptoms during periods of stress or emotional upset, absence of other systemic symptoms such as fever and weight loss, and small-volume stool without any evidence of blood.

On the other hand, the appearance of the disorder for the first time in old age, progressive course from time of onset, persistent diarrhea after a 48-h fast, and presence of nocturnal diarrhea or steatorrheal stools argue against the diagnosis of IBS.

Because the major symptoms of IBS—abdominal pain, abdominal bloating, and alteration in bowel habits—are common complaints of many GI organic disorders, the list of differential diagnoses is a long one. The quality, location, and timing of pain may be helpful to suggest specific disorders. Pain due to IBS that occurs in the epigastric or periumbilical area must be differentiated from biliary tract disease, peptic ulcer disorders, intestinal ischemia, and carcinoma of the stomach and pancreas. If pain occurs mainly in the lower abdomen, the possibility of diverticular disease of the colon, inflammatory bowel disease (including ulcerative colitis and Crohn's disease), and carcinoma of the colon must be considered. Postprandial pain accompanied by bloating, nausea, and vomiting suggests gastroparesis or partial intestinal obstruction. Intestinal infestation with *Giardia lamblia* or other parasites may cause similar symptoms. When diarrhea is the major complaint, the possibility of lactase deficiency, laxative abuse, malabsorption, celiac sprue, hyperthyroidism, inflammatory bowel disease, and infectious diarrhea must be ruled out. On the other hand, constipation may be a side effect of many different drugs, such as anticholinergic, antihypertensive, and antidepressant medications.

Endocrinopathies such as hypothyroidism and hypoparathyroidism must also be considered in the differential diagnosis of constipation, particularly if other systemic signs or symptoms of these endocrinopathies are present. In addition, acute intermittent porphyria and lead poisoning may present in a fashion similar to IBS, with painful constipation as the major complaint. These possibilities are suspected on the basis of their clinical presentations and are confirmed by appropriate serum and urine tests.

Few tests are required for patients who have typical IBS symptoms and no alarm features. Unnecessary investigations may be costly and even harmful. The American Gastroenterological Association has delineated factors to be considered when determining the aggressiveness of the diagnostic evaluation. These include the duration of symptoms, the change in symptoms over time, the age and sex of the patient, the referral status of the patient, prior diagnostic studies, a family history of colorectal malignancy, and the degree of psychosocial dysfunction. Thus, a younger individual with mild symptoms requires a minimal diagnostic evaluation, while an older person or an individual with rapidly progressive symptoms should undergo a more thorough exclusion of organic disease. Most patients should have a complete blood count and sigmoidoscopic examination; in addition, stool specimens should be examined for ova and parasites in those who have diarrhea. In patients with persistent diarrhea not responding to simple

TABLE 19-3

SENSITIVITY, SPECIFICITY, POSITIVE AND NEGATIVE PREDICTIVE VALUES, AND POSITIVE AND NEGATIVE LIKELIHOOD RATIOS FOR THE ROME AND MANNING CRITERIA FOR IRRITABLE BOWEL SYNDROME[a]

	SENSITIVITY, % (95% CI)	SPECIFICITY, % (95% CI)	POSITIVE PREDICTIVE VALUE, % (95% CI)	NEGATIVE PREDICTIVE VALUE, % (95% CI)	POSITIVE LIKELIHOOD RATIO (95% CI)	NEGATIVE LIKELIHOOD RATIO (95% CI)
Rome III criteria	17.4 (13.9–21.5)	95.6 (94.4–96.5)	49.6 (42.0–58.7)	82.1 (80.0–83.6)	3.92 (2.85–5.38)	0.86 (0.83–0.91)
Rome II criteria	23.3 (19.4–27.8)	94.5 (93.2–95.5)	51.7 (44.9–59.5)	82.9 (80.8–84.4)	4.21 (3.20–5.53)	0.81 (0.77–0.86)
Rome I criteria	24.3 (20.3–28.8)	93.9 (92.6–95.0)	50.5 (44.0–58.1)	83.0 (80.9–84.4)	4.01 (3.08–5.22)	0.81 (0.76–0.85)
Manning criteria (3 criteria)	13.7 (10.6–17.6)	97.1 (96.1–97.8)	54.1 (45.3–64.6)	81.6 (79.6–83.1)	4.66 (3.18–6.82)	0.89 (0.85–0.93)

[a]Excluding individuals reporting lower gastrointestinal alarm symptoms from the definition of irritable bowel syndrome.
Source: Adapted from AC Ford et al: *Gastroenterology* 145:1262, 2013.

antidiarrheal agents, a sigmoid colon biopsy should be performed to rule out microscopic colitis. In those age >40 years, an air-contrast barium enema or colonoscopy should also be performed. If the main symptoms are diarrhea and increased gas, the possibility of lactase deficiency should be ruled out with a hydrogen breath test or with evaluation after a 3-week lactose-free diet. Some patients with IBS-D may have undiagnosed celiac sprue. Because the symptoms of celiac sprue respond to a gluten-free diet, testing for celiac sprue in IBS may prevent years of morbidity and attendant expense. Decision-analysis studies show that serology testing for celiac sprue in patients with IBS-D has an acceptable cost when the prevalence of celiac sprue is >1% and is the dominant strategy when the prevalence is >8%. In patients with concurrent symptoms of dyspepsia, upper GI radiographs or esophagogastroduodenoscopy may be advisable. In patients with postprandial right upper quadrant pain, an ultrasonogram of the gallbladder should be obtained. Laboratory features that argue against IBS include evidence of anemia, elevated sedimentation rate, presence of leukocytes or blood in stool, and stool volume >200–300 mL/d. These findings would necessitate other diagnostic considerations.

TREATMENT Irritable Bowel Syndrome

PATIENT COUNSELING AND DIETARY ALTERATIONS Reassurance and careful explanation of the functional nature of the disorder and of how to avoid obvious food precipitants are important first steps in patient counseling and dietary change. Occasionally, a meticulous dietary history may reveal substances (such as coffee, disaccharides, legumes, and cabbage) that aggravate symptoms. Excessive fructose and artificial sweeteners, such as sorbitol or mannitol, may cause diarrhea, bloating, cramping, or flatulence. As a therapeutic trial, patients should be encouraged to eliminate any foodstuffs that appear to produce symptoms. However patients should avoid nutritionally depleted diets. A diet low in fermentable oligosaccharides, disaccharides, monosaccharides, and polyols (FODMAPs) (Table 19-4) has been shown to be helpful in IBS patients. FODMAPs are poorly absorbed by the small intestine and fermented by bacteria in the colon to produce gas and osmotically active carbohydrates. Clinical studies demonstrate that in IBS patients, ingestion of FODMAPs such as lactose, fructose, or sorbitol, alone or in combination, produce gut symptoms such as gas and diarrhea. On the other hand, a randomized controlled study showed that a diet low in FODMAPs reduced symptoms in IBS patients. This approach may be used in diarrhea-predominant IBS patients with severe gas and bloating. Durable adherence can be expected in up to 75% of patients.

Stool-bulking agents High-fiber diets and bulking agents, such as bran or hydrophilic colloid, are frequently used in treating IBS. The water-holding action of fibers may contribute to increased stool bulk because of the ability of fiber to increase fecal output of bacteria. Fiber also speeds up colonic transit in most persons. In diarrhea-prone patients, whole-colonic transit is faster than average; however, dietary fiber can delay transit. Furthermore, because of their hydrophilic properties, stool-bulking agents bind water and thus prevent both excessive hydration and dehydration of stool. The latter observation may explain the clinical experience that a high-fiber diet relieves diarrhea in some IBS patients. Fiber supplementation with psyllium has been shown to reduce perception of rectal distention, indicating that fiber may have a positive effect on visceral afferent function.

The beneficial effects of dietary fiber on colonic physiology suggest that dietary fiber should be an effective treatment for IBS patients, but controlled trials of dietary fiber have produced variable results. This is not surprising since IBS is a heterogeneous disorder, with some patients being constipated and other having predominant diarrhea. Most investigations report increases in stool weight, decreases in colonic transit times, and improvement in constipation. Others have noted benefits in patients with alternating diarrhea and constipation, pain, and bloating. However, most studies observe no responses in patients with diarrhea- or pain-predominant IBS. It is possible that different fiber preparations may have dissimilar effects on selected symptoms in IBS. A cross-over comparison of different fiber preparations found that psyllium produced greater improvements in stool pattern and abdominal pain than bran. Furthermore, psyllium preparations tend to produce less bloating and distention. Despite the equivocal data regarding efficacy, most gastroenterologists consider stool-bulking agents worth trying in patients with IBS-C. Fiber should be started at a nominal dose and slowly titrated up as tolerated over the course of several weeks to a targeted dose of 20–30 g of total dietary and supplementary fiber per day. Even when used judiciously, fiber can exacerbate bloating, flatulence, constipation, and diarrhea.

Antispasmodics Clinicians have observed that anticholinergic drugs may provide temporary relief for symptoms such as painful cramps related to intestinal spasm. Although controlled clinical trials have produced mixed results, evidence generally supports beneficial effects of anticholinergic drugs for pain. A meta-analysis of 26 double-blind clinical trials of antispasmodic agents in IBS reported better global improvement (62%) and abdominal pain reductions (64%) compared to placebo (35% and 45%, respectively), suggesting efficacy in some patients. The drugs are most effective when prescribed in anticipation of predictable pain. Physiologic studies demonstrate that anticholinergic drugs inhibit the gastrocolic reflex; hence, postprandial pain is best managed by giving antispasmodics 30 min before meals so that effective blood levels are achieved shortly before the anticipated onset of pain. Most anticholinergics contain natural belladonna alkaloids, which may cause xerostomia, urinary hesitancy and retention, blurred vision, and drowsiness. They should be used in the

TABLE 19-4

SOME COMMON FOOD SOURCES OF FODMAPs

FOOD TYPE	FREE FRUCTOSE	LACTOSE	FRUCTANS	GALACTO-OLIGOSACCHARIDES	POLYOLS
Fruits	Apple, cherry, mango, pear, watermelon		Peach, persimmon, watermelon		Apple, apricot, pear, avocado, blackberries, cherry, nectarine, plum, prune
Vegetables	Asparagus, artichokes, sugar snap peas		Artichokes, beetroot, Brussels sprout, chicory, fennel, garlic, leek, onion, peas		Cauliflower, mushroom, snow peas
Grains and cereals			Wheat, rye, barley		
Nuts and seeds			Pistachios		
Milk and milk products		Milk, yogurt, ice cream, custard, soft cheeses			
Legumes			Legumes, lentils, chickpeas	Legumes, chickpeas, lentils	
Other	Honey, high-fructose corn syrup		Chicory drinks		
Food additives			Inulin, FOS		Sorbitol, mannitol, maltitol, xylitol, isomalt

Abbreviations: FODMAPs, fermentable oligosaccharides, disaccharides, monosaccharides, and polyols; FOS, fructo-oligosaccharides
Source: Adapted from PR Gibson et al: *Am J Gastroenterol* 107:657, 2012.

elderly with caution. Some physicians prefer to use synthetic anticholinergics such as dicyclomine that have less effect on mucous membrane secretions and produce fewer undesirable side effects.

Antidiarrheal agents Peripherally acting opiate-based agents are the initial therapy of choice for IBS-D. Physiologic studies demonstrate increases in segmenting colonic contractions, delays in fecal transit, increases in anal pressures, and reductions in rectal perception with these drugs. When diarrhea is severe, especially in the painless diarrhea variant of IBS, small doses of loperamide, 2–4 mg every 4–6 h up to a maximum of 12 g/d, can be prescribed. These agents are less addictive than paregoric, codeine, or tincture of opium. In general, the intestines do not become tolerant of the antidiarrheal effect of opiates, and increasing doses are not required to maintain antidiarrheal potency. These agents are most useful if taken before anticipated stressful events that are known to cause diarrhea. However, not infrequently, a high dose of loperamide may cause cramping because of increases in segmenting colonic contractions. Another antidiarrheal agent that may be used in IBS patients is the bile acid binder cholestyramine resin.

Antidepressant drugs In addition to their mood-elevating effects, antidepressant medications have several physiologic effects that suggest they may be beneficial in IBS. In IBS-D patients, the tricyclic antidepressant imipramine slows jejunal migrating motor complex transit propagation and delays orocecal and whole-gut transit, indicative of a motor inhibitory effect. Some studies also suggest that tricyclic agents may alter visceral afferent neural function.

A number of studies indicate that tricyclic antidepressants may be effective in some IBS patients. In a 2-month study of desipramine, abdominal pain improved in 86% of patients compared to 59% given placebo. Another study of desipramine in 28 IBS patients showed improvement in stool frequency, diarrhea, pain, and depression. When stratified according to the predominant symptoms, improvements were observed in IBS-D patients, with no improvement being noted in IBS-C patients. The beneficial effects of the tricyclic compounds in the treatment of IBS appear to be independent of their effects on depression. The therapeutic benefits for the bowel symptoms occur faster and at a lower dosage. The efficacy of antidepressant agents in other chemical classes in the management of IBS is less well evaluated. In contrast to tricyclic agents, the selective serotonin reuptake inhibitor (SSRI) paroxetine accelerates orocecal transit, raising the possibility that this drug class may be useful in IBS-C patients. The SSRI citalopram blunts perception of rectal distention and reduces the magnitude of the gastrocolonic response in healthy volunteers. A small placebo-controlled study of citalopram in IBS patients reported reductions in pain. However, these findings could not be confirmed in another randomized controlled trial that showed that citalopram at 20 mg/d for 4 weeks was not superior to placebo in treating nondepressed IBS patients. Hence, the efficacy of SSRIs in the treatment of IBS needs further confirmation.

Antiflatulence therapy The management of excessive gas is seldom satisfactory, except when there is obvious aerophagia or disaccharidase deficiency. Patients should be advised to eat slowly and not chew gum or drink carbonated beverages. Bloating may decrease if an associated gut syndrome such as IBS or constipation is improved. If bloating is accompanied by diarrhea and worsens after ingesting dairy products, fresh fruits, vegetables, or juices, further investigation or a dietary exclusion trial may be worthwhile. Avoiding flatogenic foods, exercising, losing excess weight, and taking activated charcoal are safe but unproven remedies. Data regarding the use of surfactants such as simethicone are conflicting. Antibiotics may help in a subgroup of IBS patients with predominant symptoms of bloating. Beano, an over-the-counter oral β-glycosidase solution, may reduce rectal passage of gas without decreasing bloating and pain. Pancreatic enzymes reduce bloating, gas, and fullness during and after high-calorie, high-fat meal ingestion.

Modulation of gut flora Antibiotic treatment benefits a subset of IBS patients. In a double-blind, randomized, placebo-controlled study, neomycin dosed at 500 mg twice daily for 10 days was more effective than placebo at improving symptom scores among IBS patients. The nonabsorbed oral antibiotic rifaximin is the most thoroughly studied antibiotic for the treatment of IBS.

In a double-blind, placebo-controlled study, patients receiving rifaximin at a dose of 550 mg two times daily for 2 weeks experienced substantial improvement of global IBS symptoms over placebo. Rifaximin is the only antibiotic with demonstrated sustained benefit beyond therapy cessation in IBS patients. The drug has a favorable safety and tolerability profile compared with systemic antibiotics. A systematic review and meta-analysis of five studies of IBS patients found that rifaximin is more effective than placebo for global symptoms and bloating (odds ratio 1.57) with a number needed to treat (NNT) of 10.2. The modest therapeutic gain was similar to that yielded by other current available therapies for IBS. However, currently there are still insufficient data to recommend routine use of this antibiotic in the treatment of IBS.

Because altered colonic flora may contribute to the pathogenesis of IBS, this has led to great interest in using probiotics to naturally alter the flora. A meta-analysis of 10 probiotic studies in IBS patients found significant relief of pain and bloating with the use of *Bifidobacterium breve*, *B. longum*, and *Lactobacillus acidophilus* species compared to placebo. However, there was no change in stool frequency or consistency. Large-scale studies of well-phenotyped IBS patients are needed to establish the efficacy of these probiotics.

Serotonin receptor agonist and antagonists Serotonin receptor antagonists have been evaluated as therapies for IBS-D. Serotonin acting on 5-HT_3 receptors enhances the sensitivity of afferent neurons projecting from the gut. In humans, a 5-HT_3 receptor antagonist such as alosetron reduces perception of painful visceral stimulation in IBS. It also induces rectal relaxation, increases rectal compliance, and delays colonic transit. Meta-analysis of 14 randomized controlled trials of alosetron or cilansetron showed that these antagonists are more effective than placebo in achieving global improvement in IBS symptoms and relief of abdominal pain and discomfort. These agents are more likely to cause constipation in IBS patients with diarrhea alternating with constipation. Also, 0.2% of patients using 5-HT_3 antagonists developed ischemic colitis versus none in the control group. In postrelease surveillance, 84 cases of ischemic colitis were observed, including 44 cases that required surgery and 4 deaths. As a consequence, the medication was voluntarily withdrawn by the manufacturer in 2000. Alosetron has been reintroduced under a new risk-management program where patients have to sign a patient-physician agreement. This has significantly limited its usage.

Novel 5-HT_4 receptor agonists such as tegaserod exhibit prokinetic activity by stimulating peristalsis. In IBS patients with constipation, tegaserod accelerated intestinal and ascending colon transit. Clinical trials involving >4000 IBS-C patients reported reductions in discomfort and improvements in constipation and bloating, compared to placebo. Diarrhea is the major side effect. However, tegaserod has been withdrawn from the market; a meta-analysis revealed an increase in serious cardiovascular events.

Chloride channel activators Lubiprostone is a bicyclic fatty acid that stimulates chloride channels in the apical membrane of intestinal epithelial cells. Chloride secretion induces passive movement of sodium and water into the bowel lumen and improves bowel function. Oral lubiprostone was effective in the treatment of patients with constipation-predominant IBS in large phase II and phase III randomized, double-blinded, placebo-controlled multicenter trials. Responses were significantly greater in patients receiving lubiprostone 8 μg twice daily for 3 months than in those receiving placebo. In general, the drug was quite well tolerated. The major side effects are nausea and diarrhea. Lubiprostone is a new class of compounds for treatment of chronic constipation with or without IBS.

Guanylate cyclase-C agonist Linaclotide is a minimally absorbed 14-amino-acid peptide guanylate cyclase-C (GC-C) agonist that binds to and activates GC-C on the luminal surface of intestinal epithelium. Activation of GC-C results in generation of cyclic guanosine monophosphate (cGMP), which triggers secretion of fluid, sodium, and bicarbonate. In animal models, linaclotide accelerates GI transit and reduces visceral nociception. The analgesic action of linaclotide appears to be

TABLE 19-5

SPECTRUM OF SEVERITY IN IBS

	MILD	MODERATE	SEVERE
Clinical Features			
Prevalence	70%	25%	5%
Correlations with gut physiology	+++	++	+
Symptoms constant	0	+	+++
Psychosocial difficulties	0	+	+++
Health care issues	+	++	+++
Practice type	Primary	Specialty	Referral

mediated by cGMP acting on afferent pain fibers innervating the GI tract. A phase III, double-blind, controlled trial showed that linaclotide, 290 μg given once daily, significantly improved abdominal pain, bloating, and spontaneous bowel movement. The only significant side effect was diarrhea, which occurred in 4.5% of the patients. The drug has been approved for treatment of constipation in IBS-C patients.

SUMMARY The treatment strategy of IBS depends on the severity of the disorder (Table 19-5). Most IBS patients have mild symptoms. They are usually cared for in primary care practices, have little or no psychosocial difficulties, and do not seek health care often. Treatment usually involves education, reassurance, and dietary/lifestyle changes. A smaller portion have moderate symptoms that are usually intermittent and correlate with altered gut physiology, e.g., worsened with eating or stress and relieved by defecation. For IBS-D patients, treatments include gut-acting pharmacologic agents such as antispasmodics, antidiarrheals, bile acid binders, and the newer gut serotonin modulators (Table 19-6). In IBS-C patients, increased fiber intake and the use of osmotic agents such as polyethylene glycol may achieve satisfactory results. For patients with more severe constipation, a chloride channel opener (lubiprostone) or GC-C agonist (linaclotide) may be considered. For IBS patients with predominant gas and bloating, a low-FODMAP diet may provide significant relief. Some patients may benefit from probiotics and rifaximin treatment. A small proportion of IBS patients have severe and refractory symptoms, are usually seen in referral centers, and frequently have constant pain and psychosocial difficulties (Fig. 19-1). This group of patients is best managed with antidepressants and other psychological treatments (Table 19-6).

TABLE 19-6

POSSIBLE DRUGS FOR A DOMINANT SYMPTOM IN IBS

SYMPTOM	DRUG	DOSE
Diarrhea	Loperamide	2–4 mg when necessary/ maximum 12 g/d
	Cholestyramine resin	4 g with meals
	Alosetron[a]	0.5–1 mg bid (for severe IBS, women)
Constipation	Psyllium husk	3–4 g bid with meals, then adjust
	Methylcellulose	2 g bid with meals, then adjust
	Calcium polycarbophil	1 g qd to qid
	Lactulose syrup	10–20 g bid
	70% sorbitol	15 mL bid
	Polyethylene glycol 3350	17 g in 250 mL water qd
	Lubiprostone (Amitiza)	24 mg bid
	Magnesium hydroxide	30–60 mL qd
	Linaclotide	290 μg qd
Abdominal pain	Smooth-muscle relaxant	qd to qid ac
	Tricyclic antidepressants	Start 25–50 mg hs, then adjust
	Selective serotonin reuptake inhibitors	Begin small dose, increase as needed
Gas and bloating	Low FODMAP diet	
	Probiotics	qd
	Rifaximin	550 mg bid

[a]Available only in the United States.

Abbreviation: FODMAP, fermentable oligosaccharides, disaccharides, monosaccharides, and polyols.

Source: Adapted from GF Longstreth et al: *Gastroenterology* 130:1480, 2006.

CHAPTER 20

DIVERTICULAR DISEASE AND COMMON ANORECTAL DISORDERS

Rizwan Ahmed ■ Susan L. Gearhart

DIVERTICULAR DISEASE

Incidence and epidemiology

In the United States, diverticulosis affects 70% of the population above the age of 80. Fortunately, only 20% of patients with diverticulosis develop symptomatic disease, 1–2% require hospitalization, and <1% will require surgery. Diverticular disease has become the fifth most costly gastrointestinal disorder in the United States. Previously overlooked, the majority of patients with diverticular disease report a lower health-related quality of life and more depression as compared to matched controls, thus adding to health care costs. Formerly, diverticular disease was confined to developed countries; however, with the adoption of westernized diets in underdeveloped countries, diverticulosis is on the rise across the globe. Immigrants to the United States develop diverticular disease at the same rate as U.S. natives. Although the prevalence among females and males is similar, males tend to present at a younger age. The mean age at presentation of the disease is 59 years and is now shifting to affect younger populations.

Anatomy and pathophysiology

Two types of diverticula occur in the intestine: true and false (or pseudo diverticula). A true diverticulum is a saclike herniation of the entire bowel wall, whereas a pseudo diverticulum involves only a protrusion of the mucosa and submucosa through the muscularis propria of the colon (Fig. 20-1). The type of diverticulum affecting the colon is the pseudodiverticulum. Diverticula commonly affect the left and sigmoid colon; the rectum is always spared. However, in Asian populations, 70% of diverticula are seen in the right colon and cecum as well. *Diverticulitis* is inflammation of a diverticulum. Previous understanding of the pathogenesis

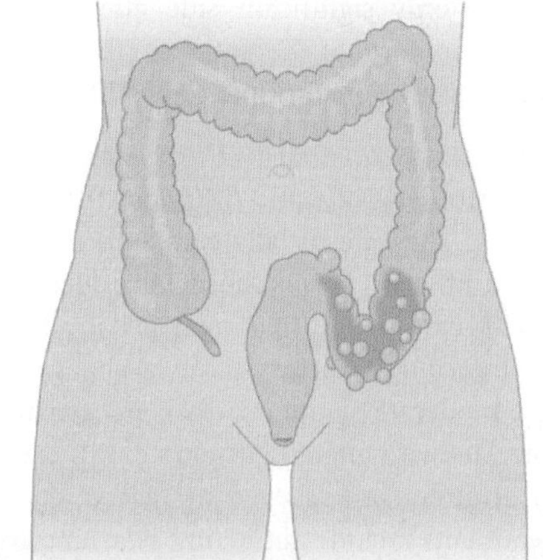

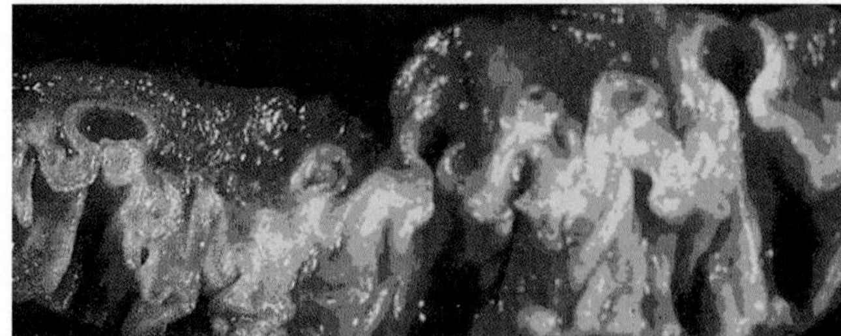

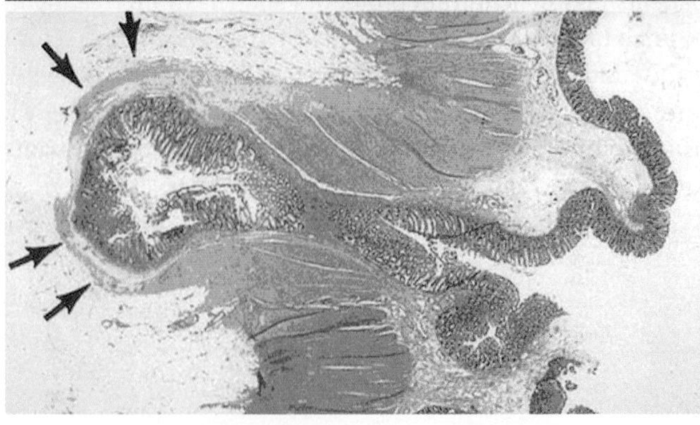

FIGURE 20-1

Gross and microscopic view of sigmoid diverticular disease. *Arrows* mark an inflamed diverticulum with the diverticular wall made up only of mucosa.

of diverticulosis attributed a low-fiber diet as the sole culprit, and onset of diverticulitis would occur acutely when these diverticula become obstructed. However, evidence now suggests that the pathogenesis is more complex and multifactorial. The diverticula occur at the point where the nutrient artery, or *vasa recti*, penetrates through the muscularis propria, resulting in a break in the integrity of the colonic wall. This anatomic restriction may be a result of the relative high-pressure zone within the muscular sigmoid colon. Thus, higher-amplitude contractions combined with constipated, high-fat-content stool within the sigmoid lumen in an area of weakness in the colonic wall results in the creation of these diverticula. Consequently, the vasa recti is either compressed or eroded, leading to either perforation or bleeding. Chronic low-grade inflammation is thought to play a key role. Furthermore, better understanding of the gut microbiota suggests that dysbiosis is an important aspect of disease.

Presentation, evaluation, and management of diverticular bleeding

Hemorrhage from a colonic diverticulum is the most common cause of hematochezia in patients >60 years, yet only 20% of patients with diverticulosis will have gastrointestinal bleeding. Patients at increased risk for bleeding tend to be hypertensive, have atherosclerosis, and regularly use aspirin and nonsteroidal anti-inflammatory agents. Most bleeds are self-limited and stop spontaneously with bowel rest. The lifetime risk of rebleeding is 25%.

Initial localization of diverticular bleeding may include colonoscopy, multiplanar computed tomography (CT) angiogram, or nuclear medicine tagged red cell scan. If the patient is stable, ongoing bleeding is best managed by angiography. If mesenteric angiography can localize the bleeding site, the vessel can be occluded successfully with a coil in 80% of cases. The patient can then be followed closely with repetitive colonoscopy, if necessary, looking for evidence of colonic ischemia. Alternatively, a segmental resection of the colon can be undertaken to eliminate the risk of further bleeding. This may be advantageous in patients on chronic anticoagulation. However, with highly selective coil embolization, the rate of colonic ischemia is <10% and the risk of acute rebleeding is <25%. Long-term results (40 months) indicate that more than 50% of patients with acute diverticular bleeds treated with highly selective angiography have had definitive treatment. As another alternative, a selective infusion of vasopressin can be given to stop the hemorrhage, although this has been associated with significant complications, including myocardial infarction and intestinal ischemia. Furthermore, bleeding recurs in 50% of patients once the infusion is stopped.

TABLE 20-1

PRESENTATION OF DIVERTICULAR DISEASE
Uncomplicated Diverticular Disease—75%
Abdominal pain
Fever
Leukocytosis
Anorexia/obstipation
Complicated Diverticular Disease—25%
Abscess 16%
Perforation 10%
Stricture 5%
Fistula 2%

If the patient is unstable or has had a 6-unit bleed within 24 h, current recommendations are that surgery should be performed. If the bleeding has been localized, a segmental resection can be performed. If the site of bleeding has not been definitively identified, a subtotal colectomy may be required. In patients without severe comorbidities, surgical resection can be performed with a primary anastomosis. A higher anastomotic leak rate has been reported in patients who received >10 units of blood.

Presentation, evaluation, and staging of diverticulitis

Acute uncomplicated diverticulitis characteristically presents with fever, anorexia, left lower quadrant abdominal pain, and obstipation (Table 20-1). In <25% of cases, patients may present with generalized peritonitis indicating the presence of a diverticular perforation. If a pericolonic abscess has formed, the patient may have abdominal distention and signs of localized peritonitis. Laboratory investigations will demonstrate a leukocytosis. Rarely, a patient may present with an air-fluid level in the left lower quadrant on plain abdominal film. This is a giant diverticulum of the sigmoid colon and is managed with resection to avoid impending perforation.

The diagnosis of diverticulitis is best made on CT with the following findings: sigmoid diverticula, thickened colonic wall >4 mm, and inflammation within the periodic fat ± the collection of contrast material or fluid. In 16% of patients, an abdominal abscess may be present. Symptoms of irritable bowel syndrome **(Chap. 19)** may mimic those of diverticulitis. Therefore, suspected diverticulitis that does not meet CT criteria or is not associated with a leukocytosis or fever is not diverticular disease. Other conditions that can mimic diverticular disease include an ovarian cyst, endometriosis, acute appendicitis, and pelvic inflammatory disease.

Although the benefit of colonoscopy in the evaluation of patients with diverticular disease has been called into question, its use is still considered important in the exclusion of colorectal cancer. The parallel epidemiology of

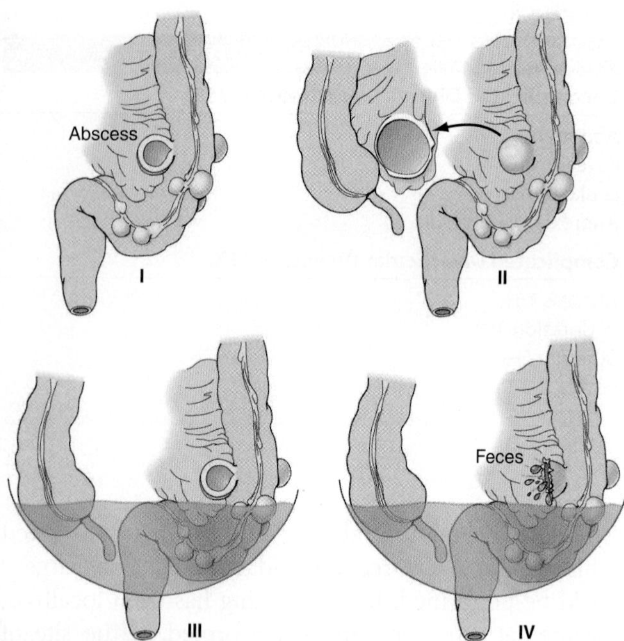

FIGURE 20-2
Hinchey classification of diverticulitis. Stage I: Perforated diverticulitis with a confined paracolic abscess. Stage II: Perforated diverticulitis that has closed spontaneously with distant abscess formation. Stage III: Noncommunicating perforated diverticulitis with fecal peritonitis (the diverticular neck is closed off, and therefore, contrast will not freely expel on radiographic images). Stage IV: Perforation and free communication with the peritoneum, resulting in fecal peritonitis.

colorectal cancer and diverticular disease provides enough concern for an endoscopic evaluation before operative management. Therefore, a colonoscopy should be performed ~6 weeks after an attack of diverticular disease.

Complicated diverticular disease is defined as diverticular disease associated with an abscess or perforation and less commonly with a fistula (Table 20-1). Perforated diverticular disease is staged using the Hinchey classification system (Fig. 20-2). This staging system was developed to predict outcomes following the surgical management of complicated diverticular disease. In complicated diverticular disease with fistula formation, common locations include cutaneous, vaginal, or vesicle fistulas. These conditions present with either passage of stool through the skin or vagina or the presence of air in the urinary stream (pneumaturia). Colovaginal fistulas are more common in women who have undergone a hysterectomy.

TREATMENT Diverticular Disease

MEDICAL MANAGEMENT Asymptomatic diverticular disease discovered on imaging studies or at the time of colonoscopy is best managed by diet alterations. Patients should be instructed to eat a fiber-enriched diet that includes 30 g of fiber each day. Supplementary fiber products such as Metamucil, Fibercon, or Citrucel are useful. The incidence of complicated diverticular disease appears to be increased in patients who smoke. Therefore, patients should be encouraged to refrain from smoking. The historical recommendation to avoid eating nuts is not based on more than anecdotal data.

Symptomatic uncomplicated diverticular disease with confirmation of inflammation and infection within the colon should be treated initially with antibiotics and bowel rest. Nearly 75% of patients hospitalized for acute diverticulitis will respond to nonoperative treatment with a suitable antimicrobial regimen. The current recommended antimicrobial coverage is trimethoprim/sulfamethoxazole or ciprofloxacin and metronidazole targeting aerobic gram-negative rods and anaerobic bacteria. Unfortunately, these agents do not cover enterococci, and the addition of ampicillin to this regimen for nonresponders is recommended. Alternatively, single-agent therapy with a third-generation penicillin such as IV piperacillin or oral penicillin/clavulanic acid may be effective. The usual course of antibiotics is 7–10 days, although this length of time is being investigated. Patients should remain on a limited diet until their pain resolves.

Once the acute attack has resolved, the mainstay medical management of diverticular disease to prevent symptoms has evolved. Newer directions are targeted at colonic inflammation and dysbiosis. Diverticular disease is now considered a functional bowel disorder associated with low-grade inflammation. Therefore, the use of anti-inflammatory medications such as mesalazine has become popular. Patients treated with mesalazine have a decreased recurrence of symptomatic disease. Randomized trials of anti-inflammatory medications are ongoing.

Treatment strategies targeting dysbiosis in diverticular disease are also beneficial. Use of the polymerase chain reaction (PCR) on stool specimens from consumers of a high-fiber diet has shown different bacterial content than stool of consumers of a low-fiber, high-fat diet. Probiotics are being increasingly used by gastroenterologists for multiple bowel disorders and have been shown to prevent recurrence of diverticulitis. Specifically probiotics containing *Lactobacillus acidophilus* and *Bifidobacterium* strains have been shown to be beneficial. Furthermore, rifaximin (a poorly absorbed broad-spectrum antibiotic), when compared to fiber alone, is associated with 30% less frequent recurrent symptoms from uncomplicated diverticular disease.

SURGICAL MANAGEMENT Preoperative risk factors influencing postoperative mortality rates include higher American Society of Anesthesiologists (ASA) physical status class (Table 20-2) and preexisting organ failure. In patients who are low risk (ASA P1 and P2), surgical therapy can be offered to those who do not rapidly improve on medical therapy. For uncomplicated diverticular disease, medical therapy can be continued beyond two attacks without an increased risk of perforation requiring a colostomy. However, patients on immunosuppressive therapy, in

TABLE 20-2

AMERICAN SOCIETY OF ANESTHESIOLOGISTS PHYSICAL STATUS CLASSIFICATION SYSTEM

P1	A normal healthy patient
P2	A patient with mild systemic disease
P3	A patient with severe systemic disease
P4	A patient with severe systemic disease that is a constant threat to life
P5	A moribund patient who is not expected to survive without the operation
P6	A declared brain-dead patient whose organs are being removed for donor purposes

chronic renal failure, or with a collagen-vascular disease have a fivefold greater risk of perforation during recurrent attacks. Surgical therapy is indicated in all low-surgical-risk patients with complicated diverticular disease.

The goals of surgical management of diverticular disease include controlling sepsis, eliminating complications such as fistula or obstruction, removing the diseased colonic segment, and restoring intestinal continuity. These goals must be obtained while minimizing morbidity rate, length of hospitalization, and cost in addition to maximizing survival and quality of life. Table 20-3 lists the operations most commonly indicated based on the Hinchey classification and the predicted morbidity and mortality rates. Surgical objectives include removal of the diseased sigmoid down to the rectosigmoid junction. Failure to do this may result in recurrent disease. The current options for uncomplicated diverticular disease include an open sigmoid resection or a laparoscopic sigmoid resection. The benefits of laparoscopic resection over open surgical techniques include early discharge (by at least 1 day), less narcotic use, less postoperative complications, and an earlier return to work.

The options for the surgical management of complicated diverticular disease (Fig. 20-3) include the following: (1) proximal diversion of the fecal stream with an ileostomy or colostomy and sutured omental patch with drainage, (2) resection with colostomy and mucous fistula or closure of distal bowel with formation of a Hartmann's pouch, (3) resection with anastomosis (coloproctostomy), or (4) resection with anastomosis and diversion (coloproctostomy with loop ileostomy or colostomy). Laparoscopic techniques have been used for complicated diverticular disease; however, higher conversion rates to open techniques have been reported.

Patients with Hinchey stages I and II disease are managed with percutaneous drainage followed by resection with anastomosis about 6 weeks later. Current guidelines put forth by the American Society of Colon and Rectal Surgeons suggest, in addition to antibiotic therapy, CT-guided percutaneous drainage of diverticular abscesses that are greater than 3 cm and have a well-defined wall. Abscesses that are less than

TABLE 20-3

OUTCOME FOLLOWING SURGICAL THERAPY FOR COMPLICATED DIVERTICULAR DISEASE

HINCHEY STAGE	OPERATIVE PROCEDURE	ANASTOMOTIC LEAK RATE, %	OVERALL MORBIDITY RATE, %
I	Resection with primary anastomosis without diverting stoma	3.8	22
II	Resection with primary anastomosis +/– diversion	3.8	30
III	Hartmann's procedure vs diverting colostomy and omental pedal graft	—	0 vs. 6 mortality
IV	Hartmann's procedure vs diverting colostomy and omental pedicle graft	—	6 vs. 2 mortality

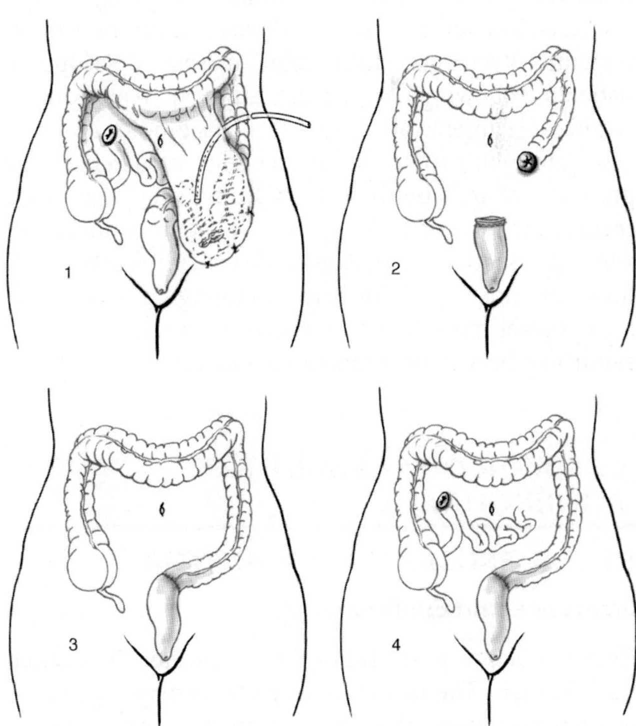

FIGURE 20-3

Methods of surgical management of complicated diverticular disease. ***(1)*** Drainage, omental pedicle graft, and proximal diversion. ***(2)*** Hartmann's procedure. ***(3)*** Sigmoid resection with coloproctostomy. ***(4)*** Sigmoid resection with coloproctostomy and proximal diversion.

3 cm may resolve with antibiotic therapy alone. Contraindications to percutaneous drainage are no percutaneous access route, pneumoperitoneum, and fecal peritonitis. Urgent operative intervention is undertaken if patients develop generalized peritonitis, and most will need to be managed with a Hartmann's procedure (resection of the sigmoid colon with end colostomy and rectal stump). In selected cases, nonoperative therapy may be considered. In one nonrandomized study, nonoperative management of isolated paracolic abscesses (Hinchey stage I) was associated with only a 20% recurrence rate at 2 years. More than 80% of patients with distant abscesses (Hinchey stage II) required surgical resection for recurrent symptoms.

Hinchey stage III disease is managed with a Hartmann's procedure or with primary anastomosis and proximal diversion. If the patient has significant comorbidities, making operative intervention risky, a limited procedure including intraoperative peritoneal lavage (irrigation), omental patch to the oversewn perforation, and proximal diversion of the fecal stream with either an ileostomy or transverse colostomy can be performed. No anastomosis of any type should be attempted in Hinchey stage IV disease. A limited approach to these patients is associated with a decreased mortality rate.

Recurrent symptoms

Recurrent abdominal symptoms following surgical resection for diverticular disease occur in 10% of patients. Recurrent diverticular disease develops in patients following inadequate surgical resection. A retained segment of diseased rectosigmoid colon is associated with twice the incidence of recurrence. The presence of irritable bowel syndrome may also cause recurrence of initial symptoms. Patients undergoing surgical resection for presumed diverticulitis and symptoms of chronic abdominal cramping and irregular loose bowel movements consistent with irritable bowel syndrome have poorer functional outcomes.

COMMON DISEASES OF THE ANORECTUM

RECTAL PROLAPSE (PROCIDENTIA)

Incidence and Epidemiology

Rectal prolapse is six times more common in women than in men. The incidence of rectal prolapse peaks in women >60 years. Women with rectal prolapse have a higher incidence of associated pelvic floor disorders including urinary incontinence, rectocele, cystocele, and enterocele. About 20% of children with rectal prolapse will have cystic fibrosis. All children presenting with prolapse should undergo a sweat chloride test. Less common associations include Ehlers-Danlos syndrome, solitary rectal ulcer syndrome, congenital hypothyroidism, Hirschsprung's disease, dementia, mental retardation, and schizophrenia.

Anatomy and pathophysiology

Rectal prolapse (procidentia) is a circumferential, full-thickness protrusion of the rectal wall through the anal orifice. It is often associated with a redundant sigmoid colon, pelvic laxity, and a deep rectovaginal septum (pouch of Douglas). Initially, rectal prolapse was felt to be the result of early internal rectal intussusception, which occurs in the upper to mid rectum. This was considered to be the first step in an inevitable progression to full-thickness external prolapse. However, only 1 of 38 patients with internal prolapse followed for >5 years developed full-thickness prolapse. Others have suggested that full-thickness prolapse is the result of damage to the nerve supply to the pelvic floor muscles or pudendal nerves from repeated stretching with straining to defecate. Damage to the pudendal nerves would weaken the pelvic floor muscles, including the external anal sphincter muscles. Bilateral pudendal nerve injury is more significantly associated with prolapse and incontinence than unilateral injury.

Presentation and evaluation

In external prolapse, the majority of patient complaints include anal mass, bleeding per rectum, and poor perianal hygiene. Prolapse of the rectum usually occurs following defecation and will spontaneously reduce or require the patient to manually reduce the prolapse. Constipation occurs in ~30–67% of patients with rectal prolapse. Differing degrees of fecal incontinence occur in 50–70% of patients. Patients with internal rectal prolapse will present with symptoms of both constipation and incontinence. Other associated findings include outlet obstruction (anismus) in 30%, colonic inertia in 10%, and solitary rectal ulcer syndrome in 12%.

Office evaluation is best performed after the patient has been given an enema, which enables the prolapse to protrude. An important distinction should be made between full-thickness rectal prolapse and isolated mucosal prolapse associated with hemorrhoidal disease (Fig. 20-4). Mucosal prolapse is known for radial grooves rather than circumferential folds around the anus and is due to increased laxity of the connective tissue between the submucosa and underlying muscle of the anal canal. The evaluation of prolapse should also include cystoproctography and colonoscopy. These examinations evaluate for associated pelvic floor disorders and rule out a malignancy or a polyp as the lead point for prolapse. If rectal prolapse is associated with chronic constipation, the patient should undergo a defecating proctogram and a sitzmark study. This will

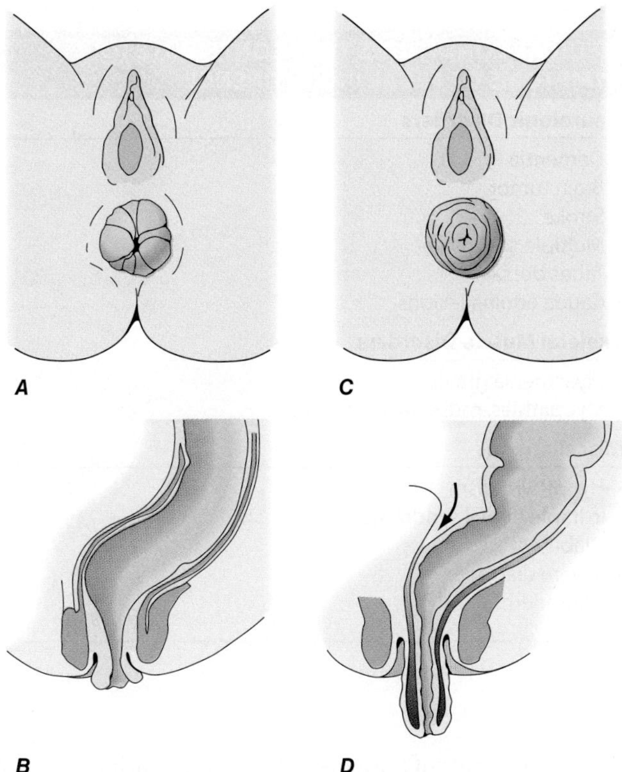

FIGURE 20-4

Degrees of rectal prolapse. Mucosal prolapse only (***A, B,*** sagittal view). Full-thickness prolapse associated with redundant rectosigmoid and deep pouch of Douglas (***C, D,*** sagittal view).

evaluate for the presence of anismus or colonic inertia. Anismus is the result of attempting to defecate against a closed pelvic floor and is also known as *nonrelaxing puborectalis*. This can be seen when straightening of the rectum fails to occur on fluoroscopy while the patient is attempting to defecate. In colonic inertia, a sitzmark study will demonstrate retention of >20% of markers on abdominal x-ray 5 days after swallowing. For patients with fecal incontinence, endoanal ultrasound and manometric evaluation, including pudendal nerve testing of their anal sphincter muscles, may be performed before surgery for prolapse (see "Fecal Incontinence," below).

TREATMENT Rectal Prolapse

The medical approach to the management of rectal prolapse is limited and includes stool-bulking agents or fiber supplementation to ease the process of evacuation. Surgical correction of rectal prolapse is the mainstay of therapy. Two approaches are commonly considered, transabdominal and transperineal. Transabdominal approaches have been associated with lower recurrence rates, but some patients with significant comorbidities are better served by a transperineal approach.

Common transperineal approaches include a transanal proctectomy (Altmeier procedure), mucosal proctectomy (Delorme procedure), or placement of a Tirsch wire encircling the anus. The goal of the transperineal approach is to remove the redundant rectosigmoid colon. Common transabdominal approaches include presacral suture or mesh rectopexy (Ripstein) with (Frykman-Goldberg) or without resection of the redundant sigmoid. Colon resection, in general, is reserved for patients with constipation and outlet obstruction. Ventral rectopexy is an effective method of abdominal repair of full-thickness prolapse that does not require sigmoid resection (see description below). This repair may have improved functional results over other abdominal repairs. Transabdominal procedures can be performed effectively with laparoscopic and, more recently, robotic techniques without increased incidence of recurrence. The goal of the transabdominal approach is to restore normal anatomy by removing redundant bowel and reattaching the supportive tissue of the rectum to the presacral fascia. The final alternative is abdominal proctectomy with end-sigmoid colostomy. If total colonic inertia is present, as defined by a history of constipation and a positive sitzmark study, a subtotal colectomy with an ileosigmoid or rectal anastomosis may be required at the time of rectopexy.

Previously, the presence of internal rectal prolapse identified on imaging studies has been considered a nonsurgical disorder and biofeedback was recommended. However, only one-third of patients will have successful resolution of symptoms from biofeedback. Two surgical procedures more effective than biofeedback are the Stapled Transanal Rectal Resection (STARR) and the Laparoscopic Ventral Rectopexy (LVR). The STARR procedure (Fig. 20-5) is performed through the anus in patients with internal prolapse.

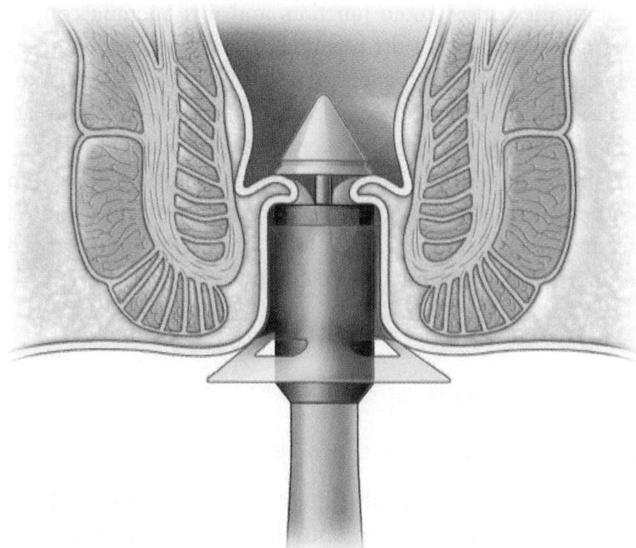

FIGURE 20-5

Stapled transanal rectal resection. Schematic of placement of the circular stapling device.

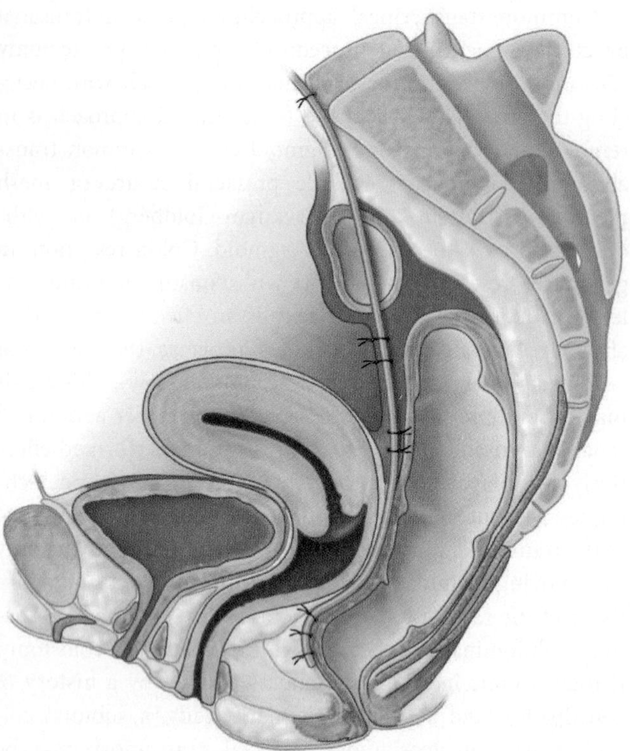

FIGURE 20-6
Laparoscopic ventral rectopexy (LVR). To reduce the internal prolapse and close any rectovaginal septal defect, the pouch of Douglas is opened and mesh is secured to the anterolateral rectum, vaginal fornix, and sacrum. *(From A D'Hoore et al: Br J Surg 91:1500, 2004.)*

A circular stapling device is inserted through the anus; the internal prolapse is identified and ligated with the stapling device. LVR (Fig. 20-6) is performed through an abdominal approach. An opening in the peritoneum is created on the left side of the rectosigmoid junction, and this opening continues down anterior on the rectum into the pouch of Douglas. No rectal mobilization is performed, thus avoiding any autonomic nerve injury. Mesh is secured to the anterior and lateral portion of the rectum, the vaginal fornix, and the sacral promontory, allowing for closure of the rectovaginal septum and correction of the internal prolapse. In both procedures, recurrence at 1 year was low (<10%) and symptoms improved in more than three-fourths of patients.

FECAL INCONTINENCE

Incidence and epidemiology

Fecal incontinence is the involuntary passage of fecal material for at least 1 month in an individual with a developmental age of at least 4 years. The prevalence of fecal incontinence in the United States is 0.5–11%. The majority of patients are women and above the age of 65. A higher incidence of incontinence is seen among parous women. One-half of patients with fecal incontinence also suffer from urinary incontinence. The majority of incontinence is a result of obstetric injury to the pelvic floor, either while carrying a fetus or during the delivery. An anatomic sphincter defect may occur in up to 32% of women following childbirth regardless of visible damage to the perineum. Risk factors at the time of delivery include prolonged labor, the use of forceps, and the need for an episiotomy. Symptoms of incontinence can present after two or more decades following obstetric injury. Medical conditions known to contribute to the development of fecal incontinence are listed in Table 20-4.

TABLE 20-4

MEDICAL CONDITIONS THAT CONTRIBUTE TO SYMPTOMS OF FECAL INCONTINENCE
Neurologic Disorders
• Dementia • Brain tumor • Stroke • Multiple sclerosis • Tabes dorsalis • Cauda equina lesions
Skeletal Muscle Disorders
• Myasthenia gravis • Myopathies, muscular dystrophy
Miscellaneous
• Hypothyroidism • Irritable bowel syndrome • Diabetes • Severe diarrhea • Scleroderma

Anatomy and pathophysiology

The anal sphincter complex is made up of the internal and external anal sphincter. The internal sphincter is smooth muscle and a continuation of the circular fibers of the rectal wall. It is innervated by the intestinal myenteric plexus and is therefore not under voluntary control. The external anal sphincter is formed in continuation with the levator ani muscles and is under voluntary control. The pudendal nerve supplies motor innervation to the external anal sphincter. Obstetric injury may result in tearing of the muscle fibers anteriorly at the time of the delivery. This results in an obvious anterior defect on endoanal ultrasound. Injury may also be the result of stretching of the pudendal nerves during pregnancy or delivery of the fetus through the birth canal.

Presentation and evaluation

Patients may suffer with varying degrees of fecal incontinence. Minor incontinence includes incontinence to flatus and occasional seepage of liquid stool. Major incontinence is frequent inability to control solid waste. As a result of fecal incontinence, patients suffer from poor perianal hygiene. Beyond the immediate problems associated with fecal incontinence, these patients are often withdrawn and suffer from depression. For this reason, quality-of-life measures are an important component in the evaluation of patients with fecal incontinence.

The evaluation of fecal incontinence should include a thorough history and physical exam including digital rectal examination (DRE). Weak sphincter tone on DRE and loss of the "anal wink" reflex (S1-level control) may indicate a neurogenic dysfunction. Perianal scars may represent surgical injury. Other studies helpful in the diagnosis of fecal incontinence include anal manometry, pudendal nerve terminal motor latency (PNTML), and endoanal ultrasound. Centers that care for patients with fecal incontinence will have an anorectal physiology laboratory that uses standardized methods of evaluating anorectal physiology. Anorectal manometry (ARM) measures resting and squeeze pressures within the anal canal using an intraluminal water-perfused catheter. Current methods of ARM include use of a three-dimensional, high-resolution system with a 12-catheter perfusion system, which allows physiologic delineation of anatomic abnormalities. Pudendal nerve studies evaluate the function of the nerves innervating the anal canal using a finger electrode placed in the anal canal. Stretch injuries to these nerves will result in a delayed response of the sphincter muscle to a stimulus, indicating a prolonged latency. Finally, endoanal ultrasound will evaluate the extent of the injury to the sphincter muscles before surgical repair. Unfortunately, all of these investigations are user-dependent, and very few studies demonstrate that these studies predict outcome following an intervention. Magnetic resonance imaging (MRI) has been used, but its routine use for imaging in fecal incontinence is not well established.

Rarely does a pelvic floor disorder exist alone. The majority of patients with fecal incontinence will have some degree of urinary incontinence. Similarly, fecal incontinence is a part of the spectrum of pelvic organ prolapse. For this reason, patients may present with symptoms of obstructed defecation as well as fecal incontinence. Careful evaluation including dynamic MRI or cinedefecography should be performed to search for other associated defects. Surgical repair of incontinence without attention to other associated defects may decrease the success of the repair.

TREATMENT Fecal Incontinence

Medical management of fecal incontinence includes strategies to bulk up the stool, which help in increasing fecal sensation. These include fiber supplementation, loperamide, diphenoxylate, and bile acid binders. These agents harden the stool and delay frequency of bowel movements and are helpful in patients with minimal to mild symptoms. Furthermore, patients can be offered a form of physical therapy called biofeedback. This therapy helps strengthen the external sphincter muscle while training the patient to relax with defecation to avoid unnecessary straining and further injury to the sphincter muscles. Biofeedback has had variable success and is dependent on the motivation of the patient. At a minimum, biofeedback is risk free and safe. Most patients will have some improvement. For this reason, it should be incorporated into the initial recommendation to all patients with fecal incontinence.

The "gold standard" for the treatment of fecal incontinence with an isolated sphincter defect has been the overlapping sphincteroplasty. The external anal sphincter muscle and scar tissue as well as any identifiable internal sphincter muscle are dissected free from the surrounding adipose and connective tissue and then an overlapping repair is performed in an attempt to rebuild the muscular ring and restore its function. Long-term results following overlapping sphincteroplasty show about a 50% failure rate over 5 years. Poorer outcome has been seen in patients with prolonged pudendal nerve terminal motor latency.

Sacral neuromodulation, collagen-enhancing injectables, radiofrequency therapy, and the artificial bowel sphincter are other options. Sacral nerve stimulation and the artificial bowel sphincter are both adaptations of procedures developed for the management of urinary incontinence. Sacral nerve stimulation is ideally suited for patients with intact but weak anal sphincters. A temporary nerve stimulator is placed on the third sacral nerve. If there is at least a 50% improvement in symptoms, a permanent nerve stimulator is placed under the skin. The artificial bowel sphincter is a cuff and reservoir apparatus that allows for manual inflation of a cuff placed around the anus, increasing anal tone. This allows the patient to manually close off the anal canal until defecation is necessary. Long-term results for sacral stimulation have been promising, with nearly 80% of patients having a reduction in incontinence episodes by at least 50%. This reduction has been sustainable in studies out to 5 years. Unfortunately, the artificial bowel sphincter has been associated with a 30% infection rate. Accordingly, implantation is performed less often.

Collagen-enhancing injectables have been around for several years. The largest open trial involved 115 incontinent patients treated with nonanimal stabilized hyaluronic acid (NASHA/DX) gel. In this study, patients underwent injections of NASHA/DX (Solesta) into the anal mucosa and were followed for 12 months. The results were promising, with over 50% achieving greater than 50% reduction in incontinence episodes, and these results were sustainable up to 2 years. This method is another less invasive therapy for patients with fecal incontinence.

Radiofrequency energy delivery to the anal canal in patients with fecal incontinence aids in the development and restructuring of collagen fibers and provides tensile strength to the sphincter muscles. The radiofrequency is delivered as an office procedure with sedation. The results have been variable, with 20–50% of patients having a sustained reduction in incontinence episodes for 5 years.

Finally, the use of stem cells to increase the bulk of the sphincter muscles is currently being tested. Stem cells can be harvested from the patient's own muscle, grown, and then implanted into their sphincter complex. Concern for cost and the need for an additional procedure dampen enthusiasm. Trial results are awaited.

HEMORRHOIDAL DISEASE

Incidence and epidemiology

Symptomatic hemorrhoids affect >1 million individuals in the Western world per year. The prevalence of hemorrhoidal disease is not selective for age or sex. However, age is known to be a risk factor. The prevalence of hemorrhoidal disease is less in underdeveloped countries. The typical low-fiber, high-fat Western diet is associated with constipation and straining and the development of symptomatic hemorrhoids.

Anatomy and pathophysiology

Hemorrhoidal cushions are a normal part of the anal canal. The vascular structures contained within this tissue aid in continence by preventing damage to the sphincter muscle. Three main hemorrhoidal complexes traverse the anal canal—the left lateral, the right anterior, and the right posterior. Engorgement and straining lead to prolapse of this tissue into the anal canal. Over time, the anatomic support system of the hemorrhoidal complex weakens, exposing this tissue to the outside of the anal canal where it is susceptible to injury. Hemorrhoids are commonly classified as external or internal. External hemorrhoids originate below the dentate line and are covered with squamous epithelium and are associated with an internal component. External hemorrhoids are painful when thrombosed. Internal hemorrhoids originate above the dentate line and are covered with mucosa and transitional zone epithelium and represent majority of hemorrhoids. The standard classification of hemorrhoidal disease is based on the progression of the disease from their normal internal location to the prolapsing external position (Table 20-5).

TABLE 20-5

THE STAGING AND TREATMENT OF HEMORRHOIDS

STAGE	DESCRIPTION OF CLASSIFICATION	TREATMENT
I	Enlargement with bleeding	Fiber supplementation Cortisone suppository Sclerotherapy
II	Protrusion with spontaneous reduction	Fiber supplementation Cortisone suppository
III	Protrusion requiring manual reduction	Fiber supplementation Cortisone suppository Banding Operative hemorrhoidectomy
IV	Irreducible protrusion	Fiber supplementation Cortisone suppository Operative hemorrhoidectomy

Presentation and evaluation

Patients commonly present to a physician for two reasons: bleeding and protrusion. Pain is less common than with fissures and, if present, is described as a dull ache from engorgement of the hemorrhoidal tissue. Severe pain may indicate a thrombosed hemorrhoid. Hemorrhoidal bleeding is described as painless bright red blood seen either in the toilet or upon wiping. Occasional patients can present with significant bleeding, which may be a cause of anemia; however, the presence of a colonic neoplasm must be ruled out in anemic patients. Patients who present with a protruding mass complain about inability to maintain perianal hygiene and are often concerned about the presence of a malignancy.

The diagnosis of hemorrhoidal disease is made on physical examination. Inspection of the perianal region for evidence of thrombosis or excoriation is performed, followed by a careful digital examination. Anoscopy is performed paying particular attention to the known position of hemorrhoidal disease. The patient is asked to strain. If this is difficult for the patient, the maneuver can be performed while sitting on a toilet. The physician is notified when the tissue prolapses. It is important to differentiate the circumferential appearance of a full-thickness rectal prolapse from the radial nature of prolapsing hemorrhoids (see "Rectal Prolapse," above). The stage and location of the hemorrhoidal complexes are defined.

TREATMENT Hemorrhoidal Disease

The treatment for bleeding hemorrhoids is based on the stage of the disease (Table 20-5). In all patients with bleeding, the possibility of other causes must be considered. In young patients without a family history of colorectal cancer, the hemorrhoidal disease may be treated first and a colonoscopic examination performed if the bleeding continues. Older patients who have not had colorectal cancer screening should undergo colonoscopy or flexible sigmoidoscopy.

With rare exceptions, the acutely thrombosed hemorrhoid can be excised within the first 72 h by performing an elliptical excision. Sitz baths, fiber, and stool softeners are prescribed. Additional therapy for bleeding hemorrhoids includes the office procedures of banding and sclerotherapy. Sensation begins at the dentate line; therefore, banding or sclerotherapy can be performed without discomfort in the office. Bands are placed around the engorged tissue, causing ischemia and fibrosis. This aids in fixing the tissue proximally in the anal canal. Patients may complain of a dull ache for 24 h following band application. During sclerotherapy, 1–2 mL of a sclerosant (usually sodium tetradecyl sulfate) is injected using a 25-gauge needle into the submucosa of the hemorrhoidal complex. Care must be taken not to inject the anal canal circumferentially, or stenosis may occur.

For surgical management of hemorrhoidal disease, excisional hemorrhoidectomy, transhemorrhoidal dearterialization (THD), or stapled hemorrhoidectomy ("the procedure for prolapse or hemorrhoids" [PPH]) is the procedure of choice. All surgical methods of management are equally effective in the treatment of symptomatic third- and fourth-degree hemorrhoids. However, because the sutured hemorrhoidectomy involves the removal of redundant tissue down to the anal verge, unpleasant anal skin tags are removed as well. The stapled hemorrhoidectomy is associated with less discomfort; however, this procedure does not remove anal skin tags. THD uses ultrasound guidance to ligate the blood supply to the anal tissue, hence reducing hemorrhoidal engorgement. No procedures on hemorrhoids should be done in patients who are immunocompromised or who have active proctitis. Furthermore, emergent hemorrhoidectomy for bleeding hemorrhoids is associated with a higher complication rate.

Acute complications associated with the treatment of hemorrhoids include pain, infection, recurrent bleeding, and urinary retention. Care should be taken to place bands properly and to avoid overhydration in patients undergoing operative hemorrhoidectomy. Late complications include fecal incontinence as a result of injury to the sphincter during the dissection. Anal stenosis may develop from overzealous excision, with loss of mucosal skin bridges for reepithelialization. Finally, an *ectropion* (prolapse of rectal mucosa from the anal canal) may develop. Patients with an ectropion complain of a "wet" anus as a result of inability to prevent soiling once the rectal mucosa is exposed below the dentate line.

ANORECTAL ABSCESS

Incidence and epidemiology

The development of a perianal abscess is more common in men than women by a ratio of 3:1. The peak incidence is in the third to fifth decade of life. Perianal pain associated with the presence of an abscess accounts for 15% of office visits to a colorectal surgeon. The disease is more prevalent in immunocompromised patients such as those with diabetes, hematologic disorders, or inflammatory bowel disease and persons who are HIV positive. These disorders should be considered in patients with recurrent perianal infections.

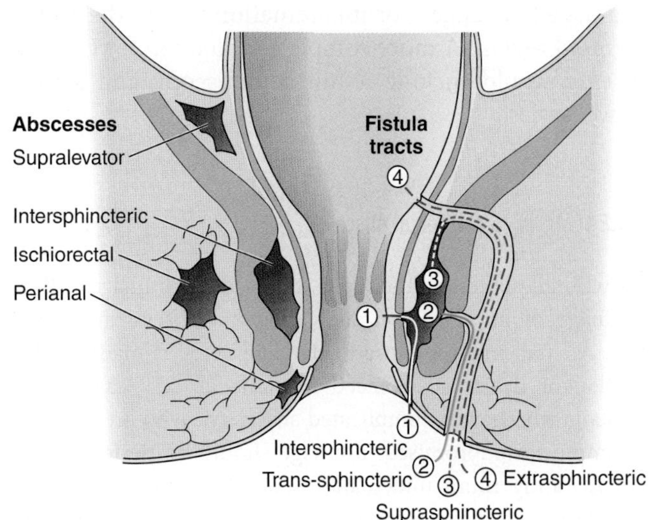

FIGURE 20-7
Common locations of anorectal abscess (*left*) and fistula in ano (***right***).

Anatomy and pathophysiology

An anorectal abscess is an abnormal fluid-containing cavity in the anorectal region. Anorectal abscess results from an infection involving the glands surrounding the anal canal. Normally, these glands release mucus into the anal canal, which aids in defecation. When stool accidentally enters the anal glands, the glands become infected and an abscess develops. Anorectal abscesses are perianal in 40–50% of patients, ischiorectal in 20–25%, intersphincteric in 2–5%, and supralevator in 2.5% (Fig. 20-7).

Presentation and evaluation

Perianal pain and fever are the hallmarks of an abscess. Patients may have difficulty voiding and have blood in the stool. A prostatic abscess may present with similar complaints, including dysuria. Patients with a prostatic abscess will often have a history of recurrent sexually transmitted diseases. On physical examination, a large fluctuant area is usually readily visible. Routine laboratory evaluation shows an elevated white blood cell count. Diagnostic procedures are rarely necessary unless evaluating a recurrent abscess. A CT scan or MRI has an accuracy of 80% in determining incomplete drainage. If there is a concern about the presence of inflammatory bowel disease, a rigid or flexible sigmoidoscopic examination may be done at the time of drainage to evaluate for inflammation within the rectosigmoid region. A more complete evaluation for Crohn's disease would include a full colonoscopy and small-bowel series.

TREATMENT **Anorectal Abscess**

As with all abscesses, the "gold standard" is drainage. Office drainage of an uncomplicated anorectal abscess may suffice. A small incision close to the anal verge is made, and a Mallenkot drain is advanced into the abscess cavity. For patients who have a complicated abscess or who are diabetic or immunocompromised, drainage should be performed in an operating room under anesthesia. These patients are at greater risk for developing necrotizing fasciitis. There is limited role of antibiotics in management of anorectal abscesses. The antibiotics are only warranted in patients who are immunocompromised or have prosthetic heart valves, artificial joints, diabetes, or inflammatory bowel disease.

FISTULA IN ANO

Incidence and epidemiology

The incidence and prevalence of fistulating perianal disease parallels the incidence of anorectal abscess, estimating to be 1 in 10,000 individuals. Some 30–40% of abscesses will give rise to fistula in ano. Although the majority of the fistulas are cryptoglandular in origin, 10% are associated with IBD, tuberculosis, malignancy, and radiation.

Anatomy and pathophysiology

A fistula in ano is defined as a communication of an abscess cavity with an identifiable internal opening within the anal canal. This identifiable opening is most commonly located at the dentate line where the anal glands enter the anal canal. Patients experiencing continuous drainage following the treatment of a perianal abscess likely have a fistula in ano. These fistulas are classified by their relationship to the anal sphincter muscles, with 70% being intersphincteric, 23% transsphincteric, 5% suprasphincteric, and 2% extrasphincteric (Fig. 20-7).

Presentation and evaluation

A patient with a fistula in ano will complain of constant drainage from the perianal region associated with a firm mass. The drainage may increase with defecation. Perianal hygiene is difficult to maintain. Examination under anesthesia is the best way to evaluate a fistula. At the time of the examination, anoscopy is performed to look for an internal opening. Diluted hydrogen peroxide will aid in identifying such an opening. In lieu of anesthesia, MRI with an endoanal coil will also identify tracts in 80% of the cases. After drainage of an abscess with insertion of a Mallenkot catheter, a fistulagram through the catheter can be obtained in search of an occult fistula tract. Goodsall's rule states that a posterior external fistula will enter the anal canal in the posterior midline, whereas an anterior fistula will enter at the nearest crypt. A fistula exiting >3 cm from the anal verge may have a complicated upward extension and may not obey Goodsall's rule.

TREATMENT **Fistula in Ano**

A newly diagnosed draining fistula is best managed with placement of a seton, a vessel loop or silk tie placed through the fistula tract, which maintains the tract open and quiets down the surrounding inflammation that occurs from repeated blockage of the tract. Once the inflammation is less, the exact relationship of the fistula tract to the anal sphincters can be ascertained. A simple fistulotomy can be performed for intersphincteric and low (less than one-third of the muscle) transsphincteric fistulas without compromising continence. For a higher transsphincteric fistula, an anorectal advancement flap in combination with a drainage catheter or fibrin glue may be used. Very long (>2 cm) and narrow tracts respond better to fibrin glue than shorter tracts. Simple ligation of the internal fistula tract (LIFT procedure) has also been used in the management of simple fistula with good success.

Patients should be maintained on stool-bulking agents, nonnarcotic pain medication, and sitz baths following surgery for a fistula. Early complications from these procedures include urinary retention and bleeding. Later complications are rare (<10%) and include temporary and permanent incontinence. Recurrence is 0–18% following fistulotomy and 20–30% following anorectal advancement flap and the LIFT procedure,

ANAL FISSURE

Incidence and epidemiology

Anal fissures occur at all ages but are more common in the third through the fifth decades. A fissure is the most common cause of rectal bleeding in infancy. The prevalence is equal in males and females. It is associated with constipation, diarrhea, infectious etiologies, perianal trauma, and Crohn's disease.

Anatomy and pathophysiology

Trauma to the anal canal occurs following defecation. This injury occurs in the anterior or, more commonly, the posterior anal canal. Irritation caused by the trauma to the anal canal results in an increased resting pressure of the internal sphincter. The blood supply to the sphincter and anal mucosa enters laterally. Therefore, increased anal sphincter tone results in a relative ischemia in the region of the fissure and leads to poor healing of the anal injury. A fissure that is not in the posterior or anterior position should raise suspicion for other causes, including tuberculosis, syphilis, Crohn's disease, and malignancy.

Presentation and evaluation

A fissure can be easily diagnosed on history alone. The classic complaint is pain, which is strongly associated with defecation and is relentless. The bright red bleeding that can be associated with a fissure is less extensive than that associated with hemorrhoids. On examination, most fissures are located in either the posterior or anterior position. A lateral fissure is worrisome because it may have a less benign nature, and systemic disorders should be ruled out. A chronic fissure is indicated by the presence of a hypertrophied anal papilla at the proximal end of the fissure and a sentinel pile or skin tag at the distal end. Often the circular fibers of the hypertrophied internal sphincter are visible within the base of the fissure. If anal manometry is performed, elevation in anal resting pressure and a sawtooth deformity with paradoxical contractions of the sphincter muscles are pathognomonic.

TREATMENT **Anal Fissure**

The management of the acute fissure is conservative. Stool softeners for those with constipation, increased dietary fiber, topical anesthetics, glucocorticoids, and sitz baths are prescribed and will heal 60–90% of fissures. Chronic fissures are those present for >6 weeks. These can be treated with modalities aimed at decreasing the anal canal resting pressure including nifedipine or nitroglycerin ointment applied three times a day and botulinum toxin type A, up to 20 units, injected into the internal sphincter on each side of the fissure. Surgical management includes anal dilatation and lateral internal sphincterotomy. Usually, one-third of the internal sphincter muscle is divided; it is easily identified because it is hypertrophied. Recurrence rates from medical therapy are higher, but this is offset by a risk of incontinence following sphincterotomy. Lateral internal sphincterotomy may lead to incontinence more commonly in women.

ACKNOWLEDGMENT

We would like to thank Cory Sandore for providing some illustrations for this chapter. Gregory Bulkley, MD, contributed to this chapter in an earlier edition and some of that material has been retained here.

CHAPTER 21

MESENTERIC VASCULAR INSUFFICIENCY

Rizwan Ahmed ■ Mahmoud Malas

INTESTINAL ISCHEMIA

INCIDENCE AND EPIDEMIOLOGY

Intestinal ischemia occurs when splanchnic perfusion fails to meet the metabolic demands of the intestines, resulting in ischemic tissue injury. Mesenteric ischemia affects 2–3 people per 100,000, and the incidence of mesenteric ischemia is bound to increase in the aging population. Delay in diagnosis and management results in a high mortality, and prompt interventions may be life-saving. Intestinal ischemia is further classified based on etiology, which dictates management: (1) arterioocclusive mesenteric ischemia, (2) nonocclusive mesenteric ischemia, and (3) mesenteric venous thrombosis.

Risk factors for arterioocclusive mesenteric ischemia are generally acute in onset and include atrial fibrillation, recent myocardial infarction, valvular heart disease, and recent cardiac or vascular catheterization, all of which result in embolic clots reaching the mesenteric circulation. Nonocclusive mesenteric ischemia, also known as "intestinal angina," is generally more insidious and most often seen in the aging population affected by atherosclerotic disease. Patients with chronic atherosclerotic disease could also suffer an acute insult from emboli leading to complete occlusion. Nonocclusive mesenteric ischemia is also seen in patients receiving high-dose vasopressor infusions, patients with cardiogenic or septic shock, and patients with cocaine overdose. Nonocclusive mesenteric ischemia is the most prevalent gastrointestinal disease complicating cardiovascular surgery. The incidence of ischemic colitis following elective aortic repair is 5–9%, and the incidence triples in patients following emergent repair. Mesenteric venous thrombosis is less common and is associated with the presence of a hypercoagulable state including protein C or S deficiency, antithrombin III deficiency, polycythemia vera, and carcinoma.

ANATOMY AND PATHOPHYSIOLOGY

The blood supply to the intestines is depicted in Fig. 21-1. To prevent ischemic injury, extensive collateralization occurs between major mesenteric trunks and branches of the mesenteric arcades. Collateral vessels within the small bowel are numerous and meet

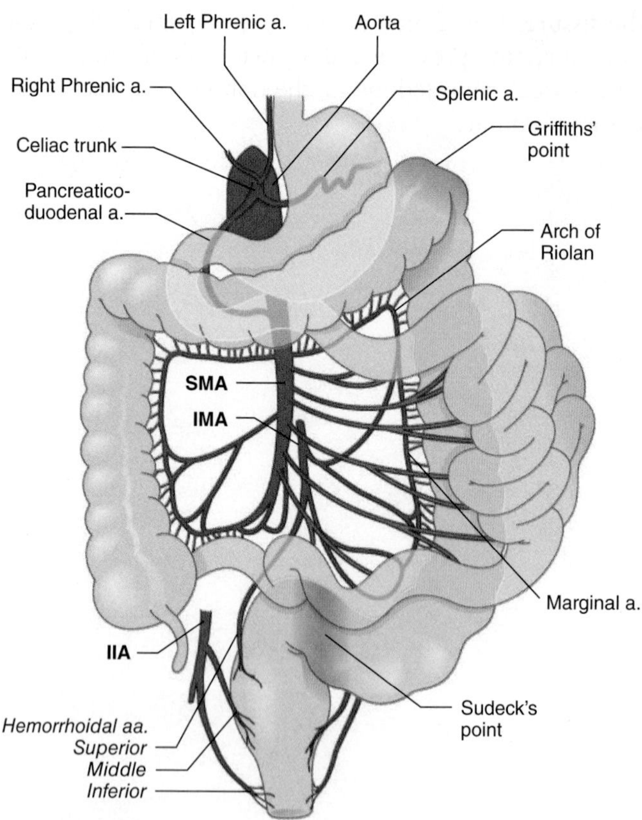

FIGURE 21-1

Blood supply to the intestines includes the celiac artery, superior mesenteric artery (SMA), inferior mesenteric artery (IMA), and branches of the internal iliac artery (IIA). Griffiths' and Sudeck's points, indicated by shaded areas, are watershed areas within the colonic blood supply and common locations for ischemia.

within the duodenum and the bed of the pancreas. Collateral vessels within the colon meet at the splenic flexure and descending/sigmoid colon. These areas, which are inherently at risk for decreased blood flow, are known as *Griffiths' point* and *Sudeck's point*, respectively, and are the most common locations for colonic ischemia (Fig. 21-1, shaded areas). The splanchnic circulation can receive up to 30% of the cardiac output. Protective responses to prevent intestinal ischemia include abundant collateralization, autoregulation of blood flow, and the ability to increase oxygen extraction from the blood.

Occlusive ischemia is a result of disruption of blood flow by an embolus or progressive thrombosis in a major artery supplying the intestine. Emboli originate from the heart in more than 75% of cases and lodge preferentially in the superior mesenteric artery just distal to the origin of the middle colic artery. Progressive thrombosis of at least two of the major vessels supplying the intestine is required for the development of chronic intestinal angina. Nonocclusive ischemia is disproportionate mesenteric vasoconstriction (arteriolar vasospasm) in response to a severe physiologic stress such as shock. If left untreated, early mucosal stress ulceration will progress to full-thickness injury. Even in the early stages of ischemia, there is translocation of bacteria across the intestinal mucosa, resulting in bacteremia that can lead to sepsis.

PRESENTATION, EVALUATION, AND MANAGEMENT

Intestinal ischemia remains one of the most challenging diagnoses. The mortality rate is greater than 50%. The most significant indicator of survival is the timeliness of diagnosis and treatment. An overview of diagnosis and management of each form of intestinal ischemia is given in Table 21-1.

Acute mesenteric ischemia resulting from arterial embolus or thrombosis presents with severe acute, nonremitting abdominal pain strikingly out of proportion to the physical findings. Associated symptoms may include nausea and vomiting, transient diarrhea, anorexia, and bloody stools. With the exception of

TABLE 21-1

OVERVIEW OF THE MANAGEMENT OF ACUTE INTESTINAL ISCHEMIA

CONDITION	KEY TO EARLY DIAGNOSIS	TREATMENT OF UNDERLYING CAUSE	TREATMENT OF SPECIFIC LESION	TREATMENT OF SYSTEMIC CONSEQUENCE
Arterioocclusive mesenteric ischemia 1. Arterial embolus	Computed tomography (CT) angiography Early laparotomy	Anticoagulation Cardioversion Proximal thrombectomy	Laparotomy Embolectomy Vascular bypass Assess viability and resect dead bowel	Ensure hydration Give antibiotics Reverse acidosis Optimize oxygen delivery Avoid vasoconstrictors
2. Arterial thrombosis	Duplex ultrasound Angiography	Anticoagulation Hydration	Endovascular approach: thrombolysis, angioplasty and stenting Endarterectomy/thrombectomy or vascular bypass Assess viability and resect dead bowel	Give antibiotics Reverse acidosis Optimize oxygen delivery Support cardiac output Avoid vasoconstrictors
Mesenteric venous thrombosis Venous thrombosis	Spiral CT Angiography with venous phase	Anticoagulation Massive hydration	Anticoagulation ± laparotomy/thrombectomy/catheter-directed thrombolysis Assess viability and resect dead bowel	Give antibiotics Reverse acidosis Optimize oxygen delivery Support cardiac output Avoid vasoconstrictors
Nonocclusive mesenteric ischemia	Vasospasm: Angiography Hypoperfusion: Spiral CT or colonoscopy	Ensure hydration Support cardiac output Avoid vasoconstrictors	Vasospasm Intraarterial vasodilators Hypoperfusion Delayed laparotomy Assess viability and resect dead bowel	Ensure hydration Give antibiotics Reverse acidosis Optimize oxygen delivery Support cardiac output Avoid vasoconstrictors

Source: Modified from GB Bulkley, in JL Cameron (ed): *Current Surgical Therapy*, 2nd ed. Toronto, BC Decker, 1986.

minimal abdominal distention and hypoactive bowel sounds, early abdominal examination is unimpressive. Later findings will demonstrate peritonitis and cardiovascular collapse. In the evaluation of acute intestinal ischemia, routine laboratory tests should be obtained, including complete blood count, serum chemistry, coagulation profile, arterial blood gas, amylase, lipase, lactic acid, blood type and cross match, and cardiac enzymes. Regardless of the need for urgent surgery, emergent admission to a monitored bed or intensive care unit is recommended for resuscitation and further evaluation. If the diagnosis of intestinal ischemia is being considered, consultation with a surgical service is necessary. Often the decision to operate is made on a high index of suspicion from the history and physical exam despite normal laboratory findings.

Other diagnostic modalities that may be useful in diagnosis but should not delay surgical therapy include electrocardiogram (ECG), echocardiogram, abdominal radiographs, computed tomography (CT), and mesenteric angiography. More recently, mesentery duplex scanning and visible light spectroscopy during colonoscopy have been demonstrated to be beneficial. The ECG may demonstrate an arrhythmia, indicating the possible source of the emboli. A plain abdominal film may show evidence of free intraperitoneal air, indicating a perforated viscus and the need for emergent exploration. Earlier features of intestinal ischemia seen on abdominal radiographs include bowel-wall edema, known as "thumbprinting." If the ischemia progresses, air can be seen within the bowel wall (*pneumatosis intestinalis*) and within the portal venous system. Other features include calcifications of the aorta and its tributaries, indicating atherosclerotic disease. With the administration of oral and IV contrast, dynamic CT angiography with three-dimensional reconstruction is a highly sensitive test for intestinal ischemia. In acute embolic disease, mesenteric angiography is best performed intraoperatively. A mesenteric duplex scan demonstrating a high peak velocity of flow in the superior mesenteric artery (SMA) is associated with an approximately 80% positive predictive value of mesenteric ischemia. More significantly, a negative duplex scan virtually precludes the diagnosis of mesenteric ischemia. Duplex imaging serves as a screening test; further investigations with angiography are needed. The biggest limitation of duplex scanning is body habitus; in obese patients, imaging is poor yield. However, in patients with chronic disease, "food fear" often leads to a decreased appetite and therefore less abdominal fat, and duplex imaging is very high yield. The endoscopic techniques using visible light spectroscopy can be used in the diagnosis of chronic ischemia. When suspecting mesenteric ischemia involving the colon, performing an endoscopy to evaluate up to the splenic flexure is high yield. This is often an excellent diagnostic tool in patients with chronic renal insufficiency who cannot tolerate IV contrast.

The "gold standard" for the diagnosis of acute arterial occlusive disease is angiography, and management is laparotomy. Surgical exploration should not be delayed if suspicion of acute occlusive mesenteric ischemia is high or evidence of clinical deterioration or frank peritonitis is present. The goal of operative exploration is to resect compromised bowel and restore blood supply. The entire length of the small and large bowel beginning at the ligament of Treitz should be evaluated. The pattern of intestinal ischemia may indicate the level of arterial occlusion. In the case of SMA occlusion where the embolus usually lies just proximal to the origin of the middle colic artery, the proximal jejunum is often spared while the remainder of the small bowel to the transverse colon will be ischemic. The surgical management of acute mesenteric ischemia of the small bowel is embolectomy via arteriotomy; a small incision is made in the artery through which the clot is retrieved. Another way to manage acute thrombosis is thrombolysis therapy and angioplasty, with stent placement. However, this approach is more commonly applied to treat chronic mesenteric ischemia. If this is unsuccessful, a bypass from the aorta or iliac artery to the SMA is performed.

Nonocclusive or vasospastic mesenteric ischemia presents with generalized abdominal pain, anorexia, bloody stools, and abdominal distention. Often these patients are obtunded, and physical findings may not assist in the diagnosis. The presence of a leukocytosis, metabolic acidosis, elevated amylase or creatinine phosphokinase levels, and/or lactic acidosis is useful in support of the diagnosis of advanced intestinal ischemia; however, these markers may not be indicative of either reversible ischemia or frank necrosis. Investigational markers for intestinal ischemia include D-dimer, glutathione *S*-transferase, platelet-activating factor (PAF), and mucosal pH monitoring. Regardless of the need for urgent surgery, emergent admission to a monitored bed or intensive care unit is recommended for resuscitation and further evaluation. Early manifestations of intestinal ischemia include fluid sequestration within the bowel wall leading to a loss of interstitial volume. Aggressive fluid resuscitation may be necessary. To optimize oxygen delivery, nasal O_2 and blood transfusions may be given. Broad-spectrum antibiotics should be given to provide sufficient coverage for enteric pathogens, including gram-negative and anaerobic organisms. Frequent monitoring of the patient's vital signs, urine output, blood gases, and lactate levels is paramount, as is frequent abdominal examination. All vasoconstricting agents should be avoided; fluid resuscitation is the intervention of choice to maintain hemodynamics.

If ischemic colitis is a concern, colonoscopy should be performed to assess the integrity of the colon mucosa. Visualization of the rectosigmoid region may demonstrate decreased mucosal integrity, associated more commonly with nonocclusive mesenteric ischemia, or, on occasion, occlusive disease as a result of acute loss of inferior mesenteric arterial flow following aortic surgery. Ischemia of the colonic mucosa is graded as *mild* with minimal mucosal erythema or as *moderate* with pale mucosal ulcerations and evidence of extension to the muscular layer of the bowel wall. *Severe* ischemic colitis presents with severe ulcerations resulting in black or green discoloration of the mucosa, consistent with full-thickness bowel-wall necrosis. The degree of reversibility can be predicted from the mucosal findings: mild erythema is nearly 100% reversible, moderate is approximately 50% reversible, and frank necrosis is simply dead bowel. Follow-up colonoscopy can be performed to rule out progression of ischemic colitis.

Laparotomy for nonocclusive mesenteric ischemia is warranted for signs of peritonitis or worsening endoscopic findings and if the patient's condition does not improve with aggressive resuscitation. Ischemic colitis is optimally treated with resection of the ischemic bowel and formation of a proximal stoma. Primary anastomosis should not be performed in patients with acute intestinal ischemia.

Patients with mesenteric venous thrombosis may present with a gradual or sudden onset. Symptoms include vague abdominal pain, nausea, and vomiting. Examination findings include abdominal distention with mild to moderate tenderness and signs of dehydration. The diagnosis of mesenteric thrombosis is frequently made on abdominal spiral CT with oral and IV contrast. Findings on CT angiography with venous phase include bowel-wall thickening and ascites. Intravenous contrast will demonstrate a delayed arterial phase and clot within the superior mesenteric vein. The goal of management is to optimize hemodynamics and correct electrolyte abnormalities with massive fluid resuscitation. Intravenous antibiotics as well as anticoagulation should be initiated. If laparotomy is performed and mesenteric venous thrombosis is suspected, heparin anticoagulation is immediately initiated, and compromised bowel is resected. Of all acute intestinal disorders, mesenteric venous insufficiency is associated with the best prognosis.

Chronic intestinal ischemia presents with intestinal angina or postprandial abdominal pain associated with need for increased blood flow to the intestine following meals. Patients report abdominal cramping and pain following ingestion of a meal. Weight loss and chronic diarrhea may also be noted. Abdominal pain without weight loss is not chronic mesenteric angina. Physical examination will often reveal a malnourished patient with an abdominal bruit as well as other manifestations of atherosclerosis. Duplex ultrasound evaluation of the mesenteric vessels has gained in popularity. It is important to perform the test fasting because the presence of increased bowel gas prevents adequate visualization of flow disturbances within the vessels or the lack of a vasodilation response to feeding during the test. This tool is frequently used as a screening test for patients with symptoms suggestive of chronic mesenteric ischemia. The gold standard for confirmation of mesenteric arterial occlusion is mesenteric angiography. Evaluation with mesenteric angiography allows for identification and possible intervention for the treatment of atherosclerosis within the vessel lumen and will also evaluate the patency of remaining mesenteric vessels. The use of mesenteric angiography may be limited in the presence of renal failure or contrast allergy. Magnetic resonance angiography is an alternative if the administration of contrast dye is contraindicated.

The management of chronic intestinal ischemia includes medical management of atherosclerotic disease by exercise, cessation of smoking, and antiplatelet and lipid-lowering medications. A full cardiac evaluation should be performed before intervention on chronic mesenteric ischemia. Newer endovascular procedures may avoid an operative intervention in selected patient populations. Angioplasty with endovascular stenting in the treatment of chronic mesenteric ischemia is associated with an 80% long-term success rate. In patients requiring surgical exploration, the approach used is determined by findings of the mesenteric angiogram. The entire length of the small and large bowel should be evaluated, beginning at the ligament of Treitz. Restoration of blood flow at the time of laparotomy is accomplished with mesenteric vessel endarterectomy or bypass.

Determination of intestinal viability intraoperatively in patients with suspected intestinal ischemia can be challenging. After revascularization, the bowel wall should be observed for return of a pink color and peristalsis. Palpation of major arterial mesenteric vessels can be performed, as well as applying a Doppler flowmeter to the antimesenteric border of the bowel wall, but neither is a definitive indicator of viability. In equivocal cases, 1 g of IV sodium fluorescein is administered, and the pattern of bowel reperfusion is observed under ultraviolet illumination with a standard (3600 A) Wood's lamp. An area of nonfluorescence >5 mm in diameter suggests nonviability. If doubt persists, reexploration performed 24–48 h following surgery will allow demarcation of nonviable bowel. Primary intestinal anastomosis in patients with ischemic bowel is always worrisome; thus, delayed bowel reconstruction and reanastomosis should be deferred to the time of second-look laparotomy.

ACKNOWLEDGMENTS

We thank Cory Sandore for providing the illustration for this chapter. Susan Gearhart contributed to this chapter in the 18th edition of Harrison's Principles of Internal Medicine.

CHAPTER 22

ACUTE INTESTINAL OBSTRUCTION

Danny O. Jacobs

EPIDEMIOLOGY

Morbidity and mortality from acute intestinal obstruction have been decreasing over the past several decades. Nevertheless, the diagnosis can still be challenging, and the type of complications that patients suffer has not changed significantly. The extent of mechanical obstruction is typically described as partial, high-grade, or complete—generally correlating with the risk of complications and the urgency with which the underlying disease process must be addressed. Obstruction is also commonly described as being either "simple" or, alternatively, "strangulated" if vascular insufficiency and intestinal ischemia are evident.

Acute intestinal obstruction occurs either *mechanically* from blockage or from intestinal dysmotility when there is no blockage. In the latter instance, the abnormality is described as being *functional*. Mechanical bowel obstruction may be caused by extrinsic processes, intrinsic abnormalities of the bowel wall, or intraluminal abnormalities (Table 22-1). Within each of these broad categories are many diseases that can impede intestinal propulsion. Intrinsic diseases that can cause intestinal obstruction are usually congenital, inflammatory, neoplastic, or traumatic in origin, although intussusception and radiation injury can also be etiologic. Primary small-bowel cancers rarely cause acute obstruction.

Acute intestinal obstruction accounts for approximately 1–3 % of all hospitalizations and a quarter of all urgent or emergent general surgery admissions. Approximately 80% of cases involve the small bowel, and about one-third of these patients show evidence of significant ischemia. The mortality rate for patients with strangulation who are operated on within 24–30 h of the onset of symptoms is approximately 8% but triples shortly thereafter.

Extrinsic diseases most commonly cause mechanical obstruction of the small intestine. In the United States and Europe, almost all cases are caused by postoperative adhesions (>50%), carcinomatosis, or herniation of the anterior abdominal wall. Carcinomatosis most often originates from the ovary, pancreas, stomach, or colon, although rarely, metastasis from distant organs like the breast and skin can occur. Adhesions are responsible for >90% of cases of early postoperative obstruction that require intervention.

TABLE 22-1

MOST COMMON CAUSES OF ACUTE INTESTINAL OBSTRUCTION
Extrinsic Disease
Adhesions (especially due to previous abdominal surgery), internal or external hernias, neoplasms (including carcinomatosis and extraintestinal malignancies, mostly commonly ovarian), endometriosis or intraperitoneal abscesses, and idiopathic sclerosis
Intrinsic Disease
Congenital (e.g., malrotation, atresia, stenosis, intestinal duplication, cyst formation, and congenital bands—the latter rarely in adults)
Inflammation (e.g., inflammatory bowel disease, especially Crohn's disease, but also diverticulitis, radiation, tuberculosis, lymphogranuloma venereum, and schistosomiasis)
Neoplasia (note: primary small-bowel cancer is rare; obstructive colon cancer may mimic small-bowel obstruction if the ileocecal valve is incompetent)
Traumatic (e.g., hematoma formation, anastomotic strictures)
Other, including intussusception (where the lead point is typically a polyp or tumor in adults), volvulus, obstruction of duodenum by superior mesenteric artery, radiation or ischemic injury, and aganglionosis, which is Hirschsprung's disease
Intraluminal Abnormalities
Bezoars, feces, foreign bodies including inspissated barium, gallstones (entering the lumen via a cholecystoenteric fistula), enteroliths

TABLE 22-2

ACUTE SMALL-INTESTINAL AND COLONIC OBSTRUCTION INCIDENCES

CAUSE	INCIDENCE
Postoperative adhesions	>50%
Neoplasms	~20%
Hernias (especially ventral or internal types, where the risk of strangulation is increased)	~10%
Inflammatory bowel disease, other inflammation (obstruction may resolve if acute inflammation and edema subside)	~5%
Intussusception, volvulus, other miscellaneous diseases	<15%

Operations of the lower abdomen, including appendectomy and colorectal and gynecologic procedures, are especially likely to create adhesions that can cause bowel obstruction (Table 22-2). Overall, small-bowel obstruction is slightly more common in women. The risk of internal herniation is increased by abdominal procedures such as laparoscopic or open Roux-en-Y gastric bypass. Although laparoscopic procedures may generate fewer postoperative adhesions compared with open surgery, the risk of obstructive adhesion formation is not eliminated.

In many patients who are successfully treated for adhesive small-bowel obstruction, obstruction will recur. The rate varies according to how patients were initially managed. Approximately 20% of patients who were treated conservatively and between 5 and 30% of patients who were managed operatively will require readmission within 10 years.

Volvulus, which occurs when bowel twists on its mesenteric axis, can cause partial or complete obstruction and vascular insufficiency. The sigmoid colon is most commonly affected, accounting for approximately two-thirds of all cases of volvulus and 4% of all cases of large-bowel obstruction. The cecum and terminal ileum can also volvulize, or the cecum alone may be involved as a cecal bascule. Risk factors include institutionalization, the presence of neuropsychiatric conditions requiring psychotropic medication, chronic constipation, and aging; patients typically present in their seventies or eighties. Colonic volvulus is more common in Eastern Europe, Russia, and Africa than it is in the United States. It is rare for adhesions or hernias to obstruct the colon. Cancer of the descending colon and rectum is responsible for approximately two-thirds of all cases, followed by diverticulitis and volvulus.

TABLE 22-3

MOST COMMON CAUSES OF ILEUS (FUNCTIONAL OR PSEUDO-OBSTRUCTION OF THE INTESTINE)

Intraabdominal procedures, lumbar spinal injuries, or surgical procedures on the lumbar spine and pelvis
Metabolic or electrolyte abnormalities, especially hypokalemia and hypomagnesemia, but also hyponatremia, uremia, and severe hyperglycemia
Drugs such as opiates, antihistamines, and some psychotropic (e.g., haloperidol, tricyclic antidepressants) and anticholinergic agents
Intestinal ischemia
Intraabdominal or retroperitoneal inflammation or hemorrhage
Lower lobe pneumonias
Intraoperative radiation (likely due to muscle damage)
Systemic sepsis
Hyperparathyroidism
Pseudo-obstruction (Ogilvie's syndrome)
Ileus secondary to hereditary or acquired visceral myopathies and neuropathies that disrupt myocellular neural coordination
Some collagen vascular diseases such as lupus erythematosus or scleroderma

Functional obstruction, also known as *ileus* and *pseudo-obstruction*, is present when dysmotility prevents intestinal contents from being propelled distally and no mechanical blockage exists. Ileus that occurs after intraabdominal surgery is the most commonly identified form of functional bowel obstruction, although there are many other causes (Table 22-3). Although postoperative ileus is most often transient, it is the most common reason why hospital discharge is delayed. Pseudo-obstruction of the colon, also known as Ogilvie's syndrome, is a relatively rare disease. Some patients with Ogilvie's syndrome have colonic dysmotility due to abnormalities of their autonomic nervous system that may be inherited.

PATHOPHYSIOLOGY

The manifestations of acute intestinal obstruction depend on the nature of the underlying disease process, its location, and changes in blood flow (Fig. 22-1). Increased intestinal contractility, which occurs proximally and distal to the obstruction, is a characteristic response. Subsequently, intestinal peristalsis slows as the intestine or stomach proximal to the point of obstruction dilates and fills with gastrointestinal secretions and swallowed air. Although swallowed air is the primary contributor to intestinal distension,

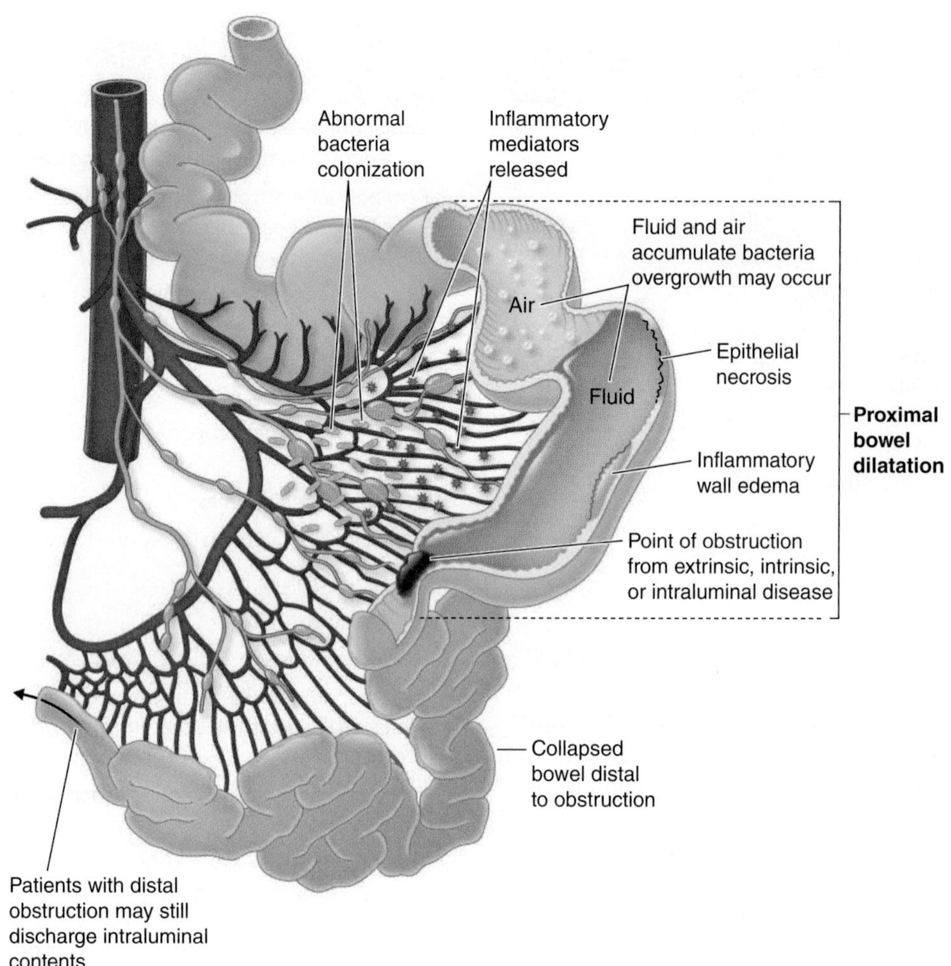

FIGURE 22-1
Pathophysiologic changes of small-bowel obstruction.

intraluminal air may also accumulate from fermentation, local carbon dioxide production, and altered gaseous diffusion.

Intraluminal dilation also increases intraluminal pressure. When luminal pressure exceeds venous pressure, venous and lymphatic drainage is impeded. Edema ensues, and the bowel wall proximal to the site of blockage may become hypoxemic. Epithelial necrosis can be identified within 12 h of obstruction. Ultimately, arterial blood supply may become so compromised that full-thickness ischemia, necrosis, and perforation result. Stasis increases the bacteria counts within the jejunum and ileum. The most commonly cultured intraluminal organisms are *Escherichia coli*, *Streptococcus faecalis*, and *Klebsiella*, which may also be recovered from mesenteric lymph nodes and other more distant sites.

Other manifestations depend on the degree of hypovolemia, the patient's metabolic response, and the presence or absence of associated intestinal ischemia. Inflammatory edema eventually increases the production of reactive oxygen species and activates neutrophils and macrophages, which accumulate within the bowel wall. Their accumulation, along with changes in innate immunity, disrupts secretory and neuromotor processes. Dehydration is caused by loss of the normal intestinal absorptive capacity as well as fluid accumulation in the gastric or intestinal wall and intraperitoneally.

Anorexia and emesis tend to exacerbate intravascular volume depletion. In the worst case scenario that is most commonly identified after distal obstruction, emesis leads to losses of gastric potassium, hydrogen, and chloride, while dehydration stimulates proximal renal tubule bicarbonate reabsorption. Intraperitoneal fluid accumulation, especially in patients with severe distal bowel obstruction, may increase intraabdominal pressure enough to elevate the diaphragm and inhibit respiration and to impede systemic venous return and promote vascular instability. Severe hemodynamic compromise may elicit a systemic inflammatory response and generalized microvascular leakage.

Closed-loop obstruction results when the proximal and distal openings of a given bowel segment are both occluded, e.g., due to volvulus or a hernia. It is the most common precursor for strangulation, but not every closed loop strangulates. The risk of vascular insufficiency, systemic inflammation, hemodynamic compromise, and irreversible intestinal ischemia is much greater in patients with closed-loop obstruction. Pathologic changes may occur more rapidly, and emergency intervention is indicated. Irreversible bowel ischemia progresses to transmural necrosis even if the obstruction is relieved. It is also important to remember that patients with high-grade distal colonic obstruction who have competent ileocecal valves may present with closed-loop obstruction. In the latter instance, the cecum may progressively dilate such that ischemic necrosis results in cecal perforation. This risk is generally greatest when the cecal diameter exceeds 12 cm, as informed by Laplace's law. Patients with distal colonic obstruction whose ileocecal valves are incompetent tend to present later in the course of disease and mimic patients with distal small-bowel obstruction.

HISTORY AND PHYSICAL FINDINGS

Even though the presenting signs and symptoms can be misleading, many patients with acute obstruction can be accurately diagnosed after a thorough history and physical examination is performed. Early recognition allows earlier treatment that decreases the risk of progression or other excess morbidity. Small-bowel obstruction with strangulation can be especially difficult to diagnosis promptly.

The cardinal signs are colicky abdominal pain, abdominal distention, emesis, and obstipation. More intraluminal fluid accumulates in patients with distal obstruction, which typically leads to greater distention, more discomfort, and delayed emesis. This emesis is feculent when there is bacterial overgrowth. Patients with more proximal obstruction commonly present with less abdominal distention but more pronounced vomiting. Elements of the history that might be helpful include any prior history of surgery, including herniorrhaphy, as well as any history of cancer or inflammatory bowel disease.

Most patients, even with simple obstruction, appear to be critically ill. Many may be oliguric, hypotensive, and tachycardic because of severe intravascular volume depletion. Fever is worrisome for strangulation or systemic inflammatory changes. Bowel sounds and bowel functional activity are notoriously difficult to interpret. Classically, many patients with early small-bowel obstruction will have high-pitched, "musical" tinkling bowel sounds and peristaltic "rushes" known as borborygmi. Later in the course of disease, the bowel sounds may be absent or hypoactive as peristaltic activity decreases. This is in contrast to the common findings in patients with ileus or pseudo-obstruction where bowel sounds are typically absent or hypoactive from the beginning. Lastly, patients with partial blockage may continue to pass flatus and stool, and those with complete blockage may evacuate bowel contents present downstream beyond their obstruction.

All surgical incisions should be examined. The presence of a tender abdominal or groin mass strongly suggests that an incarcerated hernia may be the cause of obstruction. The presence of tenderness should increase the concern about the presence of complications such as ischemia, necrosis, or peritonitis. Severe pain with localization or signs of peritoneal irritation is suspicious for strangulated or closed-loop obstruction. It is important to remember that the discomfort may be out of proportion to physical findings mimicking the complaints of patients with acute mesenteric ischemia. Every patient should have a rectal examination. Patients with colonic volvulus present with the classic manifestations of closed-loop obstruction: severe abdominal pain, vomiting, and obstipation. Asymmetrical abdominal distension and a tympanic mass may be evident.

Patients with ileus or pseudo-obstruction may have signs and symptoms similar to those of bowel obstruction. Although abdominal distention is present, colicky abdominal pain is typically absent, and patients may not have nausea or emesis. Ongoing, regular discharge of stool or flatus can sometimes help distinguish patients with ileus from those with complete mechanical bowel obstruction.

LABORATORY AND IMAGING STUDIES

Laboratory testing should include a complete blood count and serum electrolyte and creatinine measurements. Serial assessments are often useful. Mild hemoconcentration and slight elevation of the white blood cell count commonly occur after simple bowel obstruction. Emesis and dehydration may cause hypokalemia, hypochloremia, elevated blood urea nitrogen–to–creatinine ratios, and metabolic alkalosis. Patients may be hyponatremic on admission because many have attempted to rehydrate themselves with hypotonic fluids. The presence of guaiac-positive stools and iron-deficiency anemia are strongly suggestive of malignancy.

Higher white blood cell counts with the presence of immature forms or the presence of metabolic acidosis are worrisome for severe volume depletion or ischemic necrosis and sepsis. At this time, there are no laboratory tests that are especially useful for identifying the presence of simple or strangulated obstruction, although increases in serum D-lactate, creatine kinase bb isoenzymes, or intestinal fatty acid binding protein levels may be suggestive of the latter.

In all cases, when considering diagnostic imaging, the key is not to delay surgical consultation and operative intervention when the patient's signs or symptoms strongly suggest that high-grade or complete obstruction or bowel compromise is present. Plain films of the abdomen, which must include upright or cross-table lateral views, can be completed quickly and may confirm the clinical suspicion 60% of the time. Interpretation immediately after operation is difficult. A "staircasing" pattern of dilated air and fluid-filled small-bowel loops >2.5 cm in diameter with little or no air seen in the colon are classical findings in patients with small-bowel obstruction, although findings may be equivocal in some patients with documented disease. Little bowel gas appears in patients with proximal bowel obstruction or in patients whose intestinal lumens are filled with fluid. Upright plain films of the abdomen of patients with large-bowel obstruction typically show colon dilatation. Small-bowel air-fluid levels will not be obvious if the ileocecal valve is competent. Although it can be difficult to distinguish from ileus, small-bowel obstruction is more likely when air-fluid levels are seen without significant colonic distension. Free air suggests that perforation has occurred in patients who have not recently undergone surgical procedures. Radiopaque foreign bodies or enteroliths may be visualized. A gas-filled, "coffee bean"–shaped dilated shadow may be seen in patients with volvulus.

More sophisticated imaging can be beneficial when the diagnosis is unclear. Magnetic resonance imaging has been used to diagnose small-bowel obstruction, but it is more expensive and, typically, provides less spatial resolution. Ultrasonographic evaluations are especially difficult to interpret but may be sensitive and appropriate studies to evaluate patients who are pregnant or for whom x-ray exposure is otherwise contraindicated or inappropriate.

Computed tomography (CT) is the most commonly used imaging modality. Its sensitivity for detecting bowel obstruction is approximately 95% (78–100%) in patients with high-grade obstruction, with a specificity of 96% and an accuracy of ≥95%. Its accuracy in diagnosing closed-loop obstruction is much lower (60%). Examples of some CT images are reproduced in Fig. 22-2. It may also provide useful information regarding location or identify particular circumstances where surgical intervention is needed urgently. Patients who have evidence of contrast appearing within the cecum within 4–24 h of oral administration can be expected to improve with high sensitivity and specificity (~95% each). For example, contrast studies may demonstrate a "bird's beak," a "c-loop," or "whorl"

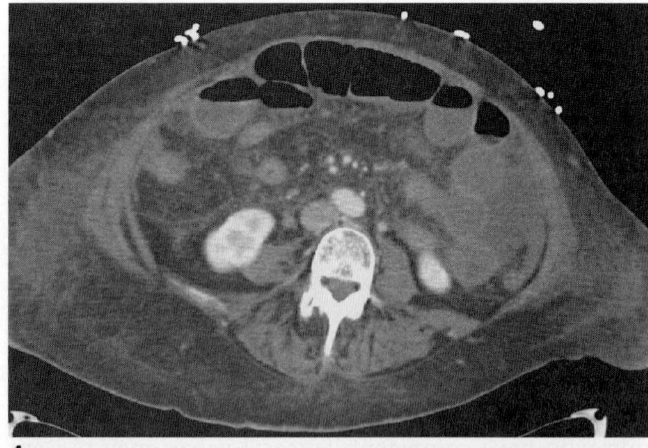

A

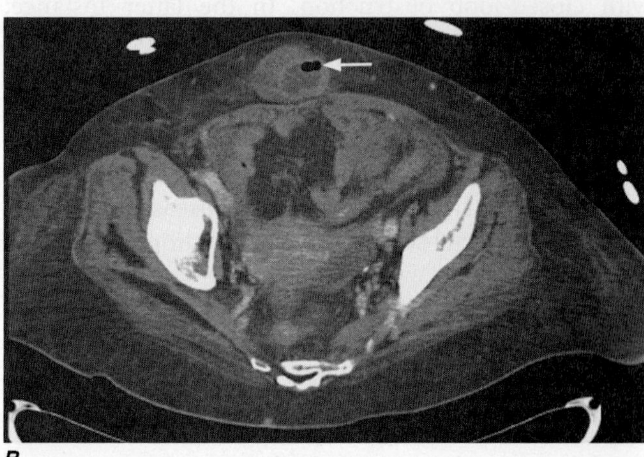

B

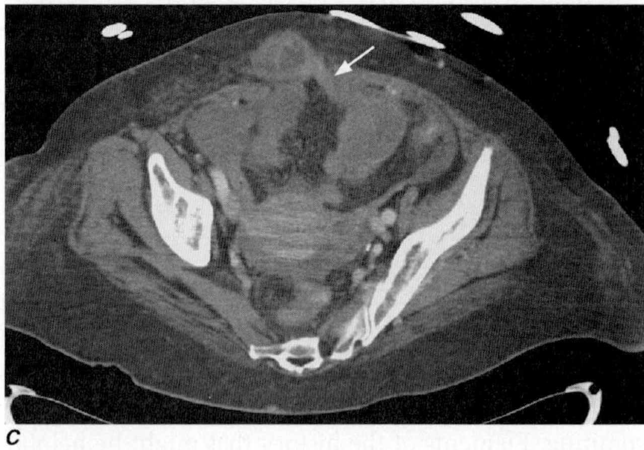

C

FIGURE 22-2

Computed tomography with oral and intravenous contrast demonstrating **(*A*)** evidence of small-bowel dilatation with air-fluid levels consistent with a small-bowel obstruction; **(*B*)** a partial small-bowel obstruction from an incarcerated ventral hernia (*arrow*); and **(*C*)** decompressed bowel seen distal to the hernia (*arrow*). *(From W Silen: Acute intestinal obstruction, in DL Longo et al [eds]: Harrison's Principles of Internal Medicine, 18th ed. New York, McGraw-Hill, 2012.)*

deformity on CT imaging at the site where twisting obstructs the lumen when a colonic volvulus is present.

CT imaging with enteral and IV contrast can also identify ischemia. Altered bowel wall enhancement is the most specific early finding, but its sensitivity is low. Mesenteric venous gas, pneumoperitoneum, and pneumatosis intestinalis are late findings indicating the presence of bowel necrosis. CT scanning after a water-soluble contrast enema may help distinguish ileus or pseudo-obstruction from distal large-bowel obstruction in patients who present with evidence of small-bowel and colonic distention. CT enteroclysis can accurately identify neoplasia as a cause of bowel obstruction. Contrast enemas or colonoscopies are almost always needed to identify causes of acute colonic obstruction.

Barium studies are generally contraindicated in patients with firm evidence of complete or high-grade bowel obstruction, especially when they present acutely. Barium should never be given orally to a patient with possible obstruction until that diagnosis has been excluded. In every other case, such investigations should only be performed in exceptional circumstances and with great caution because patients with significant obstruction may develop barium concretions as an additional source of blockage and some who would have otherwise recovered will require operative intervention. Barium opacification also renders cross-sectional imaging studies or angiography uninterpretable.

TREATMENT Acute Intestinal Obstruction

An improved understanding of the pathophysiology of bowel obstruction and the importance of fluid resuscitation, electrolyte repletion, intestinal decompression, and the selected use of antibiotics have likely contributed to a reduction in the mortality from acute bowel obstruction. Every patient should be stabilized as quickly as possible. Nasogastric tube suction decompresses the stomach, minimizes further distention from swallowed air, improves patient comfort, and reduces the risk of aspiration. Urine output should be assessed using a Foley catheter. In some cases, for example, in patients with cardiac disease, central venous pressures should be monitored. The use of antibiotics is controversial, although prophylactic administration is warranted if surgery is required. Complete bowel obstruction is an indication for intervention. Stenting may be possible and warranted for some patients with high-grade obstruction due to unresectable stage IV malignancy. Stenting may also allow elective mechanical bowel preparation before surgery is undertaken. Because treatment options are so variable, it is helpful to make as precise a diagnosis as possible preoperatively.

ILEUS Patients with ileus are treated supportively with intravenous fluids and nasogastric decompression while any underlying pathology is treated. Pharmacologic therapy is not yet proven to be efficacious or cost-effective. However, peripherally active μ-opioid receptor antagonists (e.g., alvimopan and methylnaltrexone) may accelerate gastrointestinal recovery in some patients who have undergone abdominal surgery.

COLONIC PSEUDO-OBSTRUCTION (OGILVIE'S DISEASE) Neostigmine is an acetylcholinsterase inhibitor that increases cholinergic (parasympathetic) activity, which can stimulate colonic motility. Some studies have shown it to be moderately effective in alleviating acute colonic pseudo-obstruction. It is the most common therapeutic approach and can be used once it is certain that there is no mechanical obstruction. Cardiac monitoring is required, and atropine should be immediately available. Intravenous administration induces defecation and flatus within 10 min in the majority of patients who will respond. Sympathetic blockade by epidural anesthesia can successfully ameliorate pseudo-obstruction in some patients.

VOLVULUS Patients with sigmoid volvulus can often be decompressed using a flexible tube inserted through a rigid proctoscope or using a flexible sigmoidoscope. Successful decompression results in sudden release of gas and fluid with evidence of decreased abdominal distension and allows definitive correction to be scheduled electively. Cecal volvulus most often requires laparotomy or laparoscopic correction.

INTRAOPERATIVE STRATEGIES Approximately 60–80% of selected patients with mechanical bowel obstruction can be successfully treated conservatively. Indeed, most cases of radiation-induced obstruction should also be managed nonoperatively if possible. In most circumstances, early consultation with a general surgeon is prudent when there is concern about strangulation obstruction or other abnormality that needs to be addressed urgently. Deterioration signifies a need for intervention. At this time, the decision as to whether the patient can continue to be treated nonoperatively can only be based on clinical judgment, although, as described earlier, imaging studies can sometimes be helpful. The frequency of major complications after operation ranges from 12 to 47%, with greater risk being attributed to resection therapies and the patient's overall health. Risk is increased for patients with American Society of Anesthesiologists (ASA) class III or higher.

At operation, dilation proximal to the site of blockage with distal collapse is a defining feature of bowel obstruction. Intraoperative strategies depend on the underlying problem and range from lysis of adhesions to resection with or without diverting ostomy to primary resection with anastomosis. Resection is warranted when there is concern about the bowel's viability after the obstructive process is relieved. Laparoscopic approaches can be useful for patients with early obstruction when extensive adhesions are not expected to be present. Some patients with high-grade obstruction secondary to malignant disease that is not amendable to resection will benefit from bypass procedures.

ADULT INTUSSUSCEPTION AND GALLSTONE ILEUS Primary resection is prudent. Careful manual reduction of any involved bowel may limit the amount of intestine that needs to be removed. A proximal ostomy may be required if unprepped colon is involved. Only 60% of patients with gallstone ileus obstruct in the ileum. The most common site of intestinal obstruction in patients with gallstone "ileus" is the ileum (60% of patients). The gallstone enters the intestinal tract most often via a cholecystoduodenal fistula. It can usually be removed by operative enterolithotomy. Addressing the gallbladder disease during urgent or emergent surgery is not recommended.

POSTOPERATIVE BOWEL OBSTRUCTION Early postoperative mechanical bowel obstruction is that which occurs within the first 6 weeks of operation. Most are partial and can be expected to resolve spontaneously. It tends to respond and behave differently from classic mechanical bowel obstruction and may be very difficult to distinguish from postoperative ileus. A higher index of suspicion for a definitive site of obstruction is warranted for patients who undergo laparoscopic surgical procedures. Patients who first had ileus and then subsequently develop obstructive symptoms after an initial return of normal bowel function are more likely to have true postoperative small-bowel obstruction. The longer it takes for a patient's obstructive symptoms to resolve after hospitalization, the more likely the patient is to require surgical intervention.

ACKNOWLEDGMENT

The wisdom and expertise of Dr. William Silen are gratefully acknowledged.

CHAPTER 23

ACUTE APPENDICITIS AND PERITONITIS

Danny O. Jacobs

ACUTE APPENDICITIS

INCIDENCE AND EPIDEMIOLOGY

Appendicitis occurs more frequently in Westernized societies. Although its incidence is decreasing for uncertain reasons, acute appendicitis remains the most common emergency general surgical disease affecting the abdomen, with a rate of approximately 100 per 100,000 person-years in Europe and the Americas or about 11 cases per 10,000 people annually. Approximately 9% of men and 7% of women will experience an episode during their lifetime. Appendicitis occurs most commonly in 10- to 19-year-olds, although the average age at diagnosis appears to be gradually increasing, as is the frequency of the disease in African Americans, Asians, and Native Americans. Overall, 70% of patients are less than 30 years old and most are men; the male-to-female ratio is 1.4:1.

One of the more common complications and most important causes of excess morbidity and mortality is perforation, whether it is contained and localized or unconstrained within the peritoneal cavity. In contrast to the trend observed for appendicitis and appendectomy, the incidence of perforated appendicitis (~20 cases per 100,000 person-years) is increasing. The explanation for this phenomenon is unknown. Approximately 20% of all patients have evidence of perforation at presentation, but the percentage risk is much higher in patients under 5 or over 65 years of age.

PATHOGENESIS OF APPENDICITIS AND APPENDICEAL PERFORATION

Appendicitis was first described in 1886 by Reginald Fitz. Its etiology is still not completely understood. Fecaliths, incompletely digested food residue, lymphoid hyperplasia, intraluminal scarring, tumors, bacteria, viruses, and inflammatory bowel disease have all been associated with inflammation of the appendix and appendicitis.

Although not proven, obstruction of the appendiceal lumen is believed to be an important step in the development of appendicitis. In some cases, obstruction leads to bacterial overgrowth and luminal distension, with an increase in intraluminal pressure that can inhibit the flow of lymph and blood in some cases. Then, vascular thrombosis and ischemic necrosis with perforation of the distal appendix may occur. Any perforation that occurs near the base of the appendix should raise concerns about another disease process. Most patients who will perforate do so before they are evaluated by surgeons.

Appendiceal fecaliths (or appendicoliths) are found in approximately 50% of patients with gangrenous appendicitis who perforate but are rarely identified in those who have simple disease. As mentioned earlier, the incidence of perforated, but not simple, appendicitis is increasing. The rate of perforated and nonperforated appendicitis is correlated in men but not in women. Together these observations suggest that the underlying pathophysiologic processes are different and that simple appendicitis does not always progress to perforation. Furthermore, some cases of simple acute appendicitis may resolve spontaneously or with antibiotic therapy, and recurrent disease is remotely possible. The relative frequency of these events is unknown.

When perforation occurs, the resultant leak may be contained by the omentum or other surrounding tissues to form an abscess. Free perforation normally causes severe peritonitis. These patients may also develop infective suppurative thrombosis of the portal vein and its tributaries along with intrahepatic abscesses. The prognosis of the very unfortunate patients who develop this dreaded complication is very poor.

CLINICAL MANIFESTATIONS

More refined approaches to diagnosis, supportive care, and surgical intervention are likely responsible for the

TABLE 23-1

SOME CONDITIONS THAT MIMIC APPENDICITIS	
Crohn's disease	Meckel's diverticulitis
Cholecystitis or other gall-bladder disease	Mittelschmerz
Diverticulitis	Mesenteric adenitis
Ectopic pregnancy	Omental torsion
Endometriosis	Pancreatitis
Gastroenteritis or colitis	Lower lobe pneumonia
Gastric or duodenal ulceration	Pelvic inflammatory disease
Hepatitis	Ruptured ovarian cyst or other cystic disease of the ovaries
Kidney disease, including nephrolithiasis	Small-bowel obstruction
Liver abscess	Urinary tract infection

remarkable decrease in the risk of mortality from simple appendicitis to currently less than 1%. Nevertheless, it is still important to identify patients who might have appendicitis as early as possible to minimize their risk of developing complications. Patients who have had symptoms for more than 48 h are more likely to perforate.

Appendicitis should be included in the differential diagnosis of abdominal pain for every patient in any age group unless it is certain that the organ has been previously removed (Table 23-1).

The appendix's anatomical location, which varies, directly influences how the patient presents for care. Where the appendix can be "found" ranges from local differences in how the appendiceal body and tip lie relative to its attachment to the cecum (Figs. 23-1 and 23-2), to where the appendix is actually situated in the peritoneal cavity—for example, from its typical location in the right lower quadrant, to the pelvis, right flank, right upper quadrant (as may be observed during pregnancy), or even the left side of the abdomen for patients with malrotation or who have severely redundant colons.

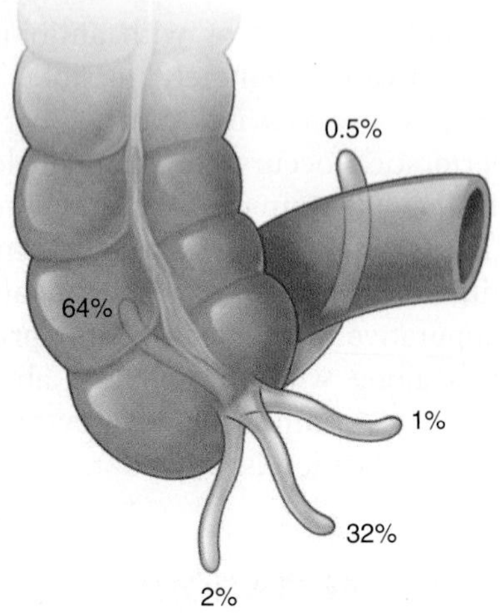

FIGURE 23-1
Regional anatomical variations of the appendix.

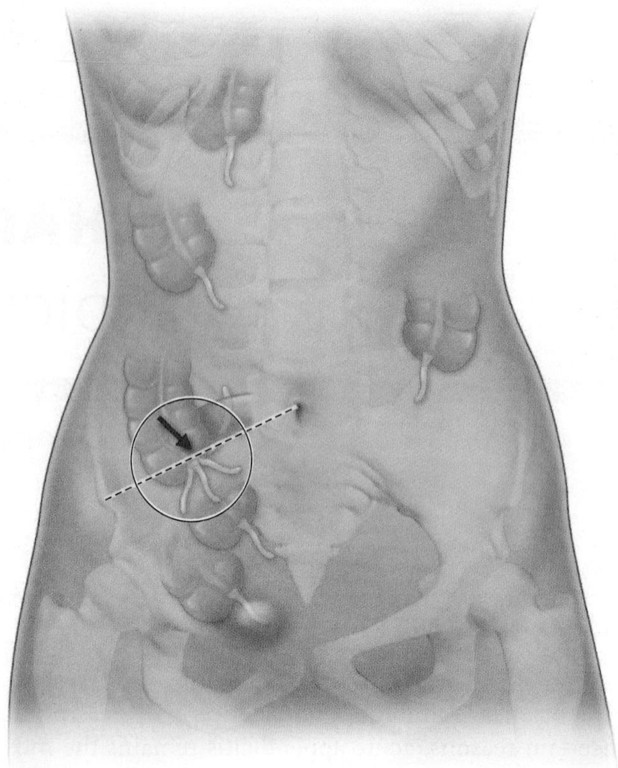

FIGURE 23-2
Locations of the appendix and cecum.

Because the differential diagnosis of appendicitis is so extensive, deciding if a patient has appendicitis can be difficult (Table 23-2). Soliciting an appropriate history requires detecting symptoms that might suggest alternative diagnoses. Patients with appendicitis may not have any abdominal discomfort early in the disease process. Furthermore, many patients may not present with the classically described history or physical findings.

TABLE 23-2

RELATIVE FREQUENCY OF COMMON PRESENTING SYMPTOMS

SYMPTOMS	FREQUENCY
Abdominal pain	>95%
Anorexia	>70%
Constipation	4–16%
Diarrhea	4–16%
Fever	10–20%
Migration of pain to right lower quadrant	50–60%
Nausea	>65%
Vomiting	50–75%

What is the classic history? Nonspecific complaints occur first. Patients may notice changes in bowel habits or malaise and vague, perhaps intermittent, crampy, abdominal pain in the epigastric or periumbilical region. The pain subsequently migrates to the right lower quadrant over 12–24 h, where it is sharper and can be definitively localized as transmural inflammation when the appendix irritates the parietal peritoneum. Parietal peritoneal irritation may be associated with local muscle rigidity and stiffness. Patients with appendicitis will most often observe that their nausea, if present, followed the development of abdominal pain, which can help distinguish them from patients with gastroenteritis, for example, where nausea occurs first. Emesis, if present, also occurs after the onset of pain and is typically mild and scant. Thus, timing of the onset of symptoms and the characteristics of the patient's pain and any associated findings must be rigorously assessed. Anorexia is so common that the diagnosis of appendicitis should be questioned in its absence.

Arriving at the correct diagnosis is even more challenging when the appendix is not located in the right lower quadrant, in women of childbearing age, and in the very young or elderly. Because the differential diagnosis of appendicitis is so broad, often the key question to answer expeditiously is whether the patient has appendicitis or some other condition that requires immediate operative intervention. A major concern is that the likelihood of a delay in diagnosis is greater if the appendix is unusually positioned. All patients should undergo a rectal examination. An inflamed appendix located behind the cecum or below the pelvic brim may prompt very little tenderness of the anterior abdominal wall.

Patients with pelvic appendicitis are more likely to present with dysuria, urinary frequency, diarrhea, or tenesmus. They may only experience pain in the suprapubic region on palpation or on rectal or pelvic examination. A pelvic examination in women is mandatory to rule out conditions affecting urogynecologic organs that can cause abdominal pain and mimic appendicitis such as pelvic inflammatory disease, ectopic pregnancy, and ovarian torsion. The relative frequencies of some presenting signs are displayed in Table 23-3.

Patients with simple appendicitis normally only appear mildly ill with a pulse and temperature that are usually only slightly above normal. The provider should be concerned about other disease processes beside appendicitis or the presence of complications such as perforation, phlegmon, or abscess formation if the temperature is >38.3°C (~101°F) and if there are rigors.

Patients with appendicitis will be found to lie quite still to avoid peritoneal irritation caused by movement, and some will report discomfort caused by a bumpy car ride on the way to the hospital or clinic, coughing, sneezing, or other actions that replicate a Valsalva maneuver. The entire abdomen should be examined systematically starting in an area where the patient does not report discomfort if possible. Classically, maximal tenderness is identified in the right lower quadrant at or near McBurney's point, which is located approximately one-third of the way along a line originating at the anterior iliac spine and running to the umbilicus. Gentle pressure in the left lower quadrant may elicit pain in the right lower quadrant if the appendix is located there. This is Rovsing's sign (Table 23-4). Evidence of parietal peritoneal irritation is often best elicited by gentle abdominal percussion, jiggling the patient's gurney or bed, or mildly bumping the feet.

Atypical presentation and pain patterns are common, especially in the very old or the very young. Diagnosing appendicitis in children can be especially challenging because they tend to respond so dramatically to stimulation and obtaining an accurate history may be difficult. In addition, it is important to remember that the smaller omentum found in children may be less likely

TABLE 23-3

RELATIVE FREQUENCY OF SOME PRESENTING SIGNS

SIGNS	FREQUENCY (%)
Abdominal tenderness	>95%
Right lower quadrant tenderness	>90%
Rebound tenderness	30–70%
Rectal tenderness	30–40%
Cervical motion tenderness	30%
Rigidity	~10%
Psoas sign	3–5%
Obturator sign	5–10%
Rovsing's sign	5%
Palpable mass	<5%

TABLE 23-4

CLASSIC SIGNS OF APPENDICITIS IN PATIENTS WITH ABDOMINAL PAIN

MANEUVER	FINDINGS
Rovsing's sign	Palpating in the left lower quadrant causes pain in the right lower quadrant
Obturator sign	Internal rotation of the hip causes pain, suggesting the possibility of an inflamed appendix located in the pelvis
Iliopsoas sign	Extending the right hip causes pain along posterolateral back and hip, suggesting retrocecal appendicitis

to wall off an appendiceal perforation. Observing the child in a quiet surrounding may be helpful.

Signs and symptoms of appendicitis can be subtle in the elderly who may not react as vigorously to appendicitis as younger people. Pain, if noticed, may be minimal and have originated in the right lower quadrant or, otherwise, where the appendix is located. It may never have been noticed to be intermittent, or there may only be significant discomfort with deep palpation. Nausea, anorexia, and emesis may be the predominant complaints. The rare patient may even present with signs and symptoms of distal bowel obstruction secondary to appendiceal inflammation and phlegmon or abscess formation.

LABORATORY TESTING

Laboratory testing does not identify patients with appendicitis but can help the clinician work through the differential diagnosis. The white blood cell count is only mildly to moderately elevated in approximately 70% of patients with simple appendicitis (with a leukocytosis of 10,000–18,000 cells/μL). A "left shift" toward immature polymorphonuclear leukocytes is present in >95% of cases. A sickle cell preparation may be prudent to obtain in those of African, Spanish, Mediterranean, or Indian ancestry. Serum amylase and lipase levels should be measured.

Urinalysis is indicated to help exclude genitourinary conditions that may mimic acute appendicitis, but a few red or white blood cells may be present as a nonspecific finding. However, an inflamed appendix that abuts the ureter or bladder may cause sterile pyuria or hematuria. Every woman of childbearing age should have a pregnancy test. Cervical cultures are indicated if pelvic inflammatory disease is suspected. Anemia and guaiac-positive stools should raise concern about the presence of other diseases or complications such as cancer.

IMAGING

Plain films of the abdomen are rarely helpful and so are not routinely obtained unless the clinician is worried about other conditions such as intestinal obstruction, perforated viscus, or ureterolithiasis. Less than 5% of patients will present with an opaque fecalith in the right lower quadrant. The presence of a fecalith is not diagnostic of appendicitis, although its presence in an appropriate location where the patient complains of pain is suggestive.

The effectiveness of ultrasonography as a tool to diagnosis appendicitis is highly operator dependent. Even in very skilled hands, the appendix may not be visualized. Its overall sensitivity is 0.86, with a specificity of 0.81. Ultrasonography, especially intravaginal techniques, appears to be most useful for identifying pelvic pathology in women. Ultrasonographic findings suggesting the presence of appendicitis include wall thickening, an increased appendiceal diameter, and the presence of free fluid.

The sensitivity and specificity of computed tomography (CT) are 0.94 and 0.95, respectively. Thus, CT imaging, given its high negative predictive value, may be helpful if the diagnosis is in doubt, although studies performed early in the course of disease may not have any typical radiographic findings. Suggestive findings on CT examination include dilatation >6 mm with wall thickening, a lumen that does not fill with enteric contrast, and fatty tissue stranding or air surrounding the appendix, which suggests inflammation (Figs. 23-3 and 23-4). The presence of luminal air or contrast is not consistent with a diagnosis of appendicitis. Furthermore, nonvisualization of the appendix is a nonspecific finding that should not be used to rule out the presence of appendiceal or periappendiceal inflammation.

SPECIAL PATIENT POPULATIONS

Appendicitis in the most common extrauterine general surgical emergency observed during pregnancy. Early symptoms of appendicitis such as nausea and anorexia may be overlooked. Diagnosing appendicitis in pregnant patients may be especially difficult because as the uterus enlarges the appendix may be pushed higher along the right flank even to the right upper quadrant or because the gravid uterus may obscure typical physical findings. Ultrasonography may facilitate early diagnosis. A high index of suspicion is required because of the effects of

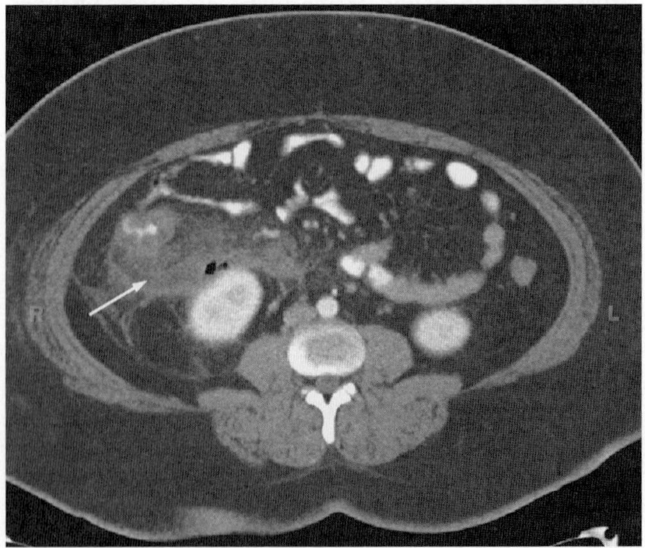

FIGURE 23-3
Computed tomography with oral and intravenous contrast of acute appendicitis. There is thickening of the wall of the appendix and periappendiceal stranding (*arrow*).

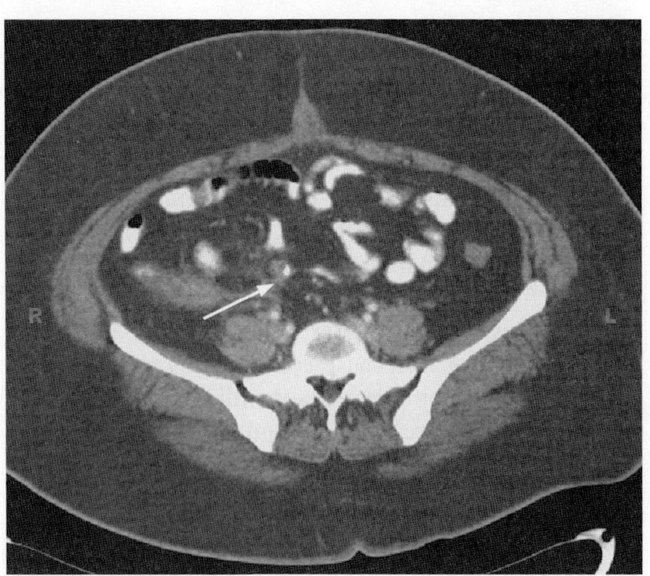

FIGURE 23-4
Appendiceal fecalith *(arrow)*.

unrecognized and untreated appendicitis on the fetus. For example, the fetal mortality rate is four times greater (from 5 to 20%) in patients with perforation.

Immunocompromised patients may present with only mild tenderness and may have many other disease processes in their differential diagnosis, including atypical infections from mycobacteria, *Cytomegalovirus*, or other fungi. Enterocolitis is a concern and may be present in patients who present with abdominal pain, fever, and neutropenia due to chemotherapy. CT imaging may be very helpful, although it is important not to be overly cautious and delay operative intervention for those patients who are believed to have appendicitis.

TREATMENT Acute Appendicitis

In the absence of contraindications, a patient who has a strongly suggestive medical history and physical examination with supportive laboratory findings should undergo appendectomy urgently. In this instance, imaging studies are not required. In patients in whom the evaluation is suggestive but not convincing, imaging and further study are appropriate. Pelvic ultrasonography is indicated in women of childbearing age. Thereafter, CT may accurately indicate the presence of appendicitis or other intraabdominal processes that warrant intervention. Whenever the diagnosis is uncertain, it is prudent to observe the patient and repeat the abdominal examination over 6–8 h. Any evidence of progression is an indication for operation. Narcotics can be given to patients with severe discomfort, especially if the first abdominal examination is completed before drugs are administered.

All patients should be fully prepared for surgery and have any fluid and electrolyte abnormalities corrected. Either laparoscopic or open appendectomy is a satisfactory choice for patients with uncomplicated appendicitis. Management of those who present with a mass representing a phlegmon or abscess can be more difficult. Such patients are best served by treatment with broad-spectrum antibiotics, drainage if there is an abscess >3 cm in diameter, and parenteral fluids and bowel rest if they appear to respond to conservative management. The appendix can then be more safely removed 6–12 weeks later when inflammation has diminished.

Laparoscopic appendectomy now accounts for approximately 60% of all appendectomies. Laparoscopic appendectomy is associated with less postoperative pain and, possibly, a shorter length of stay and faster return to normal activity. Patients who undergo laparoscopic appendectomy also appear to have fewer wound infections, although the risk of intraabdominal abscess formation may be higher. A laparoscopic approach may also be useful when the exact diagnosis is uncertain, yet direct visualization and exploration of the abdomen are needed. A laparoscopic approach may also facilitate exposure in those who are very obese. A thorough examination of the abdomen is indicated if the appendix appears normal at operation, which can be expected to occur in up to 15–20% of cases.

Absent complications, most patients can be discharged within 24–40 h of operation. The most common postoperative complications are fever and leukocytosis. Continuation of these findings beyond 5 days should raise concern for the presence of an intraabdominal abscess. The mortality rate for uncomplicated, nonperforated appendicitis is 0.1–0.5%, which approximates the overall risk of general anesthesia. The mortality rate for perforated appendicitis or other complicated disease is much higher, ranging from 3% overall to a high as 15% in the elderly.

ACUTE PERITONITIS

Acute peritonitis, or inflammation of the visceral and parietal peritoneum, is most often but not always infectious in origin, resulting from perforation of a hollow viscus. This is called *secondary peritonitis*, as opposed to *primary* or *spontaneous peritonitis*, when a specific intraabdominal source cannot be identified. In either instance, the inflammation can be localized or diffuse.

ETIOLOGY

Infective organisms may contaminate the peritoneal cavity after spillage from a hollow viscus, because of a penetrating wound of the abdominal wall, or because of the introduction of a foreign object like a peritoneal dialysis catheter or port that becomes infected. Secondary peritonitis most commonly results from perforation of the appendix, colonic diverticuli, or the stomach and duodenum. It may also occur as a complication of

TABLE 23-5

CONDITIONS LEADING TO SECONDARY BACTERIAL PERITONITIS

Bowel Perforation	Perforation or Leakage of Other Organs
Appendicitis trauma (blunt or penetrating)	Biliary leakage (e.g., after liver biopsy)
Anastomotic leakage	Cholecystitis
Adhesion	Intraperitoneal bleeding
Diverticulitis	Pancreatitis
Iatrogenic (including endoscopic perforation)	Salpingitis
Ingested foreign body	Traumatic or other rupture of urinary bladder
Inflammation	**Loss of peritoneal integrity**
Intussusception	Intraperitoneal chemotherapy
Neoplasms	Iatrogenic (e.g., postoperative foreign body)
Obstruction	Perinephric abscess
Peptic ulcer disease	Peritoneal dialysis or other indwelling devices
Strangulated hernia	Trauma
Vascular (including ischemia or embolus)	

bowel infarction or incarceration, cancer, inflammatory bowel disease, and intestinal obstruction or volvulus. Conditions that may cause secondary bacterial peritonitis and their mechanisms are listed in Table 23-5. Over 90% of the cases of primary or spontaneous bacterial peritonitis occur in patients with ascites or hypoproteinemia (<1 g/L).

Aseptic peritonitis is most commonly caused by the abnormal presence of physiologic fluids like gastric juice, bile, pancreatic enzymes, blood, or urine. It can also be caused by the effects of normally sterile foreign bodies like surgical sponges or instruments. More rarely, it occurs as a complication of systemic diseases like lupus erythematosus, porphyria, and familial Mediterranean fever. The chemical irritation caused by stomach acid and activated pancreatic enzymes is extreme and secondary bacterial infection may occur.

CLINICAL FEATURES

The cardinal signs and symptoms of peritonitis are acute, typically severe, abdominal pain with tenderness and fever. How the patient's complaints of pain are manifested depends on their overall physical health and whether the inflammation is diffuse or localized. Elderly and immunosuppressed patients may not respond as aggressively to the irritation. Diffuse, generalized peritonitis is most often recognized as diffuse abdominal tenderness with local guarding, rigidity, and other evidence of parietal peritoneal irritation. Physical findings may only be identified in a specific region of the abdomen if the intraperitoneal inflammatory process is limited or otherwise contained as may occur in patients with uncomplicated appendicitis or diverticulitis. Bowel sounds are usually absent to hypoactive.

Most patients present with tachycardia and signs of volume depletion with hypotension. Laboratory testing typically reveals a significant leukocytosis, and patients may be severely acidotic. Radiographic studies may show dilatation of the bowel and associated bowel wall edema. Free air, or other evidence of leakage, requires attention and could represent a surgical emergency. In stable patients in whom ascites is present, diagnostic paracentesis is indicated, where the fluid is tested for protein and lactate dehydrogenase and the cell count is measured.

THERAPY AND PROGNOSIS

Whereas mortality rates can be less than 10% for reasonably healthy patients with relatively uncomplicated, localized peritonitis, mortality rates >40% have been reported for the elderly or immunocompromised. Successful treatment depends on correcting any electrolyte abnormalities, restoration of fluid volume and stabilization of the cardiovascular system, appropriate antibiotic therapy, and surgical correction of any underlying abnormalities.

ACKNOWLEDGMENT

The wisdom and expertise of Dr. William Silen is gratefully acknowledged in this updated chapter on acute appendicitis and peritonitis.

SECTION IV

INFECTIONS OF THE ALIMENTARY TRACT

CHAPTER 24

ACUTE INFECTIOUS DIARRHEAL DISEASES AND BACTERIAL FOOD POISONING

Regina C. LaRocque ■ Edward T. Ryan ■ Stephen B. Calderwood

Acute diarrheal disease is a leading cause of illness globally and is associated with an estimated 1.4 million deaths per year. Among children <5 years of age, diarrheal disease is second only to lower respiratory infection as the most common infectious cause of death. The incidence rate of diarrheal disease among children in low- and middle-income countries is estimated to be 2.9 episodes per child per year, for a total of 1.7 billion episodes annually. The morbidity from diarrhea is also significant. Recurrent intestinal infections are associated with physical and mental stunting, wasting, micronutrient deficiencies, and malnutrition. In short, diarrheal disease is a driving factor in global morbidity and mortality.

The wide range of clinical manifestations of acute gastrointestinal illnesses is matched by the wide variety of infectious agents involved, including viruses, bacteria, and parasites (Table 24-1). This chapter discusses factors that enable gastrointestinal pathogens to cause disease, reviews host defense mechanisms, and delineates an approach to the evaluation and treatment of patients presenting with acute diarrhea. Individual organisms causing acute gastrointestinal illnesses are discussed in detail in subsequent chapters.

PATHOGENIC MECHANISMS

Enteric pathogens have developed a variety of tactics to overcome host defenses. Understanding the virulence factors employed by these organisms is important in the diagnosis and treatment of clinical disease.

INOCULUM SIZE

The number of microorganisms that must be ingested to cause disease varies considerably from species to species. For *Shigella*, enterohemorrhagic *Escherichia coli*, *Giardia lamblia*, or *Entamoeba*, as few as 10–100 bacteria or cysts can produce infection, while 10^5–10^8 *Vibrio cholerae* organisms must be ingested to cause disease. The infective dose of *Salmonella* varies widely, depending on the species, host, and food vehicle. The ability of organisms to overcome host defenses has important implications for transmission; *Shigella*, enterohemorrhagic *E. coli*, *Entamoeba*, and *Giardia* can spread by person-to-person contact, whereas under some circumstances *Salmonella* may have to grow in food for several hours before reaching an effective infectious dose.

ADHERENCE

Many organisms must adhere to the gastrointestinal mucosa as an initial step in the pathogenic process; thus, organisms that can compete with the normal bowel flora and colonize the mucosa have an important advantage in causing disease. Specific cell-surface proteins involved in attachment of bacteria to intestinal cells are important virulence determinants. *V. cholerae*, for example, adheres to the brush border of small-intestinal enterocytes via specific surface adhesins, including the toxin-coregulated pilus and other accessory colonization factors. Enterotoxigenic *E. coli*, which causes watery diarrhea, produces an adherence protein called *colonization factor antigen* that is necessary for colonization of the upper small intestine by the organism prior to the production of enterotoxin. Enteropathogenic *E. coli*, an agent of diarrhea in young children, and enterohemorrhagic *E. coli*, which causes hemorrhagic colitis and the hemolytic-uremic syndrome, produce virulence determinants that allow these organisms to attach to and efface the brush border of the intestinal epithelium.

TABLE 24-1

GASTROINTESTINAL PATHOGENS CAUSING ACUTE DIARRHEA				
MECHANISM	**LOCATION**	**ILLNESS**	**STOOL FINDINGS**	**EXAMPLES OF PATHOGENS INVOLVED**
Noninflammatory (enterotoxin)	Proximal small bowel	Watery diarrhea	No fecal leukocytes; mild or no increase in fecal lactoferrin	*Vibrio cholerae*, enterotoxigenic *Escherichia coli* (LT and/or ST), enteroaggregative *E. coli*, *Clostridium perfringens*, *Bacillus cereus*, *Staphylococcus aureus*, *Aeromonas hydrophila*, *Plesiomonas shigelloides*, rotavirus, norovirus, enteric adenoviruses, *Giardia lamblia*, *Cryptosporidium* spp., *Cyclospora* spp., microsporidia
Inflammatory (invasion or cytotoxin)	Colon or distal small bowel	Dysentery or inflammatory diarrhea	Fecal polymorphonuclear leukocytes; substantial increase in fecal lactoferrin	*Shigella* spp., *Salmonella* spp., *Campylobacter jejuni*, enterohemorrhagic *E. coli*, enteroinvasive *E. coli*, *Yersinia enterocolitica*, *Listeria monocytogenes*, *Vibrio parahaemolyticus*, *Clostridium difficile*, *A. hydrophila*, *P. shigelloides*, *Entamoeba histolytica*, *Klebsiella oxytoca*
Penetrating	Distal small bowel	Enteric fever	Fecal mononuclear leukocytes	*Salmonella typhi*, *Y. enterocolitica*

Abbreviations: LT, heat-labile enterotoxin; ST, heat-stable enterotoxin.

TOXIN PRODUCTION

The production of one or more exotoxins is important in the pathogenesis of numerous enteric organisms. Such toxins include *enterotoxins*, which cause watery diarrhea by acting directly on secretory mechanisms in the intestinal mucosa; *cytotoxins*, which cause destruction of mucosal cells and associated inflammatory diarrhea; and *neurotoxins*, which act directly on the central or peripheral nervous system.

The prototypical enterotoxin is cholera toxin, a heterodimeric protein composed of one A and five B subunits. The A subunit contains the enzymatic activity of the toxin, while the B subunit pentamer binds holotoxin to the enterocyte surface receptor, the ganglioside G_{M1}. After the binding of holotoxin, a fragment of the A subunit is translocated across the eukaryotic cell membrane into the cytoplasm, where it catalyzes the adenosine diphosphate ribosylation of a guanosine triphosphate–binding protein and causes persistent activation of adenylate cyclase. The end result is an increase of cyclic adenosine monophosphate in the intestinal mucosa, which increases Cl^- secretion and decreases Na^+ absorption, leading to a loss of fluid and the production of diarrhea.

Enterotoxigenic strains of *E. coli* may produce a protein called *heat-labile enterotoxin* (LT) that is similar to cholera toxin and causes secretory diarrhea by the same mechanism. Alternatively, enterotoxigenic strains of *E. coli* may produce *heat-stable enterotoxin* (ST), one form of which causes diarrhea by activation of guanylate cyclase and elevation of intracellular cyclic guanosine monophosphate. Some enterotoxigenic strains of *E. coli* produce both LT and ST.

Bacterial cytotoxins, in contrast, destroy intestinal mucosal cells and produce the syndrome of dysentery, with bloody stools containing inflammatory cells. Enteric pathogens that produce such cytotoxins include *Shigella dysenteriae* type 1, *Vibrio parahaemolyticus*, and *Clostridium difficile*. *S. dysenteriae* type 1 and Shiga toxin–producing strains of *E. coli* produce potent cytotoxins and have been associated with outbreaks of hemorrhagic colitis and hemolytic-uremic syndrome.

Neurotoxins are usually produced by bacteria outside the host and therefore cause symptoms soon after ingestion. Included are the staphylococcal and *Bacillus cereus* toxins, which act on the central nervous system to produce vomiting.

INVASION

Dysentery may result not only from the production of cytotoxins but also from bacterial invasion and destruction of intestinal mucosal cells. Infections due to *Shigella* and enteroinvasive *E. coli* are characterized by the organisms' invasion of mucosal epithelial cells, intraepithelial multiplication, and subsequent spread to adjacent cells. *Salmonella* causes inflammatory diarrhea by invasion of the bowel mucosa but generally is not associated with the destruction of enterocytes or the full clinical syndrome of dysentery. *Salmonella typhi* and *Yersinia enterocolitica* can penetrate intact intestinal mucosa, multiply intracellularly in Peyer's patches and intestinal lymph nodes, and then disseminate through the bloodstream to cause enteric fever, a syndrome characterized by fever, headache, relative bradycardia, abdominal pain, splenomegaly, and leukopenia.

HOST DEFENSES

Given the enormous number of microorganisms ingested with every meal, the normal host must combat a constant influx of potential enteric pathogens. Studies of infections in patients with alterations in defense mechanisms have led to a greater understanding of the variety of ways in which the normal host can protect itself against disease.

INTESTINAL MICROBIOTA

The large numbers of bacteria that normally inhabit the intestine (*the intestinal microbiota*) act as an important host defense mechanism, preventing colonization by potential enteric pathogens. Persons with fewer intestinal bacteria, such as infants who have not yet developed normal enteric colonization or patients receiving antibiotics, are at significantly greater risk of developing infections with enteric pathogens. The composition of the intestinal microbiota is as important as the number of organisms present. More than 99% of the normal colonic microbiota is made up of anaerobic bacteria, and the acidic pH and volatile fatty acids produced by these organisms appear to be critical elements in resistance to colonization.

GASTRIC ACID

The acidic pH of the stomach is an important barrier to enteric pathogens, and an increased frequency of infections due to *Salmonella*, *G. lamblia*, and a variety of helminths has been reported among patients who have undergone gastric surgery or are achlorhydric for some other reason. Neutralization of gastric acid with antacids, proton pump inhibitors, or H_2 blockers—a common practice in the management of hospitalized patients—similarly increases the risk of enteric colonization. In addition, some microorganisms can survive the extreme acidity of the gastric environment; rotavirus, for example, is highly stable to acidity.

INTESTINAL MOTILITY

Normal peristalsis is the major mechanism for clearance of bacteria from the proximal small intestine. When intestinal motility is impaired (e.g., by treatment with opiates or other antimotility drugs, anatomic abnormalities, or hypomotility states), the frequency of bacterial overgrowth and infection of the small bowel with enteric pathogens is increased. Some patients whose treatment for *Shigella* infection consists of diphenoxylate hydrochloride with atropine (Lomotil) experience prolonged fever and shedding of organisms, while patients treated with opiates for mild *Salmonella* gastroenteritis have a higher frequency of bacteremia than those not treated with opiates.

IMMUNITY

Both cellular immune responses and antibody production play important roles in protection from enteric infections. Humoral immunity to enteric pathogens consists of systemic IgG and IgM as well as secretory IgA. The mucosal immune system may be the first line of defense against many gastrointestinal pathogens. The binding of bacterial antigens to the luminal surface of M cells in the distal small bowel and the subsequent presentation of antigens to subepithelial lymphoid tissue lead to the proliferation of sensitized lymphocytes. These lymphocytes circulate and populate all of the mucosal tissues of the body as IgA-secreting plasma cells.

GENETIC DETERMINANTS

Host genetic variation influences susceptibility to diarrheal diseases. People with blood group O show increased susceptibility to disease due to *V. cholerae*, *Shigella*, *E. coli* O157, and norovirus. Polymorphisms in genes encoding inflammatory mediators have been associated with the outcome of infection with enteroaggregative *E. coli*, enterotoxin-producing *E. coli*, *Salmonella*, *C. difficile*, and *V. cholerae*.

APPROACH TO THE PATIENT: Infectious Diarrhea or Bacterial Food Poisoning

The approach to the patient with possible infectious diarrhea or bacterial food poisoning is shown in Fig. 24-1.

HISTORY The answers to questions with high discriminating value can quickly narrow the range of potential causes of diarrhea and help determine whether treatment is needed. Important elements of the narrative history are detailed in Fig. 24-1.

PHYSICAL EXAMINATION The examination of patients for signs of dehydration provides essential information about the severity of the diarrheal illness and the need for rapid therapy. Mild dehydration is indicated by thirst, dry mouth, decreased axillary sweat, decreased urine output, and slight weight loss. Signs of moderate dehydration include an orthostatic fall in blood pressure, skin tenting, and sunken eyes (or, in infants, a sunken fontanelle). Signs of severe dehydration include lethargy, obtundation, feeble pulse, hypotension, and frank shock.

DIAGNOSTIC APPROACH After the severity of illness is assessed, the clinician must distinguish between *inflammatory* and *noninflammatory* disease. Using the history and epidemiologic features of the case as guides, the clinician can then rapidly evaluate the need for further efforts to define a specific etiology and for therapeutic intervention. Examination of a stool sample may supplement the narrative history.

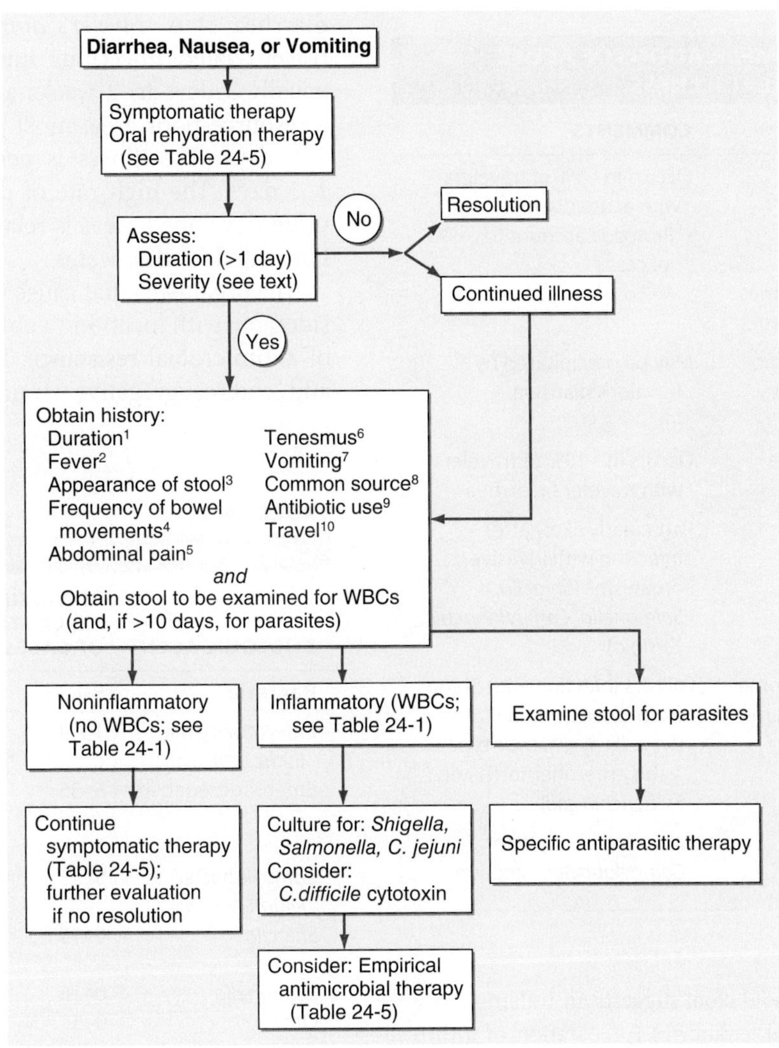

FIGURE 24-1

Clinical algorithm for the approach to patients with community-acquired infectious diarrhea or bacterial food poisoning. Key to superscripts: 1. Diarrhea lasting >2 weeks is generally defined as chronic; in such cases, many of the causes of acute diarrhea are much less likely, and a new spectrum of causes needs to be considered. 2. Fever often implies invasive disease, although fever and diarrhea may also result from infection outside the gastrointestinal tract, as in malaria. 3. Stools that contain blood or mucus indicate ulceration of the large bowel. Bloody stools without fecal leukocytes should alert the laboratory to the possibility of infection with Shiga toxin–producing enterohemorrhagic *Escherichia coli*. Bulky white stools suggest a small-intestinal process that is causing malabsorption. Profuse "rice-water" stools suggest cholera or a similar toxigenic process. 4. Frequent stools over a given period can provide the first warning of impending dehydration. 5. Abdominal pain may be most severe in inflammatory processes like those due to *Shigella*, *Campylobacter*, and necrotizing toxins. Painful abdominal muscle cramps, caused by electrolyte loss, can develop in severe cases of cholera. Bloating is common in giardiasis. An appendicitis-like syndrome should prompt a culture for *Yersinia enterocolitica* with cold enrichment. 6. Tenesmus (painful rectal spasms with a strong urge to defecate but little passage of stool) may be a feature of cases with proctitis, as in shigellosis or amebiasis. 7. Vomiting implies an acute infection (e.g., a toxin-mediated illness or food poisoning) but can also be prominent in a variety of systemic illnesses (e.g., malaria) and in intestinal obstruction. 8. Asking patients whether anyone else they know is sick is a more efficient means of identifying a common source than is constructing a list of recently eaten foods. If a common source seems likely, specific foods can be investigated. See text for a discussion of bacterial food poisoning. 9. Current antibiotic therapy or a recent history of treatment suggests *Clostridium difficile* diarrhea **(Chap. 25)**. Stop antibiotic treatment if possible and consider tests for *C. difficile* toxins. Antibiotic use may increase the risk of chronic intestinal carriage following salmonellosis. 10. See text for a discussion of traveler's diarrhea. *(After TS Steiner, RL Guerrant: Principles and syndromes of enteric infection, in Mandell, Douglas, and Bennett's Principles and Practice of Infectious Diseases, 7th ed, GL Mandell et al [eds]. Philadelphia, Churchill Livingstone, 2010, pp 1335–1351; RL Guerrant, DA Bobak: N Engl J Med 325:327, 1991; with permission.)*

TABLE 24-2

POST-DIARRHEA COMPLICATIONS OF ACUTE INFECTIOUS DIARRHEAL ILLNESS

COMPLICATION	COMMENTS
Chronic diarrhea • Lactase deficiency • Small-bowel bacterial overgrowth • Malabsorption syndromes (tropical and celiac sprue)	Occurs in ~1% of travelers with acute diarrhea • Protozoa account for ~1/3 of cases
Initial presentation or exacerbation of inflammatory bowel disease	May be precipitated by traveler's diarrhea
Irritable bowel syndrome	Occurs in ~10% of travelers with traveler's diarrhea
Reactive arthritis	Particularly likely after infection with invasive organisms (*Shigella, Salmonella, Campylobacter, Yersinia*)
Hemolytic-uremic syndrome (hemolytic anemia, thrombocytopenia, and renal failure)	Follows infection with Shiga toxin–producing bacteria (*Shigella dysenteriae* type 1 and enterohemorrhagic *Escherichia coli*)
Guillain-Barré syndrome	Particularly likely after *Campylobacter* infection

Grossly bloody or mucoid stool suggests an inflammatory process. A test for fecal leukocytes (preparation of a thin smear of stool on a glass slide, addition of a drop of methylene blue, and examination of the wet mount) can suggest inflammatory disease in patients with diarrhea, although the predictive value of this test is still debated. A test for fecal lactoferrin, which is a marker of fecal leukocytes, is more sensitive and is available in latex agglutination and enzyme-linked immunosorbent assay formats. Causes of acute infectious diarrhea, categorized as inflammatory and noninflammatory, are listed in Table 24-1.

POST-DIARRHEA COMPLICATIONS Chronic complications may follow the resolution of an acute diarrheal episode. The clinician should inquire about prior diarrheal illness if the conditions listed in Table 24-2 are observed.

EPIDEMIOLOGY

TRAVEL HISTORY

Of the several million people who travel from temperate industrialized countries to tropical regions of Asia, Africa, and Central and South America each year, 20–50% experience a sudden onset of abdominal cramps, anorexia, and watery diarrhea; thus *traveler's diarrhea* is the most common travel-related infectious illness. The time of onset is usually 3 days to 2 weeks after the traveler's arrival in a resource-poor area; most cases begin within the first 3–5 days. The illness is generally self-limited, lasting 1–5 days. The high rate of diarrhea among travelers to underdeveloped areas is related to the ingestion of contaminated food or water.

The organisms that cause traveler's diarrhea vary considerably with location (Table 24-3), as does the pattern of antimicrobial resistance. In all areas, enterotoxigenic and enteroaggregative strains of *E. coli* are the most

TABLE 24-3

CAUSES OF TRAVELER'S DIARRHEA

ETIOLOGIC AGENT	APPROXIMATE PERCENTAGE OF CASES	COMMENTS
Bacteria	**50–75**	
Enterotoxigenic *Escherichia coli*	10–45	Single most important agent
Enteroaggregative *E. coli*	5–35	Emerging enteric pathogen with worldwide distribution
Campylobacter jejuni	5–25	More common in Asia
Shigella	0–15	Major cause of dysentery
Salmonella	0–15	
Others	0–5	Including *Aeromonas*, *Plesiomonas*, and *Vibrio cholerae*
Viruses	**0–20**	
Norovirus	0–10	Associated with cruise ships
Rotavirus	0–5	Particularly common among children
Parasites	**0–10**	
Giardia lamblia	0–5	Affects hikers and campers who drink from freshwater streams
Cryptosporidium	0–5	Resistant to chlorine treatment
Entamoeba histolytica	<1	
Cyclospora	<1	
Other	**0–10**	
Acute food poisoning[a]	0–5	
No pathogen identified	10–50	

[a]For etiologic agents, see Table 24-4.

Source: After DR Hill et al: The practice of travel medicine: Guidelines by the Infectious Diseases Society of America. *Clin Infect Dis* 43:1499, 2006.

common isolates from persons with the classic secretory traveler's diarrhea syndrome. Infection with *Campylobacter jejuni* is especially common in areas of Asia.

LOCATION

Closed and semi-closed communities, including day-care centers, schools, residential facilities, and cruise ships, are important settings for outbreaks of enteric infections. Norovirus, which is highly contagious and robust in surviving on surfaces, is the most common etiologic agent associated with outbreaks of acute gastroenteritis. Other common organisms, often spread by fecal-oral contact in such communities, are *Shigella*, *C. jejuni*, and *Cryptosporidium*. Rotavirus is rarely a cause of pediatric diarrheal outbreaks in the United States since rotavirus vaccinationwas broadly recommended in 2006. Similarly, hospitals are sites in which enteric infections are concentrated. Diarrhea is one of the most common manifestations of nosocomial infections. *C. difficile* is the predominant cause of nosocomial diarrhea among adults in the United States, and outbreaks of norovirus infection are common in health care settings. *Klebsiella oxytoca* has been identified as a cause of antibiotic-associated hemorrhagic colitis. Enteropathogenic *E. coli* has been associated with outbreaks of diarrhea in nurseries for newborns. One-third of elderly patients in chronic-care institutions develop a significant diarrheal illness each year; more than one-half of these cases are caused by cytotoxin-producing *C. difficile*. Antimicrobial therapy can predispose to pseudomembranous colitis by altering the normal colonic flora and allowing the multiplication of *C. difficile* **(Chap. 25)**.

AGE

Globally, most morbidity and mortality from enteric pathogens involves children <5 years of age. Breast-fed infants are protected from contaminated food and water and derive some protection from maternal antibodies, but their risk of infection rises dramatically when they begin to eat solid foods. Exposure to rotavirus is universal, with most children experiencing their first infection in the first or second year of life if not vaccinated. Older children and adults are more commonly infected with norovirus. Other organisms with higher attack rates among children than among adults include enterotoxigenic, enteropathogenic, and enterohemorrhagic *E. coli*; *Shigella*; *C. jejuni*; and *G. lamblia*.

HOST IMMUNE STATUS

Immunocompromised hosts are at elevated risk of acute and chronic infectious diarrhea. Individuals with defects in cell-mediated immunity (including those with AIDS) are at particularly high risk of invasive enteropathies, including salmonellosis, listeriosis, and cryptosporidiosis. Individuals with hypogammaglobulinemia are at particular risk of *C. difficile* colitis and giardiasis. Patients with cancer are more likely to develop *C. difficile* infection as a result of chemotherapy and frequent hospitalizations. Infectious diarrhea can be life-threatening in immunocompromised hosts, with complications including bacteremia and metastatic seeding of infection. Furthermore, dehydration may compromise renal function and increase the toxicity of immunosuppressive drugs.

BACTERIAL FOOD POISONING

If the history and the stool examination indicate a noninflammatory etiology of diarrhea and there is evidence of a common-source outbreak, questions concerning the ingestion of specific foods and the time of onset of the diarrhea after a meal can provide clues to the bacterial cause of the illness. Potential causes of bacterial food poisoning are shown in Table 24-4.

Bacterial disease caused by an enterotoxin elaborated outside the host, such as that due to *Staphylococcus aureus* or *B. cereus*, has the shortest incubation period (1–6 h) and generally lasts <12 h. Most cases of staphylococcal food poisoning are caused by contamination from infected human carriers. Staphylococci can multiply at a wide range of temperatures; thus, if food is left to cool slowly and remains at room temperature after cooking, the organisms will have the opportunity to form enterotoxin. Outbreaks following picnics where potato salad, mayonnaise, and cream pastries have been served offer classic examples of staphylococcal food poisoning. Diarrhea, nausea, vomiting, and abdominal cramping are common, while fever is less so.

B. cereus can produce either a syndrome with a short incubation period—the *emetic* form, mediated by a staphylococcal type of enterotoxin—or one with a longer incubation period (8–16 h)—the *diarrheal* form, caused by an enterotoxin resembling *E. coli* LT, in which diarrhea and abdominal cramps are characteristic but vomiting is uncommon. The emetic form of *B. cereus* food poisoning is associated with contaminated fried rice; the organism is common in uncooked rice, and its heat-resistant spores survive boiling. If cooked rice is not refrigerated, the spores can germinate and produce toxin. Frying before serving may not destroy the preformed, heat-stable toxin.

Food poisoning due to *Clostridium perfringens* also has a slightly longer incubation period (8–14 h) and results from the survival of heat-resistant spores in inadequately cooked meat, poultry, or legumes. After ingestion, toxin is produced in the intestinal tract,

TABLE 24-4

BACTERIAL FOOD POISONING

INCUBATION PERIOD, ORGANISM	SYMPTOMS	COMMON FOOD SOURCES
1–6 h		
Staphylococcus aureus	Nausea, vomiting, diarrhea	Ham, poultry, potato or egg salad, mayonnaise, cream pastries
Bacillus cereus	Nausea, vomiting, diarrhea	Fried rice
8–16 h		
Clostridium perfringens	Abdominal cramps, diarrhea (vomiting rare)	Beef, poultry, legumes, gravies
B. cereus	Abdominal cramps, diarrhea (vomiting rare)	Meats, vegetables, dried beans, cereals
>16 h		
Vibrio cholerae	Watery diarrhea	Shellfish, water
Enterotoxigenic *Escherichia coli*	Watery diarrhea	Salads, cheese, meats, water
Enterohemorrhagic *E. coli*	Bloody diarrhea	Ground beef, roast beef, salami, raw milk, raw vegetables, apple juice
Salmonella spp.	Inflammatory diarrhea	Beef, poultry, eggs, dairy products
Campylobacter jejuni	Inflammatory diarrhea	Poultry, raw milk
Shigella spp.	Dysentery	Potato or egg salad, lettuce, raw vegetables
Vibrio parahaemolyticus	Dysentery	Mollusks, crustaceans

causing moderately severe abdominal cramps and diarrhea; vomiting is rare, as is fever. The illness is self-limited, rarely lasting >24 h.

Not all food poisoning has a bacterial cause. Nonbacterial agents of short-incubation food poisoning include capsaicin, which is found in hot peppers, and a variety of toxins found in fish and shellfish.

LABORATORY EVALUATION

Many cases of noninflammatory diarrhea are self-limited or can be treated empirically, and in these instances the clinician may not need to determine a specific etiology. Potentially pathogenic *E. coli* cannot be distinguished from normal fecal flora by routine culture, and tests to detect enterotoxins are not available in most clinical laboratories. In situations in which cholera is a concern, stool should be cultured on selective media such as thiosulfate–citrate–bile salts–sucrose (TCBS) or tellurite-taurocholate-gelatin (TTG) agar. A latex agglutination test has made the rapid detection of rotavirus in stool practical for many laboratories, while reverse-transcriptase polymerase chain reaction (PCR) and specific antigen enzyme immunoassays have been developed for the identification of norovirus. Stool specimens should be examined by immunofluorescence-based rapid assays or (less sensitive) standard microscopy for *Giardia* cysts or *Cryptosporidium* if the level of clinical suspicion regarding the involvement of these organisms is high.

All patients with fever and evidence of inflammatory disease acquired outside the hospital should have stool cultured for *Salmonella*, *Shigella*, and *Campylobacter*. *Salmonella* and *Shigella* can be selected on MacConkey agar as non-lactose-fermenting (colorless) colonies or can be grown on *Salmonella-Shigella* agar or in selenite enrichment broth, both of which inhibit most organisms except these pathogens. Evaluation of nosocomial diarrhea should initially focus on *C. difficile*; stool culture for other pathogens in this setting has an extremely low yield and is not cost-effective. Toxins A and B produced by pathogenic strains of *C. difficile* can be detected by rapid enzyme immunoassays, latex agglutination tests, or PCR **(Chap. 25)**. Isolation of *C. jejuni* requires inoculation of fresh stool onto selective growth medium and incubation at 42°C in a microaerophilic atmosphere. In many laboratories in the United States, *E. coli* O157:H7 is among the most common pathogens isolated from visibly bloody stools. Strains of this enterohemorrhagic serotype can be identified in specialized laboratories by serotyping but also can be identified presumptively in hospital laboratories as lactose-fermenting, indole-positive colonies of sorbitol nonfermenters (white colonies) on sorbitol MacConkey plates. If the clinical presentation suggests the possibility of intestinal amebiasis, stool should be examined by a rapid antigen detection assay or by (less sensitive and less specific) microscopy.

TREATMENT Infectious Diarrhea or Bacterial Food Poisoning

In many cases, a specific diagnosis is not necessary or not available to guide treatment. The clinician can proceed with the information obtained from the history, stool examination,

TABLE 24-5

TREATMENT OF TRAVELER'S DIARRHEA ON THE BASIS OF CLINICAL FEATURES[a]

CLINICAL SYNDROME	SUGGESTED THERAPY
Watery diarrhea (no blood in stool, no fever), 1 or 2 unformed stools per day without distressing enteric symptoms	Oral fluids (oral rehydration solution, Pedialyte, Lytren, or flavored mineral water) and saltine crackers
Watery diarrhea (no blood in stool, no fever), 1 or 2 unformed stools per day with distressing enteric symptoms	Bismuth subsalicylate (for adults): 30 mL or 2 tablets (262 mg/tablet) every 30 min for 8 doses; or loperamide[b]: 4 mg initially followed by 2 mg after passage of each unformed stool, not to exceed 8 tablets (16 mg) per day (prescription dose) or 4 caplets (8 mg) per day (over-the-counter dose); drugs can be taken for 2 days
Watery diarrhea (no blood in stool, no distressing abdominal pain, no fever), >2 unformed stools per day	Antibacterial drug[c] plus (for adults) loperamide[b] (see dose above)
Dysentery (passage of bloody stools) or fever (>37.8°C)	Antibacterial drug[c]
Vomiting, minimal diarrhea	Bismuth subsalicylate (for adults; see dose above)
Diarrhea in infants (<2 years old)	Fluids and electrolytes (oral rehydration solution, Pedialyte, Lytren); continue feeding, especially with breast milk; seek medical attention for moderate dehydration, fever lasting >24 h, bloody stools, or diarrhea lasting more than several days

[a]All patients should take oral fluids (Pedialyte, Lytren, or flavored mineral water) plus saltine crackers. If diarrhea becomes moderate or severe, if fever persists, or if bloody stools or dehydration develops, the patient should seek medical attention. [b]Loperamide should not be used by patients with fever or dysentery; its use may prolong diarrhea in patients with infection due to *Shigella* or other invasive organisms. [c]The recommended antibacterial drugs are as follows:

If the level of suspicion is low for fluoroquinolone-resistant *Campylobacter*:

Adults: (1) A fluoroquinolone such as ciprofloxacin, 750 mg as a single dose or 500 mg bid for 3 days; levofloxacin, 500 mg as a single dose or 500 mg qd for 3 days; or norfloxacin, 800 mg as a single dose or 400 mg bid for 3 days. (2) Azithromycin, 1000 mg as a single dose or 500 mg qd for 3 days. (3) Rifaximin, 200 mg tid or 400 mg bid for 3 days (not recommended for use in dysentery).

Children: Azithromycin, 10 mg/kg on day 1, 5 mg/kg on days 2 and 3 if diarrhea persists.

If fluoroquinolone-resistant *Campylobacter* is suspected (for example, following travel to Southeast Asia):

Adults: Azithromycin (at above dose for adults). *Children:* Same as for children traveling to other areas (see above).

Source: After DR Hill et al: The practice of travel medicine: Guidelines by the Infectious Diseases Society of America. *Clin Infect Dis* 43:1499, 2006.

and evaluation of dehydration severity. Empirical regimens for the treatment of traveler's diarrhea are listed in Table 24-5.

The mainstay of treatment is adequate rehydration. The treatment of cholera and other dehydrating diarrheal diseases was revolutionized by the promotion of oral rehydration solution (ORS), the efficacy of which depends on the fact that glucose-facilitated absorption of sodium and water in the small intestine remains intact in the presence of cholera toxin. The use of ORS has reduced mortality rates for cholera from >50% (in untreated cases) to <1%. A number of ORS formulas have been used. Initial preparations were based on the treatment of patients with cholera and included a solution containing 3.5 g of sodium chloride, 2.5 g of sodium bicarbonate (or 2.9 g of sodium citrate), 1.5 g of potassium chloride, and 20 g of glucose (or 40 g of sucrose) per liter of water. Such a preparation can still be used for the treatment of severe cholera. Many causes of secretory diarrhea, however, are associated with less electrolyte loss than occurs in cholera. Beginning in 2002, the World Health Organization recommended a "reduced-osmolarity/reduced-salt" ORS that is better tolerated and more effective than classic ORS. This preparation contains 2.6 g of sodium chloride, 2.9 g of trisodium citrate, 1.5 g of potassium chloride, and 13.5 g of glucose (or 27 g of sucrose) per liter of water. ORS formulations containing rice or cereal as the carbohydrate source may be even more effective than glucose-based solutions. Patients who are severely dehydrated or in whom vomiting precludes the use of oral therapy should receive IV solutions such as Ringer's lactate.

Although most secretory forms of traveler's diarrhea (usually due to enterotoxigenic or enteroaggregative *E. coli* or to *Campylobacter*) can be treated effectively with rehydration, bismuth subsalicylate, or antiperistaltic agents, antimicrobial agents can shorten the duration of illness from 3–4 days to 24–36 h. Changes in diet have not been shown to have an impact on the duration of illness, while the efficacy of probiotics continues to be debated. Most individuals who present with dysentery (bloody diarrhea and fever) should be treated empirically with an antimicrobial agent (e.g., a fluoroquinolone or a macrolide) pending microbiologic analysis of stool. Individuals with shigellosis should receive a 3- to 7-day course. Individuals with *Campylobacter* infection often benefit from antimicrobial treatment as well. Because of widespread resistance of *Campylobacter* to fluoroquinolones, especially in parts of Asia, a macrolide antibiotic such as erythromycin or azithromycin may be preferred for this infection.

Treatment of salmonellosis must be tailored to the individual patient. Since administration of antimicrobial agents often prolongs intestinal colonization with *Salmonella*, these drugs are usually reserved for individuals at high risk of complications from disseminated salmonellosis, such as young children, patients with prosthetic devices, elderly patients, and immunocompromised persons. Antimicrobial agents should not be administered to individuals (especially children) in whom enterohemorrhagic *E. coli* infection is suspected. Laboratory studies of enterohemorrhagic *E. coli* strains have demonstrated that a number of antibiotics induce replication of Shiga toxin–producing lambdoid bacteriophages, thereby significantly increasing toxin production by these strains. Clinical studies have supported these laboratory results, and antibiotics may increase by twentyfold the risk of hemolytic-uremic syndrome and renal failure during enterohemorrhagic *E. coli* infection. A clinical clue in the diagnosis of the latter infection is bloody diarrhea with low fever or none at all.

PROPHYLAXIS

Improvements in hygiene to limit fecal-oral spread of enteric pathogens will be necessary if the prevalence of diarrheal diseases is to be significantly reduced in developing countries. Travelers can reduce their risk of diarrhea by eating only hot, freshly cooked food; by avoiding raw vegetables, salads, and unpeeled fruit; and by drinking only boiled or treated water and avoiding ice. Historically, few travelers to tourist destinations adhere to these dietary restrictions. Bismuth subsalicylate is an inexpensive agent for the prophylaxis of traveler's diarrhea; it is taken at a dosage of 2 tablets (525 mg) four times a day. Treatment appears to be effective and safe for up to 3 weeks, but adverse events such as temporary darkening of the tongue and tinnitus can occur. A meta-analysis suggests that probiotics may lessen the likelihood of traveler's diarrhea by ~15%. Prophylactic antimicrobial agents, although effective, are not generally recommended for the prevention of traveler's diarrhea except when travelers are immunosuppressed or have other underlying illnesses that place them at high risk for morbidity from gastrointestinal infection. The risk of side effects and the possibility of developing an infection with a drug-resistant organism or with more harmful, invasive bacteria make it more reasonable to institute an empirical short course of treatment if symptoms develop. If prophylaxis is indicated, the nonabsorbed antibiotic rifaximin can be considered.

The possibility of exerting a major impact on the worldwide morbidity and mortality associated with diarrheal diseases has led to intense efforts to develop effective vaccines against the common bacterial and viral enteric pathogens. An effective rotavirus vaccine is currently available. Vaccines against *S. typhi* and *V. cholerae* also are available, although the protection they offer is incomplete and/or short lived. At present, there is no effective commercially available vaccine against *Shigella*, enterotoxigenic *E. coli*, *Campylobacter*, nontyphoidal *Salmonella*, norovirus, or intestinal parasites.

CHAPTER 25

CLOSTRIDIUM DIFFICILE INFECTION, INCLUDING PSEUDOMEMBRANOUS COLITIS

Dale N. Gerding ■ Stuart Johnson

DEFINITION

Clostridium difficile infection (CDI) is a unique colonic disease that is acquired most often in association with antimicrobial use and the consequent disruption of the normal colonic microbiota. The most commonly diagnosed diarrheal illness acquired in the hospital, CDI results from the ingestion of spores of *C. difficile* that vegetate, multiply, and secrete toxins, causing diarrhea and pseudomembranous colitis (PMC) in the most severe cases.

ETIOLOGY AND EPIDEMIOLOGY

C. difficile is an obligately anaerobic, gram-positive, spore-forming bacillus whose spores are found widely in nature, particularly in the environment of hospitals and chronic-care facilities. CDI occurs frequently in hospitals and nursing homes (or shortly after discharge from these facilities) where the level of antimicrobial use is high and the environment is contaminated by *C. difficile* spores.

Clindamycin, ampicillin, and cephalosporins were the first antibiotics associated with CDI. The second- and third-generation cephalosporins, particularly cefotaxime, ceftriaxone, cefuroxime, and ceftazidime, are frequently responsible for this condition, and the fluoroquinolones (ciprofloxacin, levofloxacin, and moxifloxacin) are the most recent drug class to be implicated in hospital outbreaks. Penicillin/β-lactamase-inhibitor combinations such as ticarcillin/clavulanate and piperacillin/tazobactam pose significantly less risk. However, all antibiotics, including vancomycin and metronidazole (the agents most commonly used to treat CDI), carry a risk of subsequent CDI. Rare cases are reported in patients without prior antibiotic exposure.

C. difficile is acquired exogenously—most frequently in the hospital or nursing home, but also possibly in the outpatient setting—and is carried in the stool of both symptomatic and asymptomatic patients. The rate of fecal colonization is often ≥20% among adult patients hospitalized for >1 week; in contrast, the rate is 1–3% among community residents. Community-onset CDI without recent hospitalization, nursing home residence, or outpatient health-care contact probably accounts for ≤10% of all cases. The risk of *C. difficile* acquisition increases in proportion to the length of hospital stay. Asymptomatic fecal carriage of *C. difficile* in healthy neonates is very common, with repeated colonization by multiple strains in infants (<1 year old), but associated disease in these infants is extremely rare if it occurs at all. Spores of *C. difficile* are found on environmental surfaces (where the organism can persist for months) and on the hands of hospital personnel who fail to practice good hand hygiene. Hospital epidemics of CDI have been attributed to a single *C. difficile* strain and to multiple strains present simultaneously. Other identified risk factors for CDI include older age, greater severity of underlying illness, gastrointestinal surgery, use of electronic rectal thermometers, enteral tube feeding, and antacid treatment. Use of proton pump inhibitors may be a risk factor, but this risk is probably modest, and no firm data have implicated these agents in patients who are not already receiving antibiotics.

PATHOLOGY AND PATHOGENESIS

Spores of toxigenic *C. difficile* are ingested, survive gastric acidity, germinate in the small bowel, and colonize the lower intestinal tract, where they elaborate two large toxins: toxin A (an enterotoxin) and toxin B (a cytotoxin). These toxins initiate processes resulting in the disruption of epithelial-cell barrier function, diarrhea, and pseudomembrane formation. Toxin A is a potent neutrophil chemoattractant, and both toxins glucosylate the guanosine triphosphate (GTP)–binding proteins of the Rho subfamily that regulate the actin cell cytoskeleton. Data from studies using molecular disruption of toxin genes in isogenic mutants suggest that toxin B is the more important virulence factor. This possibility, if confirmed, might account for the occurrence of clinical disease caused by toxin A–negative strains. Disruption of the cytoskeleton results in loss of cell shape, adherence, and tight junctions, with consequent fluid leakage. A third toxin, binary toxin CDT, was previously found in only ~6% of strains but is present in all isolates of the widely recognized epidemic NAP1/BI/027 strain (see "Global Considerations," below); this toxin is related to *C. perfringens* iota toxin. Its role in the pathogenesis of CDI has not yet been defined.

The pseudomembranes of PMC are confined to the colonic mucosa and initially appear as 1- to 2-mm whitish-yellow plaques. The intervening mucosa appears unremarkable, but, as the disease progresses, the pseudomembranes coalesce to form larger plaques and become confluent over the entire colon wall (Fig. 25-1). The whole colon is usually involved, but 10% of patients have rectal sparing. Viewed microscopically, the pseudomembranes have a mucosal attachment point and contain necrotic leukocytes, fibrin, mucus, and cellular debris. The epithelium is eroded and necrotic in focal areas, with neutrophil infiltration of the mucosa.

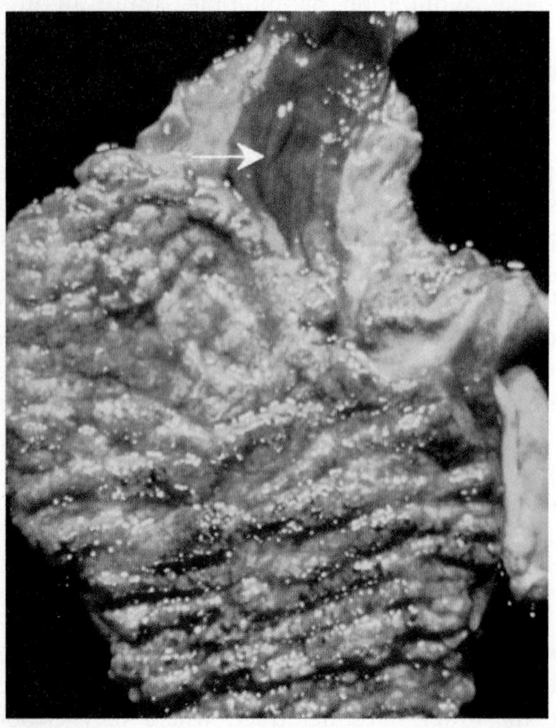

FIGURE 25-1
Autopsy specimen showing confluent pseudomembranes covering the cecum of a patient with pseudomembranous colitis. Note the sparing of the terminal ileum (*arrow*).

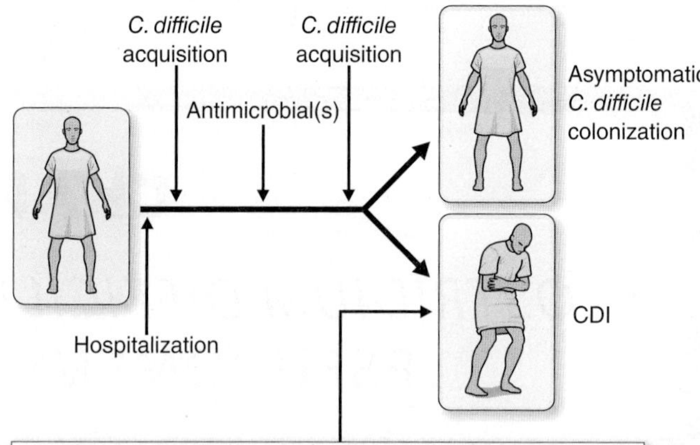

FIGURE 25-2
Pathogenesis model for hospital-acquired *Clostridium difficile* infection (CDI). At least three events are integral to *C. difficile* pathogenesis: (1) Exposure to antibiotics establishes susceptibility to infection. (2) Once susceptible, the patient may acquire nontoxigenic (nonpathogenic) or toxigenic strains of *C. difficile* as a second event. (3) Acquisition of toxigenic *C. difficile* may be followed by asymptomatic colonization or CDI, depending on one or more additional events (e.g., an inadequate host anamnestic IgG response to *C. difficile* toxin A).

Patients colonized with *C. difficile* were initially thought to be at high risk for CDI. However, four prospective studies have shown that colonized patients who have not previously had CDI actually have a decreased risk of CDI. At least three events are proposed as essential for the development of CDI (Fig. 25-2). Exposure to antimicrobial agents is the first event and establishes susceptibility to *C. difficile* infection, most likely through disruption of the normal gastrointestinal microbiota. The second event is exposure to toxigenic *C. difficile*. Given that the majority of patients do not develop CDI after the first two events, a third event is clearly essential for its occurrence. Candidate third events include exposure to a *C. difficile* strain of particular virulence, exposure to antimicrobial agents especially likely to cause CDI, and an inadequate host immune response. The host anamnestic serum IgG antibody response to toxin A of *C. difficile* is the most likely third event that determines which patients develop diarrhea and which patients remain asymptomatic. In all probability, the majority of people first develop antibody to *C. difficile* toxins when colonized asymptomatically during the first year of life or after CDI in childhood. Infants are thought not to develop symptomatic CDI because they lack suitable mucosal toxin receptors that develop later in life. In adulthood, serum levels of IgG antibody to toxin A increase more in response to infection in individuals who become asymptomatic carriers than in those who develop CDI. For persons who develop CDI, development of increasing levels of antitoxin A during treatment correlates with a lower risk of recurrence of CDI. A clinical trial using monoclonal antibodies to both toxin A and toxin B in addition to standard therapy showed rates of recurrence significantly lower than those obtained with placebo plus standard therapy.

GLOBAL CONSIDERATIONS

Rates and severity of CDI in the United States, Canada, and Europe increased markedly after the year 2000. Rates in U.S. hospitals tripled between 2000 and 2005. In 2005, hospitals in Montreal, Quebec, reported rates four times higher than the 1997 baseline, with directly attributable mortality of 6.9% (increased from 1.5%). An epidemic strain, variously known as toxinotype III, REA type BI, polymerase chain reaction (PCR) ribotype 027, and pulsed-field type NAP1 and thus collectively designated NAP1/BI/027, is thought to account for much of the increase in incidence and has been found in North America, Europe, and Asia. It is now recognized that two clones of NAP1/BI/027 originated in the United States and Canada and spread to the United Kingdom, Europe, and Asia. The epidemic organism is characterized by (1) an ability to produce 16–23 times as much toxin A and toxin B as control strains in vitro; (2) the presence of a third toxin (binary toxin CDT); and (3) high-level resistance to all fluoroquinolones. New strains have been and probably will continue to be implicated in outbreaks, including a strain (toxinotype V, ribotype 078) commonly found in food animals that also carries binary toxin and has been associated with high mortality risk in human infections. In the past 5 years, rates of CDI in the United Kingdom have markedly decreased, and the frequency of the NAP1/BI/027 strain in the countries of the European Union has likewise decreased. However, there has been no evidence of decreased rates of CDI or a decreased incidence of NAP1/BI/027 in North America; the latter strain still causes 25–35% of all CDIs in most regions of the United States.

CLINICAL MANIFESTATIONS

Diarrhea is the most common manifestation caused by *C. difficile*. Stools are almost never grossly bloody and range from soft and unformed to watery or mucoid in consistency, with a characteristic odor. Patients may have as many as 20 bowel movements per day. Clinical and laboratory findings include fever in 28% of cases, abdominal pain in 22%, and leukocytosis in 50%. When adynamic ileus (which is seen on x-ray in ~20% of cases) results in cessation of stool passage, the diagnosis of CDI is frequently overlooked. A clue to the presence of unsuspected CDI in these patients is unexplained leukocytosis, with ≥15,000 white blood cells (WBCs)/μL. Such patients are at high risk for complications of *C. difficile* infection, particularly toxic megacolon and sepsis.

C. difficile diarrhea recurs after treatment in ~15–30% of cases, and this figure may be increasing. Recurrences may represent either relapses due to the same strain or reinfections with a new strain. Susceptibility to recurrence of clinical CDI is likely a result of continued fecal-microbiota disruption caused by the antibiotic used to treat CDI.

DIAGNOSIS

The diagnosis of CDI is based on a combination of clinical criteria: (1) diarrhea (≥3 unformed stools per 24 h for ≥2 days) with no other recognized cause plus (2) toxin A or B detected in the stool, toxin-producing *C. difficile* detected in the stool by PCR or culture, or pseudomembranes seen in the colon. PMC is a more advanced form of CDI and is visualized at endoscopy in only ~50% of patients with diarrhea who have a positive stool culture and toxin assay for *C. difficile*. Endoscopy is a rapid diagnostic tool in seriously ill patients with suspected PMC and an acute abdomen, but a negative result in this examination does not rule out CDI.

Despite the array of tests available for *C. difficile* and its toxins (Table 25-1), no single traditional test has high sensitivity, high specificity, and rapid turnaround. Most laboratory tests for toxins, including enzyme immunoassays, lack sensitivity. However, testing of multiple additional stool specimens is not recommended. Nucleic acid amplification tests, including PCR assays, have now been approved for diagnostic purposes and appear to be both rapid and sensitive while retaining high specificity. Testing of asymptomatic patients is not recommended except for epidemiologic study purposes. In particular, so-called tests of cure following treatment are not recommended because >50% of patients continue to harbor the organism and toxin after diarrhea has ceased and test results do not always predict recurrence of CDI. Thus these results should not be used to restrict placement of patients in long-term-care or nursing home facilities.

TREATMENT *Clostridium Difficile* Infection

PRIMARY CDI When possible, discontinuation of any ongoing antimicrobial administration is recommended as the first step in treatment of CDI. Earlier studies indicated that 15–23% of patients respond to this simple measure. However, with the advent of the current epidemic strain and the associated rapid clinical deterioration of some patients, prompt initiation of specific CDI treatment has become the standard. Empirical

TABLE 25-1

RELATIVE SENSITIVITY AND SPECIFICITY OF DIAGNOSTIC TESTS FOR *CLOSTRIDIUM DIFFICILE* INFECTION (CDI)

TYPE OF TEST	RELATIVE SENSITIVITY[a]	RELATIVE SPECIFICITY[a]	COMMENT
Stool culture for *C. difficile*	++++	+++	Most sensitive test; specificity of ++++ if the *C. difficile* isolate tests positive for toxin; with clinical data, is diagnostic of CDI; turnaround time too slow for practical use
Cell culture cytotoxin test on stool	+++	++++	With clinical data, is diagnostic of CDI; highly specific but not as sensitive as stool culture; slow turnaround time
Enzyme immunoassay for toxin A or toxins A and B in stool	++ to +++	+++	With clinical data, is diagnostic of CDI; rapid results, but not as sensitive as stool culture or cell culture cytotoxin test
Enzyme immunoassay for *C. difficile* common antigen in stool	+++ to ++++	+++	Detects glutamate dehydrogenase found in toxigenic and nontoxigenic strains of *C. difficile* and other stool organisms; more sensitive and less specific than enzyme immunoassay for toxins; rapid results
Nucleic acid amplification tests for *C. difficile* toxin A or B gene in stool	++++	++++	Detect toxigenic *C. difficile* in stool; newly approved for clinical testing, but appears to be more sensitive than enzyme immunoassay toxin testing and at least as specific
Colonoscopy or sigmoidoscopy	+	++++	Highly specific if pseudomembranes are seen; insensitive compared with other tests

[a]According to both clinical and test-based criteria. ++++, >90%; +++, 71–90%; ++, 51–70%; +, ~50%.

treatment is appropriate if CDI is strongly suspected on clinical grounds. General treatment guidelines include hydration and the avoidance of antiperistaltic agents and opiates, which may mask symptoms and possibly worsen disease. Nevertheless, antiperistaltic agents have been used safely with vancomycin or metronidazole for mild to moderate CDI.

Oral administration of vancomycin, fidaxomicin, or metronidazole is recommended for CDI treatment. IV vancomycin is ineffective for CDI, and fidaxomicin is available only for oral administration; when IV metronidazole is administered, fecal bactericidal drug concentrations are achieved during acute diarrhea; however, in the presence of adynamic ileus, IV metronidazole treatment of CDI has failed. Two large clinical trials comparing vancomycin and fidaxomicin indicated comparable resolution of diarrhea (~90% of patients) as well as significantly reduced rates of recurrent CDI with fidaxomicin from rates with vancomycin. In previous randomized trials, diarrhea response rates to oral therapy with vancomycin or metronidazole were ≥94%, but four observational studies found that response rates for metronidazole had declined to 62–78%. Although the mean time to resolution of diarrhea is 2–4 days, the response to metronidazole may be much slower. Treatment should not be deemed a failure until a drug has been given for at least 6 days. On the basis of data for shorter courses of vancomycin and the results of two large-scale clinical trials, it is recommended that vancomycin, fidaxomicin, and metronidazole be given for at least 10 days. Metronidazole is not approved for CDI by the U.S. Food and Drug Administration (FDA), but most patients with mild to moderate illness respond to 500 mg given by mouth three times a day for 10 days; extension of the treatment period may be needed for slow responders. In addition to the reports of increases in metronidazole failures, a prospective, randomized, double-blind, placebo-controlled study has demonstrated the superiority of vancomycin over metronidazole for treatment of severe CDI. The severity assessment score in that study included age as well as laboratory parameters (elevated temperature, low albumin level, or elevated WBC count), documentation of PMC by endoscopy, and treatment of CDI in the intensive care unit. Although a validated severity score is not available, it is important to initiate treatment with oral vancomycin for patients who appear seriously ill, particularly if they have a high WBC count (>15,000/μL) or a creatinine level that is ≥1.5 times higher than the premorbid value (Table 25-2). In addition, a randomized blinded trial compared a toxin-binding polymer, tolevamer, with two antibiotic regimens for treatment of CDI and showed that vancomycin was superior to metronidazole for all patients regardless of severity. Small randomized trials of nitazoxanide, bacitracin, rifaximin, and fusidic acid for treatment of CDI have been conducted. These drugs have not been extensively studied, shown to be superior, or approved by the FDA for CDI, but they provide potential alternatives to vancomycin, fidaxomicin, and metronidazole.

RECURRENT CDI Overall, ~15–30% of successfully treated patients experience recurrences of CDI, either as relapses caused by the original organism or as reinfections following treatment. Rates of CDI recurrence are significantly lower among patients treated with fidaxomicin rather than vancomycin. Rates of recurrence are comparable with vancomycin and metronidazole. Recurrence rates are higher among patients

TABLE 25-2

RECOMMENDATIONS FOR THE TREATMENT OF *CLOSTRIDIUM DIFFICILE* INFECTION (CDI)[a]

CLINICAL SETTING	TREATMENT(S)	COMMENTS
Initial episode, mild to moderate	Metronidazole (500 mg tid × 10–14 d)	Vancomycin (125 mg qid × 10–14 d) may be more effective than metronidazole. Fidaxomicin (200 mg bid × 10 d) is another alternative.
Initial episode, severe	Vancomycin (125 mg qid × 10–14 d)	Indicators of severe disease may include leukocytosis (≥15,000 white blood cells/μL) and a creatinine level ≥1.5 times the premorbid value. Fidaxomicin is an alternative.
Initial episode, severe complicated or fulminant	Vancomycin (500 mg PO or via nasogastric tube) ***plus*** metronidazole (500 mg IV q8h) ***plus consider*** Rectal instillation of vancomycin (500 mg in 100 mL of normal saline as a retention enema q6–8h)	Severe complicated or fulminant CDI is defined as severe CDI with the addition of hypotension, shock, ileus, or toxic megacolon. The duration of treatment may need to be >2 weeks and is dictated by response. Consider using tigecycline (50 mg IV q12h after a 100-mg loading dose) in place of metronidazole.
First recurrence	Same as for initial episode	Adjust treatment if severity of CDI has changed with recurrence. Consider fidaxomicin, which significantly decreases the likelihood of additional recurrences.
Second recurrence	Vancomycin in taper/pulse regimen	Typical taper/pulse regimen: 125 mg qid × 10–14 d, then bid × 1 week, then daily × 1 week, then q2–3d for 2–8 weeks.
Multiple recurrences	Consider the following options: • Repeat vancomycin taper/pulse • Vancomycin (500 mg qid × 10 d) plus *Saccharomyces boulardii* (500 mg bid × 28 d) • Vancomycin (125 mg qid × 10–14 d); then stop vancomycin and start rifaximin (400 mg bid × 2 weeks) • Nitazoxanide (500 mg bid × 10 d) • Fecal microbiota transplantation • IV immunoglobulin (400 mg/kg)	The only controlled studies that included patients with one or more recurrent CDI episodes were with vancomycin and *S. boulardii*, which showed borderline significance compared with vancomycin plus placebo, and fecal microbiota transplantation, which was highly significant compared with a high-dose course of vancomycin. (The vancomycin taper was not compared.)

[a]All agents are given orally unless otherwise specified.

≥65 years old, those who continue to take antibiotics while being treated for CDI, and those who remain in the hospital after the initial episode of CDI. Patients who have a first recurrence of CDI have a high rate of second recurrence (33–65%). In the first recurrence, re-treatment with metronidazole is comparable to treatment with vancomycin (Table 25-2), and fidaxomicin is superior to vancomycin in reducing the risk of further recurrences in patients who have had one recurrence. Recurrent CDI, once thought to be relatively mild, has now been documented to pose a significant (11%) risk of serious complications (shock, megacolon, perforation, colectomy, or death within 30 days). There is no standard treatment for multiple recurrences, but long or repeated metronidazole courses should be avoided because of potential neurotoxicity. The use of vancomycin in tapering doses or with pulse dosing every other day for 2–8 weeks may be the most practical approach to treatment of patients with multiple recurrences. Other approaches include the administration of vancomycin followed by the yeast *Saccharomyces boulardii*; the administration of vancomycin followed by a fecal microbiota transplant given via nasoduodenal tube, colonoscope, or enema; and the intentional colonization of the patient with a nontoxigenic strain of *C. difficile*. None of these biotherapeutic approaches has been approved by the FDA for use in the United States. Other non–FDA-approved antibiotic strategies include (1) sequential treatment with vancomycin (125 mg four times daily for 10–14 days) followed by rifaximin (400 mg twice daily for 14 days) and (2) treatment with nitazoxanide (500 mg twice daily for 7 days). IV immunoglobulin, which has also been used with variable success, presumably provides antibodies to *C. difficile* toxins.

SEVERE COMPLICATED OR FULMINANT CDI Fulminant (rapidly progressive and severe) CDI presents the most difficult treatment challenge. Patients with fulminant disease often do not have diarrhea, and their illness mimics an acute surgical abdomen. Sepsis (hypotension, fever, tachycardia, leukocytosis) may result from severe CDI. An acute abdomen (with or without toxic megacolon) may include signs of obstruction, ileus, colon-wall thickening and ascites on abdominal CT, and peripheral-blood leukocytosis (≥20,000 WBCs/μL). With or without diarrhea, the differential diagnosis of an acute abdomen, sepsis, or toxic megacolon should include CDI if the patient has received antibiotics in the past 2 months. Cautious sigmoidoscopy or colonoscopy to visualize PMC and abdominal CT are the best diagnostic tests in patients without diarrhea.

Medical management of fulminant CDI is suboptimal because of the difficulty of delivering oral fidaxomicin, metronidazole, or vancomycin to the colon in the presence of ileus (Table 25-2). The combination of vancomycin (given via nasogastric tube and by retention enema) plus IV metronidazole has been used with some success in uncontrolled studies, as has IV tigecycline in small-scale uncontrolled studies. Surgical colectomy may be life-saving if there is no response to medical management. If possible, colectomy should be performed before the serum lactate level reaches 5 mmol/L. The incidence of fulminant CDI requiring colectomy appears to be increasing in the evolving epidemic; however, morbidity and death associated with colectomy may be reduced by performing instead a laparoscopic ileostomy followed by colon lavage with polyethylene glycol and vancomycin infusion into the colon via the ileostomy.

PROGNOSIS

The mortality rate attributed to CDI, previously found to be 0.6–3.5%, has reached 6.9% in recent outbreaks and rises progressively with increasing age. Most patients recover, but recurrences are common.

PREVENTION AND CONTROL

Strategies for the prevention of CDI are of two types: those aimed at preventing transmission of the organism to the patient and those aimed at reducing the risk of CDI if the organism is transmitted. Transmission of *C. difficile* in clinical practice has been prevented by gloving of personnel, elimination of the use of contaminated electronic thermometers, and use of hypochlorite (bleach) solution for environmental decontamination of patients' rooms. Hand hygiene is critical; hand washing is recommended in CDI outbreaks because alcohol hand gels are not sporicidal. CDI outbreaks have been best controlled by restricting the use of specific antibiotics, such as clindamycin and second- and third-generation cephalosporins. Outbreaks of CDI due to clindamycin-resistant strains have resolved promptly when clindamycin use is restricted. Future preventive strategies are likely to include use of monoclonal antibodies, vaccines, and biotherapeutics containing live organisms that will restore colonization protection in the microbiota.

CHAPTER 26

INTRAABDOMINAL INFECTIONS AND ABSCESSES

Miriam Baron Barshak ■ Dennis L. Kasper

Intraperitoneal infections generally arise because a normal anatomic barrier is disrupted. This disruption may occur when the appendix, a diverticulum, or an ulcer ruptures; when the bowel wall is weakened by ischemia, tumor, or inflammation (e.g., in inflammatory bowel disease); or with adjacent inflammatory processes, such as pancreatitis or pelvic inflammatory disease, in which enzymes (in the former case) or organisms (in the latter) may leak into the peritoneal cavity. Whatever the inciting event, once inflammation develops and organisms usually contained within the bowel or another organ enter the normally sterile peritoneal space, a predictable series of events takes place. Intraabdominal infections occur in two stages: peritonitis and—if the patient survives this stage and goes untreated—abscess formation. The types of microorganisms predominating in each stage of infection are responsible for the pathogenesis of disease.

PERITONITIS

Peritonitis is a life-threatening event that is often accompanied by bacteremia and sepsis syndrome. The peritoneal cavity is large but is divided into compartments. The upper and lower peritoneal cavities are divided by the transverse mesocolon; the greater omentum extends from the transverse mesocolon and from the lower pole of the stomach to line the lower peritoneal cavity. The pancreas, duodenum, and ascending and descending colon are located in the anterior retroperitoneal space; the kidneys, ureters, and adrenals are found in the posterior retroperitoneal space. The other organs, including liver, stomach, gallbladder, spleen, jejunum, ileum, transverse and sigmoid colon, cecum, and appendix, are within the peritoneal cavity. The cavity is lined with a serous membrane that can serve as a conduit for fluids—a property exploited in peritoneal dialysis (Fig. 26-1). A small amount of serous fluid is normally present in the peritoneal space, with a protein content (consisting mainly of albumin) of <30 g/L and <300 white blood cells (WBCs, generally mononuclear cells) per microliter. In bacterial infections, leukocyte recruitment into the infected peritoneal cavity consists of an early influx of polymorphonuclear leukocytes (PMNs) and a prolonged subsequent phase of mononuclear cell migration. The phenotype of the infiltrating leukocytes

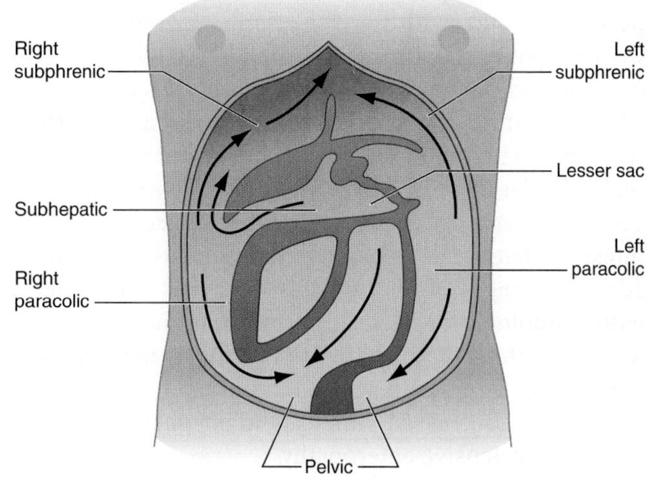

FIGURE 26-1
Diagram of the intraperitoneal spaces, showing the circulation of fluid and potential areas for abscess formation. Some compartments collect fluid or pus more often than others. These compartments include the pelvis (the lowest portion), the subphrenic spaces on the right and left sides, and Morrison's pouch, which is a posterosuperior extension of the subhepatic spaces and is the lowest part of the paravertebral groove when a patient is recumbent. The falciform ligament separating the right and left subphrenic spaces appears to act as a barrier to the spread of infection; consequently, it is unusual to find bilateral subphrenic collections. *(Reprinted with permission from B Lorber [ed]: Atlas of Infectious Diseases, vol VII: Intra-abdominal Infections, Hepatitis, and Gastroenteritis. Philadelphia, Current Medicine, 1996, p 1.13.)*

during the course of inflammation is regulated primarily by resident-cell chemokine synthesis.

PRIMARY (SPONTANEOUS) BACTERIAL PERITONITIS

Peritonitis is either primary (without an apparent source of contamination) or secondary. The types of organisms found and the clinical presentations of these two processes are different. In adults, primary bacterial peritonitis (PBP) occurs most commonly in conjunction with cirrhosis of the liver (frequently the result of alcoholism). However, the disease has been reported in adults with metastatic malignant disease, postnecrotic cirrhosis, chronic active hepatitis, acute viral hepatitis, congestive heart failure, systemic lupus erythematosus, and lymphedema as well as in patients with no underlying disease. Although PBP virtually always develops in patients with preexisting ascites, it is, in general, an uncommon event, occurring in ≤10% of cirrhotic patients. The cause of PBP has not been established definitively but is believed to involve hematogenous spread of organisms in a patient in whom a diseased liver and altered portal circulation result in a defect in the usual filtration function. Organisms multiply in ascites, a good medium for growth. The proteins of the complement cascade have been found in peritoneal fluid, with lower levels in cirrhotic patients than in patients with ascites of other etiologies. The opsonic and phagocytic properties of PMNs are diminished in patients with advanced liver disease. Cirrhosis is associated with alterations in the gut microbiota, including an increased prevalence of potentially pathogenic bacteria such as Enterobacteriaceae. Small-intestinal bacterial overgrowth is frequently present in advanced stages of liver cirrhosis and has been linked with pathologic bacterial translocation and PBP. Factors promoting these changes in cirrhosis may include deficiencies in Paneth cell defensins, reduced intestinal motility, decreased pancreatobiliary secretions, and portal-hypertensive enteropathy.

The presentation of PBP differs from that of secondary peritonitis. The most common manifestation is fever, which is reported in up to 80% of patients. Ascites is found but virtually always predates infection. Abdominal pain, an acute onset of symptoms, and peritoneal irritation during physical examination can be helpful diagnostically, but the absence of any of these findings does not exclude this often-subtle diagnosis. Nonlocalizing symptoms (such as malaise, fatigue, or encephalopathy) without another clear etiology should also prompt consideration of PBP in a susceptible patient. It is vital to sample the peritoneal fluid of any cirrhotic patient with ascites and fever. The finding of >250 PMNs/μL is diagnostic for PBP, according to Conn (*http://jac.oxfordjournals.org/cgi/content/full/47/3/369*). This criterion does not apply to secondary peritonitis (see below). The microbiology of PBP is also distinctive. While enteric gram-negative bacilli such as *Escherichia coli* are most commonly encountered, gram-positive organisms such as streptococci, enterococci, or even pneumococci are sometimes found. In an important development, widespread use of quinolones to prevent PBP in high-risk subgroups of patients, frequent hospitalizations, and exposure to broad-spectrum antibiotics have led to a change in flora of infections in patients with cirrhosis, with more gram-positive bacteria and extended-spectrum β-lactamase–producing Enterobacteriaceae in recent years. Risk factors for multiresistant infections include nosocomial origin of infection, long-term norfloxacin prophylaxis, recent infection with multiresistant bacteria, and recent use of β-lactam antibiotics. In PBP, a single organism is typically isolated; anaerobes are found less frequently in PBP than in secondary peritonitis, in which a mixed flora including anaerobes is the rule. In fact, if PBP is suspected and multiple organisms including anaerobes are recovered from the peritoneal fluid, the diagnosis must be reconsidered and a source of secondary peritonitis sought.

The diagnosis of PBP is not easy. It depends on the exclusion of a primary intraabdominal source of infection. Contrast-enhanced CT is useful in identifying an intraabdominal source for infection. It may be difficult to recover organisms from cultures of peritoneal fluid, presumably because the burden of organisms is low. However, the yield can be improved if 10 mL of peritoneal fluid is placed directly into a blood culture bottle. Because bacteremia frequently accompanies PBP, blood should be cultured simultaneously. To maximize the yield, culture samples should be collected prior to administration of antibiotics. No specific radiographic studies are helpful in the diagnosis of PBP. A plain film of the abdomen would be expected to show ascites. Chest and abdominal radiography should be performed in patients with abdominal pain to exclude free air, which signals a perforation (Fig. 26-2).

TREATMENT Primary Bacterial Peritonitis

Treatment for PBP is directed at the isolate from blood or peritoneal fluid. Gram's staining of peritoneal fluid often gives negative results in PBP. Therefore, until culture results become available, therapy should cover gram-negative aerobic bacilli and gram-positive cocci. Third-generation cephalosporins such as cefotaxime (2 g q8h, administered IV) provide reasonable initial coverage in moderately ill patients. Broad-spectrum antibiotics, such as penicillin/β-lactamase inhibitor combinations (e.g., piperacillin/tazobactam, 3.375 g q6h IV for adults with normal renal function) or ceftriaxone

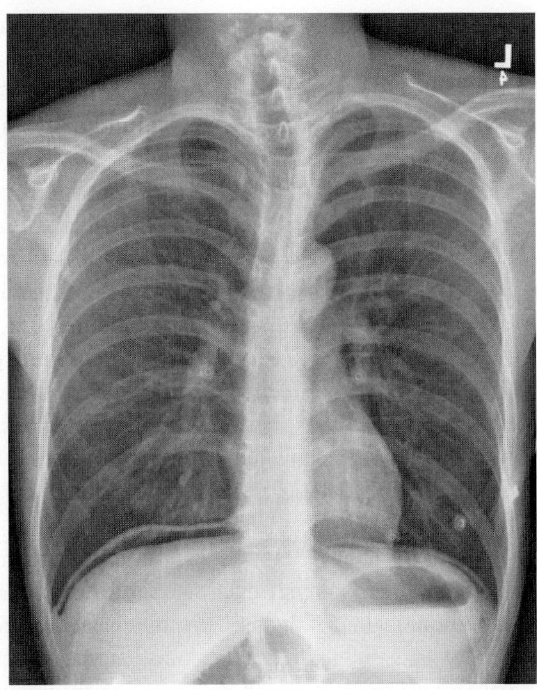

FIGURE 26-2
Pneumoperitoneum. Free air under the diaphragm on an upright chest film suggests the presence of a bowel perforation and associated peritonitis. *(Image courtesy of Dr. John Braver; with permission.)*

(2 g q24h IV), are also options. Broader empirical coverage aimed at resistant hospital-acquired gram-negative bacteria (e.g., treatment with carbapenem) may be appropriate for nosocomially acquired PBP until culture results become available. Empirical coverage for anaerobes is not necessary. A mortality benefit from albumin (1.5 g/kg of body weight within 6 h of detection and 1.0 g/kg on day 3) has been demonstrated for patients who present with serum creatinine levels ≥1 mg/dL, blood urea nitrogen levels ≥30 mg/dL, or total bilirubin levels ≥4 mg/dL but not for patients who do not meet these criteria. After the infecting organism is identified, therapy should be narrowed to target the specific pathogen. Patients with PBP usually respond within 72 h to appropriate antibiotic therapy. Antimicrobial treatment can be administered for as little as 5 days if rapid improvement occurs and blood cultures are negative, but a course of up to 2 weeks may be required for patients with bacteremia and for those whose improvement is slow. Persistence of WBCs in the ascitic fluid after therapy should prompt a search for additional diagnoses.

Prevention

Primary prevention

Several observational studies and a meta-analysis raise the concern that proton pump inhibitor therapy may increase the risk of PBP. No prospective studies have yet addressed whether avoidance of such therapy may prevent PBP. Nonselective beta blockers may prevent secondary bacterial peritonitis. A 2012 guideline from the American Association for the Study of Liver Diseases recommends chronic antibiotic prophylaxis with a regimen described in the next section for patients who are at highest risk for PBP—that is, those with an ascitic-fluid total protein level <1.5 g/dL along with impaired renal function (creatinine, ≥1.2 mg/dL; blood urea nitrogen, ≥25 mg/dL; or serum sodium, ≤130 mg/dL) and/or liver failure (Child-Pugh score, ≥9; and bilirubin, ≥3 mg/dL). A 7-day course of antibiotic prophylaxis is recommended for patients with cirrhosis and gastrointestinal bleeding.

Secondary prevention

PBP has a high rate of recurrence. Up to 70% of patients experience a recurrence within 1 year. Antibiotic prophylaxis is recommended for patients with a history of PBP to reduce this rate to <20% and improve short-term survival rates. Prophylactic regimens for adults with normal renal function include fluoroquinolones (ciprofloxacin, 750 mg weekly; norfloxacin, 400 mg/d) or trimethoprim-sulfamethoxazole (one double-strength tablet daily). However, long-term administration of broad-spectrum antibiotics in this setting has been shown to increase the risk of severe staphylococcal infections.

SECONDARY PERITONITIS

Secondary peritonitis develops when bacteria contaminate the peritoneum as a result of spillage from an intraabdominal viscus. The organisms found almost always constitute a mixed flora in which facultative gram-negative bacilli and anaerobes predominate, especially when the contaminating source is colonic. Early in the course of infection, when the host response is directed toward containment, exudate containing fibrin and PMNs is found. Early death in this setting is attributable to gram-negative bacillary sepsis and to potent endotoxins circulating in the bloodstream. Gram-negative bacilli, particularly *E. coli*, are common bloodstream isolates, but *Bacteroides fragilis* bacteremia also occurs. The severity of abdominal pain and the clinical course depend on the inciting process. The organisms isolated from the peritoneum also vary with the source of the initial process and the normal flora at that site. Secondary peritonitis can result primarily from chemical irritation and/or bacterial contamination. For example, as long as the patient is not achlorhydric, a ruptured gastric ulcer will release low-pH gastric contents that will serve as a chemical irritant. The normal flora of the stomach comprises the same organisms found in the oropharynx but in lower numbers. Thus, the bacterial burden in a ruptured ulcer is negligible compared with that in a ruptured appendix. The normal flora of the colon below the ligament of Treitz contains ~10^{11} anaerobic organisms/g of feces but only

10^8 aerobes/g; therefore, anaerobic species account for 99.9% of the bacteria. Leakage of colonic contents (pH 7–8) does not cause significant chemical peritonitis, but infection is intense because of the heavy bacterial load.

Depending on the inciting event, local symptoms may occur in secondary peritonitis—for example, epigastric pain from a ruptured gastric ulcer. In appendicitis **(Chap. 23)**, the initial presenting symptoms are often vague, with periumbilical discomfort and nausea followed in a number of hours by pain more localized to the right lower quadrant. Unusual locations of the appendix (including a retrocecal position) can complicate this presentation further. Once infection has spread to the peritoneal cavity, pain increases, particularly with infection involving the parietal peritoneum, which is innervated extensively. Patients usually lie motionless, often with knees drawn up to avoid stretching the nerve fibers of the peritoneal cavity. Coughing and sneezing, which increase pressure within the peritoneal cavity, are associated with sharp pain. There may or may not be pain localized to the infected or diseased organ from which secondary peritonitis has arisen. Patients with secondary peritonitis generally have abnormal findings on abdominal examination, with marked voluntary and involuntary guarding of the anterior abdominal musculature. Later findings include tenderness, especially rebound tenderness. In addition, there may be localized findings in the area of the inciting event. In general, patients are febrile, with marked leukocytosis and a left shift of the WBCs to band forms.

While recovery of organisms from peritoneal fluid is easier in secondary than in primary peritonitis, a tap of the abdomen is rarely the procedure of choice in secondary peritonitis. An exception is in cases involving trauma, where the possibility of a hemoperitoneum may need to be excluded early. Emergent studies (such as abdominal CT) to find the source of peritoneal contamination should be undertaken if the patient is hemodynamically stable; unstable patients may require surgical intervention without prior imaging.

TREATMENT Secondary Peritonitis

Treatment for secondary peritonitis includes early administration of antibiotics aimed particularly at aerobic gram-negative bacilli and anaerobes (see below). Mild to moderate disease can be treated with many drugs covering these organisms, including broad-spectrum penicillin/β-lactamase inhibitor combinations (e.g., ticarcillin/clavulanate, 3.1 g q4–6h IV), cefoxitin (2 g q4–6h IV), or a combination of either a fluoroquinolone (e.g., levofloxacin, 750 mg q24h IV) or a third-generation cephalosporin (e.g., ceftriaxone, 2 g q24h IV) plus metronidazole (500 mg q8h IV). Patients in intensive care units should receive imipenem (500 mg q6h IV), meropenem (1 g q8h IV), or combinations of drugs, such as ampicillin plus metronidazole plus ciprofloxacin. The role of enterococci and *Candida* species in mixed infections is controversial. Secondary peritonitis usually requires both surgical intervention to address the inciting process and antibiotics to treat early bacteremia, to decrease the incidence of abscess formation and wound infection, and to prevent distant spread of infection. Although surgery is rarely indicated in PBP in adults, it may be life-saving in secondary peritonitis. Recombinant human activated protein C (APC) was considered at one time for treatment of severe sepsis from causes including secondary peritonitis but was withdrawn from the market in 2011 after it was determined that the drug was associated with an increased risk of bleeding and that evidence for its beneficial effects was inadequate. Thus APC should not be used for sepsis or septic shock outside randomized clinical trials.

Peritonitis may develop as a complication of abdominal surgeries. These infections may be accompanied by localizing pain and/or nonlocalizing signs or symptoms such as fever, malaise, anorexia, and toxicity. As a nosocomial infection, postoperative peritonitis may be associated with organisms such as staphylococci, components of the gram-negative hospital microflora, and the microbes that cause PBP and secondary peritonitis, as described above.

PERITONITIS IN PATIENTS UNDERGOING CONTINUOUS AMBULATORY PERITONEAL DIALYSIS

A third type of peritonitis arises in patients who are undergoing continuous ambulatory peritoneal dialysis (CAPD). Unlike PBP and secondary peritonitis, which are caused by endogenous bacteria, CAPD-associated peritonitis usually involves skin organisms. The pathogenesis of infection is similar to that of intravascular device–related infection, in which skin organisms migrate along the catheter, which both serves as an entry point and exerts the effects of a foreign body. Exit-site or tunnel infection may or may not accompany CAPD-associated peritonitis. Like PBP, CAPD-associated peritonitis is usually caused by a single organism. Peritonitis is, in fact, the most common reason for discontinuation of CAPD. Improvements in equipment design, especially the Y-set connector, have resulted in a decrease from one case of peritonitis per 9 months of CAPD to one case per 24 months.

The clinical presentation of CAPD peritonitis resembles that of secondary peritonitis in that diffuse pain and peritoneal signs are common. The dialysate is usually cloudy and contains >100 WBCs/μL, >50% of which are neutrophils. However, the number of cells depends in part on dwell time. According to a guideline from the International Society for Peritoneal Dialysis (2010), for patients undergoing automated peritoneal dialysis who present during their nighttime treatment and whose dwell time is much shorter than with CAPD, the clinician should use the percentage of PMNs rather than the absolute number of WBCs to diagnose peritonitis. As the normal peritoneum has very few PMNs, a proportion above 50% is strong evidence of peritonitis even if the absolute WBC count does not reach 100/μL. Meanwhile, patients undergoing automated peritoneal dialysis without a daytime exchange who present with abdominal pain may have no fluid to withdraw, in which case 1 L of dialysate should be infused and permitted to dwell a minimum of 1–2 h, then drained, examined for turbidity, and sent for cell count with differential and culture. The differential (with a shortened dwell time) may be more useful than the absolute WBC count. In equivocal cases or in patients with systemic or abdominal symptoms in whom the effluent appears clear, a second exchange is performed, with a dwell time of at least 2 h. Clinical judgment should guide initiation of therapy.

The most common organisms are *Staphylococcus* species, which accounted for ~45% of cases in one series. Historically, coagulase-negative staphylococcal species were identified most commonly in these infections, but these isolates have more recently been decreasing in frequency. *Staphylococcus aureus* is more often involved among patients who are nasal carriers of the organism than among those who are not, and this organism is the most common pathogen in overt exit-site infections. Gram-negative bacilli and fungi such as *Candida* species are also found. Vancomycin-resistant enterococci and vancomycin-intermediate *S. aureus* have been reported to produce peritonitis in CAPD patients. The finding of more than one organism in dialysate culture should prompt evaluation for secondary peritonitis. As with PBP, culture of dialysate fluid in blood culture bottles improves the yield. To facilitate diagnosis, several hundred milliliters of removed dialysis fluid should be concentrated by centrifugation before culture.

TREATMENT CAPD Peritonitis

Empirical therapy for CAPD peritonitis should be directed at *S. aureus*, coagulase-negative *Staphylococcus*, and gram-negative bacilli until the results of cultures become available. Guidelines suggest that agents should be chosen on the basis of local experience with resistant organisms. In some centers, a first-generation cephalosporin such as cefazolin (for gram-positive bacteria) and a fluoroquinolone or a third-generation cephalosporin such as ceftazidime (for gram-negative bacteria) may be reasonable; in areas with high rates of infection with methicillin-resistant *S. aureus*, vancomycin should be used instead of cefazolin, and gram-negative coverage may need to be broadened—e.g., with an aminoglycoside, ceftazidime, cefepime, or carbapenem. Broad coverage including vancomycin should be particularly considered for toxic patients and for those with exit-site infections. Vancomycin should also be included in the regimen if the patient has a history of colonization or infection with methicillin-resistant *S. aureus* or has a history of severe allergy to penicillins and cephalosporins. Loading doses are administered intraperitoneally; doses depend on the dialysis method and the patient's renal function. Antibiotics are given either continuously (i.e., with each exchange) or intermittently (i.e., once daily, with the dose allowed to remain in the peritoneal cavity for at least 6 h). If the patient is severely ill, IV antibiotics should be added at doses appropriate for the patient's degree of renal failure. The clinical response to an empirical treatment regimen should be rapid; if the patient has not responded after 48–96 h of treatment, new samples should be collected for cell counts and cultures, and catheter removal should be considered. For patients who lack exit-site or tunnel infection, the typical duration of antibiotic treatment is 14 days. For patients with exit-site or tunnel infection, catheter removal should be considered, and a longer duration of antibiotic therapy (up to 21 days) may be appropriate. In fungal infections, the catheter should be removed immediately.

INTRAABDOMINAL ABSCESSES

INTRAPERITONEAL ABSCESSES

Abscess formation is common in untreated peritonitis if overt gram-negative sepsis either does not develop or develops but is not fatal. In experimental models of abscess formation, mixed aerobic and anaerobic organisms have been implanted intraperitoneally. Without therapy directed at anaerobes, animals develop intraabdominal abscesses. As in humans, these experimental abscesses may stud the peritoneal cavity, lie within the omentum or mesentery, or even develop on the surface of or within viscera such as the liver.

Pathogenesis and immunity

There is often disagreement about whether an abscess represents a disease state or a host response. In a sense, it represents both: while an abscess is an infection in which viable infecting organisms and PMNs are contained in a fibrous capsule, it is also a process by which the host confines microbes to a limited space, thereby preventing further spread of infection. In any event, abscesses do cause significant symptoms, and patients with abscesses can be quite ill. Experimental work has helped to define both the host cells and the bacterial virulence factors responsible—most notably in the case of *B. fragilis*. This organism, although accounting for only 0.5% of the normal colonic flora, is the anaerobe most frequently isolated from intraabdominal infections, is especially prominent in abscesses, and is the most common anaerobic bloodstream isolate. On clinical grounds, therefore, *B. fragilis* appears to be uniquely virulent. Moreover, *B. fragilis* acts alone to cause abscesses in animal models of intraabdominal infection, whereas most other *Bacteroides* species must act synergistically with a facultative organism to induce abscess formation.

Of the several virulence factors identified in *B. fragilis*, one is critical: the capsular polysaccharide complex found on the bacterial surface. This complex comprises at least eight distinct surface polysaccharides. Structural analysis of these polysaccharides has shown an unusual motif of oppositely charged sugars. Polysaccharides having these *zwitterionic* characteristics, such as polysaccharide A, evoke a host response in the peritoneal cavity that localizes bacteria into abscesses. *B. fragilis* and polysaccharide A have been found to adhere to primary mesothelial cells in vitro; this adherence, in turn, stimulates the production of tumor necrosis factor α and intercellular adhesion molecule 1 by peritoneal macrophages. Although abscesses characteristically contain PMNs, the process of abscess induction depends on the stimulation of T lymphocytes by these unique zwitterionic polysaccharides. The stimulated CD4+ T lymphocytes secrete leukoattractant cytokines and chemokines. The alternative pathway of complement and fibrinogen also participate in abscess formation.

While antibodies to the capsular polysaccharide complex enhance bloodstream clearance of *B. fragilis*, CD4+ T cells are critical in immunity to abscesses. When administered subcutaneously, *B. fragilis* polysaccharide A has immunomodulatory characteristics and stimulates CD4+ T regulatory cells via an interleukin 2–dependent mechanism to produce interleukin 10. Interleukin 10 downregulates the inflammatory response, thereby preventing abscess formation.

Clinical presentation

Of all intraabdominal abscesses, 74% are intraperitoneal or retroperitoneal and are not visceral. Most intraperitoneal abscesses result from fecal spillage from a colonic source, such as an inflamed appendix. Abscesses can also arise from other processes. They usually form within weeks of the development of peritonitis and may be found in a variety of locations from omentum to mesentery, pelvis to psoas muscles, and subphrenic space to a visceral organ such as the liver, where they may develop either on the surface of the organ or within it. Periappendiceal and diverticular abscesses occur commonly. Diverticular abscesses are least likely to rupture. Infections of the female genital tract and pancreatitis are also among the more common causative events. When abscesses occur in the female genital tract—either as a primary infection (e.g., tuboovarian abscess) or as an infection extending into the pelvic cavity or peritoneum—*B. fragilis* figures prominently among the organisms isolated. *B. fragilis* is not found in large numbers in the normal vaginal flora. For example, it is encountered less commonly in pelvic inflammatory disease and endometritis without an associated abscess. In pancreatitis with leakage of damaging pancreatic enzymes, inflammation is prominent. Therefore, clinical findings such as fever, leukocytosis, and even abdominal pain do not distinguish pancreatitis itself from complications such as pancreatic pseudocyst, pancreatic abscess **(Chap. 50)**, or intraabdominal collections of pus. Especially in cases of necrotizing pancreatitis, in which the incidence of local pancreatic infection may be as high as 30%, needle aspiration under CT guidance is performed to sample fluid for culture. Many centers prescribe preemptive antibiotics for patients with necrotizing pancreatitis. Imipenem is frequently used for this purpose because it reaches high tissue levels in the pancreas (although it is not unique in this regard). Recent randomized controlled studies have not demonstrated a benefit from this practice, and some guidelines no longer recommend preemptive antibiotics for patients with acute pancreatitis. If needle aspiration yields infected fluid in the setting of acute necrotizing pancreatitis, antibiotic treatment is appropriate in conjunction with surgical and/or percutaneous drainage of infected material. Infected pseudocysts that occur remotely from acute pancreatitis are unlikely to be associated with significant amounts of necrotic tissue and may be treated with either surgical or percutaneous catheter drainage in conjunction with appropriate antibiotic therapy.

Diagnosis

Scanning procedures have considerably facilitated the diagnosis of intraabdominal abscesses. Abdominal CT probably has the highest yield, although ultrasonography is particularly useful for the right upper quadrant, kidneys, and pelvis. Both indium-labeled WBCs and gallium tend to localize in abscesses and may be useful in finding a collection. Because gallium is taken up in the bowel, indium-labeled WBCs may have a slightly greater yield for abscesses near the bowel. Neither indium-labeled WBC nor gallium scans serve as a basis for a definitive diagnosis, however; both need to be followed by other, more specific studies, such as CT, if an area of possible abnormality is identified. Abscesses contiguous with or contained within diverticula are particularly difficult to diagnose with scanning procedures. Although barium should not be injected if a perforation is suspected, a barium enema occasionally may detect a diverticular abscess not diagnosed by other

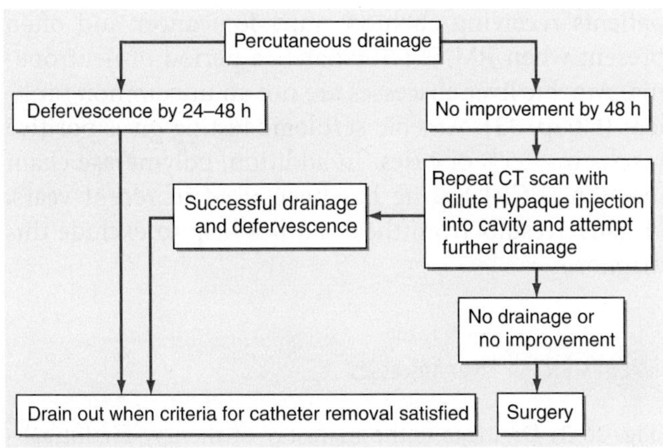

FIGURE 26-3

Algorithm for the management of patients with intraabdominal abscesses using percutaneous drainage. Antimicrobial therapy should be administered concomitantly. *(Reprinted with permission from B Lorber [ed]: Atlas of Infectious Diseases, vol VII: Intra-abdominal Infections, Hepatitis, and Gastroenteritis. Philadelphia, Current Medicine, 1996, p 1.30, as adapted from OD Rotstein, RL Simmons, in SL Gorbach et al [eds]: Infectious Diseases. Philadelphia, Saunders, 1992, p 668.)*

procedures. If one study is negative, a second study sometimes reveals a collection. Although exploratory laparotomy has been less commonly used since the advent of CT, this procedure still must be undertaken on occasion if an abscess is strongly suspected on clinical grounds.

TREATMENT Intraperitoneal Abscesses

An algorithm for the management of patients with intraabdominal (including intraperitoneal) abscesses by percutaneous drainage is presented in Fig. 26-3. The treatment of intraabdominal infections involves the determination of the initial focus of infection, the administration of broad-spectrum antibiotics targeting the organisms involved, and the performance of a drainage procedure if one or more definitive abscesses have formed. Antimicrobial therapy, in general, is adjunctive to drainage and/or surgical correction of an underlying lesion or process in intraabdominal abscesses. Unlike the intraabdominal abscesses resulting from most causes, for which drainage of some kind is generally required, abscesses associated with diverticulitis usually wall off locally after rupture of a diverticulum, so that surgical intervention is not routinely required.

A number of agents exhibit excellent activity against aerobic gram-negative bacilli. Because death in intraabdominal sepsis is linked to gram-negative bacteremia, empirical therapy for intraabdominal infection always needs to include adequate coverage of gram-negative aerobic, facultative, and anaerobic organisms. Even if anaerobes are not cultured from clinical specimens, they still must be covered by the therapeutic regimen. Empirical antibiotic therapy should be the same as that discussed above for secondary peritonitis.

VISCERAL ABSCESSES

Liver abscesses

The liver is the organ most subject to the development of abscesses. In one study of 540 intraabdominal abscesses, 26% were visceral. Liver abscesses made up 13% of the total number, or 48% of all visceral abscesses. Liver abscesses may be solitary or multiple; they may arise from hematogenous spread of bacteria or from local spread from contiguous sites of infection within the peritoneal cavity. In the past, appendicitis with rupture and subsequent spread of infection was the most common source for a liver abscess. Currently, associated disease of the biliary tract is most common. Pylephlebitis (suppurative thrombosis of the portal vein), usually arising from infection in the pelvis but sometimes from infection elsewhere in the peritoneal cavity, is another common source for bacterial seeding of the liver.

Fever is the most common presenting sign of liver abscess. Some patients, particularly those with associated disease of the biliary tract, have symptoms and signs localized to the right upper quadrant, including pain, guarding, punch tenderness, and even rebound tenderness. Nonspecific symptoms, such as chills, anorexia, weight loss, nausea, and vomiting, may also develop. Only 50% of patients with liver abscesses, however, have hepatomegaly, right-upper-quadrant tenderness, or jaundice; thus, one-half of patients have no symptoms or signs to direct attention to the liver. Fever of unknown origin may be the only manifestation of liver abscess, especially in the elderly. Diagnostic studies of the abdomen, especially the right upper quadrant, should be a part of any workup for fever of unknown origin. The single most reliable laboratory finding is an elevated serum concentration of alkaline phosphatase, which is documented in 70% of patients with liver abscesses. Other tests of liver function may yield normal results, but 50% of patients have elevated serum levels of bilirubin, and 48% have elevated concentrations of aspartate aminotransferase. Other laboratory findings include leukocytosis in 77% of patients, anemia (usually normochromic, normocytic) in 50%, and hypoalbuminemia in 33%. Concomitant bacteremia is found in one-third to one-half of patients. A liver abscess is sometimes suggested by chest radiography, especially if a new elevation of the right hemidiaphragm is seen; other suggestive findings include a right basilar infiltrate and a right pleural effusion.

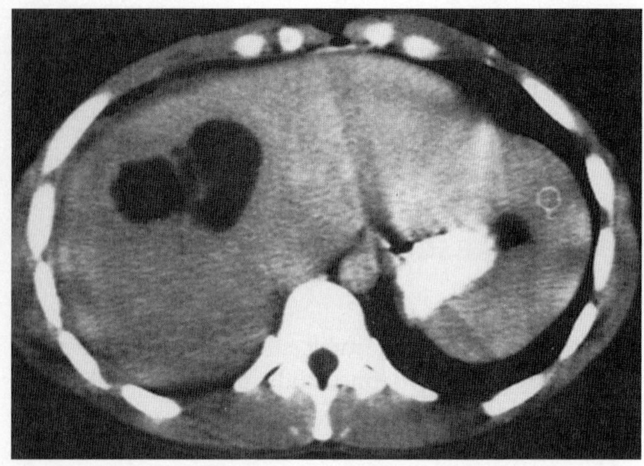

FIGURE 26-4
Multilocular liver abscess on CT scan. Multiple or multilocular abscesses are more common than solitary abscesses. *(Reprinted with permission from B Lorber [ed]: Atlas of Infectious Diseases, vol VII: Intra-abdominal Infections, Hepatitis, and Gastroenteritis. Philadelphia, Current Medicine, 1996, Fig. 1.22.)*

Imaging studies are the most reliable methods for diagnosing liver abscesses. These studies include ultrasonography, CT (Fig. 26-4), indium-labeled WBC or gallium scan, and MRI. More than one such study may be required.

Organisms recovered from liver abscesses vary with the source. In liver infection arising from the biliary tree, enteric gram-negative aerobic bacilli and enterococci are common isolates. *Klebsiella pneumoniae* liver abscess has been well described in Southeast Asia for more than 20 years and has become an emerging syndrome in North America and elsewhere. These community-acquired infections have been linked to a virulent hypermucoviscous *K. pneumoniae* phenotype and to a specific genotype. The typical syndrome includes liver abscess, bacteremia, and metastatic infection. Ampicillin/amoxicillin therapy started within the previous 30 days has been associated with increased risk for this syndrome, presumably because of selection for the causative strain. Unless previous surgery has been performed, anaerobes are not generally involved in liver abscesses arising from biliary infections. In contrast, in liver abscesses arising from pelvic and other intraperitoneal sources, a mixed flora including both aerobic and anaerobic species is common; *B. fragilis* is the species most frequently isolated. With hematogenous spread of infection, usually only a single organism is encountered; this species may be *S. aureus* or a streptococcal species such as one in the *Streptococcus milleri* group. Results of cultures obtained from drain sites are not reliable for defining the etiology of infections. Liver abscesses may also be caused by *Candida* species; such abscesses usually follow fungemia in patients receiving chemotherapy for cancer and often present when PMNs return after a period of neutropenia. Amebic liver abscesses are not an uncommon problem **(Chap. 33)**. Amebic serologic testing gives positive results in >95% of cases. In addition, polymerase chain reaction (PCR) testing has been used in recent years. Negative results from these studies help to exclude this diagnosis.

TREATMENT Liver Abscesses

(Fig. 26-3) Drainage is the mainstay of therapy for intraabdominal abscesses, including liver abscesses; the approach can be either percutaneous (with a pigtail catheter kept in place or possibly with a device that can perform pulse lavage to fragment and evacuate the semisolid contents of a liver abscess) or surgical. However, there is growing interest in medical management alone for pyogenic liver abscesses. The drugs used for empirical therapy include the same ones used in intraabdominal sepsis and secondary bacterial peritonitis. Usually, blood cultures and a diagnostic aspirate of abscess contents should be obtained before the initiation of empirical therapy, with antibiotic choices adjusted when the results of Gram's staining and culture become available. Cases treated without definitive drainage generally require longer courses of antibiotic therapy. When percutaneous drainage was compared with open surgical drainage, the average length of hospital stay for the former was almost twice that for the latter, although both the time required for fever to resolve and the mortality rate were the same for the two procedures. The mortality rate was appreciable despite treatment, averaging 15%. Several factors predict the failure of percutaneous drainage and therefore may favor primary surgical intervention. These factors include the presence of multiple, sizable abscesses; viscous abscess contents that tend to plug the catheter; associated disease (e.g., disease of the biliary tract) requiring surgery; the presence of yeast; communication with an untreated obstructed biliary tree; or the lack of a clinical response to percutaneous drainage in 4–7 days.

Treatment of candidal liver abscesses often entails initial administration of amphotericin B or liposomal amphotericin, with subsequent fluconazole therapy. In some cases, therapy with fluconazole alone (6 mg/kg daily) may be used—e.g., in clinically stable patients whose infecting isolate is susceptible to this drug.

Splenic abscesses

Splenic abscesses are much less common than liver abscesses. The incidence of splenic abscesses has ranged from 0.14% to 0.7% in various autopsy series. The clinical setting and the organisms isolated usually differ from those for liver abscesses. The degree of clinical suspicion for splenic abscess needs to be high because this condition is frequently fatal if left untreated. Even in the most recently published series, diagnosis was made only at autopsy in 37% of cases. Although splenic abscesses may arise occasionally from contiguous spread of infection or from direct trauma to the spleen, hematogenous spread of infection is more common. Bacterial endocarditis is the most common associated infection. Splenic abscesses can develop in patients who have received extensive immunosuppressive therapy (particularly those with malignancy involving the spleen) and in patients with hemoglobinopathies or other hematologic disorders (especially sickle cell anemia).

Although ~50% of patients with splenic abscesses have abdominal pain, the pain is localized to the left upper quadrant in only one-half of these cases. Splenomegaly is found in ~50% of cases. Fever and leukocytosis are generally present; the development of fever preceded diagnosis by an average of 20 days in one series. Left-sided chest findings may include abnormalities to auscultation, and chest radiographic findings may include an infiltrate or a left-sided pleural effusion. CT scan of the abdomen has been the most sensitive diagnostic tool. Ultrasonography can yield the diagnosis but is less sensitive. Liver-spleen scan or gallium scan may also be useful. Streptococcal species are the most common bacterial isolates from splenic abscesses, followed by *S. aureus*—presumably reflecting the associated endocarditis. An increase in the prevalence of gram-negative aerobic isolates from splenic abscesses has been reported; these organisms often derive from a urinary tract focus, with associated bacteremia, or from another intraabdominal source. *Salmonella* species are seen fairly commonly, especially in patients with sickle cell hemoglobinopathy. Anaerobic species accounted for only 5% of isolates in the largest collected series, but the reporting of a number of "sterile abscesses" may indicate that optimal techniques for the isolation of anaerobes were not used.

TREATMENT Splenic Abscesses

Because of the high mortality figures reported for splenic abscesses, splenectomy with adjunctive antibiotics has traditionally been considered standard treatment and remains the best approach for complex, multilocular abscesses or multiple abscesses. However, percutaneous drainage has worked well for single, small (<3-cm) abscesses in some studies and may also be useful for patients with high surgical risk. Patients undergoing splenectomy should be vaccinated against encapsulated organisms (*Streptococcus pneumoniae, Haemophilus influenzae, Neisseria meningitidis*). The most important factor in successful treatment of splenic abscesses is early diagnosis.

Perinephric and renal abscesses

Perinephric and renal abscesses are not common. The former accounted for only ~0.02% of hospital admissions and the latter for ~0.2% in Altemeier's series of 540 intraabdominal abscesses. Before antibiotics became available, most renal and perinephric abscesses were hematogenous in origin, usually complicating prolonged bacteremia, with *S. aureus* most commonly recovered. Now, in contrast, >75% of perinephric and renal abscesses arise from a urinary tract infection. Infection ascends from the bladder to the kidney, with pyelonephritis preceding abscess development. Bacteria may directly invade the renal parenchyma from medulla to cortex. Local vascular channels within the kidney may also facilitate the transport of organisms. Areas of abscess developing within the parenchyma may rupture into the perinephric space. The kidneys and adrenal glands are surrounded by a layer of perirenal fat that, in turn, is surrounded by Gerota's fascia, which extends superiorly to the diaphragm and inferiorly to the pelvic fat. Abscesses extending into the perinephric space may track through Gerota's fascia into the psoas or transversalis muscles, into the anterior peritoneal cavity, superiorly to the subdiaphragmatic space, or inferiorly to the pelvis. Of the risk factors that have been associated with the development of perinephric abscesses, the most important is concomitant nephrolithiasis obstructing urinary flow. Of patients with perinephric abscess, 20–60% have renal stones. Other structural abnormalities of the urinary tract, prior urologic surgery, trauma, and diabetes mellitus have also been identified as risk factors.

The organisms most frequently encountered in perinephric and renal abscesses are *E. coli*, *Proteus* species, and *Klebsiella* species. *E. coli*, the aerobic species most commonly found in the colonic flora, seems to have unique virulence properties in the urinary tract, including factors promoting adherence to uroepithelial cells. The urease of *Proteus* species splits urea, thereby creating a more alkaline and more hospitable environment for bacterial proliferation. *Proteus* species are frequently found in association with large struvite stones caused by the precipitation of magnesium ammonium sulfate in an alkaline environment. These stones serve as a nidus for recurrent urinary tract infection. Although a single bacterial species is usually recovered from a perinephric or renal abscess, multiple species may also be found. If a urine culture is not contaminated with periurethral flora and is found to contain more than one organism, a perinephric abscess or renal abscess should be considered in the differential diagnosis. Urine cultures may also be polymicrobial in cases of bladder diverticulum.

Candida species can cause renal abscesses. This fungus may spread to the kidney hematogenously or by ascension from the bladder. The hallmark of the latter route of infection is ureteral obstruction with large fungal balls.

The presentation of perinephric and renal abscesses is quite nonspecific. Flank pain and abdominal pain are common. At least 50% of patients are febrile. Pain may be referred to the groin or leg, particularly with extension of infection. The diagnosis of perinephric abscess, like that of splenic abscess, is frequently delayed, and the mortality rate in some series is appreciable, although lower than in the past. Perinephric or renal abscess should be most seriously considered when a patient presents with symptoms and signs of pyelonephritis and remains febrile after 4 or 5 days of treatment. Moreover, when a urine culture yields a polymicrobial flora, when a patient is known to have renal stones, or when fever and pyuria coexist with a sterile urine culture, these diagnoses should be entertained.

Renal ultrasonography and abdominal CT are the most useful diagnostic modalities. If a renal or perinephric abscess is diagnosed, nephrolithiasis should be excluded, especially when a high urinary pH suggests the presence of a urea-splitting organism.

TREATMENT Perinephric and Renal Abscesses

Treatment for perinephric and renal abscesses, like that for other intraabdominal abscesses, includes drainage of pus and antibiotic therapy directed at the organism(s) recovered. For perinephric abscesses, percutaneous drainage is usually successful.

Psoas abscesses

The psoas muscle is another location in which abscesses are encountered. Psoas abscesses may arise from a hematogenous source, by contiguous spread from an intraabdominal or pelvic process, or by contiguous spread from nearby bony structures (e.g., vertebral bodies). Associated osteomyelitis due to spread from bone to muscle or from muscle to bone is common in psoas abscesses. When Pott's disease was common, *Mycobacterium tuberculosis* was a frequent cause of psoas abscess. Currently, either *S. aureus* or a mixture of enteric organisms including aerobic and anaerobic gram-negative bacilli is usually isolated from psoas abscesses in the United States. *S. aureus* is most likely to be isolated when a psoas abscess arises from hematogenous spread or a contiguous focus of osteomyelitis; a mixed enteric flora is the most likely etiology when the abscess has an intraabdominal or pelvic source. Patients with psoas abscesses frequently present with fever, lower abdominal or back pain, or pain referred to the hip or knee. CT is the most useful diagnostic technique.

TREATMENT Psoas Abscesses

Treatment includes surgical drainage and the administration of an antibiotic regimen directed at the inciting organism(s).

Pancreatic abscesses

See Chap. 50.

ACKNOWLEDGMENT

The substantial contributions of Dori F. Zaleznik, MD, to this chapter in previous editions are gratefully acknowledged.

CHAPTER 27

HELICOBACTER PYLORI INFECTIONS

John C. Atherton ■ Martin J. Blaser

DEFINITION

Helicobacter pylori colonizes the stomach in ~50% of the world's human population, essentially for life unless eradicated by antibiotic treatment. Colonization with this organism is the main risk factor for peptic ulceration **(Chap. 15)** as well as for gastric adenocarcinoma and gastric mucosa-associated lymphoid tissue (MALT) lymphoma **(Chap. 51)**. Treatment for *H. pylori* has revolutionized the management of peptic ulcer disease, providing a permanent cure in most cases. Such treatment also represents first-line therapy for patients with low-grade gastric MALT lymphoma. Treatment of *H. pylori* is of no benefit in the treatment of gastric adenocarcinoma, but prevention of *H. pylori* colonization could potentially prevent gastric malignancy and peptic ulceration. In contrast, increasing evidence indicates that lifelong *H. pylori* colonization may offer some protection against complications of gastroesophageal reflux disease (GERD), including esophageal adenocarcinoma. Recent research has focused on whether *H. pylori* colonization is also a risk factor for some extragastric diseases and whether it is protective against some recently emergent medical problems, such as childhood-onset asthma and obesity.

ETIOLOGIC AGENT

Helicobacter pylori

H. pylori is a gram-negative bacillus that has naturally colonized humans for at least 100,000 years, and probably throughout human evolution. It lives in gastric mucus, with a small proportion of the bacteria adherent to the mucosa and possibly a very small number of the organisms entering cells or penetrating the mucosa; the organism's distribution is never systemic. Its spiral shape and flagella render *H. pylori* motile in the mucus environment. The organism has several acid-resistance mechanisms, most notably a highly expressed urease that catalyzes urea hydrolysis to produce buffering ammonia. *H. pylori* is microaerophilic (i.e., requires low levels of oxygen), is slow-growing, and requires complex growth media in vitro.

Other Helicobacter species

A very small proportion of gastric *Helicobacter* infections are due to species other than *H. pylori*, possibly acquired as zoonoses. These non-*pylori* gastric helicobacters are associated with low-level inflammation and occasionally with disease. In immunocompromised hosts, several nongastric (intestinal) *Helicobacter* species can cause disease with clinical features resembling those of *Campylobacter* infections; these species are covered in **Chap. 30**.

EPIDEMIOLOGY

Prevalence and risk factors

The prevalence of *H. pylori* among adults is <30% in most parts of the United States and in other developed countries as opposed to >80% in most developing countries. In the United States, prevalence varies with age: up to 50% of 60-year-old persons, ~20% of 30-year-old persons, and fewer than 10% of children are colonized. *H. pylori* is usually acquired in childhood. The age association is due mostly to a birth-cohort effect whereby current 60-year-olds were more commonly colonized as children than are current children. Spontaneous acquisition or loss of *H. pylori* in adulthood is uncommon. Childhood acquisition explains why the main risk factors for infection are markers of crowding and social deprivation in childhood.

Transmission

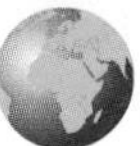

Humans are the only important reservoir of *H. pylori*. Children may acquire the organism from their parents (most often the primary caregiver) or from other children. The former is more common in developed countries and the latter in less developed countries. Whether transmission takes place more often by the fecal-oral or the oral-oral route is unknown, but *H. pylori* is easily cultured from vomitus and gastroesophageal refluxate and is less easily cultured from stool.

PATHOLOGY AND PATHOGENESIS

H. pylori colonization induces *chronic superficial gastritis*, a tissue response in the stomach that includes infiltration of the mucosa by both mononuclear and polymorphonuclear cells. (The term *gastritis* should be used specifically to describe histologic features; it has also been used to describe endoscopic appearances and even symptoms, but these features do not correlate with microscopic findings or even with the presence of *H. pylori*.) Although *H. pylori* is capable of numerous adaptations that prevent excessive stimulation of the immune system, colonization is accompanied by a considerable persistent local and systemic immune response, including the production of antibodies and cell-mediated responses. However, these responses are ineffective in clearing the bacterium. This inefficient clearing appears to be due in part to *H. pylori*'s downregulation of the immune system, which fosters its own persistence.

Most *H. pylori*–colonized persons do not develop clinical sequelae. That some persons develop overt disease whereas others do not is related to a combination of factors: bacterial strain differences, host susceptibility to disease, and environmental factors.

Bacterial virulence factors

Several *H. pylori* virulence factors are more common among strains that are associated with disease than among those that are not. The *cag* island is a group of genes that encodes a bacterial type IV secretion system. Through this system, an effector protein, CagA, is translocated into epithelial cells, where it may be transformed by phosphorylation and induces host cell signal transduction; proliferative, cytoskeletal, and inflammatory changes in the cell result. The protein at the tip of the secretory apparatus, CagL, binds to integrins on the cell surface, transducing further signaling. Finally, soluble components of the peptidoglycan cell wall enter the cell, mediated by the same secretory system. These components are recognized by the emergency intracellular bacterial receptor Nod1, which stimulates a proinflammatory cytokine response resulting in enhanced gastric inflammation. Carriage of *cag*-positive strains increases the risk of peptic ulcer or gastric adenocarcinoma. A second major virulence factor is the vacuolating cytotoxin VacA, which forms pores in cell membranes. VacA is polymorphic, and carriage of more active forms also increases the risk of disease. Other bacterial factors that are associated with increased disease risk include adhesins, such as BabA (which binds to blood group antigens on epithelial cells), and incompletely characterized factors, such as another recently described bacterial type 4 secretion system.

Host genetic and environmental factors

The best-characterized host determinants of disease are genetic polymorphisms leading to enhanced activation of the innate immune response, including polymorphisms in cytokine genes or in genes encoding bacterial recognition proteins such as Toll-like receptors. For example, colonized people with polymorphisms in the interleukin 1 gene that increase the production of this cytokine in response to *H. pylori* infection are at increased risk of gastric adenocarcinoma. In addition, environmental cofactors are important in pathogenesis. Smoking increases the risks of duodenal ulcers and gastric cancer in *H. pylori*–positive individuals. Diets high in salt and preserved foods increase cancer risk, whereas diets high in antioxidants and vitamin C are modestly protective.

Distribution of gastritis and differential disease risk

The pattern of gastric inflammation is associated with disease risk: antral-predominant gastritis is most closely linked with duodenal ulceration, whereas pan-gastritis is linked with gastric ulceration and adenocarcinoma. This difference probably explains why patients with duodenal ulceration are not at high risk of developing gastric adenocarcinoma later in life, despite being colonized by *H. pylori*.

Pathogenesis of duodenal ulceration

How gastric colonization causes duodenal ulceration is now becoming more clear. *H. pylori*–induced inflammation of the gastric antrum diminishes the number of somatostatin-producing D cells. Because somatostatin inhibits gastrin release, gastrin levels are higher than in *H. pylori*–negative persons, and these higher levels lead to increased meal-stimulated acid secretion from the relatively spared gastric corpus. How this situation increases duodenal ulcer risk remains controversial, but the increased acid secretion may contribute to the formation of the potentially protective gastric metaplasia found in the duodenum of duodenal ulcer patients. Gastric metaplasia in the duodenum may become colonized by *H. pylori* and subsequently inflamed and ulcerated.

Pathogenesis of gastric ulceration and gastric adenocarcinoma

The pathogenesis of these conditions is less well understood, although both arise in association with pan- or corpus-predominant gastritis. The hormonal changes described above still occur, but the inflammation in the gastric corpus means that it produces less acid (hypochlorhydria) despite hypergastrinemia. Gastric ulcers usually occur at the junction of antral and corpus-type mucosa, an area that is often particularly inflamed. Gastric cancer probably stems from progressive DNA damage and the survival of abnormal epithelial cell clones. The DNA damage is thought to be due principally to reactive oxygen and nitrogen species arising from inflammatory cells, perhaps in relation to other bacteria that survive in a hypochlorhydric stomach. Longitudinal analyses of gastric biopsy specimens taken years apart from the same patient show that the common *intestinal* type of gastric adenocarcinoma follows stepwise changes from simple gastritis to gastric atrophy, intestinal metaplasia, and dysplasia. A second, *diffuse* type of gastric adenocarcinoma found more commonly in younger adults may arise directly from chronic gastritis without atrophic changes.

CLINICAL MANIFESTATIONS

Essentially all *H. pylori*–colonized persons have histologic gastritis, but only ~10–15% develop associated illnesses such as peptic ulceration, gastric adenocarcinoma, or gastric lymphoma (Fig. 27-1). Rates among women are less than half of those among men for both diseases.

Peptic ulcer disease

Worldwide, >80% of duodenal ulcers and >60% of gastric ulcers are related to *H. pylori* colonization **(Chap. 15)**. However, in particular, the proportion of gastric ulcers caused by aspirin and nonsteroidal anti-inflammatory drugs (NSAIDs) is increasing, and in many developed countries these drugs have overtaken *H. pylori* as a cause of gastric ulceration. The main lines of evidence supporting an ulcer-promoting role for *H. pylori* are that (1) the presence of the organism is a risk factor for the development of ulcers, (2) non-NSAID-induced ulcers rarely develop in the absence of *H. pylori*, (3) eradication of *H. pylori* virtually abolishes long-term ulcer relapse, and (4) experimental *H. pylori* infection of gerbils can cause gastric ulceration.

Gastric adenocarcinoma and lymphoma

Prospective nested case-control studies have shown that *H. pylori* colonization is a risk factor for adenocarcinomas of the distal (noncardia) stomach **(Chap. 51)**. Long-term experimental infection of gerbils also may result in gastric adenocarcinoma. Moreover, *H. pylori* may induce primary gastric lymphoma, although this condition is much less common. Many low-grade gastric B-cell lymphomas are dependent on *H. pylori* for continuing growth and proliferation, and these tumors may regress either fully or partially after *H. pylori*

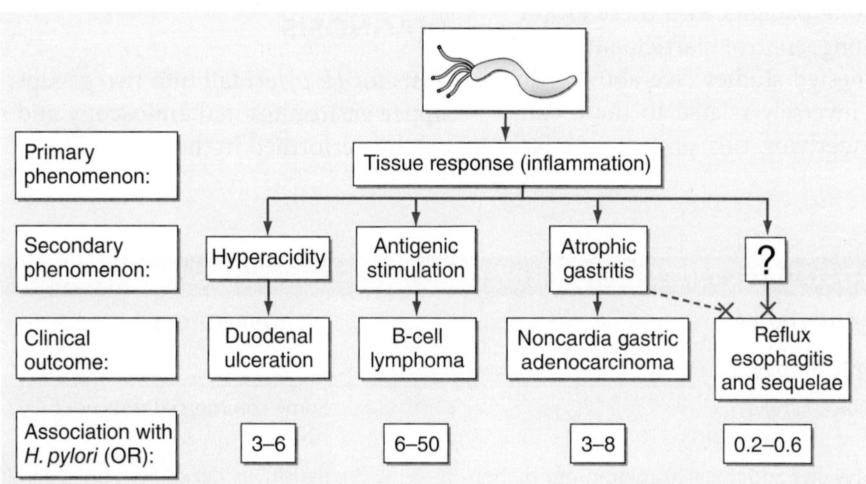

FIGURE 27-1

Schematic of the relationships between colonization with *Helicobacter pylori* and diseases of the upper gastrointestinal tract. Essentially all persons colonized with *H. pylori* develop a host response, which is generally termed *chronic gastritis*. The nature of the host's interaction with the particular bacterial population determines the clinical outcome. *H. pylori* colonization increases the lifetime risk of peptic ulcer disease, noncardia gastric cancer, and B-cell non-Hodgkin's gastric lymphoma (odds ratios [ORs] for all, >3). In contrast, a growing body of evidence indicates that *H. pylori* colonization (especially with *cagA*$^+$ strains) protects against adenocarcinoma of the esophagus (and the sometimes related gastric cardia) and premalignant lesions such as Barrett's esophagus (OR, <1). Although the incidences of peptic ulcer disease (cases not due to nonsteroidal anti-inflammatory drugs) and noncardia gastric cancer are declining in developed countries, the incidence of adenocarcinoma of the esophagus is increasing. *(Adapted from MJ Blaser: Hypothesis: The changing relationships of Helicobacter pylori and humans: Implications for health and disease. J Infect Dis 179:1523, 1999, with permission.)*

eradication. However, they require careful short- and long-term monitoring, and some necessitate additional treatment with chemotherapeutic agents.

Functional dyspepsia

Many patients have upper gastrointestinal symptoms but have normal results on upper gastrointestinal endoscopy (so-called functional or nonulcer dyspepsia; **Chap. 15**). Because *H. pylori* is common, some of these patients will be colonized with the organism. *H. pylori* eradication leads to symptom resolution a little more commonly (from 0 to 7% in different studies) than does placebo treatment. Whether such patients have peptic ulcers in remission at the time of endoscopy or whether a small subgroup of patients with "true" functional dyspepsia respond to *H. pylori* treatment is unclear.

Protection against peptic esophageal disease, including esophageal adenocarcinoma

Much interest has focused on a protective role for *H. pylori* against GERD **(Chap. 14)**, Barrett's esophagus **(Chap. 14)**, and adenocarcinoma of the esophagus and gastric cardia **(Chap. 51)**. The main lines of evidence for this role are (1) that there is a temporal relationship between a falling prevalence of gastric *H. pylori* colonization and a rising incidence of these conditions; (2) that, in most studies, the prevalence of *H. pylori* colonization (especially with proinflammatory *cagA*$^+$ strains) is significantly lower among patients with these esophageal diseases than among control participants; and (3) that, in prospective nested studies (see above), the presence of *H. pylori* is inversely related to these cancers. The mechanism underlying this protective effect is likely *H. pylori*–induced hypochlorhydria. Because, at the individual level, GERD symptoms may decrease, worsen, or remain unchanged after *H. pylori* treatment, concerns about GERD should not affect decisions about whether to treat *H. pylori* when an indication exists.

Other pathologies

H. pylori has an increasingly recognized role in other gastric pathologies. It may be one initial precipitant of autoimmune gastritis and pernicious anemia and also may predispose some patients to iron deficiency through occult blood loss and/or hypochlorhydria and reduced iron absorption. In addition, several extragastrointestinal pathologies have been linked with *H. pylori* colonization, although evidence of causality is less strong. Studies of *H. pylori* treatment in idiopathic thrombocytopenic purpura have consistently described improvement in or even normalization of platelet counts. Potentially important but even more controversial associations are with ischemic heart disease and cerebrovascular disease. However, the strength of the latter associations is reduced if confounding factors are taken into account, and most authorities consider the associations to be noncausal. Several studies have shown an inverse association of *cagA*$^+$ *H. pylori* with childhood-onset asthma, hay fever, and atopic disorders. These associations have been shown to be causal in animal models, but causality in humans and the size of any effect have not been established.

DIAGNOSIS

Tests for *H. pylori* fall into two groups: tests that require upper gastrointestinal endoscopy and simpler tests that can be performed in the clinic (Table 27-1).

TABLE 27-1

TESTS COMMONLY USED TO DETECT *HELICOBACTER PYLORI*

TEST	ADVANTAGES	DISADVANTAGES
Tests Based on Endoscopic Biopsy		
Biopsy urease test	Quick, simple	Some commercial tests not fully sensitive before 24 h
Histology	May give additional histologic information	Sensitivity dependent on experience and use of special stains
Culture	Permits determination of antibiotic susceptibility	Sensitivity dependent on experience
Noninvasive Tests		
Serology	Inexpensive and convenient; not affected by recent antibiotics or proton pump inhibitors to the same extent as breath and stool tests	Cannot be used for early follow-up after treatment; some commercial kits inaccurate, and most less accurate than urea breath test
^{13}C urea breath test	Inexpensive and simpler than endoscopy; useful for follow-up after treatment	Requires fasting; not as convenient as blood or stool tests
Stool antigen test	Inexpensive and convenient; useful for follow-up after treatment; may be useful in children	Stool-based tests are disliked by people from some cultures

Endoscopy-based tests

Endoscopy is usually unnecessary in the initial management of young patients with simple dyspepsia but is commonly used to exclude malignancy and make a positive diagnosis in older patients or those with "alarm" symptoms. If endoscopy is performed, the most convenient biopsy-based test is the biopsy urease test, in which one large or two small gastric biopsy specimens are placed into a gel containing urea and an indicator. The presence of *H. pylori* urease leads to a pH alteration and therefore to a color change, which often occurs within minutes but can require up to 24 h. Histologic examination of biopsy specimens for *H. pylori* also is accurate, provided that a special stain (e.g., a modified Giemsa or silver stain) permitting optimal visualization of the organism is used. If biopsy specimens are obtained from both antrum and corpus, histologic study yields additional information, including the degree and pattern of inflammation and the presence of any atrophy, metaplasia, or dysplasia. Microbiologic culture is most specific but may be insensitive because of difficulty with *H. pylori* isolation. Once the organism is cultured, its identity as *H. pylori* can be confirmed by its typical appearance on Gram's stain and its positive reactions in oxidase, catalase, and urease tests. Moreover, the organism's susceptibility to antibiotics can be determined, and this information can be clinically useful in difficult cases. The occasional biopsy specimens containing the less common non-*pylori* gastric helicobacters give only weakly positive results in the biopsy urease test. Positive identification of these bacteria requires visualization of the characteristic long, tight spirals in histologic sections; they cannot easily be cultured.

Noninvasive tests

Noninvasive *H. pylori* testing is the norm if gastric cancer does not need to be excluded by endoscopy. The best-established test (and a very accurate one) is the *urea breath test*. In this simple test, the patient drinks a solution of urea labeled with the nonradioactive isotope ^{13}C and then blows into a tube. If *H. pylori* urease is present, the urea is hydrolyzed, and labeled carbon dioxide is detected in breath samples. The *stool antigen test*, a simple and accurate test using monoclonal antibodies specific for *H. pylori* antigens, is more convenient and potentially less expensive than the urea breath test, but some patients dislike sampling stool. The simplest tests for ascertaining *H. pylori* status are *serologic assays* measuring specific IgG levels in serum by enzyme-linked immunosorbent assay or immunoblot. The best of these tests are as accurate as other diagnostic methods, but many commercial tests—especially rapid office tests—do not perform well.

Use of tests to assess treatment success

The urea breath test, the stool antigen test, and biopsy-based tests can all be used to assess the success of treatment (Fig. 27-2). However, because these tests are dependent on *H. pylori* load, their use <4 weeks after treatment may yield false-negative results. Furthermore, these tests are unreliable if performed within 4 weeks of intercurrent treatment with antibiotics or bismuth compounds or within 2 weeks of the discontinuation of proton pump inhibitor (PPI) treatment. In the assessment of treatment success, noninvasive tests are normally preferred; however, after gastric ulceration, endoscopy should be repeated to ensure healing and to exclude gastric carcinoma by further histologic sampling. Serologic tests are not used to monitor treatment success, as the gradual drop in titer of *H. pylori*–specific antibodies is too slow to be of practical use.

TREATMENT *Helicobacter pylori* Infection

INDICATIONS The most clear-cut indications for treatment are *H. pylori*–related duodenal or gastric ulceration or low-grade gastric B-cell lymphoma. Whether or not the ulcers are currently active, *H. pylori* should be eradicated in patients with documented ulcer disease to prevent relapse (Fig. 27-2). Testing for *H. pylori* and treatment if the results are positive also have been advocated in uninvestigated simple dyspepsia, but only when the prevalence of *H. pylori* in the community is >20% are these measures more cost-effective than simply treating the dyspepsia with PPIs. Guidelines have recommended *H. pylori* treatment in functional dyspepsia in case the patient is one of the perhaps 0–7% who will benefit from such treatment (beyond placebo effects). Some guidelines also recommend treatment of conditions not definitively known to respond to *H. pylori* eradication, including idiopathic thrombocytopenic purpura, vitamin B12 deficiency, and iron-deficiency anemia (in the last instance, only when other causes have been carefully excluded). Test-and-treat has emerged as a common clinical practice in recent years despite the lack of direct evidence that it is advantageous; whether this practice will survive the scrutiny of time and further study remains to be determined. For individuals with a strong family history of gastric cancer, treatment to eradicate *H. pylori* in the hope of reducing their cancer risk is reasonable but of unproven value. Currently, widespread community screening for and treatment of *H. pylori* as primary prophylaxis for gastric cancer and peptic ulcers are not recommended in most countries, mainly because the extent of the consequent reduction in cancer risk is not known. Several studies have found a modestly reduced cancer risk after treatment, but the period of follow-up is still fairly short and the size of the effect in different populations remains unclear. Other reasons not to treat *H. pylori* in asymptomatic populations at present include (1) the adverse side effects (which are common and can be severe in rare cases) of the multiple-antibiotic regimens used; (2) antibiotic resistance, which may emerge in

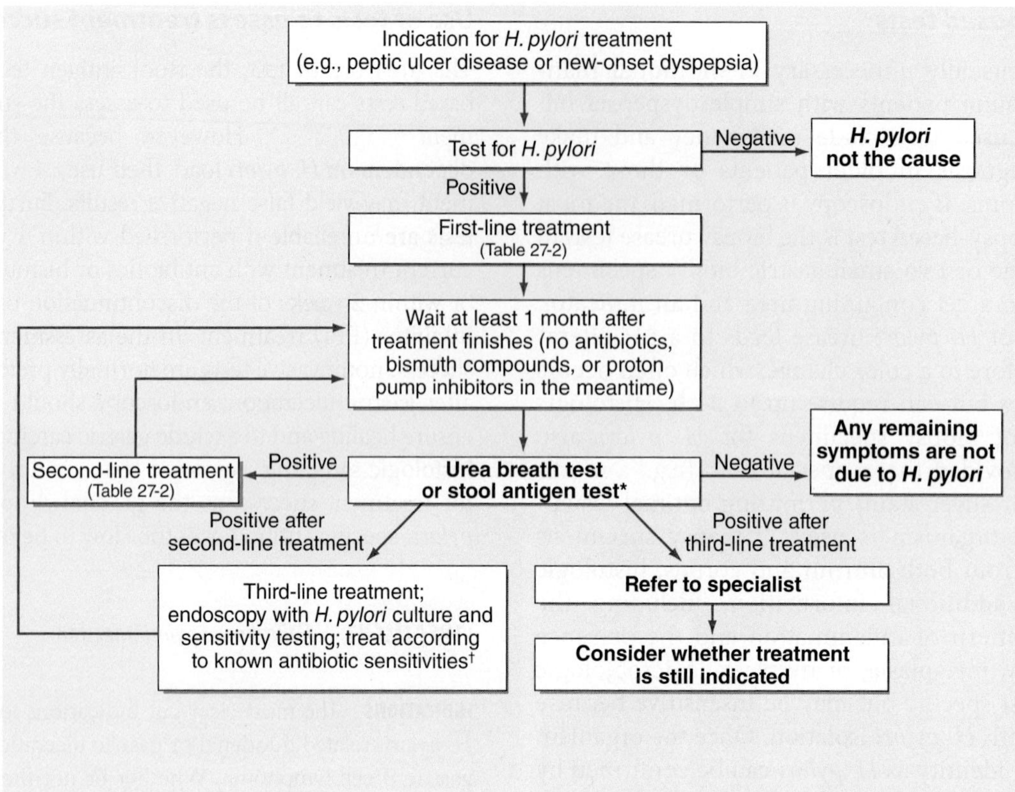

FIGURE 27-2

Algorithm for the management of *Helicobacter pylori* infection. *Note that either the urea breath test or the stool antigen test can be used in this algorithm. Occasionally, endoscopy and a biopsy-based test are used instead of either of these tests in follow-up after treatment. The main indication for these invasive tests is gastric ulceration; in this condition, as opposed to duodenal ulceration, it is important to check healing and to exclude underlying gastric adenocarcinoma. However, even in this situation, patients undergoing endoscopy may still be receiving proton pump inhibitor therapy, which precludes *H. pylori* testing. Thus a urea breath test or a stool antigen test is still required at a suitable interval after the end of therapy to determine whether treatment has been successful (see text). †Some authorities use empirical third-line regimens, of which several have been described.

H. pylori or other incidentally carried bacteria; (3) the anxiety that may arise in otherwise healthy people, especially if treatment is unsuccessful; and (4) the existence of a subset of people who will develop GERD symptoms after treatment, although, on average, *H. pylori* treatment does not affect GERD symptoms or severity. Despite the absence of screening strategies, many doctors treat *H. pylori* if it is known to be present (particularly in children and younger adults), even when the patient is asymptomatic. The rationale is that it reduces patient concern and may reduce future gastric cancer risk and that any reduction in risk is likely to be greater in younger patients. However, such practices do not factor in any potential benefits of *H. pylori* colonization. Overall, despite widespread clinical activity in this area, most treatment of asymptomatic *H. pylori* carriage is given without a firm evidence base.

REGIMENS Although *H. pylori* is susceptible to a wide range of antibiotics in vitro, monotherapy is not usually successful, probably because of inadequate antibiotic delivery to the colonization niche. Failure of monotherapy prompted the development of multidrug regimens, the most successful of which are triple and quadruple combinations. Current regimens consist of a PPI and two or three antimicrobial agents given for 7–14 days (Table 27-2). Research on optimizing drug combinations to increase efficacy continues, and guidelines are likely to change as the field develops and as countries increasingly tailor treatment to suit local antibiotic resistance patterns and economic needs.

The two most important factors in successful *H. pylori* treatment are the patient's close compliance with the regimen and the use of drugs to which the patient's strain of *H. pylori* has not acquired resistance. Treatment failure following minor lapses in compliance is common and often leads to acquired resistance to metronidazole or clarithromycin. To stress the importance of compliance, written instructions should be given to the patient, and minor side effects of the regimen should be explained. Increasing levels of *H. pylori* resistance to clarithromycin, quinolones, and—to a lesser extent—metronidazole are of growing concern and are thought to be responsible for the reduced efficacy of previously popular clarithromycin-based triple-therapy regimens worldwide. Treatment with these regimens is now virtually confined to certain northern European countries where the

TABLE 27-2

COMMONLY RECOMMENDED TREATMENT REGIMENS FOR *HELICOBACTER PYLORI*

REGIMEN[a] (DURATION)	DRUG 1	DRUG 2	DRUG 3	DRUG 4
Regimen 1: OCM (7–14 days)[b]	Omeprazole (20 mg bid[c])	Clarithromycin (500 mg bid)	Metronidazole (500 mg bid)	—
Regimen 2: OCA (7–14 days)[b]	Omeprazole (20 mg bid[c])	Clarithromycin (500 mg bid)	Amoxicillin (1 g bid)	—
Regimen 3: OBTM (14 days)[d]	Omeprazole (20 mg bid[c])	Bismuth subsalicylate (2 tabs qid)	Tetracycline HCl (500 mg qid)	Metronidazole (500 mg tid)
Regimen 4[e]: sequential (5 days + 5 days)	Omeprazole (20 mg bid[c]) Omeprazole (20 mg bid[c])	Amoxicillin (1 g bid) Clarithromycin (500 mg bid)	— Tinidazole (500 mg bid*g*)	— —
Regimen 5[f]: concomitant (14 days)	Omeprazole (20 mg bid[c])	Amoxicillin (1 g bid)	Clarithromycin (500 mg bid)	Tinidazole (500 mg bid[g])
Regimen 6[h]: OAL (10 days)	Omeprazole (20 mg bid[c])	Amoxicillin (1 g bid)	Levofloxacin (500 mg bid)	—

[a]The recommended first-line regimens for most of the world are shown in **bold** type.
[b]These regimens should be used only for populations in which the prevalence of clarithromycin-resistant strains is known to be <20%. In practice, this restriction limits the regimens' appropriate range mainly to northern Europe. Meta-analyses show that a 14-day course of therapy is slightly superior to a 7-day course.
[c]Many authorities and some guidelines recommend doubling this dose of omeprazole, as trials show resultant increased efficacy with some antibiotic combinations. Omeprazole may be replaced with any proton pump inhibitor at an equivalent dosage.
[d]Data supporting this regimen come mainly from Europe and are based on the use of bismuth subcitrate (1 tablet qid) and metronidazole (400 mg tid). This is a recommended first-line regimen in most countries and is the recommended second-line regimen in northern Europe.
[e]Data supporting this regimen come mainly from Europe. This regimen may be used as an alternative to regimen 3.
[f]This regimen may be used as an alternative to regimen 3 or 4.
[g]Metronidazole (500 mg bid) may be used as an alternative.
[h]Data supporting this regimen come mainly from Europe. It is used as second-line treatment in many countries (particularly where quadruple therapy is used as the first-line regimen) and as third-line treatment in others. This regimen may be less effective where rates of quinolone use are high.

use of clarithromycin (or azithromycin) for respiratory infections has not been widespread and resistance rates in *H. pylori* are still low. Strains of *H. pylori* with some degree of in vitro resistance to metronidazole are common but still may be eradicated with metronidazole-containing regimens, which have only slightly reduced efficacy in vivo. Assessment of antibiotic susceptibilities before treatment would be optimal but is not usually undertaken because endoscopy and mucosal biopsy are necessary to obtain *H. pylori* for culture and because most microbiology laboratories are inexperienced in *H. pylori* culture. In the absence of susceptibility information, the patient's history of (even distant) antibiotic use for other conditions should be ascertained; use of the previously administered agent(s) should then be avoided if possible, particularly in the case of clarithromycin (e.g., previous use for upper respiratory infection) and quinolones. If initial *H. pylori* treatment fails, the usual approach is empirical re-treatment with another drug regimen (Table 27-2). The third-line approach should ideally be endoscopy, biopsy, and culture plus treatment based on documented antibiotic sensitivities. However, empirical third-line therapies are often used.

Non-*pylori* gastric helicobacters are treated in the same way as *H. pylori*. However, in the absence of trials, it is unclear whether a positive outcome always represents successful treatment or whether it is sometimes due to natural clearance of the bacteria.

PREVENTION

Carriage of *H. pylori* has considerable public health significance in developed countries, where it is associated with peptic ulcer disease and gastric adenocarcinoma, and in developing countries, where gastric adenocarcinoma may be an even more common cause of cancer death late in life. If mass prevention were contemplated, vaccination would be the most obvious method, and experimental immunization of animals has given promising results. However, given that *H. pylori* has co-evolved with its human host over millennia, preventing or eliminating colonization on a population basis may have biological and clinical costs. For example, lifelong absence of *H. pylori* is a risk factor for GERD complications, including esophageal adenocarcinoma. We have speculated that the disappearance of *H. pylori* may also be associated with an increased risk of other emergent diseases reflecting aspects of the current Western lifestyle, such as childhood-onset asthma and allergy.

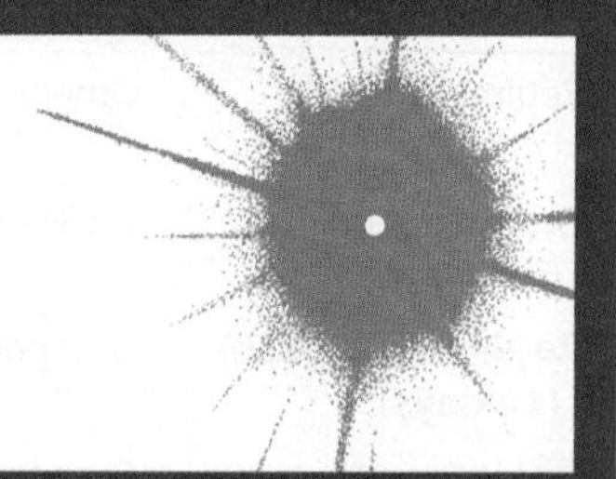

CHAPTER 28

SALMONELLOSIS

David A. Pegues ■ Samuel I. Miller

Bacteria of the genus *Salmonella* are highly adapted for growth in both humans and animals and cause a wide spectrum of disease. The growth of serotypes *Salmonella typhi* and *Salmonella paratyphi* is restricted to human hosts, in whom these organisms cause enteric (typhoid) fever. The remaining serotypes (nontyphoidal *Salmonella*, or NTS) can colonize the gastrointestinal tracts of a broad range of animals, including mammals, reptiles, birds, and insects. More than 200 serotypes of *Salmonella* are pathogenic to humans, in whom they often cause gastroenteritis and can be associated with localized infections and/or bacteremia.

ETIOLOGY

This large genus of gram-negative bacilli within the family Enterobacteriaceae consists of two species: *Salmonella enterica*, which contains six subspecies, and *Salmonella bongori*. *S. enterica* subspecies I includes almost all the serotypes pathogenic for humans. Members of the seven *Salmonella* subspecies are classified into >2500 serotypes (serovars); for simplicity, *Salmonella* serotypes (most of which are named for the city where they were identified) are often used as the species designation. For example, the full taxonomic designation *S. enterica* subspecies *enterica* serotype Typhimurium can be shortened to *Salmonella* serotype Typhimurium or simply *S. typhimurium*. Serotyping is based on the somatic O antigen (lipopolysaccharide cell-wall components), the surface Vi antigen (restricted to *S. typhi* and *S. paratyphi* C), and the flagellar H antigen.

Salmonellae are gram-negative, non-spore-forming, facultatively anaerobic bacilli that measure 2–3 μm by 0.4–0.6 μm. The initial identification of salmonellae in the clinical microbiology laboratory is based on growth characteristics. Salmonellae, like other Enterobacteriaceae, produce acid on glucose fermentation, reduce nitrates, and do not produce cytochrome oxidase. In addition, all salmonellae except *Salmonella gallinarum-pullorum* are motile by means of peritrichous flagella, and all but *S. typhi* produce gas (H_2S) on sugar fermentation. Notably, only 1% of clinical isolates ferment lactose; a high level of suspicion must be maintained to detect these rare clinical lactose-fermenting isolates.

Although serotyping of all surface antigens can be used for formal identification, most laboratories perform a few simple agglutination reactions that define specific O-antigen serogroups, designated A, B, C_1, C_2, D, and E. Strains in these six serogroups cause ~99% of *Salmonella* infections in humans and other warm-blooded animals. Molecular typing methods, including pulsed-field gel electrophoresis, polymerase chain reaction fingerprinting, and genomic DNA microarray analysis, are used in epidemiologic investigations to differentiate *Salmonella* strains of a common serotype.

PATHOGENESIS

All *Salmonella* infections begin with ingestion of organisms, most commonly in contaminated food or water. The infectious dose ranges from 200 colony-forming units (CFU) to 10^6 CFU, and the ingested dose is an important determinant of incubation period and disease severity. Conditions that decrease either stomach acidity (an age of <1 year, antacid ingestion, or achlorhydric disease) or intestinal integrity (inflammatory bowel disease, prior gastrointestinal surgery, or alteration of the intestinal flora by antibiotic administration) increase susceptibility to *Salmonella* infection.

Once *S. typhi* and *S. paratyphi* reach the small intestine, they penetrate the mucus layer of the gut and traverse the intestinal layer through phagocytic microfold (M) cells that reside within Peyer's patches. Salmonellae can trigger the formation of membrane ruffles in normally nonphagocytic epithelial cells. These ruffles reach out and enclose adherent bacteria within large vesicles by *bacterial-mediated endocytosis*. This process is dependent on the direct delivery of *Salmonella* proteins into the cytoplasm of epithelial cells by the specialized bacterial type III secretion system. These bacterial proteins mediate alterations in the actin cytoskeleton that are required for *Salmonella* uptake.

After crossing the epithelial layer of the small intestine, *S. typhi* and *S. paratyphi*, which cause enteric (typhoid) fever, are phagocytosed by macrophages. These salmonellae survive the antimicrobial environment of the macrophage by sensing environmental signals that trigger alterations in regulatory systems of the phagocytosed bacteria. For example, PhoP/PhoQ (the best-characterized regulatory system) triggers the expression of outer-membrane proteins and mediates modifications in lipopolysaccharide so that the altered bacterial surface can resist microbicidal activities and potentially alter host cell signaling. In addition, salmonellae encode a second type III secretion system that directly delivers bacterial proteins across the phagosome membrane into the macrophage cytoplasm. This secretion system functions to remodel the *Salmonella*-containing vacuole, promoting bacterial survival and replication.

Once phagocytosed, typhoidal salmonellae disseminate throughout the body in macrophages via the lymphatics and colonize reticuloendothelial tissues (liver, spleen, lymph nodes, and bone marrow). Patients have relatively few or no signs and symptoms during this initial incubation stage. Signs and symptoms, including fever and abdominal pain, probably result from secretion of cytokines by macrophages and epithelial cells in response to bacterial products that are recognized by innate immune receptors when a critical number of organisms have replicated. Over time, the development of hepatosplenomegaly is likely to be related to the recruitment of mononuclear cells and the development of a specific acquired cell-mediated immune response to *S. typhi* colonization. The recruitment of additional mononuclear cells and lymphocytes to Peyer's patches during the several weeks after initial colonization/infection can result in marked enlargement and necrosis of the Peyer's patches, which may be mediated by bacterial products that promote cell death as well as the inflammatory response.

In contrast to enteric fever, which is characterized by an infiltration of mononuclear cells into the small-bowel mucosa, NTS gastroenteritis is characterized by massive polymorphonuclear leukocyte infiltration into both the large- and small-bowel mucosa. This response appears to depend on the induction of interleukin 8, a strong neutrophil chemotactic factor, which is secreted by intestinal cells as a result of *Salmonella* colonization and translocation of bacterial proteins into host cell cytoplasm. The degranulation and release of toxic substances by neutrophils may result in damage to the intestinal mucosa, causing the inflammatory diarrhea observed with nontyphoidal gastroenteritis. An additional important factor in the persistence of nontyphoidal salmonellae in the intestinal tract and the organisms' capacity to compete with endogenous flora is the ability to utilize the sulfur-containing compound tetrathionate for metabolism in a microaerophilic environment. In the presence of intestinal inflammation, tetrathionate is generated from thiosulfate produced by epithelial cells through inflammatory cell production of reactive oxygen species.

ENTERIC (TYPHOID) FEVER

Enteric (typhoid) fever is a systemic disease characterized by fever and abdominal pain and caused by dissemination of *S. typhi* or *S. paratyphi*. The disease was initially called *typhoid fever* because of its clinical similarity to typhus. In the early 1800s, typhoid fever was clearly defined pathologically as a unique illness on the basis of its association with enlarged Peyer's patches and mesenteric lymph nodes. In 1869, given the anatomic site of infection, the term *enteric fever* was proposed as an alternative designation to distinguish typhoid fever from typhus. However, to this day, the two designations are used interchangeably.

EPIDEMIOLOGY

In contrast to other *Salmonella* serotypes, the etiologic agents of enteric fever—*S. typhi* and *S. paratyphi* serotypes A, B, and C—have no known hosts other than humans. Most commonly, food-borne or waterborne transmission results from fecal contamination by ill or asymptomatic chronic carriers. Sexual transmission between male partners has been described. Health care workers occasionally acquire enteric fever after exposure to infected patients or during processing of clinical specimens and cultures.

With improvements in food handling and water/sewage treatment, enteric fever has become rare in developed nations. Worldwide, however, there are an estimated 27 million cases of enteric fever, with 200,000–600,000 deaths annually. The annual incidence is highest (>100 cases/100,000 population) in south-central and Southeast Asia; medium (10–100 cases/100,000) in the rest of Asia, Africa, Latin America, and Oceania (excluding Australia and New Zealand); and low in other parts of the world (Fig. 28-1). A high incidence of enteric fever correlates with poor sanitation and lack of access to clean drinking water. In endemic regions, enteric fever is more common in urban than rural areas and among young children and adolescents than among other age groups. Risk factors include contaminated water or ice, flooding, food and drinks purchased from street vendors, raw fruits and vegetables

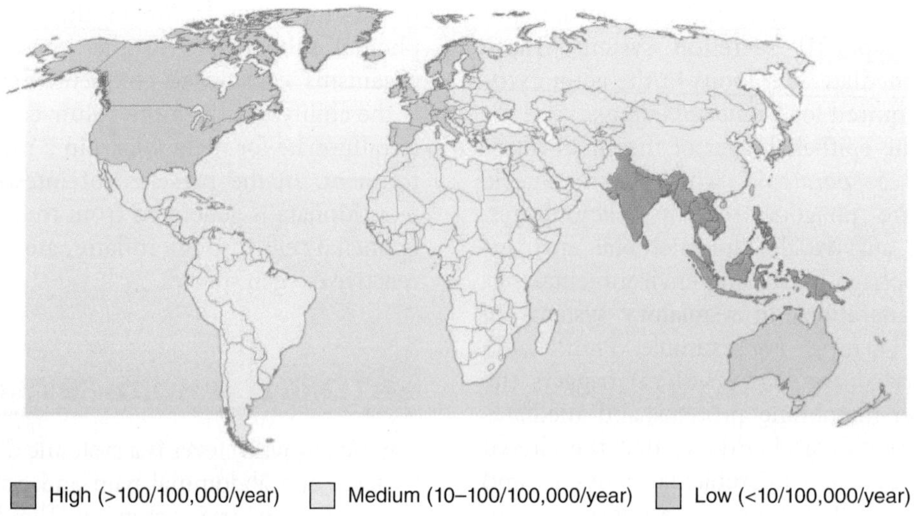

FIGURE 28-1

Annual incidence of typhoid fever per 100,000 population. *(Adapted from JA Crump et al: The global burden of typhoid fever. Bull World Health Organ 82:346, 2004.)*

grown in fields fertilized with sewage, ill household contacts, lack of hand washing and toilet access, and evidence of prior *Helicobacter pylori* infection (an association probably related to chronically reduced gastric acidity). It is estimated that there is one case of paratyphoid fever for every four cases of typhoid fever, but the incidence of infection associated with *S. paratyphi* A appears to be increasing, especially in India; this increase may be a result of vaccination for *S. typhi*.

Multidrug-resistant (MDR) strains of *S. typhi* emerged in the 1980s in China and Southeast Asia and have since disseminated widely. These strains contain plasmids encoding resistance to chloramphenicol, ampicillin, and trimethoprim—antibiotics long used to treat enteric fever. With the increased use of fluoroquinolones to treat MDR enteric fever in the 1990s, strains of *S. typhi* and *S. paratyphi* with decreased ciprofloxacin susceptibility (DCS; minimal inhibitory concentration [MIC], 0.125–0.5 μg/mL) or ciprofloxacin resistance (MIC, ≥1 μg/mL) have emerged on the Indian subcontinent, in southern Asia, and (most recently) in sub-Saharan Africa and have been associated with clinical treatment failure. Testing of isolates for resistance to the first-generation quinolone nalidixic acid detects many but not all strains with reduced susceptibility to ciprofloxacin and is no longer recommended. Strains of *S. typhi* and *S. paratyphi* producing extended-spectrum β-lactamases have emerged recently, primarily in India and Nepal.

Approximately 300 cases of typhoid and 150 cases of paratyphoid fever are reported annually in the United States. Of 1902 cases of *S. typhi*–associated enteric fever reported to the Centers for Disease Control and Prevention in 1999–2006, 79% were associated with recent international travel, most commonly to India (47%), Pakistan (10%), Bangladesh (10%), Mexico (7%), and the Philippines (4%). Only 5% of travelers diagnosed with enteric fever had received *S. typhi* vaccine. Overall, 13% of *S. typhi* isolates in the United States were resistant to ampicillin, chloramphenicol, and trimethoprim-sulfamethoxazole (TMP-SMX), and the proportion of DCS isolates increased from 19% in 1999 to 58% in 2006. Infection with DCS *S. typhi* was associated with travel to the Indian subcontinent. Of the 25–30% of reported cases of enteric fever in the United States that are domestically acquired, the majority are sporadic, but outbreaks linked to contaminated food products and previously unrecognized chronic carriers continue to occur.

CLINICAL COURSE

Enteric fever is a misnomer, in that the hallmark features of this disease—fever and abdominal pain—are variable. While fever is documented at presentation in >75% of cases, abdominal pain is reported in only 30–40%. Thus, a high index of suspicion for this potentially fatal systemic illness is necessary when a person presents with fever and a history of recent travel to a developing country.

The incubation period for *S. typhi* averages 10–14 days but ranges from 5 to 21 days, depending on the inoculum size and the host's health and immune status. The most prominent symptom is prolonged fever (38.8°–40.5°C; 101.8°–104.9°F), which can continue for up to 4 weeks if untreated. *S. paratyphi* A is thought to cause milder disease than *S. typhi*, with predominantly gastrointestinal symptoms. However, a prospective study of 669 consecutive cases of enteric fever in Kathmandu, Nepal, found that the infections caused by these organisms were clinically indistinguishable. In this series, symptoms reported on initial medical evaluation included headache (80%), chills (35–45%), cough (30%), sweating (20–25%), myalgias (20%), malaise (10%), and arthralgia (2–4%). Gastrointestinal manifestations included anorexia (55%), abdominal pain (30–40%), nausea (18–24%), vomiting (18%), and diarrhea (22–28%) more commonly than constipation (13–16%). Physical findings included coated tongue (51–56%), splenomegaly (5–6%), and abdominal tenderness (4–5%).

Early physical findings of enteric fever include rash ("rose spots"; 30%), hepatosplenomegaly (3–6%), epistaxis, and relative bradycardia at the peak of high fever (<50%). Rose spots (Fig. 28-2) make up a faint, salmon-colored, blanching, maculopapular rash located primarily on the trunk and chest. The rash is evident in ~30% of patients at the end of the first week and resolves without a trace after 2–5 days. Patients can have two or three crops of lesions, and *Salmonella* can be cultured from punch biopsies of these lesions. The faintness of the rash makes it difficult to detect in highly pigmented patients.

The development of severe disease (which occurs in ~10–15% of patients) depends on host factors (immunosuppression, antacid therapy, previous exposure, and vaccination), strain virulence and inoculum, and choice of antibiotic therapy. Gastrointestinal bleeding (10–20%) and intestinal perforation (1–3%) most commonly occur in the third and fourth weeks of illness and result from hyperplasia, ulceration, and necrosis of the ileocecal Peyer's patches at the initial site of *Salmonella* infiltration (Fig. 28-3). Both complications are life-threatening and require immediate fluid resuscitation and surgical intervention, with broadened antibiotic coverage for polymicrobial peritonitis **(Chap. 26)** and treatment of gastrointestinal hemorrhages, including bowel resection. Neurologic manifestations occur in 2–40% of patients and include meningitis, Guillain-Barré syndrome, neuritis, and neuropsychiatric symptoms (described as "muttering delirium" or "coma vigil"), with picking at bedclothes or imaginary objects.

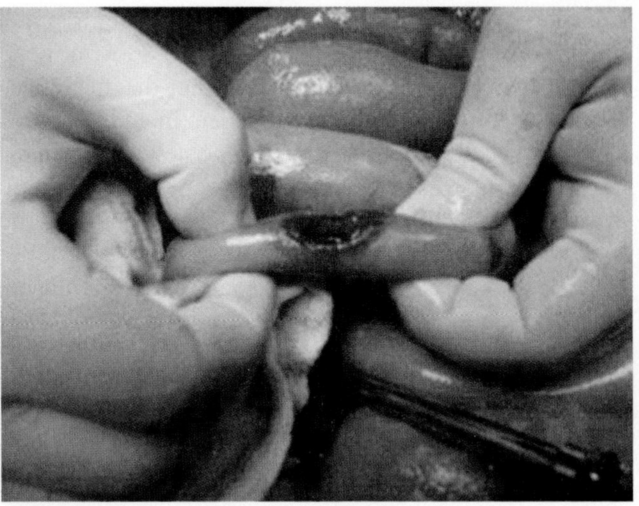

FIGURE 28-3
Typical ileal perforation associated with *Salmonella typhi* infection. *(From JM Saxe, R Cropsey: Is operative management effective in treatment of perforated typhoid? Am J Surg 189:342, 2005.)*

FIGURE 28-2
"Rose spots," the rash of enteric fever due to *Salmonella typhi* or *Salmonella paratyphi.*

Rare complications whose incidences are reduced by prompt antibiotic treatment include disseminated intravascular coagulation, hematophagocytic syndrome, pancreatitis, hepatic and splenic abscesses and granulomas, endocarditis, pericarditis, myocarditis, orchitis, hepatitis, glomerulonephritis, pyelonephritis and hemolytic-uremic syndrome, severe pneumonia, arthritis, osteomyelitis, endophthalmitis, and parotitis. Up to 10% of patients develop mild relapse, usually within 2–3 weeks of fever resolution and in association with the same strain type and susceptibility profile.

Up to 10% of untreated patients with typhoid fever excrete *S. typhi* in the feces for up to 3 months, and 1–4% develop chronic asymptomatic carriage, shedding *S. typhi* in either urine or stool for >1 year. Chronic carriage is more common among women, infants, and persons who have biliary abnormalities or concurrent bladder infection with *Schistosoma haematobium*. The anatomic abnormalities associated with the latter conditions presumably allow prolonged colonization.

DIAGNOSIS

Because the clinical presentation of enteric fever is relatively nonspecific, the diagnosis needs to be

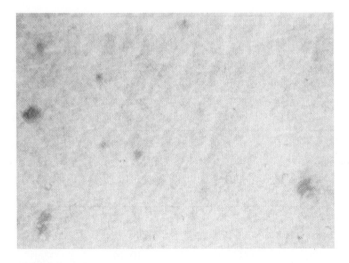

considered in any febrile traveler returning from a developing region, especially the Indian subcontinent, the Philippines, or Latin America. Other diagnoses that should be considered in these travelers include malaria, hepatitis, bacterial enteritis, dengue fever, rickettsial infections, leptospirosis, amebic liver abscesses, and acute HIV infection. Other than a positive culture, no specific laboratory test is diagnostic for enteric fever. In 15–25% of cases, leukopenia and neutropenia are detectable. Leukocytosis is more common among children, during the first 10 days of illness, and in cases complicated by intestinal perforation or secondary infection. Other nonspecific laboratory findings include moderately elevated values in liver function tests and muscle enzyme levels.

The definitive diagnosis of enteric fever requires the isolation of *S. typhi* or *S. paratyphi* from blood, bone marrow, other sterile sites, rose spots, stool, or intestinal secretions. The sensitivity of blood culture is only 40–80%, probably because of high rates of antibiotic use in endemic areas and the small number of *S. typhi* organisms (i.e., <15/mL) typically present in the blood. Because almost all *S. typhi* organisms in blood are associated with the mononuclear cell/platelet fraction, centrifugation of blood and culture of the buffy coat can substantially reduce the time to isolation of the organism but do not increase sensitivity.

Bone marrow culture is 55–90% sensitive, and, unlike that of blood culture, its yield is not reduced by up to 5 days of prior antibiotic therapy. Culture of intestinal secretions (best obtained by a noninvasive duodenal string test) can be positive despite a negative bone marrow culture. If blood, bone marrow, and intestinal secretions are all cultured, the yield is >90%. Stool cultures, although negative in 60–70% of cases during the first week, can become positive during the third week of infection in untreated patients.

Serologic tests, including the classic Widal test for "febrile agglutinins," and rapid tests to detect antibodies to outer-membrane proteins or O:9 antigen are available for detection of *S. typhi* in developing countries but have lower positive predictive values than blood culture. More sensitive antigen and nucleic acid amplification tests have been developed to detect *S. typhi* and *S. paratyphi* in blood but are not yet commercially available and remain impractical in many areas where enteric fever is endemic.

TREATMENT Enteric (Typhoid) Fever

Prompt administration of appropriate antibiotic therapy prevents severe complications of enteric fever and results in a case-fatality rate of <1%. The initial choice of antibiotics depends on the susceptibility of the *S. typhi* and *S. paratyphi* strains in the area of residence or travel (Table 28-1). For treatment of drug-susceptible

TABLE 28-1

ANTIBIOTIC THERAPY FOR ENTERIC FEVER IN ADULTS

INDICATION	AGENT	DOSAGE (ROUTE)	DURATION, DAYS
Empirical Treatment			
	Ceftriaxone[a]	2 g/d (IV)	10–14
	Azithromycin[b]	1 g/d (PO)	5
Fully Susceptible			
Optimal treatment	Ciprofloxacin[c]	500 mg bid (PO) or 400 mg q12h (IV)	5–7
	Azithromycin	1 g/d (PO)	5
Alternative treatment	Amoxicillin	1 g tid (PO) or 2 g q6h (IV)	14
	Chloramphenicol	25 mg/kg tid (PO or IV)	14–21
	Trimethoprim-sulfamethoxazole	160/800 mg bid (PO)	7–14
Multidrug-Resistant			
Optimal treatment	Ceftriaxone[a]	2 g/d (IV)	10–14
	Azithromycin	1 g/d (PO)	5
Alternative treatment	Ciprofloxacin	500 mg bid (PO) or 400 mg q12h (IV)	5–14
Quinolone-Resistant			
Optimal treatment	Ceftriaxone	2 g/d (IV)	10–14
	Azithromycin	1 g/d (PO)	5
Alternative treatment	High-dose ciprofloxacin	750 mg bid (PO) or 400 mg q8h (IV)	10–14

[a]Or another third-generation cephalosporin (e.g., cefotaxime, 2 g q8h IV; or cefixime, 400 mg bid PO).
[b]Or 1 g on day 1 followed by 500 mg/d PO for 6 days.
[c]Or ofloxacin, 400 mg bid PO for 2–5 days.

typhoid fever, fluoroquinolones are the most effective class of agents, with cure rates of ~98% and relapse and fecal carriage rates of <2%. Experience is most extensive with ciprofloxacin. Short-course ofloxacin therapy is similarly successful against infection caused by quinolone-susceptible strains. However, the increased incidence of DCS *S. typhi* in Asia, which is probably related to the widespread availability of fluoroquinolones over the counter, is now limiting the use of this drug class for empirical therapy. Patients infected with DCS *S. typhi* strains should be treated with ceftriaxone, azithromycin, or high-dose ciprofloxacin. A 7-day course of high-dose fluoroquinolone therapy for DCS enteric fever has been associated with delayed resolution of fever and high rates of fecal carriage during convalescence. Thus, for DCS strains, a 10- to 14-day course of high-dose ciprofloxacin is preferred.

Ceftriaxone, cefotaxime, and (oral) cefixime are effective for treatment of MDR enteric fever, including that caused by DCS and fluoroquinolone-resistant strains. These agents clear fever in ~1 week, with failure rates of ~5–10%, fecal carriage rates of <3%, and relapse rates of 3–6%. Oral azithromycin results in defervescence in 4–6 days, with rates of relapse and convalescent stool carriage of <3%. Against DCS strains, azithromycin is associated with lower rates of treatment failure and shorter durations of hospitalization than are fluoroquinolones. Despite efficient in vitro killing of *Salmonella*, first- and second-generation cephalosporins as well as aminoglycosides are ineffective in the treatment of clinical infections.

Most patients with uncomplicated enteric fever can be managed at home with oral antibiotics and antipyretics. Patients with persistent vomiting, diarrhea, and/or abdominal distension should be hospitalized and given supportive therapy as well as a parenteral third-generation cephalosporin or fluoroquinolone, depending on the susceptibility profile. Therapy should be administered for at least 10 days or for 5 days after fever resolution.

In a randomized, prospective, double-blind study of critically ill patients with enteric fever (i.e., those with shock and obtundation) in Indonesia in the early 1980s, the administration of dexamethasone (an initial dose of 3 mg/kg followed by eight doses of 1 mg/kg every 6 h) with chloramphenicol was associated with a substantially lower mortality rate than was treatment with chloramphenicol alone (10% vs 55%). Although this study has not been repeated in the "post-chloramphenicol era," severe enteric fever remains one of the few indications for glucocorticoid treatment of an acute bacterial infection.

The 1–5% of patients who develop chronic carriage of *Salmonella* can be treated for 4–6 weeks with an appropriate oral antibiotic. Treatment with oral amoxicillin, TMP-SMX, ciprofloxacin, or norfloxacin is ~80% effective in eradicating chronic carriage of susceptible organisms. However, in cases of anatomic abnormality (e.g., biliary or kidney stones), eradication often requires both antibiotic therapy and surgical correction.

PREVENTION AND CONTROL

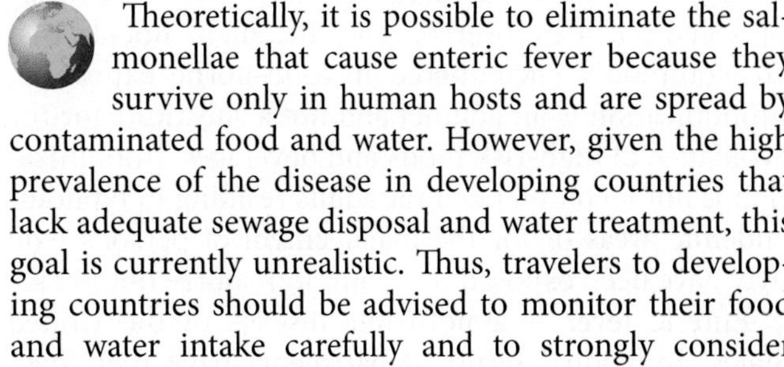

Theoretically, it is possible to eliminate the salmonellae that cause enteric fever because they survive only in human hosts and are spread by contaminated food and water. However, given the high prevalence of the disease in developing countries that lack adequate sewage disposal and water treatment, this goal is currently unrealistic. Thus, travelers to developing countries should be advised to monitor their food and water intake carefully and to strongly consider immunization against *S. typhi*.

Two typhoid vaccines are commercially available: (1) Ty21a, an oral live attenuated *S. typhi* vaccine (given on days 1, 3, 5, and 7, with a booster every 5 years); and (2) Vi CPS, a parenteral vaccine consisting of purified Vi polysaccharide from the bacterial capsule (given in a single dose, with a booster every 2 years). The old parenteral whole-cell typhoid/paratyphoid A and B vaccine is no longer licensed, largely because of significant side effects, especially fever. An acetone-killed whole-cell vaccine is available only for use by the U.S. military. The minimal age for vaccination is 6 years for Ty21a and 2 years for Vi CPS. In a recent meta-analysis of vaccines for preventing typhoid fever in populations in endemic areas, the cumulative efficacy was 48% for Ty21a at 2.5–3.5 years and 55% for Vi CPS at 3 years. Although data on typhoid vaccines in travelers are limited, some evidence suggests that efficacy rates may be substantially lower than those for local populations in endemic areas. Currently, there is no licensed vaccine for paratyphoid fever.

Vi CPS typhoid vaccine is poorly immunogenic in children <5 years of age because of T cell–independent properties. In the more recently developed Vi-rEPA vaccine, Vi is bound to a nontoxic recombinant protein that is identical to *Pseudomonas aeruginosa* exotoxin A. In 2- to 4-year-olds, two injections of Vi-rEPA induced higher T cell responses and higher levels of serum IgG antibody to Vi than did Vi CPS in 5- to 14-year-olds. In a two-dose trial in 2- to 5-year-old children in Vietnam, Vi-rEPA provided 91% efficacy at 27 months and 89% efficacy at 46 months and was very well tolerated. This vaccine is not yet commercially available in the United States. Efforts to improve the immunogenicity and reduce the number of doses of live attenuated oral vaccines are ongoing.

Typhoid vaccine is not required for international travel, but it is recommended for travelers to areas where there is a moderate to high risk of exposure to *S. typhi*, especially those who are traveling to southern Asia and other developing regions of Asia, Africa, the Caribbean, and Central and South America and who will be exposed to potentially contaminated food and drink. Typhoid vaccine should be considered even for persons planning <2 weeks of travel to high-risk areas. In addition, laboratory workers who deal with *S. typhi* and household contacts of known *S. typhi* carriers should be vaccinated. Because the protective efficacy of vaccine can be overcome by the high inocula that are commonly encountered in food-borne exposures, immunization is an adjunct and not a substitute for the avoidance of high-risk foods and beverages. Immunization is not recommended for adults residing in typhoid-endemic areas or for the management of persons who may have been exposed in a common-source outbreak.

Enteric fever is a notifiable disease in the United States. Individual health departments have their own guidelines for allowing ill or colonized food handlers or health care workers to return to their jobs. The reporting system enables public health departments to identify potential source patients and to treat chronic carriers in order to prevent further outbreaks. In addition, because 1–4% of patients with *S. typhi* infection become chronic carriers, it is important to monitor patients (especially child-care providers and food handlers) for chronic carriage and to treat this condition if indicated.

NONTYPHOIDAL SALMONELLOSIS

EPIDEMIOLOGY

In the United States, NTS causes ~12 million illnesses annually, and the incidence has remained relatively unchanged during the past two decades. In 2011, the incidence of NTS infection in this country was 16.5/100,000 persons—the highest rate among the 10 food-borne enteric pathogens under active surveillance. Five serotypes accounted for more than half of U.S. infections during the period 1996–2006: *typhimurium* (23%), *enteritidis* (16%), *newport* (10%), *heidelberg* (6%), and *javiana* (5%).

The incidence of nontyphoidal salmonellosis is highest during the rainy season in tropical climates and during the warmer months in temperate climates—a pattern coinciding with the peak in food-borne outbreaks. Rates of morbidity and mortality associated with NTS are highest among the elderly, infants, and immunocompromised individuals, including those with hemoglobinopathies, HIV infection, or infections that cause blockade of the reticuloendothelial system (e.g., bartonellosis, malaria, schistosomiasis, histoplasmosis).

Unlike *S. typhi* and *S. paratyphi*, whose only reservoir is humans, NTS can be acquired from multiple animal reservoirs. Transmission is most commonly associated with food products of animal origin (especially eggs, poultry, undercooked ground meat, and dairy products), fresh produce contaminated with animal waste, and contact with animals or their environments.

S. enteritidis infection associated with chicken eggs emerged as a major cause of food-borne disease during the 1980s and 1990s. *S. enteritidis* infection of the ovaries and upper oviduct tissue of hens results in contamination of egg contents before shell deposition. Infection is spread to egg-laying hens from breeding flocks and through contact with rodents and manure. The percentage of *Salmonella* outbreaks attributed to eggs has declined significantly in the United States, from 33% during 1998–1999 to 15% during 2006–2008. This decrease probably reflects the impact of the coordinated public health response to *S. enteritidis* infection attributed to eggs, including improved on-farm control measures, refrigeration, and education of consumers and food-service workers. Transmission via contaminated eggs can be prevented by cooking eggs until the yolk is solidified and pasteurizing egg products. Despite these control efforts, outbreaks of *S. enteritidis* infection associated with shell eggs continue to occur. In 2010, a national outbreak of *S. enteritidis* infection resulted in more than 1900 reported illnesses and the recall of 500 million eggs.

Centralization of food processing and widespread food distribution have contributed to the increased incidence of NTS in developed countries. Manufactured foods to which recent *Salmonella* outbreaks have been traced include peanut butter; milk products, including infant formula; and various processed foods, including packaged breakfast cereal, salsa, frozen prepared meals, and snack foods. Large outbreaks have also been linked to fresh produce, including alfalfa sprouts, cantaloupe, mangoes, papayas, and tomatoes; these items become contaminated by manure or water at a single site and then are widely distributed.

An estimated 6% of sporadic *Salmonella* infections in the United States are attributed to contact with reptiles or amphibians, especially iguanas, snakes, turtles, and lizards. Reptile-associated *Salmonella* infection more commonly leads to hospitalization and more frequently involves children, including infants, than do other *Salmonella* infections. Other pets, including African hedgehogs, birds, rodents, baby chicks, ducklings, dogs, and cats, are also potential sources of NTS.

Increasing antibiotic resistance in NTS species is a global problem and has been linked to the widespread use of antimicrobial agents in food animals and especially in animal feed. In the early 1990s, *S. typhimurium* definitive phage type 104 (DT104), characterized by resistance to at least five antibiotics (ampicillin, chloramphenicol, streptomycin, sulfonamides, and tetracyclines; R-type ACSSuT), emerged worldwide. In 2010, resistance to at least ACSSuT was reported in 4.3% of NTS isolates, including 18.6% of *S. typhimurium* isolates. Acquisition is associated with exposure to ill farm animals and to various meat products, including uncooked or undercooked ground beef. Although probably no more virulent than susceptible *S. typhimurium* strains, DT104 strains are associated with an increased risk of bloodstream infection and hospitalization. DCS and trimethoprim-resistant DT104 strains are emerging, especially in the United Kingdom.

Because of increased resistance to conventional antibiotics such as ampicillin and TMP-SMX, extended-spectrum cephalosporins and fluoroquinolones have emerged as the agents of choice for the treatment of MDR NTS infections. In 2010, 2.8% of all NTS strains were resistant to ceftriaxone. Most ceftriaxone-resistant isolates were from children <18 years of age, in whom ceftriaxone is the antibiotic of choice for treatment of invasive NTS infection. These strains contained plasmid-encoded AmpC β-lactamases that were probably acquired by horizontal genetic transfer from *Escherichia coli* strains in food-producing animals—an event linked to the widespread use of the veterinary cephalosporin ceftiofur.

Over the last decade, strains of DCS NTS (MIC, 0.125–1 μg/mL) have emerged and have been associated with delayed response and treatment failure. In 2009, 2.4% of NTS isolates in the United States were DCS or resistant to ciprofloxacin. These strains have diverse resistance mechanisms, including single and multiple mutations in the DNA gyrase genes *gyr*A and *gyr*B and plasmid-encoded quinolone resistance determinants that may not be reliably detected by nalidixic acid susceptibility testing. In 2012, the U.S. Clinical Laboratory Standards Institute proposed a lower ciprofloxacin susceptibility breakpoint (≥0.06 μg/mL) for all *Salmonella* species to address this issue. Currently, because commercial test systems do not contain ciprofloxacin concentrations low enough to allow use of these breakpoints, laboratories need to determine the ciprofloxacin MIC by Etest or another alternative method.

CLINICAL MANIFESTATIONS

Gastroenteritis

Infection with NTS most often results in gastroenteritis indistinguishable from that caused by other enteric pathogens. Nausea, vomiting, and diarrhea occur 6–48 h after the ingestion of contaminated food or water. Patients often experience abdominal cramping and fever (38–39°C; 100.5–102.2°F). Diarrheal stools are usually loose, nonbloody, and of moderate volume. However, large-volume watery stools, bloody stools, or symptoms of dysentery may occur. Rarely, NTS causes pseudoappendicitis or an illness that mimics inflammatory bowel disease.

Gastroenteritis caused by NTS is usually self-limited. Diarrhea resolves within 3–7 days and fever within 72 h. Stool cultures remain positive for 4–5 weeks after infection and—in rare cases of chronic carriage (<1%)—for >1 year. Antibiotic treatment usually is not recommended and may prolong fecal carriage. Neonates, the elderly, and immunosuppressed patients (e.g., transplant recipients, HIV-infected persons) with NTS gastroenteritis are especially susceptible to dehydration and dissemination and may require hospitalization and antibiotic therapy. Acute NTS gastroenteritis was associated with a threefold increased risk of dyspepsia and irritable bowel syndrome at 1 year in a study from Spain.

Bacteremia and endovascular infections

Up to 8% of patients with NTS gastroenteritis develop bacteremia; of these, 5–10% develop localized infections. Bacteremia and metastatic infection are most common with *Salmonella choleraesuis* and *Salmonella dublin* and among infants, the elderly, and immunocompromised patients, especially those with HIV infection. NTS endovascular infection should be suspected in high-grade or persistent bacteremia, especially with preexisting valvular heart disease, atherosclerotic vascular disease, prosthetic vascular graft, or aortic aneurysm. Arteritis should be suspected in elderly patients with prolonged fever and back, chest, or abdominal pain developing after an episode of gastroenteritis. Endocarditis and arteritis are rare (<1% of cases) but are associated with potentially fatal complications, including valve perforation, endomyocardial abscess, infected mural thrombus, pericarditis, mycotic aneurysms, aneurysm rupture, aortoenteric fistula, and vertebral osteomyelitis.

In some areas of sub-Saharan Africa, NTS may be among the most common causes—or even the most common cause—of bacteremia in children. NTS bacteremia among these children is not associated with diarrhea and has been associated with nutritional status and HIV infection.

Localized infections

Intraabdominal infections

Intraabdominal infections due to NTS are rare and usually manifest as hepatic or splenic abscesses or as cholecystitis. Risk factors include hepatobiliary anatomic abnormalities (e.g., gallstones), abdominal malignancy, and sickle cell disease (especially with splenic abscesses). Eradication of the infection often requires surgical correction of abnormalities and percutaneous drainage of abscesses.

Central nervous system infections

NTS meningitis most commonly develops in infants 1–4 months of age. It often results in severe sequelae (including seizures, hydrocephalus, brain infarction, and mental retardation), with death in up to 60% of cases. Other rare central nervous system infections include ventriculitis, subdural empyema, and brain abscesses.

Pulmonary infections

NTS pulmonary infections usually present as lobar pneumonia, and complications include lung abscess, empyema, and bronchopleural fistula formation. The majority of cases occur in patients with lung cancer, structural lung disease, sickle cell disease, or glucocorticoid use.

Urinary and genital tract infections

Urinary tract infections caused by NTS present as either cystitis or pyelonephritis. Risk factors include malignancy, urolithiasis, structural abnormalities, HIV infection, and renal transplantation. NTS genital infections are rare and include ovarian and testicular abscesses, prostatitis, and epididymitis. Like other focal infections, both genital and urinary tract infections can be complicated by abscess formation.

Bone, joint, and soft tissue infections

Salmonella osteomyelitis most commonly affects the femur, tibia, humerus, or lumbar vertebrae and is most often seen in association with sickle cell disease, hemoglobinopathies, or preexisting bone disease (e.g., fractures). Prolonged antibiotic treatment is recommended to decrease the risk of relapse and chronic osteomyelitis. Septic arthritis occurs in the same patient population as osteomyelitis and usually involves the knee, hip, or shoulder joints. Reactive arthritis can follow NTS gastroenteritis and is seen most frequently in persons with the HLA-B27 histocompatibility antigen. NTS rarely can cause soft tissue infections, usually at sites of local trauma in immunosuppressed patients.

DIAGNOSIS

The diagnosis of NTS infection is based on isolation of the organism from freshly passed stool or from blood or another ordinarily sterile body fluid. All salmonellae isolated in clinical laboratories should be sent to local public health departments for serotyping. Blood cultures should be done whenever a patient has prolonged or recurrent fever. Endovascular infection should be suspected if there is high-grade bacteremia (>50% of three or more positive blood cultures). Echocardiography, computed tomography (CT), and indium-labeled white cell scanning are used to identify localized infection. When another localized infection is suspected, joint fluid, abscess drainage, or cerebrospinal fluid should be cultured, as clinically indicated.

TREATMENT Nontyphoidal Salmonellosis

Antibiotics should not be used routinely to treat uncomplicated NTS gastroenteritis. The symptoms are usually self-limited, and the duration of fever and diarrhea is not significantly decreased by antibiotic therapy. In addition, antibiotic treatment has been associated with increased rates of relapse, prolonged gastrointestinal carriage, and adverse drug reactions. Dehydration secondary to diarrhea should be treated with fluid and electrolyte replacement.

Preemptive antibiotic treatment (Table 28-2) should be considered for patients at increased risk for invasive NTS infection, including neonates (probably up to 3 months of age); persons >50 years of age with suspected atherosclerosis; and patients with immunosuppression, cardiac valvular or endovascular abnormalities, or significant joint disease. Treatment should consist of an oral or IV antibiotic administered for 48–72 h or until the patient becomes afebrile. Immunocompromised persons may require up to 7–14 days of therapy. The <1% of persons who develop chronic carriage of NTS should receive a prolonged antibiotic course, as described above for chronic carriage of *S. typhi*.

Because of the increasing prevalence of antibiotic resistance, empirical therapy for life-threatening NTS bacteremia or focal NTS infection should include a third-generation cephalosporin or a fluoroquinolone (Table 28-2). If the bacteremia is low-grade (<50% of positive blood cultures), the patient should be treated for 7–14 days. Patients with HIV/AIDS and NTS bacteremia should receive 1–2 weeks of IV antibiotic therapy followed by 4 weeks of oral therapy with a fluoroquinolone. Patients whose infections relapse after this regimen should receive long-term suppressive therapy with a fluoroquinolone or TMP-SMX, as indicated by bacterial sensitivities.

If the patient has endocarditis or arteritis, treatment for 6 weeks with an IV β-lactam antibiotic (such as ceftriaxone or ampicillin) is indicated. IV ciprofloxacin followed by prolonged oral therapy is an option, but published experience is limited. Early surgical resection of infected aneurysms or other infected endovascular sites is recommended. Patients with infected prosthetic vascular grafts that cannot be resected have been maintained successfully on chronic suppressive oral therapy. For extraintestinal nonvascular infections, a 2- to 4-week course of antibiotic therapy (depending on the infection site) is usually recommended. In chronic osteomyelitis, abscess, or urinary or hepatobiliary infection associated with anatomic abnormalities, surgical resection or drainage may be required in addition to prolonged antibiotic therapy for eradication of infection.

PREVENTION AND CONTROL

Despite widespread efforts to prevent or reduce bacterial contamination of animal-derived food products and to improve food-safety education and training, recent declines in the incidence of NTS in the United States have been modest compared with those of other food-borne pathogens. This observation probably reflects the complex epidemiology of NTS. Identifying effective risk-reduction strategies requires monitoring

TABLE 28-2

ANTIBIOTIC THERAPY FOR NONTYPHOIDAL *SALMONELLA* INFECTION IN ADULTS

INDICATION	AGENT	DOSAGE (ROUTE)	DURATION, DAYS
Preemptive Treatment[a]			
	Ciprofloxacin[b]	500 mg bid (PO)	2–3
Severe Gastroenteritis[c]			
	Ciprofloxacin	500 mg bid (PO) or 400 mg q12h (IV)	3–7
	Trimethoprim-sulfamethoxazole	160/800 mg bid (PO)	
	Amoxicillin	1 g tid (PO)	
	Ceftriaxone	1–2 g/d (IV)	
Bacteremia			
	Ceftriaxone[d]	2 g/d (IV)	7–14
	Ciprofloxacin	400 mg q12h (IV), then 500 mg bid (PO)	
Endocarditis or Arteritis			
	Ceftriaxone	2 g/d (IV)	42
	Ciprofloxacin	400 mg q8h (IV), then 750 mg bid (PO)	
	Ampicillin	2 g q4h (IV)	
Meningitis			
	Ceftriaxone	2 g q12 h (IV)	14–21
	Ampicillin	2 g q4h (IV)	
Other Localized Infection			
	Ceftriaxone	2 g/d (IV)	14–28
	Ciprofloxacin	500 mg bid (PO) or 400 mg q12h (IV)	
	Ampicillin	2 g q6h (IV)	

[a]Consider for neonates; persons >50 years of age with possible atherosclerotic vascular disease; and patients with immunosuppression, endovascular graft, or joint prosthesis.

[b]Or ofloxacin, 400 mg bid (PO).

[c]Consider on an individualized basis for patients with severe diarrhea and high fever who require hospitalization.

[d]Or cefotaxime, 2 g q8h (IV).

of every step of food production, from handling of raw animal or plant products to preparation of finished foods. Contaminated food can be made safe for consumption by pasteurization, irradiation, or proper cooking. All cases of NTS infection should be reported to local public health departments because tracking and monitoring of these cases can identify the source(s) of infection and help authorities anticipate large outbreaks. Lastly, the prudent use of antimicrobial agents in both humans and animals is needed to limit the emergence of MDR *Salmonella*.

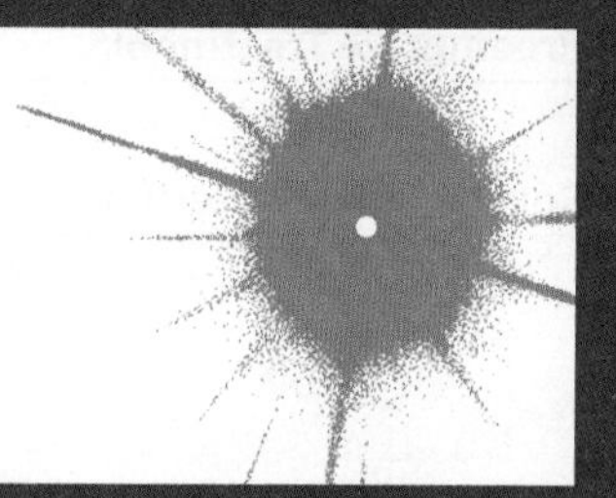

CHAPTER 29
SHIGELLOSIS

Philippe J. Sansonetti ■ Jean Bergounioux

The discovery of *Shigella* as the etiologic agent of dysentery—a clinical syndrome of fever, intestinal cramps, and frequent passage of small, bloody, mucopurulent stools—is attributed to the Japanese microbiologist Kiyoshi Shiga, who isolated the Shiga bacillus (now known as *Shigella dysenteriae* type 1) from patients' stools in 1897 during a large and devastating dysentery epidemic. *Shigella* cannot be distinguished from *Escherichia coli* by DNA hybridization and remains a separate species only on historical and clinical grounds.

DEFINITION

Shigella is a non-spore-forming, gram-negative bacterium that, unlike *E. coli*, is nonmotile and does not produce gas from sugars, decarboxylate lysine, or hydrolyze arginine. Some serovars produce indole, and occasional strains utilize sodium acetate. *Shigella dysenteriae*, *Shigella flexneri*, *Shigella boydii*, and *Shigella sonnei* (serogroups A, B, C, and D, respectively) can be differentiated on the basis of biochemical and serologic characteristics. Genome sequencing of *E. coli* K12, *S. flexneri* 2a, *S. sonnei*, *S. dysenteriae* type 1, and *S. boydii* has revealed that these species have ~93% of genes in common. The three major genomic "signatures" of *Shigella* are (1) a 215-kb virulence plasmid that carries most of the genes required for pathogenicity (particularly invasive capacity); (2) the lack or alteration of genetic sequences encoding products (e.g., lysine decarboxylase) that, if expressed, would attenuate pathogenicity; and (3) in *S. dysenteriae* type 1, the presence of genes encoding Shiga toxin, a potent cytotoxin.

EPIDEMIOLOGY

The human intestinal tract represents the major reservoir of *Shigella*, which is also found (albeit rarely) in the higher primates. Because excretion of shigellae is greatest in the acute phase of disease, the bacteria are transmitted most efficiently by the fecal-oral route via hand carriage; however, some outbreaks reflect foodborne or waterborne transmission. In impoverished areas, *Shigella* can be transmitted by flies. The high-level infectivity of *Shigella* is reflected by the very small inoculum required for experimental infection of volunteers (100 colony-forming units [CFU]), by the very high attack rates during outbreaks in day-care centers (33–73%), and by the high rates of secondary cases among family members of sick children (26–33%). Shigellosis can also be transmitted sexually.

Throughout history, *Shigella* epidemics have often occurred in settings of human crowding under conditions of poor hygiene—e.g., among soldiers in campaigning armies, inhabitants of besieged cities, groups on pilgrimages, and refugees in camps. Epidemics follow a cyclical pattern in areas such as the Indian subcontinent and sub-Saharan Africa. These devastating epidemics, which are most often caused by *S. dysenteriae* type 1, are characterized by high attack and mortality rates. In Bangladesh, for instance, an epidemic caused by *S. dysenteriae* type 1 was associated with a 42% increase in mortality rate among children 1–4 years of age. Apart from these epidemics, shigellosis is mostly an endemic disease, with 99% of cases occurring in the developing world and the highest prevalences in the most impoverished areas, where personal and general hygiene is below standard. *S. flexneri* isolates predominate in the least developed areas, whereas *S. sonnei* is more prevalent in economically emerging countries and in the industrialized world.

Prevalence in the developing world

In a review published under the auspices of the World Health Organization (WHO), the total annual number of cases in 1966–1997 was estimated at 165 million, and 69% of these cases occurred in children <5 years of age. In this review, the annual number of deaths was calculated to range between 500,000 and 1.1 million. More recent data (2000–2004) from six Asian countries indicate that, even though the incidence of shigellosis remains stable, mortality rates associated with this disease may have decreased significantly, possibly as a result of improved nutritional status. However, extensive and essentially uncontrolled use of antibiotics, which may also account for declining mortality rates, has increased the rate of emergence of multidrug-resistant *Shigella* strains. A 2013 prospective matched case-control study of children <5 years of age emphasizes the importance of *Shigella* in the burden and etiology of diarrheal diseases in developing countries. *Shigella* is one of the top four pathogens associated with moderate to severe diarrhea and is now ranked first among children 12–59 months of age. These moderate to severe cases account for an 8.5-fold increase in mortality incidence over the average diarrheal disease–related mortality. The study's authors conclude that *Shigella* remains a major pathogen to be targeted by health care programs.

An often-overlooked complication of shigellosis is the short- and long-term impairment of the nutritional status of infected children in endemic areas. Combined with anorexia, the exudative enteropathy resulting from mucosal abrasions contributes to rapid deterioration of the patient's nutritional status. Shigellosis is thus a major contributor to stunted growth among children in developing countries.

Peaking in incidence in the pediatric population, endemic shigellosis is rare among young and middle-aged adults, probably because of naturally acquired immunity. Incidence then increases again in the elderly population.

Prevalence in the industrialized world

In pediatric populations, local outbreaks occur when proper and adapted hygiene policies are not implemented in group facilities like day-care centers and institutions for the mentally retarded. In adults, as in children, sporadic cases occur among travelers returning from endemic areas, and rare outbreaks of varying size can follow waterborne or food-borne infections.

PATHOGENESIS AND PATHOLOGY

Shigella infection occurs essentially through oral contamination via direct fecal-oral transmission, the organism being poorly adapted to survive in the environment. Resistance to low-pH conditions allows shigellae to survive passage through the gastric barrier, an ability that may explain in part why a small inoculum (as few as 100 CFU) is sufficient to cause infection.

The watery diarrhea that usually precedes the dysenteric syndrome is attributable to active secretion and abnormal water reabsorption—a secretory effect at the jejunal level described in experimentally infected rhesus monkeys. This initial purge is probably due to the combined action of an enterotoxin (ShET-1) and mucosal inflammation. The dysenteric syndrome, manifested by bloody and mucopurulent stools, reflects invasion of the mucosa.

The pathogenesis of *Shigella* is essentially determined by a large virulence plasmid of 214 kb comprising ~100 genes, of which 25 encode a type III secretion system that inserts into the membrane of the host cell to allow effectors to transit from the bacterial cytoplasm to the host cell cytoplasm (Fig. 29-1). Bacteria

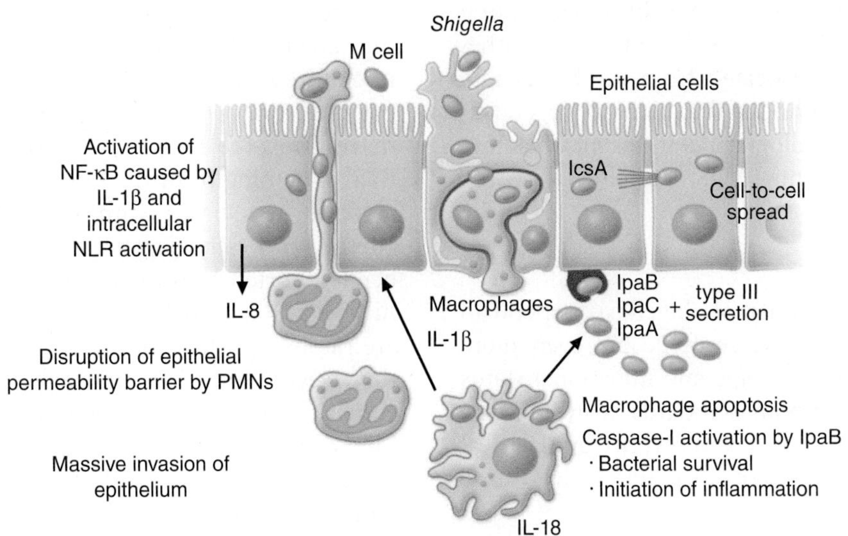

FIGURE 29-1

Invasive strategy of *Shigella flexneri*. IL, interleukin; NF-κB, nuclear factor κB; NLR, NOD-like receptor; PMN, polymorphonuclear leukocyte.

are thereby able to invade intestinal epithelial cells by inducing their own uptake after the initial crossing of the epithelial barrier through M cells (the specialized translocating epithelial cells in the follicle-associated epithelium that covers mucosal lymphoid nodules). The organisms induce apoptosis of subepithelial resident macrophages. Once inside the cytoplasm of intestinal epithelial cells, *Shigella* effectors trigger the cytoskeletal rearrangements necessary to direct uptake of the organism into the epithelial cell. The *Shigella*-containing vacuole is then quickly lysed, releasing bacteria into the cytosol.

Intracellular shigellae next use cytoskeletal components to propel themselves inside the infected cell; when the moving organism and the host cell membrane come into contact, cellular protrusions form and are engulfed by neighboring cells. This series of events permits bacterial cell-to-cell spread.

Cytokines released by a growing number of infected intestinal epithelial cells attract increased numbers of immune cells (particularly polymorphonuclear leukocytes [PMNs]) to the infected site, thus further destabilizing the epithelial barrier, exacerbating inflammation, and leading to the acute colitis that characterizes shigellosis. Evidence indicates that some type III secretion system–injected effectors can control the extent of inflammation, thus facilitating bacterial survival.

Shiga toxin produced by *S. dysenteriae* type 1 increases disease severity. This toxin belongs to a group of A1-B5 protein toxins whose B subunit binds to the receptor globotriaosylceramide on the target cell surface and whose catalytic A subunit is internalized by receptor-mediated endocytosis and interacts with the subcellular machinery to inhibit protein synthesis by expressing RNA N-glycosidase activity on 28S ribosomal RNA. This process leads to inhibition of binding of the amino-acyl-tRNA to the 60S ribosomal subunit and thus to a general shutoff of cell protein biosynthesis. Shiga toxins are translocated from the bowel into the circulation. After binding of the toxins to target cells in the kidney, pathophysiologic alterations may result in hemolytic-uremic syndrome (HUS; see below).

CLINICAL MANIFESTATIONS

The presentation and severity of shigellosis depend to some extent on the infecting serotype but even more on the age and the immunologic and nutritional status of the host. Poverty and poor standards of hygiene are strongly related to the number and severity of diarrheal episodes, especially in children <5 years old who have been weaned.

Shigellosis typically evolves through four phases: incubation, watery diarrhea, dysentery, and the postinfectious phase. The incubation period usually lasts 1–4 days but may be as long as 8 days. Typical initial manifestations are transient fever, limited watery diarrhea, malaise, and anorexia. Signs and symptoms may range from mild abdominal discomfort to severe cramps, diarrhea, fever, vomiting, and tenesmus. The manifestations are usually exacerbated in children, with temperatures up to 40°–41°C (104.0°–105.8°F) and more severe anorexia and watery diarrhea. This initial phase may represent the only clinical manifestation of shigellosis, especially in developed countries. Otherwise, dysentery follows within hours or days and is characterized by uninterrupted excretion of small volumes of bloody mucopurulent stools with increased tenesmus and abdominal cramps. At this stage, *Shigella* produces acute colitis involving mainly the distal colon and the rectum. Unlike most diarrheal syndromes, dysenteric syndromes rarely present with dehydration as a major feature. Endoscopy shows an edematous and hemorrhagic mucosa, with ulcerations and possibly overlying exudates resembling pseudomembranes. The extent of the lesions correlates with the number and frequency of stools and with the degree of protein loss by exudative mechanisms. Most episodes are self-limited and resolve without treatment in 1 week. With appropriate treatment, recovery takes place within a few days to a week, with no sequelae.

Acute life-threatening complications are seen most often in children <5 years of age (particularly those who are malnourished) and in elderly patients. Risk factors for death in a clinically severe case include nonbloody diarrhea, moderate to severe dehydration, bacteremia, absence of fever, abdominal tenderness, and rectal prolapse. Major complications are predominantly intestinal (e.g., toxic megacolon, intestinal perforations, rectal prolapse) or metabolic (e.g., hypoglycemia, hyponatremia, dehydration). Bacteremia is rare and is reported most frequently in severely malnourished and HIV-infected patients. Alterations of consciousness, including seizures, delirium, and coma, may occur, especially in children <5 years old, and are associated with a poor prognosis; fever and severe metabolic alterations are more often the major causes of altered consciousness than is meningitis or the Ekiri syndrome (toxic encephalopathy associated with bizarre posturing, cerebral edema, and fatty degeneration of viscera), which has been reported mostly in Japanese children. Pneumonia, vaginitis, and keratoconjunctivitis due to *Shigella* are rarely reported. In the absence of serious malnutrition, severe and very unusual clinical manifestations, such as meningitis, may be linked to genetic defects in innate immune functions (i.e., deficiency in interleukin 1 receptor–associated kinase 4 [IRAK-4]) and may require genetic investigation.

Two complications of particular importance are toxic megacolon and HUS. Toxic megacolon is a consequence of severe inflammation extending to the colonic smooth-muscle layer and causing paralysis and dilation. The patient presents with abdominal distention and tenderness, with or without signs of localized or generalized peritonitis. The abdominal x-ray characteristically shows marked dilation of the transverse colon (with the greatest distention in the ascending and descending segments); thumbprinting caused by mucosal inflammatory edema; and loss of the normal haustral pattern associated with pseudopolyps, often extending into the lumen. Pneumatosis coli is an occasional finding. If perforation occurs, radiographic signs of pneumoperitoneum may be apparent. Predisposing factors (e.g., hypokalemia and use of opioids, anticholinergics, loperamide, psyllium seeds, and antidepressants) should be investigated.

Shiga toxin produced by *S. dysenteriae* type 1 has been linked to HUS in developing countries but rarely in industrialized countries, where enterohemorrhagic *E. coli* (EHEC) predominates as the etiologic agent of this syndrome. HUS is an early complication that most often develops after several days of diarrhea. Clinical examination shows pallor, asthenia, and irritability and, in some cases, bleeding of the nose and gums, oliguria, and increasing edema. HUS is a nonimmune (Coombs test–negative) hemolytic anemia defined by a diagnostic triad: microangiopathic hemolytic anemia (hemoglobin level typically <80 g/L [<8 g/dL]), thrombocytopenia (mild to moderate in severity; typically <60,000 platelets/μL), and acute renal failure due to thrombosis of the glomerular capillaries (with markedly elevated creatinine levels). Anemia is severe, with fragmented red blood cells (*schizocytes*) in the peripheral smear, high serum concentrations of lactate dehydrogenase and free circulating hemoglobin, and elevated reticulocyte counts. Acute renal failure occurs in 55–70% of cases; however, renal function recovers in most of these cases (up to 70% in various series). Leukemoid reactions, with leukocyte counts of 50,000/μL, are sometimes noted in association with HUS.

The postinfectious immunologic complication known as *reactive arthritis* can develop weeks or months after shigellosis, especially in patients expressing the histocompatibility antigen HLA-B27. About 3% of patients infected with *S. flexneri* later develop this syndrome, with arthritis, ocular inflammation, and urethritis—a condition that can last for months or years and can progress to difficult-to-treat chronic arthritis. Postinfectious arthropathy occurs only after infection with *S. flexneri* and not after infection with the other *Shigella* serotypes.

LABORATORY DIAGNOSIS

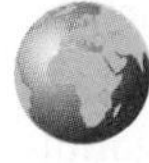

The differential diagnosis in patients with a dysenteric syndrome depends on the clinical and environmental context. In developing areas, infectious diarrhea caused by other invasive pathogenic bacteria (*Salmonella*, *Campylobacter jejuni*, *Clostridium difficile*, *Yersinia enterocolitica*) or parasites (*Entamoeba histolytica*) should be considered. Only bacteriologic and parasitologic examinations of stool can truly differentiate among these pathogens. A first flare of inflammatory bowel disease, such as Crohn's disease or ulcerative colitis **(Chap. 18)**, should be considered in patients in industrialized countries. Despite the similarity in symptoms, anamnesis discriminates between shigellosis, which usually follows recent travel in an endemic zone, and these other conditions.

Microscopic examination of stool smears shows erythrophagocytic trophozoites with very few PMNs in *E. histolytica* infection, whereas bacterial enteroinvasive infections (particularly shigellosis) are characterized by high PMN counts in each microscopic field. However, because shigellosis often manifests only as watery diarrhea, systematic attempts to isolate *Shigella* are necessary.

The "gold standard" for the diagnosis of *Shigella* infection remains the isolation and identification of the pathogen from fecal material. One major difficulty, particularly in endemic areas where laboratory facilities are not immediately available, is the fragility of *Shigella* and its common disappearance during transport, especially with rapid changes in temperature and pH. In the absence of a reliable enrichment medium, buffered glycerol saline or Cary-Blair medium can be used as a holding medium, but prompt inoculation onto isolation medium is essential. The probability of isolation is higher if the portion of stools that contains bloody and/or mucopurulent material is directly sampled. Rectal swabs can be used, as they offer the highest rate of successful isolation during the acute phase of disease. Blood cultures are positive in fewer than 5% of cases but should be done when a patient presents with a clinical picture of severe sepsis.

In addition to quick processing, the use of several media increases the likelihood of successful isolation: a nonselective medium such as bromocresol-purple agar lactose; a low-selectivity medium such as MacConkey or eosin-methylene blue; and a high-selectivity medium such as Hektoen, *Salmonella-Shigella*, or xylose-lysine-deoxycholate agar. After incubation on these media for 12–18 h at 37°C (98.6°F), shigellae appear as non-lactose-fermenting colonies that measure 0.5–1 mm in diameter and have a convex, translucent, smooth surface. Suspected colonies on nonselective or low-selectivity medium can be subcultured on a high-selectivity medium before being specifically identified or can be identified directly by standard commercial systems on the basis of four major characteristics: glucose positivity (usually without production of gas), lactose negativity, H_2S negativity, and lack of motility. The four *Shigella* serogroups (A–D) can then be differentiated by additional characteristics. This approach adds time and difficulty to the identification process; however, after presumptive diagnosis, the use of serologic methods (e.g., slide agglutination, with group- and then type-specific antisera) should be considered. Group-specific antisera are widely available; in contrast, because of the large number of serotypes and subserotypes, type-specific antisera are rare and more expensive and thus are often restricted to reference laboratories.

TREATMENT Shigellosis

ANTIBIOTIC SUSCEPTIBILITY OF *SHIGELLA*

As an enteroinvasive disease, shigellosis requires antibiotic treatment. Since the mid-1960s, however, increasing resistance to multiple drugs has been a dominant factor in treatment decisions. Resistance rates are highly dependent on the geographic area. Clonal spread of particular strains and horizontal transfer of resistance determinants, particularly via plasmids and transposons, contribute to multidrug resistance. The current global status—i.e., high rates of resistance to classic first-line antibiotics such as amoxicillin—has led to a rapid switch to quinolones such as nalidixic acid. However, resistance to such early-generation quinolones has also emerged and spread quickly as a result of chromosomal mutations affecting DNA gyrase and topoisomerase IV; this resistance has necessitated the use of later-generation quinolones as first-line antibiotics in many areas. For instance, a review of the antibiotic resistance history of *Shigella* in India found that, after their introduction in the late 1980s, the second-generation quinolones norfloxacin, ciprofloxacin, and ofloxacin were highly effective in the treatment of shigellosis, including cases caused by multidrug-resistant strains of *S. dysenteriae* type 1. However, investigations of subsequent outbreaks in India and Bangladesh detected resistance to norfloxacin, ciprofloxacin, and ofloxacin in 5% of isolates. The incidence of multidrug resistance parallels the widespread, uncontrolled use of antibiotics and calls for the rational use of effective drugs.

ANTIBIOTIC TREATMENT OF SHIGELLOSIS Because of the ready transmissibility of *Shigella*, current public health recommendations in the United States are that every case be treated with antibiotics.(Table 29-1) Ciprofloxacin is recommended as first-line treatment. A number of other drugs have been tested and shown to be effective, including ceftriaxone, azithromycin, pivmecillinam, and some fifth-generation quinolones. Whereas infections caused by non-*dysenteriae Shigella* in immunocompetent individuals are routinely treated with a 3-day course of antibiotics, it is recommended that *S. dysenteriae* type 1 infections be treated for 5 days and that *Shigella* infections in immunocompromised patients be treated for 7–10 days.

TABLE 29-1

RECOMMENDED ANTIMICROBIAL THERAPY FOR SHIGELLOSIS

ANTIMICROBIAL AGENT	TREATMENT SCHEDULE: CHILDREN	TREATMENT SCHEDULE: ADULTS	LIMITATIONS
First Line			
Ciprofloxacin	15 mg/kg 2 times per day for 3 days, PO	500 mg	
Second Line			
Pivmecillinam	20 mg/kg 4 times per day for 5 days PO	100 mg	Cost No pediatric formulation Frequent administration Emerging resistance
Ceftriaxone	50–100 mg/kg Once a day IM for 2–5 days	-	Efficacy not validated Must be injected
Azithromycin	6–20 mg/kg Once a day for 1–5 days PO	1–1.5 g	Cost Efficacy not validated Minimum inhibitory concentration near serum concentration Rapid emergence of resistance and spread to other bacteria

Source: WHO Library Cataloguing-in-Publication Data: Guidelines for the control of shigellosis, including epidemics due to *Shigella dysenteriae* type 1 (www.who.int/cholera/publications/shigellosis/en/).

Treatment for shigellosis must be adapted to the clinical context, with the recognition that the most fragile patients are children <5 years old, who represent two-thirds of all cases worldwide. There are few data on the use of quinolones in children, but *Shigella*-induced dysentery is a well-recognized indication for their use. The half-life of ciprofloxacin is longer in infants than in older individuals. The ciprofloxacin dose generally recommended for children is 30 mg/kg per day in two divided doses. Adults living in areas with high standards of hygiene are likely to develop milder, shorter-duration disease, whereas infants in endemic areas can develop severe, sometimes fatal, dysentery. In the former setting, treatment will remain minimal and bacteriologic proof of infection will often come after symptoms have resolved; in the latter setting, antibiotic treatment and more aggressive measures, possibly including resuscitation, are often required.

REHYDRATION AND NUTRITION

Shigella infection rarely causes significant dehydration. Cases requiring aggressive rehydration (particularly in industrialized countries) are uncommon. In developing countries, malnutrition remains the primary indicator for diarrhea-related death, highlighting the importance of nutrition in early management. Rehydration should be oral unless the patient is comatose or presents in shock. Because of the improved effectiveness of reduced-osmolarity oral rehydration solution (especially for children with acute non-cholera diarrhea), the WHO and UNICEF now recommend a standard solution of 245 mOsm/L (sodium, 75 mmol/L; chloride, 65 mmol/L; glucose [anhydrous], 75 mmol/L; potassium, 20 mmol/L; citrate, 10 mmol/L). In shigellosis, the coupled transport of sodium to glucose may be variably affected, but oral rehydration therapy remains the easiest and most efficient form of rehydration, especially in severe cases.Nutrition should be started as soon as possible after completion of initial rehydration. Early refeeding is safe, well tolerated, and clinically beneficial. Because breast-feeding reduces diarrheal losses and the need for oral rehydration in infants, it should be maintained in the absence of contraindications (e.g., maternal HIV infection).

NONSPECIFIC, SYMPTOM-BASED THERAPY Antimotility agents have been implicated in prolonged fever in volunteers with shigellosis. These agents are suspected of increasing the risk of toxic megacolon and are thought to have been responsible for HUS in children infected by EHEC strains. For safety reasons, it is better to avoid antimotility agents in bloody diarrhea.

TREATMENT OF COMPLICATIONS There is no consensus regarding the best treatment for toxic megacolon. The patient should be assessed frequently by both medical and surgical teams. Anemia, dehydration, and electrolyte deficits (particularly hypokalemia) may aggravate colonic atony and should be actively treated. Nasogastric aspiration helps to deflate the colon. Parenteral nutrition has not been proven to be beneficial. Fever persisting beyond 48–72 h raises the possibility of local perforation or abscess. Most studies recommend colectomy if, after 48–72 h, colonic distention persists. However, some physicians recommend continuation of medical therapy for up to 7 days if the patient seems to be improving clinically despite persistent megacolon without free perforation. Intestinal perforation, either isolated or complicating toxic megacolon, requires surgical treatment and intensive medical support.

Rectal prolapse must be treated as soon as possible. With the health care provider using surgical gloves or a soft warm wet cloth and the patient in the knee-chest position, the prolapsed rectum is gently pushed back into place. If edema of the rectal mucosa is evident (rendering reintegration difficult), it can be osmotically reduced by the application of gauze impregnated with a warm solution of saturated magnesium sulfate. Rectal prolapse often relapses but usually resolves along with the resolution of dysentery.

HUS must be treated by water restriction, including discontinuation of oral rehydration solution and potassium-rich alimentation. Hemofiltration is usually required.

PREVENTION

Hand washing after defecation or handling of children's feces and before handling of food is recommended. Stool decontamination (e.g., with sodium hypochlorite), together with a cleaning protocol for medical staff as well as for patients, has proven useful in limiting the spread of infection during *Shigella* outbreaks. Ideally, patients should have a negative stool culture before their infection is considered cured. Recurrences are rare if therapeutic and preventive measures are correctly implemented.

Although several live attenuated oral and subunit parenteral vaccine candidates have been produced and are undergoing clinical trials, no vaccine against shigellosis is currently available. Especially given the rapid progression of antibiotic resistance in *Shigella*, a vaccine is urgently needed.

CHAPTER 30

INFECTIONS DUE TO *CAMPYLOBACTER* AND RELATED ORGANISMS

Martin J. Blaser

DEFINITION

Bacteria of the genus *Campylobacter* and of the related genera *Arcobacter* and *Helicobacter* (**Chap. 27**) cause a variety of inflammatory conditions. Although acute diarrheal illnesses are most common, these organisms may cause infections in virtually all parts of the body, especially in compromised hosts, and these infections may have late nonsuppurative sequelae. The designation *Campylobacter* comes from the Greek for "curved rod" and refers to the organism's vibrio-like morphology.

ETIOLOGY

Campylobacters are motile, non-spore-forming, curved, gram-negative rods. Originally known as *Vibrio fetus*, these bacilli were reclassified as a new genus in 1973 after their dissimilarity to other vibrios was recognized. More than 15 species have since been identified. These species are currently divided into three genera: *Campylobacter, Arcobacter*, and *Helicobacter*. Not all of the species are pathogens of humans. The human pathogens fall into two major groups: those that primarily cause diarrheal disease and those that cause extraintestinal infection. The principal diarrheal pathogen is *Campylobacter jejuni*, which accounts for 80–90% of all cases of recognized illness due to campylobacters and related genera. Other organisms that cause diarrheal disease include *Campylobacter coli, Campylobacter upsaliensis, Campylobacter lari, Campylobacter hyointestinalis, Campylobacter fetus, Arcobacter butzleri, Arcobacter cryaerophilus, Helicobacter cinaedi*, and *Helicobacter fennelliae*. The two *Helicobacter* species causing diarrheal disease, *H. cinaedi* and *H. fennelliae*, are intestinal rather than gastric organisms; in terms of the clinical features of the illnesses they cause, these species most closely resemble *Campylobacter* rather than *Helicobacter pylori* (**Chap. 27**) and thus are considered in this chapter. The pathogenic roles of *Campylobacter concisus, Campylobacter ureolyticus, Campylobacter troglodytis*, and *Campylobacter pyloridis* are uncertain. A new subspecies—*C. fetus* subspecies *testudinum*—has been described, chiefly in Asian patients; its close resemblance to strains isolated from reptiles suggests a food source.

The major species causing extraintestinal illnesses is *C. fetus*. However, any of the diarrheal agents listed above may cause systemic or localized infection as well, especially in compromised hosts. Neither aerobes nor strict anaerobes, these microaerophilic organisms are adapted for survival in the gastrointestinal mucous layer. This chapter focuses on *C. jejuni* and *C. fetus* as the major pathogens in and prototypes for their groups. The key features of infection are listed by species (excluding *C. jejuni*, described in detail in the text below) in Table 30-1.

EPIDEMIOLOGY

Campylobacters are found in the gastrointestinal tract of many animals used for food (including poultry, cattle, sheep, and swine) and many household pets (including birds, dogs, and cats). These microorganisms usually do not cause illness in their animal hosts. In most cases, campylobacters are transmitted to humans in raw or undercooked food products or through direct contact with infected animals. In the United States and other developed countries, ingestion of contaminated poultry that has not been sufficiently cooked is the most common mode of acquisition (30–70% of cases). Other modes include ingestion of raw (unpasteurized) milk or untreated water, contact with infected household pets, travel to developing countries (campylobacters being among the leading causes of traveler's diarrhea), oral-anal sexual contact, and (occasionally)

TABLE 30-1

CLINICAL FEATURES ASSOCIATED WITH INFECTION DUE TO "ATYPICAL" *CAMPYLOBACTER* AND RELATED SPECIES IMPLICATED AS CAUSES OF HUMAN ILLNESS

SPECIES	COMMON CLINICAL FEATURES	LESS COMMON CLINICAL FEATURES	ADDITIONAL INFORMATION
Campylobacter coli	Fever, diarrhea, abdominal pain	Bacteremia[a]	Clinically indistinguishable from *C. jejuni*
Campylobacter fetus	Bacteremia,[a] sepsis, meningitis, vascular infections	Diarrhea, relapsing fevers	Not usually isolated from media containing cephalothin or incubated at 42°C
Campylobacter upsaliensis	Watery diarrhea, low-grade fever, abdominal pain	Bacteremia, abscesses	Difficult to isolate because of cephalothin susceptibility
Campylobacter lari	Abdominal pain, diarrhea	Colitis, appendicitis	Seagulls frequently colonized; organism often transmitted to humans via contaminated water
Campylobacter hyointestinalis	Watery or bloody diarrhea, vomiting, abdominal pain	Bacteremia	Causes proliferative enteritis in swine
Helicobacter fennelliae	Chronic mild diarrhea, abdominal cramps, proctitis	Bacteremia[a]	Best treated with fluoroquinolones
Helicobacter cinaedi	Chronic mild diarrhea, abdominal cramps, proctitis	Bacteremia[a]	Best treated with fluoroquinolones; identified in healthy hamsters
Campylobacter jejuni subspecies doylei	Diarrhea	Chronic gastritis, bacteremia[b]	Uncertain role as human pathogen
Arcobacter cryaerophilus	Diarrhea	Bacteremia	Cultured under aerobic conditions
Arcobacter butzleri	Fever, diarrhea, abdominal pain, nausea	Bacteremia, appendicitis	Cultured under aerobic conditions; enzootic in nonhuman primates
Campylobacter sputorum	Pulmonary, perianal, groin, and axillary abscesses; diarrhea	Bacteremia	Three clinically relevant biovars: *sputorum, faecalis,* and *paraureolyticus*

[a]In immunocompromised hosts, especially HIV-infected persons.
[b]In children.
Source: Adapted from BM Allos, MJ Blaser: *Clin Infect Dis* 20:1092, 1995.

contact with an index case who is incontinent of stool (e.g., a baby).

Campylobacter infections are common. Several studies indicate that, in the United States, diarrheal disease due to campylobacters is more common than that due to *Salmonella* and *Shigella* combined. Infections occur throughout the year, but their incidence peaks during summer and early autumn. Persons of all ages are affected; however, attack rates for *C. jejuni* are highest among young children and young adults, whereas those for *C. fetus* are highest at the extremes of age. Systemic infections due to *C. fetus* (and to other *Campylobacter* and related species) are most common among compromised hosts. Persons at increased risk include those with AIDS, hypogammaglobulinemia, neoplasia, liver disease, diabetes mellitus, and generalized atherosclerosis as well as neonates and pregnant women. However, apparently healthy nonpregnant persons occasionally develop transient *Campylobacter* bacteremia as part of a gastrointestinal illness.

In contrast, in many developing countries, *C. jejuni* infections are hyperendemic, with the highest rates among children <2 years old. Infection rates fall with age, as does the illness-to-infection ratio. These observations suggest that frequent exposure to *C. jejuni* leads to the acquisition of immunity.

PATHOLOGY AND PATHOGENESIS

C. jejuni infections may be subclinical, especially in hosts in developing countries who have had multiple prior infections and thus are partially immune. Symptomatic infections mostly occur within 2–4 days (range, 1–7 days) of exposure to the organism in food or water. The sites of tissue injury include the jejunum, ileum, and colon. Biopsies show an acute nonspecific inflammatory reaction, with neutrophils, monocytes, and eosinophils in the lamina propria, as well as damage to the epithelium, including loss of mucus, glandular degeneration, and crypt abscesses.

Biopsy findings may be consistent with Crohn's disease or ulcerative colitis, but these "idiopathic" chronic inflammatory diseases should not be diagnosed unless infectious colitis, *specifically including* that due to infection with *Campylobacter* species and related organisms, has been ruled out.

The high frequency of *C. jejuni* infections and their severity and recurrence among hypogammaglobulinemic patients suggest that antibodies are important in protective immunity. The pathogenesis of infection is uncertain. Both the motility of the strain and its capacity to adhere to host tissues appear to favor disease, but classic enterotoxins and cytotoxins (although they have been described and include cytolethal distending toxin, or CDT) appear not to play substantial roles in tissue injury or disease production. The organisms have been visualized within the epithelium, albeit in low numbers. The documentation of a significant tissue response and occasionally of *C. jejuni* bacteremia further suggests that tissue invasion is clinically significant, and in vitro studies are consistent with this pathogenetic feature.

The pathogenesis of *C. fetus* infections is better defined. Virtually all clinical isolates of *C. fetus* possess a proteinaceous capsule-like structure (an S-layer) that renders the organisms resistant to complement-mediated killing and opsonization. As a result, *C. fetus* can cause bacteremia and can seed sites beyond the intestinal tract. The ability of the organism to switch the S-layer proteins expressed—a phenomenon that results in antigenic variability—may contribute to the chronicity and high rate of recurrence of *C. fetus* infections in compromised hosts.

CLINICAL MANIFESTATIONS

The clinical features of infections due to *Campylobacter* and the related *Arcobacter* and intestinal *Helicobacter* species causing enteric disease appear to be highly similar. *C. jejuni* can be considered the prototype, in part because it is by far the most common enteric pathogen in the group. A prodrome of fever, headache, myalgia, and/or malaise often occurs 12–48 h before the onset of diarrheal symptoms. The most common signs and symptoms of the intestinal phase are diarrhea, abdominal pain, and fever. The degree of diarrhea varies from several loose stools to grossly bloody stools; most patients presenting for medical attention have ≥10 bowel movements on the worst day of illness. Abdominal pain usually consists of cramping and may be the most prominent symptom. Pain is usually generalized but may become localized; *C. jejuni* infection may cause pseudoappendicitis. Fever may be the only initial manifestation of *C. jejuni* infection, a situation mimicking the early stages of typhoid fever. Febrile young children may develop convulsions. *Campylobacter* enteritis is generally self-limited; however, symptoms persist for >1 week in 10–20% of patients seeking medical attention, and clinical relapses occur in 5–10% of such untreated patients. Studies of common-source epidemics indicate that milder illnesses or asymptomatic infections may commonly occur.

C. fetus may cause a diarrheal illness similar to that due to *C. jejuni*, especially in normal hosts. This organism also may cause either intermittent diarrhea or nonspecific abdominal pain without localizing signs. Sequelae are uncommon, and the outcome is benign. *C. fetus* may also cause a prolonged relapsing systemic illness (with fever, chills, and myalgias) that has no obvious primary source; this manifestation is especially common among compromised hosts. Secondary seeding of an organ (e.g., meninges, brain, bone, urinary tract, or soft tissue) complicates the course, which may be fulminant. *C. fetus* infections have a tropism for vascular sites: endocarditis, mycotic aneurysm, and septic thrombophlebitis may all occur. Infection during pregnancy often leads to fetal death. A variety of *Campylobacter* species and *H. cinaedi* can cause recurrent cellulitis with fever and bacteremia in immunocompromised hosts.

COMPLICATIONS

Except in infection with *C. fetus*, bacteremia is uncommon, developing most often in immunocompromised hosts and at the extremes of age. Three patterns of extraintestinal infection have been noted: (1) transient bacteremia in a normal host with enteritis (benign course, no specific treatment needed); (2) sustained bacteremia or focal infection in a normal host (bacteremia originating from enteritis, with patients responding well to antimicrobial therapy); and (3) sustained bacteremia or focal infection in a compromised host. Enteritis may not be clinically apparent. Antimicrobial therapy, possibly prolonged, is necessary for suppression or cure of the infection.

Campylobacter, Arcobacter, and intestinal *Helicobacter* infections in patients with AIDS or hypogammaglobulinemia may be severe, persistent, and extraintestinal; relapse after cessation of therapy is common. Hypogammaglobulinemic patients also may develop osteomyelitis and an erysipelas-like rash or cellulitis.

Local suppurative complications of infection include cholecystitis, pancreatitis, and cystitis; distant complications include meningitis, endocarditis, arthritis, peritonitis, cellulitis, and septic abortion. All these complications are rare, except in immunocompromised hosts. Hepatitis, interstitial nephritis, and the hemolytic-uremic syndrome occasionally complicate acute infection. Reactive arthritis and other rheumatologic complaints may develop several weeks after infection, especially in persons with the HLA-B27 phenotype. Guillain-Barré syndrome or its Miller Fisher (cranial polyneuropathy) variant follows *Campylobacter* infections uncommonly—i.e., in 1 of every 1000–2000 cases or, for certain *C. jejuni* serotypes (such as O19), in 1 of every 100–200 cases. Despite the low frequency of this complication, it is now estimated that *Campylobacter* infections, because of their high incidence, may trigger 20–40% of all cases of Guillain-Barré syndrome. The presence of sialylated lipopolysaccharides on *C. jejuni* strains is a form of molecular mimicry that promotes autoimmune recognition of sialylated cell surface molecules on axons. Asymptomatic *Campylobacter* infection also may trigger Guillain-Barré syndrome. Immunoproliferative small-intestinal disease (*alpha chain disease*), a form of lymphoma that originates in small-intestinal mucosa-associated lymphoid tissue, has been associated with *C. jejuni*; antimicrobial therapy has led to marked clinical improvement.

DIAGNOSIS

In patients with *Campylobacter* enteritis, peripheral leukocyte counts reflect the severity of the inflammatory process. However, stools from nearly all *Campylobacter*-infected patients presenting for medical attention in the United States contain leukocytes or erythrocytes. Gram- or Wright-stained fecal smears should be examined in all suspected cases. When the diagnosis of *Campylobacter* enteritis is suspected on the basis of findings indicating inflammatory diarrhea (fever, fecal leukocytes), clinicians can ask the microbiology laboratory to attempt the visualization of organisms with characteristic vibrioid morphology by direct microscopic examination of stools with Gram's staining or to use phase-contrast or dark-field microscopy to identify the organisms' characteristic "darting" motility. Confirmation of the diagnosis of *Campylobacter* infection is based on identification of an isolate from cultures of stool, blood, or another site. *Campylobacter*-specific media should be used to culture stools from all patients with inflammatory or bloody diarrhea. Because all *Campylobacter* species are fastidious, they will not be isolated unless selective media or other selective techniques are used. Not all media are equally useful for isolation of the broad array of campylobacters; therefore, failure to isolate campylobacters from stool does not entirely rule out their presence. Species-specific polymerase chain reaction techniques have been developed to facilitate exact diagnoses. The detection of the organisms in stool almost always implies infection; there is a brief period of postconvalescent fecal carriage and no obvious commensalism in humans. In contrast, *Campylobacter sputorum* and related organisms found in the oral cavity are commensals that only rarely have pathogenic significance. Because of the low levels of metabolic activity of *Campylobacter* species in standard blood culture media, *Campylobacter* bacteremia may be difficult to detect unless laboratorians check for low-positive results in quantitative assays.

DIFFERENTIAL DIAGNOSIS

The symptoms of *Campylobacter* enteritis are not sufficiently unusual to distinguish this illness from that due to *Salmonella, Shigella, Yersinia*, and other pathogens. The combination of fever and fecal leukocytes or erythrocytes is indicative of inflammatory diarrhea, and definitive diagnosis is based on culture or demonstration of the characteristic organisms on stained fecal smears. Similarly, extrain-testinal *Campylobacter* illness is diagnosed by culture. Infection due to *Campylobacter* should be suspected in the setting of septic abortion, and that due to *C. fetus* should be suspected specifically in the setting of septic thrombophlebitis. It is important to reiterate that (1) the presentation of *Campylobacter* enteritis may mimic that of ulcerative colitis or Crohn's disease, (2) *Campylobacter* enteritis is much more common than either of the latter (especially among young adults), and (3) biopsy may not distinguish among these entities. Thus a diagnosis of inflammatory bowel disease should not be made until *Campylobacter* infection has been ruled out, especially in persons with a history of foreign travel, significant animal contact, immunodeficiency, or exposure incurring a high risk of transmission.

TREATMENT *Campylobacter* Infection

Fluid and electrolyte replacement is central to the treatment of diarrheal illnesses **(Chap. 24)**. Even among patients presenting for medical attention with *Campylobacter* enteritis, not all clearly benefit from specific antimicrobial therapy. Indications for therapy include high fever, bloody diarrhea, severe diarrhea, persistence for >1 week, and worsening of symptoms. A 5- to 7-day course of erythromycin (250 mg orally four times daily or—for children—30–50 mg/kg per day, in divided doses) is the regimen of choice. Both clinical trials and in vitro susceptibility testing indicate that other macrolides, including azithromycin (a 1- or 3-day regimen), also are useful therapeutic agents. An alternative regimen for adults is ciprofloxacin (500 mg orally twice daily) or another fluoroquinolone for 5–7 days, but resistance to this class of agents as well as to tetracyclines is substantial; ~22% of U.S. isolates in 2010 were resistant to ciprofloxacin. Because macrolide resistance usually is much less common (<10%), these drugs are the empirical agents of choice. Patients infected with antibiotic-resistant strains are at increased risk of adverse outcomes. Use of antimotility agents, which may prolong the duration of symptoms and have been associated with toxic megacolon and with death, is not recommended.

For systemic infections, treatment with gentamicin (1.7 mg/kg IV every 8 h after a loading dose of 2 mg/kg), imipenem (500 mg IV every 6 h), or chloramphenicol (50 mg/kg IV each day in three or four divided doses) should be started empirically, but susceptibility testing should then be performed. Ciprofloxacin and amoxicillin-clavulanate are alternative agents for susceptible strains. In the absence of immunocompromise or endovascular infections, therapy should be administered for 14 days. For immunocompromised patients with systemic infections due to *C. fetus* and for patients with endovascular infections, prolonged therapy (for up to 4 weeks) is usually necessary. For recurrent infections in immunocompromised hosts, lifelong therapy/prophylaxis is sometimes necessary.

PROGNOSIS

Nearly all patients recover fully from *Campylobacter* enteritis, either spontaneously or after antimicrobial therapy. Volume depletion probably contributes to the few deaths that are reported. As stated above, occasional patients develop reactive arthritis or Guillain-Barré syndrome or its variants. Systemic infection with *C. fetus* is much more often fatal than that due to related species; this higher mortality rate reflects in part the population affected. Prognosis depends on the rapidity with which appropriate therapy is begun. Otherwise healthy hosts usually survive *C. fetus* infections without sequelae. Compromised hosts often have recurrent and/or life-threatening infections due to a variety of *Campylobacter* species.

CHAPTER 31
CHOLERA AND OTHER VIBRIOSES

Matthew K. Waldor ■ Edward T. Ryan

Members of the genus *Vibrio* cause a number of important infectious syndromes. Classic among them is cholera, a devastating diarrheal disease caused by *Vibrio cholerae* that has been responsible for seven global pandemics and much suffering over the past two centuries. Epidemic cholera remains a significant public health concern in the developing world today. Other vibrioses caused by other *Vibrio* species include syndromes of diarrhea, soft tissue infection, or primary sepsis. All *Vibrio* species are highly motile, facultatively anaerobic, curved gram-negative rods with one or more flagella. In nature, vibrios most commonly reside in tidal rivers and bays under conditions of moderate salinity. They proliferate in the summer months when water temperatures exceed 20°C. As might be expected, the illnesses they cause also increase in frequency during the warm months.

CHOLERA

DEFINITION

Cholera is an acute diarrheal disease that can, in a matter of hours, result in profound, rapidly progressive dehydration and death. Accordingly, *cholera gravis* (the severe form) is a much-feared disease, particularly in its epidemic presentation. Fortunately, prompt aggressive fluid repletion and supportive care can obviate the high mortality that is historically associated with cholera. Although the term *cholera* has occasionally been applied to any severely dehydrating secretory diarrheal illness, whether infectious in etiology or not, it now refers to disease caused by *V. cholerae* serogroup O1 or O139—i.e., the serogroups with epidemic potential.

MICROBIOLOGY AND EPIDEMIOLOGY

The species *V. cholerae* is classified into more than 200 serogroups based on the carbohydrate determinants of their lipopolysaccharide (LPS) O antigens. Although some non-O1 *V. cholerae* serogroups (strains that do not agglutinate in antisera to the O1 group antigen) have occasionally caused sporadic outbreaks of diarrhea, serogroup O1 was, until the emergence of serogroup O139 in 1992, the exclusive cause of epidemic cholera. Two biotypes of *V. cholerae* O1, classical and El Tor, are distinguished. Each biotype is further subdivided into two serotypes, termed *Inaba* and *Ogawa*.

The natural habitat of *V. cholerae* is coastal salt water and brackish estuaries, where the organism lives in close relation to plankton. *V. cholerae* can also exist in freshwater in the presence of adequate nutrients and warmth. Humans become infected incidentally but, once infected, can act as vehicles for spread. Ingestion of water contaminated by human feces is the most common means of acquisition of *V. cholerae*. Consumption of contaminated food also can contribute to spread. There is no known animal reservoir. Although the infectious dose is relatively high, it is markedly reduced in hypochlorhydric persons, in those using antacids, and when gastric acidity is buffered by a meal. Cholera is predominantly a pediatric disease in endemic areas, but it affects adults and children equally when newly introduced into a population. In endemic areas, the burden of disease is often greatest during "cholera seasons" associated with high temperatures, heavy rainfall, and flooding, but cholera can occur year-round. For unexplained reasons, susceptibility to cholera is significantly influenced by ABO blood group status; persons with type O blood are at greatest risk of severe disease if infected, whereas those with type AB are at least risk.

Cholera is native to the Ganges delta in the Indian subcontinent. Since 1817, seven global pandemics have occurred. The current (seventh) pandemic—the first due to the El Tor biotype—began in Indonesia in 1961 and spread in serial waves throughout Asia as *V. cholerae* El Tor displaced the endemic classical biotype, which is thought to have

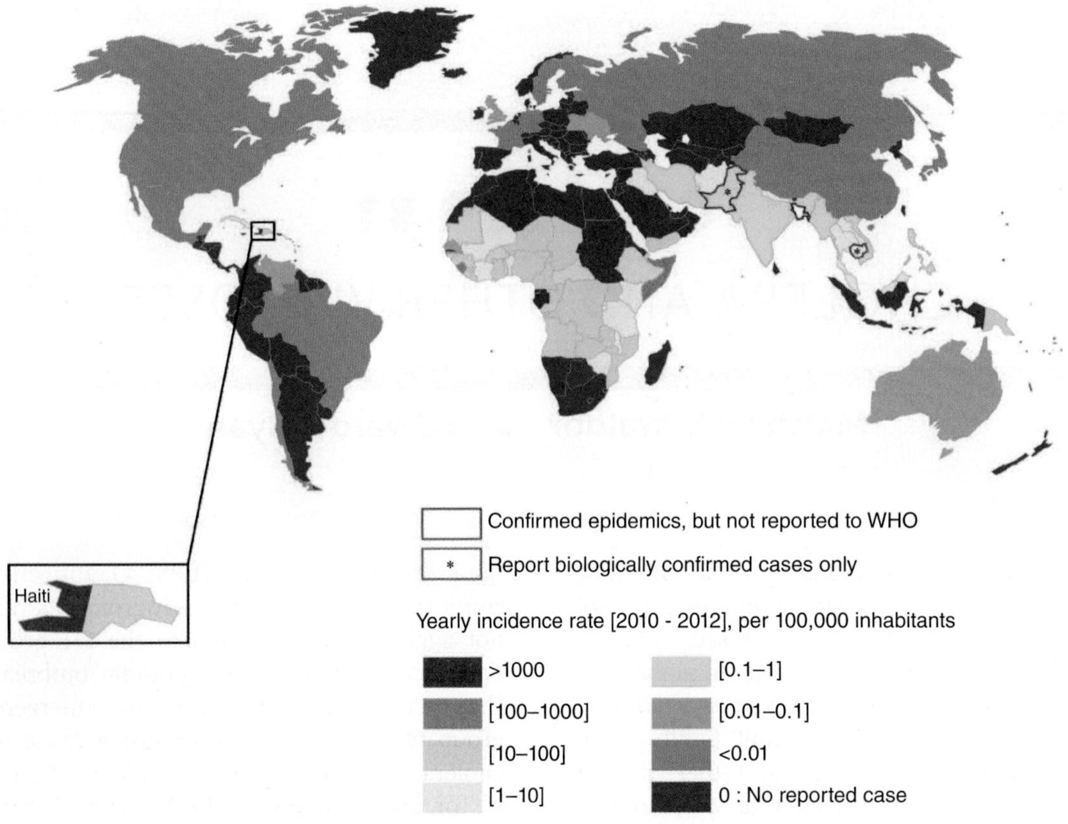

FIGURE 31-1
World distribution of cholera in 2010–2012. WHO, World Health Organization. *(Courtesy of Drs. M. and R. Piarroux, Université de la Méditerranée, France; with permission.)*

caused the previous six pandemics. In the early 1970s, El Tor cholera erupted in Africa, causing major epidemics before becoming a persistent endemic problem. Currently, >90% of cholera cases reported annually to the World Health Organization (WHO) are from Africa (Fig. 31-1), but the true burden in Africa as well as in Asia is unknown because diagnosis is often syndromic and because many countries with endemic cholera do not report cholera to the WHO. It is possible that >3 million cases of cholera occur yearly (of which only ~200,000 are reported to the WHO), resulting in >100,000 deaths annually (of which <5000 are reported to the WHO).

After a century without cholera in Latin America, the current cholera pandemic reached Central and South America in 1991. Following an initial explosive spread that affected millions, the burden of disease has markedly decreased in Latin America. In 2010, a severe cholera outbreak began in Haiti, a country with no recorded history of this disease. Several lines of evidence indicate that cholera was likely introduced into Haiti by United Nations security forces from Asia, raising the possibility that asymptomatic carriers of *V. cholerae* play an important role in transmitting cholera over long distances. To date, the outbreak has involved more than 700,000 individuals, resulting in thousands of deaths. The recent history of cholera has been punctuated by such severe outbreaks, especially among impoverished or displaced persons. These outbreaks are often precipitated by war or other circumstances that lead to the breakdown of public health measures. Such was the case in the camps for Rwandan refugees set up in 1994 around Goma, Zaire, and in 2008–2009 in Zimbabwe.

Sporadic endemic infections due to *V. cholerae* O1 strains related to the seventh-pandemic strain have been recognized along the U.S. Gulf Coast of Louisiana and Texas. These infections are typically associated with the consumption of contaminated, locally harvested shellfish. Occasionally, cases in U.S. locations remote from the Gulf Coast have been linked to shipped-in Gulf Coast seafood.

In October 1992, a large-scale outbreak of clinical cholera caused by a new serogroup, O139, occurred in southeastern India. The organism appears to be a derivative of El Tor O1 but has a distinct LPS and an immunologically related O-antigen polysaccharide capsule. (O1 organisms are not encapsulated.) After an initial spread across 11 Asian countries, *V. cholerae* O139 has once again been almost entirely replaced by O1 strains. The clinical manifestations of disease caused by *V. cholerae* O139 are indistinguishable from those of O1 cholera. Immunity to one, however, is not protective against the other.

PATHOGENESIS

In the final analysis, cholera is a toxin-mediated disease. The watery diarrhea characteristic of cholera is due to the action of cholera toxin, a potent protein enterotoxin elaborated by the organism in the small intestine. The toxin-coregulated pilus (TCP), so named because its synthesis is regulated in parallel with that of cholera toxin, is essential for *V. cholerae* to survive and multiply in (colonize) the small intestine. Cholera toxin, TCP, and several other virulence factors are coordinately regulated by ToxR. This protein modulates the expression of genes coding for virulence factors in response to environmental signals via a cascade of regulatory proteins. Additional regulatory processes, including bacterial responses to the density of the bacterial population (in a phenomenon known as *quorum sensing*), modulate the virulence of *V. cholerae.*

Once established in the human small bowel, the organism produces cholera toxin, which consists of a monomeric enzymatic moiety (the A subunit) and a pentameric binding moiety (the B subunit). The B pentamer binds to GM_1 ganglioside, a glycolipid on the surface of epithelial cells that serves as the toxin receptor and makes possible the delivery of the A subunit to its cytosolic target. The activated A subunit (A_1) irreversibly transfers ADP-ribose from nicotinamide adenine dinucleotide to its specific target protein, the GTP-binding regulatory component of adenylate cyclase. The ADP-ribosylated G protein upregulates the activity of adenylate cyclase; the result is the intracellular accumulation of high levels of cyclic AMP. In intestinal epithelial cells, cyclic AMP inhibits the absorptive sodium transport system in villus cells and activates the secretory chloride transport system in crypt cells, and these events lead to the accumulation of sodium chloride in the intestinal lumen. Because water moves passively to maintain osmolality, isotonic fluid accumulates in the lumen. When the volume of that fluid exceeds the capacity of the rest of the gut to resorb it, watery diarrhea results. Unless the wasted fluid and electrolytes are adequately replaced, shock (due to profound dehydration) and acidosis (due to loss of bicarbonate) follow. Although perturbation of the adenylate cyclase pathway is the primary mechanism by which cholera toxin causes excess fluid secretion, cholera toxin also enhances intestinal secretion via prostaglandins and/or neural histamine receptors.

The *V. cholerae* genome comprises two circular chromosomes. Lateral gene transfer has played a key role in the evolution of epidemic *V. cholerae.* The genes encoding cholera toxin (*ctxAB*) are part of the genome of a bacteriophage, CTXΦ. The receptor for this phage on the *V. cholerae* surface is the intestinal colonization factor TCP. Because *ctxAB* is part of a mobile genetic element (CTXΦ), horizontal transfer of this bacteriophage may account for the emergence of new toxigenic *V. cholerae* serogroups. Many of the other genes important for *V. cholerae* pathogenicity, including the genes encoding the biosynthesis of TCP, those encoding accessory colonization factors, and those regulating virulence gene expression, are clustered together in the *V. cholerae* pathogenicity island. Similar clustering of virulence genes is found in other bacterial pathogens. It is believed that pathogenicity islands are acquired by horizontal gene transfer. *V. cholerae* O139 is probably derived from an El Tor O1 strain that acquired the genes for O139 O-antigen synthesis by horizontal gene transfer.

CLINICAL MANIFESTATIONS

Individuals infected with *V. cholerae* O1 or O139 exhibit a range of clinical manifestations. Some individuals are asymptomatic or have only mild diarrhea; others present with the sudden onset of explosive and life-threatening diarrhea (*cholera gravis*). The reasons for the range in signs and symptoms of disease are incompletely understood but include the level of preexisting immunity, blood type, and nutritional status. In a nonimmune individual, after a 24- to 48-h incubation period, cholera characteristically begins with the sudden onset of painless watery diarrhea that may quickly become voluminous. Patients often vomit. In severe cases, volume loss can exceed 250 mL/kg in the first 24 h. If fluids and electrolytes are not replaced, hypovolemic shock and death may ensue. Fever is usually absent. Muscle cramps due to electrolyte disturbances are common. The stool has a characteristic appearance: a nonbilious, gray, slightly cloudy fluid with flecks of mucus, no blood, and a somewhat fishy, inoffensive odor. It has been called "rice-water" stool because of its resemblance to the water in which rice has been washed (Fig. 31-2). Clinical symptoms parallel volume contraction: at losses of <5% of normal body weight, thirst develops; at 5–10%, postural hypotension, weakness, tachycardia, and decreased skin turgor are documented; and at >10%, oliguria, weak or absent pulses, sunken eyes (and, in infants, sunken fontanelles), wrinkled ("washerwoman") skin, somnolence, and coma are characteristic. Complications derive exclusively from the effects of volume and electrolyte depletion and include renal failure due to acute tubular necrosis. Thus, if the patient is adequately treated with fluid and electrolytes, complications are averted and the process is self-limited, resolving in a few days.

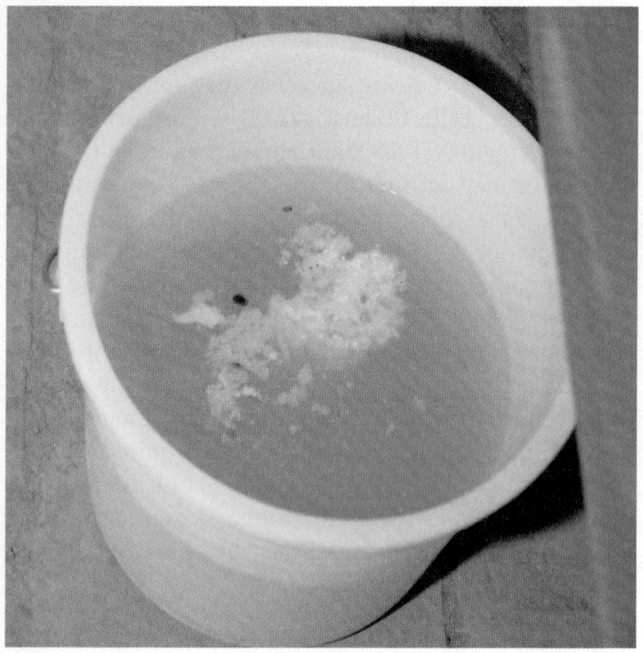

FIGURE 31-2
Rice water cholera stool. Note floating mucus and gray watery appearance. *(Courtesy of Dr. A. S. G. Faruque, International Centre for Diarrhoeal Disease Research, Dhaka; with permission.)*

Laboratory data usually reveal an elevated hematocrit (due to hemoconcentration) in nonanemic patients; mild neutrophilic leukocytosis; elevated levels of blood urea nitrogen and creatinine consistent with prerenal azotemia; normal sodium, potassium, and chloride levels; a markedly reduced bicarbonate level (<15 mmol/L); and an elevated anion gap (due to increases in serum lactate, protein, and phosphate). Arterial pH is usually low (~7.2).

DIAGNOSIS

Cholera should be suspected when a patient ≥2 years of age develops acute watery diarrhea in an area known to have cholera or when a patient ≥5 years of age develops severe dehydration or dies from acute watery diarrhea, even in an area where cholera is not known to be present. The clinical suspicion of cholera can be confirmed by the identification of *V. cholerae* in stool; however, the organism must be specifically sought. With experience, it can be detected directly by dark-field microscopy on a wet mount of fresh stool, and its serotype can be discerned by immobilization with specific antiserum. Laboratory isolation of the organism requires the use of a selective medium such as taurocholate-tellurite-gelatin (TTG) agar or thiosulfate–citrate–bile salts–sucrose (TCBS) agar. If a delay in sample processing is expected, Carey-Blair transport medium and/or alkaline-peptone water-enrichment medium may be used as well. In endemic areas, there is little need for biochemical confirmation and characterization, although these tasks may be worthwhile in places where *V. cholerae* is an uncommon isolate. Standard microbiologic biochemical testing for Enterobacteriaceae will suffice for identification of *V. cholerae*. All vibrios are oxidase-positive. A point-of-care antigen-detection cholera dipstick assay is now commercially available for use in the field or where laboratory facilities are lacking.

TREATMENT Cholera

Death from cholera is due to hypovolemic shock; thus treatment of individuals with cholera first and foremost requires fluid resuscitation and management. In light of the level of dehydration (Table 31-1) and the patient's age and weight, euvolemia should first be rapidly restored, and adequate hydration should then be maintained to replace ongoing fluid losses (Table 31-2). Administration of oral rehydration solution (ORS) takes advantage of the hexose-Na^+ co-transport mechanism to move Na^+ across the gut mucosa together with an actively transported molecule such as glucose (or galactose). Cl^- and water follow. This transport mechanism remains intact even when cholera toxin is active. ORS may be made by adding safe water to prepackaged sachets containing salts and sugar or by adding 0.5 teaspoon of table salt and 6 teaspoons of table sugar to 1 L of safe water. Potassium intake in bananas or green coconut water should be encouraged. A number of ORS formulations are available, and the WHO now recommends "low-osmolarity" ORS for treatment of individuals with dehydrating diarrhea of any cause (Table 31-3). If available, rice-based ORS is considered superior to standard ORS in the treatment of cholera. ORS can be administered via a nasogastric tube to individuals who cannot ingest fluid; however, optimal management of individuals with severe dehydration includes the administration of IV fluid and electrolytes. Because profound acidosis (pH <7.2) is common in this

TABLE 31-1

ASSESSING THE DEGREE OF DEHYDRATION IN PATIENTS WITH CHOLERA

DEGREE OF DEHYDRATION	CLINICAL FINDINGS
None or mild, but diarrhea	Thirst in some cases; <5% loss of total body weight
Moderate	Thirst, postural hypotension, weakness, tachycardia, decreased skin turgor, dry mouth/tongue, no tears; 5–10% loss of total body weight
Severe	Unconsciousness, lethargy, or "floppiness"; weak or absent pulse; inability to drink; sunken eyes (and, in infants, sunken fontanelles); >10% loss of total body weight

TABLE 31-2

TREATMENT OF CHOLERA, BASED ON DEGREE OF DEHYDRATION[a]

DEGREE OF DEHYDRATION, PATIENT'S AGE (WEIGHT)	TREATMENT[b]
None or Mild, But Diarrhea[c]	
<2 years	1/4–1/2 cup (50–100 mL) of ORS, to a maximum of 0.5 L/d
2–9 years	1/2–1 cup (100–200 mL) of ORS, to a maximum of 1 L/d
≥10 years	As much ORS as desired, to a maximum of 2 L/d
Moderate[c,d]	
<4 months (<5 kg)	200–400 mL of ORS
4–11 months (5–<8 kg)	400–600 mL of ORS
12–23 months (8–<11 kg)	600–800 mL of ORS
2–4 years (11–<16 kg)	800–1200 mL of ORS
5–14 years (16–<30 kg)	1200–2200 mL of ORS
≥15 years (≥30 kg)	2200–4000 mL of ORS
Severe[c]	
All ages and weights	Undertake IV fluid replacement with Ringer's lactate (or, if not available, normal saline). Give 100 mL/kg in the first 3-h period (or the first 6-h period for children <12 months old); start rapidly, then slow down. Give a total of 200 mL/kg in the first 24 h. Continue until the patient is awake, can ingest ORS, and no longer has a weak pulse.

[a]Adapted from World Health Organization: First steps for managing an outbreak of acute diarrhoea. Global Task Force on Cholera Control, 2009 (*www.who.int/topics/cholera*).
[b]Continue normal feeding during treatment.
[c]Reassess regularly; monitor stool and vomit output.
[d]Volumes of ORS listed should be given within the first 4 h.
Abbreviation: ORS, oral rehydration solution.

TABLE 31-3

COMPOSITION OF WORLD HEALTH ORGANIZATION REDUCED-OSMOLARITY ORAL REHYDRATION SOLUTION (ORS)[a,b]

CONSTITUENT	CONCENTRATION, MMOL/L
Na^+	75
K^+	20
Cl^-	65
Citrate[c]	10
Glucose	75
Total osmolarity	245

[a]Contains (per package, to be added to 1 L of drinking water): NaCl, 2.6 g; $Na_3C_6H_5O_7{\cdot}2H_2O$, 2.9 g; KCl, 1.5 g; and glucose (anhydrous), 13.5 g.
[b]If prepackaged ORS is unavailable, a simple homemade alternative can be prepared by combining 3.5 g (~1/2 teaspoon) of NaCl with either 50 g of precooked rice cereal or 6 teaspoons of table sugar (sucrose) in 1 L of drinking water. In that case, potassium must be supplied separately (e.g., in orange juice or coconut water).
[c]10 mmol of citrate per liter, which supplies 30 mmol HCO_3/L.

TABLE 31-4

ELECTROLYTE COMPOSITION OF CHOLERA STOOL AND OF INTRAVENOUS REHYDRATION SOLUTION

	CONCENTRATION, mmol/L			
SUBSTANCE	NA+	K+	CL−	BASE
Stool				
Adult	135	15	100	45
Child	100	25	90	30
Ringer's lactate	130	4[a]	109	28

[a]Potassium supplements, preferably administered by mouth, are required to replace the usual potassium losses from stool.

group, Ringer's lactate is the best choice among commercial products (Table 31-4); it must be used with additional potassium supplements, preferably given by mouth. The total fluid deficit in severely dehydrated patients (>10% of body weight) can be replaced safely within the first 3–4 h of therapy, half within the first hour. Transient muscle cramps and tetany are common. Thereafter, oral therapy can usually be initiated, with the goal of maintaining fluid intake equal to fluid output. However, patients with continued large-volume diarrhea may require prolonged IV treatment to match gastrointestinal fluid losses. Severe hypokalemia can develop but will respond to potassium given either IV or orally. In the absence of adequate staff to monitor the patient's progress, the oral route of rehydration and potassium replacement is safer than the IV route.

Although not necessary for cure, the use of an antibiotic to which the organism is susceptible diminishes the duration and volume of fluid loss and hastens clearance of the organism from the stool. Adjunctive antibiotics should therefore be administered to patients with moderate or severe dehydration due to cholera. In many areas, macrolides such as erythromycin (adults, 250 mg orally four times a day for 3 days; children, 12.5 mg/kg per dose four times a day for 3 days) or azithromycin (adults, a single 1-g dose; children, a single 20-mg/kg dose) are the agents of choice. Increasing resistance to tetracyclines is widespread; however, in areas with confirmed susceptibility, tetracycline (nonpregnant adults, 500 mg orally four times a day for 3 days; children >8 years old, 12.5 mg/kg per dose four times a day for 3 days) or doxycycline (nonpregnant adults, a 300-mg single dose; children >8 years old, a single dose of 4–6 mg/kg) may be used. Similarly, increasing resistance to fluoroquinolones is being reported, but in areas with confirmed susceptibility, a fluoroquinolone such as ciprofloxacin may be used (adults, 500 mg twice a day for 3 days; children, 15 mg/kg twice a day for 3 days).

PREVENTION

Provision of safe water and of facilities for sanitary disposal of feces, improved nutrition, and attention to food preparation and storage in the household can significantly reduce the incidence of cholera. In addition, precautions should be taken to prevent the spread of cholera via infected and potentially asymptomatic persons from endemic to nonendemic regions of the world (as was probably the case in the ongoing outbreak in Haiti; see "Microbiology and Epidemiology," above).

Much effort has been devoted to the development of an effective cholera vaccine over the past few decades, with a particular focus on oral vaccine strains. In an attempt to maximize mucosal responses, two types of oral cholera vaccine have been developed: oral killed vaccines and live attenuated vaccines. Currently, two oral killed cholera vaccines have been prequalified by the WHO and are available internationally. WC-rBS (Dukoral®; Crucell, Stockholm, Sweden) contains several biotypes and serotypes of *V. cholerae* O1 supplemented with 1 mg of recombinant cholera toxin B subunit per dose. BivWC (Shanchol™; Shantha Biotechnics–Sanofi Pasteur, Mumbai, India) contains several biotypes and serotypes of *V. cholerae* O1 and *V. cholerae* O139 without supplemental cholera toxin B subunit. The vaccines are administered as a two- or three-dose regimen, with doses usually separated by 14 days. They provide ~60–85% protection for the first few months. Booster immunizations of WC-rBS are recommended after 2 years for individuals ≥6 years of age and after 6 months for children 2–5 years of age. For BivWC, which was developed more recently, no formal recommendation regarding booster immunizations exists. However, BivWC was associated with ~60% protection over 5 years among recipients of all ages in a study in Kolkata, India; the rate of protection among children ≤5 years of age approximated 40%. Models predict significant herd immunity when vaccination coverage rates exceed 50%. The killed vaccines have been safely administered among populations with high rates of HIV.

Oral live attenuated vaccines for *V. cholerae* are also in development. These strains have in common the fact that they lack the genes encoding cholera toxin. One such vaccine, CVD 103-HgR, was safe and immunogenic in phase 1 and 2 studies but afforded minimal protection in a large field trial in Indonesia. Other live attenuated vaccine candidate strains have been prepared from El Tor and O139 *V. cholerae* and have been tested in studies of volunteers. A possible advantage of live attenuated cholera vaccines is that they may induce protection after a single oral dose. Conjugate and subunit cholera vaccines are also being developed. Recognizing that it may be decades before safe water and adequate sanitation become a reality for those most at risk of cholera, the WHO has now recommended incorporation of cholera vaccination into comprehensive control strategies and has established an international stockpile of oral killed cholera vaccine to assist in outbreak responses. No cholera vaccine is commercially available in the United States.

OTHER *VIBRIO* SPECIES

The genus *Vibrio* includes several human pathogens that do not cause cholera. Abundant in coastal waters throughout the world, noncholera vibrios can reach high concentrations in the tissues of filter-feeding mollusks. As a result, human infection commonly follows the ingestion of seawater or of raw or undercooked shellfish (Table 31-5). Most noncholera vibrios can be cultured on blood or MacConkey

TABLE 31-5

FEATURES OF SELECTED NONCHOLERA VIBRIOSES

ORGANISM	VEHICLE OR ACTIVITY	HOST AT RISK	SYNDROME
Vibrio parahaemolyticus	Shellfish, seawater	Normal	Gastroenteritis
	Seawater	Normal	Wound infection
Non-O1/O139 *Vibrio cholerae*	Shellfish, travel	Normal	Gastroenteritis
	Seawater	Normal	Wound infection, otitis media
Vibrio vulnificus	Shellfish	Immunosuppressed[a]	Sepsis, secondary cellulitis
	Seawater	Normal, immunosuppressed[a]	Wound infection, cellulitis
Vibrio alginolyticus	Seawater	Normal	Wound infection, cellulitis, otitis
	Seawater	Burned, other immunosuppressed	Sepsis

[a]Especially with liver disease or hemochromatosis.

Source: Table 25-3 in *Harrisons Principles of Internal Medicine,* 14th edition.

agar, which contains enough salt to support the growth of these halophilic species. In the microbiology laboratory, the species of noncholera vibrios are distinguished by standard biochemical tests. The most important of these organisms are *Vibrio parahaemolyticus* and *Vibrio vulnificus*.

The two major types of syndromes for which these species are responsible are gastrointestinal illness (due to *V. parahaemolyticus*, non-O1/O139 *V. cholerae*, *Vibrio mimicus*, *Vibrio fluvialis*, *Vibrio hollisae*, and *Vibrio furnissii*) and soft tissue infections (due to *V. vulnificus*, *Vibrio alginolyticus*, and *Vibrio damselae*). *V. vulnificus* is also a cause of primary sepsis in some compromised individuals.

SPECIES ASSOCIATED PRIMARILY WITH GASTROINTESTINAL ILLNESS

V. parahaemolyticus

Widespread in marine environments, the halophilic *V. parahaemolyticus* causes food-borne enteritis worldwide. This species was originally implicated in enteritis in Japan in 1953, accounting for 24% of reported cases in one study—a rate that presumably was due to the common practice of eating raw seafood in that country. In the United States, common-source outbreaks of diarrhea caused by this organism have been linked to the consumption of undercooked or improperly handled seafood or of other foods contaminated by seawater. Since the mid-1990s, the incidence of *V. parahaemolyticus* infections has increased in several countries, including the United States. Serotypes O3:K6, O4:K68, and O1:K-untypable, which are genetically related to one another, account in part for this increase. Serotypes O4:K12 and O4:KUT were initially unique to the Pacific Northwest but caused recent outbreaks in the eastern United States and Spain. The enteropathogenicity of *V. parahaemolyticus* is linked to its ability to cause hemolysis on Wagatsuma agar (i.e., the *Kanagawa phenomenon*). Although the mechanisms by which the organism causes diarrhea are not fully defined, the genome sequence of *V. parahaemolyticus* contains two type III secretion systems, which directly inject toxic bacterial proteins into host cells. The activity of one of these secretion systems is required for intestinal colonization and virulence in animal models. *V. parahaemolyticus* should be considered a possible etiologic agent in all cases of diarrhea that can be linked epidemiologically to seafood consumption or to the sea itself.

Infections with *V. parahaemolyticus* can result in two distinct gastrointestinal presentations. The more common of the two presentations (including nearly all cases in North America) is characterized by watery diarrhea, usually occurring in conjunction with abdominal cramps, nausea, and vomiting and accompanied in ~25% of cases by fever and chills. After an incubation period of 4 h to 4 days, symptoms develop and persist for a median of 3 days. Dysentery, the less common presentation, is characterized by severe abdominal cramps, nausea, vomiting, and bloody or mucoid stools. *V. parahaemolyticus* also causes rare cases of wound infection and otitis and very rare cases of sepsis.

Most cases of *V. parahaemolyticus*–associated gastrointestinal illness, regardless of the presentation, are self-limited. Fluid replacement should be stressed. The role of antimicrobials is uncertain, but they may be of benefit in moderate or severe disease. Doxycycline, fluoroquinolones, or macrolides are usually used. Deaths are extremely rare among immunocompetent individuals. Severe infections are associated with underlying diseases, including diabetes, preexisting liver disease, iron-overload states, or immunosuppression.

Non-01/0139 (noncholera) *V. cholerae*

The heterogeneous non-O1/O139 *V. cholerae* organisms cannot be distinguished from *V. cholerae* O1 or O139 by routine biochemical tests but do not agglutinate in O1 or O139 antiserum. Non-O1/O139 strains have caused several well-studied food-borne outbreaks of gastroenteritis and have also been responsible for sporadic cases of otitis media, wound infection, and bacteremia; although gastroenteritis outbreaks can occur, non-O1/O139 *V. cholerae* strains do not cause epidemics of cholera. Like other vibrios, non-O1/O139 *V. cholerae* organisms are widely distributed in marine environments. In most instances, recognized cases in the United States have been associated with the consumption of raw oysters or with recent travel. The broad clinical spectrum of diarrheal illness caused by these organisms is probably due to the group's heterogeneous virulence attributes.

In the United States, about half of all non-O1/O139 *V. cholerae* isolates are from stool samples. The typical incubation period for gastroenteritis due to these organisms is <2 days, and the illness lasts for ~2–7 days. Patients' stools may be copious and watery or may be partly formed, less voluminous, and bloody or mucoid. Diarrhea can result in severe dehydration. Many cases include abdominal cramps, nausea, vomiting, and fever. Like those with cholera, patients who are seriously dehydrated should receive oral or IV fluids; the value of antibiotics is not clear.

Extraintestinal infections due to non-O1/O139 *V. cholerae* commonly follow occupational or recreational exposure to seawater. Around 10% of non-O1/O139 *V. cholerae* isolates come from cases of wound infection, 10% from cases of otitis media, and 20% from cases of bacteremia (which is particularly likely to develop in patients with liver disease). Extraintestinal infections should be treated with antibiotics. Information to guide antibiotic selection and dosing is limited, but most strains are sensitive in vitro to tetracycline, ciprofloxacin, and third-generation cephalosporins.

SPECIES ASSOCIATED PRIMARILY WITH SOFT TISSUE INFECTION OR BACTEREMIA

V. vulnificus

Infection with *V. vulnificus* is rare, but this organism is the most common cause of severe *Vibrio* infections in the United States. Like most vibrios, *V. vulnificus* proliferates in the warm summer months and requires a saline environment for growth. In the United States, infections in humans typically occur in coastal states between May and October and most commonly affect men >40 years of age. *V. vulnificus* has been linked to two distinct syndromes: primary sepsis, which usually occurs in patients with underlying liver disease, and primary wound infection, which generally affects people without underlying disease. (*Vulnificus* is Latin for "wound maker.") Some authors have suggested that *V. vulnificus* also causes gastroenteritis independent of other clinical manifestations. *V. vulnificus* is endowed with a number of virulence attributes, including a capsule that confers resistance to phagocytosis and to the bactericidal activity of human serum as well as a cytolysin. Measured as the 50% lethal dose in mice, the organism's virulence is considerably increased under conditions of iron overload; this observation is consistent with the propensity of *V. vulnificus* to infect patients who have hemochromatosis.

Primary sepsis most often develops in patients who have cirrhosis or hemochromatosis. However, *V. vulnificus* bacteremia can also affect individuals who have hematopoietic disorders or chronic renal insufficiency, those who are using immunosuppressive medications or alcohol, or (in rare instances) those who have no known underlying disease. After a median incubation period of 16 h, the patient develops malaise, chills, fever, and prostration. One-third of patients develop hypotension, which is often apparent at admission. Cutaneous manifestations develop in most cases (usually within 36 h of onset) and characteristically involve the extremities (the lower more often than the upper). In a common sequence, erythematous patches are followed by ecchymoses, vesicles, and bullae. In fact, sepsis and hemorrhagic bullous skin lesions suggest the diagnosis in appropriate settings. Necrosis and sloughing may also be evident. Laboratory studies reveal leukopenia more often than leukocytosis, thrombocytopenia, or elevated levels of fibrin split products. *V. vulnificus* can be cultured from blood or cutaneous lesions. The mortality rate approaches 50%, with most deaths due to uncontrolled sepsis. Accordingly, prompt treatment is critical and should include empirical antibiotic administration, aggressive debridement, and general supportive care. *V. vulnificus* is sensitive in vitro to a number of antibiotics, including tetracycline, fluoroquinolones, and third-generation cephalosporins. Data from animal models suggest that either a fluoroquinolone or the combination of a tetracycline and a third-generation cephalosporin should be used in the treatment of *V. vulnificus* septicemia.

V. vulnificus–associated soft tissue infection can complicate either a fresh or an old wound that comes into contact with seawater; the patient may or may not have underlying disease. After a short incubation period (4 h to 4 days; mean, 12 h), the disease begins with swelling, erythema, and (in many cases) intense pain around the wound. These signs and symptoms are followed by cellulitis, which spreads rapidly and is sometimes accompanied by vesicular, bullous, or necrotic lesions. Metastatic events are uncommon. Most patients have fever and leukocytosis. *V. vulnificus* can be cultured from skin lesions and occasionally from the blood. Prompt antibiotic therapy and debridement are usually curative.

V. alginolyticus

First identified as a pathogen of humans in 1973, *V. alginolyticus* occasionally causes eye, ear, and wound infections. This species is the most salt-tolerant of the vibrios and can grow in salt concentrations of >10%. Most clinical isolates come from superinfected wounds that presumably become contaminated at the beach. Although its severity varies, *V. alginolyticus* infection tends not to be serious and generally responds well to antibiotic therapy and drainage. A few cases of otitis externa, otitis media, and conjunctivitis due to this pathogen have been described. Tetracycline treatment usually results in cure. *V. alginolyticus* is a rare cause of bacteremia in immunocompromised hosts.

Acknowledgment

The authors gratefully acknowledge the valuable contributions of Drs. Robert Deresiewicz and Gerald T. Keusch, coauthors of this chapter for previous editions.

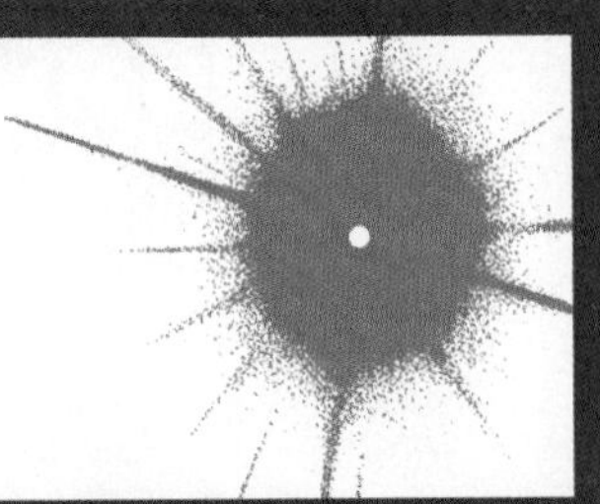

CHAPTER 32

VIRAL GASTROENTERITIS

Umesh D. Parashar ■ Roger I. Glass

Acute infectious gastroenteritis is a common illness that affects persons of all ages worldwide. It is a leading cause of mortality among children in developing countries, accounting for an estimated 0.7 million deaths each year, and is responsible for up to 10–12% of all hospitalizations among children in industrialized countries, including the United States. Elderly persons, especially those with debilitating health conditions, also are at risk of severe complications and death from acute gastroenteritis. Among healthy young adults, acute gastroenteritis is rarely fatal but incurs substantial medical and social costs, including those of time lost from work.

Several enteric viruses have been recognized as important etiologic agents of acute infectious gastroenteritis (Table 32-1, Fig. 32-1). Although most viral gastroenteritis is caused by RNA viruses, the DNA viruses that are occasionally involved (e.g., adenovirus types 40 and 41) are included in this chapter. Illness caused by these viruses is characterized by the acute onset of vomiting and/or diarrhea, which may be accompanied by fever, nausea, abdominal cramps, anorexia, and malaise. As shown in Table 32-2, several features can help distinguish gastroenteritis caused by viruses from that caused by bacterial agents. However, the distinction based on clinical and epidemiologic parameters alone is often difficult, and laboratory tests are required to confirm the diagnosis.

HUMAN CALICIVIRUSES

Etiologic agent

The Norwalk virus is the prototype strain of a group of small (27–40 nm), nonenveloped, round, icosahedral viruses with relatively amorphous surface features on visualization by electron microscopy. These viruses have been difficult to classify because they have not been adapted to growth in cell culture and no animal models are available. Molecular cloning and characterization have demonstrated that the viruses have a

TABLE 32-1

VIRAL CAUSES OF GASTROENTERITIS AMONG HUMANS

VIRUS	FAMILY	GENOME	PRIMARY AGE GROUP AT RISK	CLINICAL SEVERITY	DETECTION ASSAYS
Group A rotavirus	Reoviridae	Double-strand segmented RNA	Children <5 years	+ + +	EM, EIA (commercial), PAGE, RT-PCR
Norovirus	Caliciviridae	Positive-sense single-strand RNA	All ages	+ +	EM, RT-PCR
Sapovirus	Caliciviridae	Positive-sense single-strand RNA	Children <5 years	+	EM, RT-PCR
Astrovirus	Astroviridae	Positive-sense single-strand RNA	Children <5 years	+	EM, EIA, RT-PCR
Adenovirus (mainly types 40 and 41)	Adenoviridae	Double-strand DNA	Children <5 years	+/+ +	EM, EIA (commercial), PCR

Abbreviations: EIA, enzyme immunoassay; EM, electron microscopy; PAGE, polyacrylamide gel electrophoresis; PCR, polymerase chain reaction; RT-PCR, reverse-transcription PCR.

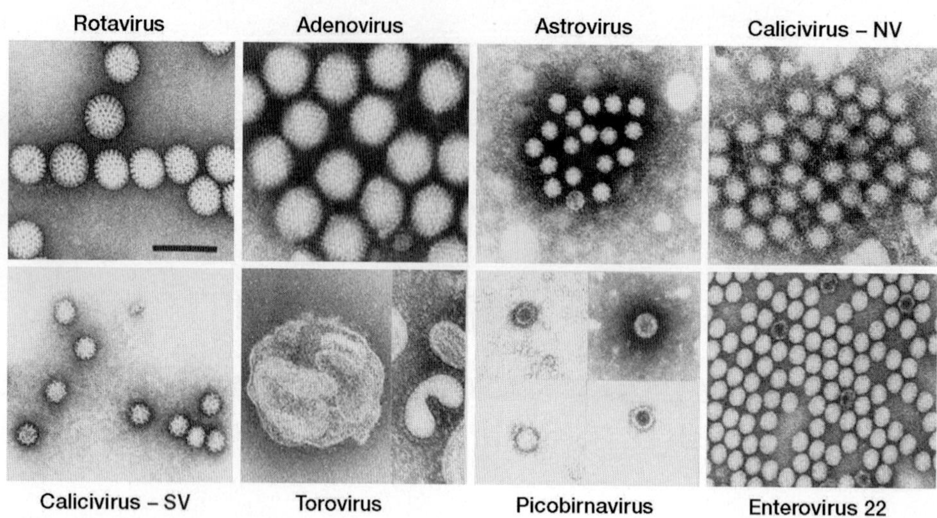

FIGURE 32-1
Viral agents of gastroenteritis. NV, norovirus; SV, sapovirus.

TABLE 32-2

CHARACTERISTICS OF GASTROENTERITIS CAUSED BY VIRAL AND BACTERIAL AGENTS

FEATURE	VIRAL GASTROENTERITIS	BACTERIAL GASTROENTERITIS
Setting	Incidence similar in developing and developed countries	More common in settings with poor hygiene and sanitation
Infectious dose	Low (10–100 viral particles) for most agents	High (>10^5 bacteria) for *Escherichia coli*, *Salmonella*, *Vibrio*; medium (10^2–10^5 bacteria) for *Campylobacter jejuni*; low (10–100 bacteria) for *Shigella*
Seasonality	In temperate climates, winter seasonality for most agents; year-round occurrence in tropical areas	More common in summer or rainy months, particularly in developing countries with a high disease burden
Incubation period	1–3 days for most agents; can be shorter for norovirus	1–7 days for common agents (e.g., *Campylobacter*, *E. coli*, *Shigella*, *Salmonella)*; a few hours for bacteria producing preformed toxins (e.g., *Staphylococcus aureus*, *Bacillus cereus*)
Reservoir	Primarily humans	Depending on species, human (e.g., *Shigella*, *Salmonella*), animal (e.g., *Campylobacter*, *Salmonella*, *E. coli*), and water (e.g., *Vibrio*) reservoirs exist
Fever	Common with rotavirus and norovirus; uncommon with other agents	Common with agents causing inflammatory diarrhea (e.g., *Salmonella*, *Shigella*)
Vomiting	Prominent and can be the only presenting feature, especially in children	Common with bacteria producing preformed toxins; less prominent in diarrhea due to other agents
Diarrhea	Common; nonbloody in almost all cases	Prominent and occasionally bloody with agents causing inflammatory diarrhea
Duration	1–3 days for norovirus and sapovirus; 2–8 days for other viruses	1–2 days for bacteria producing preformed toxins; 2–8 days for most other bacteria
Diagnosis	This is often a diagnosis of exclusion in clinical practice. Commercial enzyme immunoassays are available for detection of rotavirus and adenovirus, but identification of other agents is limited to research and public health laboratories.	Fecal examination for leukocytes and blood is helpful in differential diagnosis. Culture of stool specimens, sometimes on special media, can identify several pathogens. Molecular techniques are useful epidemiologic tools but are not routinely used in most laboratories.
Treatment	Supportive therapy to maintain adequate hydration and nutrition should be given. Antibiotics and antimotility agents are contraindicated.	Supportive hydration therapy is adequate for most patients. Antibiotics are recommended for patients with dysentery caused by *Shigella* or diarrhea caused by *Vibrio cholerae* and for some patients with *Clostridium difficile* colitis.

single, positive-strand RNA genome ~7.5 kb in length and possess a single virion-associated protein—similar to that of typical caliciviruses—with a molecular mass of 60 kDa. On the basis of these molecular characteristics, these viruses are presently classified in two genera belonging to the family Caliciviridae: the *noroviruses* and the *sapoviruses* (previously called Norwalk-like viruses and Sapporo-like viruses, respectively).

Epidemiology

Infections with the Norwalk and related human caliciviruses are common worldwide, and most adults have antibodies to these viruses. Antibody is acquired at an earlier age in developing countries—a pattern consistent with the presumed fecal-oral mode of transmission. Infections occur year-round, although, in temperate climates, a distinct increase has been noted in cold-weather months. Noroviruses may be the most common infectious agents of mild gastroenteritis in the community and affect all age groups, whereas sapoviruses primarily cause gastroenteritis in children. Noroviruses also cause traveler's diarrhea, and outbreaks have occurred among military personnel deployed to various parts of the world. The limited data available indicate that norovirus may be the second most common viral agent (after rotavirus) among young children and the most common agent among older children and adults. In the United States, with the decline in severe rotavirus disease following implementation of rotavirus vaccines, norovirus has become the leading cause of medically attended gastroenteritis in young children. Noroviruses are also recognized as the major cause of epidemics of gastroenteritis worldwide. In the United States, >90% of outbreaks of nonbacterial gastroenteritis are caused by noroviruses.

Virus is transmitted predominantly by the fecal-oral route but is also present in vomitus. Because an inoculum with very few viruses can be infectious, transmission can occur by aerosolization, by contact with contaminated fomites, and by person-to-person contact. Viral shedding and infectivity are greatest during the acute illness, but challenge studies with Norwalk virus in volunteers indicate that viral antigen may be shed by asymptomatically infected persons and also by symptomatic persons before the onset of symptoms and for several weeks after the resolution of illness. Viral shedding can be prolonged in immunocompromised individuals.

Pathogenesis

The exact sites and cellular receptors for attachment of viral particles have not been determined. Data suggest that carbohydrates that are similar to human histo-blood group antigens and are present on the gastroduodenal epithelium of individuals with the secretor phenotype may serve as ligands for the attachment of Norwalk virus. Additional studies must more fully elucidate norovirus-carbohydrate interactions, including potential strain-specific variations. After the infection of volunteers, reversible lesions are noted in the upper jejunum, with broadening and blunting of the villi, shortening of the microvilli, vacuolization of the lining epithelium, crypt hyperplasia, and infiltration of the lamina propria by polymorphonuclear neutrophils and lymphocytes. The lesions persist for at least 4 days after the resolution of symptoms and are associated with malabsorption of carbohydrates and fats and a decreased level of brush-border enzymes. Adenylate cyclase activity is not altered. No histopathologic changes are seen in the stomach or colon, but gastric motor function is delayed, and this alteration is believed to contribute to the nausea and vomiting that are typical of this illness.

Clinical manifestations

Gastroenteritis caused by Norwalk and related human caliciviruses has a sudden onset following an average incubation period of 24 h (range, 12–72 h). The illness generally lasts 12–60 h and is characterized by one or more of the following symptoms: nausea, vomiting, abdominal cramps, and diarrhea. Vomiting is more prevalent among children, whereas a greater proportion of adults develop diarrhea. Constitutional symptoms are common, including headache, fever, chills, and myalgias. The stools are characteristically loose and watery, without blood, mucus, or leukocytes. White cell counts are generally normal; rarely, leukocytosis with relative lymphopenia may be observed. Death is a rare outcome and usually results from severe dehydration in vulnerable persons (e.g., elderly patients with debilitating health conditions).

Immunity

Approximately 50% of persons challenged with Norwalk virus become ill and acquire short-term immunity against the infecting strain. Immunity to Norwalk virus appears to correlate inversely with level of antibody; i.e., persons with higher levels of preexisting antibody to Norwalk virus are more susceptible to illness. This observation suggests that some individuals have a genetic predisposition to illness. Specific ABO, Lewis, and secretor blood group phenotypes may influence susceptibility to norovirus infection.

Diagnosis

Cloning and sequencing of the genomes of Norwalk and several other human caliciviruses have allowed the development of assays based on polymerase chain reaction (PCR) for detection of virus in stool and vomitus. Virus-like particles produced by expression of capsid proteins in a recombinant baculovirus vector have been used to develop enzyme immunoassays (EIAs) for detection of virus in stool or a serologic response to a specific viral antigen. These newer diagnostic techniques are considerably more sensitive than previous detection methods, such as electron microscopy, immune electron microscopy, and EIAs based on reagents derived from humans. However, no currently available single assay can detect all human caliciviruses because of their great genetic and antigenic diversity. In addition, the assays are still cumbersome and are available primarily in research laboratories, although they are increasingly being adopted by public health laboratories for routine screening of fecal specimens from patients affected by outbreaks of gastroenteritis. Commercial EIA kits have limited sensitivity and usefulness in clinical practice and are of greatest utility in outbreaks, in which many specimens are tested and only a few need be positive to identify norovirus as the cause.

TREATMENT Infections with Norwalk and Related Human Caliciviruses

The disease is self-limited, and oral rehydration therapy is generally adequate. If severe dehydration develops, IV fluid therapy is indicated. No specific antiviral therapy is available.

Prevention

Epidemic prevention relies on situation-specific measures, such as control of contamination of food and water, exclusion of ill food handlers, and reduction of person-to-person spread through good personal hygiene and disinfection of contaminated fomites. The role of immunoprophylaxis is not clear, given the lack of long-term immunity from natural disease, but efforts to develop norovirus vaccines are ongoing. In a clinical study, a candidate virus-like particle norovirus vaccine was shown to protect against homologous viral challenge.

ROTAVIRUS

Etiologic agent

Rotaviruses are members of the family Reoviridae. The viral genome consists of 11 segments of double-strand RNA that are enclosed in a triple-layered, nonenveloped, icosahedral capsid 75 nm in diameter. Viral protein 6 (VP6), the major structural protein, is the target of commercial immunoassays and determines the group specificity of rotaviruses. There are seven major groups of rotavirus (A through G); human illness is caused primarily by group A and, to a much lesser extent, by groups B and C. Two outer-capsid proteins, VP7 (G-protein) and VP4 (P-protein), determine serotype specificity, induce neutralizing antibodies, and form the basis for binary classification of rotaviruses (G and P types). The segmented genome of rotavirus allows genetic reassortment (i.e., exchange of genome segments between viruses) during co-infection—a property that may play a role in viral evolution and that has been utilized in the development of reassortant animal-human rotavirus–based vaccines.

Epidemiology

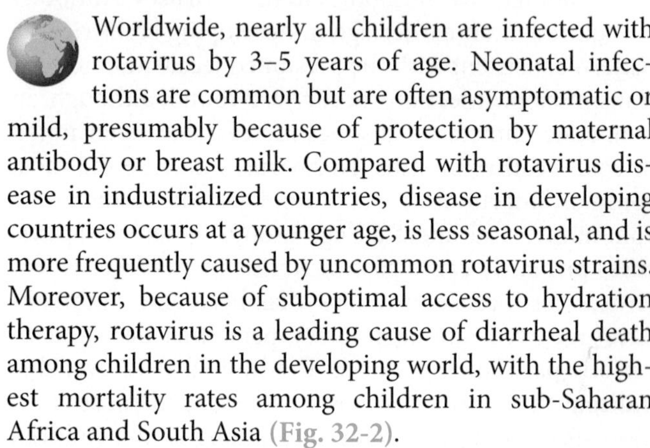

Worldwide, nearly all children are infected with rotavirus by 3–5 years of age. Neonatal infections are common but are often asymptomatic or mild, presumably because of protection by maternal antibody or breast milk. Compared with rotavirus disease in industrialized countries, disease in developing countries occurs at a younger age, is less seasonal, and is more frequently caused by uncommon rotavirus strains. Moreover, because of suboptimal access to hydration therapy, rotavirus is a leading cause of diarrheal death among children in the developing world, with the highest mortality rates among children in sub-Saharan Africa and South Asia (Fig. 32-2).

First infections after 3 months of age are likely to be symptomatic, and the incidence of disease peaks among children 4–23 months of age. Reinfections are common, but the severity of disease decreases with each repeat infection. Therefore, severe rotavirus infections are less common among older children and adults than among younger individuals. Nevertheless, rotavirus can cause illness in parents and caretakers of children with rotavirus diarrhea, immunocompromised persons, travelers, and elderly individuals and should be considered in the differential diagnosis of gastroenteritis among adults.

In tropical settings, rotavirus disease occurs year-round, with less pronounced seasonal peaks than in temperate settings, where rotavirus disease occurs predominantly during the cooler fall and winter months. Before the introduction of rotavirus vaccine in the United States, the rotavirus season each year began in the Southwest during the autumn and early winter (October through December) and migrated across the continent, peaking in the Northeast during late winter and spring (March through May). The reasons for this characteristic pattern are not clear but may be correlated with state-specific differences in birth rates, which could influence the rate of accumulation of susceptible infants after each rotavirus season. After the implementation of routine vaccination of U.S. infants against rotavirus in 2006, the characteristic prevaccine geotemporal pattern of U.S. rotavirus was dramatically altered, and these changes were accompanied by substantial

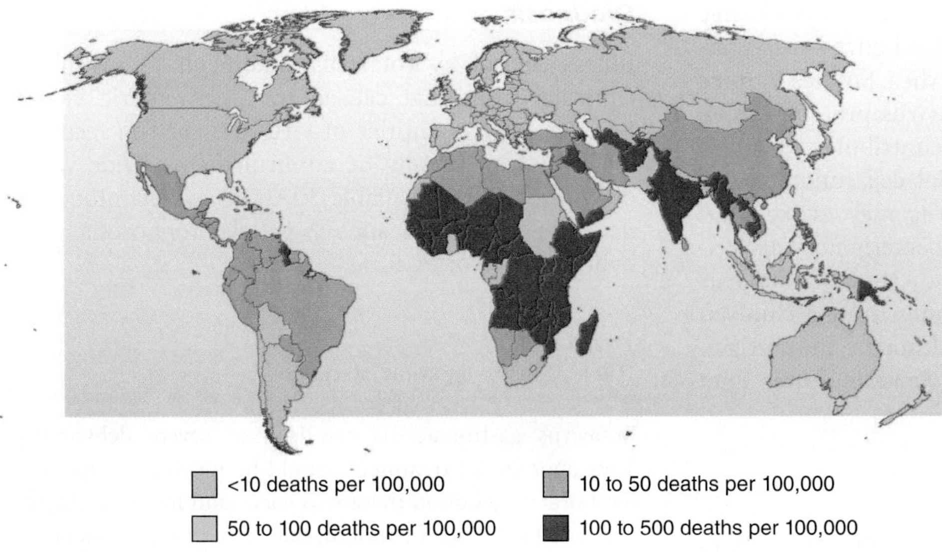

FIGURE 32-2
Rotavirus mortality rates by country, per 100,000 children <5 years of age. *(Reproduced with permission from UD Parashar et al: J Infect Dis 200:S9, 2009.)*

declines in rotavirus detections by a national network of sentinel laboratories (Fig. 32-3). During the latest two seasons with available data (spanning 2010–2012), the number of rotavirus detections declined by 74–90% from the prevaccine baseline, and the annual proportion of rotavirus tests that were positive was below 10% in both seasons (compared with a prevaccine baseline median of 26%). A pattern of biennial increases in rotavirus activity has emerged during the five postvaccine seasons (2007–2012), but activity has remained substantially below prevaccine levels in each season.

During episodes of rotavirus-associated diarrhea, virus is shed in large quantities in stool (10^7–10^{12}/g). Viral shedding detectable by EIA usually subsides within 1 week but may persist for >30 days in immunocompromised individuals; it may be detected for longer periods by sensitive molecular assays, such as PCR. The virus is transmitted predominantly through the fecal-oral route. Spread through respiratory secretions, person-to-person contact, or contaminated environmental surfaces has been postulated to explain the rapid acquisition of antibody in the first 3 years of life, regardless of sanitary conditions.

At least 10 different G serotypes of group A rotavirus have been identified in humans, but only 5 types (G1 through G4 and G9) are common. While human rotavirus strains that possess a high degree of genetic homology with animal strains have been identified, animal-to-human transmission appears to be uncommon.

Group B rotaviruses have been associated with several large epidemics of severe gastroenteritis among adults in China since 1982 and have also been identified in India. Group C rotaviruses have been associated with a small proportion of pediatric gastroenteritis cases in several countries worldwide.

FIGURE 32-3
Percentage of rotavirus tests with positive results, by week of year, July–June, 2000–2012. The maximal or minimal percentage of rotavirus-positive tests for 2000–2006 may have occurred during any of the six baseline seasons. Data are from the National Respiratory and Enteric Virus Surveillance System. *(Adapted from Centers for Disease Control and Prevention, 2012.)*

Pathogenesis

Rotaviruses infect and ultimately destroy mature enterocytes in the villous epithelium of the proximal small intestine. The loss of absorptive villous epithelium, coupled with the proliferation of secretory crypt cells, results in secretory diarrhea. Brush-border enzymes characteristic of differentiated cells are reduced, and this change leads to the accumulation of unmetabolized disaccharides and consequent osmotic diarrhea. Studies in mice indicate that a nonstructural rotavirus protein, NSP4, functions as an enterotoxin and contributes to secretory diarrhea by altering epithelial cell function and permeability. In addition, rotavirus may evoke fluid secretion through activation of the enteric nervous system in the intestinal wall. Data indicate that rotavirus antigenemia and viremia are common among children with acute rotavirus infection, although the antigen and RNA levels in serum are substantially lower than those in stool.

Clinical manifestations

The clinical spectrum of rotavirus infection ranges from subclinical infection to severe gastroenteritis leading to life-threatening dehydration. After an incubation period of 1–3 days, the illness has an abrupt onset, with vomiting frequently preceding the onset of diarrhea. Up to one-third of patients may have a temperature of >39°C. The stools are characteristically loose and watery and only infrequently contain red or white cells. Gastrointestinal symptoms generally resolve in 3–7 days.

Respiratory and neurologic features in children with rotavirus infection have been reported, but causal associations have not been proven. Moreover, rotavirus infection has been associated with a variety of other clinical conditions (e.g., sudden infant death syndrome, necrotizing enterocolitis, intussusception, Kawasaki's disease, and type 1 diabetes), but no causal relationship has been confirmed with any of these syndromes.

Rotavirus does not appear to be a major opportunistic pathogen in children with HIV infection. In severely immunodeficient children, rotavirus can cause protracted diarrhea with prolonged viral excretion and, in rare instances, can disseminate systemically. Persons who are immunosuppressed for bone marrow transplantation also are at risk for severe or even fatal rotavirus disease.

Immunity

Protection against rotavirus disease is correlated with the presence of virus-specific secretory IgA antibodies in the intestine and, to some extent, the serum. Because virus-specific IgA production at the intestinal surface is short lived, complete protection against disease is only temporary. However, each infection and subsequent reinfection confers progressively greater immunity; thus severe disease is most common among young children with first or second infections. Immunologic memory is believed to be important in the attenuation of disease severity upon reinfection.

Diagnosis

Illness caused by rotavirus is difficult to distinguish clinically from that caused by other enteric viruses. Because large quantities of virus are shed in feces, the diagnosis can usually be confirmed by a wide variety of commercially available EIAs or by techniques for detecting viral RNA, such as gel electrophoresis, probe hybridization, or PCR.

TREATMENT Rotavirus Infections

Rotavirus gastroenteritis can lead to severe dehydration. Thus appropriate treatment should be instituted early. Standard oral rehydration therapy is successful for most children who can take fluids by mouth, but IV fluid replacement may be required for patients who are severely dehydrated or are unable to tolerate oral therapy because of frequent vomiting. The therapeutic roles of probiotics, bismuth subsalicylate, enkephalinase inhibitors, and nitazoxanide have been evaluated in clinical studies but are not clearly defined. Antibiotics and antimotility agents should be avoided. In immunocompromised children with chronic symptomatic rotavirus disease, orally administered immunoglobulins or colostrum may result in the resolution of symptoms, but the best choices regarding agents and their doses have not been well studied, and treatment decisions are often empirical.

Prevention

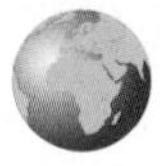

Efforts to develop rotavirus vaccines were pursued because it was apparent—given the similar rates in less developed and industrialized nations—that improvements in hygiene and sanitation were unlikely to reduce disease incidence. The first rotavirus vaccine licensed in the United States in 1998 was withdrawn from the market within 1 year because it was linked with a low incidence of intussusception, a severe bowel obstruction.

In 2006, promising safety and efficacy results for two new rotavirus vaccines were reported from large clinical trials conducted in North America, Europe, and Latin America. Both vaccines are now recommended for routine immunization of all U.S. infants, and their use has rapidly led to a >70–80% decline in rotavirus hospitalizations and emergency department visits at hospitals across the United States. Indirect benefits from vaccination (i.e., herd immunity) have also been documented in many settings. In April 2009, the World Health Organization recommended the use of rotavirus vaccines in all countries worldwide. As of May 2013, a total of 42 countries, including 5 low-income countries in Africa and Asia, have incorporated rotavirus vaccine into their national childhood immunization programs. In Mexico and in Brazil, a decline in deaths from childhood diarrhea following introduction of rotavirus vaccines has been documented. Postmarketing surveillance has identified a low risk of intussusception in some countries; however, the benefits of vaccination exceed the risks, and no changes in vaccine administration policy have been implemented.

The different epidemiology of rotavirus disease and the greater prevalence of co-infection with other enteric pathogens, of comorbidities, and of malnutrition in developing countries may adversely affect the performance of oral rotavirus vaccines, as is the case with oral vaccines against poliomyelitis, cholera, and typhoid in these regions. Therefore, evaluation of the efficacy of rotavirus vaccines in resource-poor settings of Africa and Asia was specifically recommended, and these trials have now been completed. As anticipated, the efficacy of rotavirus vaccines was moderate (50–65%) in these settings when compared with that in industrialized countries. Nevertheless, even a moderately efficacious rotavirus vaccine would be likely to have substantial public health benefits in these areas with a high disease burden.

OTHER VIRAL AGENTS OF GASTROENTERITIS

Enteric *adenoviruses* of serotypes 40 and 41 belonging to subgroup F are 70- to 80-nm viruses with double-strand DNA that cause ~2–12% of all diarrhea episodes in young children. Unlike adenoviruses that cause respiratory illness, enteric adenoviruses are difficult to cultivate in cell lines, but they can be detected with commercially available EIAs. Adenovirus types 31 and 42–49 have been linked to diarrhea in HIV-infected and other immunocompromised persons.

Astroviruses are 28- to 30-nm viruses with a characteristic icosahedral structure and a positive-sense, single-strand RNA. At least seven serotypes have been identified, of which serotype 1 is most common. Astroviruses are primarily pediatric pathogens, causing ~2–10% of cases of mild to moderate gastroenteritis in children. The availability of simple immunoassays to detect virus in fecal specimens and of molecular methods to confirm and characterize strains will permit more comprehensive assessment of the etiologic role of these agents.

Toroviruses are 100- to 140-nm, enveloped, positive-strand RNA viruses that are recognized as causes of gastroenteritis in horses (Berne virus) and cattle (Breda virus). Their role as a cause of diarrhea in humans is still unclear, but studies from Canada have demonstrated associations between torovirus excretion and both nosocomial gastroenteritis and necrotizing enterocolitis in neonates. These associations require further evaluation.

Picobirnaviruses are small, bisegmented, double-strand RNA viruses that cause gastroenteritis in a variety of animals. Their role as primary causes of gastroenteritis in humans remains unclear, but several studies have found an association between picobirnaviruses and gastroenteritis in HIV-infected adults.

Several other viruses (e.g., enteroviruses, reoviruses, pestiviruses, and parvovirus B) have been identified in the feces of patients with diarrhea, but their etiologic role in gastroenteritis has not been proven. Diarrhea has also been noted as a manifestation of infection with recently recognized viruses that primarily cause severe respiratory illness: the severe acute respiratory syndrome–associated coronavirus (SARS-CoV), influenza A/H5N1 virus, and the current pandemic strain of influenza A/H1N1 virus.

CHAPTER 33

AMEBIASIS AND INFECTION WITH FREE-LIVING AMEBAS

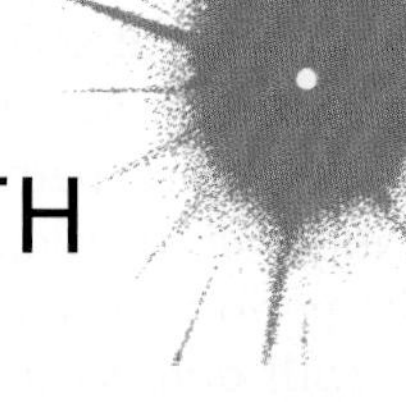

Rosa M. Andrade ■ Sharon L. Reed

AMEBIASIS

DEFINITION

Amebiasis is an infection with the intestinal protozoan *Entamoeba histolytica*. About 90% of infections are asymptomatic, and the remaining 10% produce a spectrum of clinical syndromes ranging from dysentery to abscesses of the liver or other organs.

LIFE CYCLE AND TRANSMISSION

E. histolytica is acquired by ingestion of viable cysts from fecally contaminated water, food, or hands. Food-borne exposure is most prevalent and is particularly likely when food handlers are shedding cysts or food is being grown with feces-contaminated soil, fertilizer, or water. Besides the drinking of contaminated water, less common means of transmission include oral and anal sexual practices and—in rare instances—direct rectal inoculation through colonic irrigation devices. Motile trophozoites are released from cysts in the small intestine and, in most patients, remain as harmless commensals in the large bowel. After encystation, infectious cysts are shed in the stool and can survive for several weeks in a moist environment. In some patients, the trophozoites invade either the bowel mucosa, causing symptomatic colitis, or the bloodstream, causing distant abscesses of the liver, lungs, or brain. The trophozoites may not encyst in patients with active dysentery, and motile hematophagous trophozoites are frequently present in fresh stools. Trophozoites are rapidly killed by exposure to air or stomach acid, however, and therefore cannot transmit infection.

EPIDEMIOLOGY

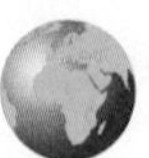

About 10% of the world's population is infected with *Entamoeba*, the majority with noninvasive *Entamoeba dispar*. Amebiasis results from infection with *E. histolytica* and is the third most common cause of death from parasitic disease (after schistosomiasis and malaria). Invasive colitis and liver abscesses are sevenfold more common among men than among women; this difference has been attributed to a disparity in complement-mediated killing. The wide spectrum of clinical disease caused by *Entamoeba* is due in part to the differences between these two infecting species. *E. histolytica* has unique isoenzymes, surface antigens, DNA markers, and virulence properties that distinguish it from other genetically related and morphologically identical species, such as *E. dispar* and *E. moshkovskii*.

Most asymptomatic carriers, including men who have sex with men (MSM) and patients with AIDS, harbor *E. dispar* and have self-limited infections. In this respect, *E. dispar* is dissimilar to other enteric pathogens such as *Cryptosporidium* and *Cystoisospora belli*, which can cause self-limited illnesses in immunocompetent hosts but devastating diarrhea in patients with AIDS. These observations indicate that *E. dispar* is incapable of causing invasive disease. Unlike *E. dispar, E. histolytica* can cause invasive disease, as demonstrated in recent reports from Korea, China, and India that suggest higher prevalences of amebic seroconversion, invasive amebiasis, and amebic liver abscesses among HIV-positive than HIV-negative patients. In another study, 10% of asymptomatic patients who were colonized with *E. histolytica* went on to develop amebic colitis, while the rest remained asymptomatic and cleared the infection within 1 year.

The potential of *E. moshkovskii* to cause diarrhea, weight loss, and colitis was recently demonstrated in a mouse model of cecal infection. However, the pathogenic potential of this species is not clear. A prospective evaluation of children from the Mirpur community of Dhaka, Bangladesh, found that most children who had diarrheal diseases associated with *E. moshkovskii* were simultaneously infected with at least one other enteric pathogen.

Areas of highest incidence of *Entamoeba* infection (due to inadequate sanitation and crowding) include most developing countries in the tropics, particularly Mexico, India, and nations of Central and South America, tropical Asia, and Africa. In a 4-year follow-up study of preschool children in a highly endemic area of Bangladesh, 80% of children had at least one episode of *E. histolytica* infection and 53% had more than one episode. Naturally acquired immunity did develop but was usually short-lived and correlated with the presence in the stool of secretory IgA antibody to the major adherence lectin galactose *N*-acetylgalactosamine (Gal/GalNAc). The main groups at risk for amebiasis in developed countries are returned travelers, recent immigrants, MSM, military personnel, and inmates of institutions. Data from the GeoSentinel Surveillance Network, which come from tropical medicine clinics on six continents, showed that, among long-term travelers (trip duration, >6 months), diarrhea due to *E. histolytica* was among the most common diagnoses.

PATHOGENESIS AND PATHOLOGY

Both trophozoites (Fig. 33-1) and cysts (Fig. 33-2) are found in the intestinal lumen, but only trophozoites of *E. histolytica* invade tissue. The trophozoite is 20–60 μm in diameter and contains vacuoles and a nucleus with a characteristic central nucleolus. In animals, depletion of intestinal mucus, diffuse inflammation, and disruption of the epithelial barrier precede trophozoite contact with the colonic mucosa. Trophozoites attach to colonic mucus and epithelial cells by their Gal/GalNAc lectin. The earliest intestinal lesions are microulcerations of the mucosa of the cecum, sigmoid colon, or rectum that release erythrocytes, inflammatory cells, and epithelial cells. Proctoscopy reveals small ulcers with heaped-up margins and normal intervening mucosa (Fig. 247-3*A*). Submucosal extension of ulcerations under viable-appearing surface mucosa causes the classic "flask-shaped" ulcer containing trophozoites at the margins of dead and viable tissues. Although neutrophilic infiltrates may accompany the early lesions in animals, human intestinal infection is marked by a paucity of inflammatory cells, probably in part because of the killing of neutrophils by trophozoites (Fig. 33-3*B*). Treated ulcers characteristically heal with little or no scarring. Occasionally, however, full-thickness necrosis and perforation occur.

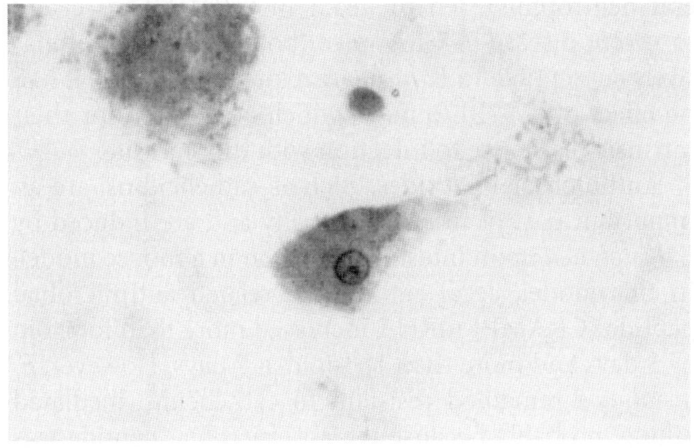

FIGURE 33-1
Trophozoite of *E. histolytica*. A single nucleus with a central, dot-like nucleolus is seen (trichrome stain).

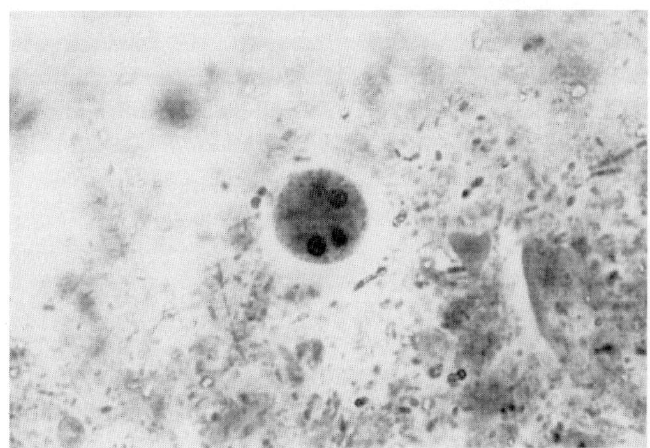

FIGURE 33-2
Cyst of *E. histolytica*. Three of the four nuclei are visible (trichrome stain).

Rarely, intestinal infection results in the formation of a mass lesion, or *ameboma*, in the bowel lumen. The overlying mucosa is usually thin and ulcerated, while other layers of the wall are thickened, edematous, and hemorrhagic; this condition results in exuberant formation of granulation tissue with little fibrous-tissue response.

A number of virulence factors have been linked to the ability of *E. histolytica* to invade through the interglandular epithelium. One factor consists of the extracellular cysteine proteinases that degrade collagen, elastin, IgA, IgG, and the anaphylatoxins C3a and C5a. Other enzymes may disrupt glycoprotein bonds between mucosal epithelial cells in the gut. Amebas can lyse neutrophils, monocytes, lymphocytes, and cells of colonic and hepatic lines. The cytolytic effect of amebas appears to require direct contact with target cells and may be linked to the release of phospholipase A and pore-forming peptides. *E. histolytica* trophozoites also cause apoptosis of human cells. Phagocytosis is a virulence factor that leads to defective parasite proliferation if inhibited. This process is potentially modulated by calmodulin-like calcium-binding protein 3, which

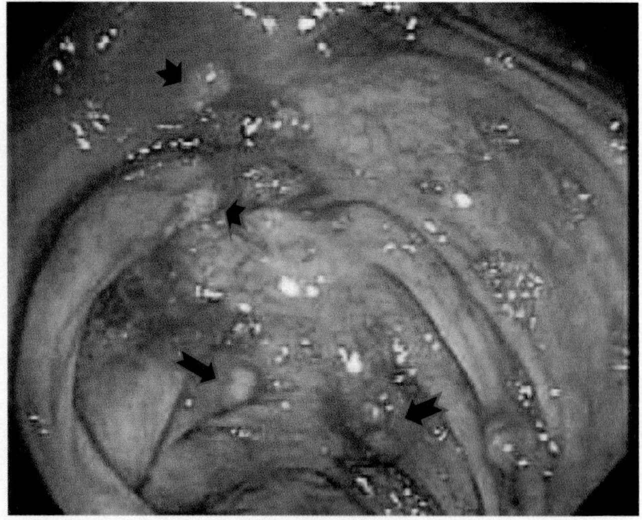

A

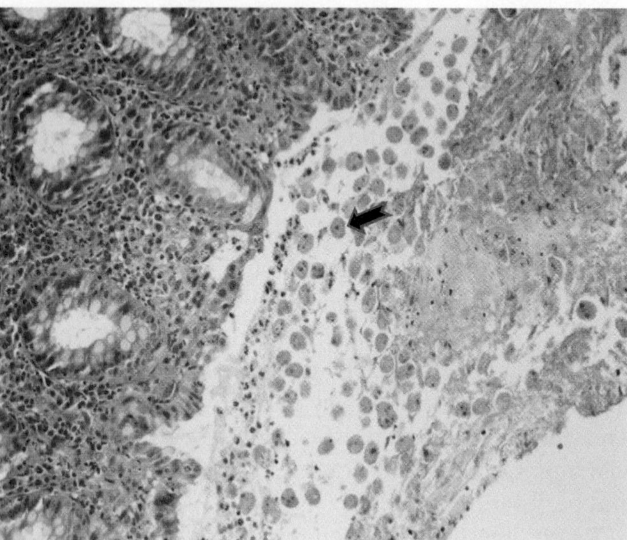

B

FIGURE 33-3

Endoscopic and histopathologic features of intestinal amebiasis. *A.* Appearance of ulcers on colonoscopy (*arrows*). ***B.*** Inflammatory infiltrate and *E. histolytica* trophozoites (*arrow*) in invasive amebic colitis (hematoxylin and eosin). *(Courtesy of the Department of Pathology and Gastroenterology, VA San Diego Medical Center.)*

pairs with actin and myosin during initiation and formation of phagosomes. Another virulence factor is the ability to resist reactive oxygen species, reactive nitrogen species such as nitric oxide, or S-nitrosothiols such as S-nitrosoglutathione (GSNO) and S-nitrosocysteine (CySNO). *E. histolytica* trophozoites are constantly exposed to reactive oxygen and nitrogen species from their own metabolism and host defenses during tissue invasion. Overexpression of hydrogen peroxide regulatory motif–binding protein appears to increase *E. histolytica* cytotoxicity. Since *E. histolytica* lacks glutathione and glutathione reductase, it relies on its thioredoxin/thioredoxin reductase system to prevent, regulate, and repair the damage caused by oxidative stress. This antioxidant system is versatile in that it can reduce reactive nitrogen species and use an alternative electron donor such as the reduced form of nicotinamide adenine dinucleotide. Metronidazole, the current standard of therapy for amebiasis, seems to exert its antiparasitic effect through the inhibition of this antioxidant system. Newer therapeutic candidates targeting this system, such as auranofin, also have demonstrated in vitro and in vivo efficacy against this parasite.

Liver abscesses are always preceded by intestinal colonization, which may be asymptomatic. Blood vessels may be compromised early by wall lysis and thrombus formation. Trophozoites invade veins to reach the liver through the portal venous system. *E. histolytica* is resistant to complement-mediated lysis—a property critical to survival in the bloodstream. In contrast, *E. dispar* is rapidly lysed by complement and is thus restricted to the bowel lumen. Inoculation of amebas into the portal system of hamsters results in an acute cellular infiltrate consisting predominantly of neutrophils. Later, the neutrophils are lysed by contact with amebas, and the release of neutrophil toxins may contribute to necrosis of hepatocytes. The liver parenchyma is replaced by necrotic material that is surrounded by a thin rim of congested liver tissue. The necrotic contents of a liver abscess are classically described as "anchovy paste," although the fluid is variable in color and is composed of bacteriologically sterile granular debris with few or no cells. Amebas, if seen, tend to be found near the capsule of the abscess.

Host innate and adaptive immunity are important factors that determine susceptibility to invasive disease and its clinical outcome. While neutrophils were thought to contribute to tissue damage in intestinal and liver amebiasis due to their cytotoxic effects on host epithelial cells, a recent report suggests that they may exert a protective effect in susceptible mice. Neutropenia, induced with an antibody to Gr-1 (i.e., to peripheral neutrophils), led to death in C3H/HeJ mice and to severe disease in CBA mice (both of which are relatively susceptible to *E. histolytica* infection), while it had no effect on C57BL/6 mice, which are known for their intrinsic resistance to infection with this parasite.

Antimicrobial peptides, such as cathelicidins, are an important part of innate immunity and are induced by *E. histolytica* upon intestinal invasion in a mouse model. In this model, cecal cathelicidin-related antimicrobial peptide (CRAMP) mRNA increased more than fourfold by 3 days and more than 100-fold at 7 days. However, *E. histolytica* remained resistant to cathelicidin-mediated killing, probably because the antimicrobial peptide was digested by amebic cysteine proteinases.

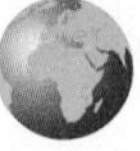

IgA plays a critical role in acquired immunity to *E. histolytica*. A study in Bangladeshi schoolchildren revealed that an intestinal IgA response to

Gal/GalNAc reduced the risk of new *E. histolytica* infection by 64%. Serum IgG antibody is not protective; titers correlate with the duration of illness rather than with the severity of disease. Indeed, Bangladeshi children with a serum IgG response were more likely than those without such a response to develop new *E. histolytica* infection. In infants from this same Bangladeshi community, passive immunity conferred by maternal parasite-specific IgA via breastfeeding resulted in a 39% reduction in risk of infection and a 64% reduction in risk of diarrheal disease from *E. histolytica* during the first year of life.

A link between nutrition and immunity is demonstrated by the elevated rate of infections due to protozoan parasites, including *E. histolytica*, among undernourished children in developing countries. Resistance to amebiasis is associated with a polymorphism in the receptor for the adipocytokine leptin. Children in a Bangladeshi cohort with a mutant R223 leptin receptor allele were nearly four times more likely to be infected with *E. histolytica* than those carrying the ancestral Q223 allele. This mutant allele is overrepresented in many geographic areas with a high prevalence of amebiasis, such as Bangladesh and India.

CLINICAL SYNDROMES

Intestinal amebiasis

The most common type of amebic infection is asymptomatic cyst passage. Even in highly endemic areas, most patients harbor *E. dispar*.

Symptomatic amebic colitis develops 2–6 weeks after the ingestion of infectious *E. histolytica* cysts. A gradual onset of lower abdominal pain and mild diarrhea is followed by malaise, weight loss, and diffuse lower abdominal or back pain. Cecal involvement may mimic acute appendicitis. Patients with full-blown dysentery may pass 10–12 stools per day. The stools contain little fecal material and consist mainly of blood and mucus. In contrast to those with bacterial diarrhea, fewer than 40% of patients with amebic dysentery are febrile. Virtually all patients have heme-positive stools.

More fulminant intestinal infection, with severe abdominal pain, high fever, and profuse diarrhea, is rare and occurs predominantly in children. Patients may develop toxic megacolon, in which there is severe bowel dilation with intramural air. Patients receiving glucocorticoids are at risk for severe amebiasis. Uncommonly, patients develop a chronic form of amebic colitis, which can be confused with inflammatory bowel disease. The association between severe amebiasis complications and glucocorticoid therapy emphasizes the importance of excluding amebiasis when inflammatory bowel disease is suspected. An occasional patient presents with only an asymptomatic or tender abdominal mass caused by an ameboma, which is easily confused with cancer on barium studies. A positive serologic test or biopsy can prevent unnecessary surgery in this setting. The syndrome of post–amebic colitis—i.e., persistent diarrhea following documented cure of amebic colitis—is controversial; no evidence of recurrent amebic infection can be found, and re-treatment usually has no effect.

Amebic liver abscess

Extraintestinal infection by *E. histolytica* most often involves the liver. Of travelers who develop an amebic liver abscess after leaving an endemic area, 95% do so within 5 months. Young patients with an amebic liver abscess are more likely than older patients to present in the acute phase with prominent symptoms of <10 days' duration. Most patients are febrile and have right-upper-quadrant pain, which may be dull or pleuritic in nature and may radiate to the shoulder. Point tenderness over the liver and right-sided pleural effusion are common. Jaundice is rare. Although the initial site of infection is the colon, fewer than one-third of patients with an amebic abscess have active diarrhea. Older patients from endemic areas are more likely to have a subacute course lasting 6 months, with weight loss and hepatomegaly. About one-third of patients with chronic presentations are febrile. Thus, the clinical diagnosis of an amebic liver abscess may be difficult to establish because the symptoms and signs are often nonspecific. Since 10–15% of patients present only with fever, amebic liver abscess must be considered in the differential diagnosis of fever of unknown origin **(Chap. 26)**.

Complications of amebic liver abscess

Pleuropulmonary involvement, which is reported in 20–30% of patients, is the most frequent complication of amebic liver abscess. Manifestations include sterile effusions, contiguous spread from the liver, and rupture into the pleural space. Sterile effusions and contiguous spread usually resolve with medical therapy, but frank rupture into the pleural space requires drainage. A hepatobronchial fistula may cause cough productive of large amounts of necrotic material that may contain amebas. This dramatic complication carries a good prognosis. Abscesses that rupture into the peritoneum may present as an indolent leak or an acute abdomen and require both percutaneous catheter drainage and medical therapy. Rupture into the pericardium, usually from abscesses of the left lobe of the liver, carries the gravest prognosis; it can occur during medical therapy and requires surgical drainage.

Other extraintestinal sites

The genitourinary tract may become involved by direct extension of amebiasis from the colon or by hematogenous spread of the infection. Painful genital ulcers, characterized by a punched-out appearance and profuse discharge, may develop secondary to extension from either the intestine or the liver. Both of these conditions respond well to medical therapy. Cerebral involvement has been reported in fewer than 0.1% of patients in large clinical series. Symptoms and prognosis depend on the size and location of the lesion.

DIAGNOSTIC TESTS

Laboratory diagnosis

Stool examinations, serologic tests, and noninvasive imaging of the liver are the most important procedures in the diagnosis of amebiasis. Fecal findings suggestive of amebic colitis include a positive test for heme, a paucity of neutrophils, and amebic cysts or trophozoites. The definitive diagnosis of amebic colitis is made by the demonstration of hematophagous trophozoites of *E. histolytica* (Fig. 33-1). Because trophozoites are killed rapidly by water, drying, or barium, it is important to examine at least three fresh stool specimens. Examination of a combination of wet mounts, iodine-stained concentrates, and trichrome-stained preparations of fresh stool and concentrates for cysts (Fig. 33-2) or trophozoites (Fig. 33-1) confirms the diagnosis in 75–95% of cases. Culture of amebas is more sensitive, but this diagnostic method is not routinely available. If stool examinations are negative, sigmoidoscopy with biopsy of the edge of ulcers may increase the yield, but this procedure is dangerous during fulminant colitis because of the risk of perforation. Trophozoites in a biopsy specimen from a colonic mass confirm the diagnosis of ameboma, but trophozoites are rare in liver aspirates because they are found in the abscess capsule and not in the readily aspirated necrotic center. Accurate diagnosis requires experience, since the trophozoites may be confused with neutrophils and the cysts must be differentiated morphologically from those of *Entamoeba hartmanni*, *Entamoeba coli*, and *Endolimax nana*, which do not cause clinical disease and do not warrant therapy. Unfortunately, the cysts of *E. histolytica* cannot be distinguished microscopically from those of *E. dispar* or *E. moshkovskii*. Therefore, the microscopic diagnosis of *E. histolytica* can be made only by the detection of *Entamoeba* trophozoites that have ingested erythrocytes. In terms of sensitivity, stool diagnostic tests based on the detection of the Gal/GalNAc lectin of *E. histolytica* compare favorably with the polymerase chain reaction and with isolation in culture followed by isoenzyme analysis.

Serology is an important addition to the methods used for parasitologic diagnosis of invasive amebiasis. Enzyme-linked immunosorbent assays and agar gel diffusion assays are positive in more than 90% of patients with colitis, amebomas, or liver abscess. Positive results in conjunction with the appropriate clinical syndrome suggest active disease because serologic findings usually revert to negative within 6–12 months. Even in highly endemic areas such as South Africa, fewer than 10% of asymptomatic individuals have a positive amebic serology. The interpretation of the indirect hemagglutination test is more difficult because titers may remain positive for as long as 10 years.

Up to 10% of patients with acute amebic liver abscess may have negative serologic findings; in suspected cases with an initially negative result, testing should be repeated in 1 week. In contrast to carriers of *E. dispar*, most asymptomatic carriers of *E. histolytica* develop antibodies. Thus, serologic tests are helpful in assessing the risk of invasive amebiasis in asymptomatic, cyst-passing individuals in nonendemic areas. Serologic tests also should be performed in patients with ulcerative colitis before the institution of glucocorticoid therapy to prevent the development of severe colitis or toxic megacolon owing to unsuspected amebiasis.

Routine hematology and chemistry tests usually are not very helpful in the diagnosis of invasive amebiasis. About three-fourths of patients with an amebic liver abscess have leukocytosis (>10,000 cells/μL); this condition is particularly likely if symptoms are acute or complications have developed. Invasive amebiasis does not elicit eosinophilia. Anemia, if present, is usually multifactorial. Even with large liver abscesses, liver enzyme levels are normal or minimally elevated. The alkaline phosphatase level is most often elevated and may remain so for months. Aminotransferase elevations suggest acute disease or a complication.

Radiographic studies

Radiographic barium studies are potentially dangerous in acute amebic colitis. Amebomas are usually identified first by a barium enema, but biopsy is necessary for differentiation from carcinoma.

Radiographic techniques such as ultrasonography, CT, and MRI are all useful for detection of the round or oval hypoechoic cyst of an amebic liver abscess. More than 80% of patients who have had symptoms for >10 days have a single abscess of the right lobe of the liver (Fig. 33-4). Approximately 50% of patients who have had symptoms for <10 days have multiple abscesses. Findings associated with complications include large abscesses (>10 cm) in the superior part of the right lobe, which may rupture into the pleural space; multiple lesions, which must be differentiated from pyogenic abscesses; and lesions of the left lobe, which may rupture into the pericardium. Because abscesses resolve slowly and may increase in size in patients who are responding clinically to therapy, frequent follow-up ultrasonography may prove confusing. Complete resolution of a liver abscess within 6 months can be anticipated in two-thirds of patients, but 10% may have persistent abnormalities for a year.

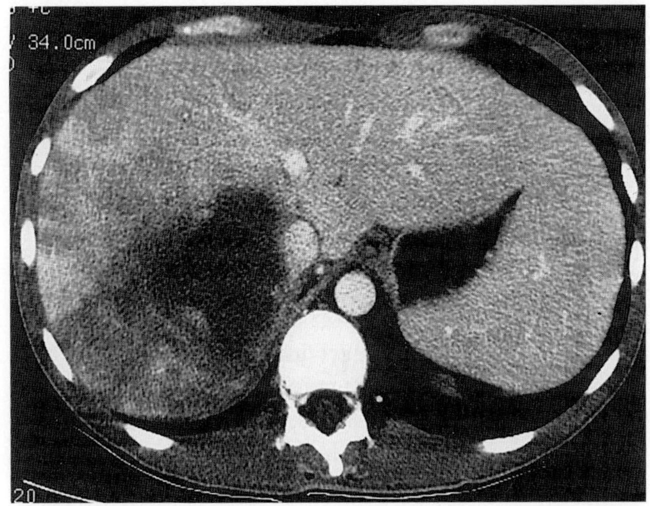

FIGURE 33-4
Abdominal CT scan of a large amebic abscess of the right lobe of the liver. *(Courtesy of the Department of Radiology, UCSD Medical Center, San Diego; with permission.)*

Differential diagnosis

The differential diagnosis of intestinal amebiasis includes bacterial diarrheas **(Chap. 24)** caused by *Campylobacter* **(Chap. 30)**; enteroinvasive *Escherichia coli* and species of *Shigella* **(Chap. 29)**, *Salmonella* **(Chap. 28)**, and *Vibrio* **(Chap. 31)**. Although the typical patient with amebic colitis has less prominent fever than in these other conditions as well as heme-positive stools with few neutrophils, correct diagnosis requires bacterial cultures, microscopic examination of stools, and amebic serologic testing. As has already been mentioned, amebiasis must be ruled out in any patient thought to have inflammatory bowel disease.

Because of the variety of presenting signs and symptoms, amebic liver abscess can easily be confused with pulmonary or gallbladder disease or with any febrile illness with few localizing signs, such as malaria or typhoid fever **(Chap. 28)**. The diagnosis should be considered in members of high-risk groups who have recently traveled outside the United States and in inmates of institutions. Once radiographic studies have identified an abscess in the liver, the most important differential diagnosis is between amebic and pyogenic abscess. Patients with pyogenic abscess typically are older and have a history of underlying bowel disease or recent surgery. Amebic serology is helpful, but aspiration of the abscess, with Gram's staining and culture of the material, may be required for differentiation of the two diseases.

TREATMENT Amebiasis

INTESTINAL DISEASE The drugs used to treat amebiasis can be classified according to their primary site of action (Table 33-1). *Luminal* amebicides are poorly absorbed; they reach high concentrations in the bowel, but their activity is limited to cysts and trophozoites close to the mucosa. Only two luminal drugs are available in the United States: iodoquinol and paromomycin. Indications for the use of luminal agents include eradication of cysts in patients with colitis or a liver abscess and treatment of asymptomatic carriers. The majority of asymptomatic individuals who pass cysts are colonized with *E. dispar*, which does not warrant specific therapy. However, it is prudent to treat asymptomatic individuals who pass cysts unless *E. dispar* colonization can be definitively demonstrated by specific antigen-detection tests.

Tissue amebicides reach high concentrations in the blood and tissue after oral or parenteral administration. The development of nitroimidazole compounds, especially metronidazole, was a major advance in the treatment of invasive amebiasis. Patients with amebic colitis should be treated with IV or oral metronidazole. Side effects include nausea, vomiting, abdominal discomfort, and a disulfiram-like reaction. Another longer-acting imidazole compound, tinidazole, is also effective and available in the United States. All patients should also receive a full course of therapy with a luminal agent, since metronidazole does not eradicate cysts. Resistance to metronidazole has been selected in the laboratory but has not been found in clinical isolates. Relapses are not uncommon and probably represent reinfection or failure to eradicate amebas from the bowel because of an inadequate dosage or duration of therapy.

AMEBIC LIVER ABSCESS Metronidazole is the drug of choice for amebic liver abscess. Longer-acting nitroimidazoles (tinidazole and ornidazole) have been effective as single-dose therapy in developing countries. With early diagnosis and therapy, mortality rates from uncomplicated amebic liver abscess are <1%. There is no evidence that combined therapy with two drugs is more effective than the single-drug regimen. Studies

TABLE 33-1

DRUG THERAPY FOR AMEBIASIS

INDICATION	THERAPY
Asymptomatic carriage	Luminal agent: iodoquinol (650-mg tablets), 650 mg tid for 20 days; *or* paromomycin (250-mg tablets), 500 mg tid for 10 days
Acute colitis	Metronidazole (250- or 500-mg tablets), 750 mg PO or IV tid for 5–10 days; *or* tinidazole, 2 g/d PO for 3 days ***plus*** Luminal agent as above
Amebic liver abscess	Metronidazole, 750 mg PO or IV for 5–10 days; *or* tinidazole, 2 g PO once; *or* ornidazole,[a] 2 g PO once ***plus*** Luminal agent as above

[a]Not available in the United States.

of South Africans with liver abscesses demonstrated that 72% of patients without intestinal symptoms had bowel infection with *E. histolytica*; thus, all treatment regimens should include a luminal agent to eradicate cysts and prevent further transmission. Amebic liver abscess recurs rarely.

More than 90% of patients respond dramatically to metronidazole therapy with decreases in both pain and fever within 72 h. Indications for aspiration of liver abscesses are (1) the need to rule out a pyogenic abscess, particularly in patients with multiple lesions; (2) the lack of a clinical response in 3–5 days; (3) the threat of imminent rupture; and (4) the need to prevent rupture of left-lobe abscesses into the pericardium. There is no evidence that aspiration, even of large abscesses (up to 10 cm), accelerates healing. Percutaneous drainage may be successful even if the liver abscess has already ruptured. Surgery should be reserved for instances of bowel perforation and rupture into the pericardium.

PREVENTION

Amebic infection is spread by ingestion of food or water contaminated with cysts. Since an asymptomatic carrier may excrete up to 15 million cysts per day, prevention of infection requires adequate sanitation and eradication of cyst carriage. In high-risk areas, infection can be minimized by the avoidance of unpeeled fruits and vegetables and the use of bottled water. Because cysts are resistant to readily attainable levels of chlorine, disinfection by iodination (tetraglycine hydroperiodide) is recommended. There is no effective prophylaxis.

INFECTION WITH FREE-LIVING AMEBAS

EPIDEMIOLOGY

Free-living amebas of the genera *Acanthamoeba* and *Naegleria* are distributed throughout the world and have been isolated from a wide variety of fresh and brackish water, including that from lakes, taps, hot springs, swimming pools, and heating and air-conditioning units, and even from the nasal passages of healthy children. Encystation may protect the protozoa from desiccation and food deprivation. The persistence of *Legionella pneumophila* in water supplies may be attributable in part to chronic infection of free-living amebas, particularly *Naegleria*. Free-living amebas of the genus *Balamuthia* have been isolated from soil samples, including a sample from a flowerpot linked to a fatal infection in a child.

NAEGLERIA INFECTIONS

Primary amebic meningoencephalitis caused by *Naegleria fowleri* follows the aspiration of water contaminated with trophozoites or cysts or the inhalation of contaminated dust, leading to invasion of the olfactory neuroepithelium. Infection is most common among otherwise healthy children or young adults, who often report recent swimming in lakes or heated swimming pools. Rarely, some cases occur when contaminated water is used for nasal irrigation. After an incubation period of 2–15 days, severe headache, high fever, nausea, vomiting, and meningismus develop. Photophobia and palsies of the third, fourth, and sixth cranial nerves are common. Rapid progression to seizures and coma may follow. The prognosis is uniformly poor: most patients die within a week. Recently, two surviving children were treated with miltefosine, an investigational drug that is available through the Centers for Disease Control and Prevention (CDC) for the treatment of *Naegleria* infections.

The diagnosis of *Naegleria* infection should be considered in any patient who has purulent meningitis without evidence of bacteria on Gram's staining, antigen detection assay, and culture. Other laboratory findings resemble those for fulminant bacterial meningitis, with elevated intracranial pressure, high white blood cell counts (up to 20,000/μL), and elevated protein concentrations and low glucose levels in cerebrospinal fluid (CSF). Diagnosis depends on the detection of motile trophozoites in wet mounts of fresh spinal fluid. Antibodies to *Naegleria* species have been detected in healthy adults; serologic testing is not useful in the diagnosis of acute infection.

ACANTHAMOEBA INFECTIONS

Granulomatous amebic encephalitis

Infection with *Acanthamoeba* species follows a more indolent course and typically occurs in chronically ill or debilitated patients. Risk factors include lymphoproliferative disorders, chemotherapy, glucocorticoid therapy, lupus erythematosus, and AIDS. Infection usually reaches the central nervous system hematogenously from a primary focus in the sinuses, skin, or lungs. In the central nervous system, the onset is insidious, and the syndrome often mimics a space-occupying lesion. Altered mental status, headache, and stiff neck may be accompanied by focal findings such as cranial nerve palsies, ataxia, and hemiparesis. Cutaneous ulcers or hard nodules containing amebas are frequently detected in AIDS patients with disseminated *Acanthamoeba* infection and can be an important diagnostic site.

Examination of the CSF for trophozoites may be diagnostically helpful, but lumbar puncture may be contraindicated because of increased intracerebral pressure. CT frequently reveals cortical and subcortical lesions of decreased density consistent with embolic infarcts. In other patients, multiple enhancing lesions with edema may mimic the computed tomographic appearance of toxoplasmosis. Demonstration of the trophozoites and cysts of *Acanthamoeba* on wet mounts or in biopsy specimens establishes the diagnosis. Culture on

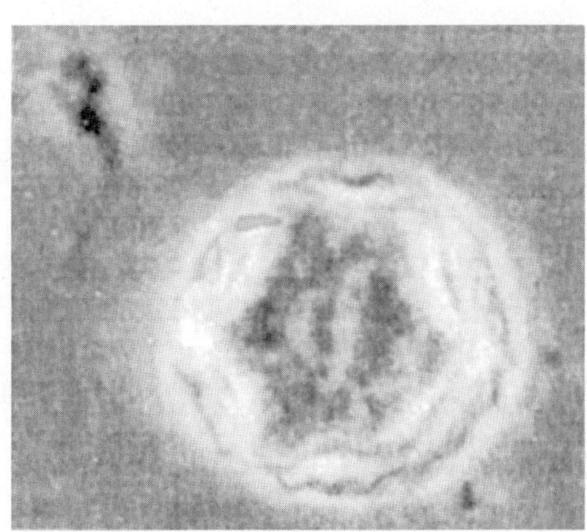

FIGURE 33-5
Double-walled cyst of *Acanthamoeba castellanii*, as seen by phase-contrast microscopy. *(From DJ Krogstad et al, in A Balows et al [eds]: Manual of Clinical Microbiology, 5th ed. Washington, DC, American Society for Microbiology, 1991.)*

nonnutrient agar plates seeded with *Escherichia coli* also may be helpful. Fluorescein-labeled antiserum is available from the CDC for the detection of protozoa in biopsy specimens. Granulomatous amebic encephalitis in patients with AIDS may have an accelerated course (with survival for only 3–40 days) because of poor granuloma formation in these individuals. Various antimicrobial agents have been used to treat *Acanthamoeba* infection, but the infection is almost uniformly fatal. The CDC has now made miltefosine available because of improved survival rates when the drug is included in treatment regimens.

Keratitis

The incidence of keratitis caused by *Acanthamoeba* has increased in the past 30 years, in part as a result of improved diagnosis. Earlier infections were associated with trauma to the eye and exposure to contaminated water. At present, most infections are linked to extended-wear contact lenses, and rare cases are associated with laser-assisted in situ keratomileusis (LASIK). Risk factors include the use of homemade saline, the wearing of lenses while swimming, and inadequate disinfection. Since contact lenses presumably cause microscopic trauma, the early corneal findings may be nonspecific. The first symptoms usually include tearing and the painful sensation of a foreign body. Once infection is established, progression is rapid; the characteristic clinical sign is an annular, paracentral corneal ring representing a corneal abscess. Deeper corneal invasion and loss of vision may follow.

The differential diagnosis includes bacterial, mycobacterial, and herpetic infection. The irregular polygonal cysts of *Acanthamoeba* (Fig. 33-5) may be identified in corneal scrapings or biopsy material, and trophozoites can be grown on special media. Cysts are resistant to available drugs, and the results of medical therapy have been disappointing. Some reports have suggested partial responses to propamidine isethionate eyedrops. Severe infections usually require keratoplasty.

Balamuthia infections

Balamuthia mandrillaris, a free-living ameba previously referred to as a leptomyxid ameba, is an important etiologic agent of amebic meningoencephalitis in immunocompetent hosts. The course is typically subacute, with focal neurologic signs, fever, seizures, and headaches leading to death within 1 week to several months after onset. Examination of CSF reveals mononuclear or neutrophilic pleocytosis, elevated protein levels, and normal to low glucose concentrations. Multiple hypodense lesions are usually detected with imaging studies (Fig. 33-6). This mixed picture of space-occupying lesions with CSF pleocytosis is suggestive of *Balamuthia*. Fluorescent antibody is available from the CDC for brain biopsy specimens. The variety of drugs used to treat the few surviving patients (i.e., fewer than five reported in the United States) includes pentamidine, flucytosine, sulfadiazine, and macrolides. The CDC recommends that miltefosine now be included, as for the other free-living amebas. The differential diagnosis includes tuberculomas and neurocysticercosis.

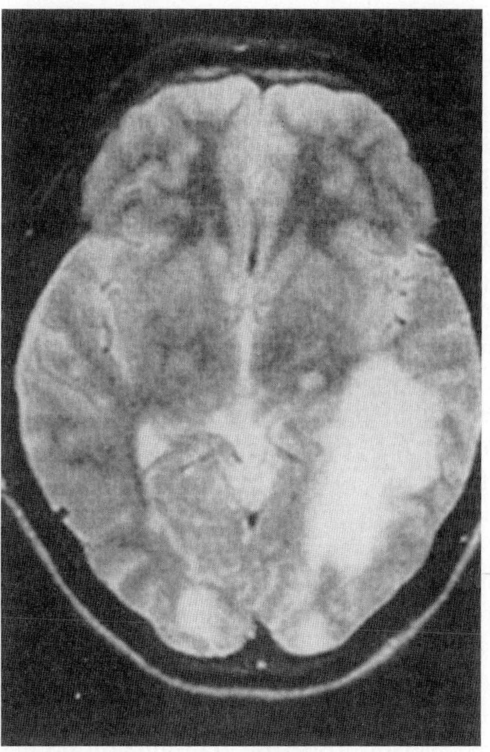

FIGURE 33-6
Brain MRI of amebic meningoencephalitis due to *Balamuthia mandrillaris.* A large lesion in the parieto-occipital lobe and other smaller lesions are seen. *(Courtesy of the Department of Radiology, UCSD Medical Center, San Diego.)*

CHAPTER 34

PROTOZOAL INTESTINAL INFECTIONS AND TRICHOMONIASIS

Peter F. Weller

PROTOZOAL INFECTIONS

GIARDIASIS

Giardia intestinalis (also known as *G. lamblia* or *G. duodenalis*) is a cosmopolitan protozoal parasite that inhabits the small intestines of humans and other mammals. Giardiasis is one of the most common parasitic diseases in both developed and developing countries worldwide, causing both endemic and epidemic intestinal disease and diarrhea.

Life cycle and epidemiology

(Fig. 34-1) Infection follows the ingestion of environmentally hardy cysts, which excyst in the small intestine, releasing flagellated trophozoites (Fig. 34-2) that multiply by binary fission. *Giardia* remains a pathogen of the proximal small bowel and does not disseminate hematogenously. Trophozoites remain free in the lumen or attach to the mucosal epithelium by means of a ventral sucking disk. As a trophozoite encounters altered conditions, it forms a morphologically distinct cyst, which is the stage of the parasite usually found in the feces. Trophozoites may be present and even predominate in loose or watery stools, but it is the resistant cyst that survives outside the body and is responsible for transmission. Cysts do not tolerate heating or desiccation, but they do remain viable for months in cold fresh water. The number of cysts excreted varies widely but can approach 10^7 per gram of stool.

Ingestion of as few as 10 cysts is sufficient to cause infection in humans. Because cysts are infectious when excreted, person-to-person transmission occurs where fecal hygiene is poor. Giardiasis is especially prevalent in day-care centers; person-to-person spread also takes place in other institutional settings with poor fecal hygiene and during anal-oral contact. If food is

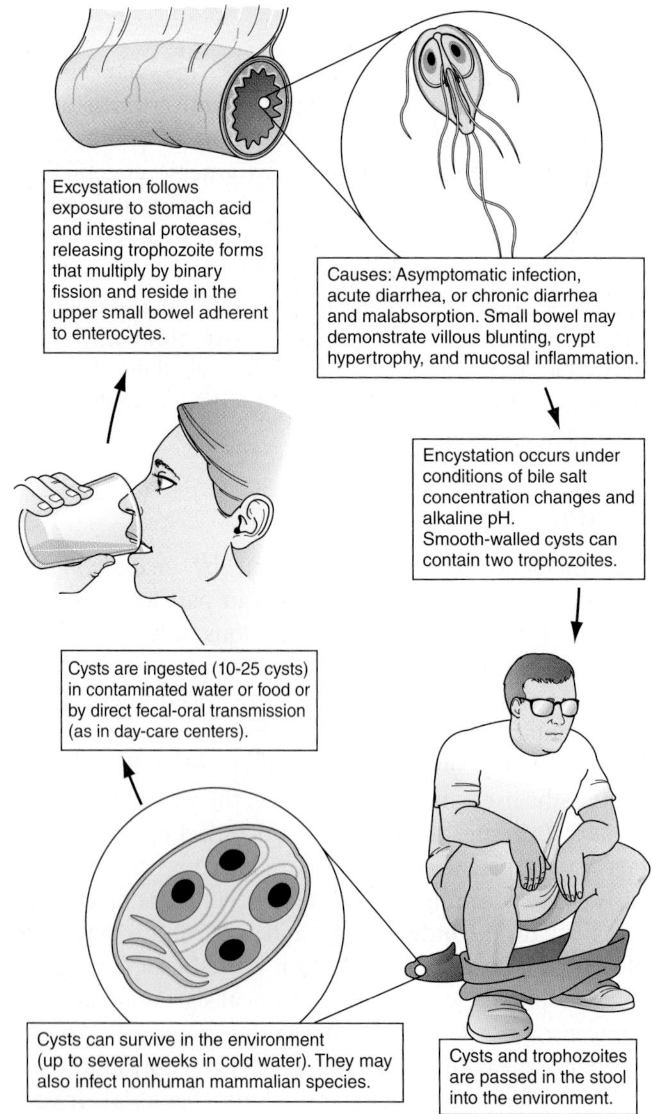

Excystation follows exposure to stomach acid and intestinal proteases, releasing trophozoite forms that multiply by binary fission and reside in the upper small bowel adherent to enterocytes.
Causes: Asymptomatic infection, acute diarrhea, or chronic diarrhea and malabsorption. Small bowel may demonstrate villous blunting, crypt hypertrophy, and mucosal inflammation.
Encystation occurs under conditions of bile salt concentration changes and alkaline pH. Smooth-walled cysts can contain two trophozoites.
Cysts are ingested (10-25 cysts) in contaminated water or food or by direct fecal-oral transmission (as in day-care centers).
Cysts can survive in the environment (up to several weeks in cold water). They may also infect nonhuman mammalian species.
Cysts and trophozoites are passed in the stool into the environment.

FIGURE 34-1

Life cycle of *Giardia*. *(Reprinted with permission from RL Guerrant et al [eds]: Tropical Infectious Diseases: Principles, Pathogens and Practice, 2nd ed, p 987. © 2006, with permission from Elsevier Science.)*

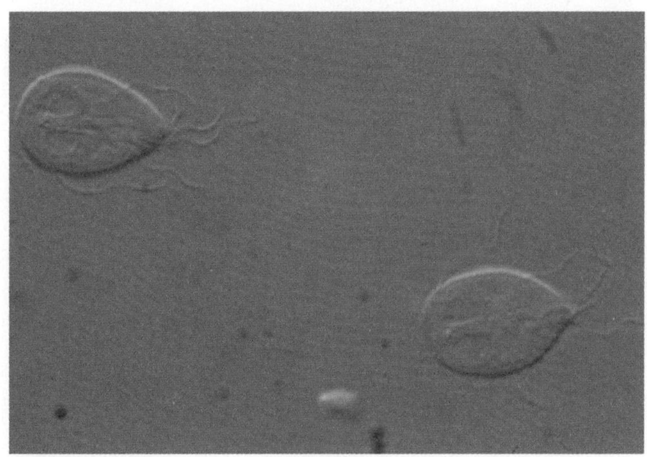

FIGURE 34-2
Flagellated, binucleate *Giardia* trophozoites.

contaminated with *Giardia* cysts after cooking or preparation, food-borne transmission can occur. Waterborne transmission accounts for episodic infections (e.g., in campers and travelers) and for major epidemics in metropolitan areas. Surface water, ranging from mountain streams to large municipal reservoirs, can become contaminated with fecally derived *Giardia* cysts. The efficacy of water as a means of transmission is enhanced by the small infectious inoculum of *Giardia*, the prolonged survival of cysts in cold water, and the resistance of cysts to killing by routine chlorination methods that are adequate for controlling bacteria. Viable cysts can be eradicated from water by either boiling or filtration.

In the United States, *Giardia* (like *Cryptosporidium*; see below) is a common cause of waterborne epidemics of gastroenteritis. *Giardia* is common in developing countries, and infections may be acquired by travelers.

There are several recognized genotypes or assemblages of *G. intestinalis*. Human infections are due to assemblages A and B, whereas other assemblages are more common in other animals, including cats and dogs. Like beavers from reservoirs implicated in epidemics, dogs and cats have been found to be infected with assemblages A and B, an observation suggesting that these animals might be sources of human infection.

Giardiasis, like cryptosporidiosis, creates a significant economic burden because of the costs incurred in the installation of water filtration systems required to prevent waterborne epidemics, in the management of epidemics that involve large communities, and in the evaluation and treatment of endemic infections.

Pathophysiology

The reasons that some, but not all, infected patients develop clinical manifestations and the mechanisms by which *Giardia* causes alterations in small-bowel function are largely unknown. Although trophozoites adhere to the epithelium, they are not invasive but may elicit apoptosis of enterocytes, epithelial barrier dysfunction, and epithelial cell malabsorption and secretion. Consequent lactose intolerance and, in a minority of infected adults and children, significant malabsorption are clinical signs of the loss of brush-border enzyme activities. In most infections, the morphology of the bowel is unaltered; however, in chronically infected, symptomatic patients, the histopathologic findings (including flattened villi) and the clinical manifestations at times resemble those of tropical sprue and gluten-sensitive enteropathy. The pathogenesis of diarrhea in giardiasis is not known.

The natural history of *Giardia* infection varies markedly. Infections may be aborted, transient, recurrent, or chronic. *G. intestinalis* parasites vary genotypically, and such variations might contribute to different courses of infection. Parasite as well as host factors may be important in determining the course of infection and disease. Both cellular and humoral responses develop in human infections, but their precise roles in disease pathogenesis and/or control of infection are unknown. Because patients with hypogammaglobulinemia suffer from prolonged, severe infections that are poorly responsive to treatment, humoral immune responses appear to be important. The greater susceptibilities of the young than of the old and of newly exposed persons than of chronically exposed populations suggest that at least partial protective immunity may develop.

Clinical manifestations

Disease manifestations of giardiasis range from asymptomatic carriage to fulminant diarrhea and malabsorption. Most infected persons are asymptomatic, but in epidemics the proportion of symptomatic cases may be higher. Symptoms may develop suddenly or gradually. In persons with acute giardiasis, symptoms develop after an incubation period that lasts at least 5–6 days and usually 1–3 weeks. Prominent early symptoms include diarrhea, abdominal pain, bloating, belching, flatus, nausea, and vomiting. Although diarrhea is common, upper intestinal manifestations such as nausea, vomiting, bloating, and abdominal pain may predominate. The duration of acute giardiasis is usually >1 week, although diarrhea often subsides. Individuals with chronic giardiasis may present with or without having experienced an antecedent acute symptomatic episode. Diarrhea is not necessarily prominent, but increased flatus, loose stools, sulfurous belching, and (in some instances) weight loss occur. Symptoms may be continual or episodic and may persist for years. Some persons who have relatively mild symptoms for long periods recognize the extent of their discomfort

TABLE 34-1

DIAGNOSIS OF INTESTINAL PROTOZOAL INFECTIONS

PARASITE	STOOL O+P[a]	FECAL ACID-FAST STAIN	FECAL ANTIGEN IMMUNOASSAYS	FECAL NAATS[b]	OTHER
Giardia	+		+	+	
Cryptosporidium	–	+	+	+	
Isospora	–	+		+	
Cyclospora	–	+		+	
Microsporidia	–			+	Special fecal stains, tissue biopsies

[a]O+P, ova and parasites.
[b]Nucleic acid amplification tests.

only in retrospect. Fever, the presence of blood and/or mucus in the stools, and other signs and symptoms of colitis are uncommon and suggest a different diagnosis or a concomitant illness. Symptoms tend to be intermittent yet recurring and gradually debilitating, in contrast with the acute disabling symptoms associated with many enteric bacterial infections. Because of the less severe illness and the propensity for chronic infections, patients may seek medical advice late in the course of the illness; however, disease can be severe, resulting in malabsorption, weight loss, growth retardation, and dehydration. A number of extraintestinal manifestations have been described, such as urticaria, anterior uveitis, and arthritis; whether these are caused by giardiasis or concomitant processes is unclear.

Giardiasis can be severe in patients with hypogammaglobulinemia and can complicate other preexisting intestinal diseases, such as that occurring in cystic fibrosis. In patients with AIDS, *Giardia* can cause enteric illness that is refractory to treatment.

Diagnosis

(Table 34-1) Giardiasis is diagnosed by detection of parasite antigens in the feces, by identification of cysts in the feces or of trophozoites in the feces or small intestines, or by nucleic acid amplification tests (NAATs). Cysts are oval, measure 8–12 μm × 7–10 μm, and characteristically contain four nuclei. Trophozoites are pear-shaped, dorsally convex, flattened parasites with two nuclei and four pairs of flagella (Fig. 34-2). The diagnosis is sometimes difficult to establish. Direct examination of fresh or properly preserved stools as well as concentration methods should be used. Because cyst excretion is variable and may be undetectable at times, repeated examination of stool, sampling of duodenal fluid, and biopsy of the small intestine may be required to detect the parasite. Tests for parasitic antigens in stool are at least as sensitive and specific as good microscopic examinations and are easier to perform. Newer NAATs are highly sensitive but are not always available for clinical use at present.

TREATMENT Giardiasis

Cure rates with metronidazole (250 mg thrice daily for 5 days) are usually >90%. Tinidazole (2 g once by mouth) may be more effective than metronidazole. Albendazole (400 mg daily for 5–10 days) is as effective as metronidazole and is associated with fewer side effects. Nitazoxanide (500 mg twice daily for 3 days) is an alternative agent for treatment of giardiasis. Paromomycin, an oral aminoglycoside that is not well absorbed, can be given to symptomatic pregnant patients, although information is limited on how effectively this agent eradicates infection.

Almost all patients respond to therapy and are cured, although some with chronic giardiasis experience delayed resolution of symptoms after eradication of *Giardia*. For many of the latter patients, residual symptoms probably reflect delayed regeneration of intestinal brush-border enzymes. Continued infection should be documented by stool examinations before treatment is repeated. Patients who remain infected after repeated treatments should be evaluated for reinfection through family members, close personal contacts, and environmental sources as well as for hypogammaglobulinemia. In cases refractory to multiple treatment courses, prolonged therapy with metronidazole (750 mg thrice daily for 21 days) or therapy with varied combinations of multiple agents has been successful.

Prevention

Giardiasis can be prevented by consumption of uncontaminated food and water and by personal hygiene during the provision of care for infected children. Boiling or filtering potentially contaminated water prevents infection.

CRYPTOSPORIDIOSIS

The coccidian parasite *Cryptosporidium* causes diarrheal disease that is self-limited in immunocompetent human hosts but can be severe in persons with AIDS or other forms of immunodeficiency. Two species of *Cryptosporidium*, *C. hominis* (especially in the United States, sub-Saharan Africa, and Asia) and *C. parvum* (in Europe), cause most human infections.

Life cycle and epidemiology

Cryptosporidium species are widely distributed in the world. Cryptosporidiosis is acquired by the consumption of oocysts (50% infectious dose: ~132 *C. parvum* oocysts in nonimmune individuals), which excyst to liberate sporozoites that in turn enter and infect intestinal epithelial cells. The parasite's further development involves both asexual and sexual cycles, which produce forms capable of infecting other epithelial cells and of generating oocysts that are passed in the feces. *Cryptosporidium* species infect a number of animals, and *C. parvum* can spread from infected animals to humans. Since oocysts are immediately infectious when passed in feces, person-to-person transmission takes place in day-care centers and among household contacts and medical providers. Waterborne transmission (especially that of *C. hominis*) accounts for infections in travelers and for common-source epidemics. Oocysts are quite hardy and resist killing by routine chlorination. Both drinking water and recreational water (e.g., pools, waterslides) have been increasingly recognized as sources of infection.

Pathophysiology

Although intestinal epithelial cells harbor cryptosporidia in an intracellular vacuole, the means by which secretory diarrhea is elicited remain uncertain. No characteristic pathologic changes are found by biopsy. The distribution of infection can be spotty within the principal site of infection, the small bowel. Cryptosporidia are found in the pharynx, stomach, and large bowel of some patients and at times in the respiratory tract. Especially in patients with AIDS, involvement of the biliary tract can cause papillary stenosis, sclerosing cholangitis, or cholecystitis.

Clinical manifestations

Asymptomatic infections can occur in both immunocompetent and immunocompromised hosts. In immunocompetent persons, symptoms develop after an incubation period of ~1 week and consist principally of watery nonbloody diarrhea, sometimes in conjunction with abdominal pain, nausea, anorexia, fever, and/or weight loss. In these hosts, the illness usually subsides after 1–2 weeks. In contrast, in immunocompromised hosts (especially those with AIDS and CD4+ T cell counts <100/μL), diarrhea can be chronic, persistent, and remarkably profuse, causing clinically significant fluid and electrolyte depletion. Stool volumes may range from 1 to 25 L/d. Weight loss, wasting, and abdominal pain may be severe. Biliary tract involvement can manifest as mid-epigastric or right-upper-quadrant pain.

Diagnosis

(Table 34-1) Evaluation starts with fecal examination for small oocysts, which are smaller (4–5 μm in diameter) than the fecal stages of most other parasites. Because conventional stool examination for ova and parasites (O+P) does not detect *Cryptosporidium*, specific testing must be requested. Detection is enhanced by evaluation of stools (obtained on multiple days) by several techniques, including modified acid-fast and direct immunofluorescent stains and enzyme immunoassays. Newer NAATs are being employed. Cryptosporidia can also be identified by light and electron microscopy at the apical surfaces of intestinal epithelium from biopsy specimens of the small bowel and, less frequently, the large bowel.

TREATMENT Cryptosporidiosis

Nitazoxanide, approved by the U.S. Food and Drug Administration (FDA) for the treatment of cryptosporidiosis, is available in tablet form for adults (500 mg twice daily for 3 days) and as an elixir for children. To date, however, this agent has not been effective for the treatment of HIV-infected patients, in whom improved immune status due to antiretroviral therapy can lead to amelioration of cryptosporidiosis. Otherwise, treatment includes supportive care with replacement of fluids and electrolytes and administration of antidiarrheal agents. Biliary tract obstruction may require papillotomy or T-tube placement. Prevention requires minimizing exposure to infectious oocysts in human or animal feces. Use of submicron water filters may minimize acquisition of infection from drinking water.

CYSTOISOSPORIASIS

The coccidian parasite *Cystoisospora belli* causes human intestinal disease. Infection is acquired by the consumption of oocysts, after which the parasite invades intestinal epithelial cells and undergoes both sexual and asexual cycles of development. Oocysts excreted in stool are not immediately infectious but must undergo further maturation.

Although *C. belli* infects many animals, little is known about the epidemiology or prevalence of this parasite in humans. It is most common in tropical and subtropical countries. Acute infections can begin abruptly with fever, abdominal pain, and watery nonbloody diarrhea and can last for weeks or months. In patients who have AIDS or are immunocompromised for other reasons, infections often are not self-limited but rather resemble cryptosporidiosis, with chronic, profuse watery diarrhea. Eosinophilia, which is not found in other enteric protozoan infections, may be detectable. The diagnosis (Table 34-1) is usually made by detection of the large (~25-μm) oocysts in stool by modified acid-fast staining. Oocyst excretion may be low-level and intermittent; if repeated stool examinations are unrevealing, sampling of duodenal contents by aspiration or small-bowel biopsy (often with electron microscopic examination) may be necessary. NAATs are promising newer diagnostic tools.

TREATMENT Cystoisosporiasis

Trimethoprim-sulfamethoxazole (TMP-SMX, 160/800 mg four times daily for 10 days; and for HIV-infected patients, then continuing three times daily for 3 weeks) is effective. For patients intolerant of sulfonamides, pyrimethamine (50–75 mg/d) can be used. Relapses can occur in persons with AIDS and necessitate maintenance therapy with TMP-SMX (160/800 mg three times per week).

CYCLOSPORIASIS

Cyclospora cayetanensis, a cause of diarrheal illness, is globally distributed: illness due to *C. cayetanensis* has been reported in the United States, Asia, Africa, Latin America, and Europe. The epidemiology of this parasite has not yet been fully defined, but waterborne transmission and food-borne transmission (e.g., by basil, sweet peas, and imported raspberries) have been recognized. The full spectrum of illness attributable to *Cyclospora* has not been delineated. Some infected patients may be without symptoms, but many have diarrhea, flulike symptoms, and flatulence and belching. The illness can be self-limited, can wax and wane, or, in many cases, can involve prolonged diarrhea, anorexia, and upper gastrointestinal symptoms, with sustained fatigue and weight loss in some instances. Diarrheal illness may persist for >1 month. *Cyclospora* can cause enteric illness in patients infected with HIV.

The parasite is detectable in epithelial cells of small-bowel biopsy samples and elicits secretory diarrhea by unknown means. The absence of fecal blood and leukocytes indicates that disease due to *Cyclospora* is not caused by destruction of the small-bowel mucosa. The diagnosis (Table 34-1) can be made by detection of spherical 8- to 10-μm oocysts in the stool, although routine stool O+P examinations are not sufficient. Specific fecal examinations must be requested to detect the oocysts, which are variably acid-fast and are fluorescent when viewed with ultraviolet light microscopy. Newer NAATs are proving to be sensitive. Cyclosporiasis should be considered in the differential diagnosis of prolonged diarrhea, with or without a history of travel by the patient to other countries.

TREATMENT Cyclosporiasis

Cyclosporiasis is treated with TMP-SMX (160/800 mg twice daily for 7–10 days). HIV-infected patients may experience relapses after such treatment and thus may require longer-term suppressive maintenance therapy.

MICROSPORIDIOSIS

Microsporidia are obligate intracellular spore-forming protozoa that infect many animals and cause disease in humans, especially as opportunistic pathogens in AIDS. Microsporidia are members of a distinct phylum, Microspora, which contains dozens of genera and hundreds of species. The various microsporidia are differentiated by their developmental life cycles, ultrastructural features, and molecular taxonomy based on ribosomal RNA. The complex life cycles of the organisms result in the production of infectious spores (Fig. 34-3). Currently, eight genera of microsporidia—*Encephalitozoon*, *Pleistophora*, *Nosema*, *Vittaforma*, *Trachipleistophora*, *Anncalia*, *Microsporidium*, and *Enterocytozoon*—are recognized as causes of human disease. Although some microsporidia are probably prevalent causes of self-limited or asymptomatic infections in immunocompetent patients, little is known about how microsporidiosis is acquired.

Microsporidiosis is most common among patients with AIDS, less common among patients with other types of immunocompromise, and rare among immunocompetent hosts. In patients with AIDS, intestinal infections with *Enterocytozoon bieneusi* and *Encephalitozoon* (formerly *Septata*) *intestinalis* are recognized to contribute to chronic diarrhea and wasting; these infections had been found in 10–40% of patients with chronic diarrhea. Both organisms have been found in the biliary tracts of patients with cholecystitis. *E. intestinalis* may also disseminate to cause fever, diarrhea, sinusitis, cholangitis, and bronchiolitis. In patients with AIDS, *Encephalitozoon hellem* has caused superficial keratoconjunctivitis as well as sinusitis, respiratory tract disease, and disseminated infection. Myositis due to *Pleistophora* has been documented.

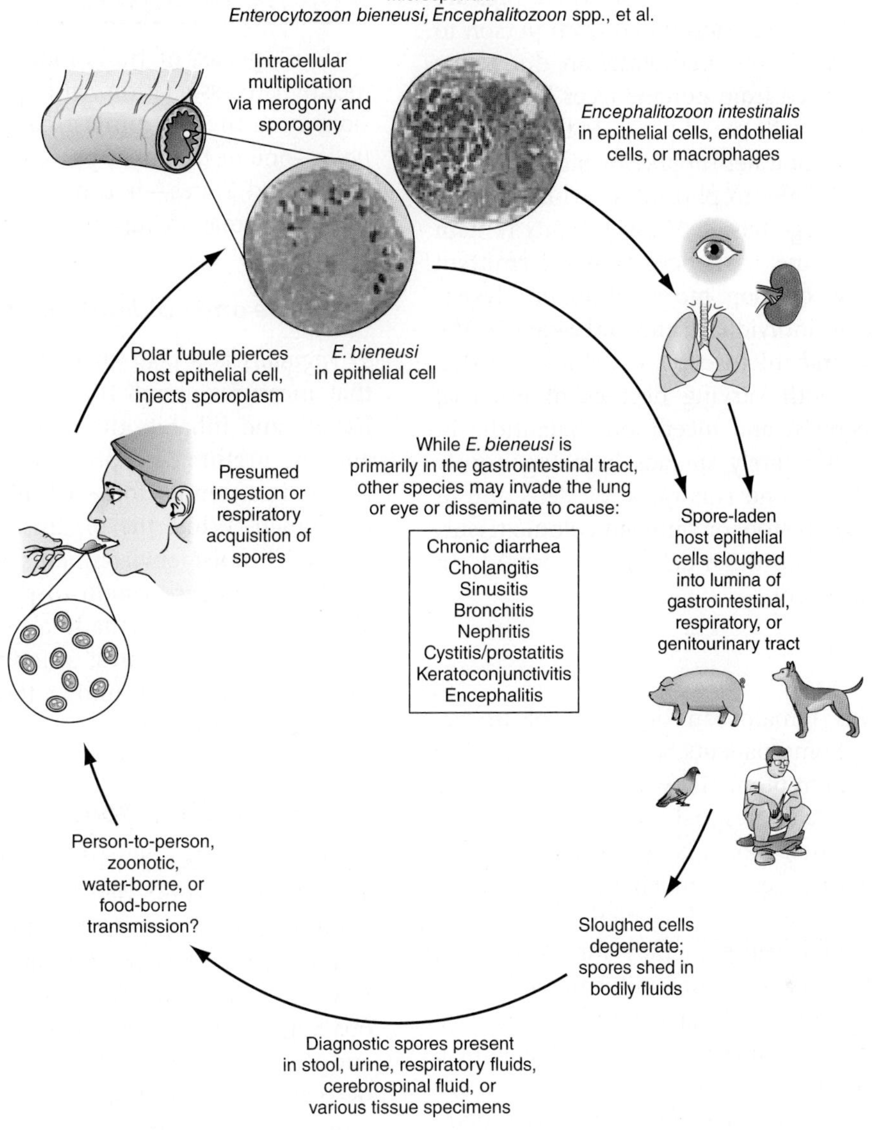
Microsporidia
Enterocytozoon bieneusi, Encephalitozoon spp., et al.
Intracellular multiplication via merogony and sporogony
Encephalitozoon intestinalis in epithelial cells, endothelial cells, or macrophages
Polar tubule pierces host epithelial cell, injects sporoplasm
E. bieneusi in epithelial cell
Presumed ingestion or respiratory acquisition of spores
While *E. bieneusi* is primarily in the gastrointestinal tract, other species may invade the lung or eye or disseminate to cause:
Chronic diarrhea
Cholangitis
Sinusitis
Bronchitis
Nephritis
Cystitis/prostatitis
Keratoconjunctivitis
Encephalitis
Spore-laden host epithelial cells sloughed into lumina of gastrointestinal, respiratory, or genitourinary tract
Person-to-person, zoonotic, water-borne, or food-borne transmission?
Sloughed cells degenerate; spores shed in bodily fluids
Diagnostic spores present in stool, urine, respiratory fluids, cerebrospinal fluid, or various tissue specimens

FIGURE 34-3

Life cycle of microsporidia. *(Reprinted with permission from RL Guerrant et al [eds]: Tropical Infectious Diseases: Principles, Pathogens and Practice, 2nd ed, p 1128. © 2006, with permission from Elsevier Science.)*

Nosema, *Vittaforma*, and *Microsporidium* have caused stromal keratitis associated with trauma in immunocompetent patients.

Microsporidia are small gram-positive organisms with mature spores measuring 0.5–2 μm × 1–4 μm. Diagnosis of microsporidial infections in tissue often requires electron microscopy, although intracellular spores can be visualized by light microscopy with hematoxylin and eosin, Giemsa, or tissue Gram's stain. For the diagnosis of intestinal microsporidiosis, modified trichrome or chromotrope 2R-based staining and Uvitex 2B or calcofluor fluorescent staining reveal spores in smears of feces or duodenal aspirates. Definitive therapies for microsporidial infections remain to be established. For superficial keratoconjunctivitis due to *E. hellem*, topical therapy with fumagillin suspension has shown promise. For enteric infections with *E. bieneusi* and *E. intestinalis* in HIV-infected patients, therapy with albendazole may be efficacious.

OTHER INTESTINAL PROTOZOA

Balantidiasis

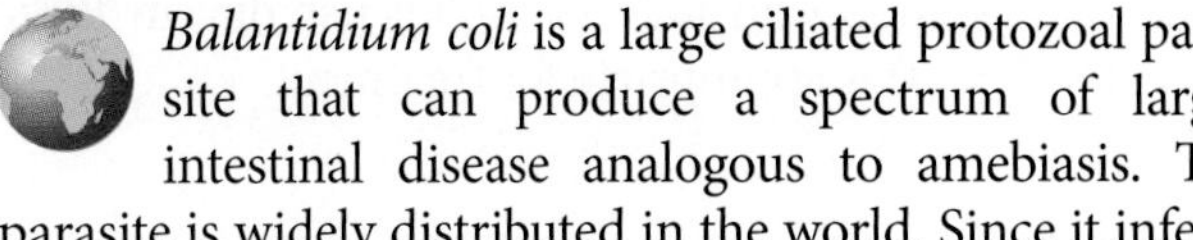

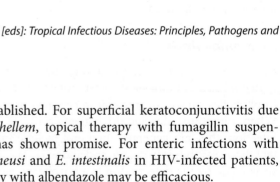

Balantidium coli is a large ciliated protozoal parasite that can produce a spectrum of large-intestinal disease analogous to amebiasis. The parasite is widely distributed in the world. Since it infects pigs, cases in humans are more common where pigs are raised. Infective cysts can be transmitted from person to person and through water, but many cases are due to the ingestion of cysts derived from porcine feces in association with slaughtering, with use of pig feces for fertilizer, or with contamination of water supplies by pig feces.

Ingested cysts liberate trophozoites, which reside and replicate in the large bowel. Many patients remain asymptomatic, but some have persisting intermittent diarrhea, and a few develop more fulminant dysentery. In symptomatic individuals, the pathology in the bowel—both gross and microscopic—is similar to that seen in amebiasis, with varying degrees of mucosal invasion, focal necrosis, and ulceration. Balantidiasis, unlike amebiasis, only rarely spreads hematogenously to other organs. The diagnosis is made by detection of the trophozoite stage in stool or sampled colonic tissue. Tetracycline (500 mg four times daily for 10 days) is an effective therapeutic agent.

Blastocystosis

Blastocystis hominis remains an organism of uncertain pathogenicity. Some patients who pass *B. hominis* in their stools are asymptomatic, whereas others have diarrhea and associated intestinal symptoms. Diligent evaluation reveals other potential bacterial, viral, or protozoal causes of diarrhea in some but not all patients with symptoms. Because the pathogenicity of *B. hominis* is uncertain and because therapy for *Blastocystis* infection is neither specific nor uniformly effective, patients with prominent intestinal symptoms should be fully evaluated for other infectious causes of diarrhea. If diarrheal symptoms associated with *Blastocystis* are prominent, either metronidazole (750 mg thrice daily for 10 days) or TMP-SMX (160 mg/800 mg twice daily for 7 days) can be used.

Dientamoebiasis

Dientamoeba fragilis is unique among intestinal protozoa in that it has a trophozoite stage but not a cyst stage. How trophozoites survive to transmit infection is not known. When symptoms develop in patients with *D. fragilis* infection, they are generally mild and include intermittent diarrhea, abdominal pain, and anorexia. The diagnosis is made by the detection of trophozoites in stool; the lability of these forms accounts for the greater yield when fecal samples are preserved immediately after collection. Since fecal excretion rates vary, examination of several samples obtained on alternate days increases the rate of detection. Iodoquinol (650 mg three times daily for 20 days) or paromomycin (25–35 mg/kg per day in three doses for 7 days) is appropriate for treatment.

TRICHOMONIASIS

Various species of trichomonads can be found in the mouth (in association with periodontitis) and occasionally in the gastrointestinal tract. *Trichomonas vaginalis*—one of the most prevalent protozoal parasites in the United States—is a pathogen of the genitourinary tract and a major cause of symptomatic vaginitis.

Life cycle and epidemiology

T. vaginalis is a pear-shaped, actively motile organism that measures about 10 × 7 μm, replicates by binary fission, and inhabits the lower genital tract of females and the urethra and prostate of males. In the United States, it accounts for ~3 million infections per year in women. While the organism can survive for a few hours in moist environments and could be acquired by direct contact, person-to-person venereal transmission accounts for virtually all cases of trichomoniasis. Its prevalence is greatest among persons with multiple sexual partners and among those with other sexually transmitted diseases.

Clinical manifestations

Many men infected with *T. vaginalis* are asymptomatic, although some develop urethritis and a few have epididymitis or prostatitis. In contrast, infection in women, which has an incubation period of 5–28 days, is usually symptomatic and manifests with malodorous vaginal discharge (often yellow), vulvar erythema and itching, dysuria or urinary frequency (in 30–50% of patients), and dyspareunia. These manifestations, however, do not clearly distinguish trichomoniasis from other types of infectious vaginitis.

Diagnosis

Detection of motile trichomonads by microscopic examination of wet mounts of vaginal or prostatic secretions has been the conventional means of diagnosis. Although this approach provides an immediate diagnosis, its sensitivity for the detection of *T. vaginalis* is only ~50–60% in routine evaluations of vaginal secretions. Direct immunofluorescent antibody staining is more sensitive (70–90%) than wet-mount examinations. *T. vaginalis* can be recovered from the urethra of both males and females and is detectable in males after prostatic massage. A new NAAT, APTIMA, is FDA approved and is highly sensitive and specific for urine and for endocervical and vaginal swabs from women.

TREATMENT Trichomoniasis

Metronidazole (either a single 2-g dose or 500-mg doses twice daily for 7 days) or tinidazole (a single 2-g dose) is effective. All sexual partners must be treated concurrently to prevent reinfection, especially from asymptomatic males. In males with persistent symptomatic urethritis after therapy for nongonococcal urethritis, metronidazole therapy should be considered for possible trichomoniasis. Alternatives to metronidazole for treatment during pregnancy are not readily available. Reinfection often accounts for apparent treatment failures, but strains of *T. vaginalis* exhibiting high-level resistance to metronidazole have been encountered. Treatment of these resistant infections with higher oral doses, parenteral doses, or concurrent oral and vaginal doses of metronidazole or with tinidazole has been successful.

CHAPTER 35

INTESTINAL NEMATODE INFECTIONS

Peter F. Weller ■ Thomas B. Nutman

More than a billion persons worldwide are infected with one or more species of intestinal nematodes. Table 35-1 summarizes biologic and clinical features of infections due to the major intestinal parasitic nematodes. These parasites are most common in regions with poor fecal sanitation, particularly in resource-poor countries in the tropics and subtropics, but they have also been seen with increasing frequency among immigrants and refugees to resource-rich countries. Although nematode infections are not usually fatal, they contribute to malnutrition and diminished work capacity. It is interesting that these helminth infections may protect some individuals from allergic disease. Humans may on occasion be infected with nematode parasites that ordinarily infect animals; these zoonotic infections produce diseases such as trichostrongyliasis, anisakiasis, capillariasis, and abdominal angiostrongyliasis.

Intestinal nematodes are roundworms; they range in length from 1 mm to many centimeters when mature (Table 35-1). Their life cycles are complex and highly varied; some species, including *Strongyloides stercoralis* and *Enterobius vermicularis*, can be transmitted directly from person to person, while others, such as *Ascaris lumbricoides*, *Necator americanus*, and *Ancylostoma duodenale*, require a soil phase for development. Because most helminth parasites do not self-replicate, the acquisition of a heavy burden of adult worms requires repeated exposure to the parasite in its infectious stage, whether larva or egg. Hence, clinical disease, as opposed to asymptomatic infection, generally develops only with prolonged residence in an endemic area and is typically related to infection intensity. In persons with marginal nutrition, intestinal helminth infections may impair growth and development. Eosinophilia and elevated serum IgE levels are features of many helminth infections and, when unexplained, should always prompt a search for intestinal helminths. Significant protective immunity to intestinal nematodes appears not to develop in humans, although mechanisms of parasite immune evasion and host immune responses to these infections have not been elucidated in detail.

ASCARIASIS

A. lumbricoides is the largest intestinal nematode parasite of humans, reaching up to 40 cm in length. Most infected individuals have low worm burdens and are asymptomatic. Clinical disease arises from larval migration in the lungs or effects of the adult worms in the intestines.

Life cycle

Adult worms live in the lumen of the small intestine. Mature female *Ascaris* worms are extraordinarily fecund, each producing up to 240,000 eggs a day, which pass with the feces. Ascarid eggs, which are remarkably resistant to environmental stresses, become infective after several weeks of maturation in the soil and can remain infective for years. After infective eggs are swallowed, larvae hatched in the intestine invade the mucosa, migrate through the circulation to the lungs, break into the alveoli, ascend the bronchial tree, and return—through swallowing—to the small intestine, where they develop into adult worms. Between 2 and 3 months elapse between initial infection and egg production. Adult worms live for 1–2 years.

Epidemiology

Ascaris is widely distributed in tropical and subtropical regions as well as in other humid areas, including the rural southeastern United States. Transmission typically occurs through fecally contaminated soil and is due either to a lack of sanitary facilities or to the use of human feces as fertilizer. With their propensity for hand-to-mouth fecal carriage, younger children are most affected. Infection outside endemic

TABLE 35-1

MAJOR HUMAN INTESTINAL PARASITIC NEMATODES

	PARASITIC NEMATODE				
FEATURE	***ASCARIS LUMBRICOIDES* (ROUNDWORM)**	***NECATOR AMERICANUS, ANCYLOSTOMA DUODENALE* (HOOKWORM)**	***STRONGYLOIDES STERCORALIS***	***TRICHURIS TRICHIURA* (WHIPWORM)**	***ENTEROBIUS VERMICULARIS* (PINWORM)**
Global prevalence in humans (millions)	807	576	100	604	209
Endemic areas	Worldwide	Hot, humid regions	Hot, humid regions	Worldwide	Worldwide
Infective stage	Egg	Filariform larva	Filariform larva	Egg	Egg
Route of infection	Oral	Percutaneous	Percutaneous or autoinfection	Oral	Oral
Gastrointestinal location of worms	Jejunal lumen	Jejunal mucosa	Small-bowel mucosa	Cecum, colonic mucosa	Cecum, appendix
Adult worm size	15–40 cm	7–12 mm	2 mm	30–50 mm	8–13 mm (female)
Pulmonary passage of larvae	Yes	Yes	Yes	No	No
Incubation period[a] (days)	60–75	40–100	17–28	70–90	35–45
Longevity	1 year	*N. americanus*: 2–5 years *A. duodenale*: 6–8 years	Decades (owing to autoinfection)	5 years	2 months
Fecundity (eggs/day/worm)	240,000	*N. americanus*: 4000–10,000 *A. duodenale*: 10,000–25,000	5000–10,000	3000–7000	2000
Principal symptoms	Rarely, biliary obstruction or, in heavy infections, gastrointestinal obstruction	Iron-deficiency anemia in heavy infection	Gastrointestinal symptoms; malabsorption or sepsis in hyperinfection	Gastrointestinal symptoms or anemia in heavy infection	Perianal pruritus
Diagnostic stage	Eggs in stool	Eggs in fresh stool, larvae in old stool	Larvae in stool or duodenal aspirate; sputum in hyperinfection	Eggs in stool	Eggs from perianal skin on cellulose acetate tape
Treatment	Mebendazole Albendazole Ivermectin	Mebendazole Albendazole	Ivermectin Albendazole	Mebendazole Albendazole Ivermectin	Mebendazole Albendazole

[a]Time from infection to egg production by mature female worm.

areas, though uncommon, can occur when eggs on transported vegetables are ingested.

Clinical features

During the lung phase of larval migration, ~9–12 days after egg ingestion, patients may develop an irritating nonproductive cough and burning substernal discomfort that is aggravated by coughing or deep inspiration. Dyspnea and blood-tinged sputum are less common. Fever is usually reported. Eosinophilia develops during this symptomatic phase and subsides slowly over weeks. Chest x-rays may reveal evidence of eosinophilic pneumonitis (Löffler's syndrome), with rounded infiltrates a few millimeters to several centimeters in size. These infiltrates may be transient and intermittent, clearing after several weeks. Where there is seasonal transmission of the parasite, seasonal pneumonitis with eosinophilia may develop in previously infected and sensitized hosts.

In established infections, adult worms in the small intestine usually cause no symptoms. In heavy infections, particularly in children, a large bolus of entangled worms can cause pain and small-bowel obstruction, sometimes complicated by perforation, intussusception, or volvulus. Single worms may cause disease when they migrate into aberrant sites. A large worm can enter and occlude the biliary tree, causing biliary colic, cholecystitis, cholangitis, pancreatitis, or (rarely) intrahepatic abscesses. Migration of an adult worm up the esophagus can provoke coughing and oral expulsion of the worm. In highly endemic areas, intestinal and biliary ascariasis can rival acute appendicitis and gallstones as causes of surgical acute abdomen.

Laboratory findings

Most cases of ascariasis can be diagnosed by microscopic detection of characteristic *Ascaris* eggs (65 by 45 μm) in fecal samples. Occasionally, patients present after passing an adult worm—identifiable by its large size and smooth cream-colored surface—in the stool or, much less commonly, through the mouth or nose. During the early transpulmonary migratory phase, when eosinophilic pneumonitis occurs, larvae can be found in sputum or gastric aspirates before diagnostic eggs appear in the stool. The eosinophilia that is prominent during this early stage usually decreases to minimal levels in established infection. Adult worms may be visualized, occasionally serendipitously, on contrast studies of the gastrointestinal tract. A plain abdominal film may reveal masses of worms in gas-filled loops of bowel in patients with intestinal obstruction. Pancreaticobiliary worms can be detected by ultrasound and endoscopic retrograde cholangiopancreatography; the latter method also has been used to extract biliary *Ascaris* worms.

TREATMENT Ascariasis

Ascariasis should always be treated to prevent potentially serious complications. Albendazole (400 mg once), mebendazole (100 g twice daily for 3 days or 500 mg once), or ivermectin (150–200 μg/kg once) is effective. These medications are contraindicated in pregnancy, however. Mild diarrhea and abdominal pain are uncommon side effects of these agents. Partial intestinal obstruction should be managed with nasogastric suction, IV fluid administration, and instillation of piperazine through the nasogastric tube, but complete obstruction and its severe complications require immediate surgical intervention.

HOOKWORM

Two hookworm species (*A. duodenale* and *N. americanus*) are responsible for human infections. Most infected individuals are asymptomatic. Hookworm disease develops from a combination of factors—a heavy worm burden, a prolonged duration of infection, and an inadequate iron intake—and results in iron-deficiency anemia and, on occasion, hypoproteinemia.

Life cycle

Adult hookworms, which are ~1 cm long, use buccal teeth (*Ancylostoma*) or cutting plates (*Necator*) to attach to the small-bowel mucosa and suck blood (0.2 mL/d per *Ancylostoma* adult) and interstitial fluid. The adult hookworms produce thousands of eggs daily. The eggs are deposited with feces in soil, where rhabditiform larvae hatch and develop over a 1-week period into infectious filariform larvae. Infective larvae penetrate the skin and reach the lungs by way of the bloodstream. There they invade alveoli and ascend the airways before being swallowed and reaching the small intestine. The prepatent period from skin invasion to appearance of eggs in the feces is ~6–8 weeks, but it may be longer with *A. duodenale*. Larvae of *A. duodenale*, if swallowed, can survive and develop directly in the intestinal mucosa. Adult hookworms may survive over a decade but usually live ~6–8 years for *A. duodenale* and 2–5 years for *N. americanus*.

Epidemiology

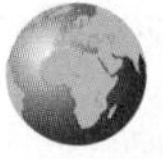

A. duodenale is prevalent in southern Europe, North Africa, and northern Asia, and *N. americanus* is the predominant species in the Western Hemisphere and equatorial Africa. The two species overlap in many tropical regions, particularly Southeast Asia. In most areas, older children have the highest incidence and greatest intensity of hookworm infection. In rural areas where fields are fertilized with human feces, older working adults also may be heavily infected.

Clinical features

Most hookworm infections are asymptomatic. Infective larvae may provoke pruritic maculopapular dermatitis ("ground itch") at the site of skin penetration as well as serpiginous tracks of subcutaneous migration (similar to those of cutaneous larva migrans; in previously sensitized hosts. Larvae migrating through the lungs occasionally cause mild transient pneumonitis, but this condition develops less frequently in hookworm infection than in ascariasis. In the early intestinal phase, infected persons may develop epigastric pain (often with postprandial accentuation), inflammatory diarrhea, or other abdominal symptoms accompanied by eosinophilia. The major consequence of chronic hookworm infection is iron deficiency. Symptoms are minimal if iron intake is adequate, but marginally nourished individuals develop symptoms of progressive iron-deficiency anemia and hypoproteinemia, including weakness and shortness of breath.

Laboratory findings

The diagnosis is established by the finding of characteristic 40- by 60-μm oval hookworm eggs in the feces.

Stool-concentration procedures may be required to detect light infections. Eggs of the two species are indistinguishable by light microscopy. In a stool sample that is not fresh, the eggs may have hatched to release rhabditiform larvae, which need to be differentiated from those of *S. stercoralis*. Hypochromic microcytic anemia, occasionally with eosinophilia or hypoalbuminemia, is characteristic of hookworm disease.

TREATMENT Hookworm Infection

Hookworm infection can be eradicated with several safe and highly effective anthelmintic drugs, including albendazole (400 mg once) and mebendazole (500 mg once). Mild iron-deficiency anemia can often be treated with oral iron alone. Severe hookworm disease with protein loss and malabsorption necessitates nutritional support and oral iron replacement along with deworming. There is some concern that the benzimidazoles (mebendazole and albendazole) are becoming less effective against human hookworms.

Ancylostoma caninum and Ancylostoma braziliense

A. caninum, the canine hookworm, has been identified as a cause of human eosinophilic enteritis, especially in northeastern Australia. In this zoonotic infection, adult hookworms attach to the small intestine (where they may be visualized by endoscopy) and elicit abdominal pain and intense local eosinophilia. Treatment with mebendazole (100 mg twice daily for 3 days) or albendazole (400 mg once) or endoscopic removal is effective. Both of these animal hookworm species can cause cutaneous larva migrans ("creeping eruption").

STRONGYLOIDIASIS

S. stercoralis is distinguished by its ability—unique among helminths (except for *Capillaria*; see below)—to replicate in the human host. This capacity permits ongoing cycles of autoinfection as infective larvae are internally produced. Strongyloidiasis can thus persist for decades without further exposure of the host to exogenous infective larvae. In immunocompromised hosts, large numbers of invasive *Strongyloides* larvae can disseminate widely and can be fatal.

Life cycle

In addition to a parasitic cycle of development, *Strongyloides* can undergo a free-living cycle of development in the soil (Fig. 35-1). This adaptability facilitates the parasite's survival in the absence of mammalian hosts. Rhabditiform larvae passed in feces can transform into infectious filariform larvae either directly or after a free-living phase of development. Humans acquire strongyloidiasis when filariform larvae in fecally contaminated soil penetrate the skin or mucous membranes. The larvae then travel through the bloodstream to the lungs, where they break into the alveolar spaces, ascend the bronchial tree, are swallowed, and thereby reach the small intestine. There the larvae mature into adult worms that penetrate the mucosa of the proximal small bowel. The minute (2-mm-long) parasitic adult female worms reproduce by parthenogenesis; adult males do not exist. Eggs hatch in the intestinal mucosa, releasing rhabditiform larvae that migrate to the lumen and pass with the feces into soil. Alternatively, rhabditiform larvae in the bowel can develop directly into filariform larvae that penetrate the colonic wall or perianal skin and enter the circulation to repeat the migration that establishes ongoing internal reinfection. This autoinfection cycle allows strongyloidiasis to persist for decades.

Epidemiology

S. stercoralis is spottily distributed in tropical areas and other hot, humid regions and is particularly common in Southeast Asia, sub-Saharan Africa, and Brazil. In the United States, the parasite is endemic in parts of the Southeast and is found in immigrants, refugees, travelers, and military personnel who have lived in endemic areas.

Clinical features

In uncomplicated strongyloidiasis, many patients are asymptomatic or have mild cutaneous and/or abdominal symptoms. Recurrent urticaria, often involving the buttocks and wrists, is the most common cutaneous manifestation. Migrating larvae can elicit a pathognomonic serpiginous eruption, *larva currens* ("running larva"). This pruritic, raised, erythematous lesion advances as rapidly as 10 cm/h along the course of larval migration. Adult parasites burrow into the duodenojejunal mucosa and can cause abdominal (usually midepigastric) pain, which resembles peptic ulcer pain except that it is aggravated by food ingestion. Nausea, diarrhea, gastrointestinal bleeding, mild chronic colitis, and weight loss can occur. Small-bowel obstruction may develop with early, heavy infection. Pulmonary symptoms are rare in uncomplicated strongyloidiasis. Eosinophilia is common, with levels fluctuating over time.

The ongoing autoinfection cycle of strongyloidiasis is normally constrained by unknown factors of the host's immune system. Abrogation of host immunity, especially with glucocorticoid therapy and much less commonly with other immunosuppressive medications, leads to

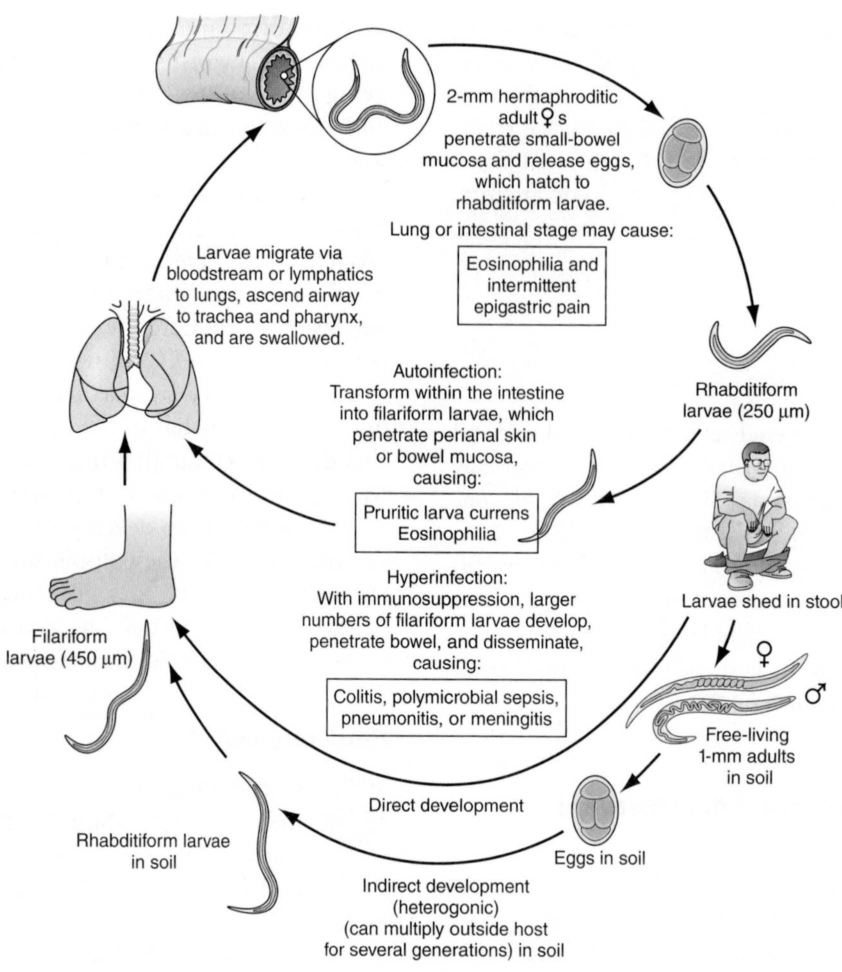

FIGURE 35-1

Life cycle of *Strongyloides stercoralis.* *(Adapted from Guerrant RL et al [eds]: Tropical Infectious Diseases: Principles, Pathogens and Practice, 2nd ed, p 1276. © 2006, with permission from Elsevier Science.)*

hyperinfection, with the generation of large numbers of filariform larvae. Colitis, enteritis, or malabsorption may develop. In disseminated strongyloidiasis, larvae may invade not only gastrointestinal tissues and the lungs but also the central nervous system, peritoneum, liver, and kidneys. Moreover, bacteremia may develop because of the passage of enteric flora through disrupted mucosal barriers. Gram-negative sepsis, pneumonia, or meningitis may complicate or dominate the clinical course. Eosinophilia is often absent in severely infected patients. Disseminated strongyloidiasis, particularly in patients with unsuspected infection who are given glucocorticoids, can be fatal. Strongyloidiasis is a frequent complication of infection with human T cell lymphotropic virus type 1, but disseminated strongyloidiasis is not common among patients infected with HIV-1.

Diagnosis

In uncomplicated strongyloidiasis, the finding of rhabditiform larvae in feces is diagnostic. Rhabditiform larvae are ~250 μm long, with a short buccal cavity that distinguishes them from hookworm larvae. In uncomplicated infections, few larvae are passed and single stool examinations detect only about one-third of cases. Serial examinations and the use of the agar plate detection method improve the sensitivity of stool diagnosis. In uncomplicated strongyloidiasis (but not in hyperinfection), stool examinations may be repeatedly negative. *Strongyloides* larvae may also be found by sampling of the duodenojejunal contents by aspiration or biopsy. An enzyme-linked immunosorbent assay for serum antibodies to antigens of *Strongyloides* is a sensitive method for diagnosing uncomplicated infections. Such serologic testing should be performed for patients whose geographic histories indicate potential exposure, especially those who exhibit eosinophilia and/or are candidates for glucocorticoid treatment of other conditions. In disseminated strongyloidiasis, filariform larvae should be sought in stool as well as in samples obtained from sites of potential larval migration, including sputum, bronchoalveolar lavage fluid, or surgical drainage fluid.

TREATMENT Strongyloidiasis

Even in the asymptomatic state, strongyloidiasis must be treated because of the potential for subsequent dissemination and fatal hyperinfection. Ivermectin (200 μg/kg daily for 2 days) is consistently more effective than albendazole (400 mg daily for 3 days). For disseminated strongyloidiasis, treatment with ivermectin should be extended for at least 5–7 days or until the parasites have been eradicated. In immunocompromised hosts, the course of ivermectin should be repeated 2 weeks after initial treatment.

TRICHURIASIS

Most infections with *Trichuris trichiura* are asymptomatic, but heavy infections may cause gastrointestinal symptoms. Like the other soil-transmitted helminths, whipworm is distributed globally in the tropics and subtropics and is most common among poor children from resource-poor regions of the world.

Life cycle

Adult *Trichuris* worms reside in the colon and cecum, the anterior portions threaded into the superficial mucosa. Thousands of eggs laid daily by adult female worms pass with the feces and mature in the soil. After ingestion, infective eggs hatch in the duodenum, releasing larvae that mature before migrating to the large bowel. The entire cycle takes ~3 months, and adult worms may live for several years.

Clinical features

Tissue reactions to *Trichuris* are mild. Most infected individuals have no symptoms or eosinophilia. Heavy infections may result in anemia, abdominal pain, anorexia, and bloody or mucoid diarrhea resembling inflammatory bowel disease. Rectal prolapse can result from massive infections in children, who often suffer from malnourishment and other diarrheal illnesses. Moderately heavy *Trichuris* burdens also contribute to growth retardation.

Diagnosis and treatment

The characteristic 50- by 20-μm lemon-shaped *Trichuris* eggs are readily detected on stool examination. Adult worms, which are 3–5 cm long, are occasionally seen on proctoscopy. Mebendazole (500 mg once) or albendazole (400 mg daily for 3 doses) is safe and moderately effective for treatment, with cure rates of 70–90%. Ivermectin (200 μg/kg daily for 3 doses) is also safe but is not quite as efficacious as the benzimidazoles.

ENTEROBIASIS (PINWORM)

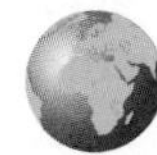

E. vermicularis is more common in temperate countries than in the tropics. In the United States, ~40 million persons are infected with pinworms, with a disproportionate number of cases among children.

Life cycle and epidemiology

Enterobius adult worms are ~1 cm long and dwell in the cecum. Gravid female worms migrate nocturnally into the perianal region and release up to 2000 immature eggs each. The eggs become infective within hours and are transmitted by hand-to-mouth passage. From ingested eggs, larvae hatch and mature into adults. This life cycle takes ~1 month, and adult worms survive for ~2 months. Self-infection results from perianal scratching and transport of infective eggs on the hands or under the nails to the mouth. Because of the ease of person-to-person spread, pinworm infections are common among family members.

Clinical features

Most pinworm infections are asymptomatic. Perianal pruritus is the cardinal symptom. The itching, which is often worse at night as a result of the nocturnal migration of the female worms, may lead to excoriation and bacterial superinfection. Heavy infections have been alleged to cause abdominal pain and weight loss. On rare occasions, pinworms invade the female genital tract, causing vulvovaginitis and pelvic or peritoneal granulomas. Eosinophilia is uncommon.

Diagnosis

Since pinworm eggs are not released in feces, the diagnosis cannot be made by conventional fecal ova and parasite tests. Instead, eggs are detected by the application of clear cellulose acetate tape to the perianal region in the morning. After the tape is transferred to a slide, microscopic examination will detect pinworm eggs, which are oval, measure 55 by 25 μm, and are flattened along one side.

TREATMENT Enterobiasis

Infected children and adults should be treated with mebendazole (100 mg once) or albendazole (400 mg once), with the same treatment repeated after 2 weeks. Treatment of household members is advocated to eliminate asymptomatic reservoirs of potential reinfection.

TRICHOSTRONGYLIASIS

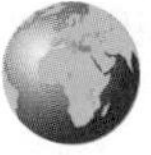

Trichostrongylus species, which are normally parasites of herbivorous animals, occasionally infect humans, particularly in Asia and Africa.

Humans acquire the infection by accidentally ingesting *Trichostrongylus* larvae on contaminated leafy vegetables. The larvae do not migrate in humans but mature directly into adult worms in the small bowel. These worms ingest far less blood than hookworms; most infected persons are asymptomatic, but heavy infections may give rise to mild anemia and eosinophilia. In stool examinations, *Trichostrongylus* eggs resemble hookworm eggs but are larger (85 by 115 μm). Treatment consists of mebendazole or albendazole.

ANISAKIASIS

Anisakiasis is a gastrointestinal infection caused by the accidental ingestion in uncooked saltwater fish of nematode larvae belonging to the family Anisakidae. The incidence of anisakiasis in the United States has increased as a result of the growing popularity of raw fish dishes. Most cases occur in Japan, the Netherlands, and Chile, where raw fish—sashimi, pickled green herring, and ceviche, respectively—are national culinary staples. Anisakid nematodes parasitize large sea mammals such as whales, dolphins, and seals. As part of a complex parasitic life cycle involving marine food chains, infectious larvae migrate to the musculature of a variety of fish. Both *Anisakis simplex* and *Pseudoterranova decipiens* have been implicated in human anisakiasis, but an identical gastric syndrome may be caused by the red larvae of eustrongylid parasites of fish-eating birds.

When humans consume infected raw fish, live larvae may be coughed up within 48 h. Alternatively, larvae may immediately penetrate the mucosa of the stomach. Within hours, violent upper abdominal pain accompanied by nausea and occasionally vomiting ensues, mimicking an acute abdomen. The diagnosis can be established by direct visualization on upper endoscopy, outlining of the worm by contrast radiographic studies, or histopathologic examination of extracted tissue. Extraction of the burrowing larvae during endoscopy is curative. In addition, larvae may pass to the small bowel, where they penetrate the mucosa and provoke a vigorous eosinophilic granulomatous response. Symptoms may appear 1–2 weeks after the infective meal, with intermittent abdominal pain, diarrhea, nausea, and fever resembling the manifestations of Crohn's disease. The diagnosis may be suggested by barium studies and confirmed by curative surgical resection of a granuloma in which the worm is embedded. Anisakid eggs are not found in the stool, since the larvae do not mature in humans. Serologic tests have been developed but are not widely available.

Anisakid larvae in saltwater fish are killed by cooking to 60°C, freezing at -20°C for 3 days, or commercial blast freezing, but usually not by salting, marinating, or cold smoking. No medical treatment is available; surgical or endoscopic removal should be undertaken.

CAPILLARIASIS

Intestinal capillariasis is caused by ingestion of raw fish infected with *Capillaria philippinensis*. Subsequent autoinfection can lead to a severe wasting syndrome. The disease occurs in the Philippines and Thailand and, on occasion, elsewhere in Asia. The natural cycle of *C. philippinensis* involves fish from fresh and brackish water. When humans eat infected raw fish, the larvae mature in the intestine into adult worms, which produce invasive larvae that cause intestinal inflammation and villus loss. Capillariasis has an insidious onset with nonspecific abdominal pain and watery diarrhea. If untreated, progressive autoinfection can lead to protein-losing enteropathy, severe malabsorption, and ultimately death from cachexia, cardiac failure, or superinfection. The diagnosis is established by identification of the characteristic peanut-shaped (20- by 40-μm) eggs on stool examination. Severely ill patients require hospitalization and supportive therapy in addition to prolonged anthelmintic treatment with albendazole (200 mg twice daily for 10 days.

ABDOMINAL ANGIOSTRONGYLIASIS

Abdominal angiostrongyliasis is found in Latin America and Africa. The zoonotic parasite *Angiostrongylus costaricensis* causes eosinophilic ileocolitis after the ingestion of contaminated vegetation. *A. costaricensis* normally parasitizes the cotton rat and other rodents, with slugs and snails serving as intermediate hosts. Humans become infected by accidentally ingesting infective larvae in mollusk slime deposited on fruits and vegetables; children are at highest risk. The larvae penetrate the gut wall and migrate to the mesenteric artery, where they develop into adult worms. Eggs deposited in the gut wall provoke an intense eosinophilic granulomatous reaction, and adult worms may cause mesenteric arteritis, thrombosis, or frank bowel infarction. Symptoms may mimic those of appendicitis, including abdominal pain and tenderness, fever, vomiting, and a palpable mass in the right iliac fossa. Leukocytosis and eosinophilia are prominent. CT with contrast medium typically shows inflamed bowel, often with concomitant obstruction, but a definitive diagnosis is usually made surgically with partial bowel resection. Pathologic study reveals a thickened bowel wall with eosinophilic granulomas surrounding the *Angiostrongylus* eggs. In nonsurgical cases, the diagnosis rests solely on clinical grounds because larvae and eggs cannot be detected in the stool. Medical therapy for abdominal angiostrongyliasis is of uncertain efficacy. Careful observation and surgical resection for severe symptoms are the mainstays of treatment.

SECTION V

EVALUATION OF THE PATIENT WITH LIVER DISEASE

CHAPTER 36

APPROACH TO THE PATIENT WITH LIVER DISEASE

Marc G. Ghany ■ Jay H. Hoofnagle

A diagnosis of liver disease usually can be made accurately by careful elicitation of the patient's history, physical examination, and application of a few laboratory tests. In some circumstances, radiologic examinations are helpful or, indeed, diagnostic. Liver biopsy is considered the criterion standard in evaluation of liver disease but is now needed less for diagnosis than for grading and staging of disease. This chapter provides an introduction to diagnosis and management of liver disease, briefly reviewing the structure and function of the liver; the major clinical manifestations of liver disease; and the use of clinical history, physical examination, laboratory tests, imaging studies, and liver biopsy.

LIVER STRUCTURE AND FUNCTION

The liver is the largest organ of the body, weighing 1–1.5 kg and representing 1.5–2.5% of the lean body mass. The size and shape of the liver vary and generally match the general body shape—long and lean or squat and square. This organ is located in the right upper quadrant of the abdomen under the right lower rib cage against the diaphragm and projects for a variable extent into the left upper quadrant. It is held in place by ligamentous attachments to the diaphragm, peritoneum, great vessels, and upper gastrointestinal organs. The liver receives a dual blood supply; ~20% of the blood flow is oxygen-rich blood from the hepatic artery, and 80% is nutrient-rich blood from the portal vein arising from the stomach, intestines, pancreas, and spleen.

The majority of cells in the liver are hepatocytes, which constitute two-thirds of the organ's mass. The remaining cell types are Kupffer cells (members of the reticuloendothelial system), stellate (Ito or fat-storing) cells, endothelial and blood vessel cells, bile ductular cells, and cells of supporting structures. Viewed by light microscopy, the liver appears to be organized in lobules, with portal areas at the periphery and central veins in the center of each lobule. However, from a functional point of view, the liver is organized into acini, with both hepatic arterial and portal venous blood entering the acinus from the portal areas (zone 1) and then flowing through the sinusoids to the terminal hepatic veins (zone 3); the intervening hepatocytes constitute zone 2. The advantage of viewing the acinus as the physiologic unit of the liver is that this perspective helps to explain the morphologic patterns and zonality of many vascular and biliary diseases not explained by the lobular arrangement.

Portal areas of the liver consist of small veins, arteries, bile ducts, and lymphatics organized in a loose stroma of supporting matrix and small amounts of collagen. Blood flowing into the portal areas is distributed through the sinusoids, passing from zone 1 to zone 3 of the acinus and draining into the terminal hepatic veins ("central veins"). Secreted bile flows in the opposite direction—i.e., in a counter-current pattern from zone 3 to zone 1. The sinusoids are lined by unique endothelial cells that have prominent fenestrae of variable sizes, allowing the free flow of plasma but not of cellular elements. The plasma is thus in direct contact with hepatocytes in the subendothelial space of Disse.

Hepatocytes have distinct polarity. The basolateral side of the hepatocyte lines the space of Disse and is richly lined with microvilli; it exhibits endocytotic and pinocytotic activity, with passive and active uptake of nutrients, proteins, and other molecules. The apical pole of the hepatocyte forms the canalicular membranes through which bile components are secreted. The canaliculi of hepatocytes form a fine network, which fuses into the bile ductular elements near the portal areas. Kupffer cells usually lie within the sinusoidal vascular space and represent the largest group of fixed macrophages in the body. The stellate cells are located in the space of Disse but are not usually prominent unless activated, when they produce collagen and matrix. Red blood cells stay in the sinusoidal space as blood flows through the lobules, but white blood cells can migrate through or around endothelial cells into the space of Disse and from there to portal areas, where they can return to the circulation through lymphatics.

Hepatocytes perform numerous and vital roles in maintaining homeostasis and health. These functions include the synthesis of most essential serum proteins (albumin, carrier proteins, coagulation factors, many hormonal and growth factors), the production of bile and its carriers (bile acids, cholesterol, lecithin, phospholipids), the regulation of nutrients (glucose, glycogen, lipids, cholesterol, amino acids), and the metabolism and conjugation of lipophilic compounds (bilirubin, anions, cations, drugs) for excretion in the bile or urine. Measurement of these activities to assess liver function is complicated by the multiplicity and variability of these functions. The most commonly used liver "function" tests are measurements of serum bilirubin, serum albumin, and prothrombin time. The serum bilirubin level is a measure of hepatic conjugation and excretion; the serum albumin level and prothrombin time are measures of protein synthesis. Abnormalities of bilirubin, albumin, and prothrombin time are typical of hepatic dysfunction. Frank liver failure is incompatible with life, and the functions of the liver are too complex and diverse to be subserved by a mechanical pump; a dialysis membrane; or a concoction of infused hormones, proteins, and growth factors.

LIVER DISEASES

While there are many causes of liver disease (Table 36-1), these disorders generally present clinically in a few distinct patterns and are usually classified as hepatocellular,

TABLE 36-1

LIVER DISEASES

Inherited hyperbilirubinemia	**Liver involvement in systemic diseases**
Gilbert's syndrome	Sarcoidosis
Crigler-Najjar syndrome, types I and II	Amyloidosis
Dubin-Johnson syndrome	Glycogen storage diseases
Rotor syndrome	Celiac disease
Viral hepatitis	Tuberculosis
Hepatitis A	*Mycobacterium avium-intracellulare* infection
Hepatitis B	**Cholestatic syndromes**
Hepatitis C	Benign postoperative cholestasis
Hepatitis D	Jaundice of sepsis
Hepatitis E	Total parenteral nutrition–induced jaundice
Others (Epstein-Barr virus [mononucleosis] herpesvirus, adenovirus hepatitis)	Cholestasis of pregnancy
Cryptogenic hepatitis	Cholangitis and cholecystitis
Immune and autoimmune liver diseases	Extrahepatic biliary obstruction (stone, stricture, cancer)
Primary biliary cirrhosis	Biliary atresia
Autoimmune hepatitis	Caroli's disease
Sclerosing cholangitis	Cryptosporidiosis
Overlap syndromes	**Drug-induced liver disease**
Graft-versus-host disease	Hepatocellular patterns (isoniazid, acetaminophen)
Allograft rejection	Cholestatic patterns (methyltestosterone)
Genetic liver diseases	Mixed patterns (sulfonamides, phenytoin)
α_1 Antitrypsin deficiency	Micro- and macrovesicular steatosis (methotrexate, fialuridine)
Hemochromatosis	**Vascular injury**
Wilson's disease	Veno-occlusive disease
Benign recurrent intrahepatic cholestasis	Budd-Chiari syndrome
Progressive familial intrahepatic cholestasis, types I–III	Ischemic hepatitis
Others (galactosemia, tyrosinemia, cystic fibrosis, Newman-Pick disease, Gaucher's disease)	Passive congestion
Alcoholic liver disease	Portal vein thrombosis
Acute fatty liver	Nodular regenerative hyperplasia
Acute alcoholic hepatitis	**Mass lesions**
Laënnec's cirrhosis	Hepatocellular carcinoma
Nonalcoholic fatty liver	Cholangiocarcinoma
Steatosis	Adenoma
Steatohepatitis	Focal nodular hyperplasia
Acute fatty liver of pregnancy	Metastatic tumors
	Abscess
	Cysts
	Hemangioma

cholestatic (obstructive), or mixed. In *hepatocellular diseases* (such as viral hepatitis and alcoholic liver disease), features of liver injury, inflammation, and necrosis predominate. In *cholestatic diseases* (such as gallstone or malignant obstruction, primary biliary cirrhosis, and some drug-induced liver diseases), features of inhibition of bile flow predominate. In a mixed pattern, features of both hepatocellular and cholestatic injury are present (such as in cholestatic forms of viral hepatitis and many drug-induced liver diseases). The pattern of onset and prominence of symptoms can rapidly suggest a diagnosis, particularly if major risk factors are considered, such as the age and sex of the patient and a history of exposure or risk behaviors.

Typical presenting symptoms of liver disease include jaundice, fatigue, itching, right-upper-quadrant pain, nausea, poor appetite, abdominal distention, and intestinal bleeding. At present, however, many patients are diagnosed with liver disease who have no symptoms and who have been found to have abnormalities in biochemical liver tests as a part of a routine physical examination or screening for blood donation or for insurance or employment. The wide availability of batteries of liver tests makes it relatively simple to demonstrate the presence of liver injury as well as to rule it out in someone in whom liver disease is suspected.

Evaluation of patients with liver disease should be directed at (1) establishing the etiologic diagnosis, (2) estimating disease severity (*grading*), and (3) establishing the disease stage (*staging*). *Diagnosis* should focus on the category of disease (hepatocellular, cholestatic, or mixed injury) as well as on the specific etiologic diagnosis. *Grading* refers to assessment of the severity or activity of disease—active or inactive as well as mild, moderate, or severe. *Staging* refers to estimation of the point in the course of the natural history of the disease, whether early or late; or precirrhotic, cirrhotic, or end-stage. This chapter introduces general, salient concepts in the evaluation of patients with liver disease that help lead to the diagnoses discussed in subsequent chapters.

CLINICAL HISTORY

The clinical history should focus on the symptoms of liver disease—their nature, patterns of onset, and progression—and on potential risk factors for liver disease. The manifestations of liver disease include constitutional symptoms such as fatigue, weakness, nausea, poor appetite, and malaise and the more liver-specific symptoms of jaundice, dark urine, light stools, itching, abdominal pain, and bloating. Symptoms can also suggest the presence of cirrhosis, end-stage liver disease, or complications of cirrhosis such as portal hypertension. Generally, the constellation of symptoms and their patterns of onset rather than a specific symptom points to an etiology.

Fatigue is the most common and most characteristic symptom of liver disease. It is variously described as lethargy, weakness, listlessness, malaise, increased need for sleep, lack of stamina, and poor energy. The fatigue of liver disease typically arises after activity or exercise and is rarely present or severe after adequate rest; i.e., it is "afternoon" rather than "morning" fatigue. Fatigue in liver disease is often intermittent and variable in severity from hour to hour and day to day. In some patients, it may not be clear whether fatigue is due to the liver disease or to other problems such as stress, anxiety, sleep disturbance, or a concurrent illness.

Nausea occurs with more severe liver disease and may accompany fatigue or be provoked by smelling food odors or eating fatty foods. Vomiting can occur but is rarely persistent or prominent. Poor appetite with weight loss occurs frequently in acute liver disease but is rare in chronic disease except when cirrhosis is present and advanced. Diarrhea is uncommon in liver disease except with severe jaundice, in which a lack of bile acids reaching the intestine can lead to steatorrhea.

Right-upper-quadrant discomfort or ache ("liver pain") occurs in many liver diseases and is usually marked by tenderness over the liver area. The pain arises from stretching or irritation of Glisson's capsule, which surrounds the liver and is rich in nerve endings. Severe pain is most typical of gallbladder disease, liver abscess, and severe veno-occlusive disease but is also an occasional accompaniment of acute hepatitis.

Itching occurs with acute liver disease, appearing early in obstructive jaundice (from biliary obstruction or drug-induced cholestasis) and somewhat later in hepatocellular disease (acute hepatitis). Itching also occurs in chronic liver diseases—typically the cholestatic forms such as primary biliary cirrhosis and sclerosing cholangitis, in which it is often the presenting symptom, preceding the onset of jaundice. However, itching can occur in any liver disease, particularly once cirrhosis develops.

Jaundice is the hallmark symptom of liver disease and perhaps the most reliable marker of severity. Patients usually report darkening of the urine before they notice scleral icterus. Jaundice is rarely detectable with a bilirubin level <43 μmol/L (2.5 mg/dL). With severe cholestasis, there will also be lightening of the color of the stools and steatorrhea. Jaundice without dark urine usually indicates indirect (unconjugated) hyperbilirubinemia and is typical of hemolytic anemia and the genetic disorders of bilirubin conjugation, the common and benign form being Gilbert's syndrome and the rare and severe form being Crigler-Najjar syndrome. Gilbert's syndrome affects up to 5% of the general population; the jaundice in this condition is more noticeable after fasting and with stress.

Major risk factors for liver disease that should be sought in the clinical history include details of alcohol use, medication use (including herbal compounds, birth control pills, and over-the-counter medications), personal habits, sexual activity, travel, exposure to jaundiced or other high-risk persons, injection drug use, recent surgery, remote or recent transfusion of blood or blood products, occupation, accidental exposure to blood or needlestick, and familial history of liver disease.

For assessing the risk of viral hepatitis, a careful history of sexual activity is of particular importance and should include the number of lifetime sexual partners and, for men, a history of having sex with men. Sexual exposure is a common mode of spread of hepatitis B but is rare for hepatitis C. A family history of hepatitis, liver disease, and liver cancer is also important. Maternal-infant transmission occurs with both hepatitis B and C. Vertical spread of hepatitis B can now be prevented by passive and active immunization of the infant at birth. Vertical spread of hepatitis C is uncommon, but there are no reliable means of prevention. Transmission is more common among HIV-co-infected mothers and is also linked to prolonged and difficult labor and delivery, early rupture of membranes, and internal fetal monitoring. A history of injection drug use, even in the remote past, is of great importance in assessing the risk for hepatitis B and C. Injection drug use is now the single most common risk factor for hepatitis C. Transfusion with blood or blood products is no longer an important risk factor for acute viral hepatitis. However, blood transfusions received before the introduction of sensitive enzyme immunoassays for antibody to hepatitis C virus in 1992 is an important risk factor for chronic hepatitis C. Blood transfusion before 1986, when screening for antibody to hepatitis B core antigen was introduced, is also a risk factor for hepatitis B. Travel to a developing area of the world, exposure to persons with jaundice, and exposure to young children in day-care centers are risk factors for hepatitis A. Tattooing and body piercing (for hepatitis B and C) and eating shellfish (for hepatitis A) are frequently mentioned but are actually types of exposure that quite rarely lead to the acquisition of hepatitis.

Hepatitis E is one of the more common causes of jaundice in Asia and Africa but is uncommon in developed nations. Recently, non-travel-related (*autochthonous*) cases of hepatitis E have been described in developed countries, including the United States. These cases appear to be due to strains of hepatitis E virus that are endemic in swine and some wild animals (genotypes 3 and 4). While occasional cases are associated with eating raw or undercooked pork or game (deer and wild boars), most cases of hepatitis E occur without known exposure, predominantly in elderly man without typical risk factors for viral hepatitis. Hepatitis E infection can become chronic in immunosuppressed individuals (such as transplant recipients, patients receiving chemotherapy, or patients with HIV infection), in whom it presents with abnormal serum enzymes in the absence of markers of hepatitis B or C.

A history of alcohol intake is important in assessing the cause of liver disease and also in planning management and recommendations. In the United States, for example, at least 70% of adults drink alcohol to some degree, but significant alcohol intake is less common; in population-based surveys, only 5% of individuals have more than two drinks per day, the average drink representing 11–15 g of alcohol. Alcohol consumption associated with an increased rate of alcoholic liver disease is probably more than two drinks (22–30 g) per day in women and three drinks (33–45 g) in men. Most patients with alcoholic cirrhosis have a much higher daily intake and have drunk excessively for ≥10 years before onset of liver disease. In assessing alcohol intake, the history should also focus on whether alcohol abuse or dependence is present. Alcoholism is usually defined by the behavioral patterns and consequences of alcohol intake, not by the amount. *Abuse* is defined by a repetitive pattern of drinking alcohol that has adverse effects on social, family, occupational, or health status. *Dependence* is defined by alcohol-seeking behavior, despite its adverse effects. Many alcoholics demonstrate both dependence and abuse, and dependence is considered the more serious and advanced form of alcoholism. A clinically helpful approach to diagnosis of alcohol dependence and abuse is the use of the CAGE questionnaire (Table 36-2), which is recommended for all medical history-taking.

Family history can be helpful in assessing liver disease. Familial causes of liver disease include Wilson's disease; hemochromatosis and α_1 antitrypsin deficiency; and the more uncommon inherited pediatric liver diseases—i.e., familial intrahepatic cholestasis, benign recurrent intrahepatic cholestasis, and Alagille syndrome. Onset of severe liver disease in childhood or adolescence in conjunction with a family history of liver disease or neuropsychiatric disturbance should lead to

TABLE 36-2

CAGE QUESTIONS[a]

ACRONYM	QUESTION
C	Have you ever felt you ought to *c*ut down on your drinking?
A	Have people *a*nnoyed you by criticizing your drinking?
G	Have you ever felt *g*uilty or bad about your drinking?
E	Have you ever had a drink first thing in the morning to steady your nerves or get rid of a hangover (*e*ye-opener)?

[a]One "yes" response should raise suspicion of an alcohol use problem, and more than one is a strong indication of abuse or dependence.

investigation for Wilson's disease. A family history of cirrhosis, diabetes, or endocrine failure and the appearance of liver disease in adulthood suggests hemochromatosis and should prompt investigation of iron status. Abnormal iron studies in adult patients warrant genotyping of the *HFE* gene for the C282Y and H63D mutations typical of genetic hemochromatosis. In children and adolescents with iron overload, other non-*HFE* causes of hemochromatosis should be sought. A family history of emphysema should provoke investigation of α_1 antitrypsin levels and, if levels are low, for protease inhibitor (Pi) genotype.

PHYSICAL EXAMINATION

The physical examination rarely uncovers evidence of liver dysfunction in a patient without symptoms or laboratory findings, nor are most signs of liver disease specific to one diagnosis. Thus, the physical examination complements rather than replaces the need for other diagnostic approaches. In many patients, the physical examination is normal unless the disease is acute or severe and advanced. Nevertheless, the physical examination is important in that it can yield the first evidence of hepatic failure, portal hypertension, and liver decompensation. In addition, the physical examination can reveal signs—related either to risk factors or to associated diseases or findings—that point to a specific diagnosis.

Typical physical findings in liver disease are icterus, hepatomegaly, hepatic tenderness, splenomegaly, spider angiomata, palmar erythema, and excoriations. Signs of advanced disease include muscle wasting, ascites, edema, dilated abdominal veins, hepatic fetor, asterixis, mental confusion, stupor, and coma. In male patients with cirrhosis, particularly that related to alcohol use, signs of hyperestrogenemia such as gynecomastia, testicular atrophy, and loss of male-pattern hair distribution may be found.

Icterus is best appreciated when the sclera is inspected under natural light. In fair-skinned individuals, a yellow tinge to the skin may be obvious. In dark-skinned individuals, examination of the mucous membranes below the tongue can demonstrate jaundice. Jaundice is rarely detectable if the serum bilirubin level is <43 μmol/L (2.5 mg/dL) but may remain detectable below this level during recovery from jaundice (because of protein and tissue binding of conjugated bilirubin).

Spider angiomata and palmar erythema occur in both acute and chronic liver disease; these manifestations may be especially prominent in persons with cirrhosis but can develop in normal individuals and are frequently found during pregnancy. Spider angiomata are superficial, tortuous arterioles and—unlike simple telangiectases—typically fill from the center outward. Spider angiomata occur only on the arms, face, and upper torso; they can be pulsatile and may be difficult to detect in dark-skinned individuals.

Hepatomegaly is not a highly reliable sign of liver disease because of variability in the liver's size and shape and the physical impediments to assessment of liver size by percussion and palpation. Marked hepatomegaly is typical of cirrhosis, veno-occlusive disease, infiltrative disorders such as amyloidosis, metastatic or primary cancers of the liver, and alcoholic hepatitis. Careful assessment of the liver edge may also reveal unusual firmness, irregularity of the surface, or frank nodules. Perhaps the most reliable physical finding in the liver examination is hepatic tenderness. Discomfort when the liver is touched or pressed upon should be carefully sought with percussive comparison of the right and left upper quadrants.

Splenomegaly, which occurs in many medical conditions, can be a subtle but significant physical finding in liver disease. The availability of ultrasound methods for assessment of the spleen allows confirmation of the physical finding.

Signs of advanced liver disease include muscle wasting and weight loss as well as hepatomegaly, bruising, ascites, and edema. Ascites is best appreciated by attempts to detect shifting dullness by careful percussion. Ultrasound examination will confirm the finding of ascites in equivocal cases. Peripheral edema can occur with or without ascites. In patients with advanced liver disease, other factors frequently contribute to edema formation, including hypoalbuminemia, venous insufficiency, heart failure, and medications.

Hepatic failure is defined as the occurrence of signs or symptoms of hepatic encephalopathy in a person with severe acute or chronic liver disease. The first signs of hepatic encephalopathy can be subtle and nonspecific—change in sleep patterns, change in personality, irritability, and mental dullness. Thereafter, confusion, disorientation, stupor, and eventually coma supervene. In acute liver failure, excitability and mania may be present. Physical findings include asterixis and flapping tremors of the body and tongue. *Fetor hepaticus* refers to the slightly sweet, ammoniacal odor that can develop in patients with liver failure, particularly if there is portal-venous shunting of blood around the liver. Other causes of coma and disorientation should be excluded, mainly electrolyte imbalances, sedative use, and renal or respiratory failure. The appearance of hepatic encephalopathy during acute hepatitis is the major criterion for diagnosis of fulminant hepatitis and indicates a poor prognosis. In chronic liver disease, encephalopathy is usually triggered by a medical complication such as gastrointestinal bleeding, over-diuresis, uremia, dehydration, electrolyte imbalance, infection, constipation, or use of narcotic analgesics.

A helpful measure of hepatic encephalopathy is a careful mental-status examination and use of the trail-making test, which consists of a series of 25 numbered circles that the patient is asked to connect as rapidly as possible using a pencil. The normal range for the connect-the-dot test is 15–30 sec; it is considerably longer in patients with early hepatic encephalopathy. Other tests include drawing of abstract objects or comparison of a signature to previous examples. More sophisticated testing—e.g., with electroencephalography and visual evoked potentials—can detect mild forms of encephalopathy but are rarely clinically useful.

Other signs of advanced liver disease include umbilical hernia from ascites, hydrothorax, prominent veins over the abdomen, and *caput medusa*, a condition that consists of collateral veins radiating from the umbilicus and results from recanulation of the umbilical vein. Widened pulse pressure and signs of a hyperdynamic circulation can occur in patients with cirrhosis as a result of fluid and sodium retention, increased cardiac output, and reduced peripheral resistance. Patients with long-standing cirrhosis and portal hypertension are prone to develop the hepatopulmonary syndrome, which is defined by the triad of liver disease, hypoxemia, and pulmonary arteriovenous shunting. The hepatopulmonary syndrome is characterized by platypnea and orthodeoxia: shortness of breath and oxygen desaturation that occur paradoxically upon the assumption of an upright position. Measurement of oxygen saturation by pulse oximetry is a reliable screening test for hepatopulmonary syndrome.

Several skin disorders and changes are common in liver disease. Hyperpigmentation is typical of advanced chronic cholestatic diseases such as primary biliary cirrhosis and sclerosing cholangitis. In these same conditions, xanthelasma and tendon xanthomata occur as a result of retention and high serum levels of lipids and cholesterol. Slate-gray pigmentation of the skin is also seen with hemochromatosis if iron levels are high for a prolonged period. Mucocutaneous vasculitis with palpable purpura, especially on the lower extremities, is typical of cryoglobulinemia of chronic hepatitis C but can also occur in chronic hepatitis B.

Some physical signs point to specific liver diseases. Kayser-Fleischer rings occur in Wilson's disease and consist of a golden-brown copper pigment deposited in Descemet's membrane at the periphery of the cornea; they are best seen by slit-lamp examination. Dupuytren contracture and parotid enlargement are suggestive of chronic alcoholism and alcoholic liver disease. In metastatic liver disease or primary hepatocellular carcinoma, signs of cachexia and wasting as well as firm hepatomegaly and a hepatic bruit may be prominent.

DIAGNOSIS OF LIVER DISEASE

The major causes of liver disease and key diagnostic features are outlined in Table 36-3, and an algorithm for evaluation of the patient with suspected liver disease is shown in Fig. 36-1. Specifics of diagnosis are discussed in later chapters. The most common causes of acute liver disease are viral hepatitis (particularly hepatitis A, B, and C), drug-induced liver injury, cholangitis, and alcoholic liver disease. Liver biopsy usually is not needed in the diagnosis and management of acute liver disease, exceptions being situations where the diagnosis remains unclear despite thorough clinical and laboratory investigation. Liver biopsy can be helpful in diagnosing drug-induced liver disease and acute alcoholic hepatitis.

TABLE 36-3

IMPORTANT DIAGNOSTIC TESTS IN COMMON LIVER DISEASES

DISEASE	DIAGNOSTIC TEST
Hepatitis A	Anti-HAV IgM
Hepatitis B	
Acute	HBsAg and anti-HBc IgM
Chronic	HBsAg and HBeAg and/or HBV DNA
Hepatitis C	Anti-HCV and HCV RNA
Hepatitis D (delta)	HBsAg and anti-HDV
Hepatitis E	Anti-HEV IgM and HEV RNA
Autoimmune hepatitis	ANA or SMA, elevated IgG levels, and compatible histology
Primary biliary cirrhosis	Mitochondrial antibody, elevated IgM levels, and compatible histology
Primary sclerosing cholangitis	P-ANCA, cholangiography
Drug-induced liver disease	History of drug ingestion
Alcoholic liver disease	History of excessive alcohol intake and compatible histology
Nonalcoholic steatohepatitis	Ultrasound or CT evidence of fatty liver and compatible histology
α_1 Antitrypsin disease	Reduced α_1 antitrypsin levels, phenotype PiZZ or PiSZ
Wilson's disease	Decreased serum ceruloplasmin and increased urinary copper; increased hepatic copper level
Hemochromatosis	Elevated iron saturation and serum ferritin; genetic testing for *HFE* gene mutations
Hepatocellular cancer	Elevated α-fetoprotein level (to >500 ng/mL); ultrasound or CT image of mass

Abbreviations: HAV, HBV, HCV, HDV, HEV: hepatitis A, B, C, D, E virus; HBsAg, hepatitis B surface antigen; anti-HBc, antibody to hepatitis B core (antigen); HBeAg, hepatitis B e antigen; ANA, antinuclear antibody; SMA, smooth-muscle antibody; P-ANCA, perinuclear antineutrophil cytoplasmic antibody.

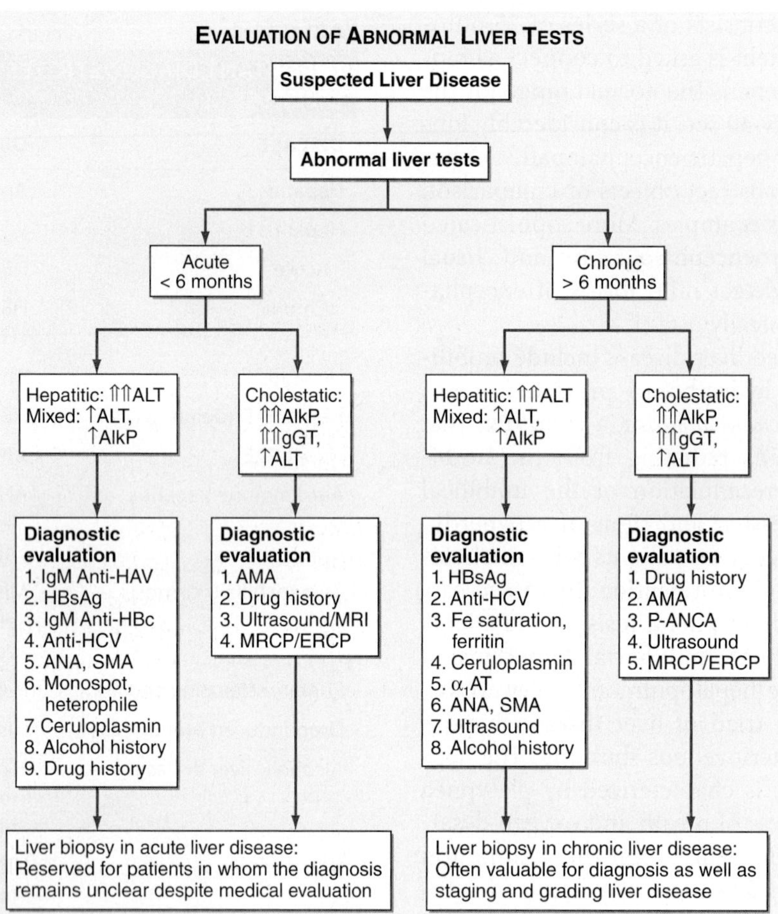

FIGURE 36-1

Algorithm for evaluation of abnormal liver tests. For patients with suspected liver disease, an appropriate approach to evaluation is initial routine liver testing—e.g., measurement of serum bilirubin, albumin, alanine aminotransferase (ALT), aspartate aminotransferase (AST), and alkaline phosphatase (AlkP). These results (sometimes complemented by testing of γ-glutamyl transpeptidase; gGT) will establish whether the pattern of abnormalities is hepatic, cholestatic, or mixed. In addition, the duration of symptoms or abnormalities will indicate whether the disease is acute or chronic. If the disease is acute and if history, laboratory tests, and imaging studies do not reveal a diagnosis, liver biopsy is appropriate to help establish the diagnosis. If the disease is chronic, liver biopsy can be helpful not only for diagnosis but also for grading of the activity and staging the progression of disease. This approach is generally applicable to patients without immune deficiency. In patients with HIV infection or recipients of bone marrow or solid organ transplants, the diagnostic evaluation should also include evaluation for opportunistic infections (e.g., with adenovirus, cytomegalovirus, *Coccidioides*, hepatitis E virus) as well as for vascular and immunologic conditions (veno-occlusive disease, graft-versus-host disease). HAV, hepatitis A virus; HCV, hepatitis C virus; HBsAg, hepatitis B surface antigen; anti-HBc, antibody to hepatitis B core (antigen); ANA, antinuclear antibody; SMA, smooth-muscle antibody; MRCP, magnetic resonance cholangiopancreatography; ERCP, endoscopic retrograde cholangiopancreatography; α_1 AT, α_1 antitrypsin; AMA; antimitochondrial antibody; P-ANCA, perinuclear antineutrophil cytoplasmic antibody.

The most common causes of chronic liver disease, in general order of frequency, are chronic hepatitis C, alcoholic liver disease, nonalcoholic steatohepatitis, chronic hepatitis B, autoimmune hepatitis, sclerosing cholangitis, primary biliary cirrhosis, hemochromatosis, and Wilson's disease. Hepatitis E virus is a rare cause of chronic hepatitis, with cases occurring mostly in persons who are immunosuppressed or immunodeficient. Strict diagnostic criteria have not been developed for most liver diseases, but liver biopsy plays an important role in the diagnosis of autoimmune hepatitis, primary biliary cirrhosis, nonalcoholic and alcoholic steatohepatitis, and Wilson's disease (with a quantitative hepatic copper level in the last instance).

Laboratory testing

Diagnosis of liver disease is greatly aided by the availability of reliable and sensitive tests of liver injury and function. A typical battery of blood tests used for initial assessment of liver disease includes measurement of levels of serum alanine and aspartate aminotransferases, alkaline phosphatase, direct and total serum bilirubin and albumin, and prothrombin time. The pattern of abnormalities generally points to hepatocellular versus cholestatic liver disease and helps determine whether the disease is acute or chronic and whether cirrhosis and hepatic failure are present. On the basis of these results, further testing over time may be necessary. Other laboratory tests may be helpful, such as γ-glutamyl transpeptidase to define whether alkaline phosphatase elevations are due to liver disease; hepatitis serology to define the type of viral hepatitis; and autoimmune markers to diagnose primary biliary cirrhosis (antimitochondrial antibody), sclerosing cholangitis (perinuclear antineutrophil cytoplasmic antibody), and autoimmune hepatitis (antinuclear, smooth-muscle, and liver-kidney microsomal antibody). A simple delineation of laboratory abnormalities and common liver diseases is given in Table 36-3.

The use and interpretation of liver function tests are summarized in Chap. 37.

Diagnostic imaging

Great advances have been made in hepatobiliary imaging, although no method is adequately accurate in demonstrating underlying cirrhosis. Of the many modalities available for imaging the liver, ultrasound, CT, and MRI are the most commonly employed and are complementary to one another. In general, ultrasound and CT are highly sensitive for detecting biliary duct dilation and are the first-line options for investigating cases of suspected obstructive jaundice. All three modalities can detect a fatty liver, which appears bright on imaging studies. Modifications of CT and MRI can be used to quantify liver fat, and this information may ultimately be valuable in monitoring therapy in patients with fatty liver disease. Magnetic resonance cholangiopancreatography (MRCP) and endoscopic retrograde cholangiopancreatography (ERCP) are the procedures of choice for visualization of the biliary tree. MRCP offers several advantages over ERCP: there is no need for contrast media or ionizing radiation, images can be acquired faster, the procedure is less operator dependent, and it carries no risk of pancreatitis. MRCP is superior to ultrasound and CT for detecting choledocholithiasis but is less specific. MRCP is useful in the diagnosis of bile duct obstruction and congenital biliary abnormalities, but ERCP is more valuable in evaluating ampullary lesions and primary sclerosing cholangitis. ERCP permits biopsy, direct visualization of the ampulla and common bile duct, and intraductal ultrasonography. It also provides several therapeutic options in patients with obstructive jaundice, such as sphincterotomy, stone extraction, and placement of nasobiliary catheters and biliary stents. Doppler ultrasound and MRI are used to assess hepatic vasculature and hemodynamics and to monitor surgically or radiologically placed vascular shunts, including transjugular intrahepatic portosystemic shunts. Multidetector or spiral CT and MRI with contrast-enhancement are the procedures of choice for the identification and evaluation of hepatic masses, the staging of liver tumors, and preoperative assessment. With regard to mass lesions, the sensitivity of hepatic imaging continues to increase; unfortunately, specificity remains a problem, and often two and sometimes three studies are needed before a diagnosis can be reached. Recently, ultrasound transient elastography has been approved for the measurement of hepatic stiffness—providing an indirect assessment of cirrhosis; this technique can eliminate the need for liver biopsy if the only indication is the assessment of disease stage. Magnetic resonance elastography is now undergoing evaluation for its ability to detect different degrees of hepatic fibrosis. Studies are ongoing to determine whether hepatic elastography is an appropriate means of monitoring fibrosis and disease progression. Finally, interventional radiologic techniques allow the biopsy of solitary lesions, the radiofrequency ablation and chemoembolization of cancerous lesions, the insertion of drains into hepatic abscesses, the measurement of portal pressure, and the creation of vascular shunts in patients with portal hypertension. Which modality to use depends on factors such as availability, cost, and experience of the radiologist with each technique.

Liver biopsy

Liver biopsy remains the criterion standard in the evaluation of patients with liver disease, particularly chronic liver disease. Liver biopsy is necessary for diagnosis in selected instances but is more often useful for assessment of the severity (grade) and stage of liver damage, prediction of prognosis, and monitoring of the response to treatment. The size of the liver biopsy sample is an important determinant of reliability; a length of 1.5–2 cm is necessary for accurate assessment of fibrosis. In the future, noninvasive means of assessing disease activity (batteries of blood tests) and fibrosis (elastography and fibrosis markers) may replace liver biopsy for the staging and grading of disease.

GRADING AND STAGING OF LIVER DISEASE

Grading refers to an assessment of the severity or activity of liver disease, whether acute or chronic; active or inactive; and mild, moderate, or severe. Liver biopsy is the most accurate means of assessing severity, particularly in chronic liver disease. Serum aminotransferase levels serve as convenient and noninvasive markers for disease activity but do not always reliably reflect disease severity. Thus, normal serum aminotransferase levels in patients with hepatitis B surface antigen in serum may indicate the inactive carrier state or may reflect mild chronic hepatitis B or hepatitis B with fluctuating disease activity. Serum testing for hepatitis B e antigen and hepatitis B virus DNA can help sort out these different patterns, but these markers can also fluctuate and change over time. Similarly, in chronic hepatitis C, serum aminotransferase levels can be normal despite moderate disease activity. Finally, in both alcoholic and nonalcoholic steatohepatitis, aminotransferase levels are quite unreliable in reflecting severity. In these conditions, liver biopsy is helpful in guiding management and identifying appropriate therapy, particularly if treatment is difficult, prolonged, and expensive, as is often the case in chronic viral hepatitis. Of the several well-verified numerical scales for grading activity in chronic liver disease, the most commonly used are the histology activity index and the Ishak histology scale.

Liver biopsy is also the most accurate means of assessing stage of disease as early or advanced, precirrhotic, and cirrhotic. Staging of disease pertains largely to chronic liver diseases in which progression to cirrhosis and end-stage disease can occur but may require years or decades. Clinical features, biochemical tests, and hepatic imaging studies are helpful in assessing stage but generally become abnormal only in the middle to late stages of cirrhosis. Noninvasive tests that suggest advanced fibrosis include mild elevations of bilirubin, prolongation of prothrombin time, slight decreases in serum albumin, and mild thrombocytopenia (which is often the first indication of worsening fibrosis). Combinations of blood test results have been used to create models for predicting advanced liver disease, but these models are not reliable enough to use on a regular basis and only separate advanced from early disease. Recently, elastography and noninvasive breath tests using ^{13}C-labeled compounds have been proposed as a means of detecting early stages of fibrosis and liver dysfunction, but their reliability and reproducibility remain to be proven. Thus, at present, mild to moderate stages of hepatic fibrosis are detectable only by liver biopsy. In the assessment of stage, the degree of fibrosis is usually used as the quantitative measure. The amount of fibrosis is generally staged on a scale of 0 to 4+ (Metavir scale) or 0 to 6+ (Ishak scale). The importance of staging relates primarily to prognosis and to optimal management of complications. Patients with cirrhosis are candidates for screening and surveillance for esophageal varices and hepatocellular carcinoma. Patients without advanced fibrosis need not undergo screening.

Cirrhosis can also be staged clinically. A reliable staging system is the modified Child-Pugh classification, with a scoring system of 5–15: scores of 5 and 6 represent Child-Pugh class A (consistent with "compensated cirrhosis"), scores of 7–9 represent class B, and scores of 10–15 represent class C (Table 36-4). This scoring system was initially devised to stratify patients into risk groups before portal decompressive surgery. The Child-Pugh score is a reasonably reliable predictor of survival in many liver diseases and predicts the likelihood of major complications of cirrhosis, such as bleeding from varices and spontaneous bacterial peritonitis. This classification scheme was used to assess prognosis in cirrhosis and to provide standard criteria for listing a patient as a candidate for liver transplantation (Child-Pugh class B). Recently, the Child-Pugh system has been replaced by the Model for End-Stage Liver Disease (MELD) system for the latter purpose. The MELD score is a prospectively derived system designed to predict the prognosis of patients with liver disease and portal hypertension. This score is calculated from three noninvasive variables: the prothrombin time expressed as the international normalized ratio (INR), the serum bilirubin level, and the serum creatinine concentration. *(http://optn.transplant.hrsa.gov/resources/MeldPeldCalculator.asp?index=98).*

The MELD system provides a more objective means of assessing disease severity and has less center-to-center variation than the Child-Pugh score as well as a wider range of values. MELD is currently used to establish priority listing for liver transplantation in the United States. A similar system, PELD (pediatric end-stage liver disease), is based on bilirubin, INR, serum albumin, age, and nutritional status and is used for children <12 years of age.

TABLE 36-4

CHILD-PUGH CLASSIFICATION OF CIRRHOSIS

		POINTS TOWARD TOTAL SCORE		
FACTOR	**UNITS**	**1**	**2**	**3**
Serum bilirubin	μmol/L	<34	34–51	>51
	mg/dL	<2.0	2.0–3.0	>3.0
Serum albumin	g/L	>35	30–35	<30
	g/dL	>3.5	3.0–3.5	<3.0
Prothrombin time	seconds prolonged	<4	4–6	>6
	INR[a]	<1.7	1.7–2.3	>2.3
Ascites		None	Easily controlled	Poorly controlled
Hepatic encephalopathy		None	Minimal	Advanced

[a]International normalized ratio.

Note: The Child-Pugh score is calculated by adding the scores for the five factors and can range from 5 to 15. The resulting Child-Pugh class can be A (a score of 5–6), B (7–9), or C (≥10). Decompensation indicates cirrhosis, with a Child-Pugh score of ≥7 (class B). This level has been the accepted criterion for listing a patient for liver transplantation.

Thus, liver biopsy is helpful not only in diagnosis but also in management of chronic liver disease and assessment of prognosis. Because liver biopsy is an invasive procedure and not without complications, it should be used only when it will contribute materially to decisions about management and therapy.

NONSPECIFIC ISSUES IN THE MANAGEMENT OF PATIENTS WITH LIVER DISEASE

Specifics on the management of different forms of acute or chronic liver disease are supplied in subsequent chapters, but certain issues are applicable to any patient with liver disease. These issues include advice regarding alcohol use, medication use, vaccination, and surveillance for complications of liver disease. Alcohol should be used sparingly, if at all, by patients with liver disease. Abstinence from alcohol should be encouraged for all patients with alcohol-related liver disease, patients with cirrhosis, and patients receiving interferon-based therapy for hepatitis B or C. With regard to vaccinations, all patients with liver disease should receive hepatitis A vaccine, and those with risk factors should receive hepatitis B vaccine as well. Influenza and pneumococcal vaccination should also be encouraged, with adherence to the recommendations of the Centers for Disease Control and Prevention. Patients with liver disease should exercise caution in using any medications other than those that are most necessary. Drug-induced hepatotoxicity can mimic many forms of liver disease and can cause exacerbations of chronic hepatitis and cirrhosis; drugs should be suspected in any situation in which the cause of exacerbation is unknown. Finally, consideration should be given to surveillance for complications of chronic liver disease such as variceal hemorrhage and hepatocellular carcinoma. Cirrhosis warrants upper endoscopy to assess the presence of varices, and the patient should receive chronic therapy with beta blockers or should be offered endoscopic obliteration if large varices are found. Moreover, cirrhosis warrants screening and long-term surveillance for development of hepatocellular carcinoma. While the optimal regimen for such surveillance has not been established, an appropriate approach is ultrasound of the liver at 6- to 12-month intervals.

CHAPTER 37

EVALUATION OF LIVER FUNCTION

Daniel S. Pratt

Several biochemical tests are useful in the evaluation and management of patients with hepatic dysfunction. These tests can be used to (1) detect the presence of liver disease, (2) distinguish among different types of liver disorders, (3) gauge the extent of known liver damage, and (4) follow the response to treatment.

Liver tests have shortcomings. They can be normal in patients with serious liver disease and abnormal in patients with diseases that do not affect the liver. Liver tests rarely suggest a specific diagnosis; rather, they suggest a general category of liver disease, such as hepatocellular or cholestatic, which then further directs the evaluation.

The liver carries out thousands of biochemical functions, most of which cannot be easily measured by blood tests. Laboratory tests measure only a limited number of these functions. In fact, many tests, such as the aminotransferases or alkaline phosphatase, do not measure liver function at all. Rather, they detect liver cell damage or interference with bile flow. Thus, no one test enables the clinician to accurately assess the liver's total functional capacity.

To increase both the sensitivity and the specificity of laboratory tests in the detection of liver disease, it is best to use them as a battery. Tests usually employed in clinical practice include the bilirubin, aminotransferases, alkaline phosphatase, albumin, and prothrombin time tests. When more than one of these tests provide abnormal findings or the findings are persistently abnormal on serial determinations, the probability of liver disease is high. When all test results are normal, the probability of missing occult liver disease is low.

When evaluating patients with liver disorders, it is helpful to group these tests into general categories as outlined below.

TESTS BASED ON DETOXIFICATION AND EXCRETORY FUNCTIONS

Serum bilirubin

(See also Chap. 8) Bilirubin, a breakdown product of the porphyrin ring of heme-containing proteins, is found in the blood in two fractions—conjugated and unconjugated. The unconjugated fraction, also termed the *indirect fraction*, is insoluble in water and is bound to albumin in the blood. The conjugated (direct) bilirubin fraction is water soluble and can therefore be excreted by the kidney. When measured by modifications of the original van den Bergh method, normal values of total serum bilirubin are reported between 1 and 1.5 mg/dL with 95% of a normal population falling between 0.2 and 0.9 mg/dL. If the direct-acting fraction is less than 15% of the total, the bilirubin can be considered to all be indirect. The most frequently reported upper limit of normal for conjugated bilirubin is 0.3 mg/dL.

Elevation of the unconjugated fraction of bilirubin is rarely due to liver disease. An isolated elevation of unconjugated bilirubin is seen primarily in hemolytic disorders and in a number of genetic conditions such as Crigler-Najjar and Gilbert's syndromes **(Chap. 8)**. Isolated unconjugated hyperbilirubinemia (bilirubin elevated but <15% direct) should prompt a workup for hemolysis (Fig. 37-1). In the absence of hemolysis, an isolated, unconjugated hyperbilirubinemia in an otherwise healthy patient can be attributed to Gilbert's syndrome, and no further evaluation is required.

In contrast, conjugated hyperbilirubinemia almost always implies liver or biliary tract disease. The rate-limiting step in bilirubin metabolism is not conjugation of bilirubin, but rather the transport of conjugated bilirubin into the bile canaliculi. Thus, elevation of the conjugated fraction may be seen in any type of liver disease. In most liver diseases, both conjugated and unconjugated fractions of the bilirubin tend to be elevated. Except in the presence of a purely unconjugated hyperbilirubinemia, fractionation of the bilirubin is rarely helpful in determining the cause of jaundice.

Although the degree of elevation of the serum bilirubin has not been critically assessed as a prognostic marker, it is important in a number of conditions. In viral hepatitis, the higher the serum bilirubin, the

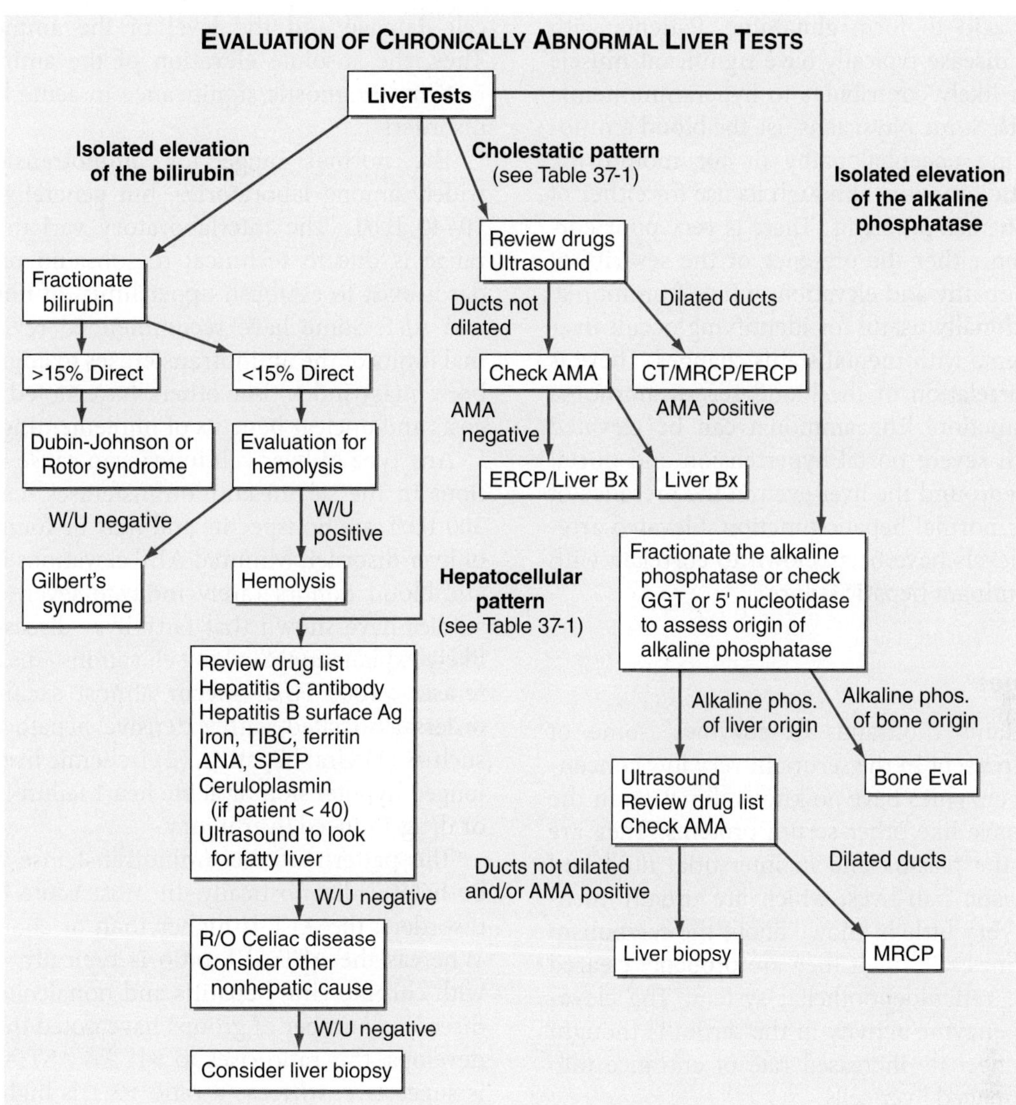

FIGURE 37-1

Algorithm for the evaluation of chronically abnormal liver tests. AMA, antimitochondrial antibody; ANA, antinuclear antibody; Bx, biopsy; CT, computed tomography; ERCP, endoscopic retrograde cholangiopancreatography; GGT, γ glutamyl transpeptidase; MRCP, magnetic resonance cholangiopancreatography; R/O, rule out; SPEP, serum protein electrophoresis; TIBC, total iron-binding capacity; W/U, workup.

greater is the hepatocellular damage. Total serum bilirubin correlates with poor outcomes in alcoholic hepatitis. It is also a critical component of the Model for End-Stage Liver Disease (MELD) score, a tool used to estimate survival of patients with end-stage liver disease and assess operative risk of patients with cirrhosis. An elevated total serum bilirubin in patients with drug-induced liver disease indicates more severe injury.

Urine bilirubin

Unconjugated bilirubin always binds to albumin in the serum and is not filtered by the kidney. Therefore, any bilirubin found in the urine is conjugated bilirubin; the presence of bilirubinuria implies the presence of liver disease. A urine dipstick test can theoretically give the same information as fractionation of the serum bilirubin. This test is almost 100% accurate. Phenothiazines may give a false-positive reading with the Ictotest tablet. In patients recovering from jaundice, the urine bilirubin clears prior to the serum bilirubin.

Blood ammonia

Ammonia is produced in the body during normal protein metabolism and by intestinal bacteria, primarily those in the colon. The liver plays a role in the detoxification of ammonia by converting it to urea, which is excreted by the kidneys. Striated muscle also plays a role in detoxification of ammonia, where it is combined with glutamic acid to form glutamine. Patients with advanced liver disease typically have significant muscle wasting, which likely contributes to hyperammonemia in these patients. Some physicians use the blood ammonia for detecting encephalopathy or for monitoring hepatic synthetic function, although its use for either of these indications has problems. There is very poor correlation between either the presence or the severity of acute encephalopathy and elevation of blood ammonia; it can be occasionally useful for identifying occult liver disease in patients with mental status changes. There is also a poor correlation of the blood serum ammonia and hepatic function. The ammonia can be elevated in patients with severe portal hypertension and portal blood shunting around the liver even in the presence of normal or near-normal hepatic function. Elevated arterial ammonia levels have been shown to correlate with outcome in fulminant hepatic failure.

Serum enzymes

The liver contains thousands of enzymes, some of which are also present in the serum in very low concentrations. These enzymes have no known function in the serum and behave like other serum proteins. They are distributed in the plasma and in interstitial fluid and have characteristic half-lives, which are usually measured in days. Very little is known about the catabolism of serum enzymes, although they are probably cleared by cells in the reticuloendothelial system. The elevation of a given enzyme activity in the serum is thought to primarily reflect its increased rate of entrance into serum from damaged liver cells.

Serum enzyme tests can be grouped into three categories: (1) enzymes whose elevation in serum reflects damage to hepatocytes, (2) enzymes whose elevation in serum reflects cholestasis, and (3) enzyme tests that do not fit precisely into either pattern.

Enzymes that reflect damage to hepatocytes

The aminotransferases (transaminases) are sensitive indicators of liver cell injury and are most helpful in recognizing acute hepatocellular diseases such as hepatitis. They include aspartate aminotransferase (AST) and alanine aminotransferase (ALT). AST is found in the liver, cardiac muscle, skeletal muscle, kidneys, brain, pancreas, lungs, leukocytes, and erythrocytes in decreasing order of concentration. ALT is found primarily in the liver and is therefore a more specific indicator of liver injury. The aminotransferases are normally present in the serum in low concentrations. These enzymes are released into the blood in greater amounts when there is damage to the liver cell membrane resulting in increased permeability. Liver cell necrosis is not required for the release of the aminotransferases, and there is a poor correlation between the degree of liver cell damage and the level of the aminotransferases. Thus, the absolute elevation of the aminotransferases is of no prognostic significance in acute hepatocellular disorders.

The normal range for aminotransferases varies widely among laboratories, but generally ranges from 10–40 IU/L. The interlaboratory variation in normal range is due to technical reasons; no reference standards exist to establish upper limits of normal for ALT and AST. Some have recommended revisions of normal limits of the aminotransferases to adjust for sex and body mass index, but others have noted the potential costs and unclear benefits of implementing this change.

Any type of liver cell injury can cause modest elevations in the serum aminotransferases. Levels of up to 300 IU/L are nonspecific and may be found in any type of liver disorder. Minimal ALT elevations in asymptomatic blood donors rarely indicate severe liver disease; studies have shown that fatty liver disease is the most likely explanation. Striking elevations—i.e., aminotransferases >1000 IU/L—occur almost exclusively in disorders associated with extensive hepatocellular injury such as (1) viral hepatitis, (2) ischemic liver injury (prolonged hypotension or acute heart failure), or (3) toxin- or drug-induced liver injury.

The pattern of the aminotransferase elevation can be helpful diagnostically. In most acute hepatocellular disorders, the ALT is higher than or equal to the AST. Whereas the AST:ALT ratio is typically <1 in patients with chronic viral hepatitis and nonalcoholic fatty liver disease, a number of groups have noted that as cirrhosis develops, this ratio rises to >1. An AST:ALT ratio >2:1 is suggestive, whereas a ratio >3:1 is highly suggestive, of alcoholic liver disease. The AST in alcoholic liver disease is rarely >300 IU/L, and the ALT is often normal. A low level of ALT in the serum is due to an alcohol-induced deficiency of pyridoxal phosphate.

The aminotransferases are usually not greatly elevated in obstructive jaundice. One notable exception occurs during the acute phase of biliary obstruction caused by the passage of a gallstone into the common bile duct. In this setting, the aminotransferases can briefly be in the 1000–2000 IU/L range. However, aminotransferase levels decrease quickly, and the liver function tests rapidly evolve into those typical of cholestasis.

Enzymes that reflect cholestasis

The activities of three enzymes—alkaline phosphatase, 5′-nucleotidase, and γ-glutamyl transpeptidase (GGT)—are usually elevated in cholestasis. Alkaline phosphatase and 5′-nucleotidase are found in or near the bile canalicular membrane of hepatocytes, whereas GGT is located in the endoplasmic reticulum and in bile duct epithelial cells. Reflecting its more diffuse localization in the liver, GGT elevation in serum is less specific for cholestasis than are elevations of alkaline phosphatase or 5′-nucleotidase. Some have advocated the use of GGT to identify patients with occult alcohol use. Its lack of specificity makes its use in this setting questionable.

The normal serum alkaline phosphatase consists of many distinct isoenzymes found in the liver; bone; placenta; and, less commonly, small intestine. Patients over age 60 can have a mildly elevated alkaline phosphatase (1–1.5 times normal), whereas individuals with blood types O and B can have an elevation of the serum alkaline phosphatase after eating a fatty meal due to the influx of intestinal alkaline phosphatase into the blood. It is also nonpathologically elevated in children and adolescents undergoing rapid bone growth because of bone alkaline phosphatase, and late in normal pregnancies due to the influx of placental alkaline phosphatase.

Elevation of liver-derived alkaline phosphatase is not totally specific for cholestasis, and a less than threefold elevation can be seen in almost any type of liver disease. Alkaline phosphatase elevations greater than four times normal occur primarily in patients with cholestatic liver disorders, infiltrative liver diseases such as cancer and amyloidosis, and bone conditions characterized by rapid bone turnover (e.g., Paget's disease). In bone diseases, the elevation is due to increased amounts of the bone isoenzymes. In liver diseases, the elevation is almost always due to increased amounts of the liver isoenzyme.

If an elevated serum alkaline phosphatase is the only abnormal finding in an apparently healthy person, or if the degree of elevation is higher than expected in the clinical setting, identification of the source of elevated isoenzymes is helpful (Fig. 37-1). This problem can be approached in two ways. First, and most precise, is the fractionation of the alkaline phosphatase by electrophoresis. The second, best substantiated, and most available approach involves the measurement of serum 5′-nucleotidase or GGT. These enzymes are rarely elevated in conditions other than liver disease.

In the absence of jaundice or elevated aminotransferases, an elevated alkaline phosphatase of liver origin often, but not always, suggests early cholestasis and, less often, hepatic infiltration by tumor or granulomata. Other conditions that cause isolated elevations of the alkaline phosphatase include Hodgkin's disease, diabetes, hyperthyroidism, congestive heart failure, amyloidosis, and inflammatory bowel disease.

The level of serum alkaline phosphatase elevation is not helpful in distinguishing between intrahepatic and extrahepatic cholestasis. There is essentially no difference among the values found in obstructive jaundice due to cancer, common duct stone, sclerosing cholangitis, or bile duct stricture. Values are similarly increased in patients with intrahepatic cholestasis due to drug-induced hepatitis; primary biliary cirrhosis; rejection of transplanted livers; and, rarely, alcohol-induced steatohepatitis. Values are also greatly elevated in hepatobiliary disorders seen in patients with AIDS (e.g., AIDS cholangiopathy due to cytomegalovirus or cryptosporidial infection and tuberculosis with hepatic involvement).

TESTS THAT MEASURE BIOSYNTHETIC FUNCTION OF THE LIVER

Serum albumin

Serum albumin is synthesized exclusively by hepatocytes. Serum albumin has a long half-life: 18–20 days, with ~4% degraded per day. Because of this slow turnover, the serum albumin is not a good indicator of acute or mild hepatic dysfunction; only minimal changes in the serum albumin are seen in acute liver conditions such as viral hepatitis, drug-related hepatotoxicity, and obstructive jaundice. In hepatitis, albumin levels <3 g/dL should raise the possibility of chronic liver disease. Hypoalbuminemia is more common in chronic liver disorders such as cirrhosis and usually reflects severe liver damage and decreased albumin synthesis. One exception is the patient with ascites in whom synthesis may be normal or even increased, but levels are low because of the increased volume of distribution. However, hypoalbuminemia is not specific for liver disease and may occur in protein malnutrition of any cause, as well as protein-losing enteropathies, nephrotic syndrome, and chronic infections that are associated with prolonged increases in levels of serum interleukin 1 and/or tumor necrosis factor, cytokines that inhibit albumin synthesis. Serum albumin should not be measured for screening in patients in whom there is no suspicion of liver disease. A general medical clinic study of consecutive patients in whom no indications were present for albumin measurement showed that although 12% of patients had abnormal test results, the finding was of clinical importance in only 0.4%.

Serum globulins

Serum globulins are a group of proteins made up of γ globulins (immunoglobulins) produced by B lymphocytes and α and β globulins produced primarily in hepatocytes. γ globulins are increased in chronic liver disease, such as chronic hepatitis and cirrhosis. In cirrhosis, the increased serum γ globulin concentration is due to the increased synthesis of antibodies, some of which are directed against intestinal bacteria. This occurs because the cirrhotic liver fails to clear bacterial antigens that normally reach the liver through the hepatic circulation.

Increases in the concentration of specific isotypes of γ globulins are often helpful in the recognition of certain chronic liver diseases. Diffuse polyclonal increases in IgG levels are common in autoimmune hepatitis; increases >100% should alert the clinician to this possibility. Increases in the IgM levels are common in primary biliary cirrhosis, whereas increases in the IgA levels occur in alcoholic liver disease.

COAGULATION FACTORS

With the exception of factor VIII, which is produced by vascular endothelial cells, the blood clotting factors are made exclusively in hepatocytes. Their serum half-lives are much shorter than albumin, ranging from 6 h for factor VII to 5 days for fibrinogen. Because of their rapid turnover, measurement of the clotting factors is the single best acute measure of hepatic synthetic function and helpful in both diagnosis and assessing the prognosis of acute parenchymal liver disease. Useful for this purpose is the *serum prothrombin time*, which collectively measures factors II, V, VII, and X. Biosynthesis of factors II, VII, IX, and X depends on vitamin K. The international normalized ratio (INR) is used to express the degree of anticoagulation on warfarin therapy. The INR standardizes prothrombin time measurement according to the characteristics of the thromboplastin reagent used in a particular lab, which is expressed as an International Sensitivity Index (ISI); the ISI is then used in calculating the INR.

The prothrombin time may be elevated in hepatitis and cirrhosis as well as in disorders that lead to vitamin K deficiency such as obstructive jaundice or fat malabsorption of any kind. Marked prolongation of the prothrombin time, >5 s above control and not corrected by parenteral vitamin K administration, is a poor prognostic sign in acute viral hepatitis and other acute and chronic liver diseases. The INR, along with the total serum bilirubin and creatinine, are components of the MELD score, which is used as a measure of hepatic decompensation and to allocate organs for liver transplantation.

OTHER DIAGNOSTIC TESTS

Although tests may direct the physician to a category of liver disease, additional radiologic testing and procedures are often necessary to make the proper diagnosis, as shown in Fig. 37-1. The most commonly used ancillary tests are reviewed here, as are the noninvasive tests available for assessing hepatic fibrosis.

Percutaneous liver biopsy

Percutaneous biopsy of the liver is a safe procedure that can be easily performed at the bedside with local anesthesia and ultrasound guidance. Liver biopsy is of proven value in the following situations: (1) hepatocellular disease of uncertain cause, (2) prolonged hepatitis with the possibility of autoimmune hepatitis, (3) unexplained hepatomegaly, (4) unexplained splenomegaly, (5) hepatic filling defects by radiologic imaging, (6) fever of unknown origin, (7) and staging of malignant lymphoma. Liver biopsy is most accurate in disorders causing diffuse changes throughout the liver and is subject to sampling error in focal infiltrative disorders such as hepatic metastases. Liver biopsy should not be the initial procedure in the diagnosis of cholestasis. The biliary tree should first be assessed for signs of obstruction. Contraindications to performing a percutaneous liver biopsy include significant ascites and prolonged INR. Under these circumstances, the biopsy can be performed via the transjugular approach.

Noninvasive tests to detect hepatic fibrosis

Although liver biopsy is the standard for the assessment of hepatic fibrosis, noninvasive measures of hepatic fibrosis have been developed and show promise. These measures include multiparameter tests aimed at detecting and staging the degree of hepatic fibrosis and imaging techniques. FibroTest (marketed as FibroSure in the United States) is the best evaluated of the multiparameter blood tests. The test incorporates haptoglobin, bilirubin, GGT, apolipoprotein A-I, and α2-macroglobulin and has been found to have high positive and negative predictive values for diagnosing advanced fibrosis in patients with chronic hepatitis C, chronic hepatitis B, and alcoholic liver disease and patients taking methotrexate for psoriasis. Transient elastography (TE), marketed as FibroScan, and magnetic resonance elastography (MRE) both have gained U.S. Food and Drug Administration approval for use in the management of patients with liver disease. TE uses ultrasound waves to measure hepatic stiffness noninvasively. TE has been shown to be accurate for identifying advanced fibrosis in patients with chronic hepatitis C, primary biliary cirrhosis, hemochromatosis, nonalcoholic fatty liver disease, and recurrent chronic hepatitis after liver transplantation. MRE has been found to be superior to TE for staging liver fibrosis in patients with a variety of chronic liver diseases, but requires access to a magnetic resonance imaging scanner.

Ultrasonography

Ultrasonography is the first diagnostic test to use in patients whose liver tests suggest cholestasis, to look for the presence of a dilated intrahepatic or extrahepatic biliary tree or to identify gallstones. In addition, it shows space-occupying lesions within the liver, enables the clinician to distinguish between cystic and solid masses, and helps direct percutaneous biopsies. Ultrasound with Doppler imaging can detect the patency of the portal vein, hepatic artery, and hepatic veins and

TABLE 37-1

LIVER TEST PATTERNS IN HEPATOBILIARY DISORDERS

TYPE OF DISORDER	BILIRUBIN	AMINOTRANSFERASES	ALKALINE PHOSPHATASE	ALBUMIN	PROTHROMBIN TIME
Hemolysis/Gilbert's syndrome	Normal to 86 μmol/L (5 mg/dL) 85% due to indirect fractions No bilirubinuria	Normal	Normal	Normal	Normal
Acute hepatocellular necrosis (viral and drug hepatitis, hepatotoxins, acute heart failure)	Both fractions may be elevated Peak usually follows aminotransferases Bilirubinuria	Elevated, often >500 IU, ALT > AST	Normal to <3× normal elevation	Normal	Usually normal. If >5× above control and not corrected by parenteral vitamin K, suggests poor prognosis
Chronic hepatocellular disorders	Both fractions may be elevated Bilirubinuria	Elevated, but usually <300 IU	Normal to <3× normal elevation	Often decreased	Often prolonged Fails to correct with parenteral vitamin K
Alcoholic hepatitis, cirrhosis	Both fractions may be elevated Bilirubinuria	AST:ALT >2 suggests alcoholic hepatitis or cirrhosis	Normal to <3× normal elevation	Often decreased	Often prolonged Fails to correct with parenteral vitamin K
Intra- and extrahepatic cholestasis	Both fractions may be elevated	Normal to moderate elevation	Elevated, often >4× normal elevation	Normal, unless chronic	Normal If prolonged, will correct with parenteral vitamin K
(Obstructive jaundice) Infiltrative diseases (tumor, granulomata); partial bile duct obstruction	Bilirubinuria Usually normal	Rarely >500 IU Normal to slight elevation	Elevated, often >4× normal elevation Fractionate, or confirm liver origin with 5'-nucleotidase or γ glutamyl transpeptidase	Normal	Normal

determine the direction of blood flow. This is the first test ordered in patients suspected of having Budd-Chiari syndrome.

USE OF LIVER TESTS

As previously noted, the best way to increase the sensitivity and specificity of laboratory tests in the detection of liver disease is to employ a battery of tests that includes the aminotransferases, alkaline phosphatase, bilirubin, albumin, and prothrombin time along with the judicious use of the other tests described in this chapter. Table 37-1 shows how patterns of liver tests can lead the clinician to a category of disease that will direct further evaluation. However, it is important to remember that no single set of liver tests will necessarily provide a diagnosis. It is often necessary to repeat these tests on several occasions over days to weeks for a diagnostic pattern to emerge. Figure 37-1 is an algorithm for the evaluation of chronically abnormal liver tests.

GLOBAL CONSIDERATIONS

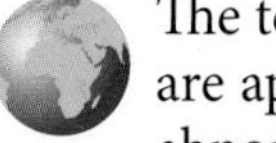

The tests and principles presented in this chapter are applicable worldwide. The causes of liver test abnormalities vary according to region. In developing nations, infectious diseases are more commonly the etiology of abnormal serum liver tests than in developed nations.

ACKNOWLEDGMENT

This chapter represents a revised version of a chapter in previous editions of Harrison's in which Marshall M. Kaplan was a co-author.

SECTION VI

DISORDERS OF THE LIVER AND BILIARY TREE

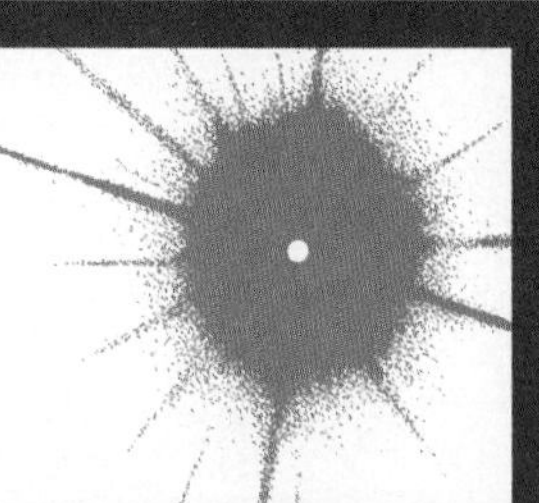

CHAPTER 38

THE HYPERBILIRUBINEMIAS

Allan W. Wolkoff

BILIRUBIN METABOLISM

The details of bilirubin metabolism are presented in **Chap. 8**. However, the hyperbilirubinemias are best understood in terms of perturbations of specific aspects of bilirubin metabolism and transport, and these will be briefly reviewed here as depicted in Fig. 38-1.

Bilirubin is the end product of heme degradation. Some 70–90% of bilirubin is derived from degradation of the hemoglobin of senescent red blood cells.

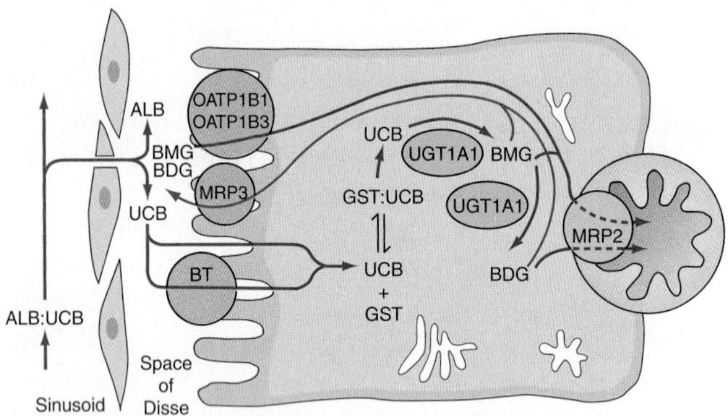

FIGURE 38-1

Hepatocellular bilirubin transport. Albumin-bound bilirubin in sinusoidal blood passes through endothelial cell fenestrae to reach the hepatocyte surface, entering the cell by both facilitated and simple diffusional processes. Within the cell, it is bound to glutathione-S-transferases and conjugated by bilirubin-UDP-glucuronosyltransferase (UGT1A1) to mono- and diglucuronides, which are actively transported across the canalicular membrane into the bile. In addition to this direct excretion of bilirubin glucuronides, a portion are transported into the portal circulation by MRP3 and subjected to reuptake into the hepatocyte by OATP1B1 and OATP1B3. ALB, albumin; BDG, bilirubin diglucuronide; BMG, bilirubin monoglucuronide; BT, proposed bilirubin transporter; GST, glutathione-S-transferase; MRP2 and MRP3, multidrug resistance–associated proteins 2 and 3; OATP1B1 and OATP1B3, organic anion transport proteins 1B1 and 1B3; UCB, unconjugated bilirubin; UGT1A1, bilirubin-UDP-glucuronosyltransferase.

Bilirubin produced in the periphery is transported to the liver within the plasma, where, due to its insolubility in aqueous solutions, it is tightly bound to albumin. Under normal circumstances, bilirubin is removed from the circulation rapidly and efficiently by hepatocytes. Transfer of bilirubin from blood to bile involves four distinct but interrelated steps (Fig. 38-1).

1. *Hepatocellular uptake:* Uptake of bilirubin by the hepatocyte has carrier-mediated kinetics. Although a number of candidate bilirubin transporters have been proposed, the actual transporter remains elusive.
2. *Intracellular binding:* Within the hepatocyte, bilirubin is kept in solution by binding as a nonsubstrate ligand to several of the glutathione-S-transferases, formerly called ligandins.
3. *Conjugation:* Bilirubin is conjugated with one or two glucuronic acid moieties by a specific UDP-glucuronosyltransferase to form bilirubin mono- and diglucuronide, respectively. Conjugation disrupts the internal hydrogen bonding that limits aqueous solubility of bilirubin, and the resulting glucuronide conjugates are highly soluble in water. Conjugation is obligatory for excretion of bilirubin across the bile canalicular membrane into bile. The UDP-glucuronosyltransferases have been classified into gene families based on the degree of homology among the mRNAs for the various isoforms. Those that conjugate bilirubin and certain other substrates have been designated the *UGT1* family. These are expressed from a single gene complex by alternative promoter usage. This gene complex contains multiple substrate-specific first exons, designated A1, A2, etc. (Fig. 38-2), each with its own promoter and each encoding the amino-terminal half of a specific isoform. In addition, there are four common exons (exons 2–5) that encode the shared carboxyl-terminal half of all of the *UGT1* isoforms. The various first exons encode the specific aglycone substrate binding sites for each isoform, while the shared exons encode

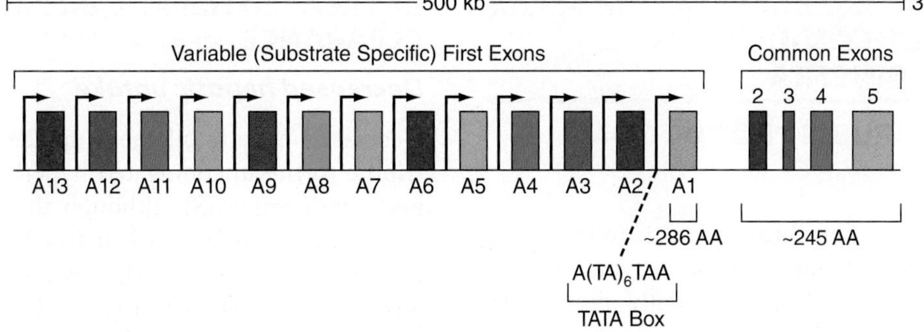

FIGURE 38-2

Structural organization of the human *UGT1* gene complex. This large complex on chromosome 2 contains at least 13 substrate-specific first exons (A1, A2, etc.). Since four of these are pseudogenes, nine UGT1 isoforms with differing substrate specificities are expressed. Each exon 1 has its own promoter and encodes the amino-terminal substrate-specific ~286 amino acids of the various *UGT1*-encoded isoforms, and common exons 2–5 that encode the 245 carboxyl-terminal amino acids common to all of the isoforms. mRNAs for specific isoforms are assembled by splicing a particular first exon such as the bilirubin-specific exon A1 to exons 2 to 5. The resulting message encodes a complete enzyme, in this particular case bilirubin-UDP-glucuronosyltransferase (UGT1A1). Mutations in a first exon affect only a single isoform. Those in exons 2–5 affect all enzymes encoded by the UGT1 complex.

the binding site for the sugar donor, UDP-glucuronic acid, and the transmembrane domain. Exon A1 and the four common exons, collectively designated the *UGT1A1* gene (Fig. 38-2), encode the physiologically critical enzyme bilirubin-UDP-glucuronosyltransferase (UGT1A1). A functional corollary of the organization of the *UGT1* gene is that a mutation in one of the first exons will affect only a single enzyme isoform. By contrast, a mutation in exons 2–5 will alter all isoforms encoded by the *UGT1* gene complex.

4. *Biliary excretion:* It has been thought until recently that bilirubin mono- and diglucuronides are excreted directly across the canalicular plasma membrane into the bile canaliculus by an ATP-dependent transport process mediated by a canalicular membrane protein called *multidrug resistance–associated protein 2* (MRP2). Mutations of MRP2 result in the Dubin-Johnson syndrome (see below). However, studies in patients with Rotor syndrome (see below) indicate that after formation, a portion of the glucuronides are transported into the portal circulation by a sinusoidal membrane protein called *multidrug resistance–associated protein 3* (MRP3) and subjected to reuptake into the hepatocyte by the sinusoidal membrane uptake transporters *organic anion transport protein 1B1* (OATP1B1) and OATP1B3.

EXTRAHEPATIC ASPECTS OF BILIRUBIN DISPOSITION

Bilirubin in the gut

Following secretion into bile, conjugated bilirubin reaches the duodenum and passes down the gastrointestinal tract without reabsorption by the intestinal mucosa. An appreciable fraction is converted by bacterial metabolism in the gut to the water-soluble colorless compound urobilinogen. Urobilinogen undergoes enterohepatic cycling. Urobilinogen not taken up by the liver reaches the systemic circulation, from which some is cleared by the kidneys. Unconjugated bilirubin ordinarily does not reach the gut except in neonates or, by ill-defined alternative pathways, in the presence of severe unconjugated hyperbilirubinemia (e.g., Crigler-Najjar syndrome, type I [CN-I]). Unconjugated bilirubin that reaches the gut is partly reabsorbed, amplifying any underlying hyperbilirubinemia. Recent reports suggest that oral administration of calcium phosphate with or without the lipase inhibitor orlistat may be an efficient means to interrupt bilirubin enterohepatic cycling to reduce serum bilirubin levels in this situation. Although orlistat administration for 4–6 weeks to 16 patients with Crigler-Najjar syndrome was associated with a 10–20% decrease in serum bilirubin in 7 patients, the cost and side effects (i.e., diarrhea) may obviate the small benefit achievable with this treatment.

Renal excretion of bilirubin conjugates

Unconjugated bilirubin is not excreted in urine, as it is too tightly bound to albumin for effective glomerular filtration and there is no tubular mechanism for its renal secretion. In contrast, the bilirubin conjugates are readily filtered at the glomerulus and can appear in urine in disorders characterized by increased bilirubin conjugates in the circulation.

DISORDERS OF BILIRUBIN METABOLISM LEADINGTO UNCONJUGATED HYPERBILIRUBINEMIA

INCREASED BILIRUBIN PRODUCTION

Hemolysis

Increased destruction of erythrocytes leads to increased bilirubin turnover and unconjugated hyperbilirubinemia; the hyperbilirubinemia is usually modest in the presence of normal liver function. In particular, the bone marrow is only capable of a sustained eight-fold increase in erythrocyte production in response to a hemolytic stress. Therefore, hemolysis alone cannot result in a sustained hyperbilirubinemia of more than ~68 μmol/L (4 mg/dL). Higher values imply concomitant hepatic dysfunction. When hemolysis is the only abnormality in an otherwise healthy individual, the result is a purely unconjugated hyperbilirubinemia, with the direct-reacting fraction as measured in a typical clinical laboratory being ≤15% of the total serum bilirubin. In the presence of systemic disease, which may include a degree of hepatic dysfunction, hemolysis may produce a component of conjugated hyperbilirubinemia in addition to an elevated unconjugated bilirubin concentration. Prolonged hemolysis may lead to the precipitation of bilirubin salts within the gallbladder or biliary tree, resulting in the formation of gallstones in which bilirubin, rather than cholesterol, is the major component. Such pigment stones may lead to acute or chronic cholecystitis, biliary obstruction, or any other biliary tract consequence of calculous disease.

Ineffective erythropoiesis

During erythroid maturation, small amounts of hemoglobin may be lost at the time of nuclear extrusion, and a fraction of developing erythroid cells is destroyed within the marrow. These processes normally account for a small proportion of bilirubin that is produced. In various disorders, including thalassemia major, megaloblastic anemias due to folate or vitamin B_{12} deficiency, congenital erythropoietic porphyria, lead poisoning, and various congenital and acquired dyserythropoietic anemias, the fraction of total bilirubin production derived from ineffective erythropoiesis is increased, reaching as much as 70% of the total. This may be sufficient to produce modest degrees of unconjugated hyperbilirubinemia.

Miscellaneous

Degradation of the hemoglobin of extravascular collections of erythrocytes, such as those seen in massive tissue infarctions or large hematomas, may lead transiently to unconjugated hyperbilirubinemia.

DECREASED HEPATIC BILIRUBIN CLEARANCE

Decreased hepatic uptake

Decreased hepatic bilirubin uptake is believed to contribute to the unconjugated hyperbilirubinemia of Gilbert syndrome (GS), although the molecular basis for this finding remains unclear (see below). Several drugs, including flavaspidic acid, novobiocin, and rifampin, as well as various cholecystographic contrast agents, have been reported to inhibit bilirubin uptake. The resulting unconjugated hyperbilirubinemia resolves with cessation of the medication.

Impaired conjugation

Physiologic neonatal jaundice

Bilirubin produced by the fetus is cleared by the placenta and eliminated by the maternal liver. Immediately after birth, the neonatal liver must assume responsibility for bilirubin clearance and excretion. However, many hepatic physiologic processes are incompletely developed at birth. Levels of UGT1A1 are low, and alternative excretory pathways allow passage of unconjugated bilirubin into the gut. Since the intestinal flora that convert bilirubin to urobilinogen are also undeveloped, an enterohepatic circulation of unconjugated bilirubin ensues. As a consequence, most neonates develop mild unconjugated hyperbilirubinemia between days 2 and 5 after birth. Peak levels are typically <85–170 μmol/L (5–10 mg/dL) and decline to normal adult concentrations within 2 weeks, as mechanisms required for bilirubin disposition mature. Prematurity, often associated with more profound immaturity of hepatic function and hemolysis, can result in higher levels of unconjugated hyperbilirubinemia. A rapidly rising unconjugated bilirubin concentration, or absolute levels >340 μmol/L (20 mg/dL), puts the infant at risk for bilirubin encephalopathy, or kernicterus. Under these circumstances, bilirubin crosses an immature blood-brain barrier and precipitates in the basal ganglia and other areas of the brain. The consequences range from appreciable neurologic deficits to death. Treatment options include phototherapy, which converts bilirubin into water-soluble photoisomers that are excreted directly into bile, and exchange transfusion. The canalicular mechanisms responsible for bilirubin excretion are also immature at birth, and their maturation may lag behind that of UGT1A1; this can lead to transient conjugated neonatal hyperbilirubinemia, especially in infants with hemolysis.

Acquired conjugation defects

A modest reduction in bilirubin conjugating capacity may be observed in advanced hepatitis or cirrhosis. However, in this setting, conjugation is better preserved than other aspects of bilirubin disposition, such as canalicular excretion. Various drugs, including pregnanediol, novobiocin, chloramphenicol, and gentamicin, may produce unconjugated hyperbilirubinemia by inhibiting UGT1A1 activity. Bilirubin conjugation may be inhibited by certain fatty acids that are present in breast milk but not serum of mothers whose infants have excessive neonatal hyperbilirubinemia (*breast milk jaundice*). Alternatively, there may be increased enterohepatic circulation of bilirubin in these infants. A recent study has correlated epidermal growth factor (EGF) content of breast milk with elevated bilirubin levels in these infants; however, a cause-and-effect relationship remains to be established. The pathogenesis of breast milk jaundice appears to differ from that of transient familial neonatal hyperbilirubinemia (Lucey-Driscoll syndrome), in which there is a UGT1A1 inhibitor in maternal serum.

HEREDITARY DEFECTS IN BILIRUBIN CONJUGATION

Three familial disorders characterized by differing degrees of unconjugated hyperbilirubinemia have long been recognized. The defining clinical features of each are described below (Table 38-1). While these disorders have been recognized for decades to reflect differing degrees of deficiency in the ability to conjugate bilirubin, recent advances in the molecular biology of the *UGT1* gene complex have elucidated their interrelationships and clarified previously puzzling features.

Crigler-Najjar syndrome, type i

CN-I is characterized by striking unconjugated hyperbilirubinemia of about 340–765 μmol/L (20–45 mg/dL) that appears in the neonatal period and persists for life. Other conventional hepatic biochemical tests such as serum aminotransferases and alkaline phosphatase are normal, and there is no evidence of hemolysis. Hepatic histology is also essentially normal except for the occasional presence of bile plugs within canaliculi. Bilirubin glucuronides are virtually absent from the bile, and there is no detectable constitutive expression of UGT1A1 activity in hepatic tissue. Neither UGT1A1 activity nor the serum bilirubin concentration responds to administration of phenobarbital or other enzyme inducers. In the absence of conjugation, unconjugated bilirubin accumulates in plasma, from which it is eliminated very slowly by alternative pathways that include direct passage into the bile and small intestine. These account for the small amounts of urobilinogen found in feces. No bilirubin is found in the urine. First described in 1952, the disorder is rare (estimated prevalence, 0.6–1.0 per million). Many patients are from geographically or socially isolated communities in which consanguinity is common, and pedigree analyses show an autosomal recessive pattern of inheritance. The majority of patients (type IA) exhibit defects in the glucuronide conjugation of a spectrum of substrates in addition to bilirubin, including various drugs and other xenobiotics. These individuals have mutations in one of the common exons (2–5) of the *UGT1* gene (Fig. 38-2). In a smaller subset (type IB), the defect is limited largely to bilirubin conjugation, and the causative mutation is in the bilirubin-specific exon A1. Estrogen glucuronidation is mediated by UGT1A1 and is defective in all CN-I patients. More than 30 different genetic lesions of *UGT1A1* responsible for CN-I have been identified, including deletions, insertions, alterations in intron

TABLE 38-1

PRINCIPAL DIFFERENTIAL CHARACTERISTICS OF GILBERT AND CRIGLER-NAJJAR SYNDROMES

FEATURE	CRIGLER-NAJJAR SYNDROME TYPE I	CRIGLER-NAJJAR SYNDROME TYPE II	GILBERT SYNDROME
Total serum bilirubin, μmol/L (mg/dL)	310–755 (usually >345) (18–45 [usually >20])	100–430 (usually ≤345)(6–25 [usually ≤20])	Typically ≤70 μmol/L (≤4 mg/dL) in absence of fasting or hemolysis
Routine liver tests	Normal	Normal	Normal
Response to phenobarbital	None	Decreases bilirubin by >25%	Decreases bilirubin to normal
Kernicterus	Usual	Rare	No
Hepatic histology	Normal	Normal	Usually normal; increased lipofuscin pigment in some
Bile characteristics			
Color	Pale or colorless	Pigmented	Normal dark color
Bilirubin fractions	>90% unconjugated	Largest fraction (mean: 57%) monoconjugates	Mainly diconjugates but monoconjugates increased (mean: 23%)
Bilirubin UDP-glucuronosyltransferase activity	Typically absent; traces in some patients	Markedly reduced: 0–10% of normal	Reduced: typically 10–33% of normal
Inheritance (all autosomal)	Recessive	Predominantly recessive	Promoter mutation: recessive Missense mutations: 7 of 8 dominant; 1 reportedly recessive

splice donor and acceptor sites, exon skipping, and point mutations that introduce premature stop codons or alter critical amino acids. Their common feature is that they all encode proteins with absent or, at most, traces of bilirubin-UDP-glucuronosyltransferase enzymatic activity.

Prior to the availability of phototherapy, most patients with CN-I died of bilirubin encephalopathy (*kernicterus*) in infancy or early childhood. A few lived as long as early adult life without overt neurologic damage, although more subtle testing usually indicated mild but progressive brain damage. In the absence of liver transplantation, death eventually supervened from late-onset bilirubin encephalopathy, which often followed a nonspecific febrile illness. Although isolated hepatocyte transplantation has been used in a small number of cases of CN-I, early liver transplantation **(Chap. 48)** remains the best hope to prevent brain injury and death.

Crigler-Najjar syndrome, type II (CN-II)

This condition was recognized as a distinct entity in 1962 and is characterized by marked unconjugated hyperbilirubinemia in the absence of abnormalities of other conventional hepatic biochemical tests, hepatic histology, or hemolysis. It differs from CN-I in several specific ways (Table 38-1): (1) Although there is considerable overlap, average bilirubin concentrations are lower in CN-II; (2) accordingly, CN-II is only infrequently associated with kernicterus; (3) bile is deeply colored, and bilirubin glucuronides are present, with a striking, characteristic increase in the proportion of monoglucuronides; (4) UGT1A1 in liver is usually present at reduced levels (typically ≤10% of normal) but may be undetectable by older, less sensitive assays; and (5) while typically detected in infancy, hyperbilirubinemia was not recognized in some cases until later in life and, in one instance, at age 34. As with CN-I, most CN-II cases exhibit abnormalities in the conjugation of other compounds, such as salicylamide and menthol, but in some instances, the defect appears limited to bilirubin. Reduction of serum bilirubin concentrations by >25% in response to enzyme inducers such as phenobarbital distinguishes CN-II from CN-I, although this response may not be elicited in early infancy and often is not accompanied by measurable UGT1A1 induction. Bilirubin concentrations during phenobarbital administration do not return to normal but are typically in the range of 51–86 μmol/L (3–5 mg/dL). Although the incidence of kernicterus in CN-II is low, instances have occurred, not only in infants but also in adolescents and adults, often in the setting of an intercurrent illness, fasting, or another factor that temporarily raises the serum bilirubin concentration above baseline and reduces serum albumin levels. For this reason, phenobarbital therapy is widely recommended, a single bedtime dose often sufficing to maintain clinically safe serum bilirubin concentrations.

Over 77 different mutations in the *UGT1* gene have been identified as causing CN-I or CN-II. It was found that missense mutations are more common in CN-II patients, as would be expected in this less severe phenotype. Their common feature is that they encode for a bilirubin-UDP-glucuronosyltransferase with markedly reduced, but detectable, enzymatic activity. The spectrum of residual enzyme activity explains the spectrum of phenotypic severity of the resulting hyperbilirubinemia. Molecular analysis has established that a large majority of CN-II patients are either homozygotes or compound heterozygotes for CN-II mutations and that individuals carrying one mutated and one entirely normal allele have normal bilirubin concentrations.

Gilbert syndrome (GS)

This syndrome is characterized by mild unconjugated hyperbilirubinemia, normal values for standard hepatic biochemical tests, and normal hepatic histology other than a modest increase of lipofuscin pigment in some patients. Serum bilirubin concentrations are most often <51 μmol/L (<3 mg/dL), although both higher and lower values are frequent. The clinical spectrum of hyperbilirubinemia fades into that of CN-II at serum bilirubin concentrations of 86–136 μmol/L (5–8 mg/dL). At the other end of the scale, the distinction between mild cases of GS and a normal state is often blurred. Bilirubin concentrations may fluctuate substantially in any given individual, and at least 25% of patients will exhibit temporarily normal values during prolonged follow-up. More elevated values are associated with stress, fatigue, alcohol use, reduced caloric intake, and intercurrent illness, while increased caloric intake or administration of enzyme-inducing agents produces lower bilirubin levels. GS is most often diagnosed at or shortly after puberty or in adult life during routine examinations that include multichannel biochemical analyses. UGT1A1 activity is typically reduced to 10–35% of normal, and bile pigments exhibit a characteristic increase in bilirubin monoglucuronides. Studies of radiobilirubin kinetics indicate that hepatic bilirubin clearance is reduced to an average of one-third of normal. Administration of phenobarbital normalizes both the serum bilirubin concentration and hepatic bilirubin clearance; however, failure of UGT1A1 activity to improve in many such instances suggests the possible coexistence of an additional defect. Compartmental analysis of bilirubin kinetic data suggests that GS patients have a defect in bilirubin uptake as well as in conjugation. Defect(s) in the hepatic uptake of other organic anions that at least partially share an uptake mechanism with bilirubin, such as sulfobromophthalein and indocyanine green (ICG), are observed in a minority of patients. The metabolism and transport of bile acids that do not utilize the bilirubin uptake mechanism are normal. The magnitude of changes in the serum bilirubin concentration induced by provocation tests such as 48 hours of fasting or the IV administration of nicotinic acid have been reported to be of help in separating GS patients from normal individuals. Other studies dispute this assertion. Moreover, on theoretical grounds, the results of such studies should provide no more information than simple measurements of the baseline serum bilirubin concentration. Family studies indicate that GS and hereditary hemolytic anemias such as hereditary spherocytosis, glucose-6-phosphate dehydrogenase deficiency, and β-thalassemia trait sort independently. Reports of hemolysis in up to 50% of GS patients are believed to reflect better case finding, since patients with both GS and hemolysis have higher bilirubin concentrations, and are more likely to be jaundiced, than patients with either defect alone.

GS is common, with many series placing its prevalence at ≥8%. Males predominate over females by reported ratios ranging from 1.5:1 to >7:1. However, these ratios may have a large artifactual component since normal males have higher mean bilirubin levels than normal females, but the diagnosis of GS is often based on comparison to normal ranges established in men. The high prevalence of GS in the general population may explain the reported frequency of mild unconjugated hyperbilirubinemia in liver transplant recipients. The disposition of most xenobiotics metabolized by glucuronidation appears to be normal in GS, as is oxidative drug metabolism in the majority of reported studies. The principal exception is the metabolism of the antitumor agent irinotecan (CPT-11), whose active metabolite (SN-38) is glucuronidated specifically by bilirubin-UDP-glucuronosyltransferase. Administration of CPT-11 to patients with GS has resulted in several toxicities, including intractable diarrhea and myelosuppression. Some reports also suggest abnormal disposition of menthol, estradiol benzoate, acetaminophen, tolbutamide, and rifamycin SV. Although some of these studies have been disputed, and there have been no reports of clinical complications from use of these agents in GS, prudence should be exercised in prescribing them, or any agents metabolized primarily by glucuronidation, in this condition. It should also be noted that the HIV protease inhibitors indinavir and atazanavir can inhibit UGT1A1, resulting in hyperbilirubinemia that is most pronounced in patients with preexisting GS.

Most older pedigree studies of GS were consistent with autosomal dominant inheritance with variable expressivity. However, studies of the *UGT1* gene in GS have indicated a variety of molecular genetic bases for the phenotypic picture and several different patterns of inheritance. Studies in Europe and the United States found that nearly all patients had normal coding regions for UGT1A1 but were homozygous for the insertion of an extra TA (i.e., $A[TA]_7TAA$ rather than $A[TA]_6TAA$) in the promoter region of the first exon. This appeared to be necessary, but not sufficient, for clinically expressed GS, since 15% of normal controls were also homozygous for this variant. While normal by standard criteria, these individuals had somewhat higher bilirubin concentrations than the rest of the controls studied. Heterozygotes for this abnormality had bilirubin concentrations identical to those homozygous for the normal $A[TA]_6TAA$ allele. The prevalence of the $A[TA]_7TAA$ allele in a general Western population is 30%, in which case 9% would be homozygotes. This is slightly higher than the prevalence of GS based on purely phenotypic parameters. It was suggested that additional variables, such as mild hemolysis or a defect in bilirubin uptake, might be among the factors enhancing phenotypic expression of the defect.

Phenotypic expression of GS due solely to the $A[TA]_7TAA$ promoter abnormality is inherited as an autosomal recessive trait. A number of CN-II kindreds have been identified in whom there is also an allele containing a normal coding region but the $A[TA]_7TAA$ promoter abnormality. CN-II heterozygotes who have the $A[TA]_6TAA$ promoter are phenotypically normal, whereas those with the $A[TA]_7TAA$ promoter express the phenotypic picture of GS. GS in such kindreds may also result from homozygosity for the $A[TA]_7TAA$ promoter abnormality. Seven different missense mutations in the *UGT1* gene that reportedly cause GS with dominant inheritance have been found in Japanese individuals. Another Japanese patient with mild unconjugated hyperbilirubinemia was homozygous for a missense mutation in exon 5. GS in her family appeared to be recessive. Missense mutations causing GS have not been reported outside of certain Asian populations.

DISORDERS OF BILIRUBIN METABOLISM LEADING TO MIXED OR PREDOMINANTLY CONJUGATED HYPERBILIRUBINEMIA

In hyperbilirubinemia due to acquired liver disease (e.g., acute hepatitis, common bile duct stone), there are usually elevations in the serum concentrations of both conjugated and unconjugated bilirubin. Although biliary tract obstruction or hepatocellular cholestatic injury may present on occasion with a predominantly conjugated hyperbilirubinemia, it is generally not possible to differentiate intrahepatic from extrahepatic causes of jaundice based on the serum levels or relative proportions of unconjugated and conjugated bilirubin. The major reason for determining the amounts of conjugated and unconjugated bilirubin in the serum is for the initial differentiation of hepatic parenchymal and obstructive disorders (mixed conjugated and unconjugated hyperbilirubinemia) from the inheritable and hemolytic disorders discussed above that are associated with unconjugated hyperbilirubinemia.

FAMILIAL DEFECTS IN HEPATIC EXCRETORY FUNCTION

Dubin-Johnson syndrome (DJS)

This benign, relatively rare disorder is characterized by low-grade, predominantly conjugated hyperbilirubinemia (Table 38-2). Total bilirubin concentrations are typically between 34 and 85 μmol/L (2 and 5 mg/dL) but on occasion can be in the normal range or as high as 340–430 μmol/L (20–25 mg/dL) and can fluctuate widely in any given patient. The degree of hyperbilirubinemia may be increased by intercurrent illness, oral contraceptive use, and pregnancy. Because the hyperbilirubinemia is due to a predominant rise in conjugated bilirubin, bilirubinuria is characteristically present. Aside from elevated serum bilirubin levels, other routine laboratory tests are normal. Physical examination is usually normal except for jaundice, although an occasional patient may have hepatosplenomegaly.

Patients with DJS are usually asymptomatic, although some may have vague constitutional symptoms. These latter patients have usually undergone extensive and often unnecessary diagnostic examinations for unexplained jaundice and have high levels of anxiety. In women, the condition may be subclinical until the patient becomes pregnant or receives oral contraceptives, at which time chemical hyperbilirubinemia becomes frank jaundice. Even in these situations, other routine liver function tests, including serum alkaline phosphatase and transaminase activities, are normal.

A cardinal feature of DJS is the accumulation in the lysosomes of centrilobular hepatocytes of dark, coarsely granular pigment. As a result, the liver may be grossly black in appearance. This pigment is thought to be derived from epinephrine metabolites that are not excreted normally. The pigment may disappear during bouts of viral hepatitis, only to reaccumulate slowly after recovery.

Biliary excretion of a number of anionic compounds is compromised in DJS. These include various cholecystographic agents, as well as sulfobromophthalein (Bromsulphalein, BSP), a synthetic dye formerly used in a test of liver function. In this test, the rate of disappearance of BSP from plasma was determined following bolus IV administration. BSP is conjugated with glutathione in the hepatocyte; the resulting conjugate is normally excreted rapidly into the bile canaliculus. Patients with DJS exhibit characteristic rises in plasma concentrations at 90 minutes after injection, due to reflux of conjugated BSP into the circulation from the hepatocyte. Dyes such as ICG that are taken up by hepatocytes but are not further metabolized prior to biliary excretion do not show this reflux phenomenon. Continuous BSP infusion studies suggest a reduction in the time to

TABLE 38-2

PRINCIPAL DIFFERENTIAL CHARACTERISTICS OF INHERITABLE DISORDERS OF BILE CANALICULAR FUNCTION

	DJS	ROTOR	PFIC1	BRIC1	PFIC2	BRIC2	PFIC3
Gene	***ABCCA***	***SLCO1B1/SLCO1B3***	***ATP8B1***	***ATP8B1***	***ABCB11***	***ABCB11***	***ABCB4***
Protein	MRP2	OATP1B1/1B3	FIC1	FIC1	BSEP	BSEP	MDR3
Cholestasis	No	No	Yes	Episodic	Yes	Episodic	Yes
Serum γ-GT	Normal	Normal	Normal	Normal	Normal	Normal	↑↑
Serum bile acids	Normal	Normal	↑↑	↑↑ during episodes	↑↑	↑↑ during episodes	↑↑
Clinical features	Mild conjugated hyperbilirubinemia; otherwise normal liver function; dark pigment in liver; characteristic pattern of urinary coproporphyrins	Mild conjugated hyperbilirubinemia; otherwise normal liver function; liver without abnormal pigmentation	Severe cholestasis beginning in childhood	Recurrent episodes of cholestasis beginning at any age	Severe cholestasis beginning in childhood	Recurrent episodes of cholestasis beginning at any age	Severe cholestasis beginning in childhood; decreased phospholipids in bile

Abbreviations: BRIC, benign recurrent intrahepatic cholestasis; BSEP, bile salt excretory protein; DJS, Dubin-Johnson syndrome; γ-GT, γ-glutamyltransferase; MRP2, multidrug resistance–associated protein 2; OATP1A/1B, organic anion transport proteins 1B1 and 1B3; PFIC, progressive familial intrahepatic cholestasis; ↑↑, increased.

maximum plasma concentration (t_{max}) for biliary excretion. Bile acid disposition, including hepatocellular uptake and biliary excretion, is normal in DJS. These patients have normal serum and biliary bile acid concentrations and do not have pruritus.

By analogy with findings in several mutant rat strains, the selective defect in biliary excretion of bilirubin conjugates and certain other classes of organic compounds, but not of bile acids, that characterizes DJS in humans was found to reflect defective expression of MRP2, an ATP-dependent canalicular membrane transporter. Several different mutations in the *MRP2* gene produce the Dubin-Johnson phenotype, which has an autosomal recessive pattern of inheritance. Although MRP2 is undoubtedly important in the biliary excretion of conjugated bilirubin, the fact that this pigment is still excreted in the absence of MRP2 suggests that other, as yet uncharacterized, transport proteins may serve in a secondary role in this process.

Patients with DJS also have a diagnostic abnormality in urinary coproporphyrin excretion. There are two naturally occurring coproporphyrin isomers, I and III. Normally, ~75% of the coproporphyrin in urine is isomer III. In urine from DJS patients, total coproporphyrin content is normal, but >80% is isomer I. Heterozygotes for the syndrome show an intermediate pattern. The molecular basis for this phenomenon remains unclear.

Rotor syndrome

This benign, autosomal recessive disorder is clinically similar to DJS (Table 38-2), although it is seen even less frequently. A major phenotypic difference is that the liver in patients with Rotor syndrome has no increased pigmentation and appears totally normal. The only abnormality in routine laboratory tests is an elevation of total serum bilirubin, due to a predominant rise in conjugated bilirubin. This is accompanied by bilirubinuria. Several additional features differentiate Rotor syndrome from DJS. In Rotor syndrome, the gallbladder is usually visualized on oral cholecystography, in contrast to the nonvisualization that is typical of DJS. The pattern of urinary coproporphyrin excretion also differs. The pattern in Rotor syndrome resembles that of many acquired disorders of hepatobiliary function, in which coproporphyrin I, the major coproporphyrin isomer in bile, refluxes from the hepatocyte back into the circulation and is excreted in urine. Thus, total urinary coproporphyrin excretion is substantially increased in Rotor syndrome, in contrast to the normal levels seen in DJS. Although the fraction of coproporphyrin I in urine is elevated, it is usually <70% of the total, compared with ≥80% in DJS. The disorders also can be distinguished by their patterns of BSP excretion. Although clearance of BSP from plasma is delayed in Rotor syndrome, there is no reflux of conjugated BSP back into the circulation as seen in DJS. Kinetic analysis of plasma BSP infusion studies suggests the presence of a defect in intrahepatocellular storage of this compound. This has never been demonstrated directly. Recent studies indicate that the molecular basis of Rotor syndrome results from simultaneous deficiency of the plasma membrane transporters OATP1B1 and OATP1B3. This results in reduced reuptake of conjugated bilirubin that has been pumped out of the cell into the portal circulation by MRP3 (Fig. 38-1).

Benign recurrent intrahepatic cholestasis (BRIC)

This rare disorder is characterized by recurrent attacks of pruritus and jaundice. The typical episode begins with mild malaise and elevations in serum aminotransferase levels, followed rapidly by rises in alkaline phosphatase and conjugated bilirubin and onset of jaundice and itching. The first one or two episodes may be misdiagnosed as acute viral hepatitis. The cholestatic episodes, which may begin in childhood or adulthood, can vary in duration from several weeks to months, followed by a complete clinical and biochemical resolution. Intervals between attacks may vary from several months to years. Between episodes, physical examination is normal, as are serum levels of bile acids, bilirubin, transaminases, and alkaline phosphatase. The disorder is familial and has an autosomal recessive pattern of inheritance. BRIC is considered a benign disorder in that it does not lead to cirrhosis or end-stage liver disease. However, the episodes of jaundice and pruritus can be prolonged and debilitating, and some patients have undergone liver transplantation to relieve the intractable and disabling symptoms. Treatment during the cholestatic episodes is symptomatic; there is no specific treatment to prevent or shorten the occurrence of episodes.

A gene termed *FIC1* was recently identified and found to be mutated in patients with BRIC. Curiously, this gene is expressed strongly in the small intestine but only weakly in the liver. The protein encoded by *FIC1* shows little similarity to those that have been shown to play a role in bile canalicular excretion of various compounds. Rather, it appears to be a member of a P-type ATPase family that transports aminophospholipids from the outer to the inner leaflet of a variety of cell membranes. Its relationship to the pathobiology of this disorder remains unclear. A second phenotypically identical form of BRIC, termed BRIC type 2, has been described resulting from mutations in the bile salt excretory protein (BSEP), the protein that is defective in progressive familial intrahepatic cholestasis type 2 (Table 38-2). How some mutations in this protein result in the episodic BRIC phenotype is unknown.

Progressive familial intrahepatic cholestasis (FIC)

This name is applied to three phenotypically related syndromes (Table 38-2). Progressive FIC type 1 (Byler disease) presents in early infancy as cholestasis that may be initially episodic. However, in contrast to BRIC, Byler disease progresses to malnutrition, growth retardation, and end-stage liver disease during childhood. This disorder is also a consequence of a *FIC1* mutation. The functional relationship of the FIC1 protein to the pathogenesis of cholestasis in these disorders is unknown. Two other types of progressive FIC (types 2 and 3) have been described. Progressive FIC type 2 is associated with a mutation in the protein originally named *sister of p-glycoprotein*, now known as *bile salt excretory protein*, which is the major bile canalicular exporter of bile acids. As noted above, some mutations of this protein are associated with BRIC type 2, rather than the progressive FIC type 2 phenotype. Progressive FIC type 3 has been associated with a mutation of MDR3, a protein that is essential for normal hepatocellular excretion of phospholipids across the bile canaliculus. Although all three types of progressive FIC have similar clinical phenotypes, only type 3 is associated with high serum levels of γ-glutamyltransferase activity. In contrast, activity of this enzyme is normal or only mildly elevated in symptomatic BRIC and progressive FIC types 1 and 2.

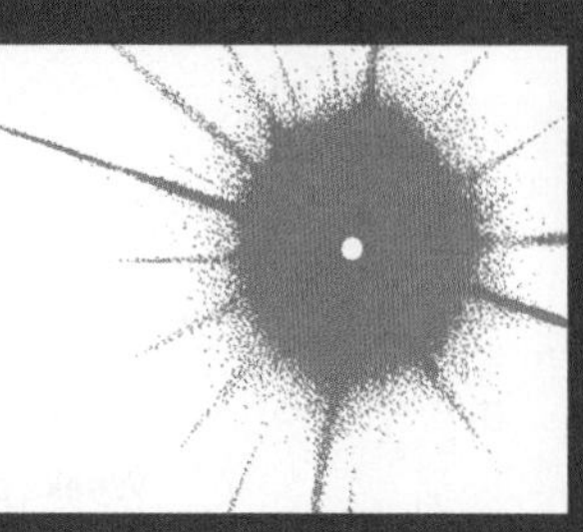

CHAPTER 39
ACUTE VIRAL HEPATITIS

Jules L. Dienstag

Acute viral hepatitis is a systemic infection affecting the liver predominantly. Almost all cases of acute viral hepatitis are caused by one of five viral agents: hepatitis A virus (HAV), hepatitis B virus (HBV), hepatitis C virus (HCV), the HBV-associated delta agent or hepatitis D virus (HDV), and hepatitis E virus (HEV). All these human hepatitis viruses are RNA viruses, except for hepatitis B, which is a DNA virus but replicates like a retrovirus. Although these agents can be distinguished by their molecular and antigenic properties, all types of viral hepatitis produce clinically similar illnesses. These range from asymptomatic and inapparent to fulminant and fatal acute infections common to all types, on the one hand, and from subclinical persistent infections to rapidly progressive chronic liver disease with cirrhosis and even hepatocellular carcinoma, common to the bloodborne types (HBV, HCV, and HDV), on the other.

VIROLOGY AND ETIOLOGY

Hepatitis A

HAV is a nonenveloped 27-nm, heat-, acid-, and ether-resistant RNA virus in the *Hepatovirus* genus of the picornavirus family (Fig. 39-1). Its virion contains four capsid polypeptides, designated VP1 to VP4, which are cleaved posttranslationally from the polyprotein product of a 7500-nucleotide genome. Inactivation of viral activity can be achieved by boiling for 1 min, by contact with formaldehyde and chlorine, or by ultraviolet irradiation. Despite nucleotide sequence variation of up to 20% among isolates of HAV, and despite the recognition of four genotypes affecting humans, all strains of this virus are immunologically indistinguishable and belong to one serotype. Hepatitis A has an incubation period of ~4 weeks. Its replication is limited to the liver, but the virus is present in the liver, bile, stools, and blood

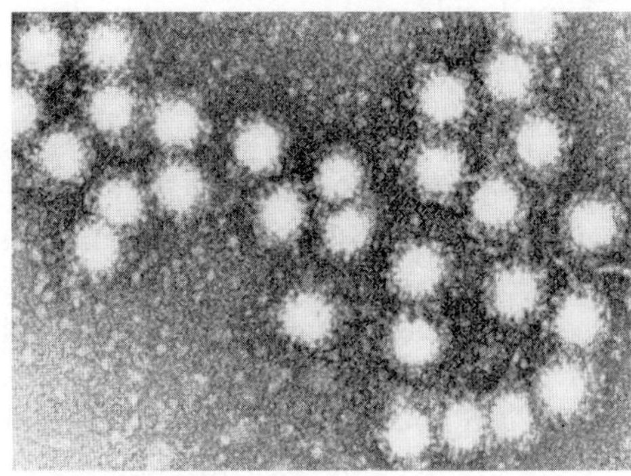

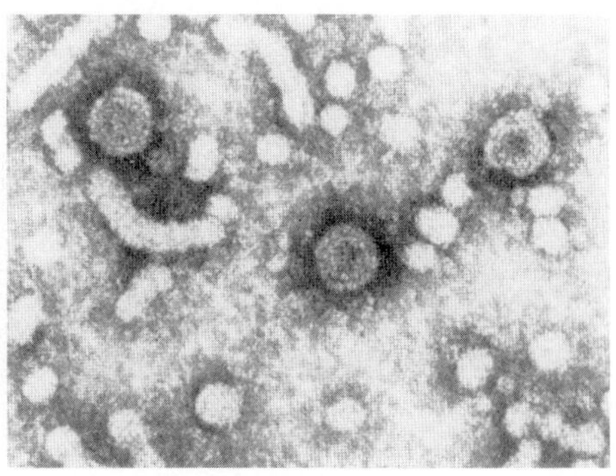

FIGURE 39-1

Electron micrographs of hepatitis A virus particles and serum from a patient with hepatitis B. ***Left:*** 27-nm hepatitis A virus particles purified from stool of a patient with acute hepatitis A and aggregated by antibody to hepatitis A virus. ***Right:*** Concentrated serum from a patient with hepatitis B, demonstrating the 42-nm virions, tubular forms, and spherical 22-nm particles of hepatitis B surface antigen. 132,000×. (Hepatitis D resembles 42-nm virions of hepatitis B but is smaller, 35–37 nm; hepatitis E resembles hepatitis A virus but is slightly larger, 32–34 nm; hepatitis C has been visualized as a 55-nm particle.)

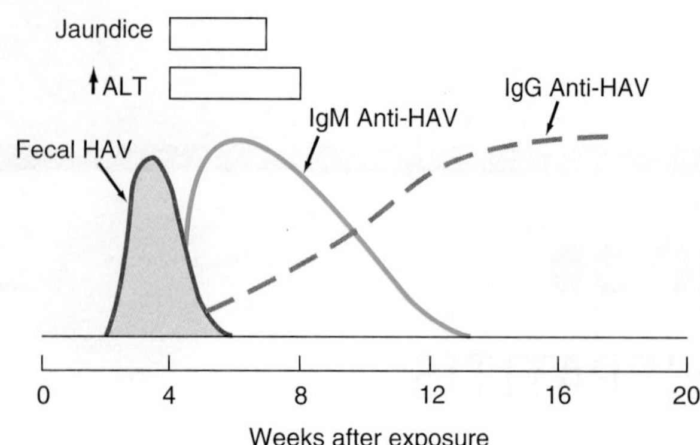

FIGURE 39-2
Scheme of typical clinical and laboratory features of hepatitis A virus (HAV). ALT, alanine aminotransferase.

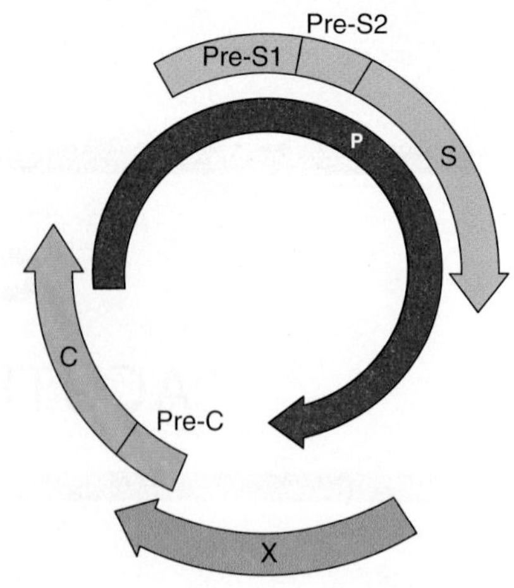

FIGURE 39-3
Compact genomic structure of hepatitis B virus (HBV). This structure, with overlapping genes, permits HBV to code for multiple proteins. The S gene codes for the "major" envelope protein, HBsAg. Pre-S1 and pre-S2, upstream of S, combine with S to code for two larger proteins, "middle" protein, the product of pre-S2 + S, and "large" protein, the product of pre-S1 + pre-S2 + S. The largest gene, P, codes for DNA polymerase. The C gene codes for two nucleocapsid proteins, HBeAg, a soluble, secreted protein (initiation from the pre-C region of the gene), and HBcAg, the intracellular core protein (initiation after pre-C). The X gene codes for HBxAg, which can transactivate the transcription of cellular and viral genes; its clinical relevance is not known, but it may contribute to carcinogenesis by binding to p53.

during the late incubation period and acute preicteric/presymptomatic phase of illness. Despite slightly longer persistence of virus in the liver, fecal shedding, viremia, and infectivity diminish rapidly once jaundice becomes apparent. HAV can be cultivated reproducibly in vitro.

Antibodies to HAV (anti-HAV) can be detected during acute illness when serum aminotransferase activity is elevated and fecal HAV shedding is still occurring. This early antibody response is predominantly of the IgM class and persists for several (~3) months, rarely for 6–12 months. During convalescence, however, anti-HAV of the IgG class becomes the predominant antibody (Fig. 39-2). Therefore, the diagnosis of hepatitis A is made during acute illness by demonstrating anti-HAV of the IgM class. After acute illness, anti-HAV of the IgG class remains detectable indefinitely, and patients with serum anti-HAV are immune to reinfection. Neutralizing antibody activity parallels the appearance of anti-HAV, and the IgG anti-HAV present in immune globulin accounts for the protection it affords against HAV infection.

Hepatitis B

HBV is a DNA virus with a remarkably compact genomic structure; despite its small, circular, 3200-bp size, HBV DNA codes for four sets of viral products with a complex, multiparticle structure. HBV achieves its genomic economy by relying on an efficient strategy of encoding proteins from four overlapping genes: S, C, P, and X (Fig. 39-3), as detailed below. Once thought to be unique among viruses, HBV is now recognized as one of a family of animal viruses, hepadnaviruses (hepatotropic DNA viruses), and is classified as hepadnavirus type 1. Similar viruses infect certain species of woodchucks, ground and tree squirrels, and Pekin ducks, to mention the most carefully characterized. Like HBV, all have the same distinctive three morphologic forms, have counterparts to the envelope and nucleocapsid virus antigens of HBV, replicate in the liver but exist in extrahepatic sites, contain their own endogenous DNA polymerase, have partially double-strand and partially single-strand genomes, are associated with acute and chronic hepatitis and hepatocellular carcinoma, and rely on a replicative strategy unique among DNA viruses but typical of retroviruses. Instead of DNA replication directly from a DNA template, hepadnaviruses rely on reverse transcription (effected by the DNA polymerase) of minus-strand DNA from a "pregenomic" RNA intermediate. Then plus-strand DNA is transcribed from the minus-strand DNA template by the DNA-dependent DNA polymerase and converted in the hepatocyte nucleus to a covalently closed circular DNA, which serves as a template for messenger RNA and pregenomic RNA. Viral proteins are translated by the messenger RNA, and the proteins and genome are packaged into virions and secreted from the hepatocyte. Although HBV is difficult to cultivate in vitro in the conventional sense from clinical material, several cell lines have been transfected with HBV DNA. Such transfected cells support in vitro replication of the intact virus and its component proteins.

Viral proteins and particles

Of the three particulate forms of HBV (Table 39-1), the most numerous are the 22-nm particles, which appear

TABLE 39-1

NOMENCLATURE AND FEATURES OF HEPATITIS VIRUSES

HEPATITIS TYPE	VIRUS PARTICLE, nm	MORPHOLOGY	GENOME[a]	CLASSIFICATION	ANTIGEN(S)	ANTIBODIES	REMARKS
HAV	27	Icosahedral nonenveloped	7.5-kb RNA, linear, ss, +	Hepatovirus	HAV	Anti-HAV	Early fecal shedding Diagnosis: IgM anti-HAV Previous infection: IgG anti-HAV
HBV	42	Double-shelled virion (surface and core) spherical	3.2-kb DNA, circular, ss/ds	Hepadnavirus	HBsAg HBcAg HBeAg	Anti-HBs Anti-HBc Anti-HBe	Bloodborne virus; carrier state Acute diagnosis: HBsAg, IgM anti-HBc Chronic diagnosis: IgG anti-HBc, HBsAg Markers of replication: HBeAg, HBV DNA Liver, lymphocytes, other organs
	27	Nucleocapsid core			HBcAg HBeAg	Anti-HBc Anti-HBe	Nucleocapsid contains DNA and DNA polymerase; present in hepatocyte nucleus; HBcAg does not circulate; HBeAg (soluble, nonparticulate) and HBV DNA circulate—correlate with infectivity and complete virions
	22	Spherical and filamentous; represents excess virus coat material			HBsAg	Anti-HBs	HBsAg detectable in >95% of patients with acute hepatitis B; found in serum, body fluids, hepatocyte cytoplasm; anti-HBs appears following infection—protective antibody
HCV	Approx. 50–80	Enveloped	9.4-kb RNA, linear, ss, +	Hepacivirus	HCV C100-3 C33c C22-3 NS5	Anti-HCV	Bloodborne agent, formerly labeled non-A, non-B hepatitis Acute diagnosis: anti-HCV (C33c, C22-3, NS5), HCV RNA Chronic diagnosis: anti-HCV (C100-3, C33c, C22-3, NS5) and HCV RNA; cytoplasmic location in hepatocytes
HDV	35–37	Enveloped hybrid particle with HBsAg coat and HDV core	1.7-kb RNA, circular, ss, –	Resembles viroids and plant satellite viruses (genus Deltavirus)	HBsAg HDAg	Anti-HBs Anti-HDV	Defective RNA virus, requires helper function of HBV (hepadnaviruses); HDV antigen (HDAg) present in hepatocyte nucleus Diagnosis: anti-HDV, HDV RNA; HBV/HDV co-infection—IgM anti-HBc and anti-HDV; HDV superinfection—IgG anti-HBc and anti-HDV
HEV	32–34	Nonenveloped icosahedral	7.6-kb RNA, linear, ss, +	Hepevirus	HEV antigen	Anti-HEV	Agent of enterically transmitted hepatitis; rare in United States; occurs in Asia, Mediterranean countries, Central America Diagnosis: IgM/IgG anti-HEV (assays not routinely available); virus in stool, bile, hepatocyte cytoplasm

[a]ss, single-strand; ss/ds, partially single-strand, partially double-strand; –, minus-strand; +, plus-strand.

Note: See text for abbreviations.

as spherical or long filamentous forms; these are antigenically indistinguishable from the outer surface or envelope protein of HBV and are thought to represent excess viral envelope protein. Outnumbered in serum by a factor of 100 or 1000 to 1 compared with the spheres and tubules are large, 42-nm, double-shelled spherical particles, which represent the intact hepatitis B virion (Fig. 39-1). The envelope protein expressed on the outer surface of the virion and on the smaller spherical and tubular structures is referred to as *hepatitis B surface antigen* (HBsAg). The concentration of HBsAg and virus particles in the blood may reach 500 μg/mL and 10 trillion particles per milliliter, respectively. The envelope protein, HBsAg, is the product of the S gene of HBV.

Envelope HBsAg subdeterminants include a common group-reactive antigen, *a*, shared by all HBsAg isolates and one of several subtype-specific antigens—*d* or *y*, *w* or *r* —as well as other specificities. Hepatitis B isolates fall into one of at least eight subtypes and ten genotypes (A–J). Geographic distribution of genotypes and subtypes varies; genotypes A (corresponding to subtype *adw*) and D (*ayw*) predominate in the United States and Europe, whereas genotypes B (*adw*) and C (*adr*) predominate in Asia. Clinical course and outcome are independent of subtype, but genotype B appears to be associated with less rapidly progressive liver disease and cirrhosis and a lower likelihood, or delayed appearance, of hepatocellular carcinoma than genotype C or D. Patients with genotype A are more likely to clear circulating viremia and to achieve HBeAg and HBsAg seroconversion, both spontaneously and in response to antiviral therapy. In addition, "precore" mutations are favored by certain genotypes (see below).

Upstream of the S gene are the pre-S genes (Fig. 39-3), which code for pre-S gene products, including receptors on the HBV surface for polymerized human serum albumin and for hepatocyte membrane proteins. The pre-S region actually consists of both pre-S1 and pre-S2. Depending on where translation is initiated, three potential HBsAg gene products are synthesized. The protein product of the S gene is HBsAg (*major protein*), the product of the S region plus the adjacent pre-S2 region is the *middle protein*, and the product of the pre-S1 plus pre-S2 plus S regions is the *large protein*. Compared with the smaller spherical and tubular particles of HBV, complete 42-nm virions are enriched in the large protein. Both pre-S proteins and their respective antibodies can be detected during HBV infection, and the period of pre-S antigenemia appears to coincide with other markers of virus replication, as detailed below; however, pre-S proteins have little clinical relevance and are not included in routine serologic testing repertoires.

The intact 42-nm virion contains a 27-nm nucleocapsid core particle. Nucleocapsid proteins are coded for by the C gene. The antigen expressed on the surface of the nucleocapsid core is *hepatitis B core antigen* (HBcAg), and its corresponding antibody is anti-HBc. A third HBV antigen is *hepatitis B e antigen* (HBeAg), a soluble, nonparticulate, nucleocapsid protein that is immunologically distinct from intact HBcAg but is a product of the same C gene. The C gene has two initiation codons, a precore and a core region (Fig. 39-3). If translation is initiated at the precore region, the protein product is HBeAg, which has a signal peptide that binds it to the smooth endoplasmic reticulum, the secretory apparatus of the cell, leading to its secretion into the circulation. If translation begins at the core region, HBcAg is the protein product; it has no signal peptide, it is not secreted, but it assembles into nucleocapsid particles, which bind to and incorporate RNA, and which, ultimately, contain HBV DNA. Also packaged within the nucleocapsid core is a DNA polymerase, which directs replication and repair of HBV DNA. When packaging within viral proteins is complete, synthesis of the incomplete plus strand stops; this accounts for the single-strand gap and for differences in the size of the gap. HBcAg particles remain in the hepatocyte, where they are readily detectable by immunohistochemical staining and are exported after encapsidation by an envelope of HBsAg. Therefore, naked core particles do not circulate in the serum. The secreted nucleocapsid protein, HBeAg, provides a convenient, readily detectable, qualitative marker of HBV replication and relative infectivity.

HBsAg-positive serum containing HBeAg is more likely to be highly infectious and to be associated with the presence of hepatitis B virions (and detectable HBV DNA, see below) than HBeAg-negative or anti-HBe-positive serum. For example, HBsAg-positive mothers who are HBeAg-positive almost invariably (>90%) transmit hepatitis B infection to their offspring, whereas HBsAg-positive mothers with anti-HBe rarely (10–15%) infect their offspring.

Early during the course of acute hepatitis B, HBeAg appears transiently; its disappearance may be a harbinger of clinical improvement and resolution of infection. Persistence of HBeAg in serum beyond the first 3 months of acute infection may be predictive of the development of chronic infection, and the presence of HBeAg during chronic hepatitis B tends to be associated with ongoing viral replication, infectivity, and inflammatory liver injury (except during the early decades after perinatally acquired HBV infection; see below).

The third and largest of the HBV genes, the P gene (Fig. 39-3), codes for HBV DNA polymerase; as noted above, this enzyme has both DNA-dependent DNA polymerase and RNA-dependent reverse transcriptase activities. The fourth gene, X, codes for a small, nonparticulate protein, *hepatitis B x antigen* (HBxAg), that is capable of transactivating the transcription of both viral and cellular genes(Fig. 39-3). In the cytoplasm, HBxAg effects calcium release (possibly from mitochondria), which activates signal-transduction pathways that lead to stimulation of HBV reverse transcription and HBV DNA replication. Such transactivation may enhance the replication of HBV, leading to the clinical association observed between the expression of HBxAg and antibodies to it in patients with severe chronic hepatitis and hepatocellular carcinoma. The transactivating activity can enhance the transcription and replication of other viruses besides HBV, such as HIV. Cellular processes transactivated by X include the human interferon γ gene and class I major histocompatibility genes; potentially, these effects could contribute to enhanced susceptibility of HBV-infected hepatocytes to cytolytic T cells. The expression of X can also induce programmed cell death (apoptosis). The clinical relevance of HBxAg is limited, however, and testing for it is not part of routine clinical practice.

Serologic and virologic markers

After a person is infected with HBV, the first virologic marker detectable in serum within 1–12 weeks, usually between 8 and 12 weeks, is HBsAg (Fig. 39-4). Circulating HBsAg precedes elevations of serum aminotransferase activity and clinical symptoms by 2–6 weeks and remains detectable during the entire icteric or symptomatic phase of acute hepatitis B and beyond. In typical cases, HBsAg becomes undetectable 1–2 months after the onset of jaundice and rarely persists beyond 6 months. After HBsAg disappears, antibody to HBsAg (anti-HBs) becomes detectable in serum and remains detectable indefinitely thereafter. Because HBcAg is intracellular and, when in the serum, sequestered within an HBsAg coat, naked core particles do not circulate in serum, and therefore, HBcAg is not detectable routinely in the serum of patients with HBV infection. By contrast, anti-HBc is readily demonstrable in serum, beginning within the first 1–2 weeks after the appearance of HBsAg and preceding detectable levels of anti-HBs by weeks to months. Because variability exists in the time of appearance of anti-HBs after HBV infection, occasionally a gap of several weeks or longer may separate the disappearance of HBsAg and the appearance of anti-HBs. During this "gap" or "window" period, anti-HBc may represent the only serologic evidence of current or recent HBV infection, and blood containing anti-HBc in the absence of HBsAg and anti-HBs has been implicated in transfusion-associated hepatitis B. In part because the sensitivity of immunoassays for HBsAg and anti-HBs has increased, however, this window period is rarely encountered. In some persons, years after HBV infection, anti-HBc may persist in the circulation longer than anti-HBs. Therefore, isolated anti-HBc does not necessarily indicate active virus replication; most instances of isolated anti-HBc represent hepatitis B infection in the remote past. Rarely, however, isolated anti-HBc represents low-level hepatitis B viremia, with HBsAg below the detection threshold, and, occasionally, isolated anti-HBc represents a cross-reacting or false-positive immunologic specificity. Recent and remote HBV infections can be distinguished by determination of the immunoglobulin class of anti-HBc. Anti-HBc of the IgM class (IgM anti-HBc) predominates during the first 6 months after acute infection, whereas IgG anti-HBc is the predominant class of anti-HBc beyond 6 months. Therefore, patients with current or recent acute hepatitis B, including those in the anti-HBc window, have IgM anti-HBc in their serum. In patients who have recovered from hepatitis B in the remote past as well as those with chronic HBV infection, anti-HBc is predominantly of the IgG class. Infrequently, in ≤1–5% of patients with acute HBV infection, levels of HBsAg are too low to be detected; in such cases, the presence of IgM anti-HBc establishes the diagnosis of acute hepatitis B. When isolated anti-HBc occurs in the rare patient with chronic hepatitis B whose HBsAg level is below the sensitivity threshold of contemporary immunoassays (a low-level carrier), anti-HBc is of the IgG class. Generally, in persons who have recovered from hepatitis B, anti-HBs and anti-HBc persist indefinitely.

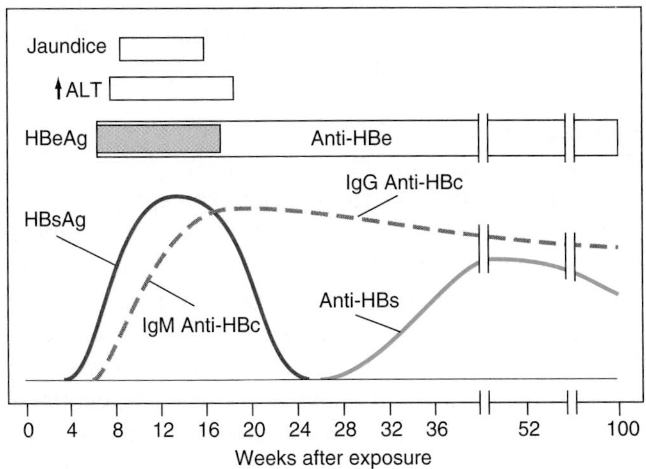

FIGURE 39-4
Scheme of typical clinical and laboratory features of acute hepatitis B. ALT, alanine aminotransferase.

The temporal association between the appearance of anti-HBs and resolution of HBV infection as well as the observation that persons with anti-HBs in serum are protected against reinfection with HBV suggests that *anti-HBs is the protective antibody*. Therefore, strategies for prevention of HBV infection are based on providing susceptible persons with circulating anti-HBs (see below). Occasionally, in ~10% of patients with chronic hepatitis B, low-level, low-affinity anti-HBs can be detected. This antibody is directed against a subtype determinant different from that represented by the patient's HBsAg; its presence is thought to reflect the stimulation of a related clone of antibody-forming cells, but it has no clinical relevance and does not signal imminent clearance of hepatitis B. These patients with

HBsAg and such nonneutralizing anti-HBs should be categorized as having chronic HBV infection.

The other readily detectable serologic marker of HBV infection, HBeAg, appears concurrently with or shortly after HBsAg. Its appearance coincides temporally with high levels of virus replication and reflects the presence of circulating intact virions and detectable HBV DNA (with the notable exception of patients with precore mutations who cannot synthesize HBeAg—see "Molecular Variants"). Pre-S1 and pre-S2 proteins are also expressed during periods of peak replication, but assays for these gene products are not routinely available. In self-limited HBV infections, HBeAg becomes undetectable shortly after peak elevations in aminotransferase activity, before the disappearance of HBsAg, and anti-HBe then becomes detectable, coinciding with a period of relatively lower infectivity (Fig. 39-4). Because markers of HBV replication appear transiently during acute infection, testing for such markers is of little clinical utility in typical cases of acute HBV infection. In contrast, markers of HBV replication provide valuable information in patients with protracted infections.

Departing from the pattern typical of acute HBV infections, in chronic HBV infection, HBsAg remains detectable beyond 6 months, anti-HBc is primarily of the IgG class, and anti-HBs is either undetectable or detectable at low levels (see "Laboratory Features") (Fig. 39-5). During early chronic HBV infection, HBV DNA can be detected both in serum and in hepatocyte nuclei, where it is present in free or episomal form. This relatively highly *replicative stage* of HBV infection is the time of maximal infectivity and liver injury; HBeAg is a qualitative marker and HBV DNA a quantitative marker of this replicative phase, during which all three forms of HBV circulate, including intact virions. Over time, the relatively replicative phase of chronic HBV infection gives way to a relatively *nonreplicative phase*. This occurs at a rate of ~10% per year and is accompanied by seroconversion from HBeAg to anti-HBe. In many cases, this seroconversion coincides with a transient, usually mild, acute hepatitis-like elevation in aminotransferase activity, believed to reflect cell-mediated immune clearance of virus-infected hepatocytes. In the nonreplicative phase of chronic infection, when HBV DNA is demonstrable in hepatocyte nuclei, it tends to be integrated into the host genome. In this phase, only spherical and tubular forms of HBV, *not intact virions*, circulate, and liver injury tends to subside. Most such patients would be characterized as *inactive HBV carriers*. In reality, the designations *replicative* and *nonreplicative* are only relative; even in the so-called nonreplicative phase, HBV replication can be detected at levels of approximately $\leq 10^3$ virions with highly sensitive amplification probes such as the polymerase chain reaction (PCR); below this replication threshold, liver injury and infectivity of HBV are limited to negligible. Still, the distinctions are pathophysiologically and clinically meaningful. Occasionally, nonreplicative HBV infection converts back to replicative infection. Such spontaneous reactivations are accompanied by reexpression of HBeAg and HBV DNA, and sometimes of IgM anti-HBc, as well as by exacerbations of liver injury. Because high-titer IgM anti-HBc can reappear during acute exacerbations of chronic hepatitis B, relying on IgM anti-HBc versus IgG anti-HBc to distinguish between acute and chronic hepatitis B infection, respectively, may not always be reliable; in such cases, patient history is invaluable in helping to distinguish de novo acute hepatitis B infection from acute exacerbation of chronic hepatitis B infection.

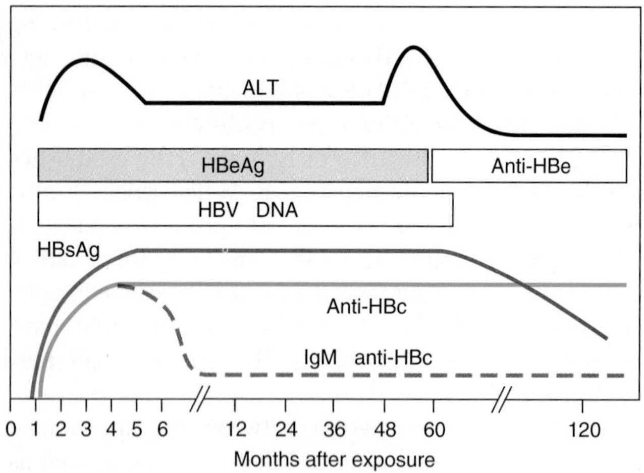

FIGURE 39-5

Scheme of typical laboratory features of wild-type chronic hepatitis B. HBeAg and hepatitis B virus (HBV) DNA can be detected in serum during the relatively *replicative phase* of chronic infection, which is associated with infectivity and liver injury. Seroconversion from the replicative phase to the relatively *nonreplicative phase* occurs at a rate of ~10% per year and is heralded by an acute hepatitis–like elevation of alanine aminotransferase (ALT) activity; during the nonreplicative phase, infectivity and liver injury are limited. In HBeAg-negative chronic hepatitis B associated with mutations in the precore region of the HBV genome, replicative chronic hepatitis B occurs in the absence of HBeAg.

Molecular variants

Variation occurs throughout the HBV genome, and clinical isolates of HBV that do not express typical viral proteins have been attributed to mutations in individual or even multiple gene locations. For example, variants have been described that lack nucleocapsid proteins (commonly), envelope proteins (very rarely), or both. Two categories of naturally occurring HBV variants have attracted the most attention. One of these was identified initially in Mediterranean countries among patients with severe chronic HBV infection and detectable HBV DNA but with anti-HBe instead of HBeAg. These patients were found to be infected with an HBV mutant that contained an alteration in the precore region rendering the virus incapable of encoding HBeAg. Although several potential mutation sites exist in the pre-C region, the region of the C gene necessary for the expression of HBeAg (see "Virology and Etiology"), the most commonly encountered in such patients is a single base substitution, from G to A in the second to last codon of the pre-C gene at nucleotide 1896. This substitution results in the replacement of the TGG tryptophan codon by a stop codon (TAG), which prevents the translation of HBeAg. Another mutation, in the core-promoter region, prevents transcription of the coding region for HBeAg and yields an HBeAg-negative phenotype. Patients with such mutations in the precore region and who are unable to secrete HBeAg may have severe liver disease that progresses more rapidly to cirrhosis, or alternatively, they are identified clinically later in the course of the natural history of chronic hepatitis B, when the disease is more advanced. Both "wild-type" HBV and precore-mutant HBV can coexist in the same patient, or mutant HBV may arise late during wild-type HBV infection. In addition, clusters of fulminant hepatitis B in Israel and Japan were attributed to common-source infection with a precore mutant. Fulminant hepatitis B in North America and western Europe, however, occurs in patients infected with wild-type HBV, in the absence of precore mutants, and both precore mutants and other mutations throughout the HBV genome occur commonly, even in patients with typical, self-limited, milder forms of HBV infection. HBeAg-negative chronic hepatitis with mutations in the precore region is now the most frequently encountered form of hepatitis B in Mediterranean countries and in Europe. In the United States, where HBV genotype A (less prone to G1896A mutation) is prevalent, precore-mutant HBV is much less common; however, as a result of immigration from Asia and Europe, the proportion of HBeAg-negative hepatitis B–infected individuals has increased in the United States, and they now represent approximately 30–40% of patients with chronic hepatitis B. Characteristic of such HBeAg-negative chronic hepatitis B are lower levels of HBV DNA (usually $\leq 10^5$ IU/mL) and one of several patterns of aminotransferase activity—persistent elevations, periodic fluctuations above the normal range, and periodic fluctuations between the normal and elevated range.

The second important category of HBV mutants consists of *escape mutants*, in which a single amino acid substitution, from glycine to arginine, occurs at position 145 of the immunodominant *a* determinant common to all HBsAg subtypes. This HBsAg alteration leads to a critical conformational change that results in a loss of neutralizing activity by anti-HBs. This specific HBV/*a* mutant has been observed in two situations, active and passive immunization, in which humoral immunologic pressure may favor evolutionary change ("escape") in the virus—in a small number of hepatitis B vaccine recipients who acquired HBV infection despite the prior appearance of neutralizing anti-HBs and in HBV-infected liver transplant recipients treated with a high-potency human monoclonal anti-HBs preparation. Although such mutants have not been recognized frequently, their existence raises a concern that may complicate vaccination strategies and serologic diagnosis.

Extrahepatic sites

Hepatitis B antigens and HBV DNA have been identified in extrahepatic sites, including lymph nodes, bone marrow, circulating lymphocytes, spleen, and pancreas. Although the virus does not appear to be associated with tissue injury in any of these extrahepatic sites, its presence in these "remote" reservoirs has been invoked (but is not necessary) to explain the recurrence of HBV infection after orthotopic liver transplantation. The clinical relevance of such extrahepatic HBV is limited.

Hepatitis D

The delta hepatitis agent, or HDV, the only member of the genus *Deltavirus*, is a defective RNA virus that coinfects with and requires the helper function of HBV (or other hepadnaviruses) for its replication and expression. Slightly smaller than HBV, HDV is a formalin-sensitive, 35- to 37-nm virus with a hybrid structure. Its nucleocapsid expresses HDV antigen (HDAg), which bears no antigenic homology with any of the HBV antigens, and contains the virus genome. The HDV core is "encapsidated" by an outer envelope of HBsAg, indistinguishable from that of HBV except in its relative compositions of major, middle, and large HBsAg component proteins. The genome is a small, 1700-nucleotide, circular, single-strand RNA of negative polarity that is nonhomologous with HBV DNA (except for a small area of the polymerase gene) but that has features and the rolling circle model of replication common to genomes of plant satellite viruses or viroids. HDV RNA contains many areas of internal complementarity; therefore, it can fold on itself by internal base pairing to form an unusual, very stable, rodlike structure that contains a very stable, self-cleaving and self-ligating ribozyme. HDV RNA requires host RNA polymerase II for its replication in the hepatocyte nucleus via RNA-directed RNA synthesis by transcription of genomic RNA to a complementary antigenomic (plus strand) RNA; the antigenomic RNA, in turn, serves as a template for subsequent genomic RNA synthesis effected by host RNA polymerase I. HDV RNA has only one open reading frame, and HDAg, a product of the antigenomic strand, is the only known HDV protein; HDAg exists in two forms: a small, 195-amino-acid species, which plays a role in facilitating HDV RNA replication, and a large, 214-amino-acid species, which appears to suppress replication but is required for assembly of the antigen into virions. HDV antigens have been shown to bind directly to RNA polymerase II, resulting in stimulation of transcription. Although complete hepatitis D virions and liver injury require the cooperative helper function of HBV, intracellular replication of HDV RNA can occur without HBV. Genomic heterogeneity among HDV isolates has been described; however, pathophysiologic and clinical consequences of this genetic diversity have not been recognized. The clinical spectrum of hepatitis D is common to all eight genotypes identified, the predominant of which is genotype 1.

HDV can either infect a person simultaneously with HBV (*co-infection*) or superinfect a person already infected with HBV (*superinfection*); when HDV infection is transmitted from a donor with one HBsAg subtype to an HBsAg-positive recipient with a different subtype, HDV assumes the HBsAg subtype of the recipient, rather than the donor. Because HDV relies absolutely on HBV, the duration of HDV infection is determined by the duration of (and cannot outlast) HBV infection. HDV replication tends to suppress HBV replication; therefore, patients with hepatitis D tend to have lower levels of HBV replication. HDV antigen is expressed primarily in hepatocyte nuclei and is occasionally detectable in serum. During acute HDV infection, anti-HDV of the IgM class predominates, and 30–40 days may elapse after symptoms appear before anti-HDV can be detected. In self-limited infection, anti-HDV is low-titer and transient, rarely remaining detectable beyond the clearance of HBsAg and HDV antigen. In chronic HDV infection, anti-HDV circulates in high titer, and both IgM and IgG anti-HDV can be detected. HDV antigen in the liver and HDV RNA in serum and liver can be detected during HDV replication.

Hepatitis C

Hepatitis C virus, which, before its identification was labeled "non-A, non-B hepatitis," is a linear, single-strand, positive-sense, 9600-nucleotide RNA virus, the genome of which is similar in organization to that of flaviviruses and pestiviruses; HCV is the only member of the genus *Hepacivirus* in the family Flaviviridae. The HCV genome contains a single, large open reading frame (gene) that codes for a virus polyprotein of ~3000 amino acids, which is cleaved after translation to yield 10 viral proteins. The 5′ end of the genome consists of an untranslated region (containing an internal ribosomal entry site, IRES) adjacent to the genes for three structural proteins, the nucleocapsid core protein, C, and two structural envelope glycoproteins, E1 and E2. The 5′ untranslated region and core gene are highly conserved among genotypes, but the envelope proteins are coded for by the hypervariable region, which varies from isolate to isolate and may allow the virus to evade host immunologic containment directed at accessible virus-envelope proteins. The 3′ end of the genome also includes an untranslated region and contains the genes for seven nonstructural (NS) proteins, p7, NS2, NS3, NS4A, NS4B, NS5A, and NS5B. p7 is a membrane ion channel protein necessary for efficient assembly and release of HCV. The NS2 cysteine protease cleaves NS3 from NS2, and the NS3-4A serine protease cleaves all the downstream proteins from the polyprotein. Important NS proteins involved in virus replication include the NS3 helicase; NS3-4A serine protease; the multifunctional membrane-associated phosphoprotein NS5A, an essential component of the viral replication membranous web (along with NS4B); and the NS5B RNA-dependent RNA polymerase (Fig. 39-6). Because HCV does not replicate via a DNA intermediate, it

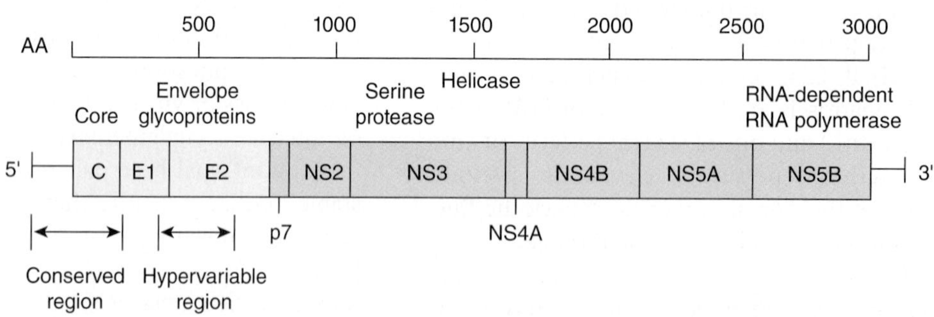

FIGURE 39-6

Organization of the hepatitis C virus genome and its associated, 3000-amino-acid (AA) proteins. The three structural genes at the 5′ end are the core region, C, which codes for the nucleocapsid, and the envelope regions, E1 and E2, which code for envelope glycoproteins. The 5′ untranslated region and the C region are highly conserved among isolates, whereas the envelope domain E2 contains the hypervariable region. At the 3′ end are seven nonstructural (NS) regions—p7, a membrane protein adjacent to the structural proteins that appears to function as an ion channel; NS2, which codes for a cysteine protease; NS3, which codes for a serine protease and an RNA helicase; NS4 and NS4B; NS5A, a multifunctional membrane-associated phosphoprotein, an essential component of the viral replication membranous web; and NS5B, which codes for an RNA-dependent RNA polymerase. After translation of the entire polyprotein, individual proteins are cleaved by both host and viral proteases.

does not integrate into the host genome. Because HCV tends to circulate in relatively low titer, 10^3–10^7 virions/mL, visualization of the 50- to 80-nm virus particles remains difficult. Still, the replication rate of HCV is very high, 10^{12} virions per day; its half-life is 2.7 h. The chimpanzee is a helpful but cumbersome animal model. Although a robust, reproducible, small animal model is lacking, HCV replication has been documented in an immunodeficient mouse model containing explants of human liver and in transgenic mouse and rat models. Although in vitro replication is difficult, replicons in hepatocellular carcinoma–derived cell lines support replication of genetically manipulated, truncated, or full-length HCV RNA (but not intact virions); infectious pseudotyped retroviral HCV particles have been shown to yield functioning envelope proteins. In 2005, complete replication of HCV and intact 55-nm virions were described in cell culture systems. HCV entry into the hepatocyte occurs via the nonliver-specific CD81 receptor and the liver-specific tight junction protein claudin-1. A growing list of additional host receptors to which HCV binds on cell entry includes occludin, low-density lipoprotein receptors, glycosaminoglycans, scavenger receptor B1, and epidermal growth factor receptor, among others. Relying on the same assembly and secretion pathway as low-density and very-low-density lipoproteins, HCV is a lipoviroparticle and masquerades as a lipoprotein, which may limit its visibility to the adaptive immune system and which may explain its ability to evade immune containment and clearance. After viral entry and uncoating, translation is initiated by the IRES on the endoplasmic reticulum membrane, and the HCV polyprotein is cleaved during translation and posttranslationally by host cellular proteases as well as HCV NS2-3 and NS3-4A proteases. Host cofactors involved in HCV replication include cyclophilin A, which binds to NS5A and yields conformational changes required for viral replication, and liver-specific host microRNA miR-122.

At least six distinct major genotypes (and a minor genotype 7), as well as >50 subtypes within genotypes, of HCV have been identified by nucleotide sequencing. Genotypes differ from one another in sequence homology by ≥30%, and subtypes differ by approximately 20%. Because divergence of HCV isolates within a genotype or subtype and within the same host may vary insufficiently to define a distinct genotype, these intragenotypic differences are referred to as *quasispecies* and differ in sequence homology by only a few percent. The genotypic and quasispecies diversity of HCV, resulting from its high mutation rate, interferes with effective humoral immunity. Neutralizing antibodies to HCV have been demonstrated, but they tend to be short lived, and HCV infection does not induce lasting immunity against reinfection with different virus isolates or even the same virus isolate. Thus, neither

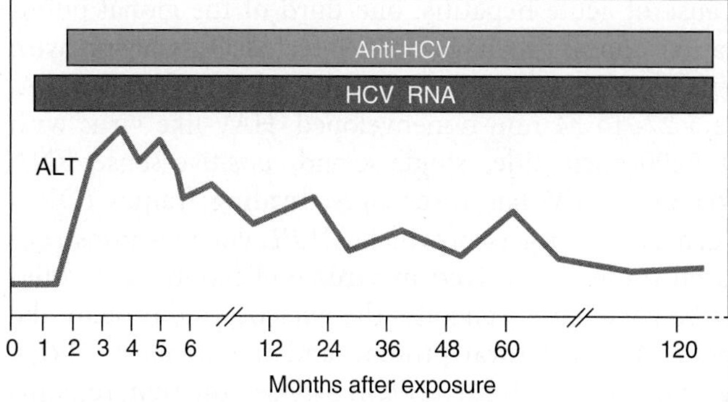

FIGURE 39-7

Scheme of typical laboratory features during acute hepatitis C progressing to chronicity. Hepatitis C virus (HCV) RNA is the first detectable event, preceding alanine aminotransferase (ALT) elevation and the appearance of anti-HCV.

heterologous nor *homologous* immunity appears to develop commonly after acute HCV infection. Some HCV genotypes are distributed worldwide, whereas others are more geographically confined (see "Epidemiology and Global Features"). In addition, differences exist among genotypes in responsiveness to antiviral therapy but not in pathogenicity or clinical progression (except for genotype 3, in which hepatic steatosis and clinical progression are more likely).

Currently available, third-generation immunoassays, which incorporate proteins from the core, NS3, and NS5 regions, detect anti-HCV antibodies during acute infection. The most sensitive indicator of HCV infection is the presence of HCV RNA, which requires molecular amplification by PCR or transcription-mediated amplification (TMA) (Fig. 39-7). To allow standardization of the quantification of HCV RNA among laboratories and commercial assays, HCV RNA is reported as international units (IUs) per milliliter; quantitative assays with a broad dynamic range are available that allow detection of HCV RNA with a sensitivity as low as 5 IU/mL. HCV RNA can be detected within a few days of exposure to HCV—well before the appearance of anti-HCV—and tends to persist for the duration of HCV infection. Application of sensitive molecular probes for HCV RNA has revealed the presence of replicative HCV in peripheral blood lymphocytes of infected persons; however, as is the case for HBV in lymphocytes, the clinical relevance of HCV lymphocyte infection is not known.

Hepatitis E

Previously labeled *epidemic* or *enterically transmitted non-A, non-B hepatitis*, HEV is an enterically transmitted virus that causes clinically apparent hepatitis primarily in India, Asia, Africa, and Central America; in those geographic areas, HEV is the most common cause of acute hepatitis; one-third of the global population appears to have been infected. This agent, with epidemiologic features resembling those of hepatitis A, is a 27- to 34-nm, nonenveloped, HAV-like virus with a 7200-nucleotide, single-strand, positive-sense RNA genome. HEV has three open reading frames (ORF) (genes), the largest of which, *ORF1*, encodes nonstructural proteins involved in virus replication. A middle-sized gene, *ORF2*, encodes the nucleocapsid protein, the major nonstructural protein, and the smallest, *ORF3*, encodes a structural protein whose function remains undetermined. All HEV isolates appear to belong to a single serotype, despite genomic heterogeneity of up to 25% and the existence of five genotypes, only four of which have been detected in humans; genotypes 1 and 2 appear to be more virulent, whereas genotypes 3 and 4 are more attenuated and account for subclinical infections. Contributing to the perpetuation of this virus are animal reservoirs, most notably in swine. No genomic or antigenic homology, however, exists between HEV and HAV or other picornaviruses; and HEV, although resembling caliciviruses, is sufficiently distinct from any known agent to merit its own classification as a unique genus, *Hepevirus*, within the family Hepeviridae. The virus has been detected in stool, bile, and liver and is excreted in the stool during the late incubation period. Both IgM anti-HEV during early acute infection and IgG anti-HEV predominating after the first 3 months can be detected. Currently, availability and reliability of serologic/virologic testing for HEV infection is limited but can be done in specialized laboratories (e.g., the Centers for Disease Control and Prevention).

PATHOGENESIS

Under ordinary circumstances, none of the hepatitis viruses is known to be directly cytopathic to hepatocytes. Evidence suggests that the clinical manifestations and outcomes after acute liver injury associated with viral hepatitis are determined by the immunologic responses of the host. Among the viral hepatitides, the immunopathogenesis of hepatitis B and C has been studied most extensively.

Hepatitis B

For HBV, the existence of inactive hepatitis B carriers with normal liver histology and function suggests that the virus is not directly cytopathic. The fact that patients with defects in cellular immune competence are more likely to remain chronically infected rather than to clear HBV supports the role of cellular immune responses in the pathogenesis of hepatitis B–related liver injury. The model that has the most experimental support involves cytolytic T cells sensitized specifically to recognize host and hepatitis B viral antigens on the liver cell surface. Nucleocapsid proteins (HBcAg and possibly HBeAg), present on the cell membrane in minute quantities, are the viral target antigens that, with host antigens, invite cytolytic T cells to destroy HBV-infected hepatocytes. Differences in the robustness and broad polyclonality of CD8+ cytolytic T cell responsiveness; in the level of HBV-specific helper CD4+ T cells; in attenuation, depletion, and exhaustion of virus-specific T cells; in viral T cell epitope escape mutations that allow the virus to evade T cell containment; and in the elaboration of antiviral cytokines by T cells have been invoked to explain differences in outcomes between those who recover after acute hepatitis and those who progress to chronic hepatitis, or between those with mild and those with severe (fulminant) acute HBV infection.

Although a robust cytolytic T cell response occurs and eliminates virus-infected liver cells during acute hepatitis B, >90% of HBV DNA has been found in experimentally infected chimpanzees to disappear from the liver and blood before maximal T cell infiltration of the liver and before most of the biochemical and histologic evidence of liver injury. This observation suggests that components of the innate immune system and inflammatory cytokines, independent of cytopathic antiviral mechanisms, participate in the early immune response to HBV infection; this effect has been shown to represent elimination of HBV replicative intermediates from the cytoplasm and covalently closed circular viral DNA from the nucleus of infected hepatocytes. In turn, the innate immune response to HBV infection is mediated largely by natural killer (NK) cell cytotoxicity, activated by immunosuppressive cytokines (e.g., interleukin [IL] 10 and transforming growth factor [TGF] β), reduced signals from inhibitory receptor expression (e.g., major histocompatibility complex), or increased signals from activating receptor expression on infected hepatocytes. In addition, NK cells reduce helper CD4+ cells, which results in reduced CD8+ cells and exhaustion of the virus-specific T cell response to HBV infection. Ultimately, HBV-HLA-specific cytolytic T cell responses of the adaptive immune system are felt to be responsible for recovery from HBV infection.

Debate continues over the relative importance of viral and host factors in the pathogenesis of HBV-associated liver injury and its outcome. As noted above, precore genetic mutants of HBV have been associated with the more severe outcomes of HBV infection (severe chronic and fulminant hepatitis), suggesting that, under certain circumstances, relative pathogenicity is a property of the virus, not the host. The fact that concomitant HDV and HBV infections are associated with more severe liver injury than HBV infection alone and the fact that cells transfected in vitro with the gene for HDV antigen express HDV antigen and then become necrotic in the absence of any immunologic influences are also consistent with a viral effect on pathogenicity.

Similarly, in patients who undergo liver transplantation for end-stage chronic hepatitis B, occasionally, rapidly progressive liver injury appears in the new liver. This clinical pattern is associated with an unusual histologic pattern in the new liver, *fibrosing cholestatic hepatitis*, which, ultrastructurally, appears to represent a choking of the cell with overwhelming quantities of HBsAg. This observation suggests that, under the influence of the potent immunosuppressive agents required to prevent allograft rejection, HBV may have a direct cytopathic effect on liver cells, independent of the immune system.

Although the precise mechanism of liver injury in HBV infection remains elusive, studies of nucleocapsid proteins have shed light on the profound immunologic tolerance to HBV of babies born to mothers with highly replicative (HBeAg-positive), chronic HBV infection. In HBeAg-expressing transgenic mice, in utero exposure to HBeAg, which is sufficiently small to traverse the placenta, induces T cell tolerance to both nucleocapsid proteins. This, in turn, may explain why, when infection occurs so early in life, immunologic clearance does not occur, and protracted, lifelong infection ensues.

An important distinction should be drawn between HBV infection acquired at birth, common in endemic areas, such as East Asia, and infection acquired in adulthood, common in the West. Infection in the neonatal period is associated with the acquisition of high-level immunologic tolerance to HBV and absence of an acute hepatitis illness, but the almost invariable establishment of chronic, often lifelong infection. Neonatally acquired HBV infection can culminate decades later in cirrhosis and hepatocellular carcinoma (see "Complications and Sequelae"). In contrast, when HBV infection is acquired during adolescence or early adulthood, the host immune response to HBV-infected hepatocytes tends to be robust, an acute hepatitis-like illness is the rule, and failure to recover is the exception. After adulthood-acquired infection, chronicity is uncommon, and the risk of hepatocellular carcinoma is very low. Based on these observations, some authorities categorize HBV infection into an "immunotolerant" phase, an "immunoreactive" phase, and an "inactive" phase. This somewhat simplistic formulation does not apply at all to the typical adult in the West with self-limited acute hepatitis B, in whom no period of immunologic tolerance occurs. Even among those with neonatally acquired HBV infection, in whom immunologic tolerance is established definitively, intermittent bursts of hepatic necroinflammatory activity punctuate the early decades of life during which liver injury appears to be quiescent (labeled by some as the "immunotolerant" phase). In addition, even when clinically apparent liver injury and progressive fibrosis emerge during later decades (the so-called immunoreactive, or immunointolerant, phase), the level of immunologic tolerance to HBV remains substantial. More accurately, in patients with neonatally acquired HBV infection, a dynamic equilibrium exists between tolerance and intolerance, the outcome of which determines the clinical expression of chronic infection. Persons infected as neonates tend to have a relatively higher level of immunologic tolerance during the early decades of life and a relatively lower level (but only rarely a loss) of tolerance in the later decades of life.

Hepatitis C

Cell-mediated immune responses and elaboration by T cells of antiviral cytokines contribute to the multicellular innate and adaptive immune responses involved in the containment of infection and pathogenesis of liver injury associated with hepatitis C. The fact that HCV is so efficient in evading these immune mechanisms is a testament to its highly evolved ability to disrupt host immune responses at multiple levels. After exposure to HCV, the host cell identifies viral product motifs (pattern recognition receptors) that distinguish the virus from "self," resulting in the elaboration of interferons and other cytokines that result in activation of innate and adaptive immune responses. Intrahepatic HLA class I restricted cytolytic T cells directed at nucleocapsid, envelope, and nonstructural viral protein antigens have been demonstrated in patients with chronic hepatitis C; however, such virus-specific cytolytic T cell responses do not correlate adequately with the degree of liver injury or with recovery. Yet, a consensus has emerged supporting a role in the pathogenesis of HCV-associated liver injury of virus-activated CD4+ helper T cells that stimulate, via the cytokines they elaborate, HCV-specific CD8+ cytotoxic T cells. These responses appear to be more robust (higher in number, more diverse in viral antigen specificity, more functionally effective, and more long lasting) in those who recover from HCV than in those who have chronic infection. Contributing to chronic infection are a CD4+ proliferative defect that results in rapid contraction of CD4+ responses, mutations in CD8+ T cell–targeted viral epitopes that allow HCV to escape immune-mediated clearance, and upregulation of inhibitory receptors on functionally impaired, exhausted T cells. Although attention has focused on adaptive immunity, HCV proteins have been shown to interfere with innate immunity by resulting in blocking of type 1 interferon responses and inhibition of interferon signaling and effector molecules in the interferon signaling cascade. Several HLA alleles have been linked with self-limited hepatitis C, the most convincing of which is the CC haplotype of the *IL28B* gene, which codes for interferon λ3, a component of innate immune antiviral defense. The *IL28B* association is even stronger when combined with HLA class II *DQB1*03:01*. The link between non-CC *IL28B* polymorphisms and failure to clear

HCV infection has been explained by a chromosome 19q13.13 frameshift variant upstream of *IL28B*, the ΔG polymorphism of which creates an ORF in a novel interferon gene (*IFN-λ4*) associated with impaired HCV clearance. Also shown to contribute to limiting HCV infection are NK cells of the innate immune system that function when HLA class I molecules required for successful adaptive immunity are underexpressed. Both peripheral and intrahepatic NK cell cytotoxicity are dysfunctional in persistent HCV infection. Adding to the complexity of the immune response, HCV core, NS4B, and NS5B have been shown to suppress the immunoregulatory nuclear factor (NF)-κB pathway, resulting in reduced antiapoptotic proteins and a resultant increased vulnerability to tumor necrosis factor (TNF) α–mediated cell death. Patients with hepatitis C and unfavorable (non-CC, associated with reduced HCV clearance) *IL28B* alleles have been shown to have depressed NK cell/innate immune function. Of note, the emergence of substantial viral quasispecies diversity and HCV sequence variation allow the virus to evade attempts by the host to contain HCV infection by both humoral and cellular immunity.

Finally, cross-reactivity between viral antigens (HCV NS3 and NS5A) and host autoantigens (cytochrome P450 2D6) has been invoked to explain the association between hepatitis C and a subset of patients with autoimmune hepatitis and antibodies to liver-kidney microsomal (LKM) antigen (anti-LKM) **(Chap. 41)**.

EXTRAHEPATIC MANIFESTATIONS

Immune complex–mediated tissue damage appears to play a pathogenetic role in the extrahepatic manifestations of acute hepatitis B. The occasional prodromal serum sickness–like syndrome observed in acute hepatitis B appears to be related to the deposition in tissue blood vessel walls of HBsAg-anti-HBs circulating immune complexes, leading to activation of the complement system and depressed serum complement levels.

In patients with chronic hepatitis B, other types of immune-complex disease may be seen. Glomerulonephritis with the nephrotic syndrome is observed occasionally; HBsAg, immunoglobulin, and C3 deposition has been found in the glomerular basement membrane. Whereas generalized vasculitis (polyarteritis nodosa) develops in considerably fewer than 1% of patients with chronic HBV infection, 20–30% of patients with polyarteritis nodosa have HBsAg in serum. In these patients, the affected small- and medium-size arterioles contain HBsAg, immunoglobulins, and complement components. Another extrahepatic manifestation of viral hepatitis, essential mixed cryoglobulinemia (EMC), was reported initially to be associated with hepatitis B. The disorder is characterized clinically by arthritis, cutaneous vasculitis (palpable purpura), and occasionally, glomerulonephritis and serologically by the presence of circulating cryoprecipitable immune complexes of more than one immunoglobulin class. Many patients with this syndrome have chronic liver disease, but the association with HBV infection is limited; instead, a substantial proportion has chronic HCV infection, with circulating immune complexes containing HCV RNA. Immune-complex glomerulonephritis is another recognized extrahepatic manifestation of chronic hepatitis C.

PATHOLOGY

The typical morphologic lesions of all types of viral hepatitis are similar and consist of panlobular infiltration with mononuclear cells, hepatic cell necrosis, hyperplasia of Kupffer cells, and variable degrees of cholestasis. Hepatic cell regeneration is present, as evidenced by numerous mitotic figures, multinucleated cells, and "rosette" or "pseudoacinar" formation. The mononuclear infiltration consists primarily of small lymphocytes, although plasma cells and eosinophils occasionally are present. Liver cell damage consists of hepatic cell degeneration and necrosis, cell dropout, ballooning of cells, and acidophilic degeneration of hepatocytes (forming so-called Councilman or apoptotic bodies). Large hepatocytes with a ground-glass appearance of the cytoplasm may be seen in chronic but not in acute HBV infection; these cells contain HBsAg and can be identified histochemically with orcein or aldehyde fuchsin. In uncomplicated viral hepatitis, the reticulin framework is preserved.

In hepatitis C, the histologic lesion is often remarkable for a relative paucity of inflammation, a marked increase in activation of sinusoidal lining cells, lymphoid aggregates, the presence of fat (more frequent in genotype 3 and linked to increased fibrosis), and, occasionally, bile duct lesions in which biliary epithelial cells appear to be piled up without interruption of the basement membrane. Occasionally, microvesicular steatosis occurs in hepatitis D. In hepatitis E, a common histologic feature is marked cholestasis. A cholestatic variant of slowly resolving acute hepatitis A also has been described.

A more severe histologic lesion, *bridging hepatic necrosis*, also termed *subacute* or *confluent necrosis* or *interface hepatitis*, is observed occasionally in acute hepatitis. "Bridging" between lobules results from large areas of hepatic cell dropout, with collapse of the reticulin framework. Characteristically, the bridge consists of condensed reticulum, inflammatory debris, and degenerating liver cells that span adjacent portal areas, portal to central veins, or central vein to central vein. This lesion had been thought to have prognostic significance;

in many of the originally described patients with this lesion, a subacute course terminated in death within several weeks to months, or severe chronic hepatitis and cirrhosis developed; however, the association between bridging necrosis and a poor prognosis in patients with acute hepatitis has not been upheld. Therefore, although demonstration of this lesion in patients with chronic hepatitis has prognostic significance **(Chap. 41)**, its demonstration during acute hepatitis is less meaningful, and liver biopsies to identify this lesion are no longer undertaken routinely in patients with acute hepatitis. In *massive hepatic necrosis* (fulminant hepatitis, "acute yellow atrophy"), the striking feature at postmortem examination is the finding of a small, shrunken, soft liver. Histologic examination reveals massive necrosis and dropout of liver cells of most lobules with extensive collapse and condensation of the reticulin framework. When histologic documentation is required in the management of fulminant or very severe hepatitis, a biopsy can be done by the angiographically guided transjugular route, which permits the performance of this invasive procedure in the presence of severe coagulopathy.

Immunohistochemical and electron-microscopic studies have localized HBsAg to the cytoplasm and plasma membrane of infected liver cells. In contrast, HBcAg predominates in the nucleus, but, occasionally, scant amounts are also seen in the cytoplasm and on the cell membrane. HDV antigen is localized to the hepatocyte nucleus, whereas HAV, HCV, and HEV antigens are localized to the cytoplasm.

EPIDEMIOLOGY AND GLOBAL FEATURES

Before the availability of serologic tests for hepatitis viruses, all viral hepatitis cases were labeled either as "infectious" or "serum" hepatitis. Modes of transmission overlap, however, and *a clear distinction among the different types of viral hepatitis cannot be made solely on the basis of clinical or epidemiologic features*(Table 39-2). The most accurate means to distinguish the various types of viral hepatitis involves specific serologic testing.

Hepatitis A

This agent is transmitted almost exclusively by the fecal-oral route. Person-to-person spread of HAV is enhanced by poor personal hygiene and overcrowding; large outbreaks as well as sporadic cases have been traced to contaminated food, water, milk, frozen raspberries and strawberries, green onions imported from Mexico, and shellfish. Intrafamily and intrainstitutional spread are also common. Early epidemiologic observations supported a predilection for hepatitis A to occur in late fall and early winter. In temperate zones, epidemic waves have been recorded every 5–20 years as new segments of nonimmune population appeared; however, in developed countries, the incidence of hepatitis A has been declining, presumably as a function of improved sanitation, and these cyclic patterns are no longer observed. No HAV carrier state has been identified after acute hepatitis A; perpetuation of the virus in nature depends presumably on nonepidemic, inapparent subclinical infection, ingestion of contaminated food or water in, or imported from, endemic areas, and/or contamination linked to environmental reservoirs.

In the general population, anti-HAV, a marker for previous HAV infection, increases in prevalence as a function of increasing age and of decreasing socioeconomic status. In the 1970s, serologic evidence of prior hepatitis A infection occurred in ~40% of urban populations in the United States, most of whose members never recalled having had a symptomatic case of hepatitis. In subsequent decades, however, the prevalence of anti-HAV has been declining in the United States. In developing countries, exposure, infection, and subsequent immunity are almost universal in childhood. As the frequency of subclinical childhood infections declines in developed countries, a susceptible cohort of adults emerges. Hepatitis A tends to be more symptomatic in adults; therefore, paradoxically, as the frequency of HAV infection declines, the likelihood of clinically apparent, even severe, HAV illnesses increases in the susceptible adult population. Travel to endemic areas is a common source of infection for adults from nonendemic areas. More recently recognized epidemiologic foci of HAV infection include child care centers, neonatal intensive care units, promiscuous men who have sex with men, injection drug users, and unvaccinated close contacts of newly arrived international adopted children, most of whom emanate from countries with intermediate-to-high hepatitis A endemicity. Although hepatitis A is rarely bloodborne, several outbreaks have been recognized in recipients of clotting-factor concentrates. In the United States, the introduction of hepatitis A vaccination programs among children from high-incidence states has resulted in a >70% reduction in the annual incidence of new HAV infections and has shifted the burden of new infections from children to young adults. In the most recent, 1999–2006 U.S. Public Health Service National Health and Nutrition Examination Survey (NHANES), the prevalence of anti-HAV in the U.S. population was 35%, representing (compared to the 1988–1994 survey) a stable frequency of infection and natural immunity in adults >19 years old but an increase in vaccine-induced immunity for children age 6–19 years.

Hepatitis B

Percutaneous inoculation has long been recognized as a major route of hepatitis B transmission, but the

TABLE 39-2

CLINICAL AND EPIDEMIOLOGIC FEATURES OF VIRAL HEPATITIS

FEATURE	HAV	HBV	HCV	HDV	HEV
Incubation (days)	15–45, mean 30	30–180, mean 60–90	15–160, mean 50	30–180, mean 60–90	14–60, mean 40
Onset	Acute	Insidious or acute	Insidious	Insidious or acute	Acute
Age preference	Children, young adults	Young adults (sexual and percutaneous), babies, toddlers	Any age, but more common in adults	Any age (similar to HBV)	Epidemic cases: young adults (20–40 years); sporadic cases: older adults (>60)
Transmission					
Fecal-oral	+++	–	–	–	+++
Percutaneous	Unusual	+++	+++	+++	–
Perinatal	–	+++	±[a]	+	–
Sexual	±	++	±[a]	++	–
Clinical					
Severity	Mild	Occasionally severe	Moderate	Occasionally severe	Mild
Fulminant	0.1%	0.1–1%	0.1%	5–20%[b]	1–2%[e]
Progression to chronicity	None	Occasional (1–10%) (90% of neonates)	Common (85%)	Common[d]	None[f]
Carrier	None	0.1–30%[c]	1.5–3.2%	Variable[g]	None
Cancer	None	+ (neonatal infection)	+	±	None
Prognosis	Excellent	Worse with age, debility	Moderate	Acute, good Chronic, poor	Good
Prophylaxis	Ig, inactivated vaccine	HBIG, recombinant vaccine	None	HBV vaccine (none for HBV carriers)	Vaccine
Therapy	None	Interferon Lamivudine Adefovir Pegylated interferon[h] Entecavir[h] Telbivudine Tenofovir[h]	Pegylated interferon ribavirin, telaprevir,[i] boceprevir,[i] simeprevir, sofosbuvir, lidipasvir paritaprevir/ritonavir ombitasvir, dasabuvir declatasvir, velpatasvir, grazoprevir, elbasvir	Pegylated interferon ±	None[j]

[a]Primarily with HIV co-infection and high-level viremia in index case; risk ~5%.
[b]Up to 5% in acute HBV/HDV co-infection; up to 20% in HDV superinfection of chronic HBV infection.
[c]Varies considerably throughout the world and in subpopulations within countries; see text.
[d]In acute HBV/HDV co-infection, the frequency of chronicity is the same as that for HBV; in HDV superinfection, chronicity is invariable.
[e]10–20% in pregnant women.
[f]Except as observed in immunosuppressed liver allograft recipients or other immunosuppressed hosts.
[g]Common in Mediterranean countries; rare in North America and western Europe.
[h]First-line agent
[i]No longer recommended
[j]Anecdotal reports and retrospective studies suggest that pegylated interferon and/or ribavirin are effective in treating chronic hepatitis E, observed in immunocompromised persons; ribavirin monotherapy has been used successfully in acute, severe hepatitis E.
Abbreviation: HBIG, hepatitis B immunoglobulin. See text for other abbreviations.

outmoded designation "serum hepatitis" is an inaccurate label for the epidemiologic spectrum of HBV infection. As detailed below, most of the hepatitis transmitted by blood transfusion is not caused by HBV; moreover, in approximately two-thirds of patients with acute type B hepatitis, no history of an identifiable percutaneous exposure can be elicited. We now recognize that many cases of hepatitis B result from less obvious modes of nonpercutaneous or covert percutaneous transmission. HBsAg has been identified in almost every body fluid from infected persons, and at least some of these body fluids—most notably semen and saliva—are infectious, albeit less so than serum, when administered percutaneously or nonpercutaneously to experimental animals. Among the nonpercutaneous modes of HBV transmission, oral ingestion has been documented as a potential but inefficient route of exposure. By contrast, the two nonpercutaneous routes considered to have the greatest impact are intimate (especially sexual) contact and perinatal transmission.

In sub-Saharan Africa, intimate contact among toddlers is considered instrumental in contributing to the maintenance of the high frequency of hepatitis B in the population. Perinatal transmission occurs primarily in infants born to mothers with chronic hepatitis B or (rarely) mothers with acute hepatitis B during the third trimester of pregnancy or during the early postpartum period. Perinatal transmission is uncommon in North America and western Europe but occurs with great frequency and is the most important mode of HBV perpetuation in East Asia and developing countries. Although the precise mode of perinatal transmission is unknown, and although ~10% of infections may be acquired in utero, epidemiologic evidence suggests that most infections occur approximately at the time of delivery and are not related to breast-feeding. The likelihood of perinatal transmission of HBV correlates with the presence of HBeAg and high-level viral replication; 90% of HBeAg-positive mothers but only 10–15% of anti-HBe-positive mothers transmit HBV infection to their offspring. In most cases, acute infection in the neonate is clinically asymptomatic, but the child is very likely to remain chronically infected.

The >350–400 million HBsAg carriers in the world constitute the main reservoir of hepatitis B in human beings. Whereas serum HBsAg is infrequent (0.1–0.5%) in normal populations in the United States and western Europe, a prevalence of up to 5–20% has been found in East Asia and in some tropical countries; in persons with Down's syndrome, lepromatous leprosy, leukemia, Hodgkin's disease, or polyarteritis nodosa; in patients with chronic renal disease on hemodialysis; and in injection drug users.

Other groups with high rates of HBV infection include spouses of acutely infected persons; sexually promiscuous persons (especially promiscuous men who have sex with men); health care workers exposed to blood; persons who require repeated transfusions especially with pooled blood-product concentrates (e.g., hemophiliacs); residents and staff of custodial institutions for the developmentally handicapped; prisoners; and, to a lesser extent, family members of chronically infected patients. In volunteer blood donors, the prevalence of anti-HBs, a reflection of previous HBV infection, ranges from 5–10%, but the prevalence is higher in lower socioeconomic strata, older age groups, and persons—including those mentioned above—exposed to blood products. Because of highly sensitive virologic screening of donor blood, the risk of acquiring HBV infection from a blood transfusion is 1 in 230,000.

Prevalence of infection, modes of transmission, and human behavior conspire to mold geographically different epidemiologic patterns of HBV infection. In East Asia and Africa, hepatitis B, a disease of the newborn and young children, is perpetuated by a cycle of maternal-neonatal spread. In North America and western Europe, hepatitis B is primarily a disease of adolescence and early adulthood, the time of life when intimate sexual contact and recreational and occupational percutaneous exposures tend to occur. To some degree, however, this dichotomy between high-prevalence and low-prevalence geographic regions has been minimized by immigration from high-prevalence to low-prevalence areas. The introduction of hepatitis B vaccine in the early 1980s and adoption of universal childhood vaccination policies in many countries resulted in a dramatic, ~90% decline in the incidence of new HBV infections in those countries as well as in the dire consequences of chronic infection, including hepatocellular carcinoma. Populations and groups for whom HBV infection screening is recommended are listed in Table 39-3.

Hepatitis D

Infection with HDV has a worldwide distribution, but two epidemiologic patterns exist. In Mediterranean countries (northern Africa, southern Europe, the Middle East), HDV infection is endemic among those with hepatitis B, and the disease is transmitted

TABLE 39-3

HIGH-RISK POPULATIONS FOR WHOM HBV INFECTION SCREENING IS RECOMMENDED
Persons born in countries/regions with a high (≥8%) and intermediate (≥2%) prevalence of HBV infection including immigrants and adopted children and including persons born in the United States who were not vaccinated as infants and whose parents emigrated from areas of high HBV endemicity
Household and sexual contacts of persons with hepatitis B
Babies born to HBsAg-positive mothers
Persons who have used injection drugs
Persons with multiple sexual contacts or a history of sexually transmitted disease
Men who have sex with men
Inmates of correctional facilities
Persons with elevated alanine or aspartate aminotransferase levels
Blood/plasma/organ/tissue/semen donors
Persons with HCV or HIV infection
Hemodialysis patients
Pregnant women
Persons who are the source of blood or body fluids that would be an indication for postexposure prophylaxis (e.g., needle-stick, mucosal exposure, sexual assault)
Persons who require immunosuppressive or cytotoxic therapy (including anti–tumor necrosis factor α therapy for rheumatologic or inflammatory bowel disorders or rituximab (anti-CD20))

predominantly by nonpercutaneous means, especially close personal contact. In nonendemic areas, such as the United States and northern Europe, HDV infection is confined to persons exposed frequently to blood and blood products, primarily injection drug users and hemophiliacs. HDV infection can be introduced into a population through drug users or by migration of persons from endemic to nonendemic areas. Thus, patterns of population migration and human behavior facilitating percutaneous contact play important roles in the introduction and amplification of HDV infection. Occasionally, the migrating epidemiology of hepatitis D is expressed in explosive outbreaks of severe hepatitis, such as those that have occurred in remote South American villages as well as in urban centers in the United States. Ultimately, such outbreaks of hepatitis D—either of co-infections with acute hepatitis B or of superinfections in those already infected with HBV—may blur the distinctions between endemic and nonendemic areas. On a global scale, HDV infection declined at the end of the 1990s. Even in Italy, an HDV-endemic area, public health measures introduced to control HBV infection resulted during the 1990s in a 1.5%/year reduction in the prevalence of HDV infection. Still, the frequency of HDV infection during the first decade of the twenty-first century has not fallen below levels reached during the 1990s; the reservoir has been sustained by survivors infected during 1970–1980 and recent immigrants from still-endemic to less-endemic countries.

Hepatitis C

Routine screening of blood donors for HBsAg and the elimination of commercial blood sources in the early 1970s reduced the frequency of, but did not eliminate, transfusion-associated hepatitis. During the 1970s, the likelihood of acquiring hepatitis after transfusion of voluntarily donated, HBsAg-screened blood was ~10% per patient (up to 0.9% per unit transfused); 90–95% of these cases were classified, based on serologic exclusion of hepatitis A and B, as "non-A, non-B" hepatitis. For patients requiring transfusion of pooled products, such as clotting factor concentrates, the risk was even higher, up to 20–30%.

During the 1980s, voluntary self-exclusion of blood donors with risk factors for AIDS and then the introduction of donor screening for anti-HIV reduced further the likelihood of transfusion-associated hepatitis to <5%. During the late 1980s and early 1990s, the introduction first of "surrogate" screening tests for non-A, non-B hepatitis (alanine aminotransferase [ALT] and anti-HBc, both shown to identify blood donors with a higher likelihood of transmitting non-A, non-B hepatitis to recipients) and, subsequently, after the discovery of HCV, first-generation immunoassays for anti-HCV reduced the frequency of transfusion-associated hepatitis even further. A prospective analysis of transfusion-associated hepatitis conducted between 1986 and 1990 showed that the frequency of transfusion-associated hepatitis at one urban university hospital fell from a baseline of 3.8% per patient (0.45% per unit transfused) to 1.5% per patient (0.19% per unit) after the introduction of surrogate testing and to 0.6% per patient (0.03% per unit) after the introduction of first-generation anti-HCV assays. The introduction of second-generation anti-HCV assays reduced the frequency of transfusion-associated hepatitis C to almost imperceptible levels—1 in 100,000—and these gains were reinforced by the application of third-generation anti-HCV assays and of automated PCR testing of donated blood for HCV RNA, which has resulted in a reduction in the risk of transfusion-associated HCV infection to 1 in 2.3 million transfusions.

In addition to being transmitted by transfusion, hepatitis C can be transmitted by other percutaneous routes, such as injection drug use. In addition, this virus can be transmitted by occupational exposure to blood, and the likelihood of infection is increased in hemodialysis units. Although the frequency of transfusion-associated hepatitis C fell as a result of blood-donor screening, the overall frequency of hepatitis C remained the same until the early 1990s, when the overall frequency fell by 80%, in parallel with a reduction in the number of new cases in injection drug users. After the exclusion of anti-HCV-positive plasma units from the donor pool, rare, sporadic instances have occurred of hepatitis C among recipients of immunoglobulin (Ig) preparations for intravenous (but not intramuscular) use.

Serologic evidence for HCV infection occurs in 90% of patients with a history of transfusion-associated hepatitis (almost all occurring before 1992, when second-generation HCV screening tests were introduced); hemophiliacs and others treated with clotting factors; injection drug users; 60–70% of patients with sporadic "non-A, non-B" hepatitis who lack identifiable risk factors; 0.5% of volunteer blood donors; and, in a survey conducted in the United States between 1999 and 2002, 1.6% of the general population in the United States, which translates into 4.1 million persons (3.2 million with viremia), the majority of whom are unaware of their infections. Moreover, such population surveys do not include higher-risk groups such as incarcerated prisoners and active injection drug users, indicating that the actual prevalence is even higher. Comparable frequencies of HCV infection occur in most countries around the world, with 170 million persons infected worldwide, but extraordinarily high prevalences of HCV infection occur in certain countries such as Egypt, where >20% of the population (as high as 50% in persons born prior to 1960) in some cities is infected. The high frequency in Egypt is attributable to contaminated equipment used for medical procedures and unsafe injection practices in the 1950s to 1980s (during a campaign to eradicate schistosomiasis with intravenous tartar emetic). In the United States, African Americans and Mexican Americans have higher frequencies of HCV infection than whites. Between 1988 and 1994, 30- to 40-year-old adult males had the highest prevalence of HCV infection; however, in a survey conducted between 1999 and 2002, the peak age decile had shifted to those age 40–49 years; an increase in hepatitis C–related mortality has paralleled this secular trend, increasing since 1995 predominantly in the 45- to 65-year age group. Thus, despite an 80% reduction in new HCV infections during the 1990s, the prevalence of HCV infection in the population was sustained by an aging cohort that had acquired their infections three to four decades earlier, during the 1960s and 1970s, as a result predominantly of self-inoculation with recreational drugs. As death resulting from HIV infection fell after 1999, age-adjusted mortality associated with HCV infection surpassed that of HIV infection in 2007; >70% of HCV-associated deaths occurred in the "baby boomer" cohort born between 1945 and 1965. Compared to the 1.6% prevalence of HCV infection in the population at large, the prevalence in the 1945–1965 birth cohort was 3.2%, representing three-quarters of all infected persons. Therefore, in 2012, the Centers for Disease Control and Prevention recommended that all persons born between 1945 and 1965 be screened for hepatitis C, without ascertainment of risk, a recommendation shown to be cost-effective and predicted to identify 800,000 infected persons. Because of the availability of highly effective antiviral therapy, such screening would have the potential to avert 200,000 cases of cirrhosis and 47,000 cases of hepatocellular carcinoma and to prevent 120,000 hepatitis-related deaths.

Hepatitis C accounts for 40% of chronic liver disease, is the most frequent indication for liver transplantation, and is estimated to account for 8000–10,000 deaths per year in the United States. The distribution of HCV genotypes varies in different parts of the world. Worldwide, genotype 1 is the most common. In the United States, genotype 1 accounts for 70% of HCV infections, whereas genotypes 2 and 3 account for the remaining 30%; among African Americans, the frequency of genotype 1 is even higher (i.e., 90%). Genotype 4 predominates in Egypt; genotype 5 is localized to South Africa, genotype 6 to Hong Kong, and genotype 7 to Central Africa. Most asymptomatic blood donors found to have anti-HCV and ~20–30% of persons with reported cases of acute hepatitis C do not fall into a recognized risk group; however, many such blood donors do recall risk-associated behaviors when questioned carefully.

As a bloodborne infection, HCV potentially can be transmitted sexually and perinatally; however, both of these modes of transmission are inefficient for hepatitis C. Although 10–15% of patients with acute hepatitis C report having potential sexual sources of infection, most studies have failed to identify sexual transmission of this agent. The chances of sexual and perinatal transmission have been estimated to be ~5% but shown in a prospective study to be only 1% between monogamous sexual partners, well below comparable rates for HIV and HBV infections. Moreover, sexual transmission appears to be confined to such subgroups as persons with multiple sexual partners and sexually transmitted diseases. Breast-feeding does not increase the risk of HCV infection between an infected mother and her infant. Infection of health workers is not dramatically higher than among the general population; however, health workers are more likely to acquire HCV infection through accidental needle punctures, the efficiency of which is ~3%. Infection of household contacts is rare as well.

Besides persons born between 1945 and 1965, other groups with an increased frequency of HCV infection are listed in Table 39-4. In immunosuppressed individuals, levels of anti-HCV may be undetectable, and a diagnosis may require testing for HCV RNA. Although new acute cases of hepatitis C are rare, newly diagnosed cases are common among otherwise healthy persons who experimented briefly with injection drugs, as noted above, three or four decades earlier. Such instances usually remain unrecognized for years, until unearthed by laboratory screening for routine medical examinations, insurance applications, and attempted blood donation. Although, overall, the annual incidence of new HCV infections has continued to fall, the rate of new infections has been increasing since 2002 in a new cohort of young injection drug users, age 15–24 years (accounting for more than two-thirds of all acute cases), who,

TABLE 39-4

HIGH-RISK POPULATIONS FOR WHOM HCV-INFECTION SCREENING IS RECOMMENDED
Persons born between 1945 and 1965
Persons who have ever used injection drugs
Persons with HIV infection
Hemophiliacs treated with clotting factor concentrates prior to 1987
Persons who have ever undergone long-term hemodialysis
Persons with unexplained elevations of aminotransferase levels
Transfusion or transplantation recipients prior to July 1992
Recipients of blood or organs from a donor found to be positive for hepatitis C
Children born to women with hepatitis C
Health care, public safety, and emergency medical personnel following needle injury or mucosal exposure to HCV-contaminated blood
Sexual partners of persons with hepatitis C infection

unlike older cohorts, had not learned to take precautions to prevent bloodborne infections.

Hepatitis E

This type of hepatitis, identified in India, Asia, Africa, the Middle East, and Central America, resembles hepatitis A in its primarily enteric mode of spread. The commonly recognized cases occur after contamination of water supplies such as after monsoon flooding, but sporadic, isolated cases occur. An epidemiologic feature that distinguishes HEV from other enteric agents is the rarity of secondary person-to-person spread from infected persons to their close contacts. Large waterborne outbreaks in endemic areas are linked to genotypes 1 and 2, arise in populations that are immune to HAV, favor young adults, and account for antibody prevalences of 30–80%. In nonendemic areas of the world, such as the United States, clinically apparent acute hepatitis E is extremely rare; however, during the 1988–1994 NHANES survey conducted by the U.S. Public Health Service, the prevalence of anti-HEV was 21%, reflecting subclinical infections, infection with genotypes 3 and 4, predominantly in older males (>60 years). In nonendemic areas, HEV accounts hardly at all for cases of sporadic hepatitis; however, cases imported from endemic areas have been found in the United States. Evidence supports a zoonotic reservoir for HEV primarily in swine, which may account for the mostly subclinical infections in nonendemic areas.

CLINICAL AND LABORATORY FEATURES

Symptoms and signs

Acute viral hepatitis occurs after an incubation period that varies according to the responsible agent. Generally, incubation periods for hepatitis A range from 15–45 days (mean, 4 weeks), for hepatitis B and D from 30–180 days (mean, 8–12 weeks), for hepatitis C from 15–160 days (mean, 7 weeks), and for hepatitis E from 14–60 days (mean, 5–6 weeks). The *prodromal symptoms* of acute viral hepatitis are systemic and quite variable. Constitutional symptoms of anorexia, nausea and vomiting, fatigue, malaise, arthralgias, myalgias, headache, photophobia, pharyngitis, cough, and coryza may precede the onset of jaundice by 1–2 weeks. The nausea, vomiting, and anorexia are frequently associated with alterations in olfaction and taste. A low-grade fever between 38° and 39°C (100°–102°F) is more often present in hepatitis A and E than in hepatitis B or C, except when hepatitis B is heralded by a serum sickness–like syndrome; rarely, a fever of 39.5°–40°C (103°–104°F) may accompany the constitutional symptoms. Dark urine and clay-colored stools may be noticed by the patient from 1–5 days before the onset of clinical jaundice.

With the onset of *clinical jaundice*, the constitutional prodromal symptoms usually diminish, but in some patients, mild weight loss (2.5–5 kg) is common and may continue during the entire icteric phase. The liver becomes enlarged and tender and may be associated with right upper quadrant pain and discomfort. Infrequently, patients present with a cholestatic picture, suggesting extrahepatic biliary obstruction. Splenomegaly and cervical adenopathy are present in 10–20% of patients with acute hepatitis. Rarely, a few spider angiomas appear during the icteric phase and disappear during convalescence. During the *recovery phase*, constitutional symptoms disappear, but usually some liver enlargement and abnormalities in liver biochemical tests are still evident. The duration of the posticteric phase is variable, ranging from 2–12 weeks, and is usually more prolonged in acute hepatitis B and C. Complete clinical and biochemical recovery is to be expected 1–2 months after all cases of hepatitis A and E and 3–4 months after the onset of jaundice in three-quarters of uncomplicated, self-limited cases of hepatitis B and C (among healthy adults, acute hepatitis B is self-limited in 95–99%, whereas hepatitis C is self-limited in only ~15%). In the remainder, biochemical recovery may be delayed. A substantial proportion of patients with viral hepatitis never become icteric.

Infection with HDV can occur in the presence of acute or chronic HBV infection; the duration of HBV infection determines the duration of HDV infection. When acute HDV and HBV infection occur simultaneously, clinical and biochemical features may be indistinguishable from those of HBV infection alone, although occasionally they are more severe. As opposed to patients with *acute* HBV infection, patients with *chronic* HBV infection can support HDV replication indefinitely, as when acute HDV infection occurs in the presence of a nonresolving acute HBV infection or, more commonly, when acute hepatitis D is superimposed on underlying chronic hepatitis B. In such cases, the HDV superinfection appears as a clinical exacerbation or an episode resembling acute viral hepatitis in someone already chronically infected with HBV. Superinfection with HDV in a patient with chronic hepatitis B often leads to clinical deterioration (see below).

In addition to superinfections with other hepatitis agents, acute hepatitis-like clinical events in persons with chronic hepatitis B may accompany spontaneous HBeAg to anti-HBe seroconversion or spontaneous reactivation (i.e., reversion from relatively nonreplicative to replicative infection). Such reactivations can occur as well in therapeutically immunosuppressed patients with chronic HBV infection when cytotoxic/immunosuppressive drugs are withdrawn; in these cases, restoration of immune competence is thought to allow resumption of previously checked cell-mediated immune cytolysis of HBV-infected hepatocytes.

Occasionally, acute clinical exacerbations of chronic hepatitis B may represent the emergence of a precore mutant (see "Virology and Etiology"), and the subsequent course in such patients may be characterized by periodic exacerbations. Cytotoxic chemotherapy can lead to reactivation of chronic hepatitis C as well, and anti-TNF-α therapy can lead to reactivation of both hepatitis B and C.

Laboratory features

The serum aminotransferases aspartate aminotransferase (AST) and alanine aminotransferase (ALT) (previously designated SGOT and SGPT) increase to a variable degree during the prodromal phase of acute viral hepatitis and precede the rise in bilirubin level (Figs. 39-2 and 39-4). The level of these enzymes, however, does not correlate well with the degree of liver cell damage. Peak levels vary from 400–4000 IU or more; these levels are usually reached at the time the patient is clinically icteric and diminish progressively during the recovery phase of acute hepatitis. The diagnosis of anicteric hepatitis is based on clinical features and on aminotransferase elevations.

Jaundice is usually visible in the sclera or skin when the serum bilirubin value is >43 μmol/L (2.5 mg/dL). When jaundice appears, the serum bilirubin typically rises to levels ranging from 85–340 μmol/L (5–20 mg/dL). The serum bilirubin may continue to rise despite falling serum aminotransferase levels. In most instances, the total bilirubin is equally divided between the conjugated and unconjugated fractions. Bilirubin levels >340 μmol/L (20 mg/dL) extending and persisting late into the course of viral hepatitis are more likely to be associated with severe disease. In certain patients with underlying hemolytic anemia, however, such as glucose-6-phosphate dehydrogenase deficiency and sickle cell anemia, a high serum bilirubin level is common, resulting from superimposed hemolysis. In such patients, bilirubin levels >513 μmol/L (30 mg/dL) have been observed and are not necessarily associated with a poor prognosis.

Neutropenia and lymphopenia are transient and are followed by a relative lymphocytosis. Atypical lymphocytes (varying between 2 and 20%) are common during the acute phase. Measurement of the prothrombin time (PT) is important in patients with acute viral hepatitis, because a prolonged value may reflect a severe hepatic synthetic defect, signify extensive hepatocellular necrosis, and indicate a worse prognosis. Occasionally, a prolonged PT may occur with only mild increases in the serum bilirubin and aminotransferase levels. Prolonged nausea and vomiting, inadequate carbohydrate intake, and poor hepatic glycogen reserves may contribute to hypoglycemia noted occasionally in patients with severe viral hepatitis. Serum alkaline phosphatase may be normal or only mildly elevated, whereas a fall in serum albumin is uncommon in uncomplicated acute viral hepatitis. In some patients, mild and transient steatorrhea has been noted, as well as slight microscopic hematuria and minimal proteinuria.

A diffuse but mild elevation of the γ globulin fraction is common during acute viral hepatitis. Serum IgG and IgM levels are elevated in about one-third of patients during the acute phase of viral hepatitis, but the serum IgM level is elevated more characteristically during acute hepatitis A. During the acute phase of viral hepatitis, antibodies to smooth muscle and other cell constituents may be present, and low titers of rheumatoid factor, nuclear antibody, and heterophile antibody can also be found occasionally. In hepatitis C and D, antibodies to LKM may occur; however, the species of LKM antibodies in the two types of hepatitis are different from each other as well as from the LKM antibody species characteristic of autoimmune hepatitis type 2 **(Chap. 41)**. The autoantibodies in viral hepatitis are nonspecific and can also be associated with other viral and systemic diseases. In contrast, virus-specific antibodies, which appear during and after hepatitis virus infection, are serologic markers of diagnostic importance.

As described above, serologic tests are available routinely with which to establish a diagnosis of hepatitis A, B, D, and C. Tests for fecal or serum HAV are not routinely available. Therefore, a diagnosis of hepatitis A is based on detection of IgM anti-HAV during acute illness (Fig. 39-2). Rheumatoid factor can give rise to false-positive results in this test.

A diagnosis of HBV infection can usually be made by detection of HBsAg in serum. Infrequently, levels of HBsAg are too low to be detected during acute HBV infection, even with contemporary, highly sensitive immunoassays. In such cases, the diagnosis can be established by the presence of IgM anti-HBc.

The titer of HBsAg bears little relation to the severity of clinical disease. Indeed, an inverse correlation exists between the serum concentration of HBsAg and the degree of liver cell damage. For example, titers are highest in immunosuppressed patients, lower in patients with chronic liver disease (but higher in mild chronic than in severe chronic hepatitis), and very low in patients with acute fulminant hepatitis. These observations suggest that, in hepatitis B, the degree of liver cell damage and the clinical course are related to variations in the patient's immune response to HBV rather than to the amount of circulating HBsAg. In immunocompetent persons, however, a correlation exists between markers of HBV *replication* and liver injury (see below).

Another important serologic marker in patients with hepatitis B is HBeAg. Its principal clinical usefulness is as an indicator of relative infectivity. Because HBeAg is invariably present during early acute hepatitis B, HBeAg testing is indicated primarily in chronic infection.

In patients with hepatitis B surface antigenemia of unknown duration (e.g., blood donors found to be HBsAg-positive) testing for IgM anti-HBc may be useful to distinguish between acute or recent infection (IgM anti-HBc-positive) and chronic HBV infection (IgM anti-HBc-negative, IgG anti-HBc-positive). A false-positive test for IgM anti-HBc may be encountered in patients with high-titer rheumatoid factor. Also, IgM anti-HBc may be reexpressed during acute reactivation of chronic hepatitis B.

Anti-HBs is rarely detectable in the presence of HBsAg in patients with *acute* hepatitis B, but 10–20% of persons with *chronic* HBV infection may harbor low-level anti-HBs. This antibody is directed not against the common group determinant, *a*, but against the heterotypic subtype determinant (e.g., HBsAg of subtype *ad* with anti-HBs of subtype *y*). In most cases, this serologic pattern cannot be attributed to infection with two different HBV subtypes, and the presence of this antibody is not a harbinger of imminent HBsAg clearance. When such antibody is detected, its presence is of no recognized clinical significance (see "Virology and Etiology").

After immunization with hepatitis B vaccine, which consists of HBsAg alone, anti-HBs is the only serologic marker to appear. The commonly encountered serologic patterns of hepatitis B and their interpretations are summarized in Table 39-5. Tests for the detection of HBV DNA in liver and serum are now available. Like HBeAg, serum HBV DNA is an indicator of HBV replication, but tests for HBV DNA are more sensitive and quantitative. First-generation hybridization assays for HBV DNA had a sensitivity of 10^5–10^6 virions/mL, a relative threshold below which infectivity and liver injury are limited and HBeAg is usually undetectable. Currently, testing for HBV DNA has shifted from insensitive hybridization assays to amplification assays (e.g., the PCR-based assay, which can detect as few as 10 or 100 virions/mL); among the commercially available PCR assays, the most useful are those with the highest sensitivity (5–10 IU/mL) and the largest dynamic range (10^0–10^9 IU/mL). With increased sensitivity, amplification assays remain reactive well below the current 10^3–10^4 IU/mL threshold for infectivity and liver injury. These markers are useful in following the course of HBV replication in patients with chronic hepatitis B receiving antiviral chemotherapy **(Chap. 41)**. Except for the early decades of life after perinatally acquired HBV infection (see above), in immunocompetent adults with chronic hepatitis B, a general correlation exists between the level of HBV replication, as reflected by the level of serum HBV DNA, and the degree of liver injury. High-serum HBV DNA levels, increased expression of viral antigens, and necroinflammatory activity in the liver go hand in hand unless immunosuppression interferes with cytolytic T cell responses to virus-infected cells; reduction of HBV replication with antiviral drugs tends to be accompanied by an improvement in liver histology. Among patients with chronic hepatitis B, high levels of HBV DNA increase the risk of cirrhosis, hepatic decompensation, and hepatocellular carcinoma (see "Complications and Sequelae").

In patients with hepatitis C, an episodic pattern of aminotransferase elevation is common. A specific serologic diagnosis of hepatitis C can be made by demonstrating the presence in serum of anti-HCV.

TABLE 39-5

COMMONLY ENCOUNTERED SEROLOGIC PATTERNS OF HEPATITIS B INFECTION

HBsAG	ANTI-HBs	ANTI-HBc	HBeAG	ANTI-HBe	INTERPRETATION
+	–	IgM	+	–	Acute hepatitis B, high infectivity[a]
+	–	IgG	+	–	Chronic hepatitis B, high infectivity
+	–	IgG	–	+	1. Late acute or chronic hepatitis B, low infectivity 2. HBeAg-negative ("precore-mutant") hepatitis B (chronic or, rarely, acute)
+	+	+	+/–	+/–	1. HBsAg of one subtype and heterotypic anti-HBs (common) 2. Process of seroconversion from HBsAg to anti-HBs (rare)
–	–	IgM	+/–	+/–	1. Acute hepatitis B[a] 2. Anti-HBc "window"
–	–	IgG	–	+/–	1. Low-level hepatitis B carrier 2. Hepatitis B in remote past
–	+	IgG	–	+/–	Recovery from hepatitis B
–	+	–	–	–	1. Immunization with HBsAg (after vaccination) 2. Hepatitis B in the remote past (?) 3. False-positive

[a]IgM anti-HBc may reappear during acute reactivation of chronic hepatitis B.
Note: See text for abbreviations.

When contemporary immunoassays are used, anti-HCV can be detected in acute hepatitis C during the initial phase of elevated aminotransferase activity and remains detectable after recovery (rare) and during chronic infection (common). Nonspecificity can confound immunoassays for anti-HCV, especially in persons with a low prior probability of infection, such as volunteer blood donors, or in persons with circulating rheumatoid factor, which can bind nonspecifically to assay reagents; testing for HCV RNA can be used in such settings to distinguish between true-positive and false-positive anti-HCV determinations. Assays for HCV RNA are the most sensitive tests for HCV infection and represent the "gold standard" in establishing a diagnosis of hepatitis C. HCV RNA can be detected even before acute elevation of aminotransferase activity and before the appearance of anti-HCV in patients with acute hepatitis C. In addition, HCV RNA remains detectable indefinitely, continuously in most but intermittently in some, in patients with chronic hepatitis C (detectable as well in some persons with normal liver tests, i.e., inactive carriers). In the very small minority of patients with hepatitis C who lack anti-HCV, a diagnosis can be supported by detection of HCV RNA. If all these tests are negative and the patient has a well-characterized case of hepatitis after percutaneous exposure to blood or blood products, a diagnosis of hepatitis caused by an unidentified agent can be entertained.

Amplification techniques are required to detect HCV RNA, and two types are available. One is a branched-chain complementary DNA (bDNA) assay, in which the detection signal (a colorimetrically detectable enzyme bound to a complementary DNA probe) is amplified. The other involves target amplification (i.e., synthesis of multiple copies of the viral genome) by PCR or TMA, in which the viral RNA is reverse transcribed to complementary DNA and then amplified by repeated cycles of DNA synthesis. Both can be used as quantitative assays and a measurement of relative "viral load"; PCR and TMA, with a sensitivity of $10–10^2$ IU/mL, are more sensitive than bDNA, with a sensitivity of 10^3 IU/mL; assays are available with a wide dynamic range ($10–10^7$ IU/mL). Determination of HCV RNA level is not a reliable marker of disease severity or prognosis but is helpful in predicting relative responsiveness to antiviral therapy. The same is true for determinations of HCV genotype **(Chap. 41)**.

A proportion of patients with hepatitis C have isolated anti-HBc in their blood, a reflection of a common risk in certain populations of exposure to multiple bloodborne hepatitis agents. The anti-HBc in such cases is almost invariably of the IgG class and usually represents HBV infection in the remote past (HBV DNA undetectable); it rarely represents current HBV infection with low-level virus carriage.

The presence of HDV infection can be identified by demonstrating intrahepatic HDV antigen or, more practically, an anti-HDV seroconversion (a rise in titer of anti-HDV or de novo appearance of anti-HDV). Circulating HDV antigen, also diagnostic of acute infection, is detectable only briefly, if at all. Because anti-HDV is often undetectable once HBsAg disappears, retrospective serodiagnosis of acute self-limited, simultaneous HBV and HDV infection is difficult. Early diagnosis of acute infection may be hampered by a delay of up to 30–40 days in the appearance of anti-HDV.

When a patient presents with acute hepatitis and has HBsAg and anti-HDV in serum, determination of the class of anti-HBc is helpful in establishing the relationship between infection with HBV and HDV. Although IgM anti-HBc does not distinguish *absolutely* between acute and chronic HBV infection, its presence is a reliable indicator of recent infection and its absence a reliable indicator of infection in the remote past. In simultaneous acute HBV and HDV infections, IgM anti-HBc will be detectable, whereas in acute HDV infection superimposed on chronic HBV infection, anti-HBc will be of the IgG class. Tests for the presence of HDV RNA are useful for determining the presence of ongoing HDV replication and relative infectivity.

The serologic/virologic course of events during acute hepatitis E is entirely analogous to that of acute hepatitis A, with brief fecal shedding of virus and viremia and an early IgM anti-HEV response that predominates during approximately the first 3 months but is eclipsed thereafter by long-lasting IgG anti-HEV. Diagnostic tests of varying reliability for hepatitis E are commercially available but used routinely primarily outside the United States; in the United States, diagnostic serologic/virologic assays can be performed at the Centers for Disease Control and Prevention or other specialized reference laboratories.

Liver biopsy is rarely necessary or indicated in acute viral hepatitis, except when the diagnosis is questionable or when clinical evidence suggests a diagnosis of chronic hepatitis.

A diagnostic algorithm can be applied in the evaluation of cases of acute viral hepatitis. A patient with acute hepatitis should undergo four serologic tests, HBsAg, IgM anti-HAV, IgM anti-HBc, and anti-HCV (Table 39-6). The presence of HBsAg, with or without IgM anti-HBc, represents HBV infection. If IgM anti-HBc is present, the HBV infection is considered acute; if IgM anti-HBc is absent, the HBV infection is considered chronic. A diagnosis of acute hepatitis B can be made in the absence of HBsAg when IgM anti-HBc is detectable. A diagnosis of acute hepatitis A is based on the presence of IgM anti-HAV. If IgM anti-HAV coexists with HBsAg, a diagnosis of simultaneous HAV and HBV infections can be made; if IgM anti-HBc (with or

TABLE 39-6

SIMPLIFIED DIAGNOSTIC APPROACH IN PATIENTS PRESENTING WITH ACUTE HEPATITIS

SEROLOGIC TESTS OF PATIENT'S SERUM				
HBsAG	**IgM ANTI-HAV**	**IgM ANTI-HBc**	**ANTI-HCV**	**DIAGNOSTIC INTERPRETATION**
+	–	+	–	Acute hepatitis B
+	–	–	–	Chronic hepatitis B
+	+	–	–	Acute hepatitis A superimposed on chronic hepatitis B
+	+	+	–	Acute hepatitis A and B
–	+	–	–	Acute hepatitis A
–	+	+	–	Acute hepatitis A and B (HBsAg below detection threshold)
–	–	+	–	Acute hepatitis B (HBsAg below detection threshold)
–	–	–	+	Acute hepatitis C

Note: See text for abbreviations.

without HBsAg) is detectable, the patient has simultaneous acute hepatitis A and B, and if IgM anti-HBc is undetectable, the patient has acute hepatitis A superimposed on chronic HBV infection. The presence of anti-HCV supports a diagnosis of acute hepatitis C. Occasionally, testing for HCV RNA or repeat anti-HCV testing later during the illness is necessary to establish the diagnosis. Absence of all serologic markers is consistent with a diagnosis of "non-A, non-B, non-C" hepatitis, if the epidemiologic setting is appropriate.

In patients with chronic hepatitis, initial testing should consist of HBsAg and anti-HCV. Anti-HCV supports and HCV RNA testing establishes the diagnosis of chronic hepatitis C. If a serologic diagnosis of chronic hepatitis B is made, testing for HBeAg and anti-HBe is indicated to evaluate relative infectivity. Testing for HBV DNA in such patients provides a more quantitative and sensitive measure of the level of virus replication and, therefore, is very helpful during antiviral therapy **(Chap. 41)**. In patients with chronic hepatitis B and normal aminotransferase activity in the absence of HBeAg, serial testing over time is often required to distinguish between inactive carriage and HBeAg-negative chronic hepatitis B with fluctuating virologic and necroinflammatory activity. In persons with hepatitis B, testing for anti-HDV is useful in those with severe and fulminant disease, with severe chronic disease, with chronic hepatitis B and acute hepatitis-like exacerbations, with frequent percutaneous exposures, and from areas where HDV infection is endemic.

PROGNOSIS

Virtually all previously healthy patients with hepatitis A recover completely with no clinical sequelae. Similarly, in acute hepatitis B, 95–99% of previously healthy adults have a favorable course and recover completely. Certain clinical and laboratory features, however, suggest a more complicated and protracted course. Patients of advanced age and with serious underlying medical disorders may have a prolonged course and are more likely to experience severe hepatitis. Initial presenting features such as ascites, peripheral edema, and symptoms of hepatic encephalopathy suggest a poorer prognosis. In addition, a prolonged PT, low serum albumin level, hypoglycemia, and very high serum bilirubin values suggest severe hepatocellular disease. Patients with these clinical and laboratory features deserve prompt hospital admission. The case fatality rate in hepatitis A and B is very low (~0.1%) but is increased by advanced age and underlying debilitating disorders. Among patients ill enough to be hospitalized for acute hepatitis B, the fatality rate is 1%. Hepatitis C is less severe during the acute phase than hepatitis B and is more likely to be anicteric; fatalities are rare, but the precise case fatality rate is not known. In outbreaks of waterborne hepatitis E in India and Asia, the case fatality rate is 1–2% and up to 10–20% in pregnant women. Contributing to fulminant hepatitis E in endemic countries are instances of acute hepatitis E superimposed on underlying chronic liver disease ("acute-on-chronic" liver disease). Patients with simultaneous acute hepatitis B and hepatitis D do not necessarily experience a higher mortality rate than do patients with acute hepatitis B alone; however, in several outbreaks of acute simultaneous HBV and HDV infection among injection drug users, the case fatality rate was ~5%. When HDV superinfection occurs in a person with chronic hepatitis B, the likelihood of fulminant hepatitis and death is increased substantially. Although the case fatality rate for hepatitis D is not known definitively, in outbreaks of severe HDV superinfection in isolated populations with a high hepatitis B carrier rate, a mortality rate >20% has been recorded.

COMPLICATIONS AND SEQUELAE

A small proportion of patients with hepatitis A experience *relapsing hepatitis* weeks to months after apparent recovery from acute hepatitis. Relapses are characterized by recurrence of symptoms, aminotransferase elevations, occasionally jaundice, and fecal excretion of

HAV. Another unusual variant of acute hepatitis A is *cholestatic hepatitis*, characterized by protracted cholestatic jaundice and pruritus. Rarely, liver test abnormalities persist for many months, even up to a year. Even when these complications occur, hepatitis A remains self-limited and does not progress to chronic liver disease. During the prodromal phase of acute hepatitis B, a serum sickness–like syndrome characterized by arthralgia or arthritis, rash, angioedema, and rarely, hematuria and proteinuria may develop in 5–10% of patients. This syndrome occurs before the onset of clinical jaundice, and these patients are often diagnosed erroneously as having rheumatologic diseases. The diagnosis can be established by measuring serum aminotransferase levels, which are almost invariably elevated, and serum HBsAg. As noted above, EMC is an immune-complex disease that can complicate chronic hepatitis C and is part of a spectrum of B cell lymphoproliferative disorders, which, in rare instances, can evolve to B cell lymphoma. Attention has been drawn as well to associations between hepatitis C and such cutaneous disorders as porphyria cutanea tarda and lichen planus. A mechanism for these associations is unknown. Finally, related to the reliance of HCV on lipoprotein secretion and assembly pathways and on interactions of HCV with glucose metabolism, HCV infection may be complicated by hepatic steatosis, hypercholesterolemia, insulin resistance (and other manifestations of the metabolic syndrome), and type 2 diabetes mellitus; both hepatic steatosis and insulin resistance appear to accelerate hepatic fibrosis and blunt responsiveness to antiviral therapy **(Chap. 41)**.

The most feared complication of viral hepatitis is *fulminant hepatitis* (massive hepatic necrosis); fortunately, this is a rare event. Fulminant hepatitis is seen primarily in hepatitis B, D, and E, but rare fulminant cases of hepatitis A occur primarily in older adults and in persons with underlying chronic liver disease, including, according to some reports, chronic hepatitis B and C. Hepatitis B accounts for >50% of fulminant cases of viral hepatitis, a sizable proportion of which are associated with HDV infection and another proportion with underlying chronic hepatitis C. Fulminant hepatitis is hardly ever seen in hepatitis C, but hepatitis E, as noted above, can be complicated by fatal fulminant hepatitis in 1–2% of all cases and in up to 20% of cases in pregnant women. Patients usually present with signs and symptoms of encephalopathy that may evolve to deep coma. The liver is usually small and the PT excessively prolonged. The combination of rapidly shrinking liver size, rapidly rising bilirubin level, and marked prolongation of the PT, even as aminotransferase levels fall, together with clinical signs of confusion, disorientation, somnolence, ascites, and edema, indicates that the patient has hepatic failure with encephalopathy. Cerebral edema is common; brainstem compression, gastrointestinal bleeding, sepsis, respiratory failure, cardiovascular collapse, and renal failure are terminal events. The mortality rate is exceedingly high (>80% in patients with deep coma), but patients who survive may have a complete biochemical and histologic recovery. If a donor liver can be located in time, liver transplantation may be life-saving in patients with fulminant hepatitis **(Chap. 48)**.

Documenting the disappearance of HBsAg after apparent clinical recovery from acute hepatitis B is particularly important. Before laboratory methods were available to distinguish between acute hepatitis and acute hepatitis-like exacerbations (*spontaneous reactivations*) of chronic hepatitis B, observations suggested that ~10% of previously healthy patients remained HBsAg-positive for >6 months after the onset of clinically apparent acute hepatitis B. One-half of these persons cleared the antigen from their circulations during the next several years, but the other 5% remained chronically HBsAg-positive. More recent observations suggest that the true rate of chronic infection after clinically apparent acute hepatitis B is as low as 1% in normal, immunocompetent, young adults. Earlier, higher estimates may have been confounded by inadvertent inclusion of acute exacerbations in chronically infected patients; these patients, chronically HBsAg-positive before exacerbation, were unlikely to seroconvert to HBsAg-negative thereafter. Whether the rate of chronicity is 10% or 1%, such patients have IgG anti-HBc in serum; anti-HBs is either undetected or detected at low titer against the opposite subtype specificity of the antigen (see "Laboratory Features"). These patients may (1) be inactive carriers; (2) have low-grade, mild chronic hepatitis; or (3) have moderate to severe chronic hepatitis with or without cirrhosis. The likelihood of remaining chronically infected after acute HBV infection is especially high among neonates, persons with Down's syndrome, chronically hemodialyzed patients, and immunosuppressed patients, including persons with HIV infection.

Chronic hepatitis is an important late complication of acute hepatitis B occurring in a small proportion of patients with acute disease but more common in those who present with chronic infection without having experienced an acute illness, as occurs typically after neonatal infection or after infection in an immunosuppressed host **(Chap. 41)**. The following clinical and laboratory features suggest progression of acute hepatitis to chronic hepatitis: (1) lack of complete resolution of clinical symptoms of anorexia, weight loss, fatigue, and the persistence of hepatomegaly; (2) the presence of bridging/interface or multilobular hepatic necrosis on liver biopsy during protracted, severe acute viral hepatitis; (3) failure of the serum aminotransferase, bilirubin, and globulin levels to return to normal within 6–12 months after the acute illness; and (4) the persistence of HBeAg for >3 months or HBsAg for >6 months after acute hepatitis.

Although acute hepatitis D infection does not increase the likelihood of chronicity of simultaneous acute hepatitis B, hepatitis D has the potential for contributing to the severity of chronic hepatitis B. Hepatitis D superinfection can transform inactive or mild chronic hepatitis B into severe, progressive chronic hepatitis and cirrhosis; it also can accelerate the course of chronic hepatitis B. Some HDV superinfections in patients with chronic hepatitis B lead to fulminant hepatitis. As defined in longitudinal studies over three decades, the annual rates of cirrhosis and hepatocellular carcinoma in patients with chronic hepatitis D are 4% and 2.8%, respectively. Although HDV and HBV infections are associated with severe liver disease, mild hepatitis and even inactive carriage have been identified in some patients, and the disease may become indolent beyond the early years of infection.

After acute HCV infection, the likelihood of remaining chronically *infected* approaches 85–90%. Although many patients with chronic hepatitis C have no symptoms, cirrhosis may develop in as many as 20% within 10–20 years of acute illness; in some series of cases reported by referral centers, cirrhosis has been reported in as many as 50% of patients with chronic hepatitis C. Although chronic hepatitis C accounts for at least 40% of cases of chronic liver disease and of patients undergoing liver transplantation for end-stage liver disease in the United States and Europe, in the majority of patients with chronic hepatitis C, morbidity and mortality are limited during the initial 20 years after the onset of infection. Progression of chronic hepatitis C may be influenced by advanced age of acquisition, long duration of infection, immunosuppression, coexisting excessive alcohol use, concomitant hepatic steatosis, other hepatitis virus infection, or HIV coinfection. In fact, instances of severe and rapidly progressive chronic hepatitis B and C are being recognized with increasing frequency in patients with HIV infection. In contrast, neither HAV nor HEV causes chronic liver disease in immunocompetent hosts; however, cases of chronic hepatitis E have been observed in immunosuppressed organ-transplant recipients, persons receiving cytotoxic chemotherapy, and persons with HIV infection.

Rare complications of viral hepatitis include pancreatitis, myocarditis, atypical pneumonia, aplastic anemia, transverse myelitis, and peripheral neuropathy. Persons with chronic hepatitis B, particularly those infected in infancy or early childhood and especially those with HBeAg and/or high-level HBV DNA, have an enhanced risk of hepatocellular carcinoma. The risk of hepatocellular carcinoma is increased as well in patients with chronic hepatitis C, almost exclusively in patients with cirrhosis, and almost always after at least several decades, usually after three decades of disease **(Chap. 53)**. In children, hepatitis B may present rarely with anicteric hepatitis, a nonpruritic papular rash of the face, buttocks, and limbs, and lymphadenopathy (papular acrodermatitis of childhood or Gianotti-Crosti syndrome).

Rarely, autoimmune hepatitis **(Chap. 41)** can be triggered by a bout of otherwise self-limited acute hepatitis, as reported after acute hepatitis A, B, and C.

DIFFERENTIAL DIAGNOSIS

Viral diseases such as infectious mononucleosis; those due to cytomegalovirus, herpes simplex, and coxsackieviruses; and toxoplasmosis may share certain clinical features with viral hepatitis and cause elevations in serum aminotransferase and, less commonly, in serum bilirubin levels. Tests such as the differential heterophile and serologic tests for these agents may be helpful in the differential diagnosis if HBsAg, anti-HBc, IgM anti-HAV, and anti-HCV determinations are negative. Aminotransferase elevations can accompany almost any systemic viral infection; other rare causes of liver injury confused with viral hepatitis are infections with *Leptospira, Candida, Brucella, Mycobacteria,* and *Pneumocystis.* A complete drug history is particularly important because many drugs and certain anesthetic agents can produce a picture of either acute hepatitis or cholestasis **(Chap. 40)**. Equally important is a past history of unexplained "repeated episodes" of acute hepatitis. This history should alert the physician to the possibility that the underlying disorder is chronic hepatitis. Alcoholic hepatitis must also be considered, but usually the serum aminotransferase levels are not as markedly elevated, and other stigmata of alcoholism may be present. The finding on liver biopsy of fatty infiltration, a neutrophilic inflammatory reaction, and "alcoholic hyaline" would be consistent with alcohol-induced rather than viral liver injury. Because acute hepatitis may present with right upper quadrant abdominal pain, nausea and vomiting, fever, and icterus, it is often confused with acute cholecystitis, common duct stone, or ascending cholangitis. Patients with acute viral hepatitis may tolerate surgery poorly; therefore, it is important to exclude this diagnosis, and in confusing cases, a percutaneous liver biopsy may be necessary before laparotomy. Viral hepatitis in the elderly is often misdiagnosed as obstructive jaundice resulting from a common duct stone or carcinoma of the pancreas. Because acute hepatitis in the elderly may be quite severe and the operative mortality high, a thorough evaluation including biochemical tests, radiographic studies of the biliary tree, and even liver biopsy may be necessary to exclude primary parenchymal liver disease. Another clinical constellation that may mimic acute hepatitis is right ventricular failure with passive hepatic congestion or hypoperfusion syndromes, such as those associated with shock, severe hypotension, and severe left ventricular failure. Also included in this general category is any disorder that interferes with venous return to the heart, such as right atrial myxoma, constrictive pericarditis, hepatic vein occlusion (Budd-Chiari syndrome), or venoocclusive disease. Clinical features are usually sufficient to distinguish among these vascular disorders and viral hepatitis. Acute fatty liver of pregnancy, cholestasis of pregnancy, eclampsia, and the HELLP (*h* emolysis, *e* levated *l* iver tests, and *l* ow *p* latelets) syndrome can be confused with viral hepatitis during pregnancy. Very rarely, malignancies metastatic to the liver can mimic acute or even fulminant viral hepatitis. Occasionally, genetic or metabolic liver disorders (e.g., Wilson's disease, α_1 antitrypsin deficiency) and nonalcoholic fatty liver disease are confused with acute viral hepatitis.

TREATMENT Acute Viral Hepatitis

Most persons with acute hepatitis (especially hepatitis A, B, and E) recover spontaneously and do not require specific antiviral therapy. In hepatitis B, among previously healthy adults who present with clinically apparent acute hepatitis, recovery occurs in ~99%; therefore, antiviral therapy is not likely to improve the rate of recovery and is not required. In rare instances of severe acute hepatitis B, treatment with a nucleoside analogue at oral doses used to treat chronic hepatitis B **(Chap. 41)** has been attempted successfully. Although clinical trials have not been done to establish the efficacy or duration of this approach, most authorities would recommend institution of antiviral therapy with a nucleoside analogue (entecavir or tenofovir, the most potent and least resistance-prone agents) for severe, but not mild–moderate, acute hepatitis B. Treatment should continue until 3 months after HBsAg seroconversion or 6 months after HBeAg seroconversion.

In typical cases of acute hepatitis C, recovery is rare (~15–20% in most experiences), progression to chronic hepatitis is the rule, and small clinical trials during the era of interferon-based regimens suggested that antiviral therapy with courses (usually 24 weeks) of standard or pegylated interferon α monotherapy reduced the rate of chronicity considerably by inducing sustained responses in 30–70% (according to a meta-analyses of published studies) and in up to 98% in a small German multicenter study (treatment initiated of patients. an average of 3 months after infection). In the current interferon-free therapy era, as of 2016, six different all-oral, brief-duration (most lasting 12 weeks), very well tolerated, highly effective (sustained virologic response rates exceeding 90–95%) combination regimens (of polymerase inhibitors, protease inhibitors, and/or NS5A inhibitors) are available to treat patients with chronic hepatitis C **(see Chap. 41)**; the same regimens are available and recommended to treat patients with acute hepatitis C. Because spontaneous recovery can occur, and because most cases of acute hepatitis C are not clinically severe or rapidly progressive, delaying antiviral therapy of acute hepatitis C for at least 12–16 weeks and even up to 6 months (after which recovery is unlikely) is a recommended approach. Patients with jaundice, those with HCV genotype 1, and women are more likely to recover from acute hepatitis C, as are persons who have genetic markers associated with spontaneous recovery (*IL28B* CC haplotype). Because of the marked reduction over the past three decades in the frequency of acute hepatitis C, opportunities to identify and treat patients with acute hepatitis C are rare, except in two population subsets: 1) In health workers who sustain hepatitis C–contaminated needle sticks (occupational accidents), monitoring for ALT elevations and the presence of HCV RNA identifies acute hepatitis C in ~3% and this group should be treated. 2) In injection drug users, the risk of acute hepatitis C has been on the rise, and the epidemic of opioid use has contributed to an amplification of HCV infection among drug users. Such patients are candidates for antiviral therapy, and efforts to combine antiviral therapy with drug-rehabilitation therapy have been very successful.

Notwithstanding these specific therapeutic considerations, in most cases of typical acute viral hepatitis, specific treatment generally is not necessary. Although hospitalization may be required for clinically severe illness, most patients do not require hospital care. Forced and prolonged bed rest is not essential for full recovery, but many patients will feel better with restricted physical activity. A high-calorie diet is desirable, and because many patients may experience nausea late in the day, the major caloric intake is best tolerated in the morning. Intravenous feeding is necessary in the acute stage if the patient has persistent vomiting and cannot maintain oral intake. Drugs capable of producing adverse reactions such as cholestasis and drugs metabolized by the liver should be avoided. If severe pruritus is present, the use of the bile salt-sequestering resin cholestyramine is helpful. Glucocorticoid therapy has no value in acute viral hepatitis, even in severe cases and may be deleterious, even increasing the risk of chronicity (e.g., of acute hepatitis B).

Physical isolation of patients with hepatitis to a single room and bathroom is rarely necessary except in the case of fecal incontinence for hepatitis A and E or uncontrolled, voluminous bleeding for hepatitis B (with or without concomitant hepatitis D) and hepatitis C. Because most patients hospitalized with hepatitis A excrete little, if any, HAV, the likelihood of HAV transmission from these patients during their hospitalization is low. Therefore, burdensome *enteric precautions are no longer recommended.* Although gloves should be worn when the bed pans or fecal material of patients with hepatitis A are handled, these precautions do not represent a departure from sensible procedure and contemporary universal precautions for all hospitalized patients. For patients with hepatitis B and hepatitis C, emphasis should be placed on blood precautions (i.e., avoiding direct, ungloved hand contact with blood and other body fluids). Enteric precautions are unnecessary. The importance of simple hygienic precautions such as hand washing cannot be overemphasized. Universal precautions that have been adopted for all patients apply to patients with viral hepatitis. Hospitalized patients may be discharged following substantial symptomatic improvement, a significant downward trend in the serum aminotransferase and bilirubin values, and a return to normal of the PT. Mild aminotransferase elevations should not be considered contraindications to the gradual resumption of normal activity.

In *fulminant hepatitis*, the goal of therapy is to support the patient by maintenance of fluid balance, support of circulation and respiration, control of bleeding, correction of hypoglycemia, and treatment of other complications of the comatose state in anticipation of liver regeneration and repair. Protein intake should be restricted, and oral lactulose or neomycin administered. Glucocorticoid therapy has been shown in controlled trials to be ineffective. Likewise, exchange transfusion, plasmapheresis, human cross-circulation, porcine liver cross-perfusion, hemoperfusion, and extracorporeal liver-assist devices have not been proven to enhance survival. Meticulous intensive care that includes prophylactic antibiotic coverage is the one factor that does appear to improve survival. Orthotopic liver transplantation is resorted to with increasing frequency, with excellent results, in patients with fulminant hepatitis **(Chap. 48)**. Fulminant hepatitis C is very rare, but in fulminant hepatitis B, oral antiviral therapy has been used successfully, as reported anecdotally. In clinically severe hepatitis E (with jaundice and coagulopathy), successful therapy with ribavirin (600 mg twice daily, 15 mg/kg) has been reported anecdotally. Unfortunately, when fulminant hepatitis E occurs in pregnant women (as it does in up to 20% of pregnant women with acute hepatitis E), ribavirin, which is teratogenic, is contraindicated.

PROPHYLAXIS

Because application of therapy for acute viral hepatitis is limited and because antiviral therapy for chronic viral hepatitis is cumbersome, costly, and not effective in all patients **(Chap. 41)**, emphasis is placed on prevention through immunization. The prophylactic approach differs for each of the types of viral hepatitis. In the past, immunoprophylaxis relied exclusively on passive immunization with antibody-containing globulin preparations purified by cold ethanol fractionation from the plasma of hundreds of normal donors. Currently, for hepatitis A, B, and E, active immunization with vaccines is the preferable approach to prevention.

Hepatitis A

Both passive immunization with IG and active immunization with killed vaccines are available. All preparations of IG contain anti-HAV concentrations sufficient to be protective. When administered before exposure or during the early incubation period, IG is effective in preventing clinically apparent hepatitis A. For post-exposure prophylaxis of intimate contacts (household, sexual, institutional) of persons with hepatitis A, the administration of 0.02 mL/kg is recommended as early after exposure as possible; it may be effective even when administered as late as 2 weeks after exposure. Prophylaxis is not necessary for those who have already received hepatitis A vaccine, for casual contacts (office, factory, school, or hospital), for most elderly persons, who are very likely to be immune, or for those known to have anti-HAV in their serum. In day care centers, recognition of hepatitis A in children or staff should provide a stimulus for immunoprophylaxis in the center and in the children's family members. By the time most common-source outbreaks of hepatitis A are recognized, it is usually too late in the incubation period for IG to be effective; however, prophylaxis may limit the frequency of secondary cases. For travelers to tropical countries, developing countries, and other areas outside standard tourist routes, IG prophylaxis had been recommended before a vaccine became available. When such travel lasted <3 months, 0.02 mL/kg was given; for longer travel or residence in these areas, a dose of 0.06 mL/kg every 4–6 months was recommended. Administration of plasma-derived globulin is safe; all contemporary lots of IG are subjected to viral inactivation steps and must be free of HCV RNA as determined by PCR testing. Administration of IM lots of IG has not been associated with transmission of HBV, HCV, or HIV.

Formalin-inactivated vaccines made from strains of HAV attenuated in tissue culture have been shown to be safe, immunogenic, and effective in preventing hepatitis A. Hepatitis A vaccines are approved for use in persons who are at least 1 year old and appear to provide adequate protection beginning 4 weeks after a primary inoculation. If it can be given within 4 weeks of an expected exposure, such as by travel to an endemic area, hepatitis A vaccine is the preferred approach to *pre-exposure* immunoprophylaxis. If travel is more imminent, IG (0.02 mL/kg) should be administered at a different injection site, along with the first dose of vaccine. Because vaccination provides long-lasting protection (protective levels of anti-HAV should last 20 years after vaccination), persons whose risk will be sustained (e.g., frequent travelers or those remaining in endemic areas for prolonged periods) should be vaccinated, and vaccine should supplant the need for repeated IG injections. Shortly after its introduction, hepatitis A vaccine was recommended for children living in communities with a high incidence of HAV infection; in 1999, this recommendation was extended to include all children living in states, counties, and communities with high rates of HAV infection. As of 2006, the Advisory Committee on Immunization Practices of the U.S. Public Health Service recommended *routine hepatitis A vaccination of all children*. Other groups considered to be at increased risk for HAV infection and who are candidates for hepatitis A vaccination include military personnel, populations with cyclic outbreaks of hepatitis A (e.g., Alaskan natives), employees of day care centers, primate handlers, laboratory workers exposed to hepatitis A or fecal specimens, and patients with chronic liver disease. Because of an increased risk of fulminant hepatitis A—observed in some experiences but not confirmed in others—among patients with chronic hepatitis C, patients with chronic hepatitis C are candidates for hepatitis A vaccination, as are persons with chronic hepatitis B. Other populations whose recognized risk of hepatitis A is increased should be vaccinated, including men who have sex with men, injection drug users, persons with clotting disorders who require frequent administration of clotting-factor concentrates, persons traveling from the United States to countries with high or intermediate hepatitis A endemicity, postexposure prophylaxis for contacts of persons with hepatitis A, and household members and other close contacts of adopted children arriving from countries with high and moderate hepatitis A endemicity. Recommendations for dose and frequency differ for the two approved vaccine preparations (Table 39-7); all injections are IM. Hepatitis A vaccine has been reported to be effective in preventing secondary household and day care center–associated cases of acute hepatitis A. Because the vaccine provides long-lasting protection and is simpler to use, in 2006, the Immunization Practices Advisory Committee of the U.S. Public Health Service favored hepatitis A vaccine to IG for postexposure prophylaxis of healthy persons age 2–40 years; for younger or older persons, for immunosuppressed patients, and for patients with chronic liver disease, IG should continue to be used. In the United States, reported mortality resulting from hepatitis A declined in parallel with hepatitis A vaccine–associated reductions in the annual incidence of new infections.

TABLE 39-7

HEPATITIS A VACCINATION SCHEDULES

AGE, YEARS	NO. OF DOSES	DOSE	SCHEDULE, MONTHS
HAVRIX (GlaxoSmithKline)[a]			
1–18	2	720 ELU[b] (0.5 mL)	0, 6–12
≥19	2	1440 ELU (1 mL)	0, 6–12
VAQTA (Merck)			
1–18	2	25 units (0.5 mL)	0, 6–18
≥19	2	50 units (1 mL)	0, 6–18

[a]A combination of this hepatitis A vaccine and hepatitis B vaccine, TWINRIX, is licensed for simultaneous protection against both of these viruses among adults (age ≥18 years). Each 1-mL dose contains 720 ELU of hepatitis A vaccine and 20 μg of hepatitis B vaccine. These doses are recommended at months 0, 1, and 6.

[b]Enzyme-linked immunoassay units.

Abbreviation: ELU, enzyme-linked immunoassay unit.

Hepatitis B

Until 1982, prevention of hepatitis B was based on *passive* immunoprophylaxis either with standard Ig, containing modest levels of anti-HBs, or hepatitis B immunoglobulin (HBIG), containing high-titer anti-HBs. The efficacy of standard IG has never been established and remains questionable; even the efficacy of HBIG, demonstrated in several clinical trials, has been challenged, and its contribution appears to be in reducing the frequency of clinical *illness*, not in preventing *infection*. The first vaccine for *active* immunization, introduced in 1982, was prepared from purified, noninfectious 22-nm spherical HBsAg particles derived from the plasma of healthy HBsAg carriers. In 1987, the plasma-derived vaccine was supplanted by a genetically engineered vaccine derived from recombinant yeast. The latter vaccine consists of HBsAg particles that are nonglycosylated but are otherwise indistinguishable from natural HBsAg; two recombinant vaccines are licensed for use in the United States. Current recommendations can be divided into those for pre-exposure and postexposure prophylaxis.

For *pre-exposure* prophylaxis against hepatitis B in settings of frequent exposure (health workers exposed to blood; first-responder public safety workers; hemodialysis patients and staff; residents and staff of custodial institutions for the developmentally handicapped; injection drug users; inmates of long-term correctional facilities; persons with multiple sexual partners or who have had a sexually transmitted disease; men who have sex with men; persons such as hemophiliacs who require long-term, high-volume therapy with blood derivatives; household and sexual contacts of persons with chronic HBV infection; persons living in or traveling extensively in endemic areas; unvaccinated children under the age of 18; unvaccinated children who are Alaskan natives, Pacific Islanders, or residents in households of first-generation immigrants from endemic countries; persons born in countries with a prevalence of HBV infection ≥2%; patients with chronic liver disease; persons <age 60 with diabetes mellitus [those ≥60 at the discretion of their physicians]; persons with end-stage renal disease; persons with HIV infection), three IM (deltoid, not gluteal) injections of hepatitis B vaccine are recommended at 0, 1, and 6 months (other, optional schedules are summarized in Table 39-8). Pregnancy is *not* a contraindication to vaccination. In areas of low HBV endemicity such as the United States, despite the availability of safe and effective hepatitis B vaccines, a strategy of vaccinating persons in high-risk

groups was not effective. The incidence of new hepatitis B cases continued to increase in the United States after the introduction of vaccines; <10% of all targeted persons in high-risk groups were actually vaccinated, and ~30% of persons with sporadic acute hepatitis B did not fall into any high-risk-group category. Therefore, to have an impact on the frequency of HBV infection in an area of low endemicity such as the United States, universal hepatitis B vaccination in childhood has been recommended. For unvaccinated children born after the implementation of universal infant vaccination, vaccination during early adolescence, at age 11–12 years, was recommended, and this recommendation has been extended to include all unvaccinated children age 0–19 years. In HBV-hyperendemic areas (e.g., Asia), universal vaccination of children has resulted in a marked (~70–90%) 30-year decline in complications of hepatitis B, including liver-related mortality and hepatocellular carcinoma.

The two available recombinant hepatitis B vaccines are comparable, one containing 10 μg of HBsAg (Recombivax-HB) and the other containing 20 μg of HBsAg (Engerix-B), and recommended doses for each injection vary for the two preparations (Table 39-8). Combinations of hepatitis B vaccine with other childhood vaccines are available as well (Table 39-8).

For unvaccinated persons sustaining an exposure to HBV, *post-exposure* prophylaxis with a combination of HBIG (for rapid achievement of high-titer circulating anti-HBs) and hepatitis B vaccine (for achievement of long-lasting immunity as well as its apparent efficacy in attenuating clinical illness after exposure) is recommended. For *perinatal* exposure of infants born to HBsAg-positive mothers, a single dose of HBIG, 0.5 mL, should be administered IM in the thigh *immediately after birth*, followed by a complete course of three injections of recombinant hepatitis B vaccine (see doses above) to be started within the first 12 h of life. For those experiencing a direct percutaneous inoculation or transmucosal exposure to HBsAg-positive blood or body fluids (e.g., accidental *needle stick*, other mucosal penetration, or ingestion), a single IM dose of HBIG, 0.06 mL/kg, administered as soon after exposure as possible, is followed by a complete course of hepatitis B vaccine to begin within the first week. For pregnant mothers with high-level HBV DNA (>2 × 10^5 IU/ml), adding antiviral nucleoside analogs (e.g., pregnancy class B tenofovir, see **Chap 40**) during the third trimester of pregnancy reduces perinatal transmission even further. For persons exposed by *sexual* contact to a patient with acute hepatitis B, a single IM dose of HBIG, 0.06 mL/kg, should be given within 14 days of exposure, to be followed by a complete course of hepatitis B vaccine. When both HBIG and hepatitis B vaccine are recommended, they may be given at the same time but at separate sites. Testing adults for anti-HBs after a course of vaccine is advisable to document the acquisition of immunity, but, because hepatitis B vaccine immunogenicity is nearly universal in infants, postvaccination anti-HBs testing of children is not recommended.

The precise duration of protection afforded by hepatitis B vaccine is unknown; however, ~80–90% of immunocompetent adult vaccinees retain protective levels of anti-HBs for at least 5 years, and 60–80% for 10 years, and protective antibody has been documented to last for at least two decades after vaccination in infancy. Thereafter and even after anti-HBs becomes undetectable, protection persists against clinical hepatitis B, hepatitis B

TABLE 39-8

PRE-EXPOSURE HEPATITIS B VACCINATION SCHEDULES

TARGET GROUP	NO. OF DOSES	DOSE	SCHEDULE, MONTHS
RECOMBIVAX-HB (MERCK)[a]			
Infants, children (<1–10 years)	3	5 μg (0.5 mL)	0, 1–2, 4–6
Adolescents (11–19 years)	3 or 4 *Or* 2	5 μg (0.5 mL) 10 μg (1 mL)	0–2, 1–4, 4–6 *or* 0, 12, 24 *or* 0, 1, 2, 12 0, 4–6 (age 11–15)
Adults (≥20 years)	3	10 μg (1 mL)	0–2, 1–4, 4–6
Hemodialysis patients[b]			
<20 years	3	5 μg (0.5 mL)	0, 1, 6
≥20 years	3	40 μg (4 mL)	0, 1, 6
ENGERIX-B (GlaxoSmithKline)[c]			
Infants, children (<1–10 years)	3 or 4	10 μg (0.5 mL)	0, 1–2, 4–6 *or* 0, 1, 2, 12
Adolescents (10–19 years)	3 or 4	10 μg (0.5 mL)	0, 1–2, 4–6 *or* 0, 12, 24 *or* 0, 1, 2, 12
Adults (≥20 years)	3 or 4	20 μg (1 mL)	0–2, 1–4, 4–6 or 0, 1, 2, 12
Hemodialysis patients[b]			
<20 years	4	10 μg (0.5 mL)	0, 1, 2, 6
≥20 years	4	40 μg (2 mL)	0, 1, 2, 6

[a]This manufacturer produces a licensed combination of hepatitis B vaccine and vaccines against *Haemophilus influenzae* type b and *Neisseria meningitides*, Comvax, for use in infants and young children. Please consult product insert for dose and schedule.

[b]This group also includes other immunocompromised persons.

[c]This manufacturer produces two licensed combination hepatitis B vaccines: (1) Twinrix, recombinant hepatitis B vaccine plus inactivated hepatitis A vaccine, is licensed for simultaneous protection against both of these viruses among adults (age ≥18 years). Each 1-mL dose contains 720 ELU of hepatitis A vaccine and 20 μg of hepatitis B vaccine. These doses are recommended at months 0, 1, and 6. (2) Pediatrix, recombinant hepatitis B vaccine plus diphtheria and tetanus toxoid, pertussis, and inactivated poliovirus, is licensed for use in infants and young children. Please consult product insert for doses and schedules.

surface antigenemia, and chronic HBV infection. Currently, *booster* immunizations are not recommended routinely, except in immunosuppressed persons who have lost detectable anti-HBs or immunocompetent persons who sustain percutaneous HBsAg-positive inoculations after losing detectable antibody. Specifically, for hemodialysis patients, annual anti-HBs testing is recommended after vaccination; booster doses are recommended when anti-HBs levels fall to <10 mIU/mL. As noted above, for persons at risk of both hepatitis A and B, a combined vaccine is available containing 720 enzyme-linked immunoassay units (ELUs) of inactivated HAV and 20 μg of recombinant HBsAg (at 0, 1, and 6 months).

Hepatitis D

Infection with hepatitis D can be prevented by vaccinating susceptible persons with hepatitis B vaccine. No product is available for immunoprophylaxis to prevent HDV superinfection in HBsAg carriers; for them, avoidance of percutaneous exposures and limitation of intimate contact with persons who have HDV infection are recommended.

Hepatitis C

IG is ineffective in preventing hepatitis C and is no longer recommended for postexposure prophylaxis in cases of perinatal, needle stick, or sexual exposure. Although prototype vaccines that induce antibodies to HCV envelope proteins have been developed, currently, hepatitis C vaccination is not feasible practically. Genotype and quasispecies viral heterogeneity as well as rapid evasion of neutralizing antibodies by this rapidly mutating virus, conspire to render HCV a difficult target for immunoprophylaxis with a vaccine. Prevention of transfusion-associated hepatitis C has been accomplished by the following successively introduced measures: exclusion of commercial blood donors and reliance on a volunteer blood supply; screening donor blood with surrogate markers such as ALT (no longer recommended) and anti-HBc, markers that identify segments of the blood donor population with an increased risk of bloodborne infections; exclusion of blood donors in high-risk groups for AIDS and the introduction of anti-HIV screening tests; and progressively sensitive serologic and virologic screening tests for HCV infection.

In the absence of active or passive immunization, prevention of hepatitis C includes behavior changes and precautions to limit exposures to infected persons. Recommendations designed to identify patients with clinically inapparent hepatitis as candidates for medical management have as a secondary benefit the identification of persons whose contacts could be at risk of becoming infected. A so-called look-back program has been recommended to identify persons who were transfused before 1992 with blood from a donor found subsequently to have hepatitis C. In addition, anti-HCV testing is recommended for persons born between 1945 and 1965, anyone who received a blood transfusion or a transplanted organ before the introduction of second-generation screening tests in 1992, those who ever used injection drugs (or took other illicit drugs by noninjection routes), chronically hemodialyzed patients, persons with clotting disorders who received clotting factors made before 1987 from pooled blood products, persons with elevated aminotransferase levels, health workers exposed to HCV-positive blood or contaminated needles, recipients of blood or organs from a donor found to be positive for hepatitis C, persons with HIV infection, health care and public safety personnel following a needle stick or other nonpercutaneous exposure to HCV-infected material, sexual partners of persons with hepatitis C, and children born to HCV-positive mothers (Table 39-4).

For stable, monogamous sexual partners, sexual transmission of hepatitis C is unlikely, and sexual barrier precautions are not recommended. For persons with multiple sexual partners or with sexually transmitted diseases, the risk of sexual transmission of hepatitis C is increased, and barrier precautions (latex condoms) are recommended. A person with hepatitis C should avoid sharing such items as razors, toothbrushes, and nail clippers with sexual partners and family members. No special precautions are recommended for babies born to mothers with hepatitis C, and breast-feeding does not have to be restricted.

Hepatitis E

Whether IG prevents hepatitis E remains undetermined. Safe and effective recombinant genotype 1 vaccines, which protect against other genotypes as well, have been developed and are available in endemic areas but not in the United States.

CHAPTER 40

TOXIC AND DRUG-INDUCED HEPATITIS

William M. Lee ■ Jules L. Dienstag

Liver injury is a possible consequence of ingestion of any xenobiotic, including industrial toxins, pharmacologic agents, and complementary and alternative medications (CAMs). Among patients with acute liver failure, drug-induced liver injury is the most common cause, and evidence for hepatotoxicity detected during clinical trials for drug development is the most common reason for failure of compounds to reach approval status. Drug-induced liver injury requires careful history taking to identify unrecognized exposure to chemicals used in work or at home, drugs taken by prescription or bought over the counter, and herbal or dietary supplement medicines. Hepatotoxic drugs can injure the hepatocyte directly, e.g., via a free-radical or metabolic intermediate that causes peroxidation of membrane lipids and that results in liver cell injury. Alternatively, a drug or its metabolite may activate components of the innate or adaptive immune system, stimulate apoptotic pathways, or initiate damage to bile excretory pathways (Fig. 40-1). Interference with bile canalicular pumps can allow endogenous bile acids, which can injure the liver, to accumulate. Such secondary injury, in turn, may lead to necrosis of hepatocytes; injure bile ducts, producing cholestasis; or block pathways of lipid movement, inhibit protein synthesis, or impair mitochondrial oxidation of fatty acids, resulting in lactic acidosis and intracellular triglyceride accumulation (expressed histologically as microvesicular steatosis). In other instances, drug metabolites sensitize hepatocytes to toxic cytokines. The differences observed between susceptible and nonsusceptible drug recipients may be attributable to HLA haplotypes that determine binding of drug-related haptens on the cell surface as well as to polymorphisms in elaboration of competing, protective cytokines, as has been suggested for acetaminophen hepatotoxicity (see below). Immune mechanisms may include cytotoxic lymphocytes or antibody-mediated cellular cytotoxicity. In addition, a role has been shown for activation of nuclear transporters, such as the constitutive androstane receptor (CAR) or, more recently, the pregnane X receptor (PXR), in the induction of drug hepatotoxicity.

DRUG METABOLISM

Most drugs, which are water-insoluble, undergo a series of metabolic steps, culminating in a water-soluble form appropriate for renal or biliary excretion. This process begins with oxidation or methylation mediated initially by the microsomal mixed-function oxygenases, cytochrome P450 (phase I reaction), followed by glucuronidation or sulfation (phase II reaction) or inactivation by glutathione. Most drug hepatotoxicity is mediated by a phase I toxic metabolite, but glutathione depletion, precluding inactivation of harmful compounds by glutathione S-transferase, can contribute as well.

LIVER INJURY CAUSED BY DRUGS

In general, two major types of chemical hepatotoxicity have been recognized: (1) direct toxic and (2) idiosyncratic. As shown in Table 40-1, direct toxic hepatitis occurs with predictable regularity in individuals exposed to the offending agent and is dose-dependent. The latent period between exposure and liver injury is usually short (often several hours), although clinical manifestations may be delayed for 24–48 h. Agents producing toxic hepatitis are generally systemic poisons or are converted in the liver to toxic metabolites. The direct hepatotoxins result in morphologic abnormalities that are reasonably characteristic and reproducible for each toxin. For example, carbon tetrachloride and trichloroethylene characteristically produce a centrilobular zonal necrosis, whereas yellow phosphorus poisoning typically results in periportal injury. The hepatotoxic octapeptides of *Amanita phalloides* usually produce massive hepatic necrosis; the lethal dose of the toxin is ~10 mg, the amount found in a single deathcap mushroom. Liver

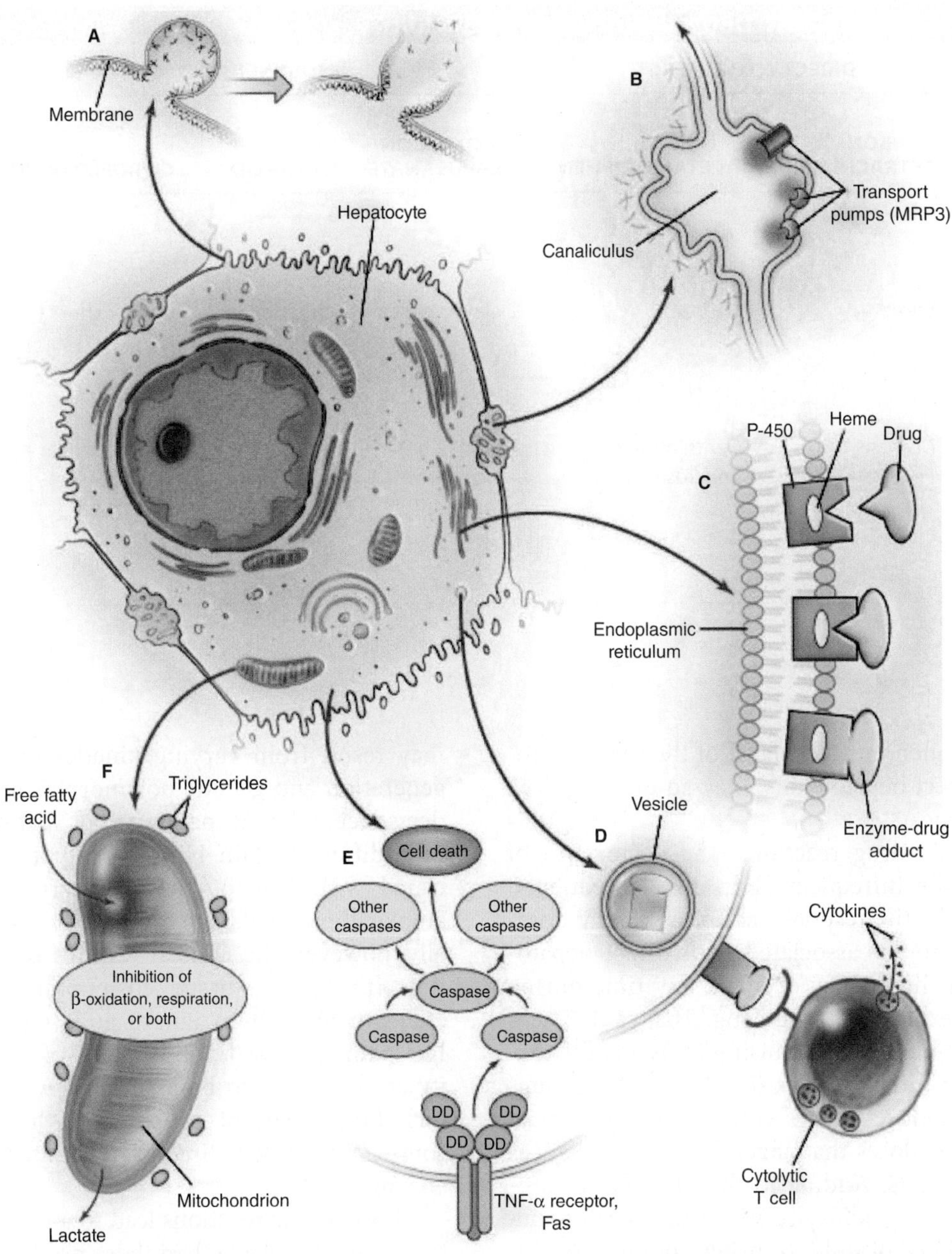

FIGURE 40-1

Potential mechanisms of drug-induced liver injury. The normal hepatocyte may be affected adversely by drugs through (***A***) disruption of intracellular calcium homeostasis that leads to the disassembly of actin fibrils at the surface of the hepatocyte, resulting in blebbing of the cell membrane, rupture, and cell lysis; (***B***) disruption of actin filaments next to the canaliculus (the specialized portion of the cell responsible for bile excretion), leading to loss of villous processes and interruption of transport pumps such as multidrug resistance–associated protein 3 (MRP3), which, in turn, prevents the excretion of bilirubin and other organic compounds; (***C***) covalent binding of the heme-containing cytochrome P450 enzyme to the drug, thus creating nonfunctioning adducts; (***D***) migration of these enzyme-drug adducts to the cell surface in vesicles to serve as target immunogens for cytolytic attack by T cells, stimulating an immune response involving cytolytic T cells and cytokines; (***E***) activation of apoptotic pathways by tumor necrosis factor α (TNF-α) receptor or Fas (DD denotes death domain), triggering the cascade of intercellular caspases, resulting in programmed cell death; or (***F***) inhibition of mitochondrial function by a dual effect on both β-oxidation and the respiratory-chain enzymes, leading to failure of free fatty acid metabolism, a lack of aerobic respiration, and accumulation of lactate and reactive oxygen species (which may disrupt mitochondrial DNA). Toxic metabolites excreted in bile may damage bile-duct epithelium (not shown). CTLs, cytolytic T lymphocytes. *(Reproduced from WM Lee: Drug-induced hepatotoxicity. N Engl J Med 349:474, 2003, with permission.)*

TABLE 40-1

SOME FEATURES OF TOXIC AND DRUG-INDUCED HEPATIC INJURY

	DIRECT TOXIC EFFECT[a]		IDIOSYNCRATIC[a]			OTHER[a]
FEATURES	**CARBON TETRACHLORIDE**	**ACETAMINOPHEN**	**AMOXICILLIN-CLAVULANATE**	**ISONIAZID**	**CIPROFLOXACIN**	**ESTROGENS/ ANDROGENIC STEROIDS**
Predictable and dose-related toxicity	+	+	0	0	0	+
Latent period	Short	Short	Delayed onset	Variable	May be short	Variable
Arthralgia, fever, rash, eosinophilia	0	0	0	0	0	0
Liver morphology	Necrosis, fatty infiltration	Centrilobular necrosis	Mixed hepatocellular/ cholestatic	Hepatocellular injury resembling viral hepatitis	Hepatocellular injury resembling viral hepatitis	Cholestasis *without* portal inflammation

[a]The drugs listed are typical examples.

injury, which is often only one facet of the toxicity produced by the direct hepatotoxins, may go unrecognized until jaundice appears.

In idiosyncratic drug reactions, the occurrence of hepatitis is usually infrequent (1 in 10^3–10^5 patients) and unpredictable; the response is not as clearly dose-dependent as is injury associated with direct hepatotoxins, and liver injury may occur at any time during or shortly after exposure to the drug. That said, recent data suggest that most agents causing idiosyncratic toxicity are given at a daily dose exceeding 100 mg, suggesting a role for dose—drugs with low potency must be given in higher doses that engender greater chances for "off-target" effects. Adding to the difficulty of predicting or identifying idiosyncratic drug hepatotoxicity is the occurrence of mild, transient, nonprogressive serum aminotransferase elevations that resolve with continued drug use. Such "adaptation," the mechanism of which is unknown, is well recognized for drugs such as isoniazid, valproate, phenytoin, and HMG-CoA reductase inhibitors (statins). Extrahepatic manifestations of hypersensitivity, such as rash, arthralgias, fever, leukocytosis, and eosinophilia, occur in about one-quarter of patients with idiosyncratic hepatotoxic drug reactions but are characteristic for certain drugs and not others. Both primary immunologic injury and direct hepatotoxicity related to idiosyncratic differences in generation of toxic metabolites have been invoked to explain idiosyncratic drug reactions. The most current data appear to implicate the adaptive immune system responding to the formation of immune stimulatory compounds resulting from phase I metabolic activation of the offending drug. Differences in host susceptibility may result from varying kinetics of toxic metabolite generation and genetic polymorphisms in downstream drug-metabolizing pathways or cytokine activation; in addition, certain HLA haplotypes have been associated with hepatotoxicity of certain drugs such as amoxicillin-clavulanate and flucloxacillin. Occasionally, however, the clinical features of an allergic reaction (prominent tissue eosinophilia, autoantibodies, etc.) are difficult to ignore and suggest activation of IgE pathways. A few instances of drug hepatotoxicity are observed to be associated with autoantibodies, including a class of antibodies to liver-kidney microsomes, anti-LKM2, directed against a cytochrome P450 enzyme.

Idiosyncratic reactions lead to a morphologic pattern that is more variable than those produced by direct toxins; a single agent is often capable of causing a variety of lesions, although certain patterns tend to predominate. Depending on the agent involved, idiosyncratic hepatitis may result in a clinical and morphologic picture indistinguishable from that of viral hepatitis (e.g., isoniazid or ciprofloxacin). So-called hepatocellular injury is the most common form, featuring spotty necrosis in the liver lobule with a predominantly lymphocytic infiltrate resembling that observed in acute hepatitis A, B, or C. Drug-induced cholestasis ranges from mild to increasingly severe: (1) bland cholestasis with limited hepatocellular injury (e.g., estrogens, 17,α-substituted androgens); (2) inflammatory cholestasis (e.g., amoxicillin-clavulanic acid [the most frequently implicated antibiotic among cases of drug-induced liver injury], oxacillin, erythromycin estolate); (3) sclerosing cholangitis (e.g., after intrahepatic infusion of the chemotherapeutic agent floxuridine for hepatic metastases from a primary colonic carcinoma); and (4) disappearance of bile ducts, "ductopenic" cholestasis, similar to that observed in chronic rejection **(Chap. 47)** following liver transplantation (e.g., carbamazepine, levofloxacin). Cholestasis may result from binding of drugs to canalicular membrane transporters, accumulation of toxic bile acids resulting from canalicular pump failure, or genetic defects in canalicular transporter proteins. Clinically, the distinction between a hepatocellular and a cholestatic reaction is indicated by the R value, the ratio of alanine aminotransferase (ALT) to alkaline phosphatase values, both expressed as multiples of the upper limit of normal. An R value of >5.0 is associated with hepatocellular injury, R <2.0 with cholestatic injury, and R between 2.0 and 5.0 with mixed hepatocellular-cholestatic injury.

Morphologic alterations may also include bridging hepatic necrosis (e.g., methyldopa) or, infrequently, hepatic granulomas (e.g., sulfonamides). Some drugs result in macrovesicular or microvesicular steatosis or steatohepatitis, which, in some cases, has been linked to mitochondrial dysfunction and lipid peroxidation. Severe hepatotoxicity associated with steatohepatitis, most likely a result of mitochondrial toxicity, is being recognized with increasing frequency among patients receiving antiretroviral therapy with reverse transcriptase inhibitors for HIV infection (e.g., zidovudine, didanosine), although many of these drugs have been withdrawn because of such hepatotoxicity. Generally, such mitochondrial hepatotoxicity of these antiretroviral agents is reversible, but dramatic, nonreversible hepatotoxicity associated with mitochondrial injury (inhibition of DNA polymerase γ) was the cause of acute liver failure encountered during early clinical trials of now-abandoned fialuridine, a fluorinated pyrimidine analogue with potent antiviral activity against hepatitis B virus. Another potential target for idiosyncratic drug hepatotoxicity is sinusoidal lining cells; when these are injured, such as by high-dose chemotherapeutic agents (e.g., cyclophosphamide, melphalan, busulfan) administered prior to bone marrow transplantation, venoocclusive disease can result. Nodular regenerative hyperplasia, a subtle form of portal hypertension, may also result from vascular injury to portal venous endothelium following systemic chemotherapy, such as with oxaliplatin, as part of adjuvant treatment for colon cancer.

Not all adverse hepatic drug reactions can be classified as either toxic or idiosyncratic. For example, oral contraceptives, which combine estrogenic and progestational compounds, may result in impairment of hepatic tests and, occasionally, jaundice; however, they do not produce necrosis or fatty change, manifestations of hypersensitivity are generally absent, and susceptibility to the development of oral contraceptive–induced cholestasis appears to be genetically determined. Such estrogen-induced cholestasis is more common in women with cholestasis of pregnancy, a disorder linked to genetic defects in multidrug resistance–associated canalicular transporter proteins.

Any idiosyncratic reaction that occurs in <1:10,000 recipients will go unrecognized in most clinical trials, which involve only several thousand recipients. The U.S. Food and Drug Administration (FDA) and pharmaceutical companies have learned to look for even subtle indications of serious toxicity and monitor regularly the number of trial subjects in whom any aminotransferase elevations develop, as a possible surrogate for more serious toxicity. Even more valid as a predictor of severe hepatotoxicity is the occurrence of jaundice in patients enrolled in a clinical drug trial, so called "Hy's Law," named after Hyman Zimmerman, one of the pioneers of the field of drug hepatotoxicity. He recognized that, if jaundice occurred during a phase III trial, more serious liver injury was likely, with a 10:1 ratio between cases of jaundice and liver failure—10 patients with jaundice to 1 patient with acute liver failure. Thus, the finding of such Hy's Law cases during drug development often portends failure of approval, particularly if any of the subjects sustains a bad outcome. Troglitazone, a peroxisome proliferator-activated receptor γ agonist, was the first in its class of thiazolidinedione insulin-sensitizing agents. Although in retrospect, Hy's Law cases of jaundice had occurred during phase III trials, no instances of liver failure were recognized until well after the drug was introduced, underlining the importance of post-marketing surveillance in identifying toxic drugs and in leading to their withdrawal from use. Fortunately, such hepatotoxicity is not characteristic of the second-generation thiazolidinedione insulin-sensitizing agents rosiglitazone and pioglitazone; in clinical trials, the frequency of aminotransferase elevations in patients treated with these medications did not differ from that in placebo recipients, and isolated reports of liver injury among recipients are extremely rare.

Proving that an episode of liver injury is caused by a drug is difficult in many cases. Drug-induced liver injury is nearly always a presumptive diagnosis, and many other disorders produce a similar clinicopathologic picture. Thus, causality may be difficult to establish and requires several separate supportive assessment variables to lead to a high level of certainty, including temporal association (time of onset, time to resolution), clinical-biochemical features, type of injury (hepatocellular versus cholestatic), extrahepatic features, likelihood that a given agent is to blame based on its past record, and exclusion of other potential causes. Scoring systems such as the Roussel-Uclaf Causality Assessment Method (RUCAM) yield residual uncertainty and have not been adopted widely. Currently, the U.S. Drug-Induced Liver Injury Network (DILIN) relies on a structured expert opinion process requiring detailed data on each case and a comprehensive review by three experts who arrive at a consensus on a five-degree scale of likelihood (definite, highly likely, probable, possible, unlikely); however, this approach is not practical for routine clinical application.

Generally, drug hepatotoxicity is not more frequent in persons with underlying chronic liver disease, although the severity of the outcome may be amplified. Reported exceptions include hepatotoxicity of aspirin, methotrexate, isoniazid (only in certain experiences), antiretroviral therapy for HIV infection, and certain drugs such as conditioning regimens for bone marrow transplantation in the presence of hepatitis C.

TREATMENT Toxic and Drug-Induced Hepatic Disease

Treatment is largely supportive, except in acetaminophen hepatotoxicity (see below). In patients with fulminant hepatitis resulting from drug hepatotoxicity, liver transplantation may be lifesaving **(Chap. 48)**. Withdrawal of the suspected agent is indicated at the first sign of an adverse reaction. A number of studies have suggested that lethal outcomes follow continued use of an agent in the face of symptoms and signs of liver injury. In the case of the direct toxins, liver involvement should not divert attention from renal or other organ involvement, which may also threaten survival. A number of agents are occasionally used but are of questionable value: glucocorticoids for drug hepatotoxicity with allergic features, silibinin for hepatotoxic mushroom poisoning, and ursodeoxycholic acid for cholestatic drug hepatotoxicity have never been shown to be effective and are not recommended.

In Table 40-2, several classes of chemical agents are listed together with examples of the pattern of liver injury produced by them. Certain drugs appear to be responsible for the development of chronic as well as acute hepatic injury. For example, nitrofurantoin, minocycline, hydralazine, and methyldopa have been associated with moderate to severe chronic hepatitis with autoimmune features. Methotrexate, tamoxifen, and amiodarone have been implicated in the development of cirrhosis. Portal hypertension in the absence of cirrhosis may result from alterations in hepatic architecture produced by vitamin A or arsenic intoxication, industrial exposure to vinyl chloride, or administration of thorium dioxide. The latter three agents have also been associated with angiosarcoma of the liver. Oral contraceptives have been implicated in the development of hepatic adenoma and, rarely, hepatocellular carcinoma and hepatic vein occlusion (Budd-Chiari syndrome). Another unusual lesion, peliosis hepatis (blood cysts of the liver), has been observed in some patients treated with anabolic or contraceptive steroids. The existence of these hepatic disorders expands the spectrum of liver injury induced by chemical agents and emphasizes the need for a thorough drug history in all patients with liver dysfunction. A helpful LiverTox website that contains up-to-date information on drug-induced liver injury is available through the National Institute of Diabetes and Digestive and Kidney Diseases and the National Library of Medicine (*www.livertox.nih.gov*).

The following are patterns of adverse hepatic reactions for some prototypic agents.

ACETAMINOPHEN HEPATOTOXICITY (DIRECT TOXIN)

Acetaminophen represents the most prevalent cause of acute liver failure in the Western world; up to 72% of patients with acetaminophen hepatotoxicity in Scandinavia—somewhat lower frequencies in the United Kingdom and the United States—progress to encephalopathy and coagulopathy. Acetaminophen causes dose-related centrilobular hepatic necrosis after single-time-point ingestions, as intentional self-harm, or over extended periods, as unintentional overdoses, when multiple drug preparations or inappropriate drug amounts are used daily for several days, e.g., for relief of pain or fever. In these instances, 8 g/d, twice the daily recommended maximum dose, over several days can readily lead to liver failure. Use of opioid-acetaminophen combinations appears to be particularly harmful, because habituation to the opioid may occur with a gradual increase in opioid-acetaminophen combination dosing over days or weeks. A single dose of 10–15 g, occasionally less, may produce clinical evidence of liver injury. Fatal fulminant disease is usually (although not invariably) associated with ingestion of ≥25 g. Blood levels of acetaminophen correlate with severity of hepatic injury (levels >300 μg/mL 4 h after ingestion are predictive of the development of severe damage; levels <150 μg/mL suggest that hepatic injury is highly unlikely). Nausea, vomiting, diarrhea, abdominal pain, and shock are early manifestations occurring 4–12 h after ingestion. Then 24–48 h later, when these features are abating, hepatic injury becomes apparent. Maximal abnormalities and hepatic failure are evident 3–5 days after ingestion, and aminotransferase levels exceeding 10,000 IU/L are not uncommon (i.e., levels far exceeding those in patients with viral hepatitis). Renal failure and myocardial injury may be present. Whether or not a clear history of overdose can be elicited, clinical suspicion of acetaminophen hepatotoxicity should be raised by the presence of the extremely high aminotransferase levels in association with low bilirubin levels that are characteristic of this hyperacute injury. This biochemical signature should trigger further questioning of the subject if possible; however, denial or altered mentation may confound

TABLE 40-2

PRINCIPAL ALTERATIONS OF HEPATIC MORPHOLOGY PRODUCED BY SOME COMMONLY USED DRUGS AND CHEMICALS[a]

PRINCIPAL MORPHOLOGIC CHANGE	CLASS OF AGENT	EXAMPLE
Cholestasis	Anabolic steroid	Methyl testosterone, many other body-building supplements
	Antibiotic	Erythromycin estolate, nitrofurantoin, rifampin, amoxicillin-clavulanic acid, oxacillin
	Anticonvulsant	Carbamazepine
	Antidepressant	Duloxetine, mirtazapine, tricyclic antidepressants
	Anti-inflammatory	Sulindac
	Antiplatelet	Clopidogrel
	Antihypertensive	Irbesartan, fosinopril
	Antithyroid	Methimazole
	Calcium channel blocker	Nifedipine, verapamil
	Immunosuppressive	Cyclosporine
	Lipid-lowering	Ezetimibe
	Oncotherapeutic	Anabolic steroids, busulfan, tamoxifen, irinotecan, cytarabine, temozolomide
	Oral contraceptive	Norethynodrel with mestranol
	Oral hypoglycemic	Chlorpropamide
	Tranquilizer	Chlorpromazine[b]
Fatty liver	Antiarrhythmic	Amiodarone
	Antibiotic	Tetracycline (high-dose, IV)
	Anticonvulsant	Valproic acid
	Antiviral	Dideoxynucleosides (e.g., zidovudine), protease inhibitors (e.g., indinavir, ritonavir)
	Oncotherapeutic	Asparaginase, methotrexate, tamoxifen
Hepatitis	Anesthetic	Halothane, fluothane
	Antiandrogen	Flutamide
	Antibiotic	Isoniazid,[c] rifampicin, nitrofurantoin, telithromycin, minocycline,[d] pyrazinamide, trovafloxacin[e]
	Anticonvulsant	Phenytoin, carbamazepine, valproic acid, phenobarbital
	Antidepressant	Iproniazid, amitriptyline, trazodone, venlafaxine, fluoxetine, paroxetine, duloxetine, sertraline, nefazodone[e]
	Antifungal	Ketoconazole, fluconazole, itraconazole
	Antihypertensive	Methyldopa,[c] captopril, enalapril, lisinopril, losartan
	Anti-inflammatory	Ibuprofen, indomethacin, diclofenac, sulindac, bromfenac
	Antipsychotic	Risperidone
	Antiviral	Zidovudine, didanosine, stavudine, nevirapine, ritonavir, indinavir, tipranavir, zalcitabine
	Calcium channel blocker	Nifedipine, verapamil, diltiazem
	Cholinesterase inhibitor	Tacrine
	Diuretic	Chlorothiazide
	Laxative	Oxyphenisatin[c,e]
	Norepinephrine-reuptake inhibitor	Atomoxetine
	Oral hypoglycemic	Troglitazone,[e] acarbose
Mixed hepatitis/ cholestatic	Antibiotic	Amoxicillin-clavulanic acid, trimethoprim-sulfamethoxazole
	Antibacterial	Clindamycin
	Antifungal	Terbinafine
	Antihistamine	Cyproheptadine
	Immunosuppressive	Azathioprine
	Lipid-lowering	Nicotinic acid, lovastatin, ezetimibe
Toxic (necrosis)	Analgesic	Acetaminophen
	Hydrocarbon	Carbon tetrachloride
	Metal	Yellow phosphorus
	Mushroom	*Amanita phalloides*
	Solvent	Dimethylformamide

(*continued*)

TABLE 40-2

PRINCIPAL ALTERATIONS OF HEPATIC MORPHOLOGY PRODUCED BY SOME COMMONLY USED DRUGS AND CHEMICALS[a] (CONTINUED)

Granulomas	Antiarrhythmic	Quinidine, diltiazem
	Antibiotic	Sulfonamides
	Anticonvulsant	Carbamazepine
	Anti-inflammatory	Phenylbutazone
	Xanthine oxidase inhibitor	Allopurinol
Vascular injury	Chemotherapeutic	Oxaliplatin, melphalan

[a]Several agents cause more than one type of liver lesion and appear under more than one category.
[b]Rarely associated with primary biliary cirrhosis–like lesion.
[c]Occasionally associated with chronic hepatitis or bridging hepatic necrosis or cirrhosis.
[d]Associated with an autoimmune hepatitis–like syndrome.
[e]Withdrawn from use because of severe hepatotoxicity.

diagnostic efforts. In this setting, a presumptive diagnosis is reasonable, and the proven antidote, *N*-acetylcysteine—both safe and presumed to be effective even when injury has already begun to evolve—should be instituted.

Acetaminophen is metabolized predominantly by a phase II reaction to innocuous sulfate and glucuronide metabolites; however, a small proportion of acetaminophen is metabolized by a phase I reaction to a hepatotoxic metabolite formed from the parent compound by the cytochrome P450 CYP2E1. This metabolite, *N*-acetyl-p-benzoquinone-imine (NAPQI), is detoxified by binding to "hepatoprotective" glutathione to become harmless, water-soluble mercapturic acid, which undergoes renal excretion. When excessive amounts of NAPQI are formed, or when glutathione levels are low, glutathione levels are depleted and overwhelmed, permitting covalent binding to nucleophilic hepatocyte macromolecules forming acetaminophen-protein "adducts." These adducts, which can be measured in serum by high-performance liquid chromatography, hold promise as diagnostic markers of acetaminophen hepatotoxicity, and a point-of-care assay for acetaminophen-Cys adducts is under development. The binding of acetaminophen to hepatocyte macromolecules is believed to lead to hepatocyte necrosis; the precise sequence and mechanism are unknown. Hepatic injury may be potentiated by prior administration of alcohol, phenobarbital, isoniazid, or other drugs; by conditions that stimulate the mixed-function oxidase system; or by conditions such as starvation (including inability to maintain oral intake during severe febrile illnesses) that reduce hepatic glutathione levels. Alcohol induces cytochrome P450 CYP2E1; consequently, increased levels of the toxic metabolite NAPQI may be produced in chronic alcoholics after acetaminophen ingestion, but the role of alcohol in potentiating acute acetaminophen injury is still debated. Alcohol also suppresses hepatic glutathione production. Therefore, in chronic alcoholics, the toxic dose of acetaminophen may be as low as 2 g, and alcoholic patients should be warned specifically about the dangers of even standard doses of this commonly used drug. In a 2006 study, aminotransferase elevations were identified in 31–44% of normal subjects treated for 14 days with the maximal recommended dose of acetaminophen, 4 g daily (administered alone or as part of an acetaminophen-opioid combination); because these changes were transient and never associated with bilirubin elevation, the clinical relevance of these findings remains to be determined. Although underlying hepatitis C virus (HCV) infection was found to be associated with an increased risk of acute liver injury in patients hospitalized for acetaminophen overdose, generally, in patients with nonalcoholic liver disease, acetaminophen taken in recommended doses is well tolerated. Acetaminophen use in cirrhotic patients has not been associated with hepatic decompensation. On the other hand, because of the link between acetaminophen use and liver injury, and because of the limited safety margin between safe and toxic doses, the FDA has recommended that the daily dose of acetaminophen be reduced from 4 g to 3 g (even lower for persons with chronic alcohol use), that all acetaminophen-containing products be labeled prominently as containing acetaminophen, and that the potential for liver injury be prominent in the packaging of acetaminophen and acetaminophen-containing products. Within opioid combination products, the limit for the acetaminophen component has been lowered to 325 mg per tablet.

TREATMENT Acetaminophen Overdosage

Treatment includes gastric lavage, supportive measures, and oral administration of activated charcoal or cholestyramine to prevent absorption of residual drug. Neither charcoal nor cholestyramine appears to be effective if given >30 min after acetaminophen ingestion; if they are used, the stomach lavage should be done before other agents are administered

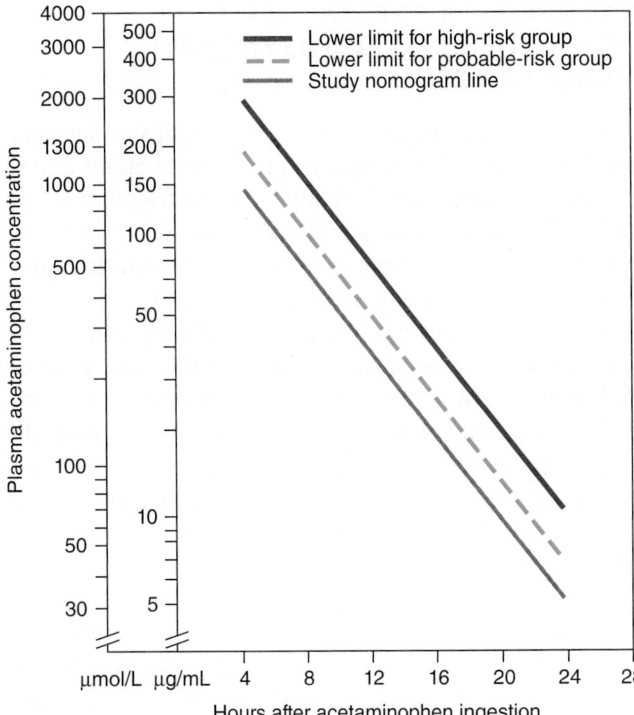

FIGURE 40-2

Nomogram to define risk of acetaminophen hepatotoxicity according to initial plasma acetaminophen concentration. *(After BH Rumack, H Matthew: Pediatrics 55:871, 1975.)*

orally. The chances of possible, probable, and high-risk hepatotoxicity can be derived from a nomogram plot (Fig. 40-2), readily available in emergency departments, as a function of measuring acetaminophen plasma levels 8 h after ingestion. In patients with high acetaminophen blood levels (>200 μg/mL measured at 4 h or >100 μg/mL at 8 h after ingestion), the administration of *N*-acetylcysteine reduces the severity of hepatic necrosis. This agent provides sulfhydryl donor groups to replete glutathione, which is required to render harmless toxic metabolites that would otherwise bind covalently via sulfhydryl linkages to cell proteins, resulting in the formation of drug metabolite-protein adducts. Therapy should be begun within 8 h of ingestion but may be at least partially effective when given as late as 24–36 h after overdose. Later administration of sulfhydryl compounds is of uncertain value. Routine use of *N*-acetylcysteine has substantially reduced the occurrence of fatal acetaminophen hepatotoxicity. *N*-acetylcysteine may be given orally but is more commonly used as an IV solution, with a loading dose of 140 mg/kg over 1 h, followed by 70 mg/kg every 4 h for 15–20 doses. Whenever a patient with potential acetaminophen hepatotoxicity is encountered, a local poison control center should be contacted. Treatment can be stopped when plasma acetaminophen levels indicate that the risk of liver damage is low. If signs of hepatic failure (e.g., progressive jaundice, coagulopathy, confusion) occur despite *N*-acetylcysteine therapy for acetaminophen hepatotoxicity, liver transplantation may be the only option. Early arterial blood lactate levels among such patients with acute liver failure may distinguish patients highly likely to require liver transplantation (lactate levels >3.5 mmol/L) from those likely to survive without liver replacement. Acute renal injury occurs in nearly 75% of patients with severe acetaminophen injury but is virtually always self-limited.

Survivors of acute acetaminophen overdose rarely, if ever, have ongoing liver injury or sequelae.

ISONIAZID HEPATOTOXICITY (TOXIC AND IDIOSYNCRATIC REACTION)

Isoniazid (INH) remains central to most antituberculous prophylactic and therapeutic regimens, despite its long-standing recognition as a hepatotoxin. In 10% of patients treated with INH, elevated serum aminotransferase levels develop during the first few weeks of therapy; however, these elevations in most cases are self-limited, mild (values for ALT <200 IU/L), and resolve despite continued drug use. This adaptive response allows continuation of the agent if symptoms and progressive enzyme elevations do not follow the initial elevations. Acute hepatocellular drug-induced liver injury secondary to INH is evident with a variable latency period up to 6 months and is more frequent in alcoholics and patients taking certain other medications, such as barbiturates, rifampin, and pyrazinamide. If the clinical threshold of encephalopathy is reached, severe hepatic injury is likely to be fatal or to require liver transplantation. Liver biopsy reveals morphologic changes similar to those of viral hepatitis or bridging hepatic necrosis. Substantial liver injury appears to be age-related, increasing substantially after age 35; the highest frequency is in patients over age 50, and the lowest is in patients under the age of 20. Even for patients >50 years of age monitored carefully during therapy, hepatotoxicity occurs in only ~2%, well below the risk estimate derived from earlier experiences. Fever, rash, eosinophilia, and other manifestations of drug allergy are distinctly unusual. Recently, antibodies to INH have been detected in INH recipients, but a link to causality of liver injury remains unclear. A clinical picture resembling chronic hepatitis has been observed in a few patients. Many public health programs that require INH prophylaxis for a positive tuberculin skin test or Quantiferon test include monthly monitoring of aminotransferase levels, although this practice has been called into question. Even more effective in limiting serious outcomes may be encouraging patients to be alert for symptoms such as nausea, fatigue, or jaundice, because most fatalities occur in the setting of continued INH use despite clinically apparent illness.

SODIUM VALPROATE HEPATOTOXICITY (TOXIC AND IDIOSYNCRATIC REACTION)

Sodium valproate, an anticonvulsant useful in the treatment of petit mal and other seizure disorders, has been associated with the development of severe hepatic toxicity and, rarely, fatalities, predominantly in children but also in adults. Among children listed as candidates for liver transplantation, valproate is the most common antiepileptic drug implicated. Asymptomatic elevations of serum aminotransferase levels have been recognized in as many as 45% of treated patients. These "adaptive" changes, however, appear to have no clinical importance, because major hepatotoxicity is not seen in the majority of patients despite continuation of drug therapy. In the rare patients in whom jaundice, encephalopathy, and evidence of hepatic failure are found, examination of liver tissue reveals microvesicular fat and bridging hepatic necrosis, predominantly in the centrilobular zone. Bile duct injury may also be apparent. Most likely, sodium valproate is not directly hepatotoxic, but its metabolite, 4-pentenoic acid, may be responsible for hepatic injury. Valproate hepatotoxicity is more common in persons with mitochondrial enzyme deficiencies and may be ameliorated by IV administration of carnitine, which valproate therapy can deplete. Recently, valproate toxicity has been linked to HLA haplotypes (*DR4* and *B*1502*) and to mutations in mitochondrial DNA polymerase gamma 1.

NITROFURANTOIN HEPATOTOXICITY (IDIOSYNCRATIC REACTION)

This commonly used antibiotic for urinary tract infections may cause an acute hepatitis leading to fatal outcome or, more frequently, chronic hepatitis of varying severity but indistinguishable from autoimmune chronic hepatitis. These two scenarios may reflect the frequent use and reuse of the drug for treatment of recurrent cystitis in women. Although most toxic agents manifest injury within 6 months of first ingestion, nitrofurantoin may have a longer latency period, in part perhaps because of its intermittent, recurrent use. Autoantibodies to nuclear components, smooth muscle, and mitochondria are seen and may subside after resolution of infection; however, glucocorticoid or other immunosuppressive medication may be necessary to resolve the autoimmune injury, and cirrhosis may be seen in cases that are not recognized quickly. Interstitial pulmonary fibrosis presenting as chronic cough and dyspnea may be present and resolve slowly with medication withdrawal. Histologic findings are identical to those of autoimmune hepatitis. A similar disease pattern can be observed with minocycline that is used repeatedly for the treatment of acne in teenagers as well as with hydralazine and alpha methyldopa.

AMOXICILLIN-CLAVULANATE HEPATOTOXICITY (IDIOSYNCRATIC MIXED REACTION)

Currently, the most common agent implicated as causing drug-induced liver injury in the United States and in Europe is amoxicillin-clavulanate (most frequent brand name: Augmentin). This medication causes a very specific syndrome of mixed or primarily cholestatic injury. Because hepatotoxicity may follow amoxicillin-clavulanate therapy after a relatively long latency period, the liver injury may begin to manifest at the time of drug withdrawal or after the drug has been withdrawn. The high prevalence of hepatotoxicity reflects in part the very frequent use of this drug for respiratory tract infections, including community-acquired pneumonia. The mechanism of hepatotoxicity is unclear, but the liver injury is thought to be caused by amoxicillin toxicity that is potentiated in some way by clavulanate, which itself appears not to be toxic. Symptoms include nausea, anorexia, fatigue, and jaundice—which may be prolonged—with pruritus. Rash is quite uncommon. On occasion, amoxicillin-clavulanate, like other cholestatic hepatotoxic drugs, causes permanent injury to small bile ducts, leading to the so-called "vanishing bile duct syndrome." In vanishing bile duct syndrome, initially, liver injury is minimal except for severe cholestasis; however, over time, histologic evidence of bile duct abnormalities is replaced by a paucity and eventual absence of discernible ducts on subsequent biopsies.

PHENYTOIN HEPATOTOXICITY (IDIOSYNCRATIC REACTION)

Phenytoin, formerly diphenylhydantoin, a mainstay in the treatment of seizure disorders, has been associated in rare instances with the development of severe hepatitis-like liver injury leading to fulminant hepatic failure. In many patients, the hepatitis is associated with striking fever, lymphadenopathy, rash (Stevens-Johnson syndrome or exfoliative dermatitis), leukocytosis, and eosinophilia, suggesting an immunologically mediated hypersensitivity mechanism. Despite these observations, evidence suggests that metabolic idiosyncrasy may be responsible for hepatic injury. In the liver, phenytoin is converted by cytochrome P450 to metabolites, including the highly reactive electrophilic arene oxides. These metabolites are normally metabolized further by epoxide hydrolases. A defect (genetic or acquired) in epoxide hydrolase activity could permit covalent binding of arene oxides to hepatic macromolecules, thereby leading to hepatic injury. Hepatic injury is usually manifest within the first 2 months after beginning phenytoin therapy. With the exception of an abundance of eosinophils in the liver, the clinical, biochemical, and histologic picture resembles that of viral hepatitis. In rare instances, bile duct injury may be the salient feature of phenytoin hepatotoxicity, with striking features of intrahepatic cholestasis. Asymptomatic elevations of aminotransferase and alkaline phosphatase levels have been observed in a sizable proportion of patients receiving long-term phenytoin therapy. These liver changes are believed by some authorities to represent the potent hepatic enzyme-inducing properties of phenytoin and are accompanied histologically by swelling of hepatocytes in the absence of necroinflammatory activity or evidence of chronic liver disease.

AMIODARONE HEPATOTOXICITY (TOXIC AND IDIOSYNCRATIC REACTION)

Therapy with this potent antiarrhythmic drug is accompanied in 15–50% of patients by modest elevations of serum aminotransferase levels that may remain stable or diminish despite continuation of the drug. Such abnormalities may appear days to many months after beginning therapy. A proportion of those with elevated aminotransferase levels have detectable hepatomegaly, and clinically important liver disease develops in <5% of patients. Features that represent a direct effect of the drug on the liver and that are common to the majority of long-term recipients are ultrastructural phospholipidosis, unaccompanied by clinical liver disease, and interference with hepatic mixed-function oxidase metabolism of other drugs. The cationic amphiphilic drug and its major metabolite desethylamiodarone accumulate in hepatocyte lysosomes and mitochondria and in bile duct epithelium. The relatively common elevations in aminotransferase levels are also considered a predictable, dose-dependent, direct hepatotoxic effect. On the other hand, in the rare patient with clinically apparent, symptomatic liver disease, liver injury resembling that seen in alcoholic liver disease is observed. The so-called pseudoalcoholic liver injury can range from steatosis to alcoholic hepatitis–like neutrophilic infiltration and Mallory's hyaline to cirrhosis. Electron-microscopic demonstration of phospholipid-laden lysosomal lamellar bodies can help to distinguish amiodarone hepatotoxicity from typical alcoholic hepatitis. This category of liver injury appears to be a metabolic idiosyncrasy that allows hepatotoxic metabolites to be generated. Rarely, an acute idiosyncratic hepatocellular injury resembling viral hepatitis or cholestatic hepatitis occurs. Hepatic granulomas have occasionally been observed. Because amiodarone has a long half-life, liver injury may persist for months after the drug is stopped.

ERYTHROMYCIN HEPATOTOXICITY (CHOLESTATIC IDIOSYNCRATIC REACTION)

The most important adverse effect associated with erythromycin, more common in children than adults, is the infrequent occurrence of a cholestatic reaction. Although most of these reactions have been associated with erythromycin estolate, other erythromycins may also be responsible. The reaction usually begins during the first 2 or 3 weeks of therapy and includes nausea, vomiting, fever, right upper quadrant abdominal pain, jaundice, leukocytosis, and moderately elevated aminotransferase and alkaline phosphatase levels. The clinical picture can resemble acute cholecystitis or bacterial cholangitis. Liver biopsy reveals variable cholestasis; portal inflammation comprising lymphocytes, polymorphonuclear leukocytes, and eosinophils; and scattered foci of hepatocyte necrosis. Symptoms and laboratory findings usually subside within a few days of drug withdrawal, and evidence of chronic liver disease has not been found on follow-up. The precise mechanism remains ill-defined.

ORAL CONTRACEPTIVE HEPATOTOXICITY (CHOLESTATIC REACTION)

The administration of oral contraceptive combinations of estrogenic and progestational steroids leads to intrahepatic cholestasis with pruritus and jaundice in a small number of patients weeks to months after taking these agents. Especially susceptible seem to be patients with recurrent idiopathic jaundice of pregnancy, severe pruritus of pregnancy, or a family history of these disorders. With the exception of liver biochemical tests, laboratory studies are normal, and extrahepatic manifestations of hypersensitivity are absent. Liver biopsy reveals cholestasis with bile plugs in dilated canaliculi and striking bilirubin staining of liver cells. In contrast to chlorpromazine-induced cholestasis, portal inflammation is absent. The lesion is reversible on withdrawal of the agent. The two steroid components appear to act synergistically on hepatic function, although the estrogen may be primarily responsible. Oral contraceptives are contraindicated in patients with a history of recurrent jaundice of pregnancy. Primarily benign, but rarely malignant, neoplasms of the liver, hepatic vein occlusion, and peripheral sinusoidal dilatation have also been associated with oral contraceptive therapy. Focal nodular hyperplasia of the liver is not more frequent among users of oral contraceptives.

ANABOLIC STEROIDS (CHOLESTATIC REACTION)

The most common form of liver injury caused by complementary and alternative medications is the profound cholestasis associated with anabolic steroids used by body builders. Unregulated agents sold in gyms and health food stores as diet supplements, which are taken by athletes to improve their performance, may contain anabolic steroids. Jaundice in a young male that is accompanied by a cholestatic, rather than a hepatitic, laboratory profile almost invariably will turn out to be caused by the use of one of a variety of androgen congeners. Such agents have the potential to injure bile transport pumps and to cause intense cholestasis; the time to onset is variable, and resolution, which is the rule, may require many weeks to months. Initially, anorexia, nausea, and malaise may occur, followed by pruritus in some but not all patients. Serum aminotransferase levels are usually <100 IU/L and serum alkaline phosphatase levels are generally moderately elevated with bilirubin levels frequently exceeding 342 μmol/L (20 mg/dL). Examination of liver tissue reveals cholestasis without substantial inflammation or necrosis. Anabolic steroids have also been used by prescription to treat bone marrow failure. In this setting, hepatic sinusoidal dilatation and peliosis hepatis have been reported in rare patients, as have hepatic adenomas and hepatocellular carcinoma.

TRIMETHOPRIM-SULFAMETHOXAZOLE HEPATOTOXICITY (IDIOSYNCRATIC REACTION)

This antibiotic combination is used routinely for urinary tract infections in immunocompetent persons and for prophylaxis against and therapy of *Pneumocystis jiroveci* pneumonia in immunosuppressed persons (transplant recipients, patients with AIDS). With its increasing use, its occasional hepatotoxicity is being recognized with growing frequency. Its likelihood is unpredictable, but when it occurs, trimethoprim-sulfamethoxazole hepatotoxicity follows a relatively uniform latency period of several weeks and is often accompanied by eosinophilia, rash, and other features of a hypersensitivity reaction. Biochemically and histologically, acute hepatocellular necrosis predominates, but cholestatic features are quite frequent. Occasionally, cholestasis without necrosis occurs, and, very rarely, a severe cholangiolytic pattern of liver injury is observed. In most cases, liver injury is self-limited, but rare fatalities have been recorded. The hepatotoxicity is attributable to the sulfamethoxazole component of the drug and is similar in features to that seen with other sulfonamides; tissue eosinophilia and granulomas may be seen. The risk of trimethoprim-sulfamethoxazole hepatotoxicity is increased in persons with HIV infection.

HMG-COA REDUCTASE INHIBITORS (STATINS) (IDIOSYNCRATIC MIXED HEPATOCELLULAR AND CHOLESTATIC REACTION)

Between 1 and 2% of patients taking lovastatin, simvastatin, pravastatin, fluvastatin, or one of the newer statin drugs for the treatment of hypercholesterolemia experience asymptomatic, reversible elevations (>threefold) of aminotransferase activity. Acute hepatitis-like histologic changes, centrilobular necrosis, and centrilobular cholestasis have been described in a very small number of cases. In a larger proportion, minor aminotransferase elevations appear during the first several weeks of therapy. Careful laboratory monitoring can distinguish between patients with minor, transitory changes, who may continue therapy and those with more profound and sustained abnormalities, who should discontinue therapy. Because clinically meaningful aminotransferase elevations are so rare after statin use and do not differ in meta-analyses from the frequency of such laboratory abnormalities in placebo recipients, a panel of liver experts recommended to the National Lipid Association's Safety Task Force that liver test monitoring was not necessary in patients treated with statins and that statin therapy need not be discontinued in patients found to have asymptomatic isolated aminotransferase elevations during therapy. Statin hepatotoxicity is not increased in patients with chronic hepatitis C, hepatic steatosis, or other underlying liver diseases, and statins can be used safely in these patients.

TOTAL PARENTERAL NUTRITION (STEATOSIS, CHOLESTASIS)

Total parenteral nutrition (TPN) is often complicated by cholestatic hepatitis attributable to steatosis, cholestasis, or gallstones (or gallbladder sludge). Steatosis or steatohepatitis may result from the excess carbohydrate calories in these nutritional supplements and is the predominant form of TPN-associated liver disorder in adults. The frequency of this complication has been reduced substantially by the introduction of balanced TPN formulas that rely on lipid as an alternative caloric source. Cholestasis and cholelithiasis, caused by the absence of stimulation of bile flow and secretion resulting from the lack of oral intake, is the predominant form of TPN-associated liver disease in infants, especially in premature neonates. Often, cholestasis in such neonates is multifactorial, contributed to by other factors such as sepsis, hypoxemia, and hypotension; occasionally, TPN-induced cholestasis in neonates culminates in chronic liver disease and liver failure. When TPN-associated liver test abnormalities occur in adults, balancing the TPN formula with more lipid is the intervention of first recourse. In infants with TPN-associated cholestasis, the addition of oral feeding may ameliorate the problem. Therapeutic interventions suggested, but not shown, to be of proven benefit, include cholecystokinin, ursodeoxycholic acid, *S*-adenosyl methionine, and taurine.

ALTERNATIVE AND COMPLEMENTARY MEDICINES (IDIOSYNCRATIC HEPATITIS, STEATOSIS)

Herbal medications that are of scientifically unproven efficacy and that lack prospective safety oversight by regulatory agencies currently account for more than 20% of drug-induced liver injury in the United States. Besides anabolic steroids, the most common category of dietary or herbal products is weight loss agents. Included among the herbal remedies associated with toxic hepatitis are Jin Bu Huan, xiao-chai-hu-tang, germander, chaparral, senna, mistletoe, skullcap, gentian, comfrey (containing pyrrolizidine alkaloids), ma huang, bee pollen, valerian root, pennyroyal oil, kava, celandine, Impila (*Callilepis laureola*), LipoKinetix, Hydroxycut, herbal nutritional supplements, and herbal teas containing *Camellia sinensis* (green tea extract). Well characterized are the acute hepatitis-like histologic lesions following Jin Bu Huan use: focal hepatocellular necrosis, mixed mononuclear portal tract infiltration, coagulative necrosis, apoptotic hepatocyte degeneration, tissue eosinophilia, and microvesicular steatosis. Megadoses of vitamin A can injure the liver, as can pyrrolizidine alkaloids, which often contaminate Chinese herbal preparations and can cause a venoocclusive injury leading to sinusoidal hepatic vein obstruction. Because some alternative medicines induce toxicity via active metabolites, alcohol and drugs that stimulate cytochrome P450 enzymes may enhance the toxicity of some of these products. Conversely, some alternative medicines also stimulate cytochrome P450 and may result in or amplify the toxicity of recognized drug hepatotoxins. Given the widespread use of such poorly defined herbal preparations, hepatotoxicity is likely to be encountered with increasing frequency; therefore, a drug history in patients with acute and chronic liver disease should include use of "alternative medicines" and other nonprescription preparations sold in so-called health food stores.

HIGHLY ACTIVE ANTIRETROVIRAL THERAPY (HAART) FOR HIV INFECTION (MITOCHONDRIAL TOXIC, IDIOSYNCRATIC, STEATOSIS; HEPATOCELLULAR, CHOLESTATIC, AND MIXED)

The recognition of drug hepatotoxicity in persons with HIV infection is complicated in this population by the many alternative causes of liver injury (chronic viral hepatitis, fatty infiltration, infiltrative disorders, mycobacterial infection, etc.), but drug hepatotoxicity associated with HAART is an emerging and common type of liver injury in HIV-infected persons. Although no one antiviral agent is recognized as a potent hepatotoxin, combination regimens including reverse transcriptase and protease inhibitors cause hepatotoxicity in ~10% of treated patients. Implicated most frequently are combinations including nucleoside analogue reverse transcriptase inhibitors zidovudine, didanosine, and, to a lesser extent, stavudine; protease inhibitors ritonavir and indinavir (and amprenavir when used together with ritonavir), as well as tipranavir; and nonnucleoside reverse transcriptase inhibitors nevirapine and, to a lesser extent, efavirenz. These drugs cause predominantly hepatocellular injury but cholestatic injury as well, and prolonged (>6 months) use of reverse transcriptase inhibitors has been associated with mitochondrial injury, steatosis, and lactic acidosis. Indirect hyperbilirubinemia, resulting from direct inhibition of bilirubin-conjugating activity by UDP-glucuronosyltransferase, usually without elevation of aminotransferase or alkaline phosphatase activities, occurs in ~10% of patients treated with the protease inhibitor indinavir. Distinguishing the impact of HAART hepatotoxicity in patients with HIV and hepatitis virus co-infection is made challenging by the following: (1) both chronic hepatitis B and hepatitis C can affect the natural history of HIV infection and the response to HAART, and (2) HAART can have an impact on chronic viral hepatitis. For example, immunologic reconstitution with HAART can result in immunologically mediated liver-cell injury in patients with chronic hepatitis B co-infection if treatment with an antiviral agent for hepatitis B (e.g., the nucleoside analogue lamivudine) is withdrawn or if nucleoside analogue resistance emerges. Infection with HIV, especially with low CD4+ T cell counts, has been reported to increase the rate of hepatic fibrosis associated with chronic hepatitis C, and HAART therapy can increase levels of serum aminotransferases and HCV RNA in patients with hepatitis C co-infection. Didanosine or stavudine should not be used with ribavirin in patients with HIV/HCV co-infection because of an increased risk of severe mitochondrial toxicity and lactic acidosis.

ACKNOWLEDGMENT

Kurt J. Isselbacher, MD, contributed to this chapter in previous editions of Harrison's.

CHAPTER 41

CHRONIC HEPATITIS

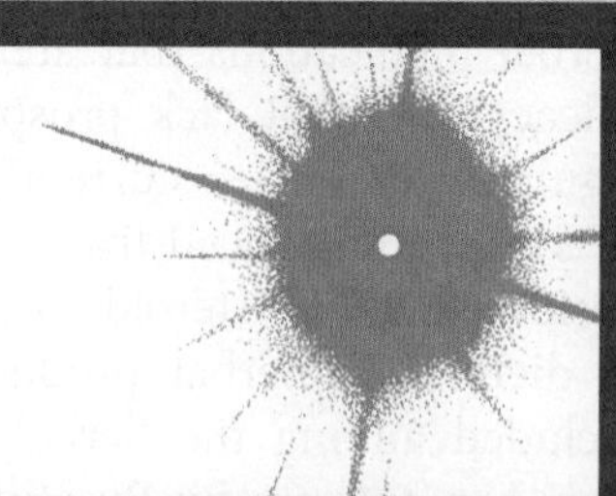

Jules L. Dienstag

Chronic hepatitis represents a series of liver disorders of varying causes and severity in which hepatic inflammation and necrosis continue for at least 6 months. Milder forms are nonprogressive or only slowly progressive, while more severe forms may be associated with scarring and architectural reorganization, which, when advanced, lead ultimately to cirrhosis. Several categories of chronic hepatitis have been recognized. These include chronic viral hepatitis, drug-induced chronic hepatitis **(Chap. 40)**, and autoimmune chronic hepatitis. In many cases, clinical and laboratory features are insufficient to allow assignment into one of these three categories; these "idiopathic" cases are also believed to represent autoimmune chronic hepatitis. Finally, clinical and laboratory features of chronic hepatitis are observed occasionally in patients with such hereditary/metabolic disorders as Wilson's disease (copper overload), α_1 antitrypsin deficiency **(Chap. 44)**, and nonalcoholic fatty liver disease **(Chap. 46)** and even occasionally in patients with alcoholic liver injury **(Chap. 42)**. Although all types of chronic hepatitis share certain clinical, laboratory, and histopathologic features, chronic viral and chronic autoimmune hepatitis are sufficiently distinct to merit separate discussions. **For discussion of acute hepatitis, see Chap. 39.**

CLASSIFICATION OF CHRONIC HEPATITIS

Common to all forms of chronic hepatitis are histopathologic distinctions based on localization and extent of liver injury. These vary from the milder forms, previously labeled *chronic persistent hepatitis* and *chronic lobular hepatitis*, to the more severe form, formerly called *chronic active hepatitis*. When first defined, these designations were believed to have prognostic implications, which were not corroborated by subsequent observations. Categorization of chronic hepatitis based primarily on histopathologic features has been replaced by a more informative classification based on a combination of clinical, serologic, and histologic variables. Classification of chronic hepatitis is based on (1) its *cause*; (2) its histologic activity, or *grade*; and (3) its degree of progression, or *stage*. Thus, neither clinical features alone nor histologic features—requiring liver biopsy—alone are sufficient to characterize and distinguish among the several categories of chronic hepatitis.

CLASSIFICATION BY CAUSE

Clinical and serologic features allow the establishment of a diagnosis of *chronic viral hepatitis*, caused by hepatitis B, hepatitis B plus D, or hepatitis C; *autoimmune hepatitis*, including several subcategories, I and II (perhaps III), based on serologic distinctions; *drug-associated chronic hepatitis*; and a category of unknown cause, or *cryptogenic chronic hepatitis* (Table 41-1). These are addressed in more detail below.

CLASSIFICATION BY GRADE

Grade, a histologic assessment of necroinflammatory activity, is based on examination of the liver biopsy. An assessment of important histologic features includes the degree of *periportal necrosis* and the disruption of the limiting plate of periportal hepatocytes by inflammatory cells (so-called *piecemeal necrosis* or *interface hepatitis*); the degree of confluent necrosis that links or forms bridges between vascular structures—between portal tract and portal tract or even more important bridges between portal tract and central vein—referred to as *bridging necrosis*; the degree of hepatocyte degeneration and focal necrosis within the lobule; and the degree of *portal inflammation*. Several scoring systems that take these histologic features into account have been devised, and the most popular are the histologic activity index (HAI), used commonly in the esions (leukocytoclastic vasculitis), immune-complex glomerulonephritis, and generalized vasculitis (polyarteritis nodosa) (**Chap. 39**).

Laboratory features of chronic hepatitis B do not distinguish adequately between histologically mild and severe hepatitis. Aminotransferase elevations tend to be modest for chronic hepatitis B but may fluctuate in the range of 100–1000 units. As is true for acute viral hepatitis B, alanine aminotransferase (ALT) tends to be more elevated than aspartate aminotransferase (AST); however, once cirrhosis is established, AST tends to exceed ALT. Levels of alkaline phosphatase activity tend to be normal or only marginally elevated. In severe cases, moderate elevations in serum bilirubin (51.3–171 μmol/L [3–10 mg/dL]) occur. Hypoalbuminemia and prolongation of the prothrombin time occur in severe or end-stage cases. Hyperglobulinemia and detectable circulating autoantibodies are distinctly absent in chronic hepatitis B (in contrast to autoimmune hepatitis). **Viral markers of chronic HBV infection are discussed in Chap. 39.**

TREATMENT Chronic Hepatitis B

Although progression to cirrhosis is more likely in severe than in mild or moderate chronic hepatitis B, all forms of chronic hepatitis B can be progressive, and progression occurs primarily in patients with active HBV replication. Moreover, in populations of patients with chronic hepatitis B who are at risk for HCC (**Chap. 53**), the risk is highest for those with continued, high-level HBV replication and lower for persons in whom initially high-level HBV DNA falls spontaneously over time. Therefore, management of chronic hepatitis B is directed at suppressing the level of virus replication. Although clinical trials tend to focus on clinical endpoints achieved over 1–2 years (e.g., suppression of HBV DNA to undetectable levels, loss of HBeAg/HBsAg, improvement in histology, normalization of ALT), these short-term gains translate into reductions in the risk of clinical progression, hepatic decompensation, and death. To date, seven drugs have been approved for treatment of chronic hepatitis B: injectable interferon (IFN) α; pegylated interferon (long-acting IFN bound to polyethylene glycol, PEG [PEG IFN]); and the oral agents lamivudine, adefovir dipivoxil, entecavir, telbivudine, and tenofovir.

Antiviral therapy for hepatitis B has evolved rapidly since the mid-1990s, as has the sensitivity of tests for HBV DNA. When IFN and lamivudine were evaluated in clinical trials, HBV DNA was measured by insensitive hybridization assays with detection thresholds of 10^5–10^6 virions/mL; when adefovir, entecavir, telbivudine, tenofovir, and PEG IFN were studied in clinical trials, HBV DNA was measured by sensitive amplification assays (polymerase chain reaction [PCR]) with detection thresholds of 10^1–10^3 viral copies/mL or IU/mL. Recognition of these distinctions is helpful when comparing results of clinical trials that established the efficacy of these therapies (reviewed below in chronological order of publication of these efficacy trials).

INTERFERON IFN-α was the first approved therapy for chronic hepatitis B. Although it is no longer used to treat hepatitis B, standard IFN is important historically, having provided important lessons about antiviral therapy in general. For immunocompetent adults with HBeAg-reactive chronic hepatitis B (who tend to have high-level HBV DNA [$>10^5$–10^6 virions/mL] and histologic evidence of chronic hepatitis on liver biopsy), a 16-week course of IFN given subcutaneously at a daily dose of 5 million units, or three times a week at a dose of 10 million units, results in a loss of HBeAg and hybridization-detectable HBV DNA (i.e., a reduction to levels below 10^5–10^6 virions/mL) in ~30% of patients, with a concomitant improvement in liver histology. Seroconversion from HBeAg to anti-HBe occurred in approximately 20%, and, in early trials, approximately 8% lost HBsAg. Successful IFN therapy and seroconversion are often accompanied by an acute hepatitis-like elevation in aminotransferase activity, which has been postulated to result from enhanced cytolytic T cell clearance of HBV-infected hepatocytes. Relapse after successful therapy is rare (1 or 2%). The likelihood of responding to IFN is higher in patients with lower levels of HBV DNA and substantial elevations of ALT. Although children can respond as well as adults, IFN therapy has not been effective in very young children infected at birth. Similarly, IFN therapy has not been effective in immunosuppressed persons, Asian patients with neonatal acquisition of infection and minimal-to-mild ALT elevations, or patients with decompensated chronic hepatitis B (in whom such therapy can actually be detrimental, sometimes precipitating decompensation, often associated with severe adverse effects). Among patients with HBeAg loss during therapy, long-term follow-up has demonstrated that 80% experience eventual loss of HBsAg (i.e., all serologic markers of infection, and normalization of ALT over a 9-year posttreatment period). In addition, improved long-term and complication-free survival as well as a reduction in the frequency of HCC have been documented among IFN responders, supporting the conclusion that successful antiviral therapy improves the natural history of chronic hepatitis B.

Initial trials of brief-duration IFN therapy in patients with *HBeAg-negative chronic hepatitis B* were disappointing, suppressing HBV replication transiently during therapy but almost never resulting in sustained antiviral responses. In subsequent IFN trials among patients with HBeAg-negative chronic hepatitis B, however, more protracted courses, lasting up to 1.5 years, have been reported to result in sustained remissions documented to last for several years, with suppressed HBV DNA and aminotransferase activity, in ~20%.

Complications of IFN therapy include systemic "flu-li symptoms; marrow suppression; emotional lability (irrit ity, depression, anxiety); autoimmune reactions (esp

TABLE 41-1

CLINICAL AND LABORATORY FEATURES OF CHRONIC HEPATITIS

TYPE OF HEPATITIS	DIAGNOSTIC TEST(S)	AUTOANTIBODIES	THERAPY
Chronic hepatitis B	HBsAg, IgG anti-HBc, HBeAg, HBV DNA	Uncommon	IFN-α, PEG IFN-α Oral agents: First-line: entecavir, tenofovir Second-line: lamivudine, adefovir, telbivudine
Chronic hepatitis C	Anti-HCV, HCV RNA	Anti-LKM1[a]	PEG IFN-α plus ribavirin Telaprevir[b] Boceprevir[b]
Chronic hepatitis D	Anti-HDV, HDV RNA, HBsAg, IgG anti-HBc	Anti-LKM3	IFN-α, PEG IFN-α[c]
Autoimmune hepatitis	ANA[d] (homogeneous), anti-LKM1 (±) Hyperglobulinemia	ANA, anti-LKM1 anti-SLA[e]	Prednisone, azathioprine
Drug-associated	—	Uncommon	Withdraw drug
Cryptogenic	All negative	None	Prednisone (?), azathioprine (?)

[a]Antibodies to liver-kidney microsomes type 1 (autoimmune hepatitis type II and some cases of hepatitis C).
[b]Administered as a triple-drug combination with PEG IFN and ribavirin. Between the writing and publication of this chapter, two additional drugs were approved for hepatitis C, simeprevir and sofosbuvir (see *www.hcvguidelines.org*).
[c]Early clinical trials suggested benefit of IFN-α therapy; PEG IFN-α is as effective, if not more so, and has supplanted standard IFN-α.
[d]Antinuclear antibody (autoimmune hepatitis type I).
[e]Antibodies to soluble liver antigen (autoimmune hepatitis type III).
Abbreviations: HBc, hepatitis B core; HBeAg, hepatitis B e antigen; HBsAg, hepatitis B surface antigen; HBV, hepatitis B virus; HCV, hepatitis C virus; HDV, hepatitis D virus; IFN-α, interferon α; IgG, immunoglobulin G; LKM, liver-kidney microsome; PEG IFN-α, pegylated interferon α; SLA, soluble liver antigen.

United States, and the METAVIR score, used in Europe (Table 41-2). Based on the presence and degree of these features of histologic activity, chronic hepatitis can be graded as mild, moderate, or severe.

CLASSIFICATION BY STAGE

The stage of chronic hepatitis, which reflects the level of progression of the disease, is based on the degree of hepatic fibrosis. When fibrosis is so extensive that fibrous septa surround parenchymal nodules and alter the normal architecture of the liver lobule, the histologic lesion is defined as *cirrhosis*. Staging is based on the degree of fibrosis as categorized on a numerical scale from 0–6 (HAI) or 0–4 (METAVIR) (Table 41-2). Several noninvasive approaches have been introduced to provide approximations of hepatic histologic stage, including serum biomarkers of fibrosis and imaging determinations of liver elasticity.

CHRONIC VIRAL HEPATITIS

Both the enterically transmitted forms of viral hepatitis, hepatitis A and E, are self-limited and do not cause chronic hepatitis (rare reports notwithstanding in which acute hepatitis A serves as a trigger for the onset of autoimmune hepatitis in genetically susceptible patients or in which hepatitis E (**Chap. 39**) can cause chronic liver disease in immunosuppressed hosts, e.g., after liver transplantation). In contrast, the entire clinicopathologic spectrum of chronic hepatitis occurs in patients with chronic viral hepatitis B and C as well as in patients with chronic hepatitis D superimposed on chronic hepatitis B.

CHRONIC HEPATITIS B

The likelihood of chronicity after acute hepatitis B varies as a function of age. Infection at birth is associated with clinically silent acute infection but a 90% chance of chronic infection, whereas infection in young adulthood in immunocompetent persons is typically associated with clinically apparent acute hepatitis but a risk of chronicity of only approximately 1%. Most cases of chronic hepatitis B among adults, however, occur in patients who never had a recognized episode of clinically apparent acute viral hepatitis. The degree of liver injury (grade) in patients with chronic hepatitis B is variable, ranging from none in inactive carriers to mild to moderate to severe. Among adults with chronic hepatitis B, histologic features are of prognostic importance. In one long-term study of patients with chronic hepatitis B, investigators found a 5-year survival rate of 97% for patients with mild chronic hepatitis, 86% for patients with moderate to severe chronic hepatitis, and autoimmune thyroiditis); and miscellaneous side effects such as alopecia, rashes, diarrhea, and numbness and tingling of the extremities. With the possible exception of autoimmune thyroiditis, all these side effects are reversible upon dose lowering or cessation of therapy.

Although no longer competitive with the newer generation of antivirals, IFN did represent the first successful antiviral approach and set a standard against which to measure subsequent drugs in the achievement of durable virologic, serologic, biochemical, and histologic responses; consolidation of virologic and biochemical benefit in the ensuing years after therapy; and improvement in the natural history of chronic hepatitis B. Standard IFN has been supplanted by long-acting PEG IFN (see below), and IFN nonresponders are now treated with one of the newer oral nucleoside analogues.

LAMIVUDINE The first of the nucleoside analogues to be approved, the dideoxynucleoside lamivudine inhibits reverse transcriptase activity of both HIV and HBV and is a potent and effective agent for patients with chronic hepatitis B. Although generally superseded by newer, more potent agents, lamivudine is still used in regions of the world where newer agents are not yet approved are or not affordable. In clinical trials among patients with HBeAg-reactive chronic hepatitis B, lamivudine therapy at daily doses of 100 mg for 48–52 weeks suppressed HBV DNA by a median of approximately 5.5 $\log_{10}$ copies/mL and to undetectable levels, as measured by PCR amplification assays, in approximately 40% of patients. Therapy was associated with HBeAg loss in 32–33%; HBeAg seroconversion (i.e., conversion from HBeAg-reactive to anti-HBe-reactive) in 16–21%; normalization of ALT in 40–75%; improvement in histology in 50–60%; retardation in fibrosis in 20–30%; and prevention of progression to cirrhosis. HBeAg responses can occur even in subgroups who are resistant to IFN (e.g., those with high-level HBV DNA) or who failed in the past to respond to it. As is true for IFN therapy of chronic hepatitis B, patients with near-normal ALT activity tend not to experience HBeAg responses (despite suppression of HBV DNA), and those with ALT levels exceeding 5 × the upper limit of normal can expect 1-year HBeAg seroconversion rates of 50–60%. Generally, HBeAg seroconversions are confined to patients who achieve suppression of HBV DNA to $<10^4$ copies/mL (equivalent to $\sim10^3$ IU/mL). Lamivudine-associated HBeAg responses are accompanied by a posttreatment HBsAg seroconversion rate comparable to that seen after IFN-induced HBeAg responses. Among Western patients who undergo HBeAg responses during a year-long course of therapy and in whom the response is sustained for 4–6 months after cessation of therapy, the response is durable thereafter in the vast majority (>80%); therefore, the achievement of an HBeAg response represents a viable stopping point in therapy. Reduced durability has been reported in Asian patients; therefore, to support the durability of HBeAg responses, patients should receive a period of consolidation therapy of ≥6 months in Western patients and ≥1 year in Asian patients after HBeAg seroconversion. Close posttreatment monitoring is necessary to identify HBV reactivation promptly and to resume therapy. If HBeAg is unaffected by lamivudine therapy, the current approach is to continue therapy until an HBeAg response occurs, but long-term therapy may be required to suppress HBV replication and, in turn, limit liver injury; HBeAg seroconversions can increase to a level of 50% after 5 years of therapy. Histologic improvement continues to accrue with therapy beyond the first year; after a cumulative course of 3 years of lamivudine therapy, necroinflammatory activity is reduced in the majority of patients, and even cirrhosis has been shown to regress to precirrhotic stages in as many as three- quarters of patients.

Losses of HBsAg have been few during the first year of lamivudine therapy, and this observation had been cited as an advantage of IFN-based over lamivudine therapy; however, in head-to-head comparisons between standard IFN and lamivudine monotherapy, HBsAg losses were rare in both groups. Trials in which lamivudine and IFN were administered in combination failed to show a benefit of combination therapy over lamivudine monotherapy for either treatment-naïve patients or prior IFN nonresponders.

In patients with *HBeAg-negative chronic hepatitis B* (i.e., in those with precore and core-promoter HBV mutations), 1 year of lamivudine therapy results in HBV DNA suppression and normalization of ALT in three-quarters of patients and in histologic improvement in approximately two-thirds. Therapy has been shown to suppress HBV DNA by approximately 4.5 $\log_{10}$ copies/mL (baseline HBV DNA levels are lower than in patients with HBeAg-reactive hepatitis B) and to undetectable levels in approximately 70%, as measured by sensitive PCR amplification assays. Lacking HBeAg at the outset, patients with HBeAg-negative chronic hepatitis B cannot achieve an HBeAg response—a stopping point in HBeAg-reactive patients; almost invariably, when therapy is discontinued, reactivation is the rule. Therefore, these patients require long-term therapy; with successive years, the proportion with suppressed HBV DNA and normal ALT increases.

Clinical and laboratory side effects of lamivudine are negligible and indistinguishable from those observed in placebo recipients. Still, lamivudine doses should be reduced in patients with reduced creatinine clearance. During lamivudine therapy, transient ALT elevations, resembling those seen during IFN therapy and during spontaneous HBeAg-to-anti-HBe seroconversions, occur in one-fourth of patients. These ALT elevations may result from restored cytolytic T cell activation permitted by suppression of HBV replication. Similar ALT elevations, however, occur at an identical frequency in placebo recipients, but ALT elevations associated with HBeAg seroconversion are confined to lamivudine-treated patients. When therapy is stopped after a year of therapy, two- to threefold ALT elevations occur in 20–30% of lamivudine-treated patients, representing renewed liver-cell injury as HBV replication returns. Although these posttreatment flares are almost always transient and mild, rare severe exacerbations, especially in cirrhotic patients, have been observed, mandating close and careful clinical and virologic monitoring after discontinuation of treatment. Many authorities caution against discontinuing therapy in patients with cirrhosis, in whom posttreatment flares could precipitate decompensation.

Long-term monotherapy with lamivudine is associated with methionine-to-valine (M204V) or methionine-to-isoleucine (M204I) mutations, primarily at amino acid 204 in the tyrosine-methionine-aspartate-aspartate (YMDD) motif of HBV DNA polymerase, analogous to mutations that occur in HIV-infected patients treated with this drug. During a year of therapy, YMDD mutations occur in 15–30% of patients; the frequency increases with each year of therapy, reaching 70% at year 5. Ultimately, patients with YMDD mutants experience degradation of clinical, biochemical, and histologic responses; therefore, if treatment is begun with lamivudine monotherapy, the emergence of lamivudine resistance, reflected clinically by a breakthrough from suppressed levels of HBV DNA and ALT, is managed by adding another antiviral to which YMDD variants are sensitive (e.g., adefovir, tenofovir; see below).

Currently, although lamivudine is very safe and still used widely in other parts of the world, in the United States and Europe, lamivudine has been eclipsed by more potent antivirals that have superior resistance profiles (see below); it is no longer recommended as first-line therapy. Still, as the first successful oral antiviral agent for use in hepatitis B, lamivudine has provided proof of the concept that polymerase inhibitors can achieve virologic, serologic, biochemical, and histologic benefits. In addition, lamivudine has been shown to be effective in the treatment of patients with decompensated hepatitis B (for whom IFN is contraindicated), in some of whom decompensation can be reversed. Moreover, among patients with cirrhosis or advanced fibrosis, lamivudine has been shown to be effective in reducing the risk of progression to hepatic decompensation and, marginally, the risk of HCC. In the half decade following the introduction in the United States of lamivudine therapy for hepatitis B, referral of patients with HBV-associated end-stage liver disease for liver transplantation was reduced by ~30%, supporting further the beneficial impact of oral antiviral therapy on the natural history of chronic hepatitis B.

Because lamivudine monotherapy can result universally in the rapid emergence of YMDD variants in persons with HIV infection, patients with chronic hepatitis B should be tested for anti-HIV prior to therapy; if HIV infection is identified, lamivudine monotherapy at the HBV daily dose of 100 mg is contraindicated. These patients should be treated for both HIV and HBV with an HIV drug regimen that includes or is supplemented by at least two drugs active against HBV; antiretroviral therapy (ART) often contains two drugs with antiviral activity against HBV (e.g., tenofovir and emtricitabine), but if lamivudine is part of the regimen, the daily dose should be 300 mg. The safety of lamivudine during pregnancy has not been established; however, the drug is not teratogenic in rodents and has been used safely in pregnant women with HIV infection and with HBV infection. Limited data even suggest that administration of lamivudine during the last months of pregnancy to mothers with high-level hepatitis B viremia (≥10^8 IU/mL) can reduce the likelihood of perinatal transmission of hepatitis B.

ADEFOVIR DIPIVOXIL At an oral daily dose of 10 mg, the acyclic nucleotide analogue adefovir dipivoxil, the prodrug of adefovir, reduces HBV DNA by approximately 3.5–4 $\log_{10}$ copies/mL and is equally effective in treatment-naïve patients and IFN nonresponders. In HBeAg-reactive chronic hepatitis B, a 48-week course of adefovir dipivoxil was shown to achieve histologic improvement (and reduce the progression of fibrosis) and normalization of ALT in just over one-half of patients, HBeAg seroconversion in 12%, HBeAg loss in 23%, and suppression to an undetectable level of HBV DNA in 13–21%, as measured by PCR. Similar to IFN and lamivudine, adefovir dipivoxil is more likely to achieve an HBeAg response in patients with high baseline ALT (e.g., among adefovir-treated patients with ALT level >5 × the upper limit of normal), and HBeAg seroconversions occurred in 25%. The durability of adefovir-induced HBeAg responses is high (91% in one study); therefore, HBeAg response can be relied upon as a stopping point for adefovir therapy, after a period of consolidation therapy, as outlined above. Although data on the impact of additional therapy beyond 1 year are limited, biochemical, serologic, and virologic outcomes improve progressively as therapy is continued.

In patients with *HBeAg-negative chronic hepatitis B*, a 48-week course of 10 mg/d of adefovir dipivoxil resulted in histologic improvement in two-thirds, normalization of ALT in three-fourths, and suppression of HBV DNA to PCR-undetectable levels in one-half to two-thirds. As was true for lamivudine, because HBeAg responses—a potential stopping point—cannot be achieved in this group, reactivation is the rule when adefovir therapy is discontinued, and indefinite, long-term therapy is required. Treatment beyond the first year consolidates the gain of the first year; after 5 years of therapy, improvement in hepatic inflammation and regression of fibrosis were observed in three-fourths of patients, ALT was normal in 70%, and HBV DNA was undetectable in almost 70%. In one study, stopping adefovir after 5 years was followed by sustained suppression of HBV DNA and ALT, but most HBeAg-negative patients are treated indefinitely unless HBsAg loss, albeit very rare, is achieved.

Adefovir contains a flexible acyclic linker instead of the L-nucleoside ring of lamivudine, avoiding steric hindrance by mutated amino acids. In addition, the molecular structure of phosphorylated adefovir is very similar to that of its natural substrate; therefore, mutations to adefovir would also affect binding of the natural substrate, dATP. Hypothetically, these are among the reasons that resistance to adefovir dipivoxil is much less likely than resistance to lamivudine; no resistance was encountered in 1 year of clinical trial therapy. In subsequent years, however, adefovir resistance

TABLE 41-1

CLINICAL AND LABORATORY FEATURES OF CHRONIC HEPATITIS

TYPE OF HEPATITIS	DIAGNOSTIC TEST(S)	AUTOANTIBODIES	THERAPY
Chronic hepatitis B	HBsAg, IgG anti-HBc, HBeAg, HBV DNA	Uncommon	IFN-α, PEG IFN-α Oral agents: First-line: entecavir, tenofovir Second-line: lamivudine, adefovir, telbivudine
Chronic hepatitis C	Anti-HCV, HCV RNA	Anti-LKM1[a]	PEG IFN-α plus ribavirin Telaprevir[b] Boceprevir[b]
Chronic hepatitis D	Anti-HDV, HDV RNA, HBsAg, IgG anti-HBc	Anti-LKM3	IFN-α, PEG IFN-α[c]
Autoimmune hepatitis	ANA[d] (homogeneous), anti-LKM1 (±) Hyperglobulinemia	ANA, anti-LKM1 anti-SLA[e]	Prednisone, azathioprine
Drug-associated	—	Uncommon	Withdraw drug
Cryptogenic	All negative	None	Prednisone (?), azathioprine (?)

[a]Antibodies to liver-kidney microsomes type 1 (autoimmune hepatitis type II and some cases of hepatitis C).
[b]Administered as a triple-drug combination with PEG IFN and ribavirin. Between the writing and publication of this chapter, two additional drugs were approved for hepatitis C, simeprevir and sofosbuvir (see *www.hcvguidelines.org*).
[c]Early clinical trials suggested benefit of IFN-α therapy; PEG IFN-α is as effective, if not more so, and has supplanted standard IFN-α.
[d]Antinuclear antibody (autoimmune hepatitis type I).
[e]Antibodies to soluble liver antigen (autoimmune hepatitis type III).
Abbreviations: HBc, hepatitis B core; HBeAg, hepatitis B e antigen; HBsAg, hepatitis B surface antigen; HBV, hepatitis B virus; HCV, hepatitis C virus; HDV, hepatitis D virus; IFN-α, interferon α; IgG, immunoglobulin G; LKM, liver-kidney microsome; PEG IFN-α, pegylated interferon α; SLA, soluble liver antigen.

United States, and the METAVIR score, used in Europe (Table 41-2). Based on the presence and degree of these features of histologic activity, chronic hepatitis can be graded as mild, moderate, or severe.

CLASSIFICATION BY STAGE

The stage of chronic hepatitis, which reflects the level of progression of the disease, is based on the degree of hepatic fibrosis. When fibrosis is so extensive that fibrous septa surround parenchymal nodules and alter the normal architecture of the liver lobule, the histologic lesion is defined as *cirrhosis*. Staging is based on the degree of fibrosis as categorized on a numerical scale from 0–6 (HAI) or 0–4 (METAVIR) (Table 41-2). Several noninvasive approaches have been introduced to provide approximations of hepatic histologic stage, including serum biomarkers of fibrosis and imaging determinations of liver elasticity.

CHRONIC VIRAL HEPATITIS

Both the enterically transmitted forms of viral hepatitis, hepatitis A and E, are self-limited and do not cause chronic hepatitis (rare reports notwithstanding in which acute hepatitis A serves as a trigger for the onset of autoimmune hepatitis in genetically susceptible patients or in which hepatitis E (**Chap. 39**) can cause chronic liver disease in immunosuppressed hosts, e.g., after liver transplantation). In contrast, the entire clinicopathologic spectrum of chronic hepatitis occurs in patients with chronic viral hepatitis B and C as well as in patients with chronic hepatitis D superimposed on chronic hepatitis B.

CHRONIC HEPATITIS B

The likelihood of chronicity after acute hepatitis B varies as a function of age. Infection at birth is associated with clinically silent acute infection but a 90% chance of chronic infection, whereas infection in young adulthood in immunocompetent persons is typically associated with clinically apparent acute hepatitis but a risk of chronicity of only approximately 1%. Most cases of chronic hepatitis B among adults, however, occur in patients who never had a recognized episode of clinically apparent acute viral hepatitis. The degree of liver injury (grade) in patients with chronic hepatitis B is variable, ranging from none in inactive carriers to mild to moderate to severe. Among adults with chronic hepatitis B, histologic features are of prognostic importance. In one long-term study of patients with chronic hepatitis B, investigators found a 5-year survival rate of 97% for patients with mild chronic hepatitis, 86% for patients with moderate to severe chronic hepatitis, and

TABLE 41-2

HISTOLOGIC GRADING AND STAGING OF CHRONIC HEPATITIS

		HISTOLOGIC ACTIVITY INDEX (HAI)[a]		METAVIR[b]	
HISTOLOGIC FEATURE		**SEVERITY**	**SCORE**	**SEVERITY**	**SCORE**
Necroinflammatory Activity (grade)					
Periportal necrosis, including piecemeal necrosis and/or bridging necrosis (BN)		None	0	None	0
		Mild	1	Mild	1
		Mild/moderate	2	Moderate	2
		Moderate	3	Severe	3
		Severe	4	Bridging necrosis	Yes
					No
Intralobular necrosis	Confluent	—None	0	None or mild	0
		—Focal	1	Moderate	1
		—Zone 3 some	2	Severe	2
		—Zone 3 most	3		
		—Zone 3 + BN few	4		
		—Zone 3 + BN multiple	5		
		—Panacinar/multiacinar	6		
	Focal	—None	0		
		—≤1 focus/10× field	1		
		—2–4 foci/10× field	2		
		—5–10 foci/10× field	3		
		—>10 foci/10× field	4		
Portal Inflammation		None	0		
		Mild	1		
		Moderate	2		
		Moderate/marked	3		
		Marked	4		
		Total	0–18		A0–A3[c]
Fibrosis (stage)					
None			0		F0
Portal fibrosis—some			1		F1
Portal fibrosis—most			2		F1
Bridging fibrosis—few			3		F2
Bridging fibrosis—many			4		F3
Incomplete cirrhosis			5		F4
Cirrhosis			6		F4
		Total	6		4

[a]Ishak K, Baptista A, Bianchi L, et al: Histologic grading and staging of chronic hepatitis. J Hepatol 22:696, 1995.
[b]Bedossa P, Poynard T, French METAVIR Cooperative Study Group: An algorithm for grading activity in chronic hepatitis C. Hepatology 24:289, 1996.
[c]Necroinflammatory grade: A0 = none; A1 = mild; A2 = moderate; A3 = severe.

only 55% for patients with chronic hepatitis and postnecrotic cirrhosis. The 15-year survival in these cohorts was 77%, 66%, and 40%, respectively. On the other hand, more recent observations do not allow us to be so sanguine about the prognosis in patients with mild chronic hepatitis; among such patients followed for 1–13 years, progression to more severe chronic hepatitis and cirrhosis has been observed in more than a quarter of cases.

More important to consider than histology alone in patients with chronic hepatitis B is the degree of hepatitis B virus (HBV) replication. As reviewed in **Chap. 39**, chronic HBV infection can occur in the presence or absence of serum hepatitis B e antigen (HBeAg), and generally, for both HBeAg-reactive and HBeAg-negative chronic hepatitis B, the level of HBV DNA correlates with the level of liver injury and risk of progression. In *HBeAg-reactive chronic hepatitis B*, two phases have been recognized based on the relative level of HBV replication. The relatively *replicative phase* is characterized by the presence in the serum of HBeAg and HBV DNA levels well in excess of 10^3–10^4 IU/mL, sometimes exceeding 10^9 IU/mL; by the presence in the liver of detectable intrahepatocyte nucleocapsid antigens (primarily hepatitis B core antigen [HBcAg]); by high infectivity; and by accompanying liver injury.

begins to emerge (asparagine to threonine at amino acid 236 [N236T] and alanine to valine or threonine at amino acid 181 [A181V/T], primarily), occurring in 2.5% after 2 years, but in 29% after 5 years of therapy (reported in HBeAg-negative patients). Among patients co-infected with HBV and HIV and who have normal CD4+ T cell counts, adefovir dipivoxil is effective in suppressing HBV dramatically (by 5 $\log_{10}$ in one study). Moreover, adefovir dipivoxil is effective in lamivudine-resistant, YMDD-mutant HBV and can be used when such lamivudine-induced variants emerge. When lamivudine resistance occurs, adding adefovir (i.e., maintaining lamivudine to preempt the emergence of adefovir resistance) is superior to switching to adefovir. Almost invariably, patients with adefovir-mutant HBV respond to lamivudine (or newer agents, such as entecavir, see below). When, in the past, adefovir had been evaluated as therapy for HIV infection, doses of 60–120 mg were required to suppress HIV, and, at these doses, the drug was nephrotoxic. Even at 30 mg/d, creatinine elevations of 44 μmol/L (0.5 mg/dL) occurred in 10% of patients; however, at the HBV-effective dose of 10 mg, such elevations of creatinine are rarely encountered. If any nephrotoxicity does occur, it rarely appears before 6–8 months of therapy. Although renal tubular injury is a rare potential side effect, and although creatinine monitoring is recommended during treatment, the therapeutic index of adefovir dipivoxil is high, and the nephrotoxicity observed in clinical trials at higher doses was reversible. For patients with underlying renal disease, frequency of administration of adefovir dipivoxil should be reduced to every 48 h for creatinine clearances of 30–49 mL/min; to every 72 h for creatinine clearances of 10–29 mL/min; and once a week, following dialysis, for patients undergoing hemodialysis. Adefovir dipivoxil is very well tolerated, and ALT elevations during and after withdrawal of therapy are similar to those observed and described above in clinical trials of lamivudine. An advantage of adefovir is its relatively favorable resistance profile; however, it is not as potent as the other approved oral agents, it does not suppress HBV DNA as rapidly or as uniformly as the others, it is the least likely of all agents to result in HBeAg seroconversion, and 20–50% of patients fail to suppress HBV DNA by 2 $\log_{10}$ ("primary nonresponders"). For these reasons, adefovir, which has been supplanted in both treatment-naïve and lamivudine-resistant patients by the more potent, less resistance-prone nucleotide analogue tenofovir (see below), is no longer recommended as first-line therapy.

PEGYLATED INTERFERON After long-acting PEG IFN was shown to be effective in the treatment of hepatitis C (see below), this more convenient drug was evaluated in the treatment of chronic hepatitis B. Once-a-week PEG IFN is more effective than the more frequently administered, standard IFN, and several large-scale trials of PEG IFN versus oral nucleoside analogues have been conducted among patients with HBeAg-reactive and HBeAg-negative chronic hepatitis B.

In HBeAg-reactive chronic hepatitis B, two large-scale studies were done. One study evaluated PEG IFN-α 2b (100 μg weekly for 32 weeks, then 50 μg weekly for another 20 weeks for a total of 52 weeks, with a comparison arm of combination PEG IFN with oral lamivudine) in 307 subjects. The other study involved PEG IFN-α 2a (180 μg weekly for 48 weeks) in 814 primarily Asian patients, three-fourths of whom had ALT ≥2 × the upper limit of normal, with comparison arms of lamivudine monotherapy and combination PEG IFN plus lamivudine. At the end of therapy (48–52 weeks) in the PEG IFN monotherapy arms, HBeAg loss occurred in approximately 30%, HBeAg seroconversion in 22–27%, undetectable HBV DNA (<400 copies/mL by PCR) in 10–25%, normal ALT in 34–39%, and a mean reduction in HBV DNA of 2 $\log_{10}$ copies/mL (PEG IFN-α 2b) to 4.5 $\log_{10}$ copies/mL (PEG IFN-α 2a). Six months after completing PEG IFN monotherapy in these trials, HBeAg losses were present in approximately 35%, HBeAg seroconversion in approximately 30%, undetectable HBV DNA in 7–14%, normal ALT in 32–41%, and a mean reduction in HBV DNA of 2–2.4 $\log_{10}$ copies/mL. Although the combination of PEG IFN and lamivudine was superior at the end of therapy in one or more serologic, virologic, or biochemical outcomes, neither the combination arm (in both studies) nor the lamivudine monotherapy arm (in the PEG IFN-α 2a trial) demonstrated any benefit compared to the PEG IFN monotherapy arms 6 months after therapy. Moreover, HBsAg seroconversion occurred in 3–7% of PEG IFN recipients (with or without lamivudine); some of these seroconversions were identified by the end of therapy, but many were identified during the posttreatment follow-up period. The likelihood of HBeAg loss in PEG IFN–treated HBeAg-reactive patients is associated with HBV genotype A > B > C > D (shown for PEG IFN-α2b but not for α-2a).

Based on these results, some authorities concluded that PEG IFN monotherapy should be the first-line therapy of choice in HBeAg-reactive chronic hepatitis B; however, this conclusion has been challenged. Although a finite, 1-year course of PEG IFN results in a higher rate of sustained response (6 months after treatment) than is achieved with oral nucleoside/nucleotide analogue therapy, the comparison is confounded by the fact that oral agents are not discontinued at the end of 1 year. Instead, taken orally and free of side effects, therapy with oral agents is extended indefinitely or until after the occurrence of an HBeAg response. The rate of HBeAg responses after 2 years of oral-agent nucleoside analogue therapy is at least as high as, if not higher than, that achieved with PEG IFN after 1 year; favoring oral agents is the absence of injections, difficult-to-tolerate side effects, and laboratory monitoring as well as lower direct and indirect medical care costs and inconvenience. The association of HBsAg responses with PEG IFN therapy occurs in such a small proportion of patients that subjecting everyone to PEG IFN for the marginal gain of HBsAg responses during or immediately after therapy in such a very small minority is questionable. Moreover, HBsAg responses occur in a comparable proportion of patients treated with early-generation nucleoside/nucleotide analogues in the years after therapy, and, with the newer, more potent nucleoside analogues, the frequency of HBsAg loss during the first year of therapy equals that of PEG IFN and is exceeded during year 2 and beyond (see below). Of course, resistance is not an issue during PEG IFN therapy, but the risk of resistance is much lower with new agents (≤1% up to 3–6 years in previously treatment-naïve, entecavir-treated and tenofovir-treated patients; see below). Finally, the level of HBV DNA inhibition that can be achieved with the newer agents, and even with lamivudine, exceeds that which can be achieved with PEG IFN, in some cases by several orders of magnitude.

In HBeAg-negative chronic hepatitis B, a trial of PEG IFN-α 2a (180 μg weekly for 48 weeks versus comparison arms of lamivudine monotherapy and of combination therapy) in 564 patients showed that PEG IFN monotherapy resulted at the end of therapy in suppression of HBV DNA by a mean of 4.1 $\log_{10}$ copies/mL, undetectable HBV DNA (<400 copies/mL by PCR) in 63%, normal ALT in 38%, and loss of HBsAg in 4%. Although lamivudine monotherapy and combination lamivudine–PEG IFN therapy were both superior to PEG IFN at the end of therapy, no advantage of lamivudine monotherapy or combination therapy was apparent over PEG IFN monotherapy 6 months after therapy—suppression of HBV DNA by a mean of 2.3 $\log_{10}$ copies/mL, undetectable HBV DNA in 19%, and normal ALT in 59%. In subjects involved in this trial followed for up to 5 years, among the two-thirds followed who had been treated initially with PEG IFN, 17% maintained HBV DNA suppression to <400 copies/mL, but ALT remained normal in only 22%; HBsAg loss increased gradually to 12%. Among the half followed who had been treated initially with lamivudine monotherapy, HBV DNA remained <400 copies/mL in 7% and ALT normal in 16%; by year 5, 3.5% had lost HBsAg. As was the case for standard IFN therapy in HBeAg-negative patients, only a small proportion maintained responsiveness after completion of PEG IFN therapy, raising questions about the relative value of a finite period of PEG IFN, versus a longer course with a potent, low-resistance oral nucleoside analogue in these patients. Moreover, the value of PEG IFN for HBeAg-negative chronic hepatitis B has not been confirmed. In the only other controlled clinical trial of PEG IFN for HBeAg-negative chronic hepatitis B, the hepatitis C regimen of PEG IFN plus ribavirin was compared to PEG IFN monotherapy. In this trial, HBV DNA suppression (<400 copies/mL) occurred in only 7.5% of the two groups combined, and no study subject lost HBsAg.

In patients treated with PEG IFN, HBeAg and HBsAg responses have been associated with *IL28B* genotype CC, the favorable genotype identified in trials of PEG IFN for chronic hepatitis C. Also, reductions in quantitative HBsAg levels have been shown to correlate with and to be predictive of responsiveness to PEG IFN in chronic hepatitis B. If HBsAg levels fail to fall within the first 12–24 weeks or to reach <20,000 IU/mL by week 24, PEG IFN therapy is unlikely to be effective and should be discontinued.

ENTECAVIR Entecavir, an oral cyclopentyl guanosine analogue polymerase inhibitor, appears to be the most potent of the HBV antivirals and is just as well tolerated as lamivudine. In a 709-subject clinical trial among HBeAg-reactive patients, oral entecavir, 0.5 mg daily, was compared to lamivudine, 100 mg daily. At 48 weeks, entecavir was superior to lamivudine in suppression of HBV DNA (mean 6.9 versus 5.5 $\log_{10}$ copies/mL), percentage with undetectable HBV DNA (<300 copies/mL by PCR; 67% versus 36%), histologic improvement (≥2-point improvement in necroinflammatory HAI score; 72% versus 62%), and normal ALT (68% versus 60%). The two treatments were indistinguishable in percentage with HBeAg loss (22% versus 20%) and seroconversion (21% versus 18%). Among patients treated with entecavir for 96 weeks, HBV DNA was undetectable cumulatively in 80% (versus 39% for lamivudine), and HBeAg seroconversions had occurred in 31% (versus 26% for lamivudine). After 3–6 years of entecavir, HBeAg seroconversions have been observed in 39–44% and HBsAg loss in 5–6%. Similarly, in a 638-subject clinical trial among HBeAg-negative patients, at week 48, oral entecavir, 0.5 mg daily, was superior to lamivudine, 100 mg daily, in suppression of HBV DNA (mean 5.0 versus 4.5 $\log_{10}$ copies/mL) and in percentage with undetectable HBV DNA (90% versus 72%), histologic improvement (70% versus 61%), and normal ALT (78% versus 71%). No resistance mutations were encountered in previously treatment-naïve, entecavir-treated patients during 96 weeks of therapy, and in a cohort of subjects treated for up to 6 years, resistance emerged in only 1.2%. Entecavir-induced HBeAg seroconversions are as durable as those achieved with other antivirals. Its high barrier to resistance coupled with its high potency renders entecavir a first-line drug for patients with chronic hepatitis B.

Entecavir is also effective against lamivudine-resistant HBV infection. In a trial of 286 lamivudine-resistant patients, entecavir, at a higher daily dose of 1 mg, was superior to lamivudine, as measured at week 48, in achieving suppression of HBV DNA (mean 5.1 versus 0.48 $\log_{10}$ copies/mL), undetectable HBV DNA (72% versus 19%), normal ALT (61% versus 15%), HBeAg loss (10% versus 3%), and HBeAg seroconversion (8% versus 3%). In this population of lamivudine-experienced patients, however, entecavir resistance emerged in 7% at 48 weeks. Although entecavir resistance requires both a YMDD mutation and a second mutation at one of several other sites (e.g., T184A, S202G/I, or M250V), resistance to entecavir in lamivudine-resistant chronic hepatitis B has been recorded to increase progressively to 43% at 4 years; therefore, entecavir is not as attractive a choice as adefovir or tenofovir for patients with lamivudine-resistant hepatitis B.

In clinical trials, entecavir has an excellent safety profile; in addition, on-treatment and posttreatment ALT flares are relatively uncommon and relatively mild in entecavir-treated patients. Doses should be reduced for patients with reduced creatinine clearance. Entecavir does have low-level antiviral activity against HIV and cannot be used as monotherapy to treat HBV infection in HIV/HBV co-infected persons.

TELBIVUDINE Telbivudine, a cytosine analogue, is similar in efficacy to entecavir but slightly less potent in suppressing HBV DNA (a slightly less profound median 6.4 $\log_{10}$ reduction in HBeAg-reactive disease and a similar 5.2 $\log_{10}$ reduction in HBeAg-negative disease). In its registration trial, telbivudine at an oral daily dose of 600 mg suppressed HBV DNA to <300 copies/mL in 60% of HBeAg-positive and 88% of HBeAg-negative patients, reduced ALT to normal in 77% of HBeAg-positive and 74% of HBeAg-negative patients, and improved histology in 65% of HBeAg-positive and 67% of HBeAg-negative patients. Although resistance to telbivudine (M204I, not M204V, mutations) was less frequent than resistance to lamivudine at the end of 1 year, resistance mutations after 2 years of treatment occurred in up to 22%. Generally well tolerated, telbivudine has been associated with a low frequency of asymptomatic creatine kinase elevations and with a very low frequency of peripheral neuropathy; frequency of administration should be reduced for patients with impaired creatinine clearance. Its excellent potency notwithstanding, the inferior resistance profile of telbivudine has limited its appeal; telbivudine is neither recommended as first-line therapy nor widely used.

TENOFOVIR Tenofovir disoproxil fumarate, an acyclic nucleotide analogue and potent antiretroviral agent used to treat HIV infection, is similar to adefovir but more potent in suppressing HBV DNA and inducing HBeAg responses; it is highly active against both wild-type and lamivudine-resistant HBV and active in patients whose response to adefovir is slow and/or limited. At an oral once-daily dose of 300 mg for 48 weeks, tenofovir suppressed HBV DNA by 6.2 $\log_{10}$ (to undetectable levels [<400 copies/mL] in 76%) in HBeAg-positive patients and by 4.6 $\log_{10}$ (to undetectable levels in 93%) in HBeAg-negative patients; reduced ALT to normal in 68% of HBeAg-positive and 76% of HBeAg-negative patients; and improved histology in 74% of HBeAg-positive and 72% of HBeAg-negative patients. In HBeAg-positive patients, HBeAg seroconversions occurred in 21% by the end of year 1, 27% by year 2, 34% by year 3, and 40% by year 5 of tenofovir treatment; HBsAg loss occurred in 3% by the end of year 1 and 6% at year 2, and 8% by year 5. After 5 years of tenofovir therapy, 87% of patients experienced histologic improvement, including reduction in fibrosis score (51%) and regression of cirrhosis (71%). The 5-year safety (negligible renal toxicity, in 1%, and mild reduction in bone density, in ~0.5%) and resistance profiles (none recorded through 5 years) of tenofovir are very favorable as well; therefore, tenofovir has supplanted adefovir both as first-line therapy for chronic hepatitis B and as add-on therapy for lamivudine-resistant chronic hepatitis B. Frequency of tenofovir administration should be reduced for patients with impaired creatinine clearance.

A comparison of the six antiviral therapies in current use appears in Table 41-3; their relative potencies in suppressing HBV DNA are shown in Fig. 41-1.

COMBINATION THERAPY Although the combination of lamivudine and PEG IFN suppresses HBV DNA more profoundly during therapy than does monotherapy with either drug alone (and is much less likely to be associated with lamivudine resistance), this combination used for a year is no better than a year of PEG IFN in achieving sustained responses. To date, combinations of oral nucleoside/nucleotide agents have not achieved an enhancement in virologic, serologic, or biochemical efficacy over that achieved by the more potent of the combined drugs given individually. In a 2-year trial of combination entecavir and tenofovir versus entecavir monotherapy, for a small subgroup of patients with very high HBV DNA levels (≥10^8 IU/mL), a reduction in HBV DNA to <50 IU/mL was higher in the combination group (79% versus 62%); however, no differences in HBeAg responses or any other endpoint were observed between the combination-therapy and monotherapy groups, even in the high-HBV DNA subgroup. On the other hand, combining agents that are not cross-resistant (e.g., lamivudine and adefovir or tenofovir) has the potential to reduce the risk or perhaps even to preempt entirely the emergence of drug resistance. In the future, the treatment paradigm may shift from the current approach of sequential monotherapy to preemptive combination therapy, perhaps not for all patients but for subsets (e.g., patients with very high levels of HBV DNA, immunosuppressed patients); however, designing and executing clinical trials that demonstrate superior efficacy and resistance profile of combination therapy over monotherapy with entecavir or tenofovir will remain challenging. For patients who already have acquired multidrug resistance (to both nucleoside analogs [lamivudine, entecavir, telbivudine] and nucleotide analogs [adefovir, tenofovir]), treatment with a combination of entecavir and tenofovir has been shown to be highly effective in suppressive HBV DNA and overcoming drug resistance.

NOVEL ANTIVIRALS AND STRATEGIES In addition to the seven approved antiviral drugs for hepatitis B, emtricitabine, a fluorinated cytosine analogue very similar to lamivudine in structure, efficacy, and resistance profile, offers no advantage over lamivudine. A combination of emtricitabine and tenofovir is approved for the treatment of HIV infection and is an appealing combination therapy for hepatitis B, especially for lamivudine-resistant disease; however, neither emtricitabine nor the combination is approved yet for hepatitis B. Several initially promising antiviral agents have been abandoned because of toxicity (e.g., clevudine, which was linked to myopathy during its clinical development). Because direct-acting antivirals have been so successful in the management of chronic hepatitis B, more unconventional approaches—e.g., immunologic (e.g., toll receptor agonists) or genetic manipulation (e.g., RNA interference—gene silencing—to reduce HBV DNA transcription)—are not likely to be competitive, unless they can be shown to go beyond current antivirals in achieving recovery (HBsAg seroconversion) from HBV infection. Finally, initial emphasis in the development of antiviral therapy for hepatitis B was placed on monotherapy; whether combination regimens will yield additive or synergistic efficacy remains to be determined.

TREATMENT RECOMMENDATIONS Several learned societies and groups of expert physicians have issued treatment

TABLE 41-3

COMPARISON OF PEGYLATED INTERFERON (PEG IFN), LAMIVUDINE, ADEFOVIR, ENTECAVIR, TELBIVUDINE, AND TENOFOVIR THERAPY FOR CHRONIC HEPATITIS B[a]

FEATURE	PEG IFN[b]	LAMIVUDINE	ADEFOVIR	ENTECAVIR	TELBIVUDINE	TENOFOVIR
Route of administration	Subcutaneous injection	Oral	Oral	Oral	Oral	Oral
Duration of therapy[c]	48–52 weeks	≥52 weeks	≥48 weeks	≥48 weeks	≥52 weeks	≥48 weeks
Tolerability	Poorly tolerated	Well tolerated	Well tolerated; creatinine monitoring recommended	Well tolerated	Well tolerated	Well tolerated; creatinine monitoring recommended
HBeAg seroconversion						
1 yr Rx	18–20%	16–21%	12%	21%	22%	21%
>1 yr Rx	NA	up to 50% @ 5 yrs	43% @ 3 yrs[d]	31% @ 2 yrs 44% @ 6 yrs	30% @ 2 yrs	40% @ 5 yrs
Log_{10} HBV DNA reduction (mean copies/mL)						
HBeAg-reactive	4.5	5.5	median 3.5–5	6.9	6.4	6.2
HBeAg-negative	4.1	4.4–4.7	median 3.5–3.9	5.0	5.2	4.6
HBV DNA PCR negative (<300–400 copies/mL; <1000 copies/mL for adefovir) at end of yr 1						
HBeAg-reactive	10–25%	36–44%	13–21%	67% (91% @ 4 yrs)	60%	76%
HBeAg-negative	63%	60–73%	48–77%	90%	88%	93%
ALT normalization at end of yr 1						
HBeAg-reactive	39%	41–75%	48–61%	68%	77%	68%
HBeAg-negative	34–38%	62–79%	48–77%	78%	74%	76%
HBsAg loss yr 1	3–4%	≤1%	0%	2%	<1%	3%
>yr 1	12% 5 yr after 1 yr of Rx	No data	5% at yr 5	6% at yr 6	No data	8% at yr 5
Histologic improvement (≥2 point reduction in HAI) at yr 1						
HBeAg-reactive	38% 6 months after	49–62%	53–68%	72%	65%	74%
HBeAg-negative	48% 6 months after	61–66%	64%	70%	67%	72%
Viral resistance	None	15–30% @ 1 yr 70% @ 5 yrs	None @ 1 yr 29% @ 5 yrs	≤1% @ 1 yr[e] 1.2% @ 6 yrs[e]	Up to 5% @ yr 1 Up to 22% @ yr 2	0% @ yr 1 0% through yr 5
Pregnancy category	C	C[f]	C	C	B	B
Cost (US$) for 1 yr	~$18,000	~$2,500	~$6,500	~$8,700[g]	~$6,000	~$6,000

[a]Generally, these comparisons are based on data on each drug tested individually versus placebo in registration clinical trials; because, with rare exception, these comparisons are not based on head-to-head testing of these drugs, relative advantages and disadvantages should be interpreted cautiously.

[b]Although standard interferon α administered daily or three times a week is approved as therapy for chronic hepatitis B, it has been supplanted by PEG IFN, which is administered once a week and is more effective. Standard interferon has no advantages over PEG IFN.

[c]Duration of therapy in clinical efficacy trials; use in clinical practice may vary.

[d]Because of a computer-generated randomization error that resulted in misallocation of drug versus placebo during the second year of clinical trial treatment, the frequency of HBeAg seroconversion beyond the first year is an estimate (Kaplan-Meier analysis) based on the small subset in whom adefovir was administered correctly.

[e]7% during a year of therapy (43% at year 4) in lamivudine-resistant patients.

[f]Despite its Class C designation, lamivudine has an extensive pregnancy safety record in women with HIV/AIDS.

[g]Approximately $17,400 for lamivudine-refractory patients.

Abbreviations: ALT, alanine aminotransferase; HAI, histologic activity index; HBeAg, hepatitis B e antigen; HBsAg, hepatitis B surface antigen; HBV, hepatitis B virus; NA, not applicable; PEG IFN, pegylated interferon; PCR, polymerase chain reaction; Rx, therapy; yr, year.

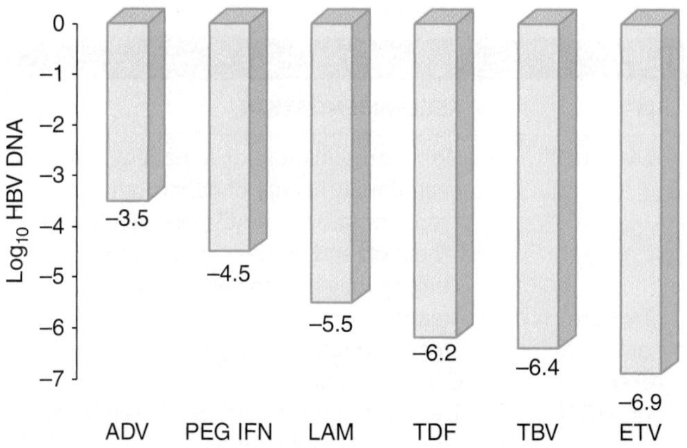

FIGURE 41-1

Relative potency of antiviral drugs for hepatitis B, as reflected by median $\log_{10}$ HBV DNA reduction in HBeAg-positive chronic hepatitis B. These data are from individual reports of large, randomized controlled registration trials that were the basis for approval of the drugs. In most instances, these data do not represent direct comparisons among the drugs, because study populations were different, baseline patient variables were not always uniform, and the sensitivity and dynamic range of the HBV DNA assays used in the trials varied. ADV, adefovir dipivoxil; ETV, entecavir; LAM, lamivudine; PEG IFN, pegylated interferon α2a; TBV, telbivudine; TDF, tenofovir disoproxil fumarate.

recommendations for patients with chronic hepatitis B; the most authoritative and updated (and free of financial support by pharmaceutical companies) are those of the American Association for the Study of Liver Diseases (AASLD) and of the European Association for the Study of the Liver (EASL). Although the recommendations differ slightly, a consensus has emerged on most of the important points (Table 41-4). No treatment is recommended or available for inactive "nonreplicative" hepatitis B carriers (undetectable HBeAg with normal ALT and HBV DNA $\leq 10^3$ IU/mL documented serially over time). In patients with detectable HBeAg and HBV DNA levels $>2 \times 10^4$ IU/mL, treatment is recommended by the AASLD for those with ALT levels above 2 × the upper limit of normal. (The EASL recommends treatment in HBeAg-positive patients for HBV DNA levels $>2 \times 10^3$ IU/mL and ALT above the upper limit of normal.) For HBeAg-positive patients with ALT ≤2 × the upper limit of normal, in whom sustained responses are not likely and who would require multiyear therapy, antiviral therapy is not recommended currently. This pattern is common during the early decades of life among Asian patients infected at birth; even in this group, therapy would be considered for those >40 years of age, ALT persistently at the high end of the twofold range, and/or with a family history of HCC, especially if the liver biopsy shows moderate to severe necroinflammatory activity or fibrosis. In this group, when, eventually, ALT becomes elevated later in life, antiviral therapy should be instituted. For patients with HBeAg-negative chronic hepatitis B, ALT >2 × the upper limit of normal (above the upper limit of normal according to EASL), and HBV DNA $>2 \times 10^3$ IU/mL, antiviral therapy is recommended. If HBV DNA is $>2 \times 10^3$ IU/mL and ALT is 1 to >2 × the upper limit of normal, liver biopsy should be considered to help in arriving at a decision to treat if substantial liver injury is present (treatment in this subset would be recommended according to EASL guidelines, because ALT is elevated).

For patients with compensated cirrhosis, because antiviral therapy has been shown to retard clinical progression, treatment is recommended regardless of HBeAg status and ALT as long as HBV DNA is detectable at $>2 \times 10^3$ IU/mL (detectable at any level according to the EASL); monitoring without therapy is recommended for those with HBV DNA $<2 \times 10^3$ IU/mL, unless ALT is elevated. For patients with decompensated cirrhosis, treatment is recommended regardless of serologic and biochemical status, as long as HBV DNA is detectable. Patients with decompensated cirrhosis should be evaluated as candidates for liver transplantation.

Among the seven available drugs for hepatitis B, PEG IFN has supplanted standard IFN, entecavir has supplanted lamivudine, and tenofovir has supplanted adefovir. PEG IFN, entecavir, or tenofovir is recommended as first-line therapy (Table 41-3). PEG IFN requires finite-duration therapy, achieves the highest rate of HBeAg responses after a year of therapy, and does not support viral mutations, but it requires subcutaneous injections and is associated with inconvenience, more intensive clinical and laboratory monitoring, and intolerability. Oral nucleoside analogues require long-term therapy in most patients, and when used alone, lamivudine and telbivudine foster the emergence of viral mutations, adefovir somewhat less so, and entecavir (except in lamivudine-experienced patients) and tenofovir rarely at all. Oral agents do not require injections or cumbersome laboratory monitoring, are very well tolerated, lead to improved histology in 50–90% of patients, suppress HBV DNA more profoundly than PEG IFN, and are effective even in patients who fail to respond to IFN-based therapy. Although oral agents are less likely to result in HBeAg responses during the first year of therapy, as compared to PEG IFN, treatment with oral agents tends to be extended beyond the first year and, by the end of the second year, yields HBeAg responses (and even HBsAg responses) comparable in frequency to those achieved after 1 year of PEG IFN (and without the associated side effects) (Table 41-5). Although adefovir and tenofovir are safe, creatinine monitoring is recommended. Substantial experience with lamivudine during pregnancy (see above) has identified no teratogenicity. Although IFNs do not appear to cause congenital anomalies, IFNs have antiproliferative properties and should be avoided during pregnancy. Adefovir during pregnancy has not been associated with birth defects; however, there may be an increased risk of spontaneous abortion. Data on the safety of entecavir during pregnancy have not been published. Sufficient data in animals and limited data in humans suggest that telbivudine and tenofovir can be used safely during pregnancy. In general, except perhaps for lamivudine, and until additional data become available, the other antivirals for hepatitis B should be avoided or used with extreme caution during pregnancy.

TABLE 41-4

RECOMMENDATIONS FOR TREATMENT OF CHRONIC HEPATITIS B[a]

HBEAG STATUS	CLINICAL	HBV DNA (IU/ML)	ALT	RECOMMENDATION
HBeAg-reactive	[b]	$>2 \times 10^4$	$\leq 2 \times$ ULN[c,d]	No treatment; monitor. In patients >40, with family history of hepatocellular carcinoma, and/or ALT persistently at the high end of the twofold range, liver biopsy may help in decision to treat
	Chronic hepatitis	$>2 \times 10^4$[d]	$>2 \times$ ULN[d]	Treat[e]
	Cirrhosis compensated	$>2 \times 10^3$	< or > ULN	Treat[e] with oral agents, not PEG IFN
		$<2 \times 10^3$	>ULN	Consider treatment[f]
	Cirrhosis decompensated	Detectable	< or > ULN	Treat[e] with oral agents[g], not PEG IFN; refer for liver transplantation
		Undetectable	< or > ULN	Observe; refer for liver transplantation
HBeAg-negative	[b]	$\leq 2 \times 10^3$	≤ULN	Inactive carrier; treatment not necessary
	Chronic hepatitis	$>10^3$	1 to $>2 \times$ ULN[d]	Consider liver biopsy; treat[h] if biopsy shows moderate to severe inflammation or fibrosis
	Chronic hepatitis	$>10^4$	$>2 \times$ ULN[d]	Treat[h,i]
	Cirrhosis compensated	$>2 \times 10^3$	< or > ULN	Treat[e] with oral agents, not PEG IFN
		$<2 \times 10^3$	>ULN	Consider treatment[f]
	Cirrhosis decompensated	Detectable	< or > ULN	Treat[h] with oral agents[g], not PEG IFN; refer for liver transplantation
		Undetectable	< or > ULN	Observe; refer for liver transplantation

[a]Based on practice guidelines of the American Association for the Study of Liver Diseases (AASLD). Except as indicated in footnotes, these guidelines are similar to those issued by the European Association for the Study of the Liver (EASL).
[b]Liver disease tends to be mild or inactive clinically; most such patients do not undergo liver biopsy.
[c]This pattern is common during early decades of life in Asian patients infected at birth.
[d]According to the EASL guidelines, treat if HBV DNA is $>2 \times 10^3$ IU/mL and ALT >ULN.
[e]One of the potent oral drugs with a high barrier to resistance (entecavir or tenofovir) or PEG IFN can be used as first-line therapy (see text). These oral agents, but not PEG IFN, should be used for interferon-refractory/intolerant and immunocompromised patients. PEG IFN is administered weekly by subcutaneous injection for a year; the oral agents are administered daily for at least a year and continued indefinitely or until at least 6 months after HBeAg seroconversion.
[f]According to EASL guidelines, patients with compensated cirrhosis and detectable HBV DNA at any level, even with normal ALT, are candidates for therapy. Most authorities would treat indefinitely, even in HBeAg-positive disease after HBeAg seroconversion.
[g]Because the emergence of resistance can lead to loss of antiviral benefit and further deterioration in decompensated cirrhosis, a low-resistance regimen is recommended—entecavir or tenofovir monotherapy or combination therapy with the more resistance-prone lamivudine (or telbivudine) plus adefovir. Therapy should be instituted urgently.
[h]Because HBeAg seroconversion is not an option, the goal of therapy is to suppress HBV DNA and maintain a normal ALT. PEG IFN is administered by subcutaneous injection weekly for a year; caution is warranted in relying on a 6-month posttreatment interval to define a sustained response, because the majority of such responses are lost thereafter. Oral agents, entecavir or tenofovir, are administered daily, usually indefinitely or until, as very rarely occurs, virologic and biochemical responses are accompanied by HBsAg seroconversion.
[i]For older patients and those with advanced fibrosis, consider lowering the HBV DNA threshold to $>2 \times 10^3$ IU/mL.
Abbreviations: AASLD, American Association for the Study of Liver Diseases; ALT, alanine aminotransferase; EASL, European Association for the Study of the Liver; HBeAg, hepatitis B e antigen; HBsAg, hepatitis B surface antigen; HBV, hepatitis B virus; PEG IFN, pegylated interferon; ULN, upper limit of normal.

As noted above, some physicians prefer to begin with PEG IFN, while other physicians and patients prefer oral agents as first-line therapy. For patients with decompensated cirrhosis, the emergence of resistance can result in further deterioration and loss of antiviral effectiveness. Therefore, in this patient subset, the threshold for relying on therapy with a very favorable resistance profile (e.g., entecavir or tenofovir) or on combination therapy is low. PEG IFN should not be used in patients with compensated or decompensated cirrhosis.

For patients with end-stage chronic hepatitis B who undergo liver transplantation, reinfection of the new liver is almost universal in the absence of antiviral therapy. The majority of patients become high-level viremic carriers with minimal liver injury. Before the availability of antiviral therapy, an unpredictable proportion experienced severe hepatitis B–related liver injury, sometimes a fulminant-like hepatitis and sometimes a rapid recapitulation of the original severe chronic hepatitis B (**Chap. 39**). Currently, however, prevention of recurrent hepatitis B after liver transplantation has been achieved definitively by *combining* hepatitis B immune globulin with one of the oral nucleoside or nucleotide analogues (**Chap. 48**); preliminary data suggest that the newer, more potent, and less resistance-prone oral agents may be used instead of hepatitis B immune globulin for post-transplantation therapy.

Patients with HBV-HIV co-infection can have progressive HBV-associated liver disease and, occasionally, a severe exacerbation of hepatitis B resulting from immunologic

TABLE 41-5

PEGYLATED INTERFERON VERSUS ORAL NUCLEOSIDE ANALOGUES FOR THE TREATMENT OF CHRONIC HEPATITIS B

	PEG IFN	NUCLEOSIDE ANALOGUES
Administration	Weekly injection	Daily, orally
Tolerability	Poorly tolerated, intensive monitoring	Well tolerated, limited monitoring
Duration of therapy	Finite 48 weeks	≥1 year, indefinite in most patients
Maximum mean HBV DNA suppression	4.5 $\log_{10}$	6.9 $\log_{10}$
Effective in high-level HBV DNA (≥10^9 IU/mL)	No	Yes
HBeAg seroconversion		
During 1 year of therapy	~30%	~20%
During >1 year of therapy	Not applicable	30% (year 2) to up to 50% (year 5)
HBeAg-negative posttreatment HBV DNA suppression	17% @ 5 years	7% @ 4 years (lamivudine)
HBsAg loss		
During 1 year of therapy	3–4%	0–3%
During >1 year of therapy	Not applicable	3–8% @ 5 years of therapy
After 1 year of therapy–HBeAg-negative	12% @ 5 years	3.5% @ 5 years
Antiviral resistance	None	Lamivudine: ~30% year 1, ~70% year 5 Adefovir: 0% year 1, ~30% year 5 Telbivudine: up to 4% year 1, 22% year 2 Entecavir: ≤1.2% through year 6 Tenofovir: 0% through year 5
Use in cirrhosis, transplantation, immunosuppressed	No	Yes
Cost, 1 year of therapy	++++	+ to ++

Abbreviations: HBV, hepatitis B virus; HBeAg, hepatitis B e antigen; HBsAg, hepatitis B surface antigen; PEG IFN, pegylated interferon.

reconstitution following ART. Lamivudine should never be used as monotherapy in patients with HBV-HIV infection because HIV resistance emerges rapidly to both viruses. Adefovir has been used successfully to treat chronic hepatitis B in HBV-HIV co-infected patients but is no longer considered a first-line agent for HBV. Entecavir has low-level activity against HIV and can result in selection of HIV resistance; therefore, it should be avoided in HBV-HIV co-infection. Tenofovir and the combination of tenofovir and emtricitabine in one pill are approved therapies for HIV and represent excellent choices for treating HBV infection in HBV-HIV co-infected patients. Generally, even for HBV-HIV co-infected patients who do not yet meet treatment criteria for HIV infection, treating for both HBV and HIV is recommended.

Patients with chronic hepatitis B who undergo cytotoxic chemotherapy for treatment of malignancies as well as patients treated with immunosuppressive, anticytokine, or antitumor necrosis factor therapies experience enhanced HBV replication and viral expression on hepatocyte membranes during chemotherapy coupled with suppression of cellular immunity. When chemotherapy is withdrawn, such patients are at risk for reactivation of hepatitis B, often severe and occasionally fatal. Such rebound reactivation represents restoration of cytolytic T cell function against a target organ enriched in HBV expression. Preemptive treatment with lamivudine prior to the initiation of chemotherapy has been shown to reduce the risk of such reactivation. The newer, more potent oral antiviral agents are even more effective in preventing hepatitis B reactivation and with a lower risk of antiviral drug resistance. The optimal duration of antiviral therapy after completion of chemotherapy is not known, but a suggested approach is 6 months for inactive hepatitis B carriers and longer-duration therapy in patients with baseline HBV DNA levels >2 × 10^3 IU/mL, until standard clinical endpoints are met (Table 41-4).

CHRONIC HEPATITIS D (DELTA HEPATITIS)

Chronic hepatitis D virus (HDV) may follow acute co-infection with HBV but at a rate no higher than the rate of chronicity of acute hepatitis B. That is, although HDV co-infection can increase the severity of acute hepatitis B, HDV does not increase the likelihood of progression to chronic hepatitis B. When, however, HDV superinfection occurs in a person who is already chronically infected with HBV, long-term HDV infection is the rule, and a worsening of the liver disease is the expected consequence. Except for severity, chronic hepatitis B plus D has similar clinical and laboratory features to those seen in chronic hepatitis B alone. Relatively severe and progressive chronic hepatitis, with or without cirrhosis, is the rule, and mild chronic hepatitis is the exception. Occasionally, however, mild hepatitis or even, rarely, inactive carriage occurs in patients with chronic hepatitis B plus D, and the disease may become indolent after several years of infection. A distinguishing serologic feature of chronic hepatitis D is the presence in the circulation of antibodies to liver-kidney microsomes (anti-LKM); however, the anti-LKM seen in hepatitis D, anti-LKM3, are directed against uridine diphosphate glucuronosyltransferase and are distinct from anti-LKM1 seen in patients with autoimmune hepatitis and in a subset of patients with chronic hepatitis C (see below). **The clinical and laboratory features of chronic HDV infection are summarized in Chap. 39.**

TREATMENT Chronic Hepatitis D

Management is not well defined. Glucocorticoids are ineffective and are not used. Preliminary experimental trials of IFN-α suggested that conventional doses and durations of therapy lower levels of HDV RNA and aminotransferase activity only transiently during treatment but have no impact on the natural history of the disease. In contrast, high-dose IFN-α (9 million units three times a week) for 12 months may be associated with a sustained loss of HDV replication and clinical improvement in up to 50% of patients. Moreover, the beneficial impact of treatment has been observed to persist for 15 years and to be associated with a reduction in grade of hepatic necrosis and inflammation, reversion of advanced fibrosis (improved stage), and clearance of HDV RNA in some patients. A suggested approach to therapy has been high-dose, long-term IFN for at least a year and, in responders, extension of therapy until HDV RNA and HBsAg clearance. PEG IFN has also been shown to be effective in the treatment of chronic hepatitis D (e.g., after 48 weeks of therapy, associated with undetectable HDV RNA, durable for at least 24 posttreatment weeks, in a quarter of patients) and is a more convenient replacement for standard IFN. None of the nucleoside analogue antiviral agents for hepatitis B are effective in hepatitis D. In patients with end-stage liver disease secondary to chronic hepatitis D, liver transplantation has been effective. If hepatitis D recurs in the new liver without the expression of hepatitis B (an unusual serologic profile in immunocompetent persons but common in transplant patients), liver injury is limited. In fact, the outcome of transplantation for chronic hepatitis D is superior to that for chronic hepatitis B; in such patients, combination hepatitis B immune globulin and nucleoside analogue therapy for hepatitis B is indicated **(Chap. 48)**.

CHRONIC HEPATITIS C

Regardless of the epidemiologic mode of acquisition of hepatitis C virus (HCV) infection, chronic hepatitis follows acute hepatitis C in 50–70% of cases; chronic infection is common even in those with a return to normal in aminotransferase levels after acute hepatitis C, adding up to an 85% likelihood of chronic HCV infection after acute hepatitis C. Few clues had emerged to explain host differences associated with chronic infection until recently, when variation in a single nucleotide polymorphism (SNP) on chromosome 19, *IL28B* (which codes for IFN-λ3), was identified that distinguished between responders and nonresponders to IFN based antiviral therapy (see below). The same variants correlated with spontaneous resolution after acute infection: 53% in genotype C/C, 30% in genotype C/T, but only 23% in genotype T/T. The association with HCV clearance after acute infection is even stronger when *IL28B* haplotype is combined with haplotype G/G of an SNP near HLA class II *DBQ1*03:01*.

In patients with chronic hepatitis C followed for 20 years, progression to cirrhosis occurs in about 20–25%. Such is the case even for patients with relatively clinically mild chronic hepatitis, including those without symptoms, with only modest elevations of aminotransferase activity, and with mild chronic hepatitis on liver biopsy. Even in cohorts of well-compensated patients with chronic hepatitis C referred for clinical research trials (no complications of chronic liver disease and with normal hepatic synthetic function), the prevalence of cirrhosis may be as high as 50%. Most cases of hepatitis C are identified initially in asymptomatic patients who have no history of acute hepatitis C (e.g., those discovered while attempting to donate blood, while undergoing lab testing as part of an application for life insurance, or as a result of routine laboratory tests). The source of HCV infection in many of these cases is not defined, although a long-forgotten percutaneous exposure (e.g., injection drug use) in the remote past can be elicited in a substantial proportion and probably accounts for most infections; most of these infections were acquired in the 1960s and 1970s, coming to clinical attention decades later.

Approximately one-third of patients with chronic hepatitis C have normal or near-normal aminotransferase activity; although one-third to one-half of these patients have chronic hepatitis on liver biopsy, the grade of liver injury and stage of fibrosis tend to be mild in the vast majority. In some cases, more severe liver injury has been reported—even, rarely, cirrhosis, most likely the result of previous histologic activity. Among patients with persistent normal aminotransferase activity sustained over ≥5–10 years, histologic progression has been shown to be rare; however, approximately one-fourth of patients with normal aminotransferase activity experience subsequent aminotransferase elevations, and histologic injury can be progressive once abnormal biochemical activity resumes. Therefore, continued clinical monitoring and antiviral therapy are indicated, even for patients with normal aminotransferase activity.

Despite this substantial rate of progression of chronic hepatitis C, and despite the fact that liver failure can result from end-stage chronic hepatitis C, the long-term prognosis over 1–2 decades for chronic hepatitis C in a majority of patients is relatively benign. Mortality over 10–20 years among patients with transfusion-associated chronic hepatitis C has been shown not to differ from mortality in a matched population of transfused patients in whom hepatitis C did not develop. Although death in the hepatitis group is more likely to result from liver failure, and although hepatic decompensation may occur in ~15% of such patients over the course of a decade, the majority (almost 60%) of patients remain asymptomatic and well compensated, with no clinical sequelae of chronic liver disease. Overall, chronic hepatitis C tends to be very slowly and insidiously progressive, if at all, in the vast majority of patients, whereas in approximately one-fourth of cases, chronic hepatitis C will progress eventually to end-stage cirrhosis. In fact, because HCV infection is so prevalent, and because a proportion of patients progress inexorably to end-stage liver disease, hepatitis C is the most frequent indication for liver transplantation **(Chap. 48)**. In the United States, hepatitis C accounts for up to 40% of all chronic liver disease; as of 2007, mortality caused by hepatitis C surpassed that associated with HIV/AIDS and as of 2012, reported deaths caused by hepatitis C surpassed those associated with all other notifiable infectious diseases (HIV, tuberculosis, hepatitis B, and 57 other infectious diseases). Moreover, because the prevalence of HCV infection is so much higher in the "baby boomer" cohort borne between 1945 and 1965, three-quarters of the mortality associated with hepatitis C occurs in this age cohort. Referral bias may account for the more severe outcomes described in cohorts of patients reported from tertiary care centers (20-year progression of ≥20%) versus the more benign outcomes in cohorts of patients monitored from initial blood-product-associated acute hepatitis or identified in community settings (20-year progression of only 4–7%). Still unexplained, however, are the wide ranges in reported progression to cirrhosis, from 2% over 17 years in a population of women with hepatitis C infection acquired from contaminated anti-D immune globulin to 30% over ≤11 years in recipients of contaminated intravenous immune globulin.

Progression of liver disease in patients with chronic hepatitis C has been reported to be more likely in patients with older age, longer duration of infection, advanced histologic stage and grade, more complex quasispecies diversity, increased hepatic iron, concomitant other liver disorders (alcoholic liver disease, chronic hepatitis B, hemochromatosis, α_1 antitrypsin deficiency, and steatohepatitis), HIV infection, and obesity. Among these variables, however, duration of infection appears to be one of the most important, and some of the others probably reflect disease duration to some extent (e.g., quasispecies diversity, hepatic iron accumulation). No other epidemiologic or clinical features of chronic hepatitis C (e.g., severity of acute hepatitis, level of aminotransferase activity, level of HCV RNA, presence or absence of jaundice during acute hepatitis) are predictive of eventual outcome. Despite the relatively benign nature of chronic hepatitis C over time in many patients, cirrhosis following chronic hepatitis C has been associated with the late development, after several decades, of HCC **(Chap. 53)**; the annual rate of HCC in cirrhotic patients with hepatitis C is 1–4%, occurring primarily in patients who have had HCV infection for 30 years or more.

Perhaps the best prognostic indicator in chronic hepatitis C is liver histology; the rate of hepatic fibrosis may be slow, moderate, or rapid. Patients with mild necrosis and inflammation as well as those with limited fibrosis have an excellent prognosis and limited progression to cirrhosis. In contrast, among patients with moderate to severe necroinflammatory activity or fibrosis, including septal or bridging fibrosis, progression to cirrhosis is highly likely over the course of 10–20 years. The pace of fibrosis progression may be accelerated by such factors as concomitant HIV infection, other causes of liver disease, excessive alcohol use, and hepatic steatosis. Among patients with compensated cirrhosis associated with hepatitis C, the 10-year survival rate is close to 80%; mortality occurs at a rate of 2–6% per year; decompensation at a rate of 4–5% per year; and, as noted above, HCC at a rate of 1–4% per year. Estimates of the natural history of chronic hepatitis C have been made, based on data available on the prevalence of HCV infection in the US population and on the rate of disease progression. Weighted primarily by the concentration of chronic hepatitis C in the baby boomer generation, the peak prevalence was estimated to have occurred in 2015. The calculated frequency of cirrhosis in US patients with hepatitis C was 5% in 1990, 25% in 2010, and is projected to be 37% in 2020. Peak mortality has been estimated to occur in 2032. **A discussion of the pathogenesis of liver injury in patients with chronic hepatitis C appears in Chap. 39.**

Clinical features of chronic hepatitis C are similar to those described above for chronic hepatitis B. Generally, fatigue is the most common symptom; jaundice is rare. Immune complex–mediated extrahepatic complications of chronic hepatitis C are less common than in chronic hepatitis B (despite the fact that assays for immune complexes are often positive in patients with chronic hepatitis C), with the exception of cryoglobulinemia **(Chap. 39)**, which is linked to cutaneous vasculitis and membranoproliferative glomerulonephritis as well as lymphoproliferative disorders such as B-cell lymphoma and unexplained monoclonal gammopathy. In addition, chronic hepatitis C has been associated with extrahepatic complications unrelated to immune-complex injury. These include Sjögren's syndrome, lichen planus, porphyria cutanea tarda, type 2 diabetes mellitus, and the metabolic syndrome (including insulin resistance and steatohepatitis).

Laboratory features of chronic hepatitis C are similar to those in patients with chronic hepatitis B, but aminotransferase levels tend to fluctuate more (the characteristic episodic pattern of aminotransferase activity) and to be lower, especially in patients with long-standing disease. An interesting and occasionally confusing finding in patients with chronic hepatitis C is the presence of autoantibodies. Rarely, patients with autoimmune hepatitis (see below) and hyperglobulinemia have false-positive immunoassays for anti-HCV. On the other hand, some patients with serologically confirmable chronic hepatitis C have circulating anti-LKM. These antibodies are anti-LKM1, as seen in patients with autoimmune hepatitis type 2 (see below), and are directed against a 33-amino-acid sequence of cytochrome P450 IID6. The occurrence of anti-LKM1 in some patients with chronic hepatitis C may result from the partial sequence homology between the epitope recognized by anti-LKM1 and two segments of the HCV polyprotein. In addition, the presence of this autoantibody in some patients with chronic hepatitis C suggests that autoimmunity may be playing a role in the pathogenesis of chronic hepatitis C.

Histopathologic features of chronic hepatitis C, especially those that distinguish hepatitis C from hepatitis B, are described in Chap. 39.

TREATMENT Chronic Hepatitis C

Therapy for chronic hepatitis C has evolved substantially in the 25 years since IFN-α was introduced for this indication in 1991. The therapeutic armamentarium grew to include PEG IFN with ribavirin and, in then, 2011, the introduction of the first protease inhibitors telaprevir and boceprevir used in combination with PEG IFN and ribavirin in patients with HCV genotype 1. The field of antiviral therapy for hepatitis C was transformed beginning in 2013, with the approval of the first nucleoside analog, sofosbuvir. As of 2016, no fewer than six, all-oral, highly effective (>95%), low-resistance, well tolerated, short-duration (usually 12 weeks) combination regimens of direct-acting antiviral drugs are available. The remarkable historical evolution of antiviral therapy for hepatitis C is instructive.

THE INTERFERON ERA (1991–2011) IFN based therapy has been supplanted by direct-acting antiviral (DAA) agents introduced in the second decade of the 21st Century; however, many important lessons about antiviral therapy for chronic hepatitis C were learned from the experience with IFN-based therapies, and many of the limitations of—and disparities in responsiveness to—IFN-based therapy have been overcome by current-generation DAA treatments.

When first approved, IFN-α was administered via subcutaneous injection three times a week for 6 months but achieved a sustained virologic response (SVR) (Fig. 41-2) (defined then as a reduction of HCV RNA to undetectable levels by PCR when measured ≥6 months after completion of therapy) below 10%. Doubling the duration of therapy—but not increasing the dose or changing IFN preparations—increased the SVR rate to ~20%, and addition to the regimen of daily ribavirin, an oral guanosine nucleoside, increased the SVR rate to 40%. When used alone, ribavirin is ineffective and does not reduce HCV RNA levels appreciably, but ribavirin enhances the efficacy of IFN by reducing the likelihood of virologic relapse after the achievement of an end-treatment response (Fig. 41-2) (response measured during, and maintained to the end of, treatment). Proposed mechanisms to explain the role of ribavirin include subtle direct reduction of HCV replication, inhibition of host inosine monophosphate dehydrogenase activity (and associated depletion of guanosine pools), immune modulation, induction of virologic

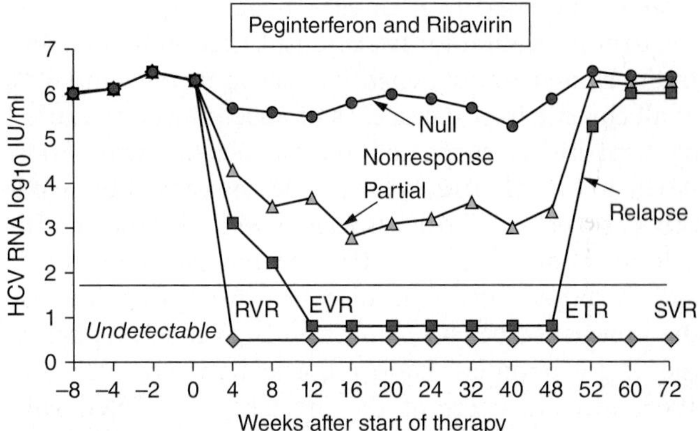

FIGURE 41-2

Classification of virologic responses based on outcomes during and after a 48-week course of pegylated interferon (PEG IFN) plus ribavirin antiviral therapy in patients with hepatitis C, genotype 1 or 4 (for genotype 2 or 3, the course would be 24 weeks). Nonresponders can be classified as null responders (hepatitis C virus [HCV] RNA reduction of <2 $\log_{10}$ IU/mL) or partial responders (HCV RNA reduction ≥2 $\log_{10}$ IU/mL but not suppressed to undetectable) by week 24 of therapy. In responders, HCV RNA can become undetectable, as shown with sensitive amplification assays, within 4 weeks (RVR, rapid virologic response); can be reduced by ≥2 $\log_{10}$ IU/mL within 12 weeks (early virologic response, EVR; if HCV RNA is undetectable at 12 weeks, the designation is "complete" EVR); or at the end of therapy, 48 weeks (ETR, end-treatment response). In responders, if HCV RNA remains undetectable for 24 weeks after ETR, week 72, the patient has a sustained virologic response (SVR), but if HCV RNA becomes detectable again, the patient is considered to have relapsed. The posttreatment week-24 SVR (SVR_{24}) has been supplanted by an SVR at week 12 (SVR_{12}), which has been shown to be equivalent to an SVR_{24} In patients treated with direct-acting antiviral therapy, RVR and EVR milestones are largely irrelevant, being met by almost all patients. *(Reproduced with permission, courtesy of Marc G. Ghany, National Institute of Diabetes and Digestive and Kidney Diseases, National Institutes of Health and the American Association for the Study of Liver Diseases. Hepatology 49:1335, 2009.)*

mutational catastrophe, and enhancement of IFN-stimulated gene expression. Ribavirin, despite its poorly understood mechanism of action) retains a modest role in supporting direct-acting antiviral agents as well (see below). IFN therapy results in activation of the JAK-STAT signal transduction pathway, which culminates in the intracellular elaboration of genes and their protein products that have antiviral properties. Hepatitis C proteins inhibit JAK-STAT signaling at several steps along the pathway, and exogenous IFN restores expression of IFN-stimulated genes and their antiviral effects.

Treatment with the combination of PEG IFN and ribavirin increased responsiveness (frequency of SVR) to as high as 55% overall, to >40% in genotypes 1 and 4, and to >80% in genotypes 2 and 3. Even in the absence of biochemical and virologic responses, histologic improvement occurred in approximately three-fourths of all treated patients. In chronic hepatitis C, ALT levels fall precipitously during therapy and up to 90% of virologic responses are achieved within the first 12 weeks of therapy; responses thereafter are rare. Most relapses occur within the first 12 weeks after treatment; therefore, an SVR at week 12 posttreatment is roughly equivalent to a 24-week SVR, and SVR_{12} has become the new standard. SVRs are very durable; normal ALT, improved histology, and absence of HCV RNA in serum and liver have been documented a decade after successful therapy, and "relapses" 2 years after sustained responses are almost unheard of. Thus, an SVR to antiviral therapy of chronic hepatitis C is tantamount to a cure, which is followed by marked improvements in liver-disease outcomes (see below).

Patient variables that correlate with sustained virologic responsiveness to IFN-based therapy include favorable genotype (genotypes 2 and 3 as opposed to genotypes 1 and 4; genotype 1b as opposed to genotype 1a); low baseline HCV RNA level (<800,000 IU/mL), low HCV quasispecies diversity, and histologically mild hepatitis and minimal fibrosis, especially absence of cirrhosis; immunocompetence, low liver iron levels, age <40; female gender; and absence of obesity, insulin resistance, type 2 diabetes mellitus, and hepatic steatosis. High levels of HCV RNA, more histologically advanced liver disease, and high quasispecies diversity all go hand in hand with advanced duration of infection and reduced IFN responsiveness. Also associated with poor responses to IFN-based therapy are African-American ethnicity (contributed to, but not explained entirely by, a higher proportion with genotype 1, slower early treatment viral kinetics, impaired HCV-specific immunity, and host genetic differences in IL28B alleles, described below), Latino ethnicity, and poor treatment adherence (<80% of IFN and ribavirin doses and <80% of prescribed duration of therapy). Ironically, patients whose disease was least likely to progress were the ones most likely to respond to IFN and vice versa. For patients treated with combination IFN-ribavirin, therapy for those with genotype 1 usually required a full 48 weeks with SVRs in the range of 40–45%, whereas in those with genotypes 2 and 3, a 24-week course of therapy sufficed with SVRs in the range of 80% (although refined tailoring of treatment duration could be indicated based on rapidity of response or associated cofactors, see below).

Genetic changes in the virus may explain differences in treatment responsiveness in some patients (e.g., among patients with genotype 1b, responsiveness to IFN is enhanced in those with amino-acid-substitution mutations in the nonstructural protein 5A gene). As described above in the discussion of spontaneous recovery from acute hepatitis C, IFN gene variants discovered in genome-wide association studies were shown to have a substantial impact on responsiveness of patients with genotype 1 to antiviral therapy. In studies of patients treated with PEG IFN and ribavirin, variants of the *IL28B* SNP that code for IFN-λ3 (a type III IFN, the receptors for which are more discretely distributed than IFN-α receptors and more concentrated in hepatocytes) correlate significantly with responsiveness. Patients homozygous for the C allele at this locus have the highest frequency of achieving an SVR (~80%), those homozygous for the T allele at this locus are least likely to achieve an SVR (~25%), and those heterozygous at this locus (C/T) have an intermediate level of responsiveness (SVRs in ~35%).

Side effects of IFN therapy are described above in the section on treatment of chronic hepatitis B. The most pronounced side effect of ribavirin therapy is hemolysis; an expected reduction in hemoglobin of up to 2–3 g or in hematocrit of 5–10% but also a small, unpredictable proportion with profound, brisk hemolysis, resulting in symptomatic anemia; therefore, close monitoring of blood counts is crucial, and ribavirin should be avoided in patients with anemia or hemoglobinopathies; in patients with coronary artery disease or cerebrovascular disease, in whom anemia can precipitate an ischemic event; in patients with renal insufficiency (the drug is excreted renally); and in pregnancy (the drug is teratogenic, mandating scrupulous use of efficient contraception during therapy in women of child-bearing age [IFNs, too, because of their antiproliferative properties, are contraindicated during pregnancy]). When symptomatic anemia occurs, ribavirin dose reductions or addition of erythropoietin to boost red blood cell levels may be required; erythropoietin was shown to improve patients' quality of life but not the likelihood of achieving an SVR. If ribavirin was stopped during therapy, SVR rates fell but responsiveness could be maintained as long as ribavirin was not stopped and the total ribavirin dose exceeded 60% of the planned dose.

Ribavirin can also cause nasal and chest congestion, pruritus, and precipitation of gout. Combination IFN-ribavirin therapy is more difficult to tolerate than IFN monotherapy and more likely to lead to dose reductions and discontinuation of therapy.

Studies of viral kinetics have shown that despite a virion half-life in serum of only 2–3 h, the level of HCV is maintained by a high replication rate of 10^{12} hepatitis C virions per day. IFN-α blocks virion production or release with an efficacy that increases with increasing drug doses; moreover, the calculated death rate for infected cells during IFN therapy is inversely related to level of HCV RNA; patients with the most rapid death rate of infected hepatocytes are more likely to achieve undetectable HCV RNA at 3 months; in practice, failure to achieve an early virologic response (EVR), a ≥2-$\log_{10}$ reduction in HCV RNA by week 12, predicts failure to experience a subsequent SVR. Similarly, patients in whom HCV RNA becomes undetectable within 4 weeks (i.e., who achieve a rapid virologic response [RVR]) have a very high likelihood of achieving an SVR(Fig. 41-2). Surprisingly, however, high-dose induction with IFN-based therapy did not yield higher SVR rates.

For the treatment of chronic hepatitis C, standard IFNs were supplanted beginning in 2001 by PEG IFNs. These have elimination times up to sevenfold longer than standard IFNs (i.e., a substantially longer half-life) and achieve prolonged concentrations, permitting administration once (rather than three times) a week. Instead of the frequent drug peaks (linked to side effects) and troughs (when drug is absent) associated with frequent administration of short-acting IFNs, administration of PEG IFNs results in drug concentrations that are more stable and sustained over time. Once-a-week PEG IFN monotherapy is twice as effective as monotherapy with its standard IFN counterpart, approaches the efficacy of combination standard IFN plus ribavirin, and is as well tolerated as standard IFNs, without more difficult-to-manage thrombocytopenia and leukopenia than standard IFNs. For most of the decade prior to 2011, when protease inhibitors were introduced for HCV genotype 1 (see below), the standard of care was a combination of PEG IFN plus ribavirin for all HCV genotypes.

Two PEG IFNs are available: PEG IFN-α2b, a 12-kD, linear PEG molecule bound to IFN-α2b, and PEG IFN-α2a a larger, 40-kD, branched PEG molecule bound to IFN-α2a; because of its larger size and smaller volume of extravascular distribution, PEG IFN-α2a can be given at a uniform dose independent of weight, whereas the dose of the smaller PEG IFN-α2b, which has a much wider volume distribution, must be weight-based. Although registration trials for the two PEG IFNs differed in design, ribavirin dose, and ascertainment of side effects, ultimately, the standard dose of PEG IFN α2a was 180 μg and of PEG IFN-α2b 1.5 μg/kg. The ribavirin dose adopted for both PEG IFNs was, for genotype 1, 1000 mg (for patients <75 kg) to 1200 mg (for patients ≥75 kg) and, for genotypes 2 and 3, 800 mg; a broader ribavirin dose/weight range was approved subsequently for PEG IFN-α2b in patients with genotype 1: <65 kg, 800 mg; 65–85 kg, 1000 mg; >85–105 kg, 1200 mg; and >105 kg, 1400 mg. For both drugs, recommended treatment durations were 48 weeks for genotype 1 and 24 weeks for genotypes 2 and 3 (somewhat more refractory, justifying a full 48 weeks especially for advanced hepatic fibrosis or cirrhosis and/or high-level HCV RNA). Between the two PEG IFNs, PEG IFN-α2a appeared to be slightly better tolerated and slightly more effective than PEG IFN-α2b in registration trials (SVRs for genotype 1: 41–51% vs 40-42%, respectively) as well as in subsequent head-to-head trials and a systematic review of randomized trials (SVR in genotypes 1–4: 48–55% vs 32–40%, respectively).

Until the 2011 introduction of protease inhibitors, unless ribavirin was contraindicated (see above), combination PEG IFN plus ribavirin was the recommended course of therapy. Even after the introduction of protease inhibitors for genotypes 1 and 4, however, PEG IFN–ribavirin remained the standard of care for patients with genotypes 2 and 3 until late 2013. For patients treated with combination PEG IFN–ribavirin, measurement of quantitative HCV RNA levels at 12 weeks was helpful in guiding therapy; if a 2-$\log_{10}$ drop in HCV RNA had not been achieved by this time, chances for an SVR were negligible, and additional therapy was futile. If the 12-week HCV RNA has fallen by 2 $\log_{10}$ (EVR), the chances for an SVR at the end of therapy were approximately two-thirds; if the 12-week HCV RNA is undetectable ("complete" EVR), the chances for an SVR exceeded 80% (Fig. 41-2).

The frequency of an SVR to PEG IFN–ribavirin therapy could be increased by tailoring therapy according to baseline variables and on-treatment virologic responsiveness. In patients with baseline variables weighing against a response (e.g., HCV RNA >800,000 IU/mL, weight >85 kg), by raising the dose of PEG IFN (e.g., to as high as 270 μg of PEG IFN-α2a) and/or the dose of ribavirin to as high as 1600 mg daily (if tolerated or supplemented by erythropoietin); by extending therapy from 48 to 72 weeks for patients with genotype 1 and a slow virologic response (i.e., failure of HCV RNA to fall rapidly to undetectable levels within 4 weeks [absence of a rapid virologic response, RVR]); and by abbreviating the duration of therapy to 24 weeks in patients with genotype 1 (and 4) who have a 4-week RVR (which occurs in ≤20%), especially in the subset with low baseline HCV RNA, yielding SVR rates of ~90%.

Responsiveness to IFN-ribavirin-based therapy was diminished in immunocompromised patients and in patients with HIV-HCV co-infection and contraindicated in patients with decompensated liver disease or end-stage renal disease. The cumbersome nature of IFN-ribavirin-based therapy (injections, complicated laboratory monitoring, side effects and poor tolerability, modest efficacy, variables and patient subsets associated with poor responsiveness, tailored therapy, futility rules, etc.) was supplanted eventually (in 2016) by direct-acting antivirals for all genotypes (see below). Most of the variables associated with poor responsiveness to IFN-based therapy became irrelevant, and difficult-to-treat patient subpopulations began to experience responses to direct-acting antivirals that were indistinguishable from responses in standard patients (see below).

Persons with chronic HCV infection have been shown to suffer increased liver-related mortality. On the other hand, successful antiviral therapy of chronic hepatitis C resulting in an SVR has been shown to improve survival (and to reduce the need for liver transplantation), to lower the risk of liver failure and liver-related death and all-cause mortality to slow the progression of chronic hepatitis C, and to reverse fibrosis and even cirrhosis. In cirrhotic patients with chronic hepatitis C, whereas the 10-year and 20-year survival in the absence of an SVR is reduced, survival at these intervals after an SVR has been found to be indistinguishable from that of the general population. Although successful treatment reduces mortality and liver failure (3–4-fold 10-year reduction) in cirrhotic patients (and those with advanced fibrosis) and reduces the need for liver transplantation and the likelihood of HCC (14-fold 10-year reduction), the risk of liver-related death and HCC persists, albeit at a much reduced level, necessitating continued clinical monitoring and cancer surveillance after SVR in cirrhotics. On the other hand, in the absence of an SVR, IFN-based therapy does not reduce the risk of HCC. Similarly, for nonresponders to PEG IFN–ribavirin therapy, three trials of long-term maintenance therapy with PEG IFN have shown no benefit in reducing the risk of histologic progression or clinical decompensation, including the development of HCC. Fortunately, PEG IFN–ribavirin nonresponders can now be retreated with direct-acting antivirals and experience SVR rates comparable to those in treatment-naïve persons (see following).

FIRST-GENERATION PROTEASE INHIBITORS (2011–2013) The HCV RNA genome encodes a single polyprotein, which is cleaved during and after translation by host and viral-encoded proteases. One protease involved in the cleavage of the viral polyprotein is an NS3-4A viral protein that has serine protease activity. Telaprevir and boceprevir are serine protease inhibitors that target NS3-4A. In 2011, telaprevir and boceprevir used in combination with PEG IFN and ribavirin were approved by the U.S. Food and Drug Administration (FDA) as the first oral direct-acting antiviral agents for the treatment of hepatitis C genotype 1 (not other genotypes) in adults with stable liver disease, both in patients who had not been treated before or who had failed previous treatment. Although now replaced by more effective, all-oral regimens, these first-in-class agents represented a breakthrough in the treatment of chronic hepatitis C and established milestones against which subsequent therapies could be measured.

Because resistance developed rapidly during monotherapy with telaprevir and boceprevir these drugs had to be used in combination with PEG IFN and ribavirin. Ribavirin in particular appeared to reduce relapse rates significantly in protease inhibitor–based regimens, such that those who could not take or were intolerant to ribavirin were unlikely to benefit from the addition of these agents. Telaprevir and boceprevir regimens consisted of periods of triple therapy (protease inhibitor plus PEG IFN plus ribavirin) and periods of dual therapy (PEG IFN plus ribavirin). Telaprevir regimens began with 12 weeks of triple therapy followed by dual therapy of a duration based on HCV RNA status at weeks 4 and 12 ("response-guided therapy") and prior treatment status. Boceprevir-based regimens consisted of a 4-week lead-in period of dual (PEG IFN–ribavirin) therapy followed by triple therapy and, in some instances, a further extension of dual therapy, with duration of response-guided therapy based on HCV RNA status at weeks 4, 8, and 24 and prior treatment status.

For patients with HCV genotype 1, protease inhibitors improved the frequency of RVRs and SVRs significantly as compared to PEG IFN plus ribavirin alone. In treatment-naïve patients telaprevir-based, SVRs were achieved in up to 79% of patients who received 12 weeks of triple therapy followed by 12–36 weeks of dual therapy, and among those with EVRs (undetectable HCV RNA at weeks 4 and 12) and response-guided therapy stopped at week 24 (12 weeks of triple therapy, then 12 weeks of dual therapy), the rate of SVRs was 83–92%. In studies with boceprevir in treatment-naïve patients, SVRs occurred in 59–66% of patients, and among those with undetectable HCV RNA at 8 weeks, the SVR rate increased to 86–88%. Adding to the complexity of treatment with these protease inhibitors were absolute stopping rules for futility, i.e., absence of HCV RNA reductions at critical treatment milestones, which were shown to be invariably predictive of nonresponse (TVR: HCV RNA >1000 IU/mL at weeks 4 or 12, or detectable at week 24; BOC: HCV RNA ≥100 IU/mL at week 12, or detectable at week 24).

In patients previously treated unsuccessfully with PEG IFN plus ribavirin, telaprevir-based treatment achieved SVRs in 83–88% of prior relapsers, 54–59% of partial responders (HCV RNA reduced by ≥2 $\log_{10}$ IU/mL but not to undetectable levels), and 29–33% of null responders (HCV RNA reduced by <2 $\log_{10}$ IU/mL). With boceprevir, a similar degradation in SVRs rate occurred as a function of prior responsiveness in 75% of prior relapsers, in 40–52% of previous partial responders; in ~30–40% of null responders. In a substantial proportion of protease inhibitor nonresponders, resistance-associated variants/substitutions (RAVs) could be identified, but these variants were not archived, and wild-type HCV reemerged in almost all cases within 1.5 to 2 years. SVRs to these protease inhibitors were highest in prior relapsers and treatment-naïve patients (white > black ethnicity), lower in prior partial responders, lower still in prior null responders, and lowest in cirrhotic prior null responders for whom no benefit accrued over PEG IFN/ribavirin treatment. Responses to protease inhibitor triple-drug regimens are higher in patients with *IL28B* C than non-C genotypes, HCV genotype 1b than genotype 1a, less advanced than more advanced fibrosis stage, whites than blacks, lower body mass index (BMI) than elevated BMI, and, for boceprevir, achievement of a >1 $\log_{10}$ HCV RNA reduction during 4 weeks of PEG IFN–ribavirin lead-in therapy. Age and HCV RNA level were less influential and insulin resistance was noninfluential on response to these antiviral agents.

Both of these protease inhibitors had substantial toxicities. Telaprevir was associated with a severe, generalized (trunk and extremities), often confluent, maculopapular, pruritic rash in ~6% of treated patients (that required careful dermatologic monitoring in all patients and systemic corticosteroid therapy in the most severely affected). Other common side effects include pruritus, rectal burning, nausea, diarrhea, fatigue, dysgeusia (altered or unpleasant taste), and anemia, which required close monitoring, could be relatively refractory, occasionally requiring transfusion. and even hospitalization (especially in cirrhotic prior nonresponders). Anemia occurred in half of boceprevir-treated patients, neutropenia in up to 30% and thrombocytopenia in 3–4%. Other side effects of boceprevir include fatigue, nausea, headache, dysgeusia, dry mouth, vomiting, and diarrhea.

Both drugs came with an inconveniently high pill burden and had to be administered every 8 hours with food (TVR with a 20-g fat meal). Use of protease inhibitors was further complicated by numerous drug-drug interactions. As telaprevir and boceprevir are both eliminated by and inhibit CYP3A4, these agents could not be administered with other medications that induce CYP3A4 or are dependent on CYP3A4 for elimination. Care had to be taken to examine for any potential interactions between these protease inhibitors and other medications the patient was taking and convenient website became available to check for such drug-drug interactions (*www.hep-druginteractions.org*).

Despite the improvement in SVRs with protease-inhibitor-based regimens for genotype 1 compared to PEG IFN/ribavirin (e.g., in treatment-naïve patients 66–79% vs 38–44%), triple-drug protease-inhibitor therapy was hampered by amplified intolerability, the complexity of response-guided regimens and futility stopping rules, the inconvenience of thrice-daily dosing with meals and a high pill burden, and the need for PEG IFN injections and ribavirin with all their intolerability, and multiple drug-drug interactions. Moreover, side effects appeared to be more severe and burdensome once these drugs entered practice, especially in cirrhotic nonreponders, in whom studies reported from Europe showed serious adverse events in up to 45% and deaths in up to 3%. All these issues, as well as rapidly accelerating progress on next-generation and all-oral direct-acting antiviral therapy (see later), conspired to temper enthusiasm for these new antivirals; after a brief stint as recommended therapy (2011–2013), these drugs became obsolete and are no longer recommended.

CONTEMPORARY DIRECT-ACTING ANTIVIRAL COMBINATION THERAPY (2013–) Since late 2013, the number of new antiviral agents for hepatitis C has expanded substantially, and, currently, PEG IFN-based treatments have been supplanted by six therapeutic regimens—all oral, IFN free, highly efficacious (>95% SVR), well tolerated, with high barriers to resistance, simple dosing and low pill burdens, treatment durations as brief as 8 to 12 weeks, and, in many cases, pangenotypic efficacy—are recommended (Table 41-6). These drugs are distributed among three classes of direct-acting antivirals: NS3/4 protease inhibitors (which cleave the single HCV polyprotein into constituent structural and nonstructural proteins), NS5B nucleoside and nonnucleoside polymerase inhibitors (which interfere with the RNA-dependent RNA polymerase [a replicase] involved in synthesis of viral RNA), and NS5A inhibitors (which interfere with a membrane-associated phosphoprotein essential to the HVC RNA replication complex).

The first of the new agents (approved in November 2013) was simeprevir, a second-generation protease inhibitor for genotype 1, followed shortly thereafter (December 2013) by sofosbuvir, a pangenotypic nucleoside polymerase inhibitor. For genotype 1, both of these agents had to be combined with PEG IFN and ribavirin; for genotypes 2 and 3, sofosbuvir was administered with ribavirin, without PEG IFN, but these treatment regimens have been supplanted by combinations of all-oral, IFN free, direct-acting antivirals (DAA), and ribavirin is rarely needed, retained only for very limited indications.

Simeprevir: When simeprevir was used with PEG IFN, its efficacy (genotype 1b > 1a) was similar to that of first-generation protease inhibitors but required only once-a-day dosing without the complexity of response-guided therapy. Like first-generation protease inhibitors, simerprevir was hampered by many drug-drug interactions and side effects (including photosensitivity, rash, and mild hyperbilirubinemia); moreover, patients, with HCV NS3 polymorphism Q80K had markedly reduced drug efficacy, necessitating pretreatment genetic testing and disqualifying a substantial proportion (~ a third) of potential treatment candidates. Little about simeprevir supported its adoption in combination with PEG IFN and ribavirin. On the other hand, the combination of simeprevir (150 mg) along with sofosbuvir (400 mg) for 12 weeks was found to be effective in treatment-naïve (97% SVR_{12}) or treatment-experienced (95% SVR_{12}) patients without cirrhosis and in treatment-naïve (88% SVR_{12}) or treatment-refractory (79% SVR_{12}) patients with cirrhosis (it remains one of the recommended regimens for genotype 1).

Sofosbuvir: Sofosbuvir, the first nonprotease inhibitor direct antiviral agent to be approved, has an excellent profile—high potency, high barrier to resistance, pangenotypic activity, very well tolerated with limited adverse effects (most commonly, generally mild fatigue, insomnia, headache, and nausea), once-daily oral administration, and relatively free from major drug-drug interactions. Sofosbuvir has efficacy in all genotypes (1 to 6); in treatment-naïve subjects and prior nonresponders to PEG IFN-based and protease-inhibitor-based therapy; with PEG IFN/RBV or in IFN-free regimens; in combination with RBV or with NS5A inhibitors; and for treatment periods as brief as 8 to 12 weeks to as long as 24 weeks. Currently, sofosbuvir is used in combination with either the protease inhibitor simeprevir (as described above) or, more commonly, with one of three NS5A inhibitors. Thus, sofosbuvir is a component of four of the six recommended regimens for genotype 1, two of the four regimens for genotype 4, and both of the regimens for genotypes 2, 3, 5, and 6 **(Table 41-6)**.

Sofosbuvir/ledipasvir: The direct-acting antiviral combination that has had a dominant role in the treatment of hepatitis C is sofosbuvir (400 mg) plus the NS5A inhibitor ledipasvir (90 mg) in a once-a day, fixed-dose, single pill, approved in October 2014 for genotypes 1, 4, and 6. Phase-III trials were conducted in treatment-naïve noncirrhotic patients, in treatment-naïve cirrhotic and noncirrhotic patients, and in treatment-experienced cirrhotic and noncirrhotic patients treated for 8,12, or 24 weeks, both with and without ribavirin. In treatment-naïve noncirrhotics, an SVR_{12} was achieved in 97–99% of subjects, and no benefit

TABLE 41-6

INDICATIONS AND RECOMMENDATIONS FOR ANTIVIRAL THERAPY OF CHRONIC HEPATITIS C[a]

Standard Indications for Therapy

All patients with chronic HCV infection (detectable HCV RNA, with or without elevated ALT) except for those with short life expectancies owing to comorbid conditions

Any stage of fibrosis; highest priority for advanced fibrosis [METAVIR stage 3]/cirrhosis [METAVIR stage 4] (pretreatment biopsy is no longer embraced and has been supplanted by noninvasive measures of fibrosis, e.g., imaging to determine liver elasticity)

Responsiveness in groups previously refractory to interferon-based therapy (HIV-HCV co-infection, renal insufficiency, African American ethnicity, IL28B non-C haplotype, obesity, insulin resistance, hepatic decompensation, etc.) is not diminished to contemporary direct-acting oral combination regimens.

Retreatment Recommended

Relapsers, partial responders, or nonresponders after a previous course of interferon-based therapy or prior direct-acting antiviral therapy (see genotype-specific recommendations below).

Antiviral Therapy Not Recommended

Pregnancy (teratogenicity of ribavirin unknown safety of direct-acting antiviral combinations)

Contraindications to use of antiviral medications

Therapeutic Regimens (based on AASLD-IDSA recommendations, www.hcvguidelines.org)[b]

TREATMENT-NAÏVE OR RELAPSED AFTER PRIOR PEG IFN/RIBAVIRIN THERAPY

Genotype 1a

ledipasvir + sofosbuvir 12 weeks

paritaprevir/ritonavir + ombitasvir + dasabuvir + RBV 12 weeks (no cirrhosis) or 24 weeks (cirrhosis)

sofosbuvir + simeprevir 12 weeks (no cirrhosis) or ± RBV 24 weeks (cirrhosis)

daclatasvir + sofosbuvir 12 weeks (no cirrhosis) or ± RBV 24 weeks (cirrhosis)

grazoprevir + elbasvir 12 weeks (no cirrhosis or cirrhosis sans ELB NS5A RAVs) or + RBV x 16 weeks (ELB NS5A RAVs)

sofosbuvir + velpatasvir 12 weeks

Genotype 1b

ledipasvir + sofosbuvir 12 weeks

paritaprevir/ritonavir + ombitasvir + dasabuvir 12 weeks

sofosbuvir + simeprevir 12 weeks (no cirrhosis) or ± RBV 24 weeks (cirrhosis)

daclatasvir + sofosbuvir 12 weeks (no cirrhosis) or ± RBV 24 weeks (cirrhosis)

grazoprevir + elbasvir 12 weeks

sofosbuvir + velpatasvir 12 weeks

Genotype 2

sofosbuvir + velpatasvir 12 weeks

daclatasvir + sofosbuvir (no cirrhosis) 12 weeks or 16-24 weeks (cirrhosis)

Genotype 3

sofosbuvir + velpatasvir 12 weeks

daclatasvir + sofosbuvir 12 weeks (no cirrhosis) or ± RBV 24 weeks (cirrhosis)

Genotype 4

sofosbuvir + velpatasvir 12 weeks

ledipasvir + sofosbuvir 12 weeks

paritaprevir/r + ombitasvir + RBV 12 weeks (no dasabuvir)

grazoprevir + elbasvir 12 weeks

Genotypes 5, 6

sofosbuvir + velpatasvir 12 weeks

ledipasvir + sofosbuvir 12 weeks

FAILED PRIOR PEG IFN/RIBAVIRIN THERAPY, NO CIRRHOSIS

Genotype 1a

ledipasvir + sofosbuvir 12 weeks

paritaprevir/ritonavir + ombitasvir + dasabuvir + RBV 12 weeks

sofosbuvir + simeprevir 12 weeks

daclatasvir + sofosbuvir 12 weeks

grezoprevir + elbasvir 12 weeks (without ELB NS5A RAVs) or + RBV x 16 weeks (ELB NS5A RAVs)

sofosbuvir + velpatasvir 12 weeks

Genotype 1b

ledipasvir + sofosbuvir 12 weeks

paritaprevir/ritonavir + ombitasvir + dasabuvir 12 weeks

sofosbuvir + simeprevir 12 weeks

daclatasvir + sofosbuvir 12 weeks

(continued)

TABLE 41-6

INDICATIONS AND RECOMMENDATIONS FOR ANTIVIRAL THERAPY OF CHRONIC HEPATITIS C[a] (*CONTINUED*)

grazoprevir + elbasvir 12 weeks
sofosbuvir + velpatasvir 12 weeks
Genotype 2
Sofosbuvir + Velpatasvir 12 weeks
Daclatasvir + Sofosbuvir 12 weeks
Genotype 3
Sofosbuvir + Velpatasvir 12 weeks
Daclatasvir + Sofosbuvir 12 weeks
Genotype 4
Sofosbuvir + Velpatasvir 12 weeks
Ledipasvir + Sofosbuvir 12 weeks
Paritaprevir/r + Ombitasvir + RBV 12 weeks (no dasabuvir)
Grazoprevir + Elbasvir 12 weeks (prior relapse) or + RBV 16 weeks (prior nonresponse)
Genotypes 5, 6
Sofosbuvir + Velpatasvir 12 weeks
Ledipasvir + Sofosbuvir 12 weeks
FAILED PRIOR PEG IFN/RIBAVIRIN THERAPY, COMPENSATED CIRRHOSIS
Genotype 1a
ledipasvir + sofosbuvir + RBV 12 weeks
ledipasvir + sofosbuvir 24 weeks
sofosbuvir + velpatasvir 12 weeks
grazoprevir + elbasvir 12 weeks (without ELB NS5A RAVs) or + RBV x 16 weeks (ELB NS5A RAVs)
paritaprevir/ritonavir + ombitasvir + dasabuvir + RBV 24 weeks
sofosbuvir + simeprevir ± RBV 24 weeks (no Q80K variant)
daclatasvir + sofosbuvir ± RBV 24 weeks
Genotype 1b
ledipasvir + sofosbuvir + RBV 12 weeks
ledipasvir + sofosbuvir 24 weeks
sofosbuvir + velpatasvir 12 weeks
grazoprevir + elbasvir 12 weeks
paritaprevir/ritonavir + ombitasvir + dasabuvir 12 weeks
sofosbuvir + simeprevir ± RBV 24 weeks
daclatasvir + sofosbuvir ± RBV 24 weeks
Genotype 2
sofosbuvir + velpatasvir 12 weeks
sofosbuvir + declatasvir 16 or 24 weeks
Genotype 3
sofosbuvir + velpatasvir 12 weeks
daclatasvir + sofosbuvir + RBV 24 weeks
Genotype 4
sofosbuvir + velpatasvir 12 weeks
ledipasvir + sofosbuvir + RBV 12 weeks
paritaprevir/ritonavir + ombitasvir + RBV 12 weeks (no dasabuvir)
grazoprevir + elbasvir 12 weeks (prior relapse) or + RBV 16 weeks (prior nonresponse)
ledepasvir + sofosbuvir 24 weeks
Genotypes 5, 6
sofosbuvir + velpatasvir 12 weeks
ledipasvir + sofosbuvir 12 weeks

Features Associated with Reduced Responsiveness to Direct-Acting Antiviral Combination Therapy
Genotype and subtype (genotype 1a less responsive than genotype 1b for several drugs)
Treatment experience
Advanced fibrosis (bridging fibrosis, cirrhosis)
Reduced adherence

[a]Rapidly evolving new recommendations; for up-to-date treatment recommendations, please see *www.hcvguidelines.org*.
[b]Class-I recommendations in *Italic* font, all others are Class-II recommendations.

Drug doses: sofosbuvir 400 mg; ledipasvir 90 mg; paritaprevir 150 mg; ritonavir 100 mg; ombitasvir 25 mg; dasabuvir 250 mg; ribavirin, weight-based: 1,000 mg (<75Kg)-1,200 mg (≥75 Kg); simeprevir 150 mg; daclatasvir 60 mg; elbasvir 50 mg; grazoprevir 100 mg; valpatasvir 100 mg.

Abbreviations: AASLD, American Association for the Study of Liver Diseases; ALT, alanine aminotransferase; ELB NS5A RAVs, elbasvir NS5A resistance-associated variants/substitutions; HCV, hepatitis C virus; IFN, interferon; IDSA, Infectious Diseases Society of America PEG IFN, pegylated interferon; IU, international units (1 IU/mL is equivalent to ~2.5 copies/mL). RBV, ribavirin was observed by extending therapy from 12 to 24 weeks or by adding ribavirin. Moreover, for treatment-naïve, noncirrhotic patients with baseline HCV RNA <6 × 10^6 IU/ml, a treatment duration of 8 weeks was as effective as one of 12 weeks (94–95% SVR_{12}), which may be a consideration for a proportion of patients. In cirrhotic patients, SVR_{12} was achieved in 97–100% of treatment-naïve subjects (no advantage of extending therapy from 12 to 24 weeks or of adding ribavirin); however, for cirrhotic prior nonresponders to IFN based therapy, 12 weeks of therapy was inferior (86% SVR_{12}) to 24 weeks of therapy (100% SVR_{12}). This combination, which is equally effective in patients with HIV-HCV co-infection and in African American patients, has been shown to be highly effective in patients with decompensated cirrhosis and in patients with hepatitis C after liver transplantation. On the other hand, the safety and efficacy of sofosbuvir/ledipasvir in patients with advanced renal failure have not been established, and all sofosbuvir-containing regimens can be associated with severe bradycardia in patients taking amiodarone, especially along with beta-blockers; sofosbuvir-containing combinations are contraindicated with amiodarone. Drug-drug interactions are few, but P-gp inducers, like St. John's wort and rifampin, and proton-pump gastric acid inhibitors, like omeprazole, may reduce sofosbuvir/ledipasvir concentrations. Responsiveness to sofosbuvir/ledipasvir is not reduced in patients with baseline RAVs to these agents.

Paritaprevir/ritonavir, ombitasvir, and dasabuvir: The combination of ritonavir (100 mg)-boosted paritaprevir (150 mg), a protease inhibitor, ombitasvir (25 mg), an NS5A inhibitor, dasabuvir (250 mg), a nonnucleoside polymerase inhibitor, ± weight-based ribavirin (total of five drugs) was approved in December 2014 for genotypes 1 and 4. Paritaprevir/ritonavir and ombitasvir, formulated in a single tablet, are taken once daily, and both dasabuvir (a separate pill) and weight-based ribavirin (when included in the regimen) are taken twice daily. In clinical trials, this combination achieved SVR_{12} rates of 87–100% in treatment-naïve and treatment-experienced patients with genotype 1; without ribavirin, this combination in genotype 1a is approximately 7% less responsive than genotype 1b. Therefore, in treatment-naïve patients with genotype 1a, this combination is administered *with* ribavirin for 12 weeks in the absence of cirrhosis (95–97% SVR_{12}) or for 24 weeks in the presence of compensated cirrhosis (94% SVR_{12}), while in patients with genotype 1b, the combination does not require ribavirin, and the duration of therapy is 12 weeks for both noncirrhotics and cirrhotics (99–100% SVR_{12}). In prior nonresponders without cirrhosis, the combination is administered for 12 weeks, *with* ribarivin in genotype 1a (96% SVR_{12}), *without* ribavirin in genotype 1b (100% SVR_{12}). In prior nonresponders with cirrhosis, the combination is administered for 24 weeks *with* ribavirin in genotype 1a (SVR_{12} 100% in prior relapsers and partial responders, 95% in prior null responders [in whom treatment without ribavirin was associated with an 80% SVR_{12}]), but only for 12 weeks and *without* ribavirin in genotype 1b (100% SVR_{12}). For genotype 4, the regimen is given for 12 weeks with ribavirin but without dasabuvir in treatment-naïve and treatment-experienced patients (100% SVR_{12}), including those with compensated cirrhosis. In July 2016, the FDA approved a long-acting formulation of dasabuvir, allowing once-a-day instead of twice-a-day treatment; for genotype 1a, twice-daily ribavirin dosing remains.

This combination is well tolerated with generally mild side effects, e.g., fatigue, asthenia, insomnia, headache, and pruritus. Hyperbilirubinemia (primarily unconjugated) and elevations in alanine aminotransferase activity may occur but resolve during or shortly after treatment. Because of occasional hyperbilirubinemia and potential hepatotoxicity (FDA warning letter issued October 2015 regarding hepatic failure/decompensation reported in treated cirrhotic patients), this combination is not recommended in patients with decompensated cirrhosis, and treated cirrhotic patients should be monitored closely for decompensation; however, the safety and efficacy of this combination have been demonstrated for patients with advanced renal insufficiency. Similar to other regimens containing protease inhibitors, drug-drug interactions are common with other drugs that induce CYP3A4 or are dependent on CYP3A4 for elimination. Checking for potential drug-drug interactions is important prior to initiating therapy with this drug combination (www.hep-druginteractions.org).

Compared to sofosbuvir/ledipasvir, this regimen has the disadvantage of requiring twice-a-day therapy ribavirin for genotype 1a and a contraindication in decompensated cirrhosis but the advantage of a 12-week, ribavirin-free regimen for prior null responders with cirrhosis and an indication in renal failure.

Sofosbuvir and Daclatasvir: Daclatasvir, an NS5A inhibitor, along with the polymerase inhibitor sofosbuvir, was approved by the FDA in July 2015 for genotype 3 and in February 2016 for genotype 1. At the time of its approval for genotype 3, daclatasvir filled a need inadequately met by other available combination direct-acting antivirals. Although data on genotype 3 are the most robust, clinical trials of this combination in genotypes 1 and 2 support its efficacy and recommendations for first-line (genotype 1) and alternative (genotype 2) treatment, in some cases with ribavirin (**Table 41-6**). Daclatasvir, a 60-mg tablet, and sofosbuvir, a separate 400 mg tablet are taken once a day for 12 to 24 weeks.

In clinical trials among treatment-naïve or treatment-experienced patients, SVR_{12} rates for 12 weeks of daclatasvir plus sofosbuvir were 98% with genotype 1 (comparable results in genotypes 1a and 1b), 92% for genotype 2, and 89% for genotype 3. For noncirrhotic patients, the addition of ribavirin or the extension of therapy to 24 weeks did not improve efficacy. In patients with compensated cirrhosis limited prospective data and data from observational cohorts suggested that extending therapy to 24 weeks, with or without ribavirin, improved efficacy. In cirrhotics, SVR_{12} was achieved in 93% with Child Class-Pugh A and B but in only 56% with Class-C decompensated cirrhosis. For patients with genotype 3 and cirrhosis, the combination was effective in treatment-naïve patients (94% SVR_{12}) but less so in prior nonresponders (69% SVR_{12}). Outcomes in patients with HIV-HCV co-infection were comparable.

Like other sofosbuvir-NS5A inhibitor combinations, declatasvir plus sofosbuvir is well tolerated (mild fatigue, headache, nausea, diarrhea in 5-14%) but can cause severe bradycardia when administered with amiodarone (contraindicated), especially along with beta blockers. Because daclatasvir is a substrate for CYP3A, CYP3A inducers can reduce daclatasvir levels, and CYP3A inhibitors reduce daclatasvir levels. Similarly, daclatasvir, an inhibitor of P-gp, OATP1B1 and 1B3, and BCP, can increase the levels of drugs that are substrates of these transporters. As noted above for other direct-acting antivirals, checking for potential drug-drug interactions is advisable prior to initiating therapy (www.hep-druginteractions.org).

Although daclatasvir-sofosbuvir is approved for genotypes 1 and 3 and recommended as an alternative for genotype 2, better documented efficacy and simplicity of other regimens have limited the popularity of this drug combination.

Elbasvir/Grazoprevir: Elbasvir (50 mg), an NS5A inhibitor, combined in a single, fixed-dose pill with grazoprevir (100 mg), an NS3/4 protease inhibitor was approved in January 2016 as a once-a-day (with or without food) treatment for genotypes 1 and 4. In clinical trials, a 12-week course was effective in treatment-naïve and treatment-experienced patients without cirrhosis or with compensated cirrhosis. In treatment-naïve patients, this combination yielded an SVR_{12} in 92% of patients with genotype 1a, 99% with genotype 1b, and 100% with genotype 4 (very small numbers, however); 10 patients with genotype 6 were included, but only 80% achieved SVR_{12}. Cirrhotic and noncirrhotic patients had comparable rates of SVR_{12}, 97% and 94%, respectively. For this drug combination, however, approximately 11% of patients with genotype 1a harbor NS5A polymorphisms, i.e., RAVs, at baseline. If present, these NS5A RAVs reduce efficacy of elbasvir/grazoprevir (unlike baseline RAVs to the other combination regiments described above and below) from 99% to 58% in treatment-naïve patients. Therefore, all patients with genotype 1a require baseline RAV testing; if these RAVs are present, treatment extension to 16 weeks and the addition of weight-based ribavirin brings the SVR_{12} up to expected levels of close to 100%. In treatment-experienced patients, both extending treatment to 16 weeks and adding ribavirin were studied; however, generally, in the absence of baseline NS5A RAVs, SVR_{12} rates were not increased over those without ribavirin for 12 weeks (94–97%). For genotype 1a, among prior nonresponders to PEG IFN/ribavirin, 12 weeks of elbasvir/grazoprevir suffices without ribavirin except for patients with baseline NS5A RAVs, who require 16 weeks of therapy and ribavirin. Among nonresponders to prior protease-inhibitor therapy, even in the absence of baseline NS5A RAVs, ribavirin should be added to a 12-week regimen; in the presence of baseline NS5A RAVs, treatment should be extended to 16 weeks and ribavirin added. For genotype 1b, NS5A RAVs are not an issue, and the only subgroup requiring modification of a 12 week course of therapy are prior nonreponders to protease-inhibitor regimens, for whom ribavirin is added. For genotype 4, the recommended regimen for all prior nonresponders (whether to PEG IFN/ribavirin or protease inhibitor regimens) is 16 weeks of elbasvir/grazoprevir plus ribavirin **(Table 41-6)**.

This combination is just as effective in patients with HIV-HCV co-infection and in patients with advanced renal failure (including those requiring hemodialysis) but contraindicated in decompensated cirrhosis. Like other protease inhibitor regimens, elbasvir/grazoprevir can be associated with aminotransferase elevations and potential hepatotoxicity; because these drugs are excreted by the liver, in decompensated liver disease, plasma drug concentrations may become elevated substantially. Therefore, all treated patients should have alanine aminotransferase screening periodically during therapy, and the drug should be stopped for elevations exceeding 10 fold or for elevations of conjugated bilirubin, alkaline phosphatase, or prothrombin time.

Elbasvir/grazoprevir is well tolerated, with only low levels of mild adverse effects (fatigue, headache, nausea in 5–11%) seen just as frequently in placebo recipients. Both elbasvir and grazoprevir are substrates for CYP3A and are subject to multiple potential drug-drug interactions. Therefore, this combination should not be used with potent CYP3A inducers; conversely, CYP3A and OATP1B1 inhibitors can lead to untoward elevations of plasma elbasvir/grazoprevir concentrations. Checking for potential drug-drug interactions is advisable prior to initiating therapy (www.hep-druginteractions.org).

Compared to other available regimens for genotypes 1 and 4, elbasvir/grazoprevir has the disadvantage/inconvenience of requiring baseline NS5A RAV testing but the advantages of a comparable regimen for cirrhotics and noncirrhotics, for treatment-naïve and treatment-experienced patients, and for patients with normal renal function and with renal failure.

Sofosbuvir/velpatasvir: The combination in a single, fixed-dose pill of velpatasvir (100 mg), a highly potent, pangenotypic NS5A inhibitor, along with the polymerase inhibitor sofosbuvir (400 mg) was approved in June 2016 for genotypes 1-6, in treatment-naïve and treatment-experienced noncirrhotics and cirrhotics. Ribavirin is not required, including in patients with genotypes 2 and 3, except in patients with decompensated cirrhosis.

In a series of clinical trials, this combination for 12 weeks in the absence of ribavirin was shown to yield 99% SVR_{12} (range 97–100%) in genotypes 1, 2, 4, 5, and 6 and 95% in genotype 3. Baseline NS5A RAVs had no impact on responsiveness.

Prior to the availability of this drug combination, patients with genotype 3, especially those with cirrhosis and prior null response to other therapies, proved to be the most refractory subset of patients. In treatment-naïve patients with genotype 3, 12 weeks of sofosbuvir/velpatasvir (95% SVR_{12}) was superior to 24 weeks of sofosbuvir plus ribavirin (80% SVR_{12}). In patients with genotype 3, the combination of sofosbuvir/velpatasvir for 12 weeks was comparable in noncirrhotics (97% SVR_{12}) and cirrhotics (91% SVR_{12}) and in treatment-naïve

(97% SVR_{12}) and treatment-experienced (90% SVR_{12}) patients, superior in all these categories to 24 weeks of sofosbuvir plus ribavirin (87%, 66%, 86%, and 63%, respectively). In cirrhotic null responders, most available IFN free regimens (including daclatasvir plus sofosbuvir, approved specifically for this genotype) achieved SVR_{12} rates in the range of ~60-75%, while the combination of PEG IFN, ribavirin, and sofosbuvir could boost SVR_{12} to the mid-80% range. For sofosbuvir/velpatasvir, in treatment-experienced patients, noncirrhotics and cirrhotics had similarly high efficacy (91% and 89% SVR_{12}, respectively), the highest recorded SVR_{12} for cirrhotic null responders treated with IFN free regimens. Finally, in patients with genotypes 1-4 and 6 and with decompensated, Class-B cirrhosis (55% treatment-experienced), sofosbuvir/velpatasvir plus ribavirin for 12 weeks yielded an SVR_{12} in 94%, better than sofosbuvir/velpatasvir without ribavirin for 12 weeks (83% SVR_{12}) or 24 weeks (86% SVR_{12}).

Like other all-oral direct-acting antivirals, sofosbuvir/valpatasvir was very well tolerated (in noncirrhotic and compensated cirrhotic patients, mild headache and fatigue in over 10%, occurring in a comparable proportion of placebo recipients; in decompensated cirrhosis, mild fatigue, headache, nausea, insomnia, diarrhea, and anemia [ribavirin part of the regimen] in over 10%). Like other sofosbuvir-containing regimens, sofosbuvir/valpatasvir should not be administered along with amiodarone (potential serious bradycardia), and P-gp inducers and moderate-to-potent CYP3A inducers can reduce plasma levels of sofosbuvir and/or velpatasvir. Checking for drug-drug interactions prior to therapy is advisable (www.hep-druginteractions.org). Baseline RAVs do not influence responsiveness to this combination.

FUTURE DIRECT-ACTING ANTIVIRAL COMBINATION THERAPY (2017)
Most treatment needs have been met by contemporary direct-acting antiviral regimens described above; however, several additional, highly potent, pangenotypic drug combinations are in development. For example, an investigative protease inhibitor ("GS-9857") added to the polymerase inhibitor/NS5A inhibitor combination of sofosbuvir/velpatasvir yields a very well tolerated *triple-drug* combination with 97% SVR_{12} across all HCV genotypes and patient subgroups (noncirrhotic/cirrhotic, treatment-naïve/treatment-experienced [including prior NS5A treatment and independent of the number of prior direct-acting antiviral drug classes received], no effect of baseline NS5A RAVs). Several experimental combinations may allow even briefer durations of therapy. In a small, exploratory trial, a *6-week* combination of sofosbuvir plus an experimental pangenotypic, very high potency, very low resistance NS5A inhibitor achieved SVR_{12} in 100% of 12 patients. In phase-II clinical trials, an experimental combination of two high-potency, pangenotypic direct-acting antivirals, a protease inhibitor ("ABT-493") plus an NS5A inhibitor ("ABT-530") for 8 weeks yielded 100% SVR_{12} in treatment-naïve noncirrhotic patients with genotypes 1, 2, and 3; in cirrhotics with genotype 3, and in patients with genotypes 4, 5, and 6, 100% efficacy of this combination was observed with 12 weeks of therapy. In patients with prior direct-acting antiviral treatment failure, 12 weeks without ribavirin sufficed to achieve a ≥95% SVR_{12}; neither baseline NS5A nor protease inhibitor RAVs influenced SVR_{12} rates. No safety issues have been encountered, and the potential for drug-drug interactions is limited. These promising combinations are undergoing phase-III trials.

Less advanced is development of inhibitors of host proteins, such as oral, nonimmunosuppressive inhibitors of cyclophilin A (which interacts with NS5A during HCV replication) and subcutaneous antisense antagonists of host liver-expressed micro-RNA-122 (which promotes HCV replication). Given the accelerated progress of all-oral, short-treatment-duration, high-efficacy, direct-acting antivirals, these alternative approaches may not be practical or competitive; moreover, development of both approaches has been retarded by emerging toxicities (pancreatitis associated with cyclophilin inhibitors and jaundice associated with micro-RNA-122).

Although data on the impact of direct-acting antivirals on the natural history of chronic hepatitis C are still limited, preliminary findings are that successful therapy is associated with a gradual reduction in fibrosis progression and a regression of advanced fibrosis (cirrhosis), improvement in survival among patients with decompensated cirrhosis, and a decline in the number of patients with hepatitis C being referred for liver transplantation. Based on the known prevalence, natural history, and rate of progression of chronic hepatitis C; and on the efficacy of direct-acting antiviral therapies and their impact on the complications of hepatitis C; modeling estimates have suggested that the availability and application of these therapies have the potential to reduce the hepatitis C-associated disease burden (liver-related death, hepatocellular carcinoma, decompensated cirrhosis, liver transplantation) by 50-70% between 2015 and 2050.

TREATMENT RECOMMENDATIONS Because the pace of new drug development and approval has been so rapid, the American Association for the Study of Liver Disease (AASLD) and the Infectious Diseases Society of America (IDSA) have been providing a consensus of updated treatment recommendations for patients with hepatitis C; these recommendations, which continue to be revised regularly based on new data, are available online at www.hcvguidelines.org and should be consulted before initiating therapy **(Table 41-6)**. The European Association for the Study of the Liver (EASL) issues similar (but not identical) treatment recommendations periodically for hepatitis C (www.easl.eu), most recently in September 2016.

Prior to therapy, HCV genotype should be determined, because the genotype dictates which treatment regimens are indicated **(Table 41-6)**. Monitoring of serum HCV RNA levels pretreatment, during treatment, and post-treatment is crucial in assessing response to therapy; moreover, the baseline level may contribute to determining the duration of therapy (e.g., in noncirrhotic patients with genotype 1 and HCV RNA $<6 \times 10^6$ IU/mL, 8 (instead of the usual 12) weeks of sofosbuvir/ledipasvir may be a consideration). The goal of treatment is to eradicate HCV RNA during therapy and to document that the virus remains undetectable for at least 12 weeks after completion of therapy (SVR_{12}).

INDICATIONS FOR ANTIVIRAL THERAPY Patients with chronic hepatitis C who have detectable HCV RNA in serum, whether or not aminotransferase levels are increased, and chronic hepatitis of any grade and stage (portal or bridging fibrosis) are candidates for antiviral therapy with direct-acting antiviral agents. The only exception would be patients with short life expectancies, for whom treating hepatitis C would have no influence on longevity. Certainly, for patients with advanced liver disease, early treatment merits a high priority. Although patients with persistently normal aminotransferase activity tend to progress histologically very slowly or not at all, they respond to antiviral therapy just as well as do patients with elevated aminotrasferase levels; therefore, although observation without therapy is an option, such patients are potential candidates for antiviral therapy. As noted above, antiviral therapy has been shown to improve survival and complication-free survival and to slow progression of (and to reverse) fibrosis.

HCV genotype determines the regimen to be selected (**Table 41-6**). Similarly, the absence or presence of cirrhosis/advanced fibrosis determines the treatment options from which to select, including the antiviral agents to be used, the duration of therapy, and the need for ribavirin (**Table 41-6**). A pretreatment liver biopsy to assess histologic grade and stage provides substantial information about progression of hepatitis C in the past, has prognostic value for future progression, and can identify such histologic factors as steatosis and stage of fibrosis, which can influence responsiveness to therapy. As therapy has improved for patients with a broad range of histologic severity, and as noninvasive measures of fibrosis stage (e.g., assessment of liver elasticity by imaging) have gained in accuracy and popularity, noninvasive approaches have supplanted histology in most cases, If cirrhosis/advanced fibrosis is present prior to therapy, the risk of hepatocellular carcinoma (HCC), although reduced substantially by successful therapy, is not eliminated, and twice yearly posttreatment imaging HCC surveillance (and endoscopic surveillance for esophageal varices at intervals of 1–3 years) is indicated even after an SVR. In patients with low-level fibrosis at baseline, achievement of an SVR allows the cessation of such surveillance.

Patients who have relapsed after, or failed to respond to, a course of IFN-based or direct-acting antiviral agent-based therapy are candidates for retreatment with a direct-acting antiviral therapy regimen (**Table 41-6**). For patients who have failed to respond to a direct-acting antiviral combination, options include increasing the duration of therapy with the failed regimen, adding ribavirin, or changing the drug class (e.g., after failed protease and polymerase inhibitors, switching to an NS5A-containing combination). In the presence of cirrhosis or a need for urgent retreatment, patients who have failed protease inhibitor plus polymerase inhibitor combination therapy or who have failed an NS5A combination are candidates for RAV testing and tailored therapy based on such resistance testing. Additional details for treatment of such patient subgroups can be found at www.hcvguidelines.org.

Persons with acute hepatitis C are also candidates for antiviral therapy (**Chap 39**) with the same direct-acting antiviral agents approved for chronic hepatitis C; delaying the initiation of therapy for an observation period of 12–16 weeks (and even up to 6 months) has been recommended to allow for spontaneous recovery, especially in light of the fact that most cases of acute hepatitis C are not clinically severe or rapidly progressive. The duration of therapy for acute hepatitis C has not been determined, but in a small study of 20 patients, 6 weeks of sofosbuvir/ledipasvir sufficed for a 100% SVR_{12}. In patients with biochemically and histologically mild chronic hepatitis C, the rate of progression is slow, and monitoring without therapy is an option; however, such patients respond just as well to antiviral therapy as those with elevated aminotransferase levels and more histologically severe hepatitis. Because of the high cost of direct-acting antiviral treatments, initially a higher priority was assigned to patients with advanced fibrosis/cirrhosis; however, this controversial approach was relied upon by some medical insurers and pharmacy benefit management organizations to withhold therapy from patients with low-level fibrosis. Unfortunately, delaying therapy until fibrosis becomes advanced misses the opportunity to prevent all the dire consequences of chronic hepatitis C (liver failure, death/transplantation, hepatocellular carcinoma), which can be reduced but not eliminated completely once advanced fibrosis is established. Therefore, therapy for patients with mild disease is justified (as it is cost-effective).

Patients with compensated cirrhosis can respond to therapy, and their likelihood of a sustained response with direct-acting antivirals is comparable to that in noncirrhotics. Patients with decompensated cirrhosis, who were not candidates for IFN-based antiviral therapy, respond well to direct-acting antiviral therapy combinations of polymerase inhibitors and NS5A inhibitors (e.g., sofosbuvir/ledipasir, sofosbuvir/valpatasvir), but protease-inhibitor-containing combinations have been associated with potential hepatotoxicity and hepatic decompensation and are contraindicated in this patient subset. Patients with decompensated cirrhosis should be referred to a liver transplantation center. Direct-acting antivirals are highly effective not only for patients with end-stage liver disease awaiting liver transplantation but also for patients with recurrent hepatitis C after liver transplantation. Ideally, patients should be treated prior to liver transplantation; however, a concern is that eradication of HCV infection will disqualify such patients from accepting donor livers from persons with HCV infection, contracting the potential donor pool and limiting accessibility to donor organs and timely transplantation. Therefore, advocacy has been expressed for postponing direct-acting antiviral therapy in patients with HCV-associated end-stage liver disease until after liver transplantation for end-stage liver disease caused by hepatitis C; whether to treat pretransplantation or posttransplantation should be individualized thoughtfully for each patient. The cutaneous and renal vasculitis of HCV-associated cryoglobulinemia may respond to antiviral therapy, but sustained responses were rare after discontinuation of therapy in the IFN era, and prolonged, potentially indefinite, therapy was recommended. Now that more effective direct-acting antivirals are available, a 12-week course of sofosbuvir-based therapy has been shown to yield and SVR_{12} rate exceeding 80% in cryoglobulinemic vasculitis. Anecdotal reports suggest that IFN based antiviral therapy may be effective in porphyria cutanea tarda or lichen planus associated with hepatitis C; whether the more appealing direct-acting antivirals are effective in these groups remains to be determined.

In patients with HCV/HIV co-infection, hepatitis C is more progressive and severe than in HCV-monoinfected patients. Although patients with HCV/HIV co-infection responded less well to IFN based antiviral therapy for hepatitis C, they respond as well as patients with HCV infection alone to direct-acting antiviral combination regimens.

In HCV/HIV-infected patients, ribavirin can potentiate the toxicity of didanosine (e.g., lactic acidosis) and the lipoatrophy of stavudine, and zidovudine can exacerbate ribavirin-associated hemolytic anemia; therefore, these drug combinations should be avoided.

Patients with a history of injection drug use and alcoholism can be treated successfully for chronic hepatitis C, preferably in conjunction with drug and alcohol treatment programs. Moreover, because injection-drug users, as a source of transmission to others, account disproportionately for perpetuating the spread of HCV infection in the population, the impact of treating active injection-drug users is amplified by reducing such transmission. The approved oral combinations of direct-acting antivirals are effective in patients with mild-modest renal failure and require no dose adjustments, but in patients with severe renal impairment (creatinine clearances <30 ml/minute), data are limited on the use of sofosbuvir-containing combinations. For such patients, including those undergoing hemodialysis, recommended combinations for genotypes 1a, 1b, and 4 are elbasvir/grazoprevir or for 12 weeks. In genotype 1a, the addition to paritaprevir/ritonavir, ombitasvir, and dasabuvir of 200 mg/day of ribavirin, if the hemoglobin level exceeds 10 g/dl, is an alternative regimen but requires vigilance for ribavirin-induced hemolytic anemia. For patients with severe renal impairment and HCV genotypes 2, 3, 5, or 6, PEG IFN with low-dose ribavirin (200 mg daily, if the hemoglobin exceeds 10 g/dl) is recommended. After renal transplantation, levels of SVR_{12} in patients treated with any of the approved oral combinations have approached 100%.

Choosing among available treatment options: The large number of recommended all-oral direct-acting antiviral combinations can be daunting to treating clinicians. In some instances, the combination approved is determined by insurance payers, but, cost considerations aside, how is the clinician to choose among the options? The most popular of the regimens has been fixed-dose, single-pill sofosbuvir/ledipasvir, which is effective for all genotypes except 2 and 3, and which can be used in noncirrhotic patients with genotype 1 and low-level viremia for as brief a period as 8 weeks. For genotypes 2 and 3, fixed-dose, single-pill sofosbuvir/valpatasvir appears to be the combination of choice; because this combination is so effective across all genotypes, in the future, for simplicity, clinicians may resort to a "one-size-fits-all" regimen like this one in all patients (except for those with advanced renal failure). As noted above, protease-inhibitor-containing direct-acting antiviral regimens (elbasvir/grazoprevir; paritaprevir/ritonavir, ombitasvir, and dasabuvir; simeprevir and sofosbuvir) are contraindicated in decompensated cirrhosis. For advanced renal failure, safety and efficacy have been documented for elbasvir/grazoprevir and paritaprevir/ritonavir, ombitasvir, and dasabuvir, not for sofosbuvir-NS5A combinations.

AUTOIMMUNE HEPATITIS

DEFINITION

Autoimmune hepatitis is a chronic disorder characterized by continuing hepatocellular necrosis and inflammation, usually with fibrosis, which can progress to cirrhosis and liver failure. When fulfilling criteria of severity, this type of chronic hepatitis, when untreated, may have a 6-month mortality of as high as 40%. Based on contemporary estimates of the natural history of autoimmune hepatitis, the 10-year survival is 80–98% for treated and 67% for untreated patients. The prominence of extrahepatic features of autoimmunity and seroimmunologic abnormalities in this disorder supports an autoimmune process in its pathogenesis; this concept is reflected in the prior labels *lupoid* and *plasma cell hepatitis*. Autoantibodies and other typical features of autoimmunity, however, do not occur in all cases; among the broader categories of "idiopathic" or cryptogenic chronic hepatitis, many, perhaps the majority, are probably autoimmune in origin. Cases in which hepatotropic viruses, metabolic/genetic derangements (including nonalcoholic fatty liver disease), and hepatotoxic drugs have been excluded represent a spectrum of heterogeneous liver disorders of unknown cause, a proportion of which are most likely autoimmune hepatitis.

IMMUNOPATHOGENESIS

The weight of evidence suggests that the progressive liver injury in patients with autoimmune hepatitis is the result of a cell-mediated immunologic attack directed against liver cells. In all likelihood, predisposition to autoimmunity is inherited, whereas the liver

specificity of this injury is triggered by environmental (e.g., chemical, drug [e.g., minocycline], or viral) factors. For example, patients have been described in whom apparently self-limited cases of acute hepatitis A, B, or C led to autoimmune hepatitis, presumably because of genetic susceptibility or predisposition. Evidence to support an autoimmune pathogenesis in this type of hepatitis includes the following: (1) In the liver, the histopathologic lesions are composed predominantly of cytotoxic T cells and plasma cells; (2) circulating autoantibodies (nuclear, smooth muscle, thyroid, etc.; see below), rheumatoid factor, and hyperglobulinemia are common; (3) other autoimmune disorders—such as thyroiditis, rheumatoid arthritis, autoimmune hemolytic anemia, ulcerative colitis, membranoproliferative glomerulonephritis, juvenile diabetes mellitus, celiac disease, and Sjögren's syndrome—occur with increased frequency in patients and in their relatives who have autoimmune hepatitis; (4) histocompatibility haplotypes associated with autoimmune diseases, such as HLA-B1, -B8, -DR3, and -DR4 as well as extended haplotype *DRB1*0301* and *DRB1*0401* alleles, are common in patients with autoimmune hepatitis; and (5) this type of chronic hepatitis is responsive to glucocorticoid/immunosuppressive therapy, effective in a variety of autoimmune disorders.

Cellular immune mechanisms appear to be important in the pathogenesis of autoimmune hepatitis. In vitro studies have suggested that in patients with this disorder, $CD4^+$ T lymphocytes are capable of becoming sensitized to hepatocyte membrane proteins and of destroying liver cells. Molecular mimicry by cross-reacting antigens that contain epitopes similar to liver antigens is postulated to activate these T cells, which infiltrate, and result in injury to, the liver. Abnormalities of immunoregulatory control over cytotoxic lymphocytes (impaired regulatory CD4+CD25+ T cell influences) may play a role as well. Studies of genetic predisposition to autoimmune hepatitis demonstrate that certain haplotypes are associated with the disorder, as enumerated above, as are polymorphisms in cytotoxic T lymphocyte antigens (*CTLA-4*) and tumor necrosis factor α (*TNFA*2*). The precise triggering factors, genetic influences, and cytotoxic and immunoregulatory mechanisms involved in this type of liver injury remain incompletely defined.

Intriguing clues into the pathogenesis of autoimmune hepatitis come from the observation that circulating autoantibodies are prevalent in patients with this disorder. Among the autoantibodies described in these patients are antibodies to nuclei (so-called antinuclear antibodies [ANAs], primarily in a homogeneous pattern) and smooth muscle (so-called anti-smooth-muscle antibodies, directed at actin, vimentin, and skeletin), antibodies to F-actin, antibodies to liver-kidney microsomes (anti-LKM, see below), antibodies to "soluble liver antigen" (directed against a uracil-guanine-adenine transfer RNA suppressor protein), antibodies to α-actinin, and antibodies to the liver-specific asialoglycoprotein receptor (or "hepatic lectin") and other hepatocyte membrane proteins. Although some of these provide helpful diagnostic markers, their involvement in the pathogenesis of autoimmune hepatitis has not been established.

Humoral immune mechanisms have been shown to play a role in the extrahepatic manifestations of autoimmune and idiopathic hepatitis. Arthralgias, arthritis, cutaneous vasculitis, and glomerulonephritis occurring in patients with autoimmune hepatitis appear to be mediated by the deposition of circulating immune complexes in affected tissue vessels, followed by complement activation, inflammation, and tissue injury. While specific viral antigen-antibody complexes can be identified in acute and chronic viral hepatitis, the nature of the immune complexes in autoimmune hepatitis has not been defined.

CLINICAL FEATURES

Many of the *clinical features* of autoimmune hepatitis are similar to those described for chronic viral hepatitis. The onset of disease may be insidious or abrupt; the disease may present initially like, and be confused with, acute viral hepatitis; a history of recurrent bouts of what had been labeled *acute hepatitis* is not uncommon. In approximately a quarter of patients, the diagnosis is made in the absence of symptoms, based on abnormal liver laboratory tests. A subset of patients with autoimmune hepatitis has distinct features. Such patients are predominantly young to middle-aged women with marked hyperglobulinemia and high-titer circulating ANAs. This is the group with positive lupus erythematosus (LE) preparations (initially labeled "*lupoid*" hepatitis) in whom other autoimmune features are common. Fatigue, malaise, anorexia, amenorrhea, acne, arthralgias, and jaundice are common. Occasionally, arthritis, maculopapular eruptions (including cutaneous vasculitis), erythema nodosum, colitis, pleurisy, pericarditis, anemia, azotemia, and sicca syndrome (keratoconjunctivitis, xerostomia) occur. In some patients, complications of cirrhosis, such as ascites and edema (associated with portal hypertension and hypoalbuminemia), encephalopathy, hypersplenism, coagulopathy, or variceal bleeding may bring the patient to initial medical attention.

The course of autoimmune hepatitis may be variable. In patients with mild disease or limited histologic lesions (e.g., piecemeal necrosis without bridging), progression to cirrhosis is limited, but, even in this subset, clinical monitoring is important to identify progression;

up to half left untreated can progress to cirrhosis over the course of 15 years. In North America, cirrhosis at presentation is more common in African Americans than in whites. In those with severe symptomatic autoimmune hepatitis (aminotransferase levels >10 times normal, marked hyperglobulinemia, "aggressive" histologic lesions—bridging necrosis or multilobular collapse, cirrhosis), the 6-month mortality without therapy may be as high as 40%. Such severe disease accounts for only 20% of cases; the natural history of milder disease is variable, often accentuated by spontaneous remissions and exacerbations. Especially poor prognostic signs include the presence histologically of multilobular collapse at the time of initial presentation and failure of serum bilirubin to improve after 2 weeks of therapy. Death may result from hepatic failure, hepatic coma, other complications of cirrhosis (e.g., variceal hemorrhage), and intercurrent infection. In patients with established cirrhosis, HCC may be a late complication **(Chap. 53)** but occurs less frequently than in cirrhosis associated with viral hepatitis.

Laboratory features of autoimmune hepatitis are similar to those seen in chronic viral hepatitis. Liver biochemical tests are invariably abnormal but may not correlate with the clinical severity or histopathologic features in individual cases. Many patients with autoimmune hepatitis have normal serum bilirubin, alkaline phosphatase, and globulin levels with only minimal aminotransferase elevations. Serum AST and ALT levels are increased and fluctuate in the range of 100–1000 units. In severe cases, the serum bilirubin level is moderately elevated (51–171 μmol/L [3–10 mg/dL]). Hypoalbuminemia occurs in patients with very active or advanced disease. Serum alkaline phosphatase levels may be moderately elevated or near normal. In a small proportion of patients, marked elevations of alkaline phosphatase activity occur; in such patients, clinical and laboratory features overlap with those of primary biliary cirrhosis **(Chap. 44)**. The prothrombin time is often prolonged, particularly late in the disease or during active phases.

Hypergammaglobulinemia (>2.5 g/dL) is common in autoimmune hepatitis, as is the presence of rheumatoid factor. As noted above, circulating autoantibodies are also prevalent, most characteristically ANAs in a homogeneous staining pattern. Smooth-muscle antibodies are less specific, seen just as frequently in chronic viral hepatitis. Because of the high levels of globulins achieved in the circulation of some patients with autoimmune hepatitis, occasionally the globulins may bind nonspecifically in solid-phase binding immunoassays for viral antibodies. This has been recognized most commonly in tests for antibodies to hepatitis C virus, as noted above. In fact, studies of autoantibodies in autoimmune hepatitis have led to the recognition of new categories of autoimmune hepatitis. *Type I autoimmune hepatitis* is the classic syndrome prevalent in North America and northern Europe occurring in young women, associated with marked hyperglobulinemia, lupoid features, circulating ANAs, and HLA- DR3 or HLA-DR4 (especially *B8-DRB1*03*). Also associated with type I autoimmune hepatitis are autoantibodies against actin and atypical perinuclear antineutrophilic cytoplasmic antibodies (pANCA).

Type II autoimmune hepatitis, often seen in children, more common in Mediterranean populations, and linked to HLA- DRB1 and HLA-DQB1 haplotypes, is associated not with ANA but with anti-LKM. Actually, anti-LKM represent a heterogeneous group of antibodies. In type II autoimmune hepatitis, the antibody is anti-LKM1, directed against cytochrome P450 2D6. This is the same anti-LKM seen in some patients with chronic hepatitis C. Anti-LKM2 is seen in drug-induced hepatitis, and anti-LKM3 (directed against uridine diphosphate glucuronyltransferases) is seen in patients with chronic hepatitis D. Another autoantibody observed in type II autoimmune hepatitis is directed against liver cytosol formiminotransferase cyclodeaminase (anti-liver cytosol 1). More controversial is whether or not a third category of autoimmune hepatitis exists, *type III autoimmune hepatitis*. These patients lack ANA and anti-LKM1 but have circulating antibodies to soluble liver antigen. Most of these patients are women and have clinical features similar to, perhaps more severe than, those of patients with type I autoimmune hepatitis. Type III autoimmune hepatitis does not appear to represent a distinct category but, instead, is part of the spectrum of type I autoimmune hepatitis; this subcategory has not been adopted by a consensus of international experts.

Liver biopsy abnormalities are similar to those described for chronic viral hepatitis. Expanding portal tracts and extending beyond the plate of periportal hepatocytes into the parenchyma (designated *interface hepatitis* or *piecemeal necrosis*) is a mononuclear cell infiltrate that, in autoimmune hepatitis, may include the presence of plasma cells. Necroinflammatory activity characterizes the lobular parenchyma, and evidence of hepatocellular regeneration is reflected by "rosette" formation, the occurrence of thickened liver cell plates, and regenerative "pseudolobules." Septal fibrosis, bridging fibrosis, and cirrhosis are frequent. In patients with early autoimmune hepatitis presenting as an acute-hepatitis-like illness, lobular and centrilobular (as opposed to the more common periportal) necrosis has been reported. Bile duct injury and granulomas are uncommon; however, a subgroup of patients with autoimmune hepatitis has histologic, biochemical, and serologic features overlapping those of primary biliary cirrhosis **(Chap. 44)**.

DIAGNOSTIC CRITERIA

An international group has suggested a set of criteria for establishing a diagnosis of autoimmune hepatitis. Exclusion of liver disease caused by genetic disorders, viral hepatitis, drug hepatotoxicity, and alcohol are linked with such inclusive diagnostic criteria as hyperglobulinemia, autoantibodies, and characteristic histologic features. This international group has also suggested a comprehensive diagnostic scoring system that, rarely required for typical cases, may be helpful when typical features are not present. Factors that weigh in favor of the diagnosis include female gender; predominant aminotransferase elevation; presence and level of globulin elevation; presence of nuclear, smooth muscle, LKM1, and other autoantibodies; concurrent other autoimmune diseases; characteristic histologic features (interface hepatitis, plasma cells, rosettes); HLA-DR3 or -DR4 markers; and response to treatment (see below). A more simplified, more specific scoring system relies on four variables: autoantibodies, serum IgG level, typical or compatible histologic features, and absence of viral hepatitis markers. Weighing against the diagnosis are predominant alkaline phosphatase elevation, mitochondrial antibodies, markers of viral hepatitis, history of hepatotoxic drugs or excessive alcohol, histologic evidence of bile duct injury, or such atypical histologic features as fatty infiltration, iron overload, and viral inclusions.

DIFFERENTIAL DIAGNOSIS

Early during the course of chronic hepatitis, autoimmune hepatitis may resemble typical *acute viral hepatitis* **(Chap. 39)**. Without histologic assessment, severe chronic hepatitis cannot be readily distinguished based on clinical or biochemical criteria from mild chronic hepatitis. In adolescence, *Wilson's disease* **(Chap. 44)** may present with features of chronic hepatitis long before neurologic manifestations become apparent and before the formation of Kayser-Fleischer rings (copper deposition in Descemet's membrane in the periphery of the cornea). In this age group, serum ceruloplasmin and serum and urinary copper determinations plus measurement of liver copper levels establish the correct diagnosis. *Postnecrotic* or *cryptogenic cirrhosis* and *primary biliary cirrhosis* **(Chap. 44)** share clinical features with autoimmune hepatitis, and both alcoholic hepatitis **(Chap. 42)** and nonalcoholic steatohepatitis **(Chap. 46)** may present with many features common to autoimmune hepatitis; historic, biochemical, serologic, and histologic assessments are usually sufficient to allow these entities to be distinguished from autoimmune hepatitis. Of course, the distinction between autoimmune and chronic viral hepatitis is not always straightforward, especially when viral antibodies occur in patients with autoimmune disease or when autoantibodies occur in patients with viral disease. Furthermore, the presence of extrahepatic features such as arthritis, cutaneous vasculitis, or pleuritis—not to mention the presence of circulating autoantibodies—may cause confusion with *rheumatologic disorders* such as rheumatoid arthritis and systemic lupus erythematosus. The existence of clinical and biochemical features of progressive necroinflammatory liver disease distinguishes chronic hepatitis from these other disorders, which are not associated with severe liver disease. Rarely, hepatic venous outflow obstruction (Budd-Chiari syndrome) may present with features suggestive of autoimmune hepatitis, but painful hepatomegaly, ascites, and vascular imaging provide distinguishing diagnostic clues. Other diagnostic considerations would include celiac disease and ischemic liver disease, which would be readily distinguishable by clinical and laboratory features from autoimmune hepatitis.

Finally, occasionally, features of autoimmune hepatitis overlap with features of autoimmune biliary disorders such as primary biliary cirrhosis, primary sclerosing cholangitis **(Chaps. 44 and 48)**, or, even more rarely, mitochondrial antibody-negative autoimmune cholangitis. Such overlap syndromes are difficult to categorize, and often response to therapy may be the distinguishing factor that establishes the diagnosis.

TREATMENT Autoimmune Hepatitis

The mainstay of management in autoimmune hepatitis is glucocorticoid therapy. Several controlled clinical trials have documented that such therapy leads to symptomatic, clinical, biochemical, and histologic improvement as well as increased survival. A therapeutic response can be expected in up to 80% of patients. Unfortunately, therapy has not been shown in clinical trials to prevent ultimate progression to cirrhosis; however, instances of reversal of fibrosis and cirrhosis have been reported in patients responding to treatment, and rapid treatment responses within 1 year do translate into a reduction in progression to cirrhosis. Although some advocate the use of prednisolone (the hepatic metabolite of prednisone), prednisone is just as effective and is favored by most authorities. Therapy may be initiated at 20 mg/d, but a popular regimen in the United States relies on an initiation dose of 60 mg/d. This high dose is tapered successively over the course of a month down to a maintenance level of 20 mg/d. An alternative, but equally effective, approach is to begin with half the prednisone dose (30 mg/d) along with azathioprine (50 mg/d). With azathioprine maintained at 50 mg/d, the prednisone dose is tapered over the course of a month down to a maintenance level of 10 mg/d. The advantage of the combination approach is a reduction, over the span of an 18-month course of therapy, in serious, life-threatening complications of steroid therapy (e.g., cushingoid features, hypertension, diabetes, osteoporosis) from 66% down to under 20%. Genetic analysis for thiopurine S-methyltransferase allelic variants does not correlate with azathioprine-associated cytopenias or efficacy and is not assessed routinely in patients with autoimmune hepatitis. In combination regimens, 6-mercaptopurine may be substituted for its prodrug azathioprine, but this is rarely required. Azathioprine alone, however, is not effective in achieving remission, nor is alternate-day glucocorticoid therapy. Limited experience with budesonide in noncirrhotic patients suggests that this steroid side effect–sparing drug may be effective. Although therapy has been shown to be effective for severe autoimmune hepatitis (AST ≥10 × the upper limit of normal or ≥5 × the upper limit of normal in conjunction with serum globulin greater than or equal to twice normal; bridging necrosis or multilobular necrosis on liver biopsy; presence of symptoms), therapy is not indicated for mild forms of chronic hepatitis, and the efficacy of therapy in mild or asymptomatic autoimmune hepatitis has not been established.

Improvement of fatigue, anorexia, malaise, and jaundice tends to occur within days to several weeks; biochemical improvement occurs over the course of several weeks to months, with a fall in serum bilirubin and globulin levels and an increase in serum albumin. Serum aminotransferase levels usually drop promptly, but improvements in AST and ALT alone do not appear to be reliable markers of recovery in individual patients; histologic improvement, characterized by a decrease in mononuclear infiltration and in hepatocellular necrosis, may be delayed for 6–24 months. Still, if interpreted cautiously, aminotransferase levels are valuable indicators of relative disease activity, and many authorities do *not* advocate for serial liver biopsies to assess therapeutic success or to guide decisions to alter or stop therapy. Rapidity of response is more common in older patients (≥69 years) and those with HLA *DBR1*04*; although rapid responders may progress less slowly to cirrhosis and liver transplantation, they are no less likely than slower responders to relapse after therapy. Therapy should continue for at least 12–18 months. After tapering and cessation of therapy, the likelihood of relapse is at least 50%, even if posttreatment histology has improved to show mild chronic hepatitis, and the majority of patients require therapy at maintenance doses indefinitely. Continuing azathioprine alone (2 mg/kg body weight daily) after cessation of prednisone therapy has been shown to reduce the frequency of relapse. Long-term maintenance with low-dose prednisone (≤10 mg daily) has also been shown to keep autoimmune hepatitis in check, but maintenance azathioprine is more effective in maintaining remission.

In medically refractory cases, an attempt should be made to intensify treatment with high-dose glucocorticoid monotherapy(60 mg daily) or combination glucocorticoid (30 mg daily) plus high-dose azathioprine (150 mg daily) therapy. After a month, doses of prednisone can be reduced by 10 mg a month, and doses of azathioprine can be reduced by 50 mg a month toward ultimate, conventional maintenance doses. Patients refractory to this regimen may be treated with cyclosporine, tacrolimus, or mycophenolate mofetil; however, to date, only limited anecdotal reports support these approaches. If medical therapy fails, or when chronic hepatitis progresses to cirrhosis and is associated with life-threatening complications of liver decompensation, liver transplantation is the only recourse **(Chap. 48)**; failure of the bilirubin to improve after 2 weeks of therapy should prompt early consideration of the patient for liver transplantation. Recurrence of autoimmune hepatitis in the new liver occurs rarely in most experiences but in as many as 35–40% of cases in others.

Like all patients with chronic liver disease, patients with autoimmune hepatitis should be vaccinated against hepatitis A and B, ideally before immunosuppressive therapy is begun, if practical.

ACKNOWLEDGMENT

Kurt J. Isselbacher, MD, contributed to this chapter in previous editions of Harrison's.

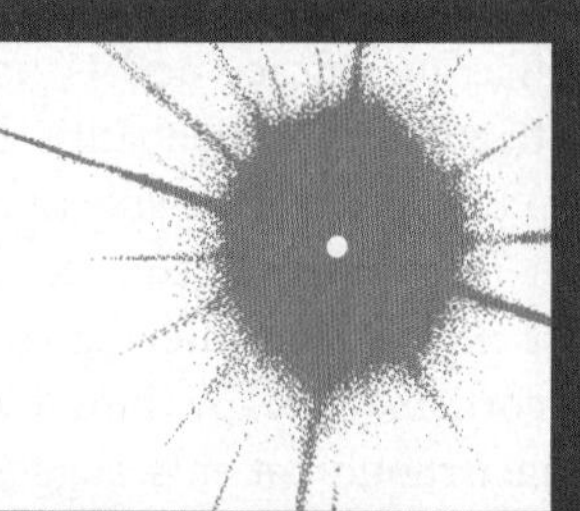

CHAPTER 42

ALCOHOLIC LIVER DISEASE

Mark E. Mailliard ■ Michael F. Sorrell

Chronic and excessive alcohol ingestion is one of the major causes of liver disease. The pathology of alcoholic liver disease consists of three major lesions, with the progressive injury rarely existing in a pure form: (1) fatty liver, (2) alcoholic hepatitis, and (3) cirrhosis. Fatty liver is present in >90% of daily as well as binge drinkers. A much smaller percentage of heavy drinkers will progress to alcoholic hepatitis, thought to be a precursor to cirrhosis. The prognosis of severe alcoholic liver disease is dismal; the mortality of patients with alcoholic hepatitis concurrent with cirrhosis is nearly 60% at 4 years. Although alcohol is considered a direct hepatotoxin, only between 10 and 20% of alcoholics will develop alcoholic hepatitis. The explanation for this apparent paradox is unclear but involves the complex interaction of facilitating factors, such as drinking patterns, diet, obesity, and gender. There are no diagnostic tools that can predict individual susceptibility to alcoholic liver disease.

GLOBAL CONSIDERATIONS

Alcohol is the world's third largest risk factor for disease burden. The harmful use of alcohol results in 2.5 million deaths each year. Most of the mortality attributed to alcohol is secondary to cirrhosis. Mortality from cirrhosis is declining in most Western countries, concurrent with a reduction in alcohol consumption, with the exceptions of the United Kingdom, Russia, Romania, and Hungary. These increases in cirrhosis and its complications are closely correlated with increased volume of alcohol consumed per capita population and are regardless of gender.

ETIOLOGY AND PATHOGENESIS

Quantity and duration of alcohol intake are the most important risk factors involved in the development of alcoholic liver disease (Table 42-1). The roles of beverage type(s), i.e. wine, beer, or spirits, and pattern of drinking (daily versus binge drinking) are less clear. Progress beyond the fatty liver stage seems to require additional risk factors that remain incompletely defined. Although there are genetic predispositions for alcoholism, gender is a strong determinant for alcoholic liver disease. Women are more susceptible to alcoholic liver injury when compared to men. They develop advanced liver disease with substantially less alcohol intake. In general, the time it takes to develop liver disease is directly related to the amount of alcohol consumed. It is useful in estimating alcohol consumption to understand that one beer, four ounces of wine, or one ounce of 80% spirits all contain ~12 g of alcohol. The threshold for developing alcoholic liver disease is higher in men, while women are at increased risk for

TABLE 42-1

RISK FACTORS FOR ALCOHOLIC LIVER DISEASE

RISK FACTOR	COMMENT
Quantity	In men, 40–80 g/d of ethanol produces fatty liver; 160 g/d for 10–20 years causes hepatitis or cirrhosis. Only 15% of alcoholics develop alcoholic liver disease.
Gender	Women exhibit increased susceptibility to alcoholic liver disease at amounts >20 g/d; two drinks per day is probably safe.
Hepatitis C	HCV infection concurrent with alcoholic liver disease is associated with younger age for severity, more advanced histology, and decreased survival.
Genetics	Patatin-like phospholipase domain-containing protein 3 (PNPLA3) has been associated with alcoholiccirrhosis.
Fatty liver	Alcohol injury does not require malnutrition, but obesity and nonalcoholic fatty liver are risk factors. Patients should receive vigorous attention to nutritional support.

developing similar degrees of liver injury by consuming significantly less. Gender-dependent differences result from poorly understood effects of estrogen, proportion of body fat, and the gastric metabolism of alcohol. Obesity, a high-fat diet, and the protective effect of coffee have been postulated to play a part in the development of the pathogenic process.

Chronic infection with hepatitis C virus (HCV) **(Chap. 41)** is an important comorbidity in the progression of alcoholic liver disease to cirrhosis in chronic and excessive drinkers. Even moderate alcohol intake of 20–50 g/d increases the risk of cirrhosis and hepatocellular cancer in HCV-infected individuals. Patients with both alcoholic liver injury and HCV infection develop decompensated liver disease at a younger age and have poorer overall survival. Increased liver iron stores and, rarely, porphyria cutanea tarda can occur as a consequence of the overlapping injurious processes secondary to alcohol abuse and HCV infection. In addition, alcohol intake of >50 g/d by HCV-infected patients decreases the efficacy of interferon-based antiviral therapy.

The pathogenesis of alcoholic liver injury is unclear. The present conceptual foundation is that alcohol acts as a direct hepatotoxin and that malnutrition does not have a major role. Ingestion of alcohol initiates an inflammatory cascade by its metabolism to acetaldehyde, resulting in a variety of metabolic responses. Steatosis from lipogenesis, fatty acid synthesis, and depression of fatty acid oxidation appears secondary to effects on sterol regulatory transcription factor and peroxisome proliferator-activated receptor α (PPAR-α). Intestinal-derived endotoxin initiates a pathogenic process through toll-like receptor 4 and tumor necrosis factor α (TNF-α) that facilitates hepatocyte apoptosis and necrosis. The cell injury and endotoxin release initiated by ethanol and its metabolites also activate innate and adaptive immunity pathways releasing proinflammatory cytokines (e.g., TNF-α), chemokines, and proliferation of T and B cells. The production of toxic protein-aldehyde adducts, generation of reducing equivalents, and oxidative stress also contribute to the liver injury. Hepatocyte injury and impaired regeneration following chronic alcohol ingestion are ultimately associated with stellate cell activation and collagen production, which are key events in fibrogenesis. The resulting fibrosis from continuing alcohol use determines the architectural derangement of the liver and associated pathophysiology.

PATHOLOGY

The liver has a limited repertoire in response to injury. Fatty liver is the initial and most common histologic response to hepatotoxic stimuli, including excessive alcohol ingestion. The accumulation of fat within the perivenular hepatocytes coincides with the location of alcohol dehydrogenase, the major enzyme responsible for alcohol metabolism. Continuing alcohol ingestion results in fat accumulation throughout the entire hepatic lobule. Despite extensive fatty change and distortion of the hepatocytes with macrovesicular fat, the cessation of drinking results in normalization of hepatic architecture and fat content. Alcoholic fatty liver has traditionally been regarded as entirely benign, but similar to the spectrum of nonalcoholic fatty liver disease **(Chap. 46)**, the appearance of steatohepatitis and certain pathologic features such as giant mitochondria, perivenular fibrosis, and macrovesicular fat may be associated with progressive liver injury.

The transition between fatty liver and the development of alcoholic hepatitis is blurred. The hallmark of alcoholic hepatitis is hepatocyte injury characterized by ballooning degeneration, spotty necrosis, polymorphonuclear infiltrate, and fibrosis in the perivenular and perisinusoidal space of Disse. Mallory-Denk bodies are often present in florid cases but are neither specific nor necessary to establish the diagnosis. Alcoholic hepatitis is thought to be a precursor to the development of cirrhosis. However, like fatty liver, it is potentially reversible with cessation of drinking. Cirrhosis is present in up to 50% of patients with biopsy-proven alcoholic hepatitis, and its regression is uncertain, even with abstention.

CLINICAL FEATURES

The clinical manifestations of alcoholic fatty liver are subtle and characteristically detected as a consequence of the patient's visit for a seemingly unrelated matter. Previously unsuspected hepatomegaly is often the only clinical finding. Occasionally, patients with fatty liver will present with right upper quadrant discomfort, nausea, and, rarely, jaundice. Differentiation of alcoholic fatty liver from nonalcoholic fatty liver is difficult unless an accurate drinking history is ascertained. In every instance where liver disease is present, a thoughtful and sensitive drinking history should be obtained. Standard, validated questions accurately detect alcohol-related problems. Alcoholic hepatitis is associated with a wide gamut of clinical features. Fever, spider nevi, jaundice, and abdominal pain simulating an acute abdomen represent the extreme end of the spectrum, while many patients will be entirely asymptomatic. Portal hypertension, ascites, or variceal bleeding can occur in the absence of cirrhosis. Recognition of the clinical features of alcoholic hepatitis is central to the initiation of an effective and appropriate diagnostic and therapeutic strategy. It is important to recognize that patients with alcoholic cirrhosis often exhibit clinical features identical to other causes of cirrhosis.

LABORATORY FEATURES

Patients with alcoholic liver disease are often identified through routine screening tests. The typical laboratory abnormalities seen in fatty liver are nonspecific and include modest elevations of aspartate aminotransferase (AST), alanine aminotransferase (ALT), and γ-glutamyl transpeptidase (GGTP), often accompanied by hypertriglyceridemia and hyperbilirubinemia. In alcoholic hepatitis and in contrast to other causes of fatty liver, AST and ALT are usually elevated two- to sevenfold. They are rarely >400 IU, and the AST/ALT ratio is >1 (Table 42-2). Hyperbilirubinemia is accompanied by modest increases in the alkaline phosphatase level. Derangement in hepatocyte synthetic function indicates more serious disease. Hypoalbuminemia and coagulopathy are common in advanced liver injury. Ultrasonography is useful in detecting fatty infiltration of the liver and determining liver size. The demonstration by ultrasound of portal vein flow reversal, ascites, and intraabdominal venous collaterals indicates serious liver injury with less potential for complete reversal.

PROGNOSIS

Critically ill patients with alcoholic hepatitis have short-term (30-day) mortality rates >50%. Severe alcoholic hepatitis is heralded by coagulopathy (prothrombin time increased >5 s), anemia, serum albumin concentrations <25 g/L (2.5 mg/dL), serum bilirubin levels >137 μmol/L (8 mg/dL), renal failure, and ascites. A discriminant function calculated as 4.6 X (the prolongation of the prothrombin time above control [seconds]) + serum bilirubin (mg/dL) can identify patients with a poor prognosis (discriminant function >32). A Model for End-Stage Liver Disease (MELD) score **(Chap. 48)** ≥21 also is associated with significant mortality in alcoholic hepatitis. The presence of ascites, variceal hemorrhage, deep encephalopathy, or hepatorenal syndrome predicts a dismal prognosis. The pathologic stage of the injury can be helpful in predicting prognosis. Liver biopsy should be performed whenever possible to establish the diagnosis and to guide the therapeutic decisions.

TABLE 42-2

LABORATORY DIAGNOSIS OF ALCOHOLIC FATTY LIVER AND ALCOHOLIC HEPATITIS

TEST	COMMENT
AST	Increased two- to sevenfold, <400 IU/L, greaterthan ALT
ALT	Increased two- to sevenfold, <400 IU/L
AST/ALT	Usually >1
GGTP	Not specific to alcohol, easily inducible, elevated in all forms of fatty liver
Bilirubin	May be markedly increased in alcoholic hepatitis despite modest elevation in alkaline phosphatase

Abbreviations: ALT, alanine aminotransferase; AST, aspartate aminotransferase; GGTP, γ-glutamyl transpeptidase.

TREATMENT Alcoholic Liver Disease

Complete abstinence from alcohol is the cornerstone in the treatment of alcoholic liver disease. Improved survival and the potential for reversal of histologic injury regardless of the initial clinical presentation are associated with total avoidance of alcohol ingestion. Referral of patients to experienced alcohol counselors and/or alcohol treatment programs should be routine in the management of patients with alcoholic liver disease. Attention should be directed to the nutritional and psychosocial states during the evaluation and treatment periods. Because of data suggesting that the pathogenic mechanisms in alcoholic hepatitis involve cytokine release and the perpetuation of injury by immunologic processes, glucocorticoids have been extensively evaluated in the treatment of alcoholic hepatitis. Patients with severe alcoholic hepatitis, defined as a discriminant function >32 or MELD >20, should be given prednisone, 40 mg/d, or prednisolone, 32 mg/d, for 4 weeks, followed by a steroid taper (Fig. 42-1). Exclusion criteria include active gastrointestinal bleeding, renal failure, or pancreatitis. Women with encephalopathy from severe alcoholic hepatitis may be particularly good candidates for glucocorticoids. A Lille score >0.45, at *http://www.lillemodel.com*, uses pretreatment variables plus the change in total bilirubin at day 7 of glucocorticoids to identify patients unresponsive to therapy.

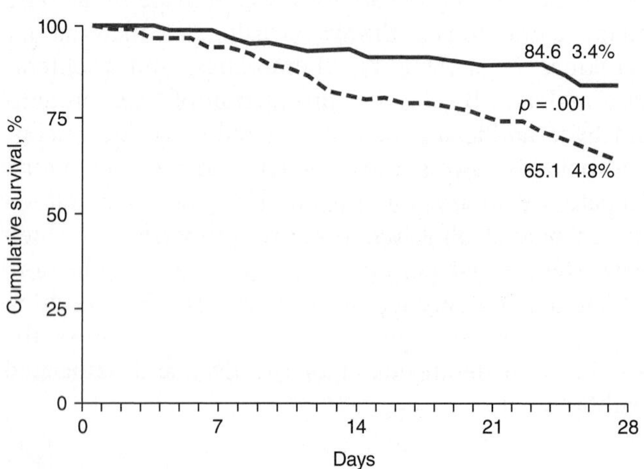

FIGURE 42-1

Effect of glucocorticoid therapy of severe alcoholic hepatitis on short-term survival: the result of a meta-analysis of individual data from three studies. Prednisolone, solid line; placebo, dotted line. *(Adapted from P Mathurin et al: J Hepatol 36:480, 2002, with permission from Elsevier Science.)*

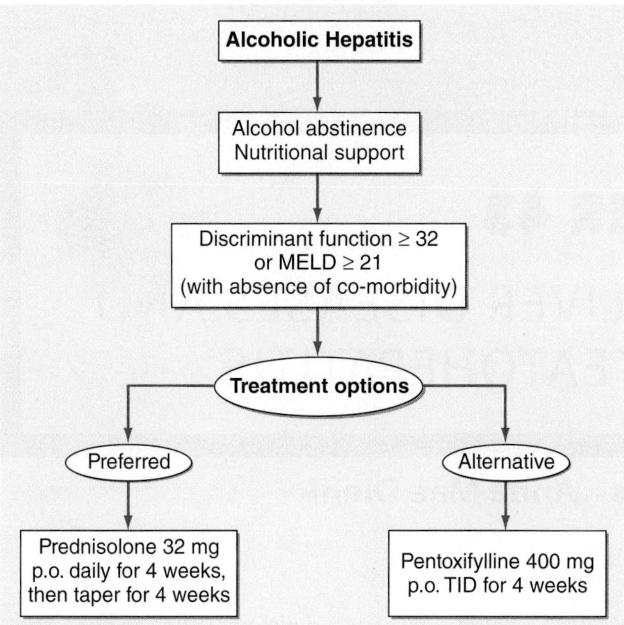

FIGURE 42-2

Treatment algorithm for alcoholic hepatitis. As identified by a calculated discriminant function >32 (see text), patients with severe alcoholic hepatitis, without the presence of gastrointestinal bleeding or infection, would be candidates for either glucocorticoids or pentoxifylline administration.

The role of TNF-α expression and receptor activity in alcoholic liver injury has led to an examination of TNF inhibition as an alternative to glucocorticoids for severe alcoholic hepatitis. The nonspecific TNF inhibitor, pentoxifylline, demonstrated improved survival in the therapy of severe alcoholic hepatitis, primarily due to a decrease in hepatorenal syndrome (Fig. 42-2). Monoclonal antibodies that neutralize serum TNF-α should not be used in alcoholic hepatitis because of studies reporting increased deaths secondary to infection and renal failure.

Liver transplantation is an accepted indication for treatment in selected and motivated patients with end-stage cirrhosis. Outcomes are equal or superior to other indications for transplantation. In general, transplant candidacy should be reevaluated after a defined period of sobriety. Patients presenting with alcoholic hepatitis have been largely excluded from transplant candidacy because of the perceived risk of increased surgical mortality and high rates of recidivism following transplantation. Recently, a European multidisciplinary group has reported excellent long-term transplant outcomes in highly selected patients with florid alcoholic hepatitis. General application of transplantation in such patients must await confirmatory outcomes by others.

CHAPTER 43

NONALCOHOLIC FATTY LIVER DISEASES AND NONALCOHOLIC STEATOHEPATITIS

Manal F. Abdelmalek ■ Anna Mae Diehl

INCIDENCE, PREVALENCE, AND NATURAL HISTORY

Nonalcoholic fatty liver disease (NAFLD) is the most common chronic liver disease in many parts of the world, including the United States. Population-based abdominal imaging studies have demonstrated fatty liver in at least 25% of American adults. Because the vast majority of these subjects deny hazardous levels of alcohol consumption (defined as greater than one drink per day in women or two drinks per day in men), they are considered to have NAFLD. NAFLD is strongly associated with overweight/obesity and insulin resistance. However, it can also occur in lean individuals and is particularly common in those with a paucity of adipose depots (i.e., lipodystrophy). Ethnic/racial factors also appear to influence liver fat accumulation; the documented prevalence of NAFLD is lowest in African Americans (~25%), highest in Americans of Hispanic ancestry (~50%), and intermediate in American whites (~33%).

NAFLD encompasses a spectrum of liver pathology with different clinical prognoses. The simple accumulation of triglyceride within hepatocytes (hepatic steatosis) is on the most clinically benign extreme of the spectrum. On the opposite, most clinically ominous extreme, are cirrhosis **(Chap. 44)** and primary liver cancer **(Chap. 53)**. The risk of developing cirrhosis is extremely low in individuals with chronic hepatic steatosis, but increases as steatosis becomes complicated by histologically conspicuous hepatocyte death and inflammation (i.e., nonalcoholic steatohepatitis [NASH]). NASH itself is also a heterogeneous condition; sometimes it improves to steatosis or normal histology, sometimes it remains relatively stable for years, but sometimes it results in progressive accumulation of fibrous scar that eventuates in cirrhosis. Once NAFLD-related cirrhosis develops, the annual incidence of primary liver cancer is 1%.

Abdominal imaging is not able to determine which individuals with NAFLD have associated liver cell death and inflammation (i.e., NASH), and specific blood tests to diagnose NASH are not yet available. However, population-based studies that have used elevated serum ALT as a marker of liver injury indicate that about 6–8% of American adults have serum ALT elevations that cannot be explained by excessive alcohol consumption, other known causes of fatty liver disease (Table 43-1), viral hepatitis, or drug-induced or congenital liver diseases. Because the prevalence of such "cryptogenic" ALT elevations increases with body mass index, it is presumed that they are due to NASH. Hence, at any given point in time, NASH is present in about 25% of individuals who have NAFLD (i.e., about 6% of the general U.S. adult population has NASH). Smaller cross-sectional studies in which liver biopsies have been performed on NASH patients at tertiary referral centers consistently demonstrate advanced fibrosis or cirrhosis in about 25% of those cohorts. By extrapolation, therefore, cirrhosis develops in about 6% of individuals with NAFLD (i.e., in about 1.5–2% of the general U.S. population). The risk for advanced liver fibrosis is highest in individuals with NASH who are older than 45–50 years of age and overweight/obese or afflicted with type 2 diabetes.

To put these data in perspective, it is helpful to recall that the prevalence of hepatitis C–related cirrhosis in the United States is about 0.5%. Thus, NAFLD-related cirrhosis is about three to four times more common than cirrhosis caused by chronic hepatitis C infection. Consistent with these data, experts have predicted that NAFLD will surpass hepatitis C as the leading indication for liver transplantation in the United States within

TABLE 43-1

ALTERNATIVE CAUSES OF HEPATIC STEATOSIS

- Alcoholic liver disease
- Hepatitis C (particularly genotype 3)
- Inborn errors of metabolism
  - Abetalipoproteinemia
  - Cholesterol ester storage disease
  - Galactosemia
  - Glycogen storage disease
  - Hereditary fructose intolerance
  - Homocystinuria
  - Systemic carnitine deficiency
  - Tyrosinemia
  - Weber-Christian syndrome
  - Wilson's disease
  - Wolman's disease
- Medications (see Table 43–2)
- Miscellaneous
  - Industrial exposure to petrochemical
  - Inflammatory bowel disease
  - Lipodystrophy
  - Bacterial overgrowth
  - Starvation
  - Parenteral nutrition
- Surgical procedures
  - Bilopancreatic diversion
  - Extensive small-bowel resection
  - Gastric bypass
  - Jejunoileal bypass
- Reye's syndrome
- Acute fatty liver of pregnancy
- HELLP syndrome (*h*emolytic anemia, *e*levated *l*iver enzymes, *l*ow *p*latelet count)

TABLE 43-2

MEDICATIONS ASSOCIATED WITH HEPATIC STEATOSIS

- Cytotoxic and cytostatic drugs
  - l-Asparaginase
  - Azacitidine
  - Azaserine
  - Bleomycin
  - Methotrexate
  - Puromycin
  - Tetracycline
  - Doxycycline
- Metals
  - Antimony
  - Barium salts
  - Chromates
  - Phosphorus
  - Rare earths of low atomic number
  - Thallium compounds
  - Uranium compounds
- Other drugs and toxins
  - Amiodarone
  - 4,4′-Diethylaminoethoxyhexesterol
  - Ethionine
  - Ethyl bromide
  - Estrogens
  - Glucocorticoids
  - Highly active antiretroviral therapy
  - Hydralazine
  - Hypoglycin
  - Orotate
  - Perhexiline maleate
  - Safrole
  - Tamoxifen

the next decade. Similar to cirrhosis caused by other liver diseases, cirrhosis caused by NAFLD increases the risk for primary liver cancer. Both hepatocellular carcinoma and intrahepatic cholangiocarcinoma (ICC) have also been reported to occur in NAFLD patients without cirrhosis, suggesting that NAFLD per se may be a premalignant condition. NAFLD, NASH, and NAFLD-related cirrhosis are not limited to adults. All have been well documented in children. As in adults, obesity and insulin resistance are the main risk factors for pediatric NAFLD. Thus, the rising incidence and prevalence of childhood obesity suggests that NAFLD is likely to become an even greater contributor to society's burden of liver disease in the future.

PATHOGENESIS

The mechanisms underlying the pathogenesis and progression of NAFLD are not entirely clear. The best-understood mechanisms pertain to hepatic steatosis. This is proven to result when hepatocyte mechanisms for triglyceride synthesis (e.g., lipid uptake and de novo lipogenesis) overwhelm mechanisms for triglyceride disposal (e.g., degradative metabolism and lipoprotein export), leading to accumulation of fat (i.e., triglyceride) within hepatocytes. Obesity stimulates hepatocyte triglyceride accumulation by altering the intestinal microbiota to enhance both energy harvest from dietary sources and intestinal permeability. Reduced intestinal barrier function increases hepatic exposure to gut-derived products, which stimulate liver cells to generate inflammatory mediators that inhibit insulin actions. Obese adipose depots also produce excessive soluble factors (adipokines) that inhibit tissue insulin sensitivity. Insulin resistance promotes hyperglycemia. This drives the pancreas to produce more insulin to maintain glucose homeostasis. However, hyperinsulinemia also promotes lipid uptake, fat synthesis, and fat storage. The net result is hepatic triglyceride accumulation (i.e., steatosis).

Triglyceride per se is not hepatotoxic. However, its precursors (e.g., fatty acids and diacylglycerols) and metabolic by-products (e.g., reactive oxygen species) may damage hepatocytes, leading to hepatocyte lipotoxicity. Lipotoxicity also triggers the generation of other factors (e.g., inflammatory cytokines, hormonal mediators) that deregulate systems that normally maintain hepatocyte viability. The net result is increased hepatocyte death. Dying hepatocytes, in turn, release various factors that trigger wound healing responses that aim to replace (regenerate) lost hepatocytes. Such repair involves transient expansion of other cell types, such as myofibroblasts and progenitor cells, that make and degrade matrix, remodel the vasculature, and generate replacement hepatocytes, as well as the recruitment of immune cells that release factors that modulate liver injury and repair. NASH is the morphologic manifestation of lipotoxicity and resultant wound healing responses. Because the severity and duration of lipotoxic liver injury dictate the intensity and duration of repair, the histologic features and outcomes of NASH are variable. Cirrhosis and liver cancer are potential outcomes of chronic NASH. Cirrhosis results from futile repair, i.e., progressive accumulation of wound healing cells, fibrous matrix, and abnormal vasculature (scarring), rather than efficient reconstruction/regeneration of healthy hepatic parenchyma. Primary liver cancers develop when malignantly transformed liver cells escape mechanisms that normally control regenerative growth. The mechanisms responsible for futile repair (cirrhosis) and liver carcinogenesis are not well understood. Because normal liver regeneration is a very complex process, there are multiple opportunities for deregulation and, thus, pathogenic heterogeneity. To date, this heterogeneity has confounded development of both diagnostic tests and treatments for defective/deregulated liver repair (i.e., cirrhosis and cancer). Hence, current strategies focus on circumventing misrepair by preventing and/or reducing lipotoxic liver injury.

DIAGNOSIS

Diagnosing NAFLD requires demonstration of increased liver fat in the absence of hazardous levels of alcohol consumption. Thresholds for potentially dangerous alcohol ingestion have been set at more than one drink per day in women and two drinks per day in men based on epidemiologic evidence that the prevalence of serum aminotransferase elevations increases when alcohol consumption habitually exceeds these levels. In those studies, one drink was defined as having 10 g of ethanol and, thus, is equivalent to one can of beer, 4 ounces of wine, or 1.5 ounces (one shot) of distilled spirits. Other causes of liver fat accumulation (particularly exposure to certain drugs; Table 43-2) and liver injury (e.g., viral hepatitis, autoimmune liver disease, iron or copper overload, α_1 antitrypsin deficiency) must also be excluded. Thus, establishing the diagnosis of NAFLD does not require invasive testing: it can be accomplished by history and physical examination, liver imaging (ultrasound is an acceptable first-line test; computed tomography [CT] or magnetic resonance imaging [MRI] enhances sensitivity for liver fat detection but adds expense), and blood tests to exclude other liver diseases. It is important to emphasize that the liver may not be enlarged, and serum aminotransferases and liver function tests (e.g., bilirubin, albumin, prothrombin time) may be completely normal, in individuals with NAFLD. Because there is yet no one specific blood test for NAFLD, confidence in the diagnosis of NAFLD is increased by identification of NAFLD risk factors. The latter include increased body mass index, insulin resistance/type 2 diabetes mellitus, and other parameters indicative of the metabolic syndrome (e.g., systemic hypertension, dyslipidemia, hyperuricemia/gout, cardiovascular disease; **Chap. 63**) in the patient or family members.

Establishing the severity of NAFLD-related liver injury and related scarring (i.e., staging NAFLD) is more difficult than simply diagnosing NAFLD. Staging is critically important, however, because it is necessary to define prognosis and thereby determine treatment recommendations. The goal of staging is to distinguish patients with NASH from those with simple steatosis and to identify which of the NASH patients have advanced fibrosis. The 10-year probability of developing liver-related morbidity or mortality in steatosis is negligible, and hence, this subgroup of NAFLD patients tends to be managed conservatively (see below). In contrast, more intensive follow-up and therapy are justified in NASH patients, and the subgroup with advanced fibrosis merits the most intensive scrutiny and intervention because their 10-year risk of liver-related morbidity and mortality is clearly increased.

Staging approaches can be separated into noninvasive testing (i.e., blood testing, physical examination, and imaging) and invasive approaches (i.e., liver biopsy). Blood test evidence of hepatic dysfunction (e.g., hyperbilirubinemia, hypoalbuminemia, prothrombin time prolongation) or portal hypertension (e.g., thrombocytopenia) and stigmata of portal hypertension on physical examination (e.g., spider angiomata, palmar erythema, splenomegaly, ascites, clubbing, encephalopathy) suggest a diagnosis of advanced NAFLD. Currently, however, liver biopsy is the gold standard for establishing the severity of liver injury and fibrosis because it is both more sensitive and specific than these other tests for establishing NAFLD severity. Although invasive, liver biopsy is seldom complicated by serious adverse sequelae such as significant bleeding, pain, or inadvertent puncture of other organs and thus is relatively safe. However, biopsy suffers from potential sampling error unless tissue cores of 2 cm or longer are acquired. Also, examination of tissue at a single point in time is not reliable for determining whether the pathologic processes are progressing or regressing. The risk of serial liver biopsies within short time intervals is generally deemed as unacceptable outside of research studies. These limitations of liver biopsy have stimulated efforts to develop noninvasive approaches to stage NAFLD. As is true for many other types of chronic liver disease, in NAFLD the levels of serum aminotransferases (aspartate aminotransferase [AST] and alanine aminotransferase [ALT]) do not reliably reflect the severity of liver cell injury, extent of liver cell death, or related liver inflammation and fibrosis. Thus, they are imperfect for determining which individuals with NAFLD have NASH. This has stimulated research to identify superior markers of liver injury. Serum levels of keratin 8 and keratin 18 appear to be promising surrogates. Keratins 8 and 18 (K8/18) are epithelial cytoskeletal proteins that undergo cleavage during programmed cell death (apoptosis). Both cleaved and full-length K8/18 are released into the blood as hepatocytes die, and studies suggest that serum levels of K8/18 differentiate individuals with NASH from those with simple steatosis or normal livers more reliably than do serum aminotransferase levels. Moreover, K8/18 levels appear to parallel the severity of liver fibrosis, with higher levels marking individuals who are likely to have worse scarring (i.e., advanced liver fibrosis or cirrhosis). While promising, testing for K8/18 has not yet become standard clinical practice. Other blood tests and imaging approaches that quantify liver fibrosis are also being developed. Recently, the U.S. Food and Drug Administration (FDA) approved an ultrasound-based test that measures liver stiffness as a surrogate marker of fibrosis (FibroScan®) (**Chap. 37**). This new tool will likely be used serially to monitor fibrosis progression and regression in NAFLD patients. Studies that compare the receiver operator characteristics of K8/18 plus FibroScan versus liver biopsy for monitoring NAFLD evolution are forthcoming.

CLINICAL FEATURES OF NAFLD

Most subjects with NAFLD are asymptomatic. The diagnosis is often made when abnormal liver aminotransferases or features of fatty liver are noted during an evaluation performed for other reasons. NAFLD may also be diagnosed during the workup of vague right upper quadrant abdominal pain, hepatomegaly, or an abnormal-appearing liver at time of abdominal surgery. Obesity is present in 50–90% of subjects. Most patients with NAFLD also have other features of the metabolic syndrome (**Chap. 63**). Some have subtle stigmata of chronic liver disease, such as spider angiomata, palmer erythema, or splenomegaly. In a small minority of patients with advanced NAFLD, complications of end-stage liver disease (e.g., jaundice, features of portal hypertension such as ascites or variceal hemorrhage) may be the initial findings.

The association of NAFLD with obesity, diabetes, hypertriglyceridemia, hypertension, and cardiovascular disease is well known. Other associations include chronic fatigue, mood alterations, obstructive sleep apnea, thyroid dysfunction, and chronic pain syndrome. NAFLD is an independent risk factor for metabolic syndrome (**Chap. 63**). Longitudinal studies suggest that patients with NASH are at two- to threefold increased risk for the development of metabolic syndrome. Similarly, studies have shown that patients with NASH have a higher risk for the development of hypertension and diabetes mellitus. The presence of NAFLD is also independently associated with endothelial dysfunction, increased carotid intimal thickness, and the number of plaques in carotid and coronary arteries. Such data indicate that NAFLD has many deleterious effects on health in general.

TREATMENT OF NAFLD

Treatment of NAFLD can be divided into three components: (1) specific therapy of NAFLD-related liver disease; (2) treatment of NAFLD-associated comorbidities; and (3) treatment of the complications of advanced NAFLD. The subsequent discussion focuses on specific therapies for NAFLD, with some mention of their impact on major NAFLD comorbidities (insulin resistance/diabetes, obesity, and dyslipidemia). Treatment of the complications of advanced NAFLD involves management of the complications of cirrhosis and portal hypertension, including primary liver cancers. Approaches to accomplish these objectives are similar to those used in other chronic liver diseases and are covered elsewhere in the textbook (**Chaps. 44 and 53**).

At present, there are no FDA-approved therapies for the treatment of NAFLD. Thus, the current approach to NAFLD management focuses on treatment to improve the risk factors for NASH (i.e., obesity, insulin resistance, metabolic syndrome, dyslipidemia). Based on our understanding of the natural history of NAFLD, only patients with NASH or those with features of hepatic fibrosis on liver biopsy are considered currently for targeted pharmacologic therapies. This approach may change as our understanding of disease pathophysiology improves and potential targets of therapy evolve.

Diet and exercise

Lifestyle changes and dietary modification are the foundation for NAFLD treatment. Many studies indicate that lifestyle modification can improve serum aminotransferases and hepatic steatosis, with loss of at least 3–5% of body weight improving steatosis, but greater weight loss (up to 10%) necessary to improve steatohepatitis. The benefits of different dietary macronutrient contents (e.g., low-carbohydrate vs low-fat diets, saturated vs unsaturated fat diets) and different intensities of calorie restriction appear to be comparable. In adults with NAFLD, exercise regimens that improve fitness may be sufficient to reduce hepatic steatosis, but their impact on other aspects of liver histology remains unknown. Unfortunately, most NAFLD patients are unable to achieve sustained weight loss. Although pharmacologic therapies such as orlistat, topiramate, and phentermine to facilitate weight loss are available, their role in the treatment of NAFLD remains experimental.

Pharmacologic therapies

Several drug therapies have been tried in both research and clinical settings. No agent has yet been approved by the FDA for the treatment of NAFLD. Hence, this remains an area of active research. Because NAFLD is strongly associated with the metabolic syndrome and type 2 diabetes, the efficacy of various insulin-sensitizing agents has been examined. *Metformin*, an agent that mainly improves hepatic insulin sensitivity, has been evaluated in several small, open-label studies in adults and a recent larger, prospectively randomized trial in children (dubbed the TONIC study). Although several of the adult NASH studies suggested improvements in aminotransferases and/or liver histology, metformin did not improve liver histology in the TONIC study of children with NASH. Thus, it is not currently recommended as a treatment for NASH. Uncontrolled open-label studies have also investigated *thiazolidinediones (pioglitazone and rosiglitazone)* in adults with NASH. This class of drugs is known to improve systemic insulin resistance. Both pioglitazone and rosiglitazone reduced aminotransferases and improved some of the histologic features of NASH in small, uncontrolled studies. A large, National Institutes of Health–sponsored, randomized placebo-controlled clinical trial, the PIVENs Study (Pioglitazone vs Vitamin E vs Placebo for the Treatment of 247 Nondiabetic Adults with NASH), demonstrated that resolution of histologic NASH occurred more often in subjects treated with pioglitazone (30 mg/d) than with placebo for 18 months (47 vs 21%, p = .001). However, many subjects in the pioglitazone group gained weight, and liver fibrosis did not improve. Also, it should be noted that the long-term safety and efficacy of thiazolidinediones in patients with NASH has not been established. Five-year follow-up of subjects treated with rosiglitazone demonstrated no reduction in liver fibrosis, and rosiglitazone has been associated with increased long-term risk for cardiovascular mortality. Hence, it is not recommended as a treatment for NAFLD. Pioglitazone may be safer because in a recent large meta-analysis it was associated with reduced overall morality, myocardial infarction, and stroke. However, caution must be exercised when considering its use in patients with impaired myocardial function.

Antioxidants have also been evaluated for the treatment of NAFLD because oxidant stress is thought to contribute to the pathogenesis of NASH. *Vitamin E*, an inexpensive yet potent antioxidant, has been examined in several small pediatric and adult studies with varying results. In all of those studies, vitamin E was well tolerated, and most showed modest improvements in aminotransferase levels, radiographic features of hepatic steatosis, and/or histologic features of NASH. Vitamin E (800 IU/d) was also compared to placebo in the PIVENs and TONIC studies. In PIVENs, vitamin E was the only agent that achieved the predetermined primary endpoint (i.e., improvement in steatohepatitis, lobular inflammation, and steatosis score, without an increase in the fibrosis score). This endpoint was met in 43% of patients in the vitamin E group (p = .001 vs placebo), 34% in the pioglitazone group (p = .04 vs placebo), and 19% in the placebo group. Vitamin E also improved NASH histology in pediatric patients with NASH (TONIC trial). However, a recent population-based study suggested that chronic vitamin E therapy may increase the risk for cardiovascular mortality. Thus, vitamin E should only be considered as a first-line pharmacotherapy for nondiabetic NASH patients. Also, given its potentially negative effects on cardiovascular health, caution should be exercised until the risk-to-benefit ratio and long-term therapeutic efficacy of vitamin E are better defined. Ursodeoxycholic acid (a bile acid that improves certain cholestatic liver diseases) and *betaine* (metabolite of choline that raises SAM levels and decreases cellular oxidative damage) offer no histologic benefit over placebo in patients with NASH. Experimental evidence to support the use of *omega-3 fatty acids* in NAFLD exists; however, a recent large, multicenter, placebo-controlled study failed to demonstrate a histologic benefit. Other pharmacotherapies are also being evaluated in NAFLD (e.g., *probiotics, farnesoid X receptor agonists, anticytokine agents, glucagon-like peptide agonists, dipeptidyl IV antagonists*); however, sufficient data do not yet exist to justify their use as NASH treatments in standard clinical practice.

Statins are an important class of agents to treat dyslipidemia and decrease cardiovascular risk. There is no evidence to suggest that statins cause liver failure in patients with any chronic liver disease, including NAFLD. The incidence of liver enzyme elevations in NAFLD patients taking statins is also no different than that of healthy controls or patients with other chronic liver diseases. Moreover, several studies have suggested that statins may improve aminotransferases and histology in patients with NASH. Yet, there is continued reluctance to use statins in patients with NAFLD. The lack of evidence that statins harm the liver in NAFLD patients, combined with the increase risk for cardiovascular morbidity and mortality in NAFLD patients, warrants the use of statins to treat dyslipidemia in patients with NAFLD/NASH.

Bariatric surgery

Although interest in bariatric surgery as a treatment for NAFLD exists, a recently published Cochrane review concluded that lack of randomized clinical trials or adequate clinical studies prevents definitive assessment of benefits and harms of bariatric surgery as a treatment for NASH. Most studies of bariatric surgery have shown that bariatric surgery is generally safe in individuals with well-compensated chronic liver disease and improves hepatic steatosis and necroinflammation (i.e., features of NAFLD/NASH); however, effects on hepatic fibrosis have been variable. Concern lingers because some of the largest prospective studies suggest that hepatic fibrosis might progress after bariatric surgery. Thus, the Cochrane review deemed it premature to recommend bariatric surgery as a primary treatment for NASH. There is also general agreement that patients with NAFLD-related cirrhosis and portal hypertension should be excluded as candidates for bariatric surgery. However, given growing evidence for the benefits of bariatric surgery on metabolic syndrome complications in individuals with refractory obesity, it is not contraindicated in otherwise eligible patients with NAFLD or NASH.

Liver transplantation

Patients with NAFLD in whom end-stage liver disease develops should be evaluated for liver transplantation **(Chap. 48)**. The outcomes of liver transplantation in well-selected patients with NAFLD are generally good, but comorbid medical conditions associated with NAFLD, such as diabetes mellitus, obesity, and cardiovascular disease, often limit transplant candidacy. NAFLD may recur after liver transplantation. The risk factors for recurrent or de novo NAFLD after liver transplantation are multifactorial and include hypertriglyceridemia, obesity, diabetes mellitus, and immunosuppressive therapies, particularly glucocorticoids.

GLOBAL HEALTH CONSIDERATIONS

The epidemic of obesity is now a global and accelerating phenomenon. Worldwide, there are over 1 billion overweight adults, of whom at least 300 million are obese. In the wake of the obesity epidemic follow numerous comorbidities, including NAFLD. NAFLD is the most common liver disease identified in Western countries and the fastest rising form of chronic liver disease worldwide. Present understanding of NAFLD natural history is based mainly on studies in whites who became overweight/obese and developed the metabolic syndrome in adulthood. The impact of the global childhood obesity epidemic on NAFLD pathogenesis/progression is unknown. Emerging evidence demonstrates that advanced NAFLD, including cirrhosis and primary liver cancer, can occur in children, prompting concerns that childhood-onset NAFLD might follow a more aggressive course than typical adult-acquired NAFLD. Some of the most populated parts of the world are in the midst of industrial revolutions, and certain environmental pollutants seem to exacerbate NAFLD. Some studies also suggest that the risk for NASH and NAFLD-related cirrhosis may be higher in certain ethnic groups such as Asians, certain Hispanics, and Native Americans and lower in others such as African Americans, compared with whites. Although all of these variables confound efforts to predict the net impact of this obesity-related liver disease on global health, it seems likely that NAFLD will remain a major cause of chronic liver disease worldwide for the foreseeable future.

CHAPTER 44

CIRRHOSIS AND ITS COMPLICATIONS

Bruce R. Bacon

Cirrhosis is a condition that is defined histopathologically and has a variety of clinical manifestations and complications, some of which can be life-threatening. In the past, it has been thought that cirrhosis was never reversible; however, it has become apparent that when the underlying insult that has caused the cirrhosis has been removed, there can be reversal of fibrosis. This is most apparent with the successful treatment of chronic hepatitis C; however, reversal of fibrosis is also seen in patients with hemochromatosis who have been successfully treated and in patients with alcoholic liver disease who have discontinued alcohol use.

Regardless of the cause of cirrhosis, the pathologic features consist of the development of fibrosis to the point that there is architectural distortion with the formation of regenerative nodules. This results in a decrease in hepatocellular mass, and thus function, and an alteration of blood flow. The induction of fibrosis occurs with activation of hepatic stellate cells, resulting in the formation of increased amounts of collagen and other components of the extracellular matrix.

Clinical features of cirrhosis are the result of pathologic changes and mirror the severity of the liver disease. Most hepatic pathologists provide an assessment of grading and staging when evaluating liver biopsy samples. These grading and staging schemes vary between disease states and have been developed for most conditions, including chronic viral hepatitis, nonalcoholic fatty liver disease, and primary biliary cirrhosis. Advanced fibrosis usually includes bridging fibrosis with nodularity designated as stage 3 and cirrhosis designated as stage 4. Patients who have cirrhosis have varying degrees of compensated liver function, and clinicians need to differentiate between those who have stable, compensated cirrhosis and those who have decompensated cirrhosis. Patients who have developed complications of their liver disease and have become decompensated should be considered for liver transplantation. Many of the complications of cirrhosis will require specific therapy. *Portal hypertension* is a significant complicating feature of decompensated cirrhosis and is responsible for the development of ascites and bleeding from esophagogastric varices, two complications that signify decompensated cirrhosis. Loss of hepatocellular function results in jaundice, coagulation disorders, and hypoalbuminemia and contributes to the causes of portosystemic encephalopathy. The complications of cirrhosis are basically the same regardless of the etiology. Nonetheless, it is useful to classify patients by the cause of their liver disease (Table 44-1); patients can be divided into broad groups with alcoholic cirrhosis, cirrhosis due to chronic viral hepatitis, biliary cirrhosis, and other, less common causes such as cardiac cirrhosis, cryptogenic cirrhosis, and other miscellaneous causes.

ALCOHOLIC CIRRHOSIS

Excessive chronic alcohol use can cause several different types of chronic liver disease, including alcoholic fatty liver, alcoholic hepatitis, and alcoholic cirrhosis.

TABLE 44-1

CAUSES OF CIRRHOSIS

Alcoholism	Cardiac cirrhosis
Chronic viral hepatitis	Inherited metabolic liver disease
Hepatitis B	Hemochromatosis
Hepatitis C	Wilson's disease
Autoimmune hepatitis	α_1 Antitrypsin deficiency
Nonalcoholic steatohepatitis	Cystic fibrosis
Biliary cirrhosis	Cryptogenic cirrhosis
Primary biliary cirrhosis	
Primary sclerosing cholangitis	
Autoimmune cholangiopathy	

Furthermore, use of excessive alcohol can contribute to liver damage in patients with other liver diseases, such as hepatitis C, hemochromatosis, and fatty liver disease related to obesity. Chronic alcohol use can produce fibrosis in the absence of accompanying inflammation and/or necrosis. Fibrosis can be centrilobular, pericellular, or periportal. When fibrosis reaches a certain degree, there is disruption of the normal liver architecture and replacement of liver cells by regenerative nodules. In alcoholic cirrhosis, the nodules are usually <3 mm in diameter; this form of cirrhosis is referred to as *micronodular*. With cessation of alcohol use, larger nodules may form, resulting in a mixed micronodular and macronodular cirrhosis.

Pathogenesis

Alcohol is the most commonly used drug in the United States, and more than two-thirds of adults drink alcohol each year. Thirty percent have had a binge within the past month, and over 7% of adults regularly consume more than two drinks per day. Unfortunately, more than 14 million adults in the United States meet the diagnostic criteria for alcohol abuse or dependence. In the United States, chronic liver disease is the tenth most common cause of death in adults, and alcoholic cirrhosis accounts for approximately 40% of deaths due to cirrhosis.

Ethanol is mainly absorbed by the small intestine and, to a lesser degree, through the stomach. Gastric alcohol dehydrogenase (ADH) initiates alcohol metabolism. Three enzyme systems account for metabolism of alcohol in the liver. These include cytosolic ADH, the microsomal ethanol oxidizing system (MEOS), and peroxisomal catalase. The majority of ethanol oxidation occurs via ADH to form acetaldehyde, which is a highly reactive molecule that may have multiple effects. Ultimately, acetaldehyde is metabolized to acetate by aldehyde dehydrogenase (ALDH). Intake of ethanol increases intracellular accumulation of triglycerides by increasing fatty acid uptake and by reducing fatty acid oxidation and lipoprotein secretion. Protein synthesis, glycosylation, and secretion are impaired. Oxidative damage to hepatocyte membranes occurs due to the formation of reactive oxygen species; acetaldehyde is a highly reactive molecule that combines with proteins to form protein-acetaldehyde adducts. These adducts may interfere with specific enzyme activities, including microtubular formation and hepatic protein trafficking. With acetaldehyde-mediated hepatocyte damage, certain reactive oxygen species can result in Kupffer cell activation. As a result, profibrogenic cytokines are produced that initiate and perpetuate stellate cell activation, with the resultant production of excess collagen and extracellular matrix. Connective tissue appears in both periportal and pericentral zones and eventually connects portal triads with central veins forming regenerative nodules. Hepatocyte loss occurs, and with increased collagen production and deposition, together with continuing hepatocyte destruction, the liver contracts and shrinks in size. This process generally takes from years to decades to occur and requires repeated insults.

Clinical features

The diagnosis of alcoholic liver disease requires an accurate history regarding both amount and duration of alcohol consumption. Patients with alcoholic liver disease can present with nonspecific symptoms such as vague right upper quadrant abdominal pain, fever, nausea and vomiting, diarrhea, anorexia, and malaise. Alternatively, they may present with more specific complications of chronic liver disease, including ascites, edema, or upper gastrointestinal (GI) hemorrhage. Many cases present incidentally at the time of autopsy or elective surgery. Other clinical manifestations include the development of jaundice or encephalopathy. The abrupt onset of any of these complications may be the first event prompting the patient to seek medical attention. Other patients may be identified in the course of an evaluation of routine laboratory studies that are found to be abnormal. On physical examination, the liver and spleen may be enlarged, with the liver edge being firm and nodular. Other frequent findings include scleral icterus, palmar erythema (Fig. 44-1), spider angiomas (Fig. 44-2), parotid gland enlargement, digital clubbing, muscle wasting, or the development of edema and ascites. Men may have decreased body hair and gynecomastia as well as testicular atrophy, which may be a consequence of hormonal abnormalities or a direct toxic effect of alcohol on the testes.

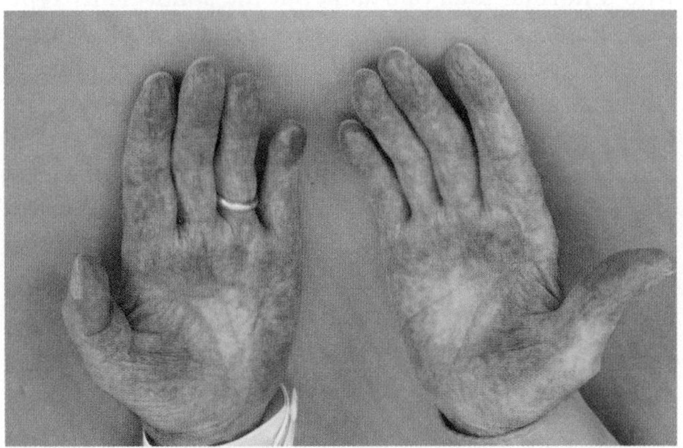

FIGURE 44-1
Palmar erythema. This figure shows palmar erythema in a patient with alcoholic cirrhosis. The erythema is peripheral over the palm with central pallor.

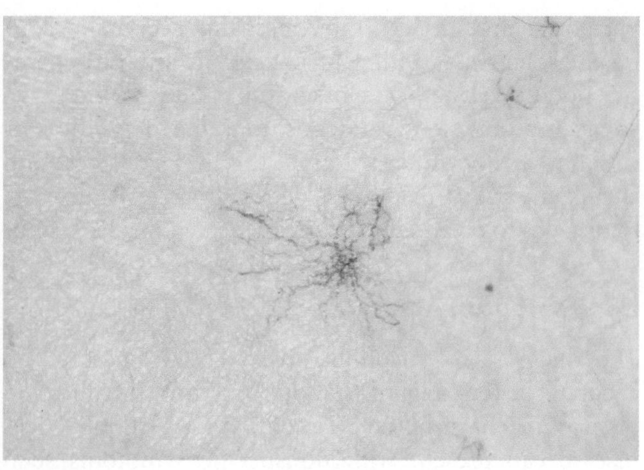

FIGURE 44-2
Spider angioma. This figure shows a spider angioma in a patient with hepatitis C cirrhosis. With release of central compression, the arteriole fills from the center and spreads out peripherally.

In women with advanced alcoholic cirrhosis, menstrual irregularities usually occur, and some women may be amenorrheic. These changes are often reversible following cessation of alcohol.

Laboratory tests may be completely normal in patients with early compensated alcoholic cirrhosis. Alternatively, in advanced liver disease, many abnormalities usually are present. Patients may be anemic either from chronic GI blood loss, nutritional deficiencies, or hypersplenism related to portal hypertension, or as a direct suppressive effect of alcohol on the bone marrow. A unique form of hemolytic anemia (with spur cells and acanthocytes) called *Zieve's syndrome* can occur in patients with severe alcoholic hepatitis. Platelet counts are often reduced early in the disease, reflective of portal hypertension with hypersplenism. Serum total bilirubin can be normal or elevated with advanced disease. Direct bilirubin is frequently mildly elevated in patients with a normal total bilirubin, but the abnormality typically progresses as the disease worsens. Prothrombin times are often prolonged and usually do not respond to administration of parenteral vitamin K. Serum sodium levels are usually normal unless patients have ascites and then can be depressed, largely due to ingestion of excess free water. Serum alanine and aspartate aminotransferases (ALT, AST) are typically elevated, particularly in patients who continue to drink, with AST levels being higher than ALT levels, usually by a 2:1 ratio.

Diagnosis

Patients who have any of the above-mentioned clinical features, physical examination findings, or laboratory studies should be considered to have alcoholic liver disease. The diagnosis, however, requires accurate knowledge that the patient is continuing to use and abuse alcohol. Furthermore, other forms of chronic liver disease (e.g., chronic viral hepatitis or metabolic or autoimmune liver diseases) must be considered or ruled out, or if present, an estimate of relative causality along with the alcohol use should be determined. Liver biopsy can be helpful to confirm a diagnosis, but generally when patients present with alcoholic hepatitis and are still drinking, liver biopsy is withheld until abstinence has been maintained for at least 6 months to determine residual, nonreversible disease.

In patients who have had complications of cirrhosis and who continue to drink, there is a <50% 5-year survival. In contrast, in patients who are able to remain abstinent, the prognosis is significantly improved. In patients with advanced liver disease, the prognosis remains poor; however, in individuals who are able to remain abstinent, liver transplantation is a viable option.

TREATMENT Alcoholic Cirrhosis

Abstinence is the cornerstone of therapy for patients with alcoholic liver disease. In addition, patients require good nutrition and long-term medical supervision to manage underlying complications that may develop. Complications such as the development of ascites and edema, variceal hemorrhage, or portosystemic encephalopathy all require specific management and treatment. Glucocorticoids are occasionally used in patients with severe alcoholic hepatitis in the absence of infection. Survival has been shown to improve in certain studies. Treatment is restricted to patients with a discriminant function (DF) value of >32. The DF is calculated as the serum total bilirubin plus the difference in the patient's prothrombin time compared to control (in seconds) multiplied by 4.6. In patients for whom this value is >32, there is improved survival at 28 days with the use of glucocorticoids.

Other therapies that have been used include oral pentoxifylline, which decreases the production of tumor necrosis factor α (TNF-α) and other proinflammatory cytokines. In contrast to glucocorticoids, with which complications can occur, pentoxifylline is relatively easy to administer and has few, if any, side effects. A variety of nutritional therapies have been tried with either parenteral or enteral feedings; however, it is unclear whether any of these modalities have significantly improved survival.

Recent studies have used parenterally administered inhibitors of TNF-α such as infliximab or etanercept. Early results have shown no adverse events; however, there was no clear-cut improvement in survival. Anabolic steroids, propylthiouracil, antioxidants, colchicine, and penicillamine have all been used but do not show clear-cut benefits and are not recommended.

As mentioned above, the cornerstone to treatment is cessation of alcohol use. Recent experience with medications that reduce craving for alcohol, such as acamprosate calcium, has been favorable. Patients may take other necessary medications even in the presence of cirrhosis. Acetaminophen use is often discouraged in patients with liver disease; however, if no more than 2 g of acetaminophen per day are consumed, there generally are no problems.

CIRRHOSIS DUE TO CHRONIC VIRAL HEPATITIS B OR C

Of patients exposed to the hepatitis C virus (HCV), approximately 80% develop chronic hepatitis C, and of those, about 20–30% will develop cirrhosis over 20–30 years. Many of these patients have had concomitant alcohol use, and the true incidence of cirrhosis due to hepatitis C alone is unknown. Nonetheless, this represents a significant number of patients. It is expected that an even higher percentage will go on to develop cirrhosis over longer periods of time. In the United States, approximately 5 to 6 million people have been exposed to HCV, with about 4 million who are chronically viremic. Worldwide, about 170 million individuals have hepatitis C, with some areas of the world (e.g., Egypt) having up to 15% of the population infected. HCV is a noncytopathic virus, and liver damage is probably immune-mediated. Progression of liver disease due to chronic hepatitis C is characterized by portal-based fibrosis with bridging fibrosis and nodularity developing, ultimately culminating in the development of cirrhosis. In cirrhosis due to chronic hepatitis C, the liver is small and shrunken with characteristic features of a mixed micro- and macronodular cirrhosis seen on liver biopsy. In addition to the increased fibrosis that is seen in cirrhosis due to hepatitis C, an inflammatory infiltrate is found in portal areas with interface hepatitis and occasionally some lobular hepatocellular injury and inflammation. In patients with HCV genotype 3, steatosis is often present.

Similar findings are seen in patients with cirrhosis due to chronic hepatitis B. Of adult patients exposed to hepatitis B, about 5% develop chronic hepatitis B, and about 20% of those patients will go on to develop cirrhosis. Special stains for hepatitis B core (HBc) and hepatitis B surface (HBs) antigen will be positive, and ground-glass hepatocytes signifying hepatitis B surface antigen (HBsAg) may be present. In the United States, there are about 2 million carriers of hepatitis B, whereas in other parts of the world where hepatitis B virus (HBV) is endemic (i.e., Asia, Southeast Asia, sub-Saharan Africa), up to 15% of the population may be infected, having acquired the infection vertically at the time of birth. Thus, over 300–400 million individuals are thought to have hepatitis B worldwide. Approximately 25% of these individuals may ultimately develop cirrhosis.

Clinical features and diagnosis

Patients with cirrhosis due to either chronic hepatitis C or B can present with the usual symptoms and signs of chronic liver disease. Fatigue, malaise, vague right upper quadrant pain, and laboratory abnormalities are frequent presenting features. Diagnosis requires a thorough laboratory evaluation, including quantitative HCV RNA testing and analysis for HCV genotype, or hepatitis B serologies to include HBsAg, anti-HBs, HBeAg (hepatitis B e antigen), anti-HBe, and quantitative HBV DNA levels.

TREATMENT Cirrhosis Due to Chronic Viral Hepatitis B or C

Management of complications of cirrhosis revolves around specific therapy for treatment of whatever complications occur (e.g., esophageal variceal hemorrhage, development of ascites and edema, or encephalopathy). In patients with chronic hepatitis B, numerous studies have shown beneficial effects of antiviral therapy, which is effective at viral suppression, as evidenced by reducing aminotransferase levels and HBV DNA levels, and improving histology by reducing inflammation and fibrosis. Several clinical trials and case series have demonstrated that patients with decompensated liver disease can become compensated with the use of antiviral therapy directed against hepatitis B. Currently available therapy includes lamivudine, adefovir, telbivudine, entecavir, and tenofovir. Interferon α can also be used for treating hepatitis B, but it should not be used in cirrhotics.

Treatment of patients with cirrhosis due to hepatitis C is a little more difficult because the side effects of pegylated interferon and ribavirin therapy are often difficult to manage. Dose-limiting cytopenias (platelets, white blood cells, red blood cells) or severe side effects can result in discontinuation of treatment. Nonetheless, if patients can tolerate treatment, and if it is successful, the benefit is great and disease progression is reduced. Recent studies have shown that if platelets are <100,000, albumin is <3.5 g/dL, and Model for End-Stage Liver Disease (MELD) score is >10, the risk of severe complications of interferon-based antiviral therapy is significant. Recent approval of Direct Acting Antivirals (DAAs) has led to improved efficacy of treatment with regimens that are safe and well tolerated.

CIRRHOSIS FROM AUTOIMMUNE HEPATITIS AND NONALCOHOLIC FATTY LIVER DISEASE

Other causes of posthepatitic cirrhosis include autoimmune hepatitis and cirrhosis due to nonalcoholic steatohepatitis. Many patients with autoimmune hepatitis (AIH) present with cirrhosis that is already established.

Typically, these patients will not benefit from immunosuppressive therapy with glucocorticoids or azathioprine because the AIH is "burned out." In this situation, liver biopsy does not show a significant inflammatory infiltrate. Diagnosis in this setting requires positive autoimmune markers such as antinuclear antibody (ANA) or anti-smooth-muscle antibody (ASMA). When patients with AIH present with cirrhosis and active inflammation accompanied by elevated liver enzymes, there can be considerable benefit from the use of immunosuppressive therapy.

Patients with nonalcoholic steatohepatitis are increasingly being found to have progressed to cirrhosis. With the epidemic of obesity that continues in Western countries, more and more patients are identified with nonalcoholic fatty liver disease **(Chap. 43)**. Of these, a significant subset has nonalcoholic steatohepatitis and can progress to increased fibrosis and cirrhosis. Over the past several years, it has been increasingly recognized that many patients who were thought to have cryptogenic cirrhosis in fact have nonalcoholic steatohepatitis. As their cirrhosis progresses, they become catabolic and then lose the telltale signs of steatosis seen on biopsy. Management of complications of cirrhosis due to either AIH or nonalcoholic steatohepatitis is similar to that for other forms of cirrhosis.

BILIARY CIRRHOSIS

Biliary cirrhosis has pathologic features that are different from either alcoholic cirrhosis or posthepatitic cirrhosis, yet the manifestations of end-stage liver disease are the same. Cholestatic liver disease may result from necroinflammatory lesions, congenital or metabolic processes, or external bile duct compression. Thus, two broad categories reflect the anatomic sites of abnormal bile retention: *intrahepatic* and *extrahepatic*. The distinction is important for obvious therapeutic reasons. Extrahepatic obstruction may benefit from surgical or endoscopic biliary tract decompression, whereas intrahepatic cholestatic processes will not improve with such interventions and require a different approach.

The major causes of chronic cholestatic syndromes are primary biliary cirrhosis (PBC), autoimmune cholangitis (AIC), primary sclerosing cholangitis (PSC), and idiopathic adulthood ductopenia. These syndromes are usually clinically distinguished from each other by antibody testing, cholangiographic findings, and clinical presentation. However, they all share the histopathologic features of chronic cholestasis, such as cholate stasis; copper deposition; xanthomatous transformation of hepatocytes; and irregular, so-called biliary fibrosis. In addition, there may be chronic portal inflammation, interface activity, and chronic lobular inflammation. Ductopenia is a result of this progressive disease as patients develop cirrhosis.

PRIMARY BILIARY CIRRHOSIS

PBC is seen in about 100–200 individuals per million, with a strong female preponderance and a median age of around 50 years at the time of diagnosis. The cause of PBC is unknown; it is characterized by portal inflammation and necrosis of cholangiocytes in small- and medium-sized bile ducts. Cholestatic features prevail, and biliary cirrhosis is characterized by an elevated bilirubin level and progressive liver failure. Liver transplantation is the treatment of choice for patients with decompensated cirrhosis due to PBC. A variety of therapies have been proposed, but ursodeoxycholic acid (UDCA) is the only approved treatment that has some degree of efficacy by slowing the rate of progression of the disease.

Antimitochondrial antibodies (AMA) are present in about 90% of patients with PBC. These autoantibodies recognize intermitochondrial membrane proteins that are enzymes of the pyruvate dehydrogenase complex (PDC), the branched-chain 2-oxoacid dehydrogenase complex, and the 2-oxogluterate dehydrogenase complex. Most relate to pyruvate dehydrogenase. These autoantibodies are not pathogenic but rather are useful markers for making a diagnosis of PBC.

Pathology

Histopathologic analyses of liver biopsies of patients with PBC have resulted in identifying four distinct stages of the disease as it progresses. The earliest lesion is termed *chronic nonsuppurative destructive cholangitis* and is a necrotizing inflammatory process of the portal tracts. Medium and small bile ducts are infiltrated with lymphocytes and undergo duct destruction. Mild fibrosis and sometimes bile stasis can occur. With progression, the inflammatory infil-trate becomes less prominent, but the number of bile ducts is reduced and there is proliferation of smaller bile ductules. Increased fibrosis ensues with the expansion of periportal fibrosis to bridging fibrosis. Finally, cirrhosis, which may be micronodular or macronodular, develops.

Clinical features

Currently, most patients with PBC are diagnosed well before the end-stage manifestations of the disease are present, and, as such, most patients are actually asymptomatic. When symptoms are present, they most prominently include a significant degree of fatigue out of proportion to what would be expected for either the severity of the liver disease or the age of the patient. Pruritus is seen in approximately 50% of patients at the time of diagnosis, and it can be debilitating. It might be intermittent and usually is most bothersome in the evening. In some patients, pruritus can develop toward the end of pregnancy, and there are examples of patients having been diagnosed with cholestasis of pregnancy rather than PBC. Pruritus that presents prior to the development of jaundice indicates severe disease and a poor prognosis.

Physical examination can show jaundice and other complications of chronic liver disease, including hepatomegaly, splenomegaly, ascites, and edema. Other features that are unique to PBC include hyperpigmentation, xanthelasma, and xanthomata, which are related to the altered cholesterol metabolism seen in this disease. Hyperpigmentation is evident on the trunk and the arms and is seen in areas of exfoliation and lichenification associated with progressive scratching related to the pruritus. Bone pain resulting from osteopenia or osteoporosis is occasionally seen at the time of diagnosis.

Laboratory findings

Laboratory findings in PBC show cholestatic liver enzyme abnormalities with an elevation in γ-glutamyl transpeptidase and alkaline phosphatase (ALP) along with mild elevations in aminotransferases (ALT and AST). Immunoglobulins, particularly IgM, are typically increased. Hyperbilirubinemia usually is seen once cirrhosis has developed. Thrombocytopenia, leukopenia, and anemia may be seen in patients with portal hypertension and hypersplenism. Liver biopsy shows characteristic features as described above and should be evident to any experienced hepatopathologist. Up to 10% of patients with characteristic PBC will have features of AIH as well and are defined as having "overlap" syndrome. These patients are usually treated as PBC patients and may progress to cirrhosis with the same frequency as typical PBC patients. Some patients require immunosuppressive medications as well.

Diagnosis

PBC should be considered in patients with chronic cholestatic liver enzyme abnormalities. It is most often seen in middle-aged women. AMA testing may be negative, and it should be remembered that as many as 10% of patients with PBC may be AMA-negative. Liver biopsy is most important in this setting of AMA-negative PBC. In patients who are AMA-negative with cholestatic liver enzymes, PSC should be ruled out by way of cholangiography.

TREATMENT Primary Biliary Cirrhosis

Treatment of the typical manifestations of cirrhosis are no different for PBC than for other forms of cirrhosis. UDCA has been shown to improve both biochemical and histologic features of the disease. Improvement is greatest when therapy is initiated early; the likelihood of significant improvement with UDCA is low in patients with PBC who present with manifestations of cirrhosis. UDCA is given in doses of 13–15 mg/kg per day; the medication is usually well-tolerated, although some patients have worsening pruritus with initiation of therapy. A small proportion of patients may have diarrhea or headache as a side effect of the drug. UDCA has been shown to slow the rate of progression of PBC, but it does not reverse or cure the disease. Patients with PBC require long-term follow-up by a physician experienced with the disease. Certain patients may need to be considered for liver transplantation should their liver disease decompensate.

The main symptoms of PBC are fatigue and pruritus, and symptom management is important. Several therapies have been tried for treatment of fatigue, but none of them have been successful; frequent naps should be encouraged. Pruritus is treated with antihistamines, narcotic receptor antagonists (naltrexone), and rifampin. Cholestyramine, a bile salt–sequestering agent, has been helpful in some patients but is somewhat tedious and difficult to take. Plasmapheresis has been used rarely in patients with severe intractable pruritus. There is an increased incidence of osteopenia and osteoporosis in patients with cholestatic liver disease, and bone density testing should be performed. Treatment with a bisphosphonate should be instituted when bone disease is identified.

PRIMARY SCLEROSING CHOLANGITIS

As in PBC, the cause of PSC remains unknown. PSC is a chronic cholestatic syndrome that is characterized by diffuse inflammation and fibrosis involving the entire biliary tree, resulting in chronic cholestasis. This pathologic process ultimately results in obliteration of both the intra- and extrahepatic biliary tree, leading to biliary cirrhosis, portal hypertension, and liver failure. The cause of PSC remains unknown despite extensive investigation into various mechanisms related to bacterial and viral infections, toxins, genetic predisposition, and immunologic mechanisms, all of which have been postulated to contribute to the pathogenesis and progression of this syndrome.

Pathologic changes that can occur in PSC show bile duct proliferation as well as ductopenia and fibrous cholangitis (pericholangitis). Often, liver biopsy changes in PSC are not pathognomonic, and establishing the diagnosis of PSC must involve imaging of the biliary tree. Periductal fibrosis is occasionally seen on biopsy specimens and can be quite helpful in making the diagnosis. As the disease progresses, biliary cirrhosis is the final, end-stage manifestation of PSC.

Clinical features

The usual clinical features of PSC are those found in cholestatic liver disease, with fatigue, pruritus, steatorrhea, deficiencies of fat-soluble vitamins, and the associated consequences. As in PBC, the fatigue is profound and nonspecific. Pruritus can often be debilitating and is related to the cholestasis. The severity of pruritus does not correlate with the severity of the disease. Metabolic bone disease, as seen in PBC, can occur with PSC and should be treated (see above).

Laboratory findings

Patients with PSC typically are identified in the course of an evaluation of abnormal liver enzymes. Most patients have at least a twofold increase in ALP and may have elevated aminotransferases as well. Albumin levels may be decreased, and prothrombin times are prolonged in a substantial proportion of patients at the time of diagnosis. Some degree of correction of a prolonged prothrombin time may occur with parenteral vitamin K. A small subset of patients have aminotransferase elevations greater than five times the upper limit of normal and may have features of AIH on biopsy. These individuals are thought to have an overlap syndrome between PSC and AIH. Autoantibodies are frequently positive in patients with the overlap syndrome but are typically negative in patients who only have PSC. One autoantibody, the perinuclear antineutrophil cytoplasmic antibody (p-ANCA), is positive in about 65% of patients with PSC. Over 50% of patients with PSC also have ulcerative colitis (UC); accordingly, once a diagnosis of PSC is established, colonoscopy should be performed to look for evidence of UC.

Diagnosis

The definitive diagnosis of PSC requires cholangiographic imaging. Over the last several years, magnetic resonance imaging (MRI) with magnetic resonance cholangiopancreatography (MRCP) has been used as the imaging technique of choice for initial evaluation. Once patients are screened in this manner, some investigators feel that endoscopic retrograde cholangiopancreatography (ERCP) should also be performed to be certain whether or not a dominant stricture is present. Typical cholangiographic findings in PSC are multifocal stricturing and beading involving both the intrahepatic and extrahepatic biliary tree. However, although involvement may be of the intrahepatic bile ducts alone or of the extrahepatic bile ducts alone, more commonly, both are involved. These strictures are typically short and with intervening segments of normal or slightly dilated bile ducts that are distributed diffusely, producing the classic beaded appearance. The gallbladder and cystic duct can be involved in up to 15% of cases. Patients with high-grade, diffuse stricturing of the intrahepatic bile ducts have an overall poor prognosis. Gradually, biliary cirrhosis develops, and patients will progress to decompensated liver disease with all the manifestations of ascites, esophageal variceal hemorrhage, and encephalopathy.

TREATMENT Primary Sclerosing Cholangitis

There is no specific proven treatment for PSC. A recently completed study of high-dose (20 mg/kg per day) UDCA was found to be harmful. Some clinicians use UDCA at "PBC dosages" of 13–15 mg/kg per day with anecdotal improvement. Endoscopic dilatation of dominant strictures can be helpful, but the ultimate treatment is liver transplantation. A dreaded complication of PSC is the development of cholangiocarcinoma, which is a relative contraindication to liver transplantation. Symptoms of pruritus are common, and the approach is as mentioned previously for this problem in patients with PBC (see above).

CARDIAC CIRRHOSIS

Definition

Patients with long-standing right-sided congestive heart failure may develop chronic liver injury and cardiac cirrhosis. This is an increasingly uncommon, if not rare, cause of chronic liver disease given the advances made in the care of patients with heart failure.

Etiology and pathology

In the case of long-term right-sided heart failure, there is an elevated venous pressure transmitted via the inferior vena cava and hepatic veins to the sinusoids of the liver, which become dilated and engorged with blood. The liver becomes enlarged and swollen, and with long-term passive congestion and relative ischemia due to poor circulation, centrilobular hepatocytes can become necrotic, leading to pericentral fibrosis. This fibrotic pattern can extend to the periphery of the lobule outward until a unique pattern of fibrosis causing cirrhosis can occur.

Clinical features

Patients typically have signs of congestive heart failure and will manifest an enlarged firm liver on physical examination. ALP levels are characteristically elevated, and aminotransferases may be normal or slightly increased with AST usually higher than ALT. It is unlikely that patients will develop variceal hemorrhage or encephalopathy.

Diagnosis

The diagnosis is usually made in someone with clear-cut cardiac disease who has an elevated ALP and an enlarged liver. Liver biopsy shows a pattern of fibrosis that can be recognized by an experienced hepatopathologist. Differentiation from Budd-Chiari syndrome (BCS) can be made by seeing extravasation of red blood cells in BCS, but not in cardiac hepatopathy. Venoocclusive disease can also affect hepatic outflow and has characteristic features on liver biopsy. Venoocclusive disease can be seen under the circumstances of conditioning for bone marrow transplant with radiation and chemotherapy; it can also be seen with the ingestion of certain herbal teas as well as pyrrolizidine alkaloids. This is typically seen in Caribbean countries and rarely in the United States. Treatment is based on management of the underlying cardiac disease.

OTHER TYPES OF CIRRHOSIS

There are several other less common causes of chronic liver disease that can progress to cirrhosis. These include inherited metabolic liver diseases such as hemochromatosis, Wilson's disease, α_1 antitrypsin (α_1AT) deficiency, and cystic fibrosis. For all of these disorders, the manifestations of cirrhosis are similar, with some minor variations, to those seen in other patients with other causes of cirrhosis.

Hemochromatosis is an inherited disorder of iron metabolism that results in a progressive increase in hepatic iron deposition, which, over time, can lead to a portal-based fibrosis progressing to cirrhosis, liver failure, and hepatocellular cancer. While the frequency of hemochromatosis is relatively common, with genetic susceptibility occurring in 1 in 250 individuals, the frequency of end-stage manifestations due to the disease is relatively low, and fewer than 5% of those patients who are genotypically susceptible will go on to develop severe liver disease from hemochromatosis. Diagnosis is made with serum iron studies showing an elevated transferrin saturation and an elevated ferritin level, along with abnormalities identified by *HFE* mutation analysis. Treatment is straightforward, with regular therapeutic phlebotomy.

Wilson's disease is an inherited disorder of copper homeostasis with failure to excrete excess amounts of copper, leading to an accumulation in the liver. This disorder is relatively uncommon, affecting 1 in 30,000 individuals. Wilson's disease typically affects adolescents and young adults. Prompt diagnosis before end-stage manifestations become irreversible can lead to significant clinical improvement. Diagnosis requires determination of ceruloplasmin levels, which are low; 24-h urine copper levels, which are elevated; typical physical examination findings, including Kayser-Fleischer corneal rings; and characteristic liver biopsy findings. Treatment consists of copper-chelating medications.

α_1 AT deficiency results from an inherited disorder that causes abnormal folding of the α_1AT protein, resulting in failure of secretion of that protein from the liver. It is unknown how the retained protein leads to liver disease. Patients with α_1AT deficiency at greatest risk for developing chronic liver disease have the ZZ phenotype, but only about 10–20% of such individuals will develop chronic liver disease. Diagnosis is made by determining α_1AT levels and phenotype. Characteristic periodic acid–Schiff (PAS)-positive, diastase-resistant globules are seen on liver biopsy. The only effective treatment is liver transplantation, which is curative.

Cystic fibrosis is an uncommon inherited disorder affecting whites of northern European descent. A biliary-type cirrhosis can occur, and some patients derive benefit from the chronic use of UDCA.

MAJOR COMPLICATIONS OF CIRRHOSIS

The clinical course of patients with advanced cirrhosis is often complicated by a number of important sequelae that can occur regardless of the underlying cause of the liver disease. These include portal hypertension and its consequences of gastroesophageal variceal hemorrhage, splenomegaly, ascites, hepatic encephalopathy, spontaneous bacterial peritonitis (SBP), hepatorenal syndrome, and hepatocellular carcinoma (Table 44-2).

TABLE 44-2

COMPLICATIONS OF CIRRHOSIS

Portal hypertension	Coagulopathy
Gastroesophageal varices	Factor deficiency
Portal hypertensive gastropathy	Fibrinolysis
Splenomegaly, hypersplenism	Thrombocytopenia
Ascites	Bone disease
Spontaneous bacterial peritonitis	Osteopenia
	Osteoporosis
Hepatorenal syndrome	Osteomalacia
Type 1	Hematologic abnormalities
Type 2	
Hepatic encephalopathy	Anemia
Hepatopulmonary syndrome	Hemolysis
Portopulmonary hypertension	Thrombocytopenia
Malnutrition	Neutropenia

PORTAL HYPERTENSION

Portal hypertension is defined as the elevation of the hepatic venous pressure gradient (HVPG) to >5 mmHg. Portal hypertension is caused by a combination of two simultaneously occurring hemodynamic processes: (1) increased intrahepatic resistance to the passage of blood flow through the liver due to cirrhosis and regenerative nodules, and (2) increased splanchnic blood flow secondary to vasodilation within the splanchnic vascular bed. Portal hypertension is directly responsible for the two major complications of cirrhosis: variceal hemorrhage and ascites. *Variceal hemorrhage* is an immediate life-threatening problem with a 20–30% mortality rate associated with each episode of bleeding. The portal venous system normally drains blood from the stomach, intestines, spleen, pancreas, and gallbladder, and the portal vein is formed by the confluence of the superior mesenteric and splenic veins. Deoxygenated blood from the small bowel drains into the superior mesenteric vein along with blood from the head of the pancreas, the ascending colon, and part of the transverse colon. Conversely, the splenic vein drains the spleen and the pancreas and is joined by the inferior mesenteric vein, which brings blood from the transverse and descending colon as well as from the superior two-thirds of the rectum. Thus, the portal vein normally receives blood from almost the entire GI tract.

The causes of portal hypertension are usually subcategorized as prehepatic, intrahepatic, and posthepatic (Table 44-3). Prehepatic causes of portal hypertension are those affecting the portal venous system before it enters the liver; they include portal vein thrombosis and splenic vein thrombosis. Posthepatic causes encompass those affecting the hepatic veins and venous drainage to the heart; they include BCS, venoocclusive disease, and chronic right-sided cardiac congestion. Intrahepatic causes account for over 95% of cases of portal hypertension and are represented by the major forms of cirrhosis. Intrahepatic causes of portal hypertension can be further subdivided into presinusoidal, sinusoidal, and postsinusoidal causes. Postsinusoidal causes include venoocclusive disease, whereas presinusoidal causes include congenital hepatic fibrosis and schistosomiasis. Sinusoidal causes are related to cirrhosis from various causes.

Cirrhosis is the most common cause of portal hypertension in the United States, and clinically significant portal hypertension is present in >60% of patients with cirrhosis. Portal vein obstruction may be idiopathic or can occur in association with cirrhosis or with infection, pancreatitis, or abdominal trauma.

Coagulation disorders that can lead to the development of portal vein thrombosis include polycythemia vera; essential thrombocytosis; deficiencies in protein C, protein S, antithrombin 3, and factor V Leiden; and abnormalities in the gene-regulating prothrombin production. Some patients may have a subclinical myeloproliferative disorder.

TABLE 44-3

CLASSIFICATION OF PORTAL HYPERTENSION
Prehepatic
Portal vein thrombosis
Splenic vein thrombosis
Massive splenomegaly (Banti's syndrome)
Hepatic
Presinusoidal
Schistosomiasis
Congenital hepatic fibrosis
Sinusoidal
Cirrhosis—many causes
Alcoholic hepatitis
Postsinusoidal
Hepatic sinusoidal obstruction (venoocclusive syndrome)
Posthepatic
Budd-Chiari syndrome
Inferior vena caval webs
Cardiac causes
Restrictive cardiomyopathy
Constrictive pericarditis
Severe congestive heart failure

Clinical features

The three primary complications of portal hypertension are gastroesophageal varices with hemorrhage, ascites, and hypersplenism. Thus, patients may present with upper GI bleeding, which, on endoscopy, is found to be due to esophageal or gastric varices; with the development of ascites along with peripheral edema; or with an enlarged spleen with associated reduction in platelets and white blood cells on routine laboratory testing.

Esophageal varices

Over the last decade, it has become common practice to screen known cirrhotics with endoscopy to look for esophageal varices. Such screening studies have shown that approximately one-third of patients with histologically confirmed cirrhosis have varices. Approximately 5–15% of cirrhotics per year develop varices, and it is estimated that the majority of patients with cirrhosis will develop varices over their lifetimes. Furthermore, it is anticipated that roughly one-third of patients with varices will develop bleeding. Several factors predict the risk of bleeding, including the severity of cirrhosis (Child's class, MELD score); the height of wedged-hepatic vein pressure; the size of the varix; the location of the varix; and certain endoscopic stigmata, including red wale signs, hematocystic spots, diffuse erythema, bluish color, cherry red spots, or white-nipple spots. Patients with tense ascites are also at increased risk for bleeding from varices.

Diagnosis

In patients with cirrhosis who are being followed chronically, the development of portal hypertension is usually revealed by the presence of thrombocytopenia; the appearance of an enlarged spleen; or the development of ascites, encephalopathy, and/or esophageal varices with or without bleeding. In previously undiagnosed patients, any of these features should prompt further evaluation to determine the presence of portal hypertension and liver disease. Varices should be identified by endoscopy. Abdominal imaging, either by computed tomography (CT) or MRI, can be helpful in demonstrating a nodular liver and in finding changes of portal hypertension with intraabdominal collateral circulation. If necessary, interventional radiologic procedures can be performed to determine wedged and free hepatic vein pressures that will allow for the calculation of a wedged-to-free gradient, which is equivalent to the portal pressure. The average normal wedged-to-free gradient is 5 mmHg, and patients with a gradient >12 mmHg are at risk for variceal hemorrhage.

TREATMENT Variceal Hemorrhage

Treatment for variceal hemorrhage as a complication of portal hypertension is divided into two main categories: (1) primary prophylaxis and (2) prevention of rebleeding once there has been an initial variceal hemorrhage. Primary prophylaxis requires routine screening by endoscopy of all patients with cirrhosis. Once varices that are at increased risk for bleeding are identified, primary prophylaxis can be achieved either through nonselective beta blockade or by variceal band ligation. Numerous placebo-controlled clinical trials of either propranolol or nadolol have been reported in the literature. The most rigorous studies were those that only included patients with significantly enlarged varices or with hepatic vein pressure gradients >12 mmHg. Patients treated with beta blockers have a lower risk of variceal hemorrhage than those treated with placebo over 1 and 2 years of follow-up. There is also a decrease in mortality related to variceal hemorrhage. Unfortunately, overall survival was improved in only one study. Further studies have demonstrated that the degree of reduction of portal pressure is a significant feature to determine success of therapy. Therefore, it has been suggested that repeat measurements of hepatic vein pressure gradients may be used to guide pharmacologic therapy; however, this may be cost-prohibitive. Several studies have evaluated variceal band ligation and variceal sclerotherapy as methods for providing primary prophylaxis.

Endoscopic variceal ligation (EVL) has achieved a level of success and comfort with most gastroenterologists who see patients with these complications of portal hypertension. Thus, in patients with cirrhosis who are screened for portal hypertension and are found to have large varices, it is recommended that they receive either beta blockade or primary prophylaxis with EVL.

The approach to patients once they have had a variceal bleed is first to treat the acute bleed, which can be life-threatening, and then to prevent further bleeding. Prevention of further bleeding is usually accomplished with repeated variceal band ligation until varices are obliterated. Treatment of acute bleeding requires both fluid and blood-product replacement as well as prevention of subsequent bleeding with EVL.

The medical management of acute variceal hemorrhage includes the use of vasoconstricting agents, usually somatostatin or octreotide. Vasopressin was used in the past but is no longer commonly used. Balloon tamponade (Sengstaken-Blakemore tube or Minnesota tube) can be used in patients who cannot get endoscopic therapy immediately or who need stabilization prior to endoscopic therapy. Control of bleeding can be achieved in the vast majority of cases; however, bleeding recurs in the majority of patients if definitive endoscopic therapy has not been instituted. Octreotide, a direct splanchnic vasoconstrictor, is given at dosages of 50–100 μg/h by continuous infusion. Endoscopic intervention is used as first-line treatment to control bleeding acutely. Some endoscopists will use variceal injection therapy (sclerotherapy) as initial therapy, particularly when bleeding is vigorous. Variceal band ligation is used to control acute bleeding in over 90% of cases and should be repeated until obliteration of all varices is accomplished. When esophageal varices extend into the proximal stomach, band ligation is less successful. In these situations, when bleeding continues from gastric varices, consideration for a transjugular intrahepatic portosystemic shunt (TIPS) should be made. This technique creates a portosystemic shunt by a percutaneous approach using an expandable metal stent, which is advanced under angiographic guidance to the hepatic veins and then through the substance of the liver to create a direct portocaval shunt. This offers an alternative to surgery for acute decompression of portal hypertension. Encephalopathy can occur in as many as 20% of patients after TIPS and is particularly problematic in elderly patients and in patients with preexisting encephalopathy. TIPS should be reserved for individuals who fail endoscopic or medical management or who are poor surgical risks. TIPS can sometimes be used as a bridge to transplantation. Surgical esophageal transsection is a procedure that is rarely used and generally is associated with a poor outcome.

PREVENTION OF RECURRENT BLEEDING (FIG. 44-3) Once patients have had an acute bleed and have been managed successfully, attention should be paid to preventing recurrent bleeding. This usually requires repeated variceal band ligation until varices are obliterated. Beta blockade may be of adjunctive benefit in patients who are having recurrent variceal band ligation; however, once varices have been obliterated, the need for beta blockade is lessened. Despite successful variceal obliteration, many patients will still have portal hypertensive gastropathy from which bleeding can occur. Nonselective beta blockade

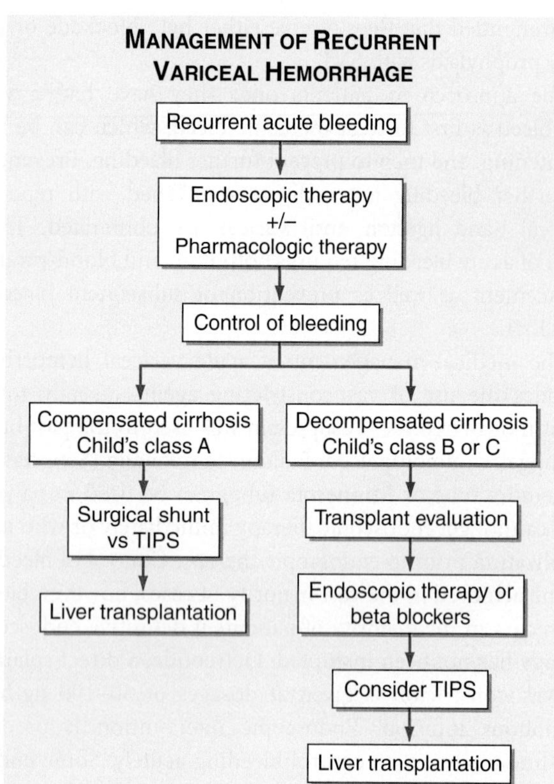

FIGURE 44-3

Management of recurrent variceal hemorrhage. This algorithm describes an approach to management of patients who have recurrent bleeding from esophageal varices. Initial therapy is generally with endoscopic therapy often supplemented by pharmacologic therapy. With control of bleeding, a decision needs to be made as to whether patients should go on to a surgical shunt or TIPS (if they are Child's class A) and be considered for transplant, or if they should have TIPS and be considered for transplant (if they are Child's class B or C). TIPS, transjugular intrahepatic portosystemic shunt.

may be helpful to prevent further bleeding from portal hypertensive gastropathy once varices have been obliterated.

Portosystemic shunt surgery is less commonly performed with the advent of TIPS; nonetheless, this procedure should be considered for patients with good hepatic synthetic function who could benefit by having portal decompressive surgery.

SPLENOMEGALY AND HYPERSPLENISM

Congestive splenomegaly is common in patients with portal hypertension. Clinical features include the presence of an enlarged spleen on physical examination and the development of thrombocytopenia and leukopenia in patients who have cirrhosis. Some patients will have fairly significant left-sided and left upper quadrant abdominal pain related to an enlarged and engorged spleen. Splenomegaly itself usually requires no specific treatment, although splenectomy can be successfully performed under very special circumstances.

Hypersplenism with the development of thrombocytopenia is a common feature of patients with cirrhosis and is usually the first indication of portal hypertension.

ASCITES

Definition

Ascites is the accumulation of fluid within the peritoneal cavity. Overwhelmingly, the most common cause of ascites is portal hypertension related to cirrhosis; however, clinicians should remember that malignant or infectious causes of ascites can be present as well, and careful differentiation of these other causes are obviously important for patient care.

Pathogenesis

The presence of portal hypertension contributes to the development of ascites in patients who have cirrhosis (Fig. 44-4). There is an increase in intrahepatic resistance, causing increased portal pressure, but there is also vasodilation of the splanchnic arterial system, which, in turn, results in an increase in portal venous inflow. Both of these abnormalities result in increased production of splanchnic lymph. Vasodilating factors such as nitric oxide are responsible for the vasodilatory effect. These hemodynamic changes result in sodium retention by causing activation of the renin-angiotensin-aldosterone system with the development

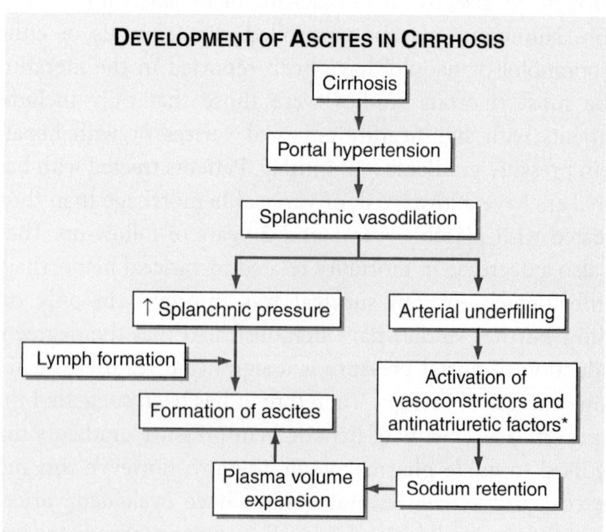

FIGURE 44-4

Development of ascites in cirrhosis. This flow diagram illustrates the importance of portal hypertension with splanchnic vasodilation in the development of ascites.

*Antinatriuretic factors include the renin-angiotensin-aldosterone system and the sympathetic nervous system.

of hyperaldosteronism. The renal effects of increased aldosterone leading to sodium retention also contribute to the development of ascites. Sodium retention causes fluid accumulation and expansion of the extracellular fluid volume, which results in the formation of peripheral edema and ascites. Sodium retention is the consequence of a homeostatic response caused by underfilling of the arterial circulation secondary to arterial vasodilation in the splanchnic vascular bed. Because the retained fluid is constantly leaking out of the intravascular compartment into the peritoneal cavity, the sensation of vascular filling is not achieved, and the process continues. Hypoalbuminemia and reduced plasma oncotic pressure also contribute to the loss of fluid from the vascular compartment into the peritoneal cavity. Hypoalbuminemia is due to decreased synthetic function in a cirrhotic liver.

Clinical features

Patients typically note an increase in abdominal girth that is often accompanied by the development of peripheral edema. The development of ascites is often insidious, and it is surprising that some patients wait so long and become so distended before seeking medical attention. Patients usually have at least 1–2 L of fluid in the abdomen before they are aware that there is an increase. If ascitic fluid is massive, respiratory function can be compromised, and patients will complain of shortness of breath. Hepatic hydrothorax may also occur in this setting, contributing to respiratory symptoms. Patients with massive ascites are often malnourished and have muscle wasting and excessive fatigue and weakness.

Diagnosis

Diagnosis of ascites is by physical examination and is often aided by abdominal imaging. Patients will have bulging flanks, may have a fluid wave, or may have the presence of shifting dullness. This is determined by taking patients from a supine position to lying on either their left or right side and noting the movement of the dullness to percussion. Subtle amounts of ascites can be detected by ultrasound or CT scanning. Hepatic hydrothorax is more common on the right side and implicates a rent in the diaphragm with free flow of ascitic fluid into the thoracic cavity.

When patients present with ascites for the first time, it is recommended that a diagnostic paracentesis be performed to characterize the fluid. This should include the determination of total protein and albumin content, blood cell counts with differential, and cultures. In the appropriate setting, amylase may be measured and cytology performed. In patients with cirrhosis, the protein concentration of the ascitic fluid is quite low, with the majority of patients having an ascitic fluid protein concentration <1 g/dL. The development of the serum ascites-to-albumin gradient (SAAG) has replaced the description of exudative or transudative fluid. When the gradient between the serum albumin level and the ascitic fluid albumin level is >1.1 g/dL, the cause of the ascites is most likely due to portal hypertension; this is usually in the setting of cirrhosis. When the gradient is <1.1 g/dL, infectious or malignant causes of ascites should be considered. When levels of ascitic fluid proteins are very low, patients are at increased risk for developing SBP. A high level of red blood cells in the ascitic fluid signifies a traumatic tap or perhaps a hepatocellular cancer or a ruptured omental varix. When the absolute level of polymorphonuclear leukocytes is >250/μL, the question of ascitic fluid infection should be strongly considered. Ascitic fluid cultures should be obtained using bedside inoculation of culture media.

TREATMENT Ascites

Patients with small amounts of ascites can usually be managed with dietary sodium restriction alone. Most average diets in the United States contain 6–8 g of sodium per day, and if patients eat at restaurants or fast-food outlets, the amount of sodium in their diet can exceed this amount. Thus, it is often extremely difficult to get patients to change their dietary habits to ingest <2 g of sodium per day, which is the recommended amount. Patients are frequently surprised to realize how much sodium is in the standard U.S. diet; thus, it is important to make educational pamphlets available to the patient. Often, a simple recommendation is to eat fresh or frozen foods, avoiding canned or processed foods, which are usually preserved with sodium. When a moderate amount of ascites is present, diuretic therapy is usually necessary. Traditionally, spironolactone at 100–200 mg/d as a single dose is started, and furosemide may be added at 40–80 mg/d, particularly in patients who have peripheral edema. In patients who have never received diuretics before, the failure of the above-mentioned dosages suggests that they are not being compliant with a low-sodium diet. If compliance is confirmed and ascitic fluid is not being mobilized, spironolactone can be increased to 400–600 mg/d and furosemide increased to 120–160 mg/d. If ascites is still present with these dosages of diuretics in patients who are compliant with a low-sodium diet, then they are defined as having *refractory ascites*, and alternative treatment modalities including repeated large-volume paracentesis or a TIPS procedure should be considered (Fig. 44-5). Recent studies have shown that TIPS, while managing the ascites, does not improve survival in these patients. Unfortunately, TIPS is often associated with an increased frequency of hepatic encephalopathy and must be considered carefully on a case-by-case basis. The prognosis for patients with cirrhosis with ascites is poor,

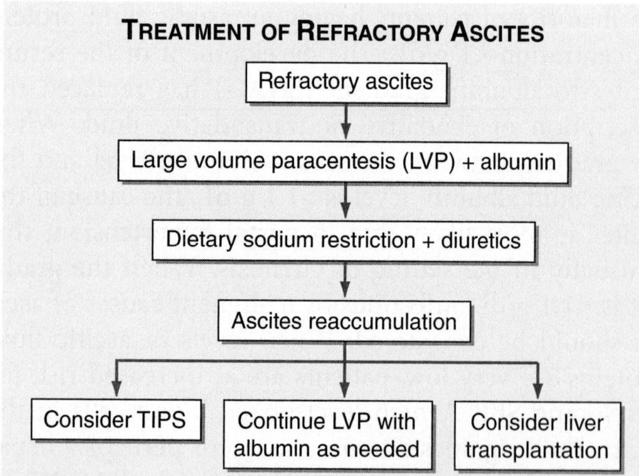

FIGURE 44-5

Treatment of refractory ascites. In patients who develop azotemia in the course of receiving diuretics in the management of their ascites, some will require repeated large-volume paracentesis (LVP), some may be considered for transjugular intrahepatic portosystemic shunt (TIPS), and some would be good candidates for liver transplantation. These decisions are all individualized.

and some studies have shown that <50% of patients survive 2 years after the onset of ascites. Thus, there should be consideration for liver transplantation in patients with the onset of ascites.

SPONTANEOUS BACTERIAL PERITONITIS

SBP is a common and severe complication of ascites characterized by spontaneous infection of the ascitic fluid without an intraabdominal source. In patients with cirrhosis and ascites severe enough for hospitalization, SBP can occur in up to 30% of individuals and can have a 25% in-hospital mortality rate. Bacterial translocation is the presumed mechanism for development of SBP, with gut flora traversing the intestine into mesenteric lymph nodes, leading to bacteremia and seeding of the ascitic fluid. The most common organisms are *Escherichia coli* and other gut bacteria; however, gram-positive bacteria, including *Streptococcus viridans, Staphylococcus aureus,* and *Enterococcus* sp., can also be found. If more than two organisms are identified, secondary bacterial peritonitis due to a perforated viscus should be considered. The diagnosis of SBP is made when the fluid sample has an absolute neutrophil count >250/μL. Bedside cultures should be obtained when ascitic fluid is tapped. Patients with ascites may present with fever, altered mental status, elevated white blood cell count, and abdominal pain or discomfort, or they may present without any of these features. Therefore, it is necessary to have a high degree of clinical suspicion, and peritoneal taps are important for making the diagnosis. Treatment is with a third-generation cephalosporin, with cefotaxime being the most commonly used antibiotic. In patients with variceal hemorrhage, the frequency of SBP is significantly increased, and prophylaxis against SBP is recommended when a patient presents with upper GI bleeding. Furthermore, in patients who have had an episode(s) of SBP and recovered, once-weekly administration of antibiotics is used as prophylaxis for recurrent SBP.

HEPATORENAL SYNDROME

The hepatorenal syndrome (HRS) is a form of functional renal failure without renal pathology that occurs in about 10% of patients with advanced cirrhosis or acute liver failure. There are marked disturbances in the arterial renal circulation in patients with HRS; these include an increase in vascular resistance accompanied by a reduction in systemic vascular resistance. The reason for renal vasoconstriction is most likely multifactorial and is poorly understood. The diagnosis is made usually in the presence of a large amount of ascites in patients who have a stepwise progressive increase in creatinine. Type 1 HRS is characterized by a progressive impairment in renal function and a significant reduction in creatinine clearance within 1–2 weeks of presentation. Type 2 HRS is characterized by a reduction in glomerular filtration rate with an elevation of serum creatinine level, but it is fairly stable and is associated with a better outcome than that of type 1 HRS.

HRS is often seen in patients with refractory ascites and requires exclusion of other causes of acute renal failure. Treatment has, unfortunately, been difficult, and in the past, dopamine or prostaglandin analogues were used as renal vasodilating medications. Carefully performed studies have failed to show clear-cut benefit from these therapeutic approaches. Currently, patients are treated with midodrine, an α-agonist, along with octreotide and intravenous albumin. The best therapy for HRS is liver transplantation; recovery of renal function is typical in this setting. In patients with either type 1 or type 2 HRS, the prognosis is poor unless transplant can be achieved within a short period of time.

HEPATIC ENCEPHALOPATHY

Portosystemic encephalopathy is a serious complication of chronic liver disease and is broadly defined as an alteration in mental status and cognitive function occurring in the presence of liver failure. In acute liver injury with fulminant hepatic failure, the development of encephalopathy is a requirement for a diagnosis of fulminant failure. Encephalopathy is much more commonly seen in patients with chronic liver disease. Gut-derived neurotoxins that are not removed by the liver because of vascular shunting and decreased hepatic mass get to the brain and cause the symptoms that we know of as hepatic encephalopathy. Ammonia levels are typically elevated in patients with hepatic encephalopathy, but the correlation between severity of liver disease and height of ammonia levels is often poor, and most hepatologists do not rely on ammonia levels to make a diagnosis. Other compounds and metabolites that may contribute to the development of encephalopathy include certain false neurotransmitters and mercaptans.

CLINICAL FEATURES

In acute liver failure, changes in mental status can occur within weeks to months. Brain edema can be seen in these patients, with severe encephalopathy associated with swelling of the gray matter. Cerebral herniation is a feared complication of brain edema in acute liver failure, and treatment is meant to decrease edema with mannitol and judicious use of intravenous fluids.

In patients with cirrhosis, encephalopathy is often found as a result of certain precipitating events such as hypokalemia, infection, an increased dietary protein load, or electrolyte disturbances. Patients may be confused or exhibit a change in personality. They may actually be quite violent and difficult to manage; alternatively, patients may be very sleepy and difficult to rouse. Because precipitating events are so commonly found, they should be sought carefully. If patients have ascites, this should be tapped to rule out infection. Evidence of GI bleeding should be sought, and patients should be appropriately hydrated. Electrolytes should be measured and abnormalities corrected. In patients presenting with encephalopathy, asterixis is often present. Asterixis can be elicited by having patients extend their arms and bend their wrists back. In this maneuver, patients who are encephalopathic have a "liver flap"—i.e., a sudden forward movement of the wrist. This requires patients to be able to cooperate with the examiner and obviously cannot be elicited in patients who are severely encephalopathic or in hepatic coma.

The diagnosis of hepatic encephalopathy is clinical and requires an experienced clinician to recognize and put together all of the various features. Often when patients have encephalopathy for the first time, they are unaware of what is transpiring, but once they have been through the experience for the first time, they can identify when this is developing in subsequent situations and can often self-medicate to impair the development or worsening of encephalopathy.

TREATMENT Hepatic Encephalopathy

Treatment is multifactorial and includes management of the above-mentioned precipitating factors. Sometimes hydration and correction of electrolyte imbalance are all that is necessary. In the past, restriction of dietary protein was considered for patients with encephalopathy; however, the negative impact of that maneuver on overall nutrition is thought to outweigh the benefit when treating encephalopathy, and it is thus discouraged. There may be some benefit to replacing animal-based protein with vegetable-based protein in some patients with encephalopathy that is difficult to manage. The mainstay of treatment for encephalopathy, in addition to correcting precipitating factors, is to use lactulose, a nonabsorbable disaccharide, which results in colonic acidification. Catharsis ensues, contributing to the elimination of nitrogenous products in the gut that are responsible for the development of encephalopathy. The goal of lactulose therapy is to promote 2–3 soft stools per day. Patients are asked to titrate their amount of ingested lactulose to achieve the desired effect. Poorly absorbed antibiotics are often used as adjunctive therapies for patients who have had a difficult time with lactulose. The alternating administration of neomycin and metronidazole has commonly been used to reduce the individual side effects of each: neomycin for renal insufficiency and ototoxicity and metronidazole for peripheral neuropathy. More recently, rifaximin at 550 mg twice daily has been very effective in treating encephalopathy without the known side effects of neomycin or metronidazole. Zinc supplementation is sometimes helpful in patients with encephalopathy and is relatively harmless. The development of encephalopathy in patients with chronic liver disease is a poor prognostic sign, but this complication can be managed in the vast majority of patients.

MALNUTRITION IN CIRRHOSIS

Because the liver is principally involved in the regulation of protein and energy metabolism in the body, it is not surprising that patients with advanced liver disease are commonly malnourished. Once patients become cirrhotic, they are more catabolic, and muscle protein is metabolized. There are multiple factors that contribute to the malnutrition of cirrhosis, including poor dietary intake, alterations in gut nutrient absorption, and alterations in protein metabolism. Dietary supplementation for patients with cirrhosis is helpful in preventing patients from becoming catabolic.

ABNORMALITIES IN COAGULATION

Coagulopathy is almost universal in patients with cirrhosis. There is decreased synthesis of clotting factors and impaired clearance of anticoagulants. In addition, patients may have thrombocytopenia from hypersplenism due to portal hypertension. Vitamin K–dependent clotting factors are factors II, VII, IX, and X. Vitamin K requires biliary excretion for its subsequent absorption; thus, in patients with chronic cholestatic syndromes, vitamin K absorption is frequently diminished. Intravenous or intramuscular vitamin K can quickly correct this abnormality. More commonly, the synthesis of vitamin K–dependent clotting factors is diminished because of a decrease in hepatic mass, and, under these circumstances, administration of parenteral vitamin K does not improve the clotting factors or the prothrombin time. Platelet function is often abnormal in patients with chronic liver disease, in addition to decreases in platelet levels due to hypersplenism.

BONE DISEASE IN CIRRHOSIS

Osteoporosis is common in patients with chronic cholestatic liver disease because of malabsorption of vitamin D and decreased calcium ingestion. The rate of bone resorption exceeds that of new bone formation in patients with cirrhosis, resulting in bone loss. Dual x-ray absorptiometry (DEXA) is a useful method for determining osteoporosis or osteopenia in patients with chronic liver disease. When a DEXA scan shows decreased bone mass, treatment should be administered with bisphosphonates that are effective at inhibiting resorption of bone and efficacious in the treatment of osteoporosis.

HEMATOLOGIC ABNORMALITIES IN CIRRHOSIS

Numerous hematologic manifestations of cirrhosis are present, including anemia from a variety of causes including hypersplenism, hemolysis, iron deficiency, and perhaps folate deficiency from malnutrition. Macrocytosis is a common abnormality in red blood cell morphology seen in patients with chronic liver disease, and neutropenia may be seen as a result of hypersplenism.

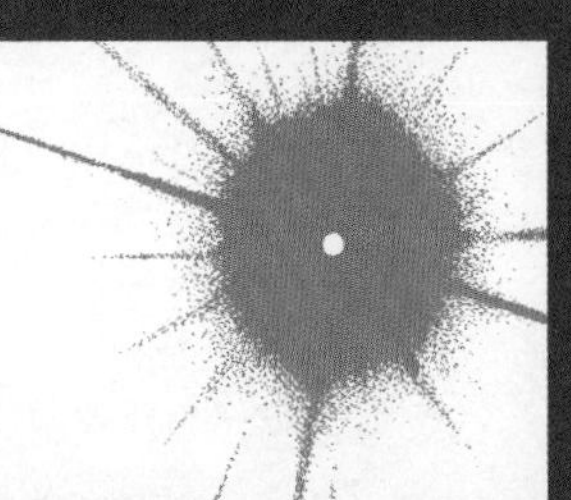

CHAPTER 45

ATLAS OF LIVER BIOPSIES

Jules L. Dienstag ■ Atul K. Bhan

Although clinical and laboratory features yield clues to the extent of inflammatory processes (disease grade), the degree of scarring and architectural distortion (disease stage), and the nature of the disease process, the liver biopsy is felt to represent the gold standard for assessing the degree of liver injury and fibrosis. Examination of liver histology provides not only a basis for quantitative scoring of disease activity and progression but also a wealth of qualitative information that can direct and inform diagnosis and management.

A normal liver lobule consists of portal (zone 1), lobular (midzonal or zone 2), and central (zone 3) zones. The portal tract contains the hepatic artery (HA) and portal vein (PV), which represent the dual vascular supply to the liver, as well as the bile duct (BD). The lobular area contains cords of liver cells surrounded by vascular sinusoids, and the central zone consists of the central vein (CV), the terminal branch of the hepatic vein (see figure below).

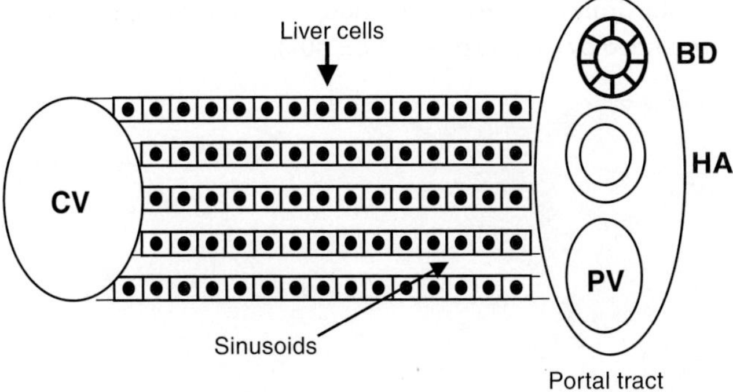

Included in this atlas of liver biopsies are examples of common morphologic features of acute and chronic liver disorders, some involving the lobular areas (e.g., the lobular inflammatory changes of acute hepatitis, apoptotic hepatocyte degeneration in acute and chronic hepatitis, virus antigen localization in hepatocyte cytoplasm and/or nuclei, viral inclusion bodies, copper or iron deposition, other inclusion bodies) and others involving the portal tracts (e.g., the portal mononuclear infiltrate that expands and spills over beyond the border of periportal hepatocytes in chronic hepatitis C, autoimmune hepatitis, and liver allograft rejection) or centrizonal areas (e.g., acute acetaminophen hepatotoxicity). Other histologic features of importance include hepatic steatosis (observed in alcoholic liver injury, nonalcoholic fatty liver disorders, and metabolic disorders–including mitochondrial injury–and in patients with chronic viral hepatitis); injury of bile ducts in the portal tract, an important diagnostic hallmark of primary biliary cirrhosis, primary sclerosing cholangitis, and liver allograft rejection; cholestasis in intrahepatic or extrahepatic biliary obstruction or in infiltrative disorders; ductular proliferation in the setting of marked hepatocellular necrosis; plasma cell infiltration common in autoimmune hepatitis; portal inflammation affecting portal veins ("endothelialitis") in liver allograft rejection; and mild-to-severe fibrosis, in varying distribution and pattern, as a consequence of liver injury common to many disorders. (All magnifications reflect the objective lens used.)

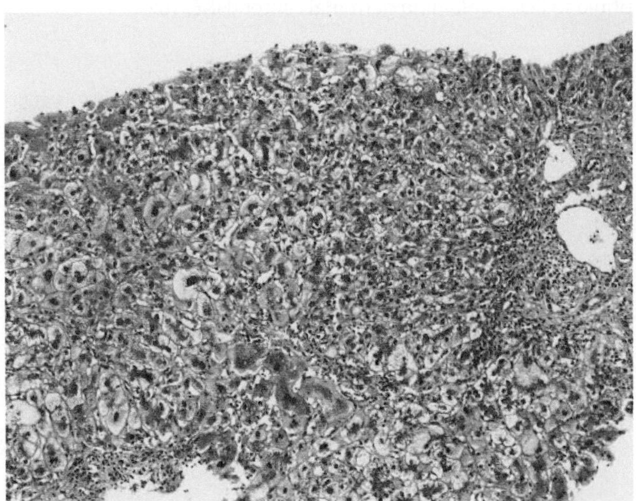

FIGURE 45-1
Acute hepatitis with lobular inflammation and hepatocellular ballooning (hematoxylin and eosin [H&E], 10×).

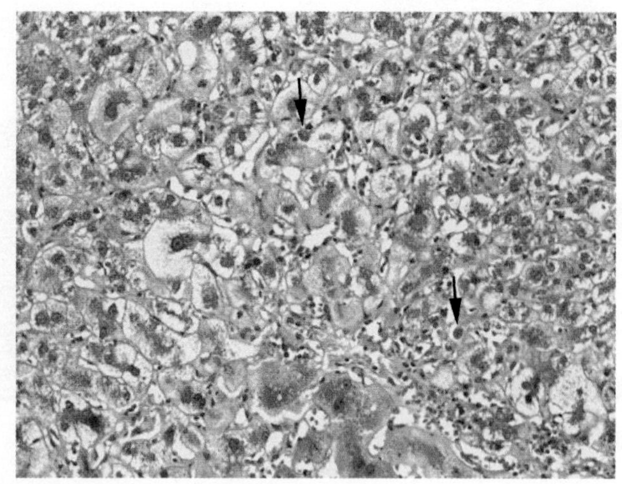

FIGURE 45-2
Acute hepatitis, higher magnification, showing lobular inflammation, hepatocellular ballooning, and acidophilic bodies (*arrows*) (H&E, 20×).

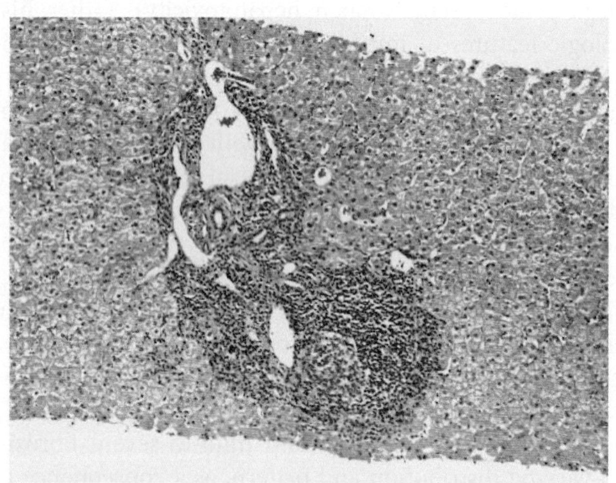

FIGURE 45-3
Chronic hepatitis C with portal lymphoid infiltrate and lymphoid follicle containing germinal center (H&E, 10×).

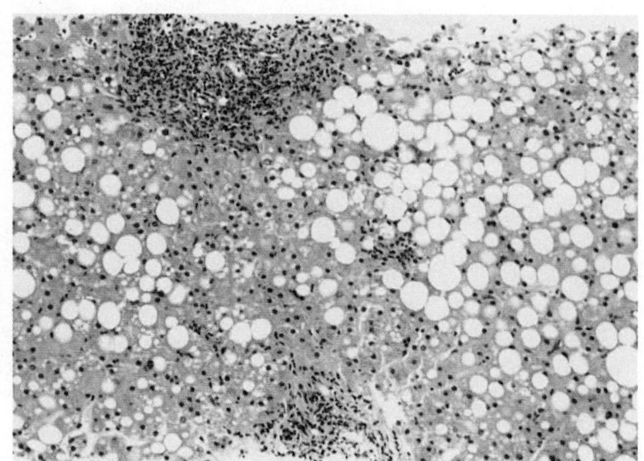

FIGURE 45-4
Chronic hepatitis C with portal and lobular inflammation and steatosis (H&E, 10×).

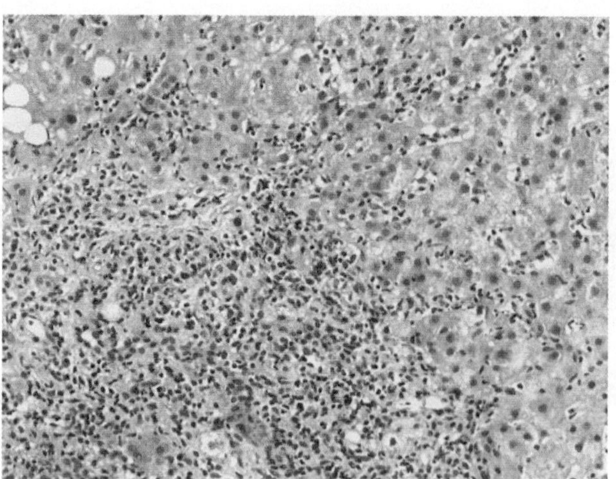

FIGURE 45-5
Chronic hepatitis C with portal inflammation and interface hepatitis (erosion of the limiting plate of periportal hepatocytes by infiltrating mononuclear cells) (H&E, 20×).

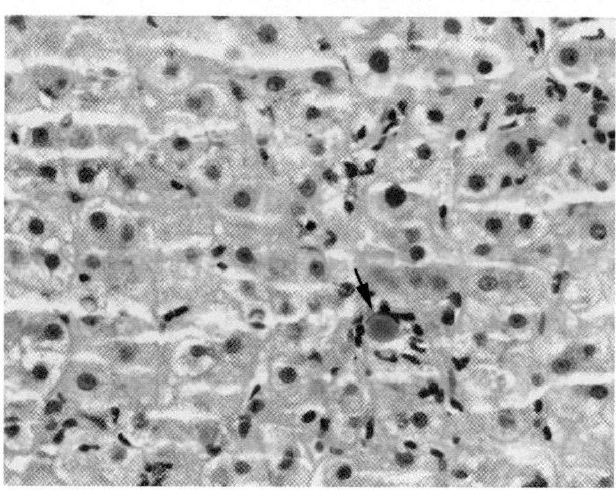

FIGURE 45-6
Lobular inflammation with acidophilic body (apoptotic body) surrounded by lymphoid cells (H&E, 40×).

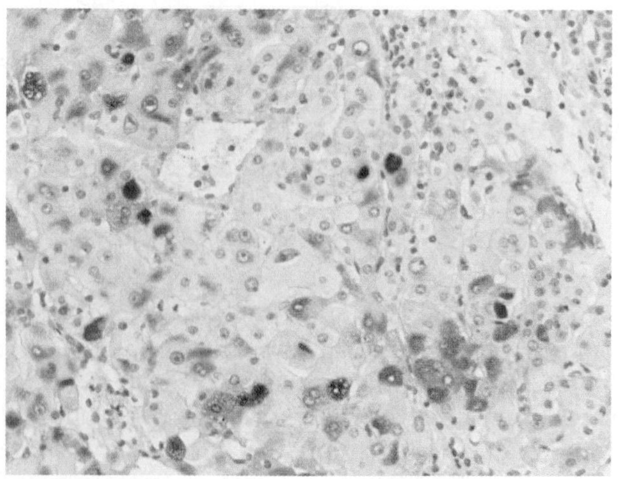

FIGURE 45-7
Chronic hepatitis B with hepatocellular cytoplasmic staining for hepatitis B surface antigen (immunoperoxidase, 20×).

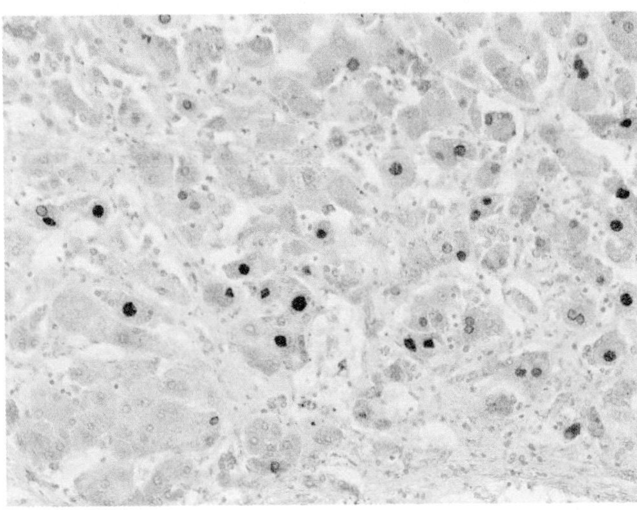

FIGURE 45-8
Chronic hepatitis B with hepatocellular nuclear staining for hepatitis B core antigen (immunoperoxidase, 20×).

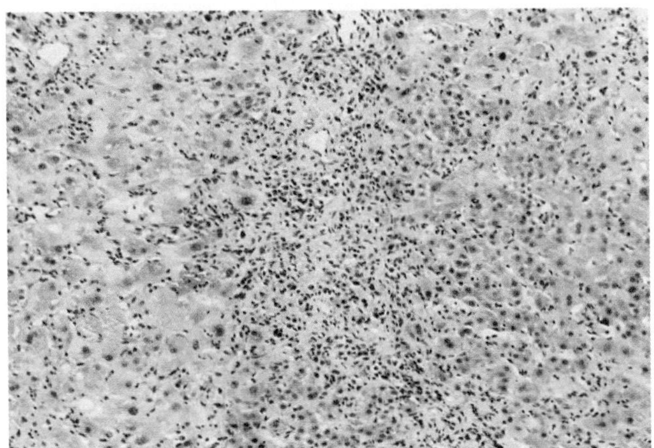

FIGURE 45-9
Autoimmune hepatitis with portal and lobular inflammation, interface hepatitis, and cholestasis (H&E, 10×).

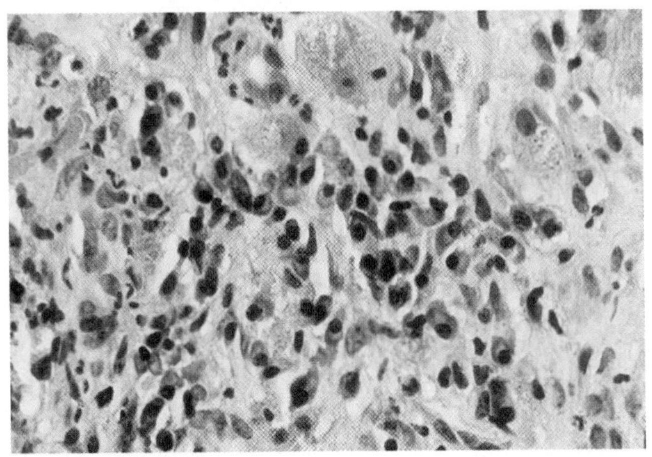

FIGURE 45-10
Autoimmune hepatitis, higher magnification, showing dense plasma cell infiltrate in the portal and periportal regions (H&E, 40×).

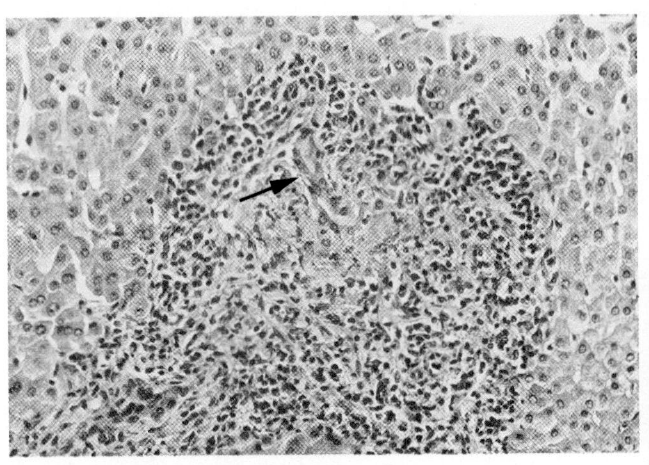

FIGURE 45-11
Primary biliary cirrhosis with degenerating bile duct epithelium ("florid ductular lesion") (*arrow*) surrounded by epithelioid granulomatous reaction and lymphoplasmacytic infiltrate (H&E, 40×).

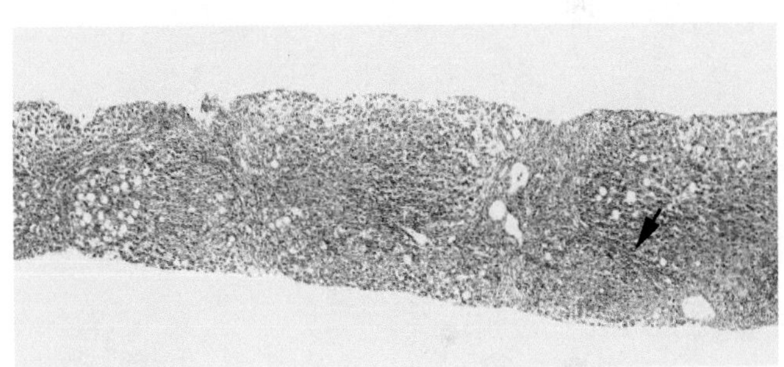

FIGURE 45-12
Chronic hepatitis C with bridging fibrosis (*arrow*) (Masson trichrome, 10×).

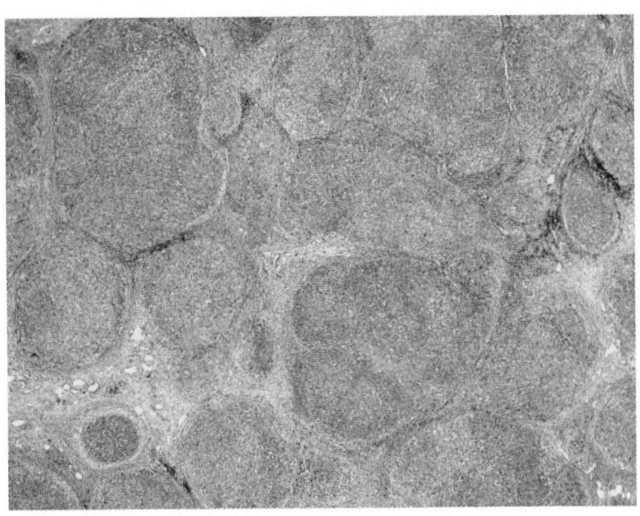

FIGURE 45-13
Cirrhosis with architectural alteration resulting from fibrosis and nodular hepatocellular regeneration (Masson trichrome, 2×).

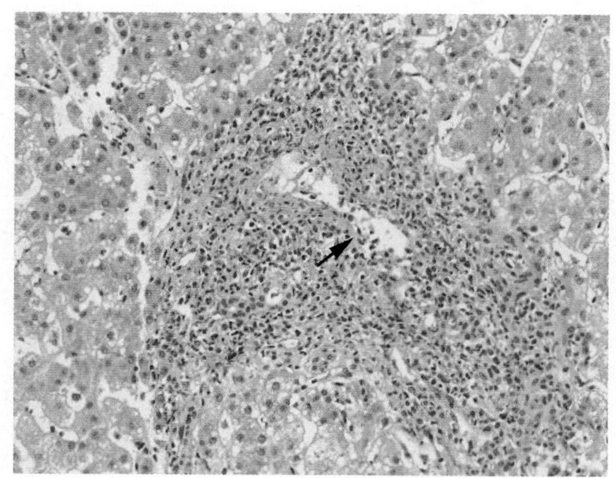

FIGURE 45-14
Acute cellular rejection of orthotopic liver allograft demonstrating a mixed inflammatory cell infiltrate (lymphoid cells, eosinophils, neutrophils) of the portal tract as well as endothelialitis of the portal vein (*arrow*) and bile duct injury (H&E, 10×).

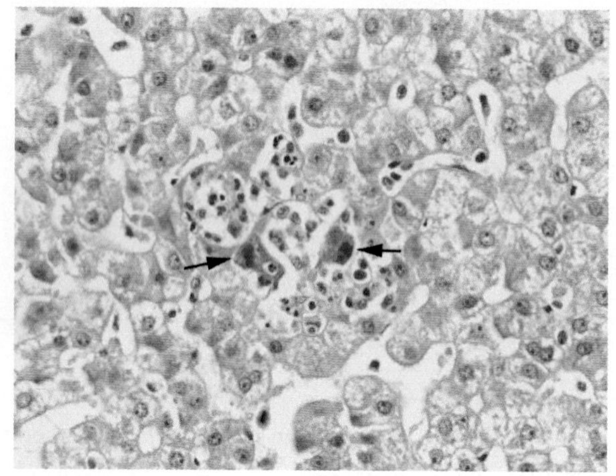

FIGURE 45-15
Liver allograft with cytomegalovirus infection showing hepatocytes with nuclear inclusions (*arrows*) surrounded by a neutrophilic and lymphoid infiltrate (H&E, 10×).

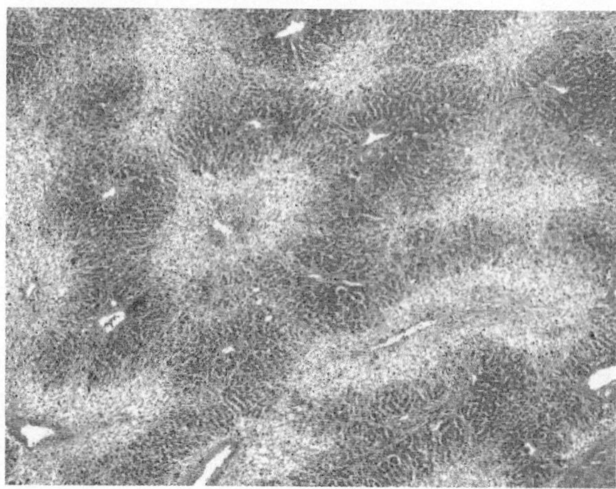

FIGURE 45-16
Combined acetaminophen hepatotoxicity and alcoholic liver injury with extensive centrilobular areas of necrosis (H&E, 4×).

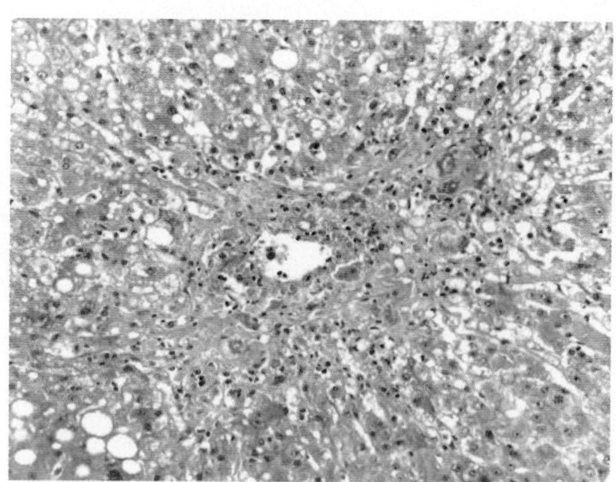

FIGURE 45-17
Combined acetaminophen hepatotoxicity and alcoholic liver injury at higher magnification showing necrotic centrilobular area with Mallory bodies (H&E 20×).

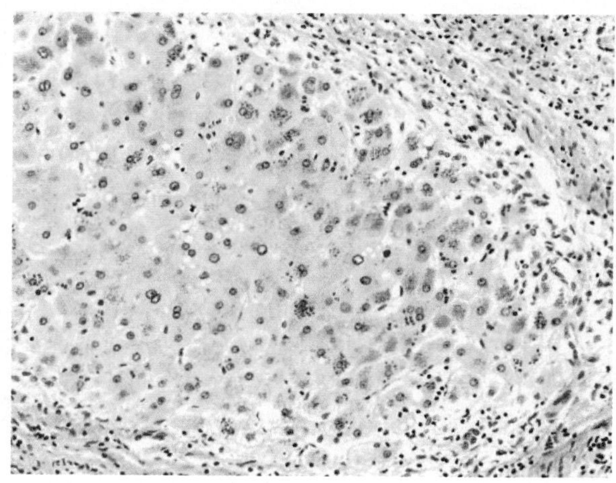

FIGURE 45-18
α_1 **Antitrypsin deficiency** with cytoplasmic periodic acid–Schiff (PAS)-positive, diastase-resistant globules in many hepatocytes, predominantly at the periphery of a cirrhotic nodule (PAS, 20×).

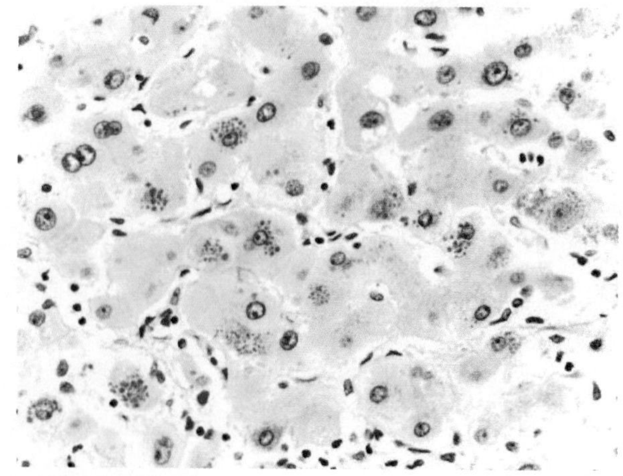

FIGURE 45-19
α_1 **Antitrypsin deficiency** with higher magnification of PAS-positive, diastase-resistant globules (PAS, 40×).

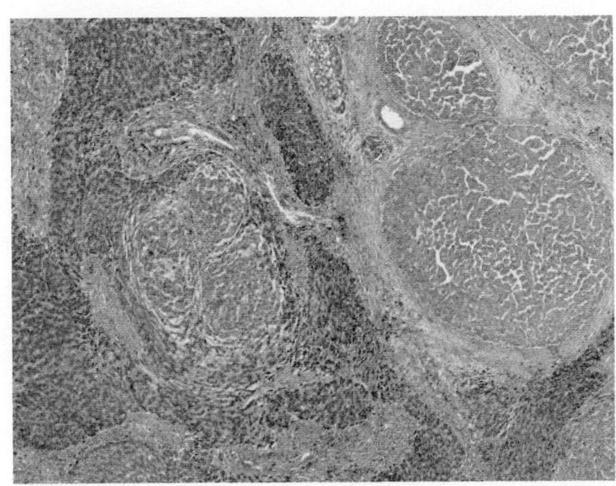

FIGURE 45-20
Cirrhosis secondary to hemochromatosis with hepatocellular carcinoma; brown hemosiderin pigment (iron) is present in the cirrhotic liver, while the hepatocellular carcinoma nodules are hemosiderin-free (H&E, 4×).

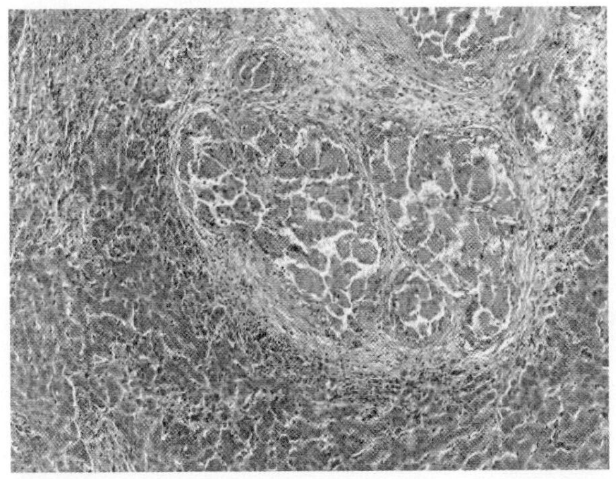

FIGURE 45-21
Cirrhosis secondary to hemochromatosis with hepatocellular carcinoma at higher magnification, demonstrating nodules of large malignant cells with highly disorganized architecture (H&E, 10×).

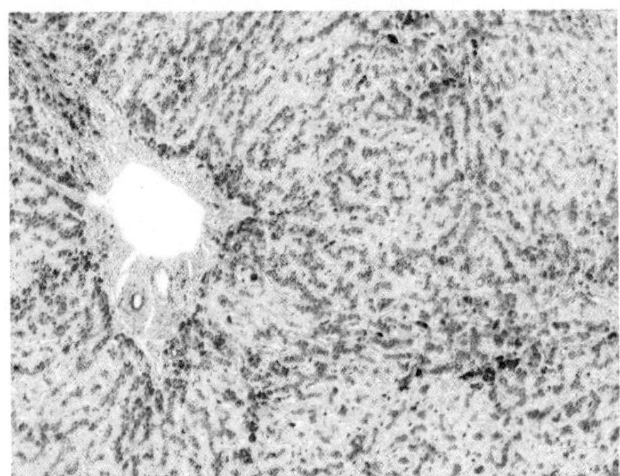

FIGURE 45-22
Hemochromatosis with iron stain demonstrating extensive iron deposition and characteristic pattern of pericanalicular distribution of iron (iron stain, 10×).

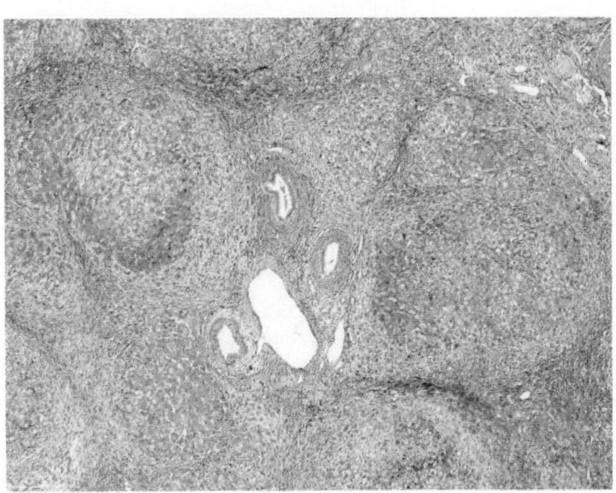

FIGURE 45-23
Primary sclerosing cholangitis showing cirrhosis and periductular fibrosis (Masson trichrome, 4×).

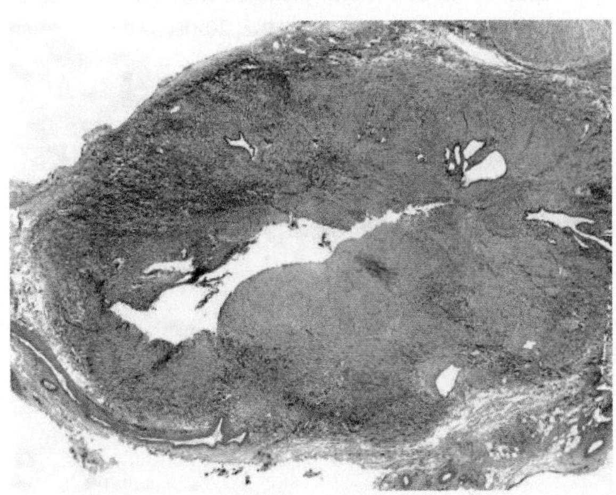

FIGURE 45-24
Primary sclerosing cholangitis showing the extrahepatic bile duct (in a liver explant obtained at the time of hepatectomy for orthotopic liver transplantation) with marked mural chronic inflammation and fibrosis as well as peribiliary glands (H&E, 2×).

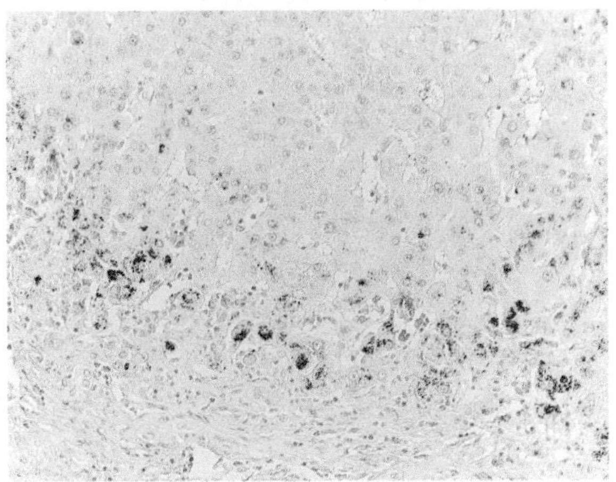

FIGURE 45-25
Primary sclerosing cholangitis showing peripheral cholestasis (*green*) and cytoplasmic red granular staining of hepatocytes for copper (rhodamine copper stain, 20×).

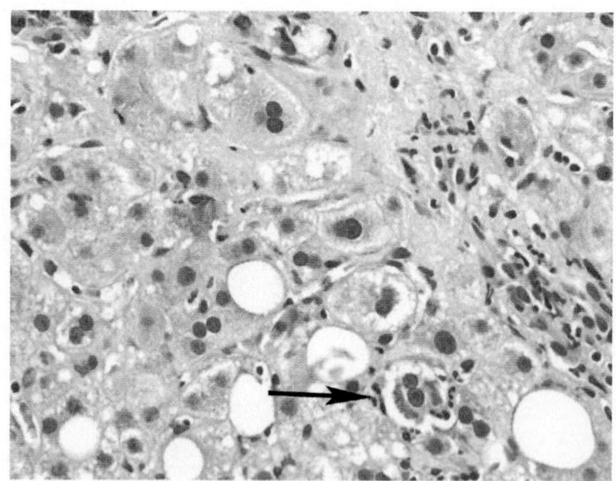

FIGURE 45-26
Nonalcoholic steatohepatitis (NASH) showing steatosis, ballooned hepatocytes, and Mallory bodies with surrounding polymorphonuclear leukocytes (*arrow*) (H&E, 20×).

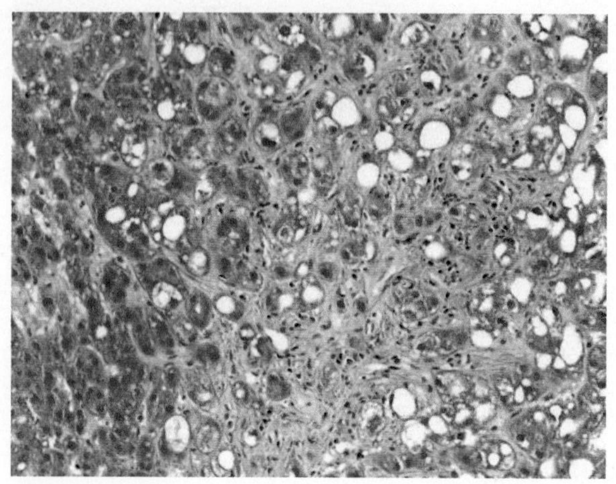

FIGURE 45-27
Nonalcoholic steatohepatitis (NASH) showing steatosis with perisinusoidal and pericellular fibrosis (H&E, 20×).

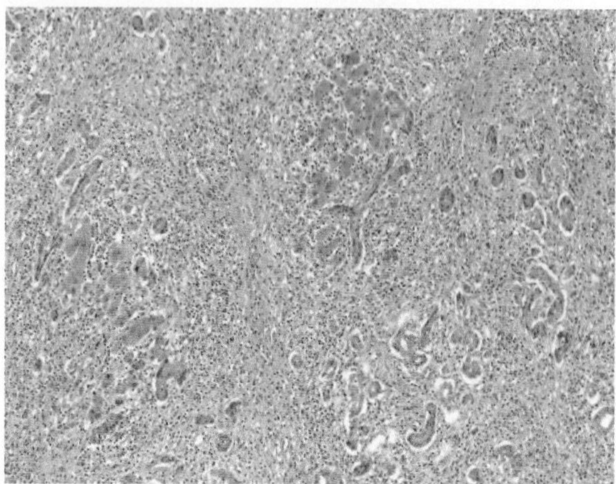

FIGURE 45-28
Acute hepatitis with submassive hepatic necrosis with marked parenchymal collapse, remnant islands of surviving hepatocytes, and a marked ductular reaction (H&E, 10×).

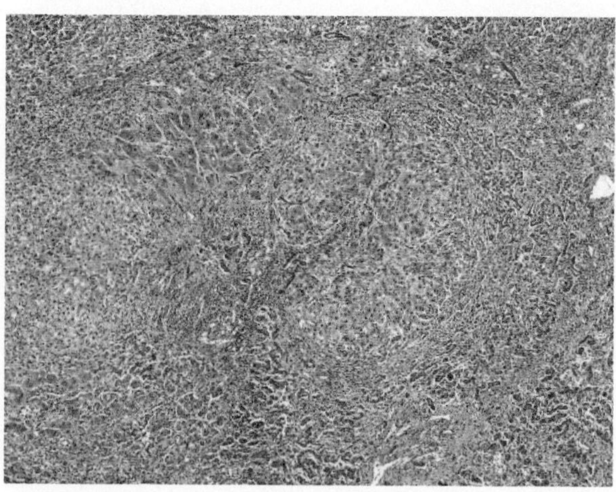

FIGURE 45-29
Wilson's disease showing cirrhosis, extensive collapse, and ductular reaction in a teenager with an acute presentation (H&E, 4×).

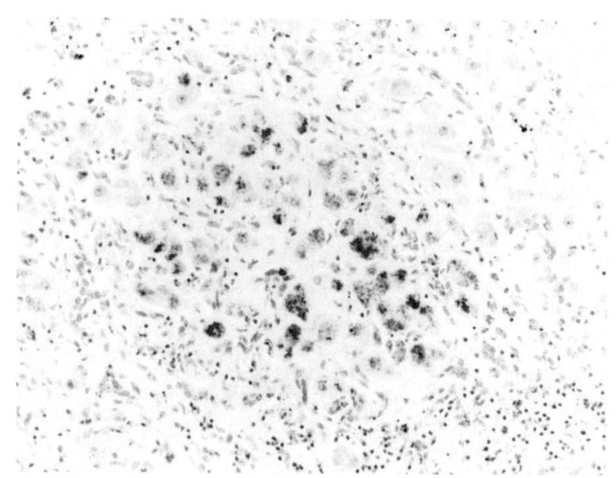

FIGURE 45-30
Wilson's disease showing extensive hepatocyte cytoplasmic red granular staining for copper in a cirrhotic nodule (rhodanine copper stain, 20×).

CHAPTER 46

GENETIC, METABOLIC, AND INFILTRATIVE DISEASES AFFECTING THE LIVER

Bruce R. Bacon

There are a number of disorders of the liver that fit within the categories of genetic, metabolic, and infiltrative disorders (Table 46-1). Inherited disorders include hemochromatosis, Wilson's disease, α_1 antitrypsin (α_1AT) deficiency, and cystic fibrosis (CF). Hemochromatosis is the most common inherited disorder affecting white populations, with the genetic susceptibility for the disease being identified in 1 in 250 individuals. Over the past 15 years, it has become increasingly apparent that nonalcoholic fatty liver disease (NAFLD) is the most common cause of elevated liver enzymes found in the U.S. population. This disorder is discussed in greater detail in **Chap. 43.** Infiltrative disorders of the liver are relatively rare.

TABLE 46-1

GENETIC, METABOLIC, AND INFILTRATIVE DISEASES AFFECTING THE LIVER
Genetic • Hereditary hemochromatosis • Wilson's disease • α_1 Antitrypsin deficiency • Cystic fibrosis

Metabolic
• Nonalcoholic fatty liver disease
• Lipid storage diseases
  • Gaucher's
  • Niemann-Pick
  • Tangier
  • Fabry's
• Porphyrias
  • Porphyria cutanea tarda

Infiltrative disorders • Amyloidosis • Granulomas • Sarcoidosis • Lymphoma

GENETIC LIVER DISEASES

Hereditary hemochromatosis

Hereditary hemochromatosis (HH) is a common inherited disorder of iron metabolism. Our knowledge of the disease and its phenotypic expression has changed since 1996, when the gene for HH, called *HFE*, was identified, allowing for genetic testing for the two major mutations (C282Y and H63D) that are responsible for *HFE*-related HH. Subsequently, several additional genes/proteins involved in the regulation of iron homeostasis have been identified, contributing to a better understanding of cellular iron uptake and release and the characterization of additional causes of inherited iron overload (Table 46-2).

Most patients with HH are asymptomatic; however, when patients present with symptoms, they are frequently nonspecific and include weakness, fatigue, lethargy, and weight loss. Specific, organ-related symptoms include abdominal pain, arthralgias, and symptoms and signs of chronic liver disease. Increasingly, most patients are now identified before they have symptoms, either through family studies or from the performance of screening iron studies. Several prospective population studies have shown that C282Y homozygosity is found in about 1 in 250 individuals of northern European descent, with the heterozygote frequency seen in approximately 1 in 10 individuals. It is important to consider HH in patients who present with the symptoms and signs known to occur in established HH. When confronted with abnormal serum iron studies, clinicians should not wait for typical symptoms or findings of HH to appear before considering the diagnosis. However, once the diagnosis of HH is considered, either by an evaluation of abnormal screening iron studies in the context of family studies, in a patient with an abnormal genetic test, or in the evaluation of a patient

TABLE 46-2

CLASSIFICATION OF IRON OVERLOAD SYNDROMES
Hereditary Hemochromatosis (HH)
HFE-related (type 1)
C282Y/C282Y
C282Y/H63D
Other *HFE* mutations
Non-*HFE*-related
Juvenile HH
HJV—hemojuvelin (type 2a)
HAMP—hepcidin (type 2b)
TfR2-related HH (type 3)
Ferroportin-related HH (type 4)
African iron overload
Secondary Iron Overload
Iron-loading anemias
Parenteral iron overload
Chronic liver disease
Miscellaneous
Neonatal iron overload
Aceruloplasminemia
Congenital atransferrinemia

Abbreviations: HAMP, hepcidin; HJV, hemojuvelin; TfR2, transferrin receptor 2.

with any of the typical symptoms (Table 46-3) or clinical findings (Table 46-4), definitive diagnosis is relatively straightforward. Transferrin saturation (serum iron divided by total iron-binding capacity [TIBC] or transferrin, times 100%) and ferritin levels should be obtained. Both of these will be elevated in a symptomatic patient. It must be remembered that ferritin is an acute-phase reactant and can be elevated in a number of other inflammatory disorders, such as rheumatoid arthritis, or in various neoplastic diseases, such as lymphoma or other cancers. Also, serum ferritin is elevated in a majority of patients with nonalcoholic steatohepatitis (NASH), hepatitis C, and alcoholic liver disease in the absence of iron overload.

TABLE 46-3

SYMPTOMS OF HEREDITARY HEMOCHROMATOSIS

SYMPTOM	%
Weakness, lethargy, fatigue	40–85
Apathy, lack of interest	40–85
Abdominal pain	30–60
Weight loss	30–60
Arthralgias	40–60
Loss of libido, impotence	30–60
Amenorrhea	20–60
Congestive heart failure symptoms	0–40

TABLE 46-4

PHYSICAL FINDINGS IN HEREDITARY HEMOCHROMATOSIS

FINDING	%
Hepatomegaly	60–85
Cirrhosis	50–95
Skin pigmentation	40–80
Arthritis (second, third metacarpophalangeal joints)	40–60
Clinical diabetes	10–60
Splenomegaly	10–40
Loss of body hair	10–30
Testicular atrophy	10–30
Dilated cardiomyopathy	0–30

At present, if patients have an elevated transferrin saturation or ferritin level, genetic testing should be performed; if they are a C282Y homozygote or a compound heterozygote (C282Y/H63D), the diagnosis is confirmed. If liver enzymes (alanine aminotransferase [ALT], aspartate aminotransferase [AST]) are elevated or the ferritin is >1000 μg/L, the patient should be considered for liver biopsy because there is an increased frequency of advanced fibrosis in these individuals. If liver biopsy is performed, iron deposition is found in a periportal distribution with a periportal to pericentral gradient; iron is found predominantly in parenchymal cells, and Kupffer cells are spared.

TREATMENT Hereditary Hemochromatosis

Treatment of HH is relatively straightforward with weekly phlebotomy aimed to reduce iron stores, recognizing that each unit of blood contains 200–250 mg of iron. If patients are diagnosed and treated before the development of hepatic fibrosis, all complications of the disease can be avoided. Maintenance phlebotomy is required in most patients and usually can be achieved with 1 unit of blood removed every 2–3 months. Family studies should be performed with transferrin saturation, ferritin, and genetic testing offered to all first-degree relatives.

Wilson's disease

Wilson's disease is an inherited disorder of copper homeostasis first described in 1912. The Wilson's disease gene was discovered in 1993, with the identification of *ATP7B*. This P-type ATPase is involved in copper transport and is necessary for the export of copper from the hepatocyte. Thus, in patients with mutations in *ATP7B*, copper is retained in the liver, leading to increased copper storage and ultimately liver disease as a result.

The clinical presentation of Wilson's disease is variable and includes chronic hepatitis, hepatic steatosis, and cirrhosis in adolescents and young adults. Neurologic manifestations indicate that liver disease is present and include speech disorders and various movement disorders. Diagnosis includes the demonstration of a reduced ceruloplasmin level, increased urinary excretion of copper, the presence of Kayser-Fleischer rings in the corneas of the eyes, and an elevated hepatic copper level, in the appropriate clinical setting. The genetic diagnosis of Wilson's disease is difficult because >500 mutations in *ATP7B* have been described with different degrees of frequency and penetration in certain populations.

TREATMENT Wilson's Disease

Treatment consists of copper-chelating medications such as D-penicillamine and trientine. A role for zinc acetate has also been established. Medical treatment is lifelong, and severe relapses leading to liver failure and death can occur with cessation of therapy. Liver transplantation is curative with respect to the underlying metabolic defect and restores the normal phenotype with respect to copper homeostasis.

α_1 Antitrypsin deficiency

α_1AT deficiency was first described in the late 1960s in patients with severe pulmonary disease. α_1AT is a 52-kDa glycoprotein produced in hepatocytes, phagocytes, and epithelial cells in the lungs, which inhibits serine proteases, primarily neutrophil elastase. In α_1AT deficiency, increased amounts of neutrophil elastase can result in progressive lung injury from degradation of elastin, leading to premature emphysema. In the 1970s, α_1AT deficiency was discovered as a cause of neonatal liver disease, so-called "neonatal hepatitis." It is now known to be a cause of liver disease in infancy, early childhood, and adolescence, and in adults.

In α_1AT deficiency, variants in the proteinase inhibitor (Pi) gene located on chromosome 14 alter α_1AT structure, interfering with hepatocellular export. Aggregated, deformed polymers of α_1AT accumulate in the hepatocyte endoplasmic reticulum. There are over 75 different α_1AT variants. Conventional nomenclature identifies normal variants as PiMM; these individuals have normal blood levels of α_1AT. The most common abnormal variants are called S and Z. Individuals homozygous for the Z mutation (PiZZ) have low levels of α_1AT (about 15% of normal), and these patients are susceptible to liver and/or lung disease, yet only a proportion (about 25%) of PiZZ patients develop disease manifestations. Null variants have undetectable levels of α_1AT and are susceptible to premature lung disease.

α_1AT deficiency has been identified in all populations; however, the disorder is most common in patients of northern European and Iberian descent. The disorder affects about 1 in 1500 to 2000 individuals in North America. The natural history of α_1AT deficiency is quite variable because many individuals with the PiZZ variant never develop disease, whereas others can develop childhood cirrhosis leading to liver transplantation.

In adults, the diagnosis often comes in the course of evaluation of patients with abnormal liver test abnormalities or in a workup for cirrhosis. A hint to diagnosis may be coexistent lung disease at a relatively young age or a family history of liver and/or lung disease. Patients may have symptoms of pulmonary disease with cough and dyspnea. Liver disease may be asymptomatic other than fatigue, or patients may present with complications of decompensated liver disease.

Diagnosis of α_1AT deficiency is confirmed by blood tests showing reduced levels of serum α_1AT, accompanied by Pi determinations. Most patients with liver disease have either PiZZ or PiSZ; occasionally, patients with PiMZ have reduced levels of α_1AT, but they usually do not have a low enough level to cause disease. Liver biopsy is often performed to determine stage of hepatic fibrosis and shows characteristic PAS-positive, diastase-resistant globules in the periphery of the hepatic lobule.

TREATMENT α_1 Antitrypsin Deficiency

Treatment of α_1AT deficiency is usually nonspecific and supportive. For patients with liver involvement, other sources of liver injury, such as alcohol, should be avoided. Evidence for other liver diseases (e.g., viral hepatitis B and C, hemochromatosis, NAFLD) should be sought and treated if possible. Smoking can worsen lung disease progression in α_1AT deficiency and should be discontinued. Patients with lung disease may be eligible to receive infusions of α_1AT, which has been shown to halt further damage to the lungs. If liver disease becomes decompensated, transplantation should be pursued and is curative. Following transplant, patients express the Pi phenotype of the donor. Finally, risk of hepatocellular carcinoma is significantly increased in patients with cirrhosis due to α_1AT deficiency.

Cystic fibrosis

CF should also be considered as an inherited form of chronic liver disease, although the principal manifestations of CF include chronic lung disease and pancreatic insufficiency. A small percentage of patients with CF who survive to adulthood have a form of biliary cirrhosis characterized by cholestatic liver enzyme abnormalities and the development of chronic liver disease. Ursodeoxycholic acid is occasionally helpful in improving liver test abnormalities and in reducing symptoms. The disease is slowly progressive.

METABOLIC LIVER DISEASES

Nonalcoholic fatty liver disease

NAFLD and NASH are common liver diseases causing abnormal liver test results and progressing to cirrhosis. **NAFLD and NASH are discussed in detail in Chap. 43**.

Lipid storage diseases

There are a number of rare lipid storage diseases that involve the liver, including the inherited disorders of Gaucher's disease and Niemann-Pick disease. Other rare disorders include abetalipoproteinemia, Tangier disease, Fabry's disease, and types I and V hyperlipoproteinemia (Table 46-5). Hepatomegaly is present due to increased fat deposition, and increased glycogen is found in the liver.

Porphyrias

The porphyrias are a group of metabolic disorders in which there are defects in the biosynthesis of heme necessary for incorporation into numerous hemoproteins such as hemoglobin, myoglobin, catalase, and the cytochromes. Porphyrias can present as either acute or chronic diseases, with the acute disorder causing recurring bouts of abdominal pain, and the chronic disorders characterized by painful skin lesions. Porphyria cutanea tarda (PCT) is the most commonly encountered porphyria. Patients present with characteristic vesicular lesions on sun-exposed areas of the skin, principally the dorsum of the hands, the tips of the ears, or the cheeks. About 40% of patients with PCT have mutations in the gene for hemochromatosis (*HFE*), and ~50% have hepatitis C; thus, iron studies and *HFE* mutation analysis as well as hepatitis C testing should be considered in all patients who present with PCT. PCT is also associated with excess alcohol use and some medications, most notably estrogens.

TABLE 46-5

LIPID STORAGE DISEASES
Gaucher's
Niemann-Pick
Abetalipoproteinemia
Tangier
Fabry's
Types I and IV hyperlipoproteinemia

TREATMENT Porphyrias

The mainstay of treatment of PCT is iron reduction by therapeutic phlebotomy, which is successful in reversing the skin lesions in the majority of patients. If hepatitis C is present, this should be treated as well. Acute intermittent porphyria presents with abdominal pain, with the diagnosis made by avoidance of certain precipitating factors such as starvation or certain diets. Intravenous heme as hematin has been used for treatment.

INFILTRATIVE DISORDERS

Amyloidosis

Amyloidosis is a metabolic storage disease that results from deposition of insoluble proteins that are aberrantly folded and assembled and then deposited in a variety of tissues. Amyloidosis is divided into two types, primary and secondary, based on the broad concepts of association with myeloma (primary) or chronic inflammatory illnesses (secondary). The disease is generally considered rare, although, in certain disease states or in certain populations, it can be more common. For example, when associated with familial Mediterranean fever, it is seen in high frequency in Sephardic Jews and Armenians living in Armenia and less frequently in Ashkenazi Jews, Turks, and Arabs. Amyloidosis frequently affects patients suffering from tuberculosis and leprosy and can be seen in upwards of 10–15% of patients with ankylosing spondylitis, rheumatoid arthritis, or Crohn's disease. In one surgical pathology series, amyloid was found in <1% of cases. The liver is commonly involved in cases of systemic amyloidosis, but it is frequently not clinically apparent and only documented at autopsy. Pathologic findings in the liver include positive staining with the Congo red histochemical stain where there is an apple-green birefringence noted under polarizing light.

Granulomas

Granulomas are frequently found in the liver when patients are being evaluated for cholestatic liver enzyme abnormalities. Granulomas can be seen in primary biliary cirrhosis, but there are other characteristic clinical (e.g., pruritus, fatigue) and laboratory findings (cholestatic liver tests, antimitochondrial antibody) that allow for a definitive diagnosis of that disorder. Granulomatous infiltration can also be seen as the principal hepatic manifestation of sarcoidosis, and this is the most common presentation of hepatic granulomas. The vast majority of these patients do not require any specific treatment other than what would normally be used for treatment of their sarcoidosis. A small subset, however, can develop a particularly bothersome desmoplastic reaction with a significant increase in fibrosis, which can progress to cirrhosis and liver failure. These patients may require treatment with immunosuppressive therapy and may require liver transplantation. In patients who have granulomas in the liver not associated with sarcoidosis, treatment is rarely needed.

Diagnosis requires liver biopsy, and it is important to establish a diagnosis so that a cause for the elevated liver enzymes is carefully identified. Some medications can cause granulomatous infiltration of the liver, the most notable of which is allopurinol.

Lymphoma

Involvement of the liver with lymphoma can sometimes be with bulky mass lesions but can also be as a difficult-to-diagnose infiltrative disorder that does not show any characteristic findings on abdominal imaging studies. Patients may present with severe liver disease, jaundice, hypoalbuminemia, mild to moderately elevated aminotransferases, and an elevated alkaline phosphatase.

A liver biopsy is required for diagnosis and should be considered when routine blood testing does not lead to a diagnosis of the liver dysfunction.

CHAPTER 47

DISEASES OF THE GALLBLADDER AND BILE DUCTS

Norton J. Greenberger ■ Gustav Paumgartner

PHYSIOLOGY OF BILE PRODUCTION AND FLOW

BILE SECRETION AND COMPOSITION

Bile formed in the hepatic lobules is secreted into a complex network of canaliculi, small bile ductules, and larger bile ducts that run with lymphatics and branches of the portal vein and hepatic artery in portal tracts situated between hepatic lobules. These interlobular bile ducts coalesce to form larger septal bile ducts that join to form the right and left hepatic ducts, which in turn, unite to form the common hepatic duct. The common hepatic duct is joined by the cystic duct of the gallbladder to form the common bile duct (CBD), which enters the duodenum (often after joining the main pancreatic duct) throughthe ampulla of Vater.

Hepatic bile is an isotonic fluid with an electrolyte composition resembling blood plasma. The electrolyte composition of gallbladder bile differs from that of hepatic bile because most of the inorganic anions, chloride and bicarbonate, have been removed by reabsorption across the gallbladder epithelium. As a result of water reabsorption, total solute concentration of bile increases from 3–4 g/dL in hepatic bile to 10–15 g/dL in gallbladder bile.

Major solute components of bile by moles percent include bile acids (80%), lecithin and traces of other phospholipids (16%), and unesterified cholesterol (4.0%). In the lithogenic state, the cholesterol value can be as high as 8–10%. Other constituents include conjugated bilirubin; proteins (all immunoglobulins, albumin, metabolites of hormones, and other proteins metabolized in the liver); electrolytes; mucus; and, often, drugs and their metabolites.

The total daily basal secretion of hepatic bile is ~500–600 mL. Many substances taken up or synthesized by the hepatocyte are secreted into the bile canaliculi. The canalicular membrane forms microvilli and is associated with microfilaments of actin, microtubules, and other contractile elements. Prior to their secretion into the bile, many substances are taken up into the hepatocyte, while others, such as phospholipids, a portion of primary bile acids, and some cholesterol, are synthesized de novo in the hepatocyte. Three mechanisms are important in regulating bile flow: (1) active transport of bile acids from hepatocytes into the bile canaliculi, (2) active transport of other organic anions, and(3) cholangiocellular secretion. The last is a secretin-mediated and cyclic AMP–dependent mechanism that results in the secretion of a sodium- and bicarbonate-rich fluid into the bile ducts.

Active vectorial secretion of biliary constituents from the portal blood into the bile canaliculi is driven by a set of polarized transport systems at the basolateral (sinusoidal) and the canalicular apical plasma membrane domains of the hepatocyte. Two sinusoidal bile salt uptake systems have been cloned in humans, the Na^+/taurocholate cotransporter (NTCP, SLC10A1) and the organic anion–transporting proteins (OATPs), which also transport a large variety of non-bile salt organic anions. Several ATP-dependent canalicular transport systems, "export pumps," (ATP-binding cassette transport proteins, also known as ABC transporters) have been identified, the most important of which are: the bile salt export pump (BSEP, ABCB11); the anionic conjugate export pump (MRP2, ABCC2), which mediates the canalicular excretion of various amphiphilic conjugates formed by phase II conjugation (e.g., bilirubin mono- and diglucuronides and drugs); the multidrug export pump (MDR1, ABCB1) for hydrophobic cationic compounds; and the phospholipid export pump (MDR3, ABCB4). Two hemitransporters ABCG5/G8, functioning as a couple, constitute the canalicular cholesterol and phytosterol transporter.

F1C1 (ATP8B1) is an aminophospholipid transferase ("flippase") essential for maintaining the lipid asymmetry of the canalicular membrane. The canalicular membrane also contains ATP-independent transport systems such as the Cl/HCO_3 anion exchanger isoform 2 (AE2, SLC4A2) for canalicular bicarbonate secretion. For most of these transporters, genetic defects have been identified that are associated with various forms of cholestasis or defects of biliary excretion. F1C1 is defective in progressive familial intrahepatic cholestasis type 1 (PFIC1) and benign recurrent intrahepatic cholestasis type 1 (BRIC1) and results in ablation of all other ATP-dependent transporter functions. BSEP is defective in PFIC2 and BRIC2. Mutations of MRP2 (ABCC2) cause the Dubin-Johnson syndrome, an inherited form of conjugated hyperbilirubinemia **(Chap. 38)**. A defective MDR3 (ABCB4) results in PFIC3. ABCG5/G8, the canalicular half transporters for cholesterol and other neutral sterols, are defective in sitosterolemia. The cystic fibrosis transmembrane regulator (CFTR, ABCC7) located on bile duct epithelial cells but not on canalicular membranes is defective in cystic fibrosis, which is associated with impaired cholangiocellular pH regulation during ductular bile formation and chronic cholestatic liver disease, occasionally resulting in biliary cirrhosis.

THE BILE ACIDS

The primary bile acids, cholic acid and chenodeoxycholic acid (CDCA), are synthesized from cholesterol in the liver, conjugated with glycine or taurine, and secreted into the bile. Secondary bile acids, including deoxycholate and lithocholate, are formed in the colon as bacterial metabolites of the primary bile acids. However, lithocholic acid is much less efficiently absorbed from the colon than deoxycholic acid. Another secondary bile acid, found in low concentration, is ursodeoxycholic acid (UDCA), a stereoisomer of CDCA. In healthy subjects, the ratio of glycine to taurine conjugates in bile is ~3:1.

Bile acids are detergent-like molecules that in aqueous solutions and above a critical concentration of about 2 m*M* form molecular aggregates called *micelles.* Cholesterol alone is sparingly soluble in aqueous environments, and its solubility in bile depends on both the total lipid concentration and the relative molar percentages of bile acids and lecithin. Normal ratios of these constituents favor the formation of solubilizing *mixed micelles*, while abnormal ratios promote the precipitation of cholesterol crystals in bile via an intermediate liquid crystal phase.

In addition to facilitating the biliary excretion of cholesterol, bile acids facilitate the normal intestinal absorption of dietary fats, mainly cholesterol and fat-soluble vitamins, via a micellar transport mechanism. Bile acids also serve as a major physiologic driving force for hepatic bile flow and aid in water and electrolyte transport in the small bowel and colon.

ENTEROHEPATIC CIRCULATION

Bile acids are efficiently conserved under normal conditions. Unconjugated, and to a lesser degree also conjugated, bile acids are absorbed by *passive diffusion* along the entire gut. Quantitatively much more important for bile salt recirculation, however, is the *active transport* mechanism for conjugated bile acids in the distal ileum. The reabsorbed bile acids enter the portal bloodstream and are taken up rapidly by hepatocytes, reconjugated, and resecreted into bile (enterohepatic circulation).

The normal bile acid pool size is approximately 2–4 g. During digestion of a meal, the bile acid pool undergoes at least one or more enterohepatic cycles, depending on the size and composition of the meal. Normally, the bile acid pool circulates ~5–10 times daily. Intestinal reabsorption of the pool is about 95% efficient; therefore, fecal loss of bile acids is in the range of 0.2–0.4 g/d. In the steady state, this fecal loss is compensated by an equal daily synthesis of bile acids by the liver, and, thus, the size of the bile acid pool is maintained. Bile acids in the intestine release fibroblast growth factor 19 (FGF19) into the circulation, which is transported to the liver where it suppresses synthesis of bile acids from cholesterol by inhibiting the rate-limiting enzyme cytochrome P450 7A1 (CYP7A1) and also promotes gallbladder relaxation. While the loss of bile salts in stool is usually matched by increased hepatic synthesis, the maximum rate of synthesis is ~5 g/d, which may be insufficient to replete the bile acid pool size when there is pronounced impairment of intestinal bile salt reabsorption.

The expression of ABC transporters in the enterohepatic circulation and of the rate-limiting enzymes of bile acid and cholesterol synthesis are regulated in a coordinated fashion by nuclear receptors, which are ligand-activated transcription factors. The hepatic BSEP (ABCB11) is upregulated by the farnesoid X receptor (FXR), a bile acid sensor that also represses bile acid synthesis. The expression of the cholesterol transporter, ABCG5/G8, is upregulated by the liver X receptor (LXR), which is an oxysterol sensor.

GALLBLADDER AND SPHINCTERIC FUNCTIONS

In the fasting state, the sphincter of Oddi offers a high-pressure zone of resistance to bile flow from the CBD into the duodenum. Its tonic contraction serves to (1) prevent reflux of duodenal contents into the pancreatic and bile ducts and (2) promote filling of the gallbladder. The major factor controlling the evacuation of the gallbladder is the peptide hormone cholecystokinin (CCK), which is released from the duodenal mucosa in response to the ingestion of fats and amino acids. CCK produces (1) powerful contraction of the gallbladder, (2) decreased resistance of the sphincter of Oddi, and (3) enhanced flow of biliary contents into the duodenum.

Hepatic bile is "concentrated" within the gallbladder by energy-dependent transmucosal absorption of water and electrolytes. Almost the entire bile acid pool may be sequestered in the gallbladder following an overnight fast for delivery into the duodenum with the first meal of the day. The normal capacity of the gallbladder is ~30 mL of bile.

DISEASES OF THE GALLBLADDER

CONGENITAL ANOMALIES

Anomalies of the biliary tract are not uncommon and include abnormalities in number, size, and shape (e.g., agenesis of the gallbladder, duplications, rudimentary or oversized "giant" gallbladders, and diverticula). *Phrygian cap* is a clinically innocuous entity in which a partial or complete septum (or fold) separates the fundus from the body. Anomalies of position or suspension are not uncommon and include left-sided gallbladder, intrahepatic gallbladder, retrodisplacement of the gallbladder, and "floating" gallbladder. The latter condition predisposes to acute torsion, volvulus, or herniation of the gallbladder.

GALLSTONES

Epidemiology and pathogenesis

Gallstones are quite prevalent in most Western countries. Gallstone formation increases after age 50. In the United States, the third National Health and Nutrition Examination Survey (NHANES III) has revealed an overall prevalence of gallstones of 7.9% in men and 16.6% in women. The prevalence was high in Mexican Americans (8.9% in men, 26.7% in women), intermediate for non-Hispanic whites (8.6% in men, 16.6% in women), and low for African Americans (5.3% in men, 13.9% in women).

Gallstones are formed because of abnormal bile composition. They are divided into two major types: cholesterol stones and pigment stones. Cholesterol stones account for more than 90% of all gallstones in Western industrialized countries. Cholesterol gallstones usually contain >50% cholesterol monohydrate plus an admixture of calcium salts, bile pigments, proteins, and fatty acids. Pigment stones are composed primarily of calcium bilirubinate; they contain <20% cholesterol and are classified into "black" and "brown" types, the latter forming secondary to chronic biliary infection.

Cholesterol stones and biliary sludge

Cholesterol is essentially water insoluble and requires aqueous dispersion into either micelles or vesicles, both of which require the presence of a second lipid to solubilize the cholesterol. Cholesterol and phospholipids are secreted into bile as unilamellar bilayered vesicles, which are converted into mixed micelles consisting of bile acids, phospholipids, and cholesterol by the action of bile acids. If there is an excess of cholesterol in relation to phospholipids and bile acids, unstable, cholesterol-rich vesicles remain, which aggregate into large multilamellar vesicles from which cholesterol crystals precipitate (Fig. 47-1).

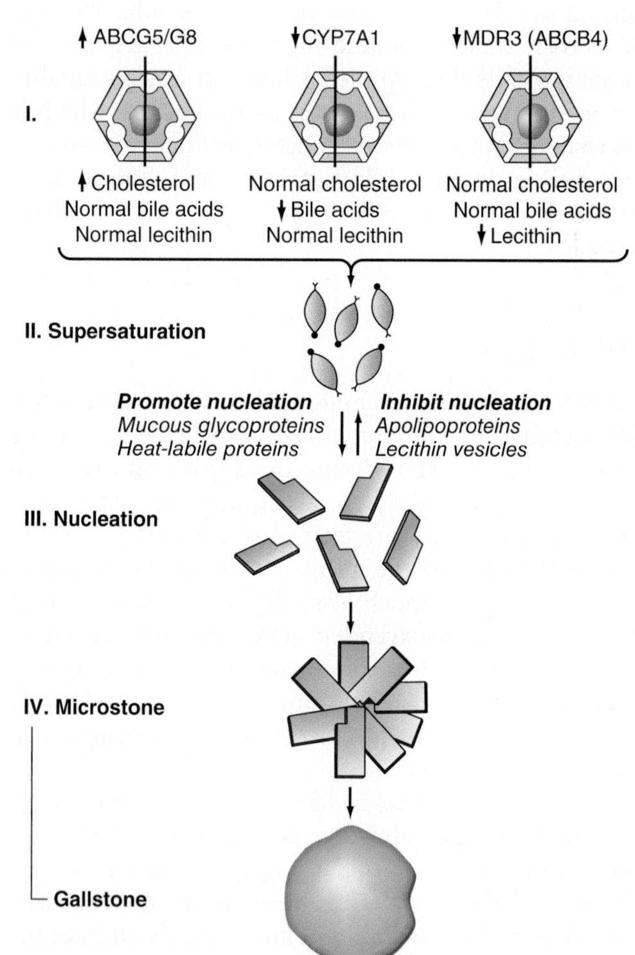

FIGURE 47-1

Scheme showing pathogenesis of cholesterol gallstone formation. Conditions or factors that increase the ratio of cholesterol to bile acids and phospholipids (lecithin) favor gallstone formation. ABCB4, ATP-binding cassette transporter; ABCG5/8, ATP-binding cassette (ABC) transporter G5/G8; CYP7A1, cytochrome P450 7A1; MDR3, multidrug resistance protein 3, also called phospholipid export pump.

There are several important mechanisms in the formation of lithogenic (stone-forming) bile. The most important is increased biliary secretion of cholesterol. This may occur in association with obesity, the metabolic syndrome, high-caloric and cholesterol-rich diets, or drugs (e.g., clofibrate) and may result from increased activity of hydroxymethylglutaryl-coenzyme A (HMG-CoA) reductase, the rate-limiting enzyme of hepatic cholesterol synthesis, and increased hepatic uptake of cholesterol from blood. In patients with gallstones, dietary cholesterol *increases* biliary cholesterol secretion. This does not occur in non-gallstone patients on high-cholesterol diets. In addition to environmental factors such as high-caloric and cholesterol-rich diets, genetic factors play an important role in gallstone disease. A large study of symptomatic gallstones in Swedish twins provided strong evidence for a role of genetic factors in gallstone pathogenesis. Genetic factors accounted for 25%, shared environmental factors for 13%, and individual environmental factors for 62% of the phenotypic variation among monozygotic twins. A single nucleotide polymorphism of the gene encoding the hepatic cholesterol transporter ABCG5/G8 has been found in 21% of patients with gallstones, but only in 9% of the general population. It is thought to cause a gain of function of the cholesterol transporter and to contribute to cholesterol hypersecretion. A high prevalence of gallstones is found among first-degree relatives of gallstone carriers and in certain ethnic populations such as American Indians, Chilean Indians, and Chilean Hispanics. A common genetic trait has been identified for some of these populations by mitochondrial DNA analysis. In some patients, impaired hepatic conversion of cholesterol to bile acids may also occur, resulting in an increase of the lithogenic cholesterol/bile acid ratio. Although most cholesterol stones have a polygenic basis, there are rare monogenic (Mendelian) causes. Recently, a mutation in the *CYP7A1* gene has described that results in a deficiency of the enzyme cholesterol 7-hydroxylase, which catalyzes the initial step in cholesterol catabolism and bile acid synthesis. The homozygous state is associated with hypercholesterolemia and gallstones. Because the phenotype is expressed in the heterozygote state, mutations in the *CYP7A1* gene may contribute to the susceptibility to cholesterol gallstone disease in the population. Mutations in the *MDR3* (ABCB4) gene, which encodes the phospholipid export pump in the canalicular membrane of the hepatocyte, may cause defective phospholipid secretion into bile, resulting in cholesterol supersaturation of bile and formation of cholesterol gallstones in the gallbladder and in the bile ducts. Thus, an excess of biliary cholesterol in relation to bile acids and phospholipids is primarily due to hypersecretion of cholesterol, but hyposecretion of bile acids or phospholipids may contribute. An additional disturbance of bile acid metabolism that is likely to contribute to supersaturation of bile with cholesterol is enhanced conversion of cholic acid to deoxycholic acid, with replacement of the cholic acid pool by an expanded deoxycholic acid pool. It may result from enhanced dehydroxylation of cholic acid and increased absorption of newly formed deoxycholic acid. An increased deoxycholate secretion is associated with hypersecretion of cholesterol into bile.

While supersaturation of bile with cholesterol is an important prerequisite for gallstone formation, it is generally not sufficient by itself to produce cholesterol precipitation in vivo. Most individuals with supersaturated bile do not develop stones because the time required for cholesterol crystals to nucleate and grow is longer than the time bile remains in the gallbladder.

An important mechanism is *nucleation* of cholesterol monohydrate crystals, which is greatly accelerated in human lithogenic bile. Accelerated nucleation of cholesterol monohydrate in bile may be due to either an *excess of pronucleating factors* or a *deficiency of antinucleating factors*. Mucin and certain nonmucin glycoproteins, principally immunoglobulins, appear to be pronucleating factors, while apolipoproteins A-I and A-II and other glycoproteins appear to be antinucleating factors. Pigment particles may possibly play a role as nucleating factors. In a genome-wide analysis of serum bilirubin levels, the uridine diphosphate-glucuronyltransferase 1A1 (*UGT1A1*) Gilbert's syndrome gene variant was associated with the presence of gallstone disease. Because most gallstones associated with the *UGT1A1* variant were cholesterol stones, this finding points to the role of pigment particles in the pathogenesis of gallbladder stones. Cholesterol monohydrate crystal nucleation and crystal growth probably occur within the mucin gel layer. Vesicle fusion leads to liquid crystals, which, in turn, nucleate into solid cholesterol monohydrate crystals. Continued growth of the crystals occurs by direct nucleation of cholesterol molecules from supersaturated unilamellar or multilamellar biliary vesicles.

A third important mechanism in cholesterol gallstone formation is *gallbladder hypomotility*. If the gallbladder emptied all supersaturated or crystal-containing bile completely, stones would not be able to grow. A high percentage of patients with gallstones exhibit abnormalities of gallbladder emptying. Ultrasonographic studies show that gallstone patients display an increased gallbladder volume during fasting and also after a test meal (residual volume) and that fractional emptying after gallbladder stimulation is decreased. The incidence of gallstones is increased in conditions associated with infrequent or impaired gallbladder emptying such as fasting, parenteral nutrition, or pregnancy and in patients using drugs that inhibit gallbladder motility.

Biliary sludge is a thick, mucous material that, upon microscopic examination, reveals lecithin-cholesterol liquid crystals, cholesterol monohydrate crystals, calcium bilirubinate, and mucin gels. Biliary sludge typically forms a crescent-like layer in the most dependent portion of the gallbladder and is recognized by characteristic echoes on ultrasonography (see below). The presence of biliary sludge implies two abnormalities: (1) the normal balance between gallbladder mucin secretion and elimination has become deranged, and (2) nucleation of biliary solutes has occurred. That biliary sludge may be a precursor form of gallstone disease is evident from several observations. In one study, 96 patients with gallbladder sludge were followed prospectively by serial ultrasound studies. In 18%, biliary sludge disappeared and did not recur for at least 2 years. In 60%, biliary sludge disappeared and reappeared; in 14%, gallstones (8% asymptomatic, 6% symptomatic) developed; and in 6%, severe biliary pain with or without acute pancreatitis occurred. In 12 patients, cholecystectomies were performed, 6 for gallstone-associated biliary pain and 3 in symptomatic patients with sludge but without gallstones who had prior attacks of pancreatitis; the latter did not recur after cholecystectomy. It should be emphasized that biliary sludge can develop with disorders that cause gallbladder hypomotility; i.e., surgery, burns, total parenteral nutrition, pregnancy, and oral contraceptives—all of which are associated with gallstone formation. However, the presence of biliary sludge implies supersaturation of bile with either cholesterol or calcium bilirubinate.

Two other conditions are associated with cholesterol-stone orbiliary-sludge formation: pregnancy and rapid weight reduction through a very-low-calorie diet. There appear to be two key changes during pregnancy that contribute to a "cholelithogenic state": (1) a marked increase in cholesterol saturation of bile during the third trimester and (2) sluggish gallbladder contraction in response to a standard meal, resulting in impaired gallbladder emptying. That these changes are related to pregnancy per se is supported by several studies that show reversal of these abnormalities quite rapidly after delivery. During pregnancy, gallbladder sludge develops in 20–30% of women and gallstones in 5–12%. Although biliary sludge is a common finding during pregnancy, it is usually asymptomatic and often resolves spontaneously after delivery. Gallstones, which are less common than sludge and frequently associated with biliary colic, may also disappear after delivery because of spontaneous dissolution related to bile becoming unsaturated with cholesterol postpartum.

Approximately 10–20% of persons with rapid weight reduction achieved through very-low-calorie dieting develop gallstones. In a study involving 600 patients who completed a 3-month, 520-kcal/d diet, UDCA in a dosage of 600 mg/d proved highly effective in preventing gallstone formation; gallstones developed in only 3% of UDCA recipients, compared to 28% of placebo-treated patients. In obese patients treated by gastric banding, 500 mg/d of UDCA reduced the risk of gallstone formation from 30% to 8% within a follow-up of 6 months.

To summarize, cholesterol gallstone disease occurs because of several defects, which include (1) bile supersaturation with cholesterol, (2) nucleation of cholesterol monohydrate with subsequent crystal retention and stone growth, and (3) abnormal gallbladder motor function with delayed emptying and stasis. Other important factors known to predispose to cholesterol-stone formation are summarized in Table 47-1.

Pigment stones

Black pigment stones are composed of either pure calcium bilirubinate or polymer-like complexes with calcium and mucin glycoproteins. They are more common in patients who have chronic hemolytic states (with increased conjugated bilirubin in bile), liver cirrhosis, Gilbert's syndrome, or cystic fibrosis. Gallbladder stones in patients with ileal diseases, ileal resection, or ileal bypass generally are also black pigment stones. Enterohepatic recycling of bilirubin in ileal disease states contributes to their pathogenesis. Brown pigment stones are composed of calcium salts of unconjugated bilirubin with varying amounts of cholesterol and protein. They are caused by the presence of increased amounts of unconjugated, insoluble bilirubin in bile that precipitates to form stones. Deconjugation of an excess of soluble bilirubin mono- and diglucuronides may be mediated by endogenous β-glucuronidase but may also occur by spontaneous hydrolysis. Sometimes, the enzyme is also produced when bile is chronically infected by bacteria, and such stones are brown. Pigment stone formation is frequent in Asia and is often associated with infections in the gallbladder and biliary tree (Table 47-1).

Diagnosis

Procedures of potential use in the diagnosis of cholelithiasis and other diseases of the gallbladder are detailed in Table 47-2. Ultrasonography of the gallbladder is very accurate in the identification of cholelithiasis and has replaced oral cholecystography (Fig. 47-2A). Stones as small as 1.5 mm in diameter may be confidently identified provided that firm criteria are used (e.g., acoustic "shadowing" of opacities that are within the gallbladder lumen and that change with the patient's position [by gravity]). In major medical centers, the false-negative and false-positive rates for ultrasound

TABLE 47-1

PREDISPOSING FACTORS FOR CHOLESTEROL AND PIGMENT GALLSTONE FORMATION

Cholesterol Stones

1. Demographic/genetic factors: Prevalence highest in North American Indians, Chilean Indians, and Chilean Hispanics, greater in Northern Europe and North America than in Asia, lowest in Japan; familialdisposition; hereditary aspects
2. Obesity, metabolic syndrome: Normal bile acid pool and secretion but increased biliary secretion of cholesterol
3. Weight loss: Mobilization of tissue cholesterol leads to increased biliary cholesterol secretion while enterohepatic circulation of bile acids is decreased
4. Female sex hormones
   a. Estrogens stimulate hepatic lipoprotein receptors, increase uptake of dietary cholesterol, and increase biliary cholesterol secretion
   b. Natural estrogens, other estrogens, and oral contraceptives lead to decreased bile salt secretion and decreased conversion of cholesterol to cholesteryl esters
5. Pregnancy: Impaired gallbladder emptying caused by progesterone combined with the influence of estrogens, which increase biliary cholesterol secretion
6. Increasing age: Increased biliary secretion of cholesterol, decreased size of bile acid pool, decreased secretion of bile salts
7. Gallbladder hypomotility leading to stasis and formation of sludge
   a. Prolonged parenteral nutrition
   b. Fasting
   c. Pregnancy
   d. Drugs such as octreotide
8. Clofibrate therapy: Increased biliary secretion of cholesterol
9. Decreased bile acid secretion
   a. Primary biliary cirrhosis
   b. Genetic defect of the *CYP7A1* gene
10. Decreased phospholipid secretion: Genetic defect of the *MDR3* gene
11. Miscellaneous
   a. High-calorie, high-fat diet
   b. Spinal cord injury

Pigment Stones

1. Demographic/genetic factors: Asia, rural setting
2. Chronic hemolysis
3. Alcoholic liver cirrhosis
4. Pernicious anemia
5. Cystic fibrosis
6. Chronic biliary tract infection, parasite infections
6. Increasing age
7. Ileal disease, ileal resection or bypass

in gallstone patients are ~2–4%. Biliary sludge is material of low echogenic activity that typically forms a layer in the most dependent position of the gallbladder. This layer shifts with postural changes but fails to produce acoustic shadowing; these two characteristics distinguish sludges from gallstones. Ultrasound can also be used to assess the emptying function of the gallbladder.

The plain abdominal film may detect gallstones containing sufficient calcium to be radiopaque (10–15% of cholesterol and ~50% of pigment stones). Plain radiography may also be of use in the diagnosis of emphysematous cholecystitis, porcelain gallbladder, limey bile, and gallstone ileus.

Oral cholecystography (OCG) has historically been a useful procedure for the diagnosis of gallstones but has been replaced by ultrasound and is regarded as obsolete. It may be used to assess the patency of the cystic duct and gallbladder emptying function. Further, OCG can also delineate the size and number of gallstones and determine whether they are calcified.

Radiopharmaceuticals such as ^{99m}Tc-labeled *N*-substituted iminodiacetic acids (HIDA, DIDA, DISIDA, etc.) are rapidly extracted from the blood and are excreted into the biliary tree in high concentration even in the presence of mild to moderate serum bilirubin elevations. Failure to image the gallbladder in the presence of biliary ductal visualization may indicate cystic duct obstruction, acute or chronic cholecystitis, or surgical absence of the organ. Such scans have some application in the diagnosis of acute cholecystitis.

Symptoms of gallstone disease

Gallstones usually produce symptoms by causing inflammation or obstruction following their migration into the cystic duct or CBD. The most specific and characteristic symptom of gallstone disease is biliary colic that is a constant and often long-lasting pain (see below). Obstruction of the cystic duct or CBD by a stone produces increased intraluminal pressure and distention of the viscus that cannot be relieved by repetitive biliary contractions. The resultant visceral pain is characteristically a severe, steady ache or fullness in the epigastrium or right upper quadrant (RUQ) of the abdomen with frequent radiation to the interscapular area, right scapula, or shoulder.

Biliary colic begins quite suddenly and may persist with severe intensity for 30 min to 5 h, subsiding gradually or rapidly. It is steady rather than intermittent, as would be suggested by the word *colic*, which must be regarded as a misnomer, although it is in widespread use. An episode of biliary pain persisting beyond 5 h should raise the suspicion of acute cholecystitis (see below). Nausea and vomiting frequently accompany episodes of biliary pain. An elevated level of serum bilirubin and/or alkaline phosphatase suggests a common duct stone. Fever or chills (rigors) with biliary pain usually imply a complication, i.e., cholecystitis, pancreatitis, or cholangitis. Complaints of short-lasting, vague

TABLE 47-2

DIAGNOSTIC EVALUATION OF THE GALLBLADDER

DIAGNOSTIC ADVANTAGES	DIAGNOSTIC LIMITATIONS	COMMENT
Gallbladder Ultrasound		
Rapid Accurate identification of gallstones (>95%) Simultaneous scanning of GB, liver, bile ducts, pancreas "Real-time" scanning allows assessment of GB volume, contractility Not limited by jaundice, pregnancy May detect very small stones	Bowel gas Massive obesity Ascites	Procedure of choice for detection of stones
Plain Abdominal X-Ray		
Low cost Readily available	Relatively low yield ? Contraindicated in pregnancy	Pathognomonic findings in: calcified gallstones Limey bile, porcelain GB Emphysematous cholecystitis Gallstone ileus
Radioisotope Scans (HIDA, DIDA, etc.)		
Accurate identification of cystic duct obstruction Simultaneous assessment of bile ducts	? Contraindicated in pregnancy Serum bilirubin >103–205 μmol/L (6–12 mg/dL) Cholecystogram of low resolution	Indicated for confirmation of suspected acute cholecystitis; less sensitive and less specific in chronic cholecystitis; useful indiagnosis of acalculous cholecystopathy, especially if given with CCK to assess gallbladder emptying

Abbreviations: CCK, cholecystokinin; GB, gallbladder.

epigastric fullness, dyspepsia, eructation, or flatulence, especially following a fatty meal, should not be confused with biliary pain. Such symptoms are frequently elicited from patients with or without gallstone disease but are not specific for biliary calculi. Biliary colic may be precipitated by eating a fatty meal, by consumption of a large meal following a period of prolonged fasting, or by eating a normal meal; it is frequently nocturnal, occurring within a few hours of retiring.

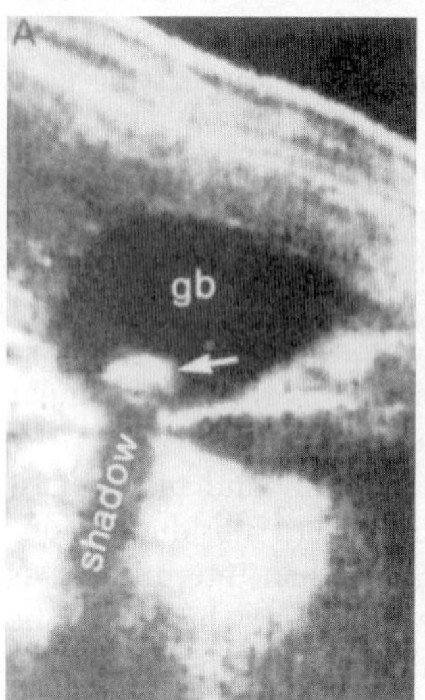

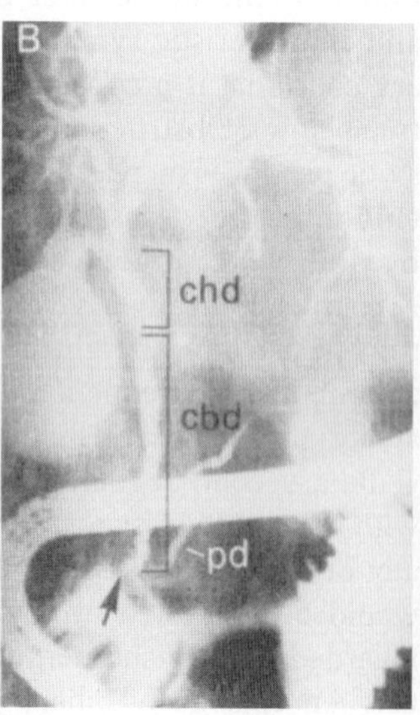

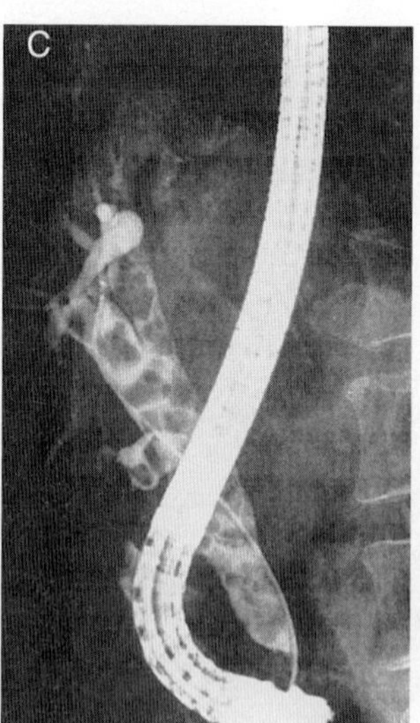

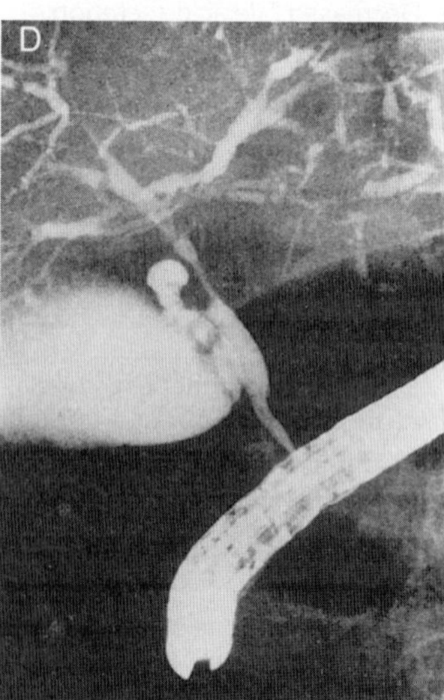

FIGURE 47-2

Examples of ultrasound and radiologic studies of the biliary tract. *A.* An ultrasound study showing a distended gallbladder (GB) containing a single large stone (*arrow*), which casts an acoustic shadow. ***B.*** Endoscopic retrograde cholangiopancreatogram (ERCP) showing normal biliary tract anatomy. In addition to the endoscope and large vertical gallbladder filled with contrast dye, the common hepatic duct (CHD), common bile duct (CBD), and pancreatic duct (PD) are shown. The *arrow* points to the ampulla of Vater. ***C.*** Endoscopic retrograde cholangiogram (ERC) showing choledocholithiasis. The biliary tract is dilated and contains multiple radiolucent calculi. ***D.*** ERCP showing sclerosing cholangitis. The common bile duct shows areas that are strictured and narrowed.

Natural history

Gallstone disease discovered in an asymptomatic patient or in a patient whose symptoms are not referable to cholelithiasis is a common clinical problem. Sixty to 80% of persons with asymptomatic gallstones remain asymptomatic over follow-up periods of up to 25 years. The probability of developing symptoms within5 years after diagnosis is 2–4% per year and decreases in the years thereafter to 1–2%. The yearly incidence of complications is about 0.1–0.3%. Patients remaining asymptomatic for 15 years were found to be unlikely to develop symptoms during further follow-up, and most patients who did develop complications from their gallstones experienced *prior* warning symptoms. Similar conclusions apply to diabetic patients with silent gallstones. Decision analysis has suggested that (1) the cumulative risk of death due to gallstone disease while on expectant management is small, and (2) prophylactic cholecystectomy is not warranted.

Complications requiring cholecystectomy are much more common in gallstone patients who have developed symptoms of biliary pain. Patients found to have gallstones at a young age are more likely to develop symptoms from cholelithiasis than are patients >60 years at the time of initial diagnosis. Patients with diabetes mellitus and gallstones may be somewhat more susceptible to septic complications, but the magnitude of risk of septic biliary complications in diabetic patients is incompletely defined.

TREATMENT Gallstones

SURGICAL THERAPY In asymptomatic gallstone patients, the risk of developing symptoms or complications requiring surgery is quite small (see above). Thus, a recommendation for cholecystectomy in a patient with gallstones should probably be based on assessment of three factors: (1) the presence of symptoms that are frequent enough or severe enough to interfere with the patient's general routine; (2) the presence of a prior complication of gallstone disease, i.e., history of acute cholecystitis, pancreatitis, gallstone fistula, etc.; or (3) the presence of an underlying condition predisposing the patient to increased risk of gallstone complications (e.g., calcified or porcelain gallbladder and/or a previous attack of acute cholecystitis regardless of current symptomatic status). Patients with very large gallstones (>3 cm in diameter) and patients harboring gallstones in a congenitally anomalous gallbladder might also be considered for prophylactic cholecystectomy. Although young age is a worrisome factor in asymptomatic gallstone patients, few authorities would now recommend routine cholecystectomy in all young patients with silent stones. Laparoscopic cholecystectomy is a minimal-access approach for the removal of the gallbladder together with its stones. Its advantages include a markedly shortened hospital stay, minimal disability, and decreased cost, and it is the procedure of choice for most patients referred for elective cholecystectomy.

From several studies involving >4000 patients undergoing laparoscopic cholecystectomy, the following key points emerge:(1) complications develop in ~4% of patients, (2) conversion to laparotomy occurs in 5%, (3) the death rate is remarkably low (i.e., <0.1%), and (4) the rate of bile duct injuries is low (i.e., 0.2–0.6%) and comparable with open cholecystectomy. These data indicate why laparoscopic cholecystectomy has become the "gold standard" for treating symptomatic cholelithiasis.

MEDICAL THERAPY—GALLSTONE DISSOLUTION In carefully selected patients with a functioning gallbladder and with radiolucent stones <10 mm in diameter, complete dissolution can be achieved in ~50% of patients within 6 months to 2 years. For good results within a reasonable time period, this therapy should be limited to radiolucent stones smaller than 5 mm in diameter. The dose of UDCA should be 10–15 mg/kg per day. Stones larger than 10 mm in size rarely dissolve. Pigment stones are not responsive to UDCA therapy. Probably ≤10% of patients with *symptomatic* cholelithiasis are candidates for such treatment. However, in addition to the vexing problem of recurrent stones (30–50% over 3–5 years of follow-up), there is also the factor of taking an expensive drug for up to 2 years. The advantages and success of laparoscopic cholecystectomy have largely reduced the role of gallstone dissolution to patients who wish to avoid or are not candidates for elective cholecystectomy. However, patients with cholesterol gallstone disease who develop recurrent choledocholithiasis after cholecystectomy should be on long-term treatment with UDCA.

ACUTE AND CHRONIC CHOLECYSTITIS

Acute cholecystitis

Acute inflammation of the gallbladder wall usually follows obstruction of the cystic duct by a stone. Inflammatory response can be evoked by three factors: (1) *mechanical inflammation* produced by increased intraluminal pressure and distention with resulting ischemia of the gallbladder mucosa and wall, (2) *chemical inflammation* caused by the release of lysolecithin (due to the action of phospholipase on lecithin in bile) and other local tissue factors, and (3) *bacterial inflammation*, which may play a role in 50–85% of patients with acute cholecystitis. The organisms most frequently isolated by culture of gallbladder bile in these patients include *Escherichia coli*, *Klebsiella* spp., *Streptococcus* spp., and *Clostridium* spp.

Acute cholecystitis often begins as an attack of biliary pain that progressively worsens. Approximately 60–70% of patients report having experienced prior attacks that resolved spontaneously. As the episode progresses, however, the pain of acute cholecystitis becomes more generalized in the right upper abdomen. As with biliary colic, the pain of cholecystitis may radiate to the interscapular area, right scapula, or shoulder. Peritoneal signs of inflammation such as increased pain with jarring or on deep respiration may be apparent. The patient is anorectic and often nauseated. Vomiting is relatively common and may produce symptoms and signs of vascular and extracellular volume depletion. Jaundice is unusual early in the course of acute cholecystitis but may occur when edematous inflammatory changes involve the bile ducts and surrounding lymph nodes.

A low-grade fever is characteristically present, but shaking chills or rigors are not uncommon. The RUQ of the abdomen is almost invariably tender to palpation. An enlarged, tense gallbladder is palpable in 25–50% of patients. Deep inspiration or cough during subcostal palpation of the RUQ usually produces increased pain and inspiratory arrest (Murphy's sign). Localized rebound tenderness in the RUQ is common, as are abdominal distention and hypoactive bowel sounds from paralytic ileus, but generalized peritoneal signs and abdominal rigidity are usually lacking, in the absence of perforation.

The diagnosis of acute cholecystitis is usually made on the basis of a characteristic history and physical examination. The triad of sudden onset of RUQ tenderness, fever, and leukocytosis is highly suggestive. Typically, leukocytosis in the range of 10,000–15,000 cells per microliter with a left shift on differential count is found. The serum bilirubin is mildly elevated (<85.5 μmol/L [5 mg/dL]) in fewer than half of patients, whereas about one-fourth have modest elevations in serum aminotransferases (usually less than a fivefold elevation). Ultrasound will demonstrate calculi in 90–95% of cases and is useful for detection of signs of gallbladder inflammation including thickening of the wall, pericholecystic fluid, and dilatation of the bile duct. The radionuclide (e.g., HIDA) biliary scan may be confirmatory if bile duct imaging is seen without visualization of the gallbladder.

Approximately 75% of patients treated medically have remission of acute symptoms within 2–7 days following hospitalization. In 25%, however, a complication of acute cholecystitis will occur despite conservative treatment (see below). In this setting, prompt surgical intervention is required. Of the 75% of patients with acute cholecystitis who undergo remission of symptoms, ~25% will experience a recurrence of cholecystitis within 1 year, and 60% will have at least one recurrent bout within 6 years. In view of the natural history of the disease, acute cholecystitis is best treated by early surgery whenever possible.

Mirizzi's syndrome is a rare complication in which a gallstone becomes impacted in the cystic duct or neck of the gallbladder causing compression of the CBD, resulting in CBD obstruction and jaundice. Ultrasound shows gallstone(s) lying outside the hepatic duct. Endoscopic retrograde cholangiopancreatography (ERCP) (Fig. 47-2*B*), percutaneous transhepatic cholangiography (PTC), or magnetic resonance cholangiopancreatography (MRCP) will usually demonstrate the characteristic extrinsic compression of the CBD. Surgery consists of removing the cystic duct, diseased gallbladder, and the impacted stone. The preoperative diagnosis of Mirizzi's syndrome is important to avoid CBD injury.

Acalculous cholecystitis

In 5–10% of patients with acute cholecystitis, calculi obstructing the cystic duct are not found at surgery. In >50% of such cases, an underlying explanation for acalculous inflammation is not found. An increased risk for the development of acalculous cholecystitis is especially associated with serious trauma or burns, with the postpartum period following prolonged labor, and with orthopedic and other nonbiliary major surgical operations in the postoperative period. It may possibly complicate periods of prolonged parenteral hyperalimentation. For some of these cases, biliary sludge in the cystic duct may be responsible. Other precipitating factors include vasculitis, obstructing adenocarcinoma of the gallbladder, diabetes mellitus, torsion of the gallbladder, "unusual" bacterial infections of the gallbladder (e.g., *Leptospira*, *Streptococcus*, *Salmonella*, or *Vibrio cholerae*), and parasitic infestation of the gallbladder. Acalculous cholecystitis may also be seen with a variety of other systemic disease processes (e.g., sarcoidosis, cardiovascular disease, tuberculosis, syphilis, actinomycosis).

Although the clinical manifestations of acalculous cholecystitis are indistinguishable from those of calculous cholecystitis, the setting of acute gallbladder inflammation complicating severe underlying illness is characteristic of acalculous disease. Ultrasound or computed tomography (CT) examinations demonstrating a large, tense, static gallbladder without stones and with evidence of poor emptying over a prolonged period may be diagnostically useful in some cases. The complication rate for acalculous cholecystitis exceeds that for calculous cholecystitis. Successful management of acute acalculous cholecystitis appears to depend primarily on early diagnosis and surgical intervention, with meticulous attention to postoperative care.

Acalculous cholecystopathy

Disordered motility of the gallbladder can produce recurrent biliary pain in patients without gallstones. Infusion of an octapeptide of CCK can be used to measure the gallbladder ejection fraction during cholescintigraphy. The surgical findings have included abnormalities such as chronic cholecystitis, gallbladder muscle hypertrophy, and/or a markedly narrowed cystic duct. Some of these patients may well have had antecedent gallbladder disease. The following criteria can be used to identify patients with acalculous cholecystopathy: (1) recurrent episodes of typical RUQ pain characteristic of biliary tract pain, (2) abnormal CCK cholescintigraphy demonstrating a gallbladder ejection fraction of <40%, and (3) infusion of CCK reproducing the patient's pain. An additional clue would be the identification of a large gallbladder on ultrasound examination. Finally, it should be noted that sphincter of Oddi dysfunction can also give rise to recurrent RUQ pain and CCK-scintigraphic abnormalities.

Emphysematous cholecystitis

So-called emphysematous cholecystitis is thought to begin with acute cholecystitis (calculous or acalculous) followed by ischemia or gangrene of the gallbladder wall and infection by gas-producing organisms. Bacteria most frequently cultured in this setting include anaerobes, such as *Clostridium welchii* or *Clostridium perfringens*, and aerobes, such as *E. coli*. This condition occurs most frequently in elderly men and in patients with diabetes mellitus. The clinical manifestations are essentially indistinguishable from those of nongaseous cholecystitis. The diagnosis is usually made on plain abdominal film by finding gas within the gallbladder lumen, dissecting within the gallbladder wall to form a gaseous ring, or in the pericholecystic tissues. The morbidity and mortality rates with emphysematous cholecystitis are considerable. Prompt surgical intervention coupled with appropriate antibiotics is mandatory.

Chronic cholecystitis

Chronic inflammation of the gallbladder wall is almost always associated with the presence of gallstones and is thought to result from repeated bouts of subacute or acute cholecystitis or from persistent mechanical irritation of the gallbladder wall by gallstones. The presence of bacteria in the bile occurs in >25% of patients with chronic cholecystitis. The presence of infected bile in a patient with *chronic* cholecystitis undergoing elective cholecystectomy probably adds little to the operative risk. Chronic cholecystitis may be asymptomatic for years, may progress to symptomatic gallbladder disease or to acute cholecystitis, or may present with complications (see below).

Complications of cholecystitis

Empyema and hydrops

Empyema of the gallbladder usually results from progression of acute cholecystitis with persistent cystic duct obstruction to superinfection of the stagnant bile with a pus-forming bacterial organism. The clinical picture resembles that of cholangitis with high fever; severe RUQ pain; marked leukocytosis; and often, prostration. Empyema of the gallbladder carries a high risk of gram-negative sepsis and/or perforation. Emergency surgical intervention with proper antibiotic coverage is required as soon as the diagnosis is suspected.

Hydrops or mucocele of the gallbladder may also result from prolonged obstruction of the cystic duct, usually by a large solitary calculus. In this instance, the obstructed gallbladder lumen is progressively distended, over a period of time, by mucus (mucocele) or by a clear transudate (hydrops) produced by mucosal epithelial cells. A visible, easily palpable, nontender mass sometimes extending from the RUQ into the right iliac fossa may be found on physical examination. The patient with hydrops of the gallbladder frequently remains asymptomatic, although chronic RUQ pain may also occur. Cholecystectomy is indicated, because empyema, perforation, or gangrene may complicate the condition.

Gangrene and perforation

Gangrene of the gallbladder results from ischemia of the wall and patchy or complete tissue necrosis. Underlying conditions often include marked distention of the gallbladder, vasculitis, diabetes mellitus, empyema, or torsion resulting in arterial occlusion. Gangrene usually predisposes to perforation of the gallbladder, but perforation may also occur in chronic cholecystitis without premonitory warning symptoms. *Localized perforations* are usually contained by the omentum or by adhesions produced by recurrent inflammation of the gallbladder. Bacterial superinfection of the walled-off gallbladder contents results in abscess formation. Most patients are best treated with cholecystectomy, but some seriously ill patients may be managed with cholecystostomy and drainage of the abscess. *Free perforation* is less common but is associated with a mortality rate of ~30%. Such patients may experience a sudden transient relief of RUQ pain as the distended gallbladder decompresses; this is followed by signs of generalized peritonitis.

Fistula formation and gallstone ileus

Fistula formation into an adjacent organ adherent to the gallbladder wall may result from inflammation and adhesion formation. Fistulas into the duodenum are most common, followed in frequency by those involving the hepatic flexure of the colon, stomach or jejunum, abdominal wall, and renal pelvis. Clinically "silent" biliary-enteric fistulas occurring as a complication of acute cholecystitis have been found in up to 5% of patients undergoing cholecystectomy. Asymptomatic cholecystoenteric fistulas may sometimes be diagnosed by finding gas in the biliary tree on plain abdominal films. Barium contrast studies or endoscopy of the upper gastrointestinal tract or colon may demonstrate the fistula. Treatment in the symptomatic patient usually consists of cholecystectomy, CBD exploration, and closure of the fistulous tract.

Gallstone ileus refers to mechanical intestinal obstruction resulting from the passage of a large gallstone into the bowel lumen. The stone customarily enters the duodenum through a cholecystoenteric fistula at that level. The site of obstruction by the impacted gallstone is usually at the ileocecal valve, provided that the more proximal small bowel is of normal caliber. The majority of patients do not give a history of either prior biliary tract symptoms or complaints suggestive of acute cholecystitis or fistula formation. Large stones, >2.5 cm in diameter, are thought to predispose to fistula formation by gradual erosion through the gallbladder fundus. Diagnostic confirmation may occasionally be found on the plain abdominal film (e.g., small-intestinal obstruction with gas in the biliary tree and a calcified, ectopic gallstone) or following an upper gastrointestinal series (cholecystoduodenal fistula with small-bowel obstruction at the ileocecal valve). Laparotomy with stone extraction (or propulsion into the colon) remains the procedure of choice to relieve obstruction. Evacuation of large stones within the gallbladder should also be performed. In general, the gallbladder and its attachment to the intestines should be left alone.

Limey (milk of calcium) bile and porcelain gallbladder

Calcium salts in the lumen of the gallbladder in sufficient concentration may produce calcium precipitation and diffuse, hazy opacification of bile or a layering effect on plain abdominal roentgenography. This so-called limey bile, or milk of calcium bile, is usually clinically innocuous, but cholecystectomy is recommended, especially when it occurs in a hydropic gallbladder. In the entity called *porcelain gallbladder*, calcium salt deposition within the wall of a chronically inflamed gallbladder may be detected on the plain abdominal film. Cholecystectomy is advised in all patients with porcelain gallbladder because in a high percentage of cases this finding appears to be associated with the development of carcinoma of the gallbladder.

TREATMENT Acute Cholecystitis

MEDICAL THERAPY Although surgical intervention remains the mainstay of therapy for acute cholecystitis and its complications, a period of in-hospital stabilization may be required before cholecystectomy. Oral intake is eliminated, nasogastric suction may be indicated, and extracellular volume depletion and electrolyte abnormalities are repaired. Meperidine or nonsteroidal anti-inflammatory drugs (NSAIDs) are usually employed for analgesia because they may produce less spasm of the sphincter of Oddi than drugs such as morphine. Intravenous antibiotic therapy is usually indicated in patients with severe acute cholecystitis, even though bacterial superinfection of bile may not have occurred in the early stages of the inflammatory process. Antibiotic therapy is guided by the most common organisms likely to be present, which are *E. coli*, *Klebsiella* spp., and *Streptococcus* spp. Effective antibiotics include ureidopenicillins such as piperacillin or mezlocillin, ampicillin sulbactam, ciprofloxacin, moxifloxacin, and third-generation cephalosporins. Anaerobic coverage by a drug such as metronidazole should be added if gangrenous or emphysematous cholecystitis is suspected. Imipenem and meropenem represent potent parenteral antibiotics that cover the whole spectrum of bacteria causing ascending cholangitis. They should, however, be reserved for the most severe, life-threatening infections when other regimens have failed. Postoperative complications of wound infection, abscess formation, and sepsis are reduced in antibiotic-treated patients.

SURGICAL THERAPY The optimal timing of surgical intervention in patients with acute cholecystitis depends on stabilization of the patient. The clear trend is toward earlier surgery, and this is due in part to requirements for shorter hospital stays. Urgent (emergency) cholecystectomy or cholecystostomy is probably appropriate in most patients in whom a complication of acute cholecystitis such as empyema, emphysematous cholecystitis, or perforation is suspected or confirmed. Patients with uncomplicated acute cholecystitis should undergo early elective laparoscopic cholecystectomy, ideally within 48–72 h after diagnosis. The complication rate is not increased in patients undergoing early as opposed to delayed (>6 weeks after diagnosis) cholecystectomy. Delayed surgical intervention is probably best reserved for (1) patients in whom the overall medical condition imposes an unacceptable risk for early surgery and (2) patients in whom the diagnosis of acute cholecystitis is in doubt. Thus, early cholecystectomy (within 72 h) is the treatment of choice for most patients with acute cholecystitis. Mortality figures for emergency cholecystectomy in most centers range from 1–3%, whereas the mortality risk for early elective cholecystectomy is ~0.5% in patients under age 60. Of course, the operative risks increase with age-related diseases of other organ systems and with the presence of long- or short-term complications of gallbladder disease. Seriously ill or debilitated patients with cholecystitis may be managed with cholecystostomy and tube drainage of the gallbladder. Elective cholecystectomy may then be done at a later date.

Postcholecystectomy complications

Early complications following cholecystectomy include atelectasis and other pulmonary disorders, abscess formation (often subphrenic), external or internal hemorrhage, biliary-enteric fistula, and bile leaks. Jaundice may indicate absorption of bile from an intraabdominal collection following a biliary leak or mechanical obstruction of the CBD by retained calculi, intraductal blood clots, or extrinsic compression.

Overall, cholecystectomy is a very successful operation that provides total or near-total relief of preoperative symptoms in 75–90% of patients. The most common cause of persistent postcholecystectomy symptoms is an overlooked symptomatic nonbiliary disorder (e.g., reflux esophagitis, peptic ulceration, pancreatitis, or—most often—irritable bowel syndrome). In a small percentage of patients, however, a disorder of the extrahepatic bile ducts may result in persistent symptomatology. These so-called postcholecystectomy syndromes may be due to (1) biliary strictures, (2) retained biliary calculi, (3) cystic duct stump syndrome, (4) stenosis or dyskinesia of the sphincter of Oddi, or (5) bile salt–induced diarrhea or gastritis.

Cystic duct stump syndrome

In the absence of cholangiographically demonstrable retained stones, symptoms resembling biliary pain or cholecystitis in the postcholecystectomy patient have frequently been attributed to disease in a long (>1 cm) cystic duct remnant (cystic duct stump syndrome). Careful analysis, however, reveals that postcholecystectomy complaints are attributable to other causes in almost all patients in whom the symptom complex was originally thought to result from the existence of a long cystic duct stump. Accordingly, considerable care should be taken to investigate the possible role of other factors in the production of postcholecystectomy symptoms before attributing them to cystic duct stump syndrome.

Papillary dysfunction, papillary stenosis, spasm of the sphincter of oddi, and biliary dyskinesia

Symptoms of biliary colic accompanied by signs of recurrent, intermittent biliary obstruction may be produced by acalculous cholecystopathy, papillary stenosis, papillary dysfunction, spasm of the sphincter of Oddi, and biliary dyskinesia. Papillary stenosis is thought to result from acute or chronic inflammation of the papilla of Vater or from glandular hyperplasia of the papillary segment. Five criteria have been used to define papillary stenosis: (1) upper abdominal pain, usually RUQ or epigastric; (2) abnormal liver tests; (3) dilatation of the CBD upon ERCP examination; (4) delayed (>45 min) drainage of contrast material from the duct; and (5) increased basal pressure of the sphincter of Oddi, a finding that may be of only minor significance. An alternative to ERCP is magnetic resonance cholangiography (MRC) if ERCP and/or biliary manometry are either unavailable or not feasible. After exclusion of acalculous cholecystopathy, treatment consists of endoscopic or surgical sphincteroplasty to ensure wide patency of the distal portions of both the bile and pancreatic ducts. The greater the number of the preceding criteria present, the greater is the likelihood that a patient does have a degree of papillary stenosis sufficient to justify correction. The factors usually considered as indications for sphincterotomy include (1) prolonged duration of symptoms, (2) lack of response to symptomatic treatment, (3) presence of severe disability, and (4) the patient's choice of sphincterotomy over surgery (given a clear understanding on his or her part of the risks involved in both procedures).

Criteria for diagnosing dyskinesia of the sphincter of Oddi are even more controversial than those for papillary stenosis. Proposed mechanisms include spasm of the sphincter, denervation sensitivity resulting in hypertonicity, and abnormalities of the sequencing or frequency rates of sphincteric-contraction waves. When thorough evaluation has failed to demonstrate another cause for the pain, and when cholangiographic and manometric criteria suggest a diagnosis of biliary dyskinesia, medical treatment with nitrites or anticholinergics to attempt pharmacologic relaxation of the sphincter has been proposed. Endoscopic biliary sphincterotomy (EBS) or surgical sphincteroplasty may be indicated in patients who fail to respond to a 2- to 3-month trial of medical therapy, especially if basal sphincter of Oddi pressures are elevated. EBS has become the procedure of choice for removing bile duct stones and for other biliary and pancreatic problems.

Bile salt–induced diarrhea and gastritis

Postcholecystectomy patients may develop symptoms of dyspepsia, which have been attributed to duodenogastric reflux of bile. However, firm data linking these symptoms to bile gastritis after surgical removal of the gallbladder are lacking. Cholecystectomy induces persistent changes in gut transit, and these changes effect a noticeable modification of bowel habits. Cholecystectomy shortens gut transit time by accelerating passage of the fecal bolus through the colon with marked acceleration in the right colon, thus causing an increase in colonic bile acid output and a shift in bile acid composition toward the more diarrheagenic secondary bile acids, i.e. deoxycholic acid. Diarrhea that is severe enough, i.e., three or more watery movements per day, can be classified as postcholecystectomy diarrhea, and this occurs in 5–10% of patients undergoing elective cholecystectomy. Treatment with bile acid–sequestering agents such as cholestyramine or colestipol is often effective in ameliorating troublesome diarrhea.

THE HYPERPLASTIC CHOLECYSTOSES

The term *hyperplastic cholecystoses* is used to denote a group of disorders of the gallbladder characterized by excessive proliferation of normal tissue components.

Adenomyomatosis is characterized by a benign proliferation of gallbladder surface epithelium with glandlike formations, extramural sinuses, transverse strictures, and/or fundal nodule ("adenoma" or "adenomyoma") formation.

Cholesterolosis is characterized by abnormal deposition of lipid, especially cholesteryl esters, within macrophages in the lamina propria of the gallbladder wall. In its diffuse form ("strawberry gallbladder"), the gallbladder mucosa is brick red and speckled with bright yellow flecks of lipid. The localized form shows solitary or multiple "cholesterol polyps" studding the gallbladder wall. Cholesterol stones of the gallbladder are found in nearly half the cases. Cholecystectomy is indicated in both adenomyomatosis and cholesterolosis when symptomatic or when cholelithiasis is present.

The prevalence of gallbladder polyps in the adult population is ~5%, with a marked male predominance. Few significant changes have been found over a 5-year period in asymptomatic patients with gallbladder polyps <10 mm in diameter. Cholecystectomy is recommended in symptomatic patients, as well as in asymptomatic patients >50 years of age, or in those whose polyps are >10 mm in diameter or associated with gallstones or polyp growth on serial ultrasonography.

DISEASES OF THE BILE DUCTS

CONGENITAL ANOMALIES

Biliary atresia and hypoplasia

Atretic and hypoplastic lesions of the extrahepatic and large intrahepatic bile ducts are the most common biliary anomalies of clinical relevance encountered in infancy. The clinical picture is one of severe obstructive jaundice during the first month of life, with pale stools. When biliary atresia is suspected on the basis of clinical, laboratory, and imaging findings, the diagnosis is confirmed by surgical exploration and operative cholangiography. Approximately 10% of cases of biliary atresia are treatable withRoux-en-Y choledochojejunostomy, with the Kasai procedure (hepatic portoenterostomy) being attempted in the remainder in an effort to restore some bile flow. Most patients, even those having successful biliary-enteric anastomoses, eventually develop chronic cholangitis, extensive hepatic fibrosis, and portal hypertension.

Choledochal cysts

Cystic dilatation may involve the free portion of the CBD, i.e., choledochal cyst, or may present as diverticulum formation in the intraduodenal segment. In the latter situation, chronic reflux of pancreatic juice into the biliary tree can produce inflammation and stenosis of the extrahepatic bile ducts leading to cholangitis or biliary obstruction. Because the process may be gradual, ~50% of patients present with onset of symptoms after age 10. The diagnosis may be made by ultrasound, abdominal CT, MRC, or cholangiography. Only one-third of patients show the classic triad of abdominal pain, jaundice, and an abdominal mass. Ultrasonographic detection of a cyst separate from the gallbladder should suggest the diagnosis of choledochal cyst, which can be confirmed by demonstrating the entrance of extrahepatic bile ducts into the cyst. Surgical treatment involves excision of the "cyst" and biliary-enteric anastomosis. Patients with choledochal cysts are at increased risk for the subsequent development of cholangiocarcinoma.

Congenital biliary ectasia

Dilatation of intrahepatic bile ducts may involve either the major intrahepatic radicles (Caroli's disease), the inter- and intralobular ducts (congenital hepatic fibrosis), or both. In Caroli's disease, clinical manifestations include recurrent cholangitis, abscess formation in and around the affected ducts, and, often, brown pigment gallstone formation within portions of ectatic intrahepatic biliary radicles. Ultrasound, MRC, and CT are of great diagnostic value in demonstrating cystic dilatation of the intrahepatic bile ducts. Treatment with ongoing antibiotic therapy is usually undertaken in an effort to limit the frequency and severity of recurrent bouts of cholangitis. Progression to secondary biliary cirrhosis with portal hypertension, extrahepatic biliary obstruction, cholangiocarcinoma, or recurrent episodes of sepsis with hepatic abscess formation is common.

CHOLEDOCHOLITHIASIS

Pathophysiology and clinical manifestations

Passage of gallstones into the CBD occurs in ~10–15% of patients with cholelithiasis. The incidence of common duct stones increases with increasing age of the patient, so that up to 25% of elderly patients may have calculi in the common duct at the time of cholecystectomy. Undetected duct stones are left behind in ~1–5% of cholecystectomy patients. The overwhelming majority of bile duct stones are cholesterol stones formed in the gallbladder, which then migrate into the extrahepatic biliary tree through the cystic duct. Primary calculi arising de novo in the ducts are usually brown pigment stones developing in patients with (1) hepatobiliary parasitism or chronic, recurrent cholangitis; (2) congenital anomalies of the bile ducts (especially Caroli's disease); (3) dilated, sclerosed, or strictured ducts; or (4) an *MDR3* (ABCB4) gene defect leading to impaired biliary phospholipids secretion (low phospholipid-associated cholesterol cholelithiasis). Common duct stones may remain asymptomatic for years, may pass spontaneously into the duodenum, or (most often) may present with biliary colic or a complication.

Complications

Cholangitis

Cholangitis may be acute or chronic, and symptoms result from inflammation, which usually is caused by at least partial obstruction to the flow of bile. Bacteria are present on bile culture in ~75% of patients with acute cholangitis early in the symptomatic course. The characteristic presentation of acute cholangitis involves biliary pain, jaundice, and spiking fevers with chills (Charcot's triad). Blood cultures are frequently positive, and leukocytosis is typical. *Nonsuppurative acute cholangitis* is most common and may respond relatively rapidly to supportive measures and to treatment with antibiotics. In *suppurative acute cholangitis*, however, the presence of pus under pressure in a completely obstructed ductal system leads to symptoms of severe toxicity—mental confusion, bacteremia, and septic shock. Response to antibiotics alone in this setting is relatively poor, multiple hepatic abscesses are often present, and the mortality rate approaches 100% unless prompt endoscopic or surgical relief of the obstruction and drainage of infected bile are carried out. Endoscopic management of bacterial cholangitis is as effective as surgical intervention. ERCP with endoscopic sphincterotomy is safe and the preferred initial procedure for both establishing a definitive diagnosis and providing effective therapy.

Obstructive jaundice

Gradual obstruction of the CBD over a period of weeks or months usually leads to initial manifestations of jaundice or pruritus without associated symptoms of biliary colic or cholangitis. Painless jaundice may occur in patients with choledocholithiasis, but is much more characteristic of biliary obstruction secondary to malignancy of the head of the pancreas, bile ducts, or ampulla of Vater.

In patients whose obstruction is secondary to choledocholithiasis, associated chronic calculous cholecystitis is very common, and the gallbladder in this setting may be unable to distend. The absence of a palpable gallbladder in most patients with biliary obstruction from duct stones is the basis for Courvoisier's law, i.e., that the presence of a palpably enlarged gallbladder suggests that the biliary obstruction is secondary to an underlying malignancy rather than to calculous disease. Biliary obstruction causes progressive dilatation of the intrahepatic bile ducts as intrabiliary pressures rise. Hepatic bile flow is suppressed, and reabsorption and regurgitation of conjugated bilirubin into the bloodstream lead to jaundice accompanied by dark urine (bilirubinuria) and light-colored (acholic) stools.

CBD stones should be suspected in any patient with cholecystitis whose serum bilirubin level is >85.5 μmol/L (5 mg/dL). The maximum bilirubin level is seldom >256.5 μmol/L (15.0 mg/dL) in patients with choledocholithiasis unless concomitant hepatic or renal disease or another factor leading to marked hyperbilirubinemia exists. Serum bilirubin levels ≥342.0 μmol/L (20 mg/dL) should suggest the possibility of neoplastic obstruction. The serum alkaline phosphatase level is almost always elevated in biliary obstruction. A rise in alkaline phosphatase often precedes clinical jaundice and may be the only abnormality in routine liver function tests. There may be a two- to tenfold elevation of serum aminotransferases, especially in association with acute obstruction. Following relief of the obstructing process, serum aminotransferase elevations usually return rapidly to normal, while the serum bilirubin level may take 1–2 weeks to return to normal. The alkaline phosphatase level usually falls slowly, lagging behind the decrease in serum bilirubin.

Pancreatitis

The most common associated entity discovered in patients with nonalcoholic acute pancreatitis is biliary tract disease. Biochemical evidence of pancreatic inflammation complicates acute cholecystitis in 15% of cases and choledocholithiasis in >30%, and the common factor appears to be the passage of gallstones through the common duct. Coexisting pancreatitis should be suspected in patients with symptoms of cholecystitis who develop (1) back pain or pain to the left of the abdominal midline, (2) prolonged vomiting with paralytic ileus, or (3) a pleural effusion, especially on the left side. Surgical treatment of gallstone disease is usually associated with resolution of the pancreatitis.

Secondary biliary cirrhosis

Secondary biliary cirrhosis may complicate prolonged or intermittent duct obstruction with or without recurrent cholangitis. Although this complication may be seen in patients with choledocholithiasis, it is more common in cases of prolonged obstruction from stricture or neoplasm. Once established, secondary biliary cirrhosis may be progressive even after correction of the obstructing process, and increasingly severe hepatic cirrhosis may lead to portal hypertension or to hepatic failure and death. Prolonged biliary obstruction may also be associated with clinically relevant deficiencies of the fat-soluble vitamins A, D, E, and K.

Diagnosis and treatment

The diagnosis of choledocholithiasis is usually made by cholangiography (Table 47-3), either preoperatively by endoscopic retrograde cholangiogram (ERC) (Fig. 47-2C) or MRCP or intraoperatively at the time

TABLE 47-3

DIAGNOSTIC EVALUATION OF THE BILE DUCTS

DIAGNOSTIC ADVANTAGES	DIAGNOSTIC LIMITATIONS	CONTRAINDICATIONS	COMPLICATIONS	COMMENT
Hepatobiliary Ultrasound				
Rapid Simultaneous scanning of GB, liver, bile ducts, pancreas Accurate identification of dilated bile ducts Not limited by jaundice, pregnancy Guidance for fine-needle biopsy	Bowel gas Massive obesity Ascites Barium Partial bile duct obstruction Poor visualization of distal CBD	None	None	Initial procedure of choice in investigating possible biliary tract obstruction
Computed Tomography				
Simultaneous scanning of GB, liver, bile ducts, pancreas Accurate identification of dilat-edbile ducts, masses Not limited by jaundice, gas, obesity, ascites High-resolution image Guidance for fine-needle biopsy	Extreme cachexia Movement artifact Ileus Partial bile duct obstruction	Pregnancy	Reaction to iodinated contrast, if used	Indicated for evaluation of hepatic or pancreatic masses Procedure of choice in investigating possible biliary obstruction if diagnosticlimitations prevent HBUS
Magnetic Resonance Cholangiopancreatography				
Useful modality for visualizing-pancreatic and biliary ducts Has excellent sensitivity for bile-duct dilatation, biliary stricture, and intraductal abnormalities Can identify pancreatic duct dilatation or stricture, pancreatic duct stenosis, and pancreas divisum	Cannot offer therapeutic intervention High cost	Claustrophobia Certain metals (iron)	None	
Endoscopic Retrograde Cholangiopancreatography				
Simultaneous pancreatography Best visualization of distal biliary tract Bile or pancreatic cytology Endoscopic sphincterotomy and stone removal Biliary manometry	Gastroduodenal obstruction ? Roux-en-Y biliary-enteric anastomosis	Pregnancy ? Acute pancreatitis ? Severe cardiopulmonary disease	Pancreatitis Cholangitis, sepsis Infected pancreatic pseudocyst Perforation (rare) Hypoxemia, aspiration	Cholangiogram of choice in: Absence of dilated ducts ? Pancreatic, ampullary or gastroduodenal disease Prior biliary surgery Endoscopic sphincterotomy a treatment possibility
Percutaneous Transhepatic Cholangiogram				
Extremely successful when bile-ducts dilated Best visualization of proximal biliary tract Bile cytology/culture Percutaneous transhepatic drainage	Nondilated or sclerosed ducts	Pregnancy Uncorrectable coagulopathy Massive ascites ? Hepatic abscess	Bleeding Hemobilia Bile peritonitis Bacteremia, sepsis	Indicated when ERCP is contraindicated or failed
Endoscopic Ultrasound				
Most sensitive method to detect ampullary stones				

Abbreviations: CBD, common bile duct; ERCP, endoscopic retrograde cholangiopancreatography; GB, gallbladder; HBUS, hepatobiliary ultrasound.

of cholecystectomy. As many as 15% of patients undergoing cholecystectomy will prove to have CBD stones. When CBD stones are suspected prior to laparoscopic cholecystectomy, preoperative ERCP with endoscopic papillotomy and stone extraction is the preferred approach. It not only provides stone clearance but also defines the anatomy of the biliary tree in relationship to the cystic duct. CBD stones should be suspected in gallstone patients who have any of the following risk factors: (1) a history of jaundice or pancreatitis, (2) abnormal tests of liver function, and(3) ultrasonographic or MRCP evidence of a dilated CBD or stones in the duct. Alternatively, if intraoperative cholangiography reveals retained stones, postoperative ERCP can be carried out. The need for preoperative ERCP is expected to decrease further as laparoscopic techniques for bile duct exploration improve.

The widespread use of laparoscopic cholecystectomy and ERCP has decreased the incidence of complicated biliary tract disease and the need for choledocholithotomy and T-tube drainage of the bile ducts. EBS followed by spontaneous passage or stone extraction is the treatment of choice in the management of patients with common duct stones, especially in elderly or poor-risk patients.

TRAUMA, STRICTURES, AND HEMOBILIA

Most benign strictures of the extrahepatic bile ducts result from surgical trauma and occur in about 1 in 500 cholecystectomies. Strictures may present with bile leak or abscess formation in the immediate postoperative period or with biliary obstruction or cholangitis as long as 2 years or more following the inciting trauma. The diagnosis is established by percutaneous or endoscopic cholangiography. Endoscopic brushing of biliary strictures may be helpful in establishing the nature of the lesion and is more accurate than bile cytology alone. When positive exfoliative cytology is obtained, the diagnosis of a neoplastic stricture is established. This procedure is especially important in patients with primary sclerosing cholangitis (PSC) who are predisposed to the development of cholangiocarcinomas. Successful operative correction of non-PSC bile duct strictures by a skillful surgeon with duct-to-bowel anastomosis is usually possible, although mortality rates from surgical complications, recurrent cholangitis, or secondary biliary cirrhosis are high.

Hemobilia may follow traumatic or operative injury to the liver or bile ducts, intraductal rupture of a hepatic abscess or aneurysm of the hepatic artery, biliary or hepatic tumor hemorrhage, or mechanical complications of choledocholithiasis or hepatobiliary parasitism. Diagnostic procedures such as liver biopsy, PTC, and transhepatic biliary drainage catheter placement may also be complicated by hemobilia. Patients often present with a classic triad of biliary pain, obstructive jaundice, and melena or occult blood in the stools. The diagnosis is sometimes made by cholangiographic evidence of blood clot in the biliary tree, but selective angiographic verification may be required. Although minor episodes of hemobilia may resolve without operative intervention, surgical ligation of the bleeding vessel is frequently required.

EXTRINSIC COMPRESSION OF THE BILE DUCTS

Partial or complete biliary obstruction may be produced by extrinsic compression of the ducts. The most common cause of this form of obstructive jaundice is carcinoma of the head of the pancreas. Biliary obstruction may also occur as a complication of either acute or chronic pancreatitis or involvement of lymph nodes in the porta hepatis by lymphoma or metastatic carcinoma. The latter should be distinguished from cholestasis resulting from massive replacement of the liver by tumor.

HEPATOBILIARY PARASITISM

Infestation of the biliary tract by adult helminths or their ova may produce a chronic, recurrent pyogenic cholangitis with or without multiple hepatic abscesses, ductal stones, or biliary obstruction. This condition is relatively rare but does occur in inhabitants of southern China and elsewhere in Southeast Asia. The organisms most commonly involved are trematodes or flukes, including *Clonorchis sinensis*, *Opisthorchis viverrini* or *Opisthorchis felineus*, and *Fasciola hepatica*. The biliary tract also may be involved by intraductal migration of adult *Ascaris lumbricoides* from the duodenum or by intrabiliary rupture of hydatid cysts of the liver produced by *Echinococcus* spp. The diagnosis is made by cholangiography and the presence of characteristic ova on stool examination. When obstruction is present, the treatment of choice is laparotomy under antibiotic coverage, with common duct exploration and a biliary drainage procedure.

SCLEROSING CHOLANGITIS

Primary or idiopathic sclerosing cholangitis is characterized by a progressive, inflammatory, sclerosing, and obliterative process affecting the extrahepatic and/or the intrahepatic bile ducts. The disorder occurs up to 75% in association with inflammatory bowel disease, especially ulcerative colitis. It may also be associated with autoimmune pancreatitis; multifocal fibrosclerosis syndromes such as retroperitoneal, mediastinal, and/or periureteral fibrosis; Riedel's struma; or pseudotumor of the orbit.

Immunoglobulin G4 (IgG4)–associated cholangitis is a recently described biliary disease of unknown etiology that presents with biochemical and cholangiographic features indistinguishable from PSC, is often associated with autoimmune pancreatitis and other fibrosing conditions, and is characterized by elevated serum IgG4 and infiltration of IgG4-positive plasma cells in bile ducts and liver tissue. In contrast to PSC, it is not associated with inflammatory bowel disease and should be suspected if associated with increased serum IgG4 and unexplained pancreatic disease. Glucocorticoids are regarded as the initial treatment of choice. Relapse is common after steroid withdrawal, especially with proximal strictures. Long-term treatment with glucocorticoids and/or azathioprine may be needed after relapse or for inadequate response **(Chap. 50)**.

Patients with primary sclerosing cholangitis often present with signs and symptoms of chronic or intermittent biliary obstruction: RUQ abdominal pain, pruritus, jaundice, or acute cholangitis. Late in the course, complete biliary obstruction, secondary biliary cirrhosis, hepatic failure, or portal hypertension with bleeding varices may occur. The diagnosis is usually established by finding multifocal, diffusely distributed strictures with intervening segments of normal or dilated ducts, producing a beaded appearance on cholangiography (Fig. 47-2*D*). The cholangiographic techniques of choice in suspected cases are MRCP and ERCP. When a diagnosis of sclerosing cholangitis has been established, a search for associated diseases, especially for chronic inflammatory bowel disease, should be carried out.

A recent study describes the natural history and outcome for 305 patients of Swedish descent with primary sclerosing cholangitis; 134 (44%) of the patients were asymptomatic at the time of diagnosis and, not surprisingly, had a significantly higher survival rate. The independent predictors of a bad prognosis were advanced age, serum bilirubin concentration, and liver histologic changes. Cholangiocarcinoma was found in 24 patients (8%). Inflammatory bowel disease was closely associated with primary sclerosing cholangitis and had a prevalence of 81% in this study population.

Small duct PSC is defined by the presence of chronic cholestasis and hepatic histology consistent with PSC but with normal findings on cholangiography. Small duct PSC is found in ~5% of patients with PSC and may represent an earlier stage of PSC associated with a significantly better long-term prognosis. However, such patients may progress to classic PSC and/or end-stage liver disease with consequent necessity of liver transplantation.

In patients with AIDS, cholangiopancreatography may demonstrate a broad range of biliary tract changes as well as pancreatic duct obstruction and occasionally pancreatitis. Further, biliary tract lesions in AIDS include infection and cholangiopancreatographic changes similar to those of PSC. Changes noted include: (1) diffuse involvement of intrahepatic bile ducts alone, (2) involvement of both intra- and extrahepatic bile ducts, (3) ampullary stenosis, (4) stricture of the intrapancreatic portion of the CBD, and (5) pancreatic duct involvement. Associated infectious organisms include *Cryptosporidium*, *Mycobacterium avium-intracellulare*, cytomegalovirus, *Microsporidia*, and *Isospora*. In addition, acalculous cholecystitis occurs in up to 10% of patients. ERCP sphincterotomy, while not without risk, provides significant pain reduction in patients with AIDS-associated papillary stenosis. Secondary sclerosing cholangitis may occur as a long-term complication of choledocholithiasis, cholangiocarcinoma, operative or traumatic biliary injury, or contiguous inflammatory processes.

TREATMENT Sclerosing Cholangitis

Therapy with cholestyramine may help control symptoms of pruritus, and antibiotics are useful when cholangitis complicates the clinical picture. Vitamin D and calcium supplementation may help prevent the loss of bone mass frequently seen in patients with chronic cholestasis. Glucocorticoids, methotrexate, and cyclosporine have not been shown to be efficacious in PSC. UDCA in high dosage (20 mg/kg) improves serum liver tests, but an effect on survival has not been documented. In cases where high-grade biliary obstruction (dominant strictures) has occurred, balloon dilatation or stenting may be appropriate. Only rarely is surgical intervention indicated. Efforts at biliary-enteric anastomosis or stent placement may, however, be complicated by recurrent cholangitis and further progression of the stenosing process. The prognosis is unfavorable, with a median survival of 9–12 years following the diagnosis, regardless of therapy. Four variables (age, serum bilirubin level, histologic stage, and splenomegaly) predict survival in patients with PSC and serve as the basis for a risk score. PSC is one of the most common indications for liver transplantation.

SECTION VII

LIVER TRANSPLANTATION

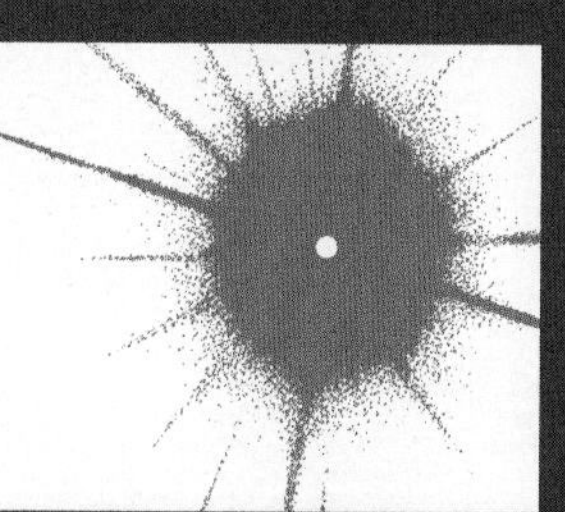

CHAPTER 48
LIVER TRANSPLANTATION

Raymond T. Chung ■ Jules L. Dienstag

Liver transplantation—the replacement of the native, diseased liver by a normal organ (allograft)—has matured from an experimental procedure reserved for desperately ill patients to an accepted, lifesaving operation applied more optimally in the natural history of end-stage liver disease. The preferred and technically most advanced approach is *orthotopic transplantation*, in which the native organ is removed and the donor organ is inserted in the same anatomic location. Pioneered in the 1960s by Thomas Starzl at the University of Colorado and, later, at the University of Pittsburgh and by Roy Calne in Cambridge, England, liver transplantation is now performed routinely worldwide. Success measured as 1-year survival has improved from ~30% in the 1970s to >90% today. These improved prospects for prolonged survival resulted from refinements in operative technique, improvements in organ procurement and preservation, advances in immunosuppressive therapy, and, perhaps most influentially, more enlightened patient selection and timing. Despite the perioperative morbidity and mortality, the technical and management challenges of the procedure, and its costs, liver transplantation has become the approach of choice for selected patients whose chronic or acute liver disease is progressive, life-threatening, and unresponsive to medical therapy. Based on the current level of success, the number of liver transplants has continued to grow each year; in 2012, 6256 patients received liver allografts in the United States. Still, the demand for new livers continues to outpace availability; as of mid-2013, 15,806 patients in the United States were on a waiting list for a donor liver. In response to this drastic shortage of donor organs, many transplantation centers supplement cadaver-organ liver transplantation with living-donor transplantation.

INDICATIONS

Potential candidates for liver transplantation are children and adults who, in the absence of contraindications (see below), suffer from severe, irreversible liver disease for which alternative medical or surgical treatments have been exhausted or are unavailable. *Timing of the operation is of critical importance.* Indeed, improved timing and better patient selection are felt to have contributed more to the increased success of liver transplantation in the 1980s and beyond than all the impressive technical and immunologic advances combined. Although the disease should be advanced, and although opportunities for spontaneous or medically induced stabilization or recovery should be allowed, the procedure should be done sufficiently early to give the surgical procedure a fair chance for success. Ideally, transplantation should be considered in patients with end-stage liver disease who are experiencing or have experienced a life-threatening complication of hepatic decompensation or whose quality of life has deteriorated to unacceptable levels. Although patients with well-compensated cirrhosis can survive for many years, many patients with quasi-stable chronic liver disease have much more advanced disease than may be apparent. As discussed below, the better the status of the patient prior to transplantation, the higher will be its anticipated success rate. The decision about *when* to transplant is complex and requires the combined judgment of an experienced team of hepatologists, transplant surgeons, anesthesiologists, and specialists in support services, not to mention the well-informed consent of the patient and the patient's family.

TRANSPLANTATION IN CHILDREN

Indications for transplantation in children are listed in Table 48-1. The most common is *biliary atresia. Inherited or genetic disorders of metabolism* associated with liver failure constitute another major indication for transplantation in children and adolescents. In Crigler-Najjar disease type I and in certain hereditary disorders of the urea cycle and of amino acid or lactate-pyruvate metabolism, transplantation may be the only way to prevent impending deterioration of central nervous system function, despite the fact that the native liver is structurally normal. Combined heart and liver transplantation has yielded dramatic improvement in cardiac function and in cholesterol levels in children with homozygous familial hypercholesterolemia; combined liver and kidney transplantation has been successful in patients with primary hyperoxaluria type I. In hemophiliacs with transfusion-associated hepatitis and liver failure, liver transplantation has been associated with recovery of normal factor VIII synthesis.

TRANSPLANTATION IN ADULTS

Liver transplantation is indicated for end-stage *cirrhosis* of all causes (Table 48-1). In *sclerosing cholangitis* and *Caroli's disease* (multiple cystic dilatations of the intrahepatic biliary tree), recurrent infections and sepsis associated with inflammatory and fibrotic obstruction of the biliary tree may be an indication for transplantation. Because prior biliary surgery complicates and is a relative contraindication for liver transplantation, surgical diversion of the biliary tree has been all but abandoned for patients with sclerosing cholangitis. In patients who undergo transplantation for *hepatic vein thrombosis* (*Budd-Chiari syndrome*), postoperative anticoagulation is essential; underlying myeloproliferative disorders may have to be treated but are not a contraindication to liver transplantation. If a donor organ can be located quickly, before life-threatening complications—including cerebral edema—set in, patients with acute liver failure are candidates for liver transplantation. Routine candidates for liver transplantation are patients with *alcoholic cirrhosis*, *chronic viral hepatitis*, and *primary hepatocellular malignancies*. Although all three of these categories are considered to be high risk, liver transplantation can be offered to carefully selected patients. Currently, chronic hepatitis C and alcoholic liver disease are the most common indications for liver transplantation, accounting for over 40% of all adult candidates who undergo the procedure. Patients with alcoholic cirrhosis can be considered as candidates for transplantation if they meet strict criteria for abstinence and reform; however, these criteria still do not prevent recidivism in up to a quarter of cases. In highly selected cases in a limited number of centers, transplantation for severe *acute* alcoholic hepatitis has been performed with success; however, because patients with acute alcoholic hepatitis are still actively using alcohol, and because continued alcohol abuse remains a concern, acute alcoholic hepatitis is not a routine indication for liver transplantation. Patients with chronic hepatitis C have early allograft and patient survival comparable to those of other subsets of patients after transplantation; however, reinfection in the donor organ is universal, recurrent hepatitis C is insidiously progressive, allograft cirrhosis develops in 20–30% at 5 years, and cirrhosis and late organ failure occur at a higher frequency beyond 5 years. With the introduction of highly effective direct acting antiviral agents targeting HCV, it is expected that allograft outcomes will improve significantly in the coming years. In patients with chronic hepatitis B, in the absence of measures to prevent recurrent hepatitis B, survival after transplantation is reduced by approximately 10–20%; however, prophylactic use of hepatitis B immune globulin (HBIg) during and after transplantation increases the success of transplantation to a level comparable to that seen in patients with nonviral causes of liver decompensation. Specific oral antiviral drugs (e.g., entecavir, tenofovir disoproxil fumarate) **(Chap. 41)** can be used both for prophylaxis against and for treatment of recurrent hepatitis B,

TABLE 48-1

INDICATIONS FOR LIVER TRANSPLANTATION

CHILDREN	ADULTS
Biliary atresia	Primary biliary cirrhosis
Neonatal hepatitis	Secondary biliary cirrhosis
Congenital hepatic fibrosis	Primary sclerosing cholangitis
Alagille's syndrome[a]	Autoimmune hepatitis
Byler's disease[b]	Caroli's disease[c]
α_1-Antitrypsin deficiency	Cryptogenic cirrhosis
Inherited disorders of metabolism	Chronic hepatitis with cirrhosis
Wilson's disease	Hepatic vein thrombosis
Tyrosinemia	Fulminant hepatitis
Glycogen storage diseases	Alcoholic cirrhosis
Lysosomal storage diseases	Chronic viral hepatitis
Protoporphyria	Primary hepatocellular malignancies
Crigler-Najjar disease type I	Hepatic adenomas
Familial hypercholesterolemia	Nonalcoholic steatohepatitis
Primary hyperoxaluria type I	Familial amyloid polyneuropathy
Hemophilia	

[a]Arteriohepatic dysplasia, with paucity of bile ducts, and congenital malformations, including pulmonary stenosis.
[b]Intrahepatic cholestasis, progressive liver failure, and mental and growth retardation.
[c]Multiple cystic dilatations of the intrahepatic biliary tree.

facilitating further the management of patients undergoing liver transplantation for end-stage hepatitis B; most transplantation centers rely on antiviral drugs with or without HBIg to manage patients with hepatitis B. Issues of disease recurrence are discussed in more detail below. Patients with nonmetastatic primary hepatobiliary tumors—primary hepatocellular carcinoma (HCC), cholangiocarcinoma, hepatoblastoma, angiosarcoma, epithelioid hemangioendothelioma, and multiple or massive hepatic adenomata—have undergone liver transplantation; however, for some hepatobiliary malignancies, overall survival is significantly lower than that for other categories of liver disease. Most transplantation centers have reported 5-year recurrence-free survival rates in patients with unresectable HCC for single tumors <5 cm in diameter or for three or fewer lesions all <3 cm comparable to those seen in patients undergoing transplantation for nonmalignant indications. Consequently, liver transplantation is currently restricted to patients whose hepatic malignancies meet these criteria. Expanded criteria for patients with HCC continue to be evaluated. Because the likelihood of recurrent cholangiocarcinoma is very high, only highly selected patients with limited disease are being evaluated for transplantation after intensive chemotherapy and radiation.

CONTRAINDICATIONS

Absolute contraindications for transplantation include life-threatening systemic diseases, uncontrolled extrahepatic bacterial or fungal infections, preexisting advanced cardiovascular or pulmonary disease, multiple uncorrectable life-threatening congenital anomalies, metastatic malignancy, and active drug or alcohol abuse (Table 48–2). Because carefully selected patients in their sixties and even seventies have undergone transplantation successfully, advanced age per se is no longer considered an absolute contraindication; however, in older patients a more thorough preoperative evaluation should be undertaken to exclude ischemic cardiac disease and other comorbid conditions. Advanced age (>70 years), however, should be considered a *relative contraindication*—that is, a factor to be taken into account with other relative contraindications. Other relative contraindications include portal vein thrombosis, HIV infection, preexisting renal disease not associated with liver disease (which may prompt consideration of combined liver and kidney transplantation), intrahepatic or biliary sepsis, severe hypoxemia (Po_2 <50 mmHg) resulting from right-to-left intrapulmonary shunts, portopulmonary hypertension with high mean pulmonary artery pressures (>35 mmHg), previous extensive hepatobiliary surgery, any uncontrolled serious psychiatric disorder, and lack of sufficient social supports. Any one of these relative contraindications is insufficient in and of itself to preclude transplantation. For example, the problem of portal vein thrombosis can be overcome by constructing a graft from the donor liver portal vein to the recipient's superior mesenteric vein. Now that highly active antiretroviral therapy has dramatically improved the survival of persons with HIV infection, and because end-stage liver disease caused by chronic hepatitis C and B has emerged as a serious source of morbidity and mortality in the HIV-infected population, liver transplantation has now been performed successfully in selected HIV-positive persons who have excellent control of HIV infection. Selected patients with CD4± T cell counts >100/μL and with pharmacologic suppression of HIV viremia have undergone transplantation for end-stage liver disease. HIV-infected persons who have received liver allografts for end-stage liver disease resulting from chronic hepatitis B have experienced survival rates compared to those of HIV-negative persons undergoing transplantation for the same indication. In contrast, recurrent hepatitis C

TABLE 48-2

CONTRAINDICATIONS TO LIVER TRANSPLANTATION

ABSOLUTE	RELATIVE
Uncontrolled extrahepato biliary infection	Age >70
Active, untreated sepsis	Prior extensive hepatobiliary surgery
Uncorrectable, life-limiting congenital anomalies	Portal vein thrombosis
Active substance or alcohol abuse	Renal failure not attributable to liver disease
Advanced cardiopulmonary disease	Previous extrahepatic malignancy (not including nonmelanoma skin cancer)
Extrahepatobiliary malignancy (not including nonmelanoma malignancy skin cancer)	Severe obesity
Metastatic malignancy to the liver	Severe malnutrition/wasting
Cholangiocarcinoma	Medical noncompliance
AIDS	HIV seropositivity with failure to control HIV viremia or CD4 <100/μL
Life-threatening systemic diseases	Intrahepatic sepsis Severe hypoxemia secondary to right-to-left intrapulmonary shunts (Po_2 <50 mmHg) Severe pulmonary hypertension (mean pulmonary artery pressure >35 mmHg) Uncontrolled psychiatric disorder

virus (HCV) in the allograft has limited long-term success in persons with HCV-related end-stage liver disease. Again, it is expected that the availability of direct acting antiviral agents targeting HCV, will significantly improve allograft outcomes.

TECHNICAL CONSIDERATIONS

CADAVER DONOR SELECTION

Cadaver donor livers for transplantation are procured primarily from victims of head trauma. Organs from brain-dead donors up to age 60 are acceptable if the following criteria are met: hemodynamic stability, adequate oxygenation, absence of bacterial or fungal infection, absence of abdominal trauma, absence of hepatic dysfunction, and serologic exclusion of hepatitis B (HBV) and C viruses and HIV. Occasionally, organs from donors with hepatitis B and C are used (e.g., for recipients with prior hepatitis B and C, respectively). Organs from donors with antibodies to hepatitis B core antigen (anti-HBc) can also be used when the need is especially urgent, and recipients of these organs are treated prophylactically with antiviral drugs. Cardiovascular and respiratory functions are maintained artificially until the liver can be removed. Transplantation of organs procured from deceased donors who have succumbed to cardiac death can be performed successfully under selected circumstances, when ischemic time is minimized and liver histology preserved. Compatibility in ABO blood group and organ size between donor and recipient are important considerations in donor selection; however, ABO-incompatible, split liver, or reduced-donor-organ transplants can be performed in emergencies or marked donor scarcity. Tissue typing for human leukocyte antigen (HLA) matching is not required, and preformed cytotoxic HLA antibodies do not preclude liver transplantation. Following perfusion with cold electrolyte solution, the donor liver is removed and packed in ice. The use of University of Wisconsin (UW) solution, rich in lactobionate and raffinose, has permitted the extension of cold ischemic time up to 20 h; however, 12 h may be a more reasonable limit. Improved techniques for harvesting multiple organs from the same donor have increased the availability of donor livers, but the availability of donor livers is far outstripped by the demand. Currently in the United States, all donor livers are distributed through a nationwide organ-sharing network (United Network for Organ Sharing [UNOS]) designed to allocate available organs based on regional considerations and recipient acuity. Recipients who have the highest disease severity generally have the highest priority, but allocation strategies that balance highest urgency against best outcomes continue to evolve to distribute cadaver organs most effectively. Allocation based on the Child-Turcotte-Pugh (CTP) score, which uses five clinical variables (encephalopathy stage, ascites, bilirubin, albumin, and prothrombin time) and waiting time, has been replaced by allocation based on urgency alone, calculated by the Model for End-Stage Liver Disease (MELD) score. The MELD score is based on a mathematical model that includes bilirubin, creatinine, and prothrombin time expressed as international normalized ratio (INR) (Table 48-3). Neither waiting time (except as a tie breaker between two potential recipients with the same MELD scores) nor posttransplantation outcome is taken into account, but use of the MELD score has been shown to reduce waiting list mortality, to reduce waiting time prior to transplantation, to be the best predictor of pretransplantation mortality, to satisfy the prevailing view that medical need should be the decisive determinant, and to eliminate both the subjectivity inherent in the CTP scoring system (presence and degree of ascites and hepatic encephalopathy) and the differences in waiting times among different regions of the country. Recent data indicate that liver recipients with MELD scores <15 experienced higher posttransplantation mortality rates than similarly classified

TABLE 48-3

UNITED NETWORK FOR ORGAN SHARING (UNOS) LIVER TRANSPLANTATION WAITING LIST CRITERIA	
Status 1	Fulminant hepatic failure (including primary graft nonfunction and hepatic artery thrombosis within 7 days after transplantation as well as acute decompensated Wilson's disease)[a]
The Model for End-Stage Liver Disease (MELD) score, on a continuous scale,[b] determines allocation of the remainder of donor organs. This model is based on the following calculation:	
$3.78 \times \log_e$ bilirubin (mg/100 mL) $\pm$ $11.2 \times \log_e$ international normalized ratio (INR) $\pm$ $9.57 \times \log_e$ creatinine (mg/100 mL) $\pm$ 6.43 (v 0 for alcoholic and cholestatic liver disease, $\times$ 1 for all other types of liver disease).[c,d,e]	
Online calculators to determine MELD scores are available, such as the following: *http://optn.transplant.hrsa.gov/resources/professionalresources.asp?index=9.*	

[a]For children <18 years of age, status 1 includes acute or chronic liver failure plus hospitalization in an intensive care unit or inborn errors of metabolism. Status 1 is retained for those persons with fulminant hepatic failure and supersedes the MELD score.

[b]The MELD scale is continuous, with 34 levels ranging between 6 and 40. Donor organs usually do not become available unless the MELD score exceeds 20.

[c]Patients with stage T2 hepatocellular carcinoma receive 22 disease-specific points.

[d]Creatinine is included because renal function is a validated predictor of survival in patients with liver disease. For adults undergoing dialysis twice a week, the creatinine in the equation is set to 4 mg/100 mL.

[e]For children <18 years of age, the Pediatric End-Stage Liver Disease (PELD) scale is used. This scale is based on albumin, bilirubin, INR, growth failure, and age. Status 1 is retained.

patients who remained on the wait list. This observation led to the modification of UNOS policy to allocate donor organs to candidates with MELD scores exceeding 15 within the local or regional procurement organization before offering the organ to local patients whose scores are <15. In addition, serum sodium, another important predictor of survival in liver transplantation candidates, is taken into consideration in allocating donor livers.

The highest priority (status 1) continues to be reserved for patients with fulminant hepatic failure or primary graft nonfunction. Because candidates for liver transplantation who have HCC may not be sufficiently decompensated to compete for donor organs based on urgency criteria alone, and because protracted waiting for cadaver donor organs often results in tumor growth beyond acceptable limits for transplantation, such patients are assigned disease-specific MELD points (Table 48-3). Other disease-specific MELD exceptions include portopulmonary hypertension, hepatopulmonary syndrome, familial amyloid polyneuropathy, primary hyperoxaluria (necessitating liver-kidney transplantation), cystic fibrosis liver disease, and highly selected cases of hilar cholangiocarcinoma.

LIVING DONOR TRANSPLANTATION

Occasionally, especially for liver transplantation in children, one cadaver organ can be split between two recipients (one adult and one child). A more viable alternative, transplantation of the right lobe of the liver from a healthy adult donor into an adult recipient, has gained increased popularity. Living donor transplantation of the left lobe (left lateral segment), introduced in the early 1990s to alleviate the extreme shortage of donor organs for small children, accounts currently for approximately one-third of all liver transplantation procedures in children. Driven by the shortage of cadaver organs, living donor transplantation involving the more sizable right lobe is being considered with increasing frequency in adults; however, living donor liver transplantation cannot be expected to solve the donor organ shortage; 246 such procedures were done in 2012, representing only about 4% of all liver transplant operations done in the United States.

Living donor transplantation can reduce waiting time and cold-ischemia time; is done under elective, rather than emergency, circumstances; and may be lifesaving in recipients who cannot afford to wait for a cadaver donor. The downside, of course, is the risk to the healthy donor (a mean of 10 weeks of medical disability; biliary complications in ~5%; postoperative complications such as wound infection, small-bowel obstruction, and incisional hernias in 9–19%; and even, in 0.2–0.4%, death) as well as the increased frequency of biliary (15–32%) and vascular (10%) complications in the recipient. Potential donors must participate voluntarily without coercion, and transplantation teams should go to great lengths to exclude subtle coercive or inappropriate psychological factors as well as outline carefully to both donor and recipient the potential benefits and risks of the procedure. Donors for the procedure should be 18–60 years old; have a compatible blood type with the recipient; have no chronic medical problems or history of major abdominal surgery; be related genetically or emotionally to the recipient; and pass an exhaustive series of clinical, biochemical, and serologic evaluations to unearth disqualifying medical disorders. The recipient should meet the same UNOS criteria for liver transplantation as recipients of a cadaver donor allograft. Comprehensive outcome data on adult-to-adult living donor liver transplantation are being collected (*www.nih-a2all.org*).

SURGICAL TECHNIQUE

Removal of the recipient's native liver is technically difficult, particularly in the presence of portal hypertension with its associated collateral circulation and extensive varices and especially in the presence of scarring from previous abdominal operations. The combination of portal hypertension and coagulopathy (elevated prothrombin time and thrombocytopenia) may translate into large blood product transfusion requirements. After the portal vein and infrahepatic and suprahepatic inferior vena cavae are dissected, the hepatic artery and common bile duct are dissected. Then the native liver is removed and the donor organ inserted. During the anhepatic phase, coagulopathy, hypoglycemia, hypocalcemia, and hypothermia are encountered and must be managed by the anesthesiology team. Caval, portal vein, hepatic artery, and bile duct anastomoses are performed in succession, the last by end-to-end suturing of the donor and recipient common bile ducts (Fig. 48-1) or by choledochojejunostomy to a Roux-en-Y loop if the recipient common bile duct cannot be used for reconstruction (e.g., in sclerosing cholangitis). A typical transplant operation lasts 8 h, with a range of 6–18 h. Because of excessive bleeding, large volumes of blood, blood products, and volume expanders may be required during surgery; however, blood requirements have fallen sharply with improvements in surgical technique, blood-salvage interventions, and experience.

As noted above, emerging alternatives to orthotopic liver transplantation include split-liver grafts, in which one donor organ is divided and inserted into two recipients; and living donor procedures, in which part of the left (for children), the left (for children or small adults), or the right (for adults) lobe of the liver is harvested from a living donor for transplantation into the

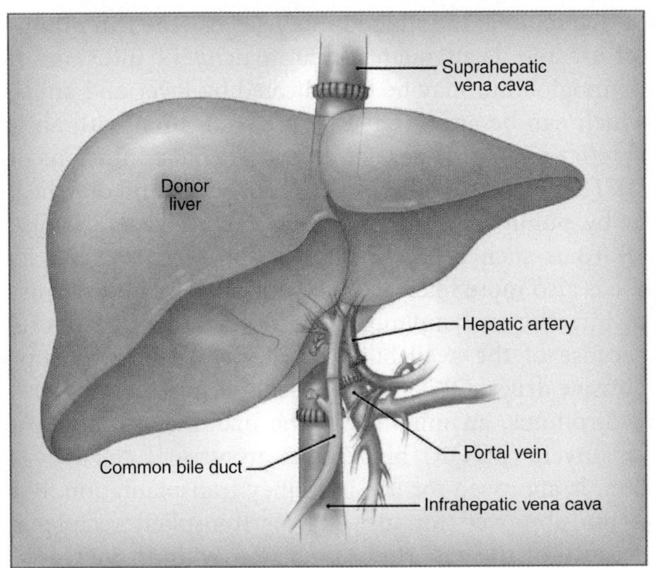

FIGURE 48-1
The anastomoses in orthotopic liver transplantation. The anastomoses are performed in the following sequence: (1) suprahepatic and infrahepatic vena cava, (2) portal vein, (3) hepatic artery, and (4) common bile duct-to-duct anastomosis. *(Adapted from JL Dienstag, AB Cosimi: N Engl J Med 367:1483, 2012.)*

recipient. In the adult procedure, once the right lobe is removed from the donor, the donor right hepatic vein is anastomosed to the recipient right hepatic vein remnant, followed by donor-to-recipient anastomoses of the portal vein and then the hepatic artery. Finally, the biliary anastomosis is performed, duct-to-duct if practical or via Roux-en-Y anastomosis. Heterotopic liver transplantation, in which the donor liver is inserted without removal of the native liver, has met with very limited success and acceptance, except in a very small number of centers. In attempts to support desperately ill patients until a suitable donor organ can be identified, several transplantation centers are studying extracorporeal perfusion with bioartificial liver cartridges constructed from hepatocytes bound to hollow fiber systems and used as temporary hepatic-assist devices, but their efficacy remains to be established. Areas of research with the potential to overcome the shortage of donor organs include hepatocyte transplantation and xenotransplantation with genetically modified organs of nonhuman origin (e.g., swine).

POSTOPERATIVE COURSE AND MANAGEMENT

IMMUNOSUPPRESSIVE THERAPY

The introduction in 1980 of cyclosporine as an immunosuppressive agent contributed substantially to the improvement in survival after liver transplantation. Cyclosporine, a calcineurin inhibitor, blocks early activation of T cells and is specific for T cell functions that result from the interaction of the T cell with its receptor and that involve the calcium-dependent signal transduction pathway. As a result, the activity of cyclosporine leads to inhibition of lymphokine gene activation, blocking interleukins 2, 3, and 4, tumor necrosis factor a, and other lymphokines. Cyclosporine also inhibits B cell functions. This process occurs without affecting rapidly dividing cells in the bone marrow, which may account for the reduced frequency of posttransplantation systemic infections. The most common and important side effect of cyclosporine therapy is nephrotoxicity. Cyclosporine causes dose-dependent renal tubular injury and direct renal artery vasospasm. Following renal function is therefore important in monitoring cyclosporine therapy, perhaps even a more reliable indicator than blood levels of the drug. Nephrotoxicity is reversible and can be managed by dose reduction. Other adverse effects of cyclosporine therapy include hypertension, hyperkalemia, tremor, hirsutism, glucose intolerance, and gingival hyperplasia.

Tacrolimus, a macrolide lactone antibiotic isolated from a Japanese soil fungus, *Streptomyces tsukubaensis*, has the same mechanism of action as cyclosporine but is 10–100 times more potent. Initially applied as "rescue" therapy for patients in whom rejection occurred despite the use of cyclosporine, tacrolimus was shown to be associated with a reduced frequency of acute, refractory, and chronic rejection. Although patient and graft survival are the same with these two drugs, the advantage of tacrolimus in minimizing episodes of rejection, reducing the need for additional glucocorticoid doses, and reducing the likelihood of bacterial and cytomegalovirus (CMV) infection has simplified the management of patients undergoing liver transplantation. In addition, the oral absorption of tacrolimus is more predictable than that of cyclosporine, especially during the early postoperative period when T-tube drainage interferes with the enterohepatic circulation of cyclosporine. As a result, in most transplantation centers, tacrolimus has now supplanted cyclosporine for primary immunosuppression, and many centers rely on oral rather than IV administration from the outset. For transplantation centers that prefer cyclosporine, a better-absorbed microemulsion preparation is available.

Although more potent than cyclosporine, tacrolimus is also more toxic and more likely to be discontinued for adverse events. The toxicity of tacrolimus is similar to that of cyclosporine; nephrotoxicity and neurotoxicity are the most commonly encountered adverse effects, and neurotoxicity (tremor, seizures, hallucinations, psychoses, coma) is more likely and more severe in tacrolimus-treated patients. Both drugs can cause diabetes mellitus, but tacrolimus does not cause hirsutism or gingival hyperplasia. Because of overlapping toxicity between cyclosporine and tacrolimus, especially nephrotoxicity, and because tacrolimus reduces cyclosporine clearance, these two drugs should not be used together. Because 99% of tacrolimus is metabolized by the liver, hepatic dysfunction reduces its clearance; in primary graft nonfunction (when, for technical reasons or because of ischemic damage prior to its insertion, the allograft is defective and does not function normally from the outset), tacrolimus doses have to be reduced substantially, especially in children. Both cyclosporine and tacrolimus are metabolized by the cytochrome P450 IIIA system, and, therefore, drugs that induce cytochrome P450 (e.g., phenytoin, phenobarbital, carbamazepine, rifampin) reduce available levels of cyclosporine and tacrolimus; and drugs that inhibit cytochrome P450 (e.g., erythromycin, fluconazole, ketoconazole, clotrimazole, itraconazole, verapamil, diltiazem, danazol, metoclopramide, the HIV protease inhibitor ritonavir, and the HCV protease inhibitors telaprevir and boceprevir) increase cyclosporine and tacrolimus blood levels. Indeed, itraconazole is used occasionally to help boost tacrolimus levels. Like azathioprine, cyclosporine and tacrolimus appear to be associated with a risk of lymphoproliferative malignancies (see below), which may occur earlier after cyclosporine or tacrolimus than after azathioprine therapy. Because of these side effects, combinations of cyclosporine or tacrolimus with prednisone and an antimetabolite (azathioprine or mycophenolic acid, see below)—all at reduced doses—are preferable regimens for immunosuppressive therapy.

Mycophenolic acid, a nonnucleoside purine metabolism inhibitor derived as a fermentation product from several *Penicillium* species, is another immunosuppressive drug being used for patients undergoing liver transplantation. Mycophenolate has been shown to be better than azathioprine, when used with other standard immunosuppressive drugs, in preventing rejection after renal transplantation and has been adopted widely as well for use in liver transplantation. The most common adverse effects of mycophenolate are bone marrow suppression and gastrointestinal complaints.

In patients with pretransplantation renal dysfunction or renal deterioration that occurs intraoperatively or immediately postoperatively, tacrolimus or cyclosporine therapy may not be practical; under these circumstances, induction or maintenance of immunosuppression with antithymocyte globulin (ATG, thymoglobulin) or monoclonal antibodies to T cells, OKT3, may be appropriate. Therapy with these agents has been especially effective in reversing acute rejection in the posttransplantation period and is the standard treatment for acute rejection that fails to respond to methylprednisolone boluses. Available data support the use of thymoglobulin induction to delay calcineurin inhibitor use and its attendant nephrotoxicity. IV infusions of thymoglobulin may be complicated by fever and chills, which can be ameliorated by premedication with antipyretics and a low dose of glucocorticoids. Infusions of OKT3 may be complicated by fever, chills, and diarrhea, or by pulmonary edema, which can be fatal. Because OKT3 is such a potent immunosuppressive agent, its use is also more likely to be complicated by opportunistic infection or lymphoproliferative disorders; therefore, because of the availability of alternative immunosuppressive drugs, OKT3 is now used sparingly.

Sirolimus, an inhibitor of the mammalian target of rapamycin (mTOR), blocks later events in T cell activation, is approved for use in kidney transplantation, but is not approved for use in liver transplant recipients because of the reported association with an increased frequency of hepatic artery thrombosis in the first month posttransplantation. In patients with calcineurin inhibitor–related nephrotoxicity, conversion to sirolimus has been demonstrated to be effective in preventing rejection with accompanying improvements in renal function. Because of its profound antiproliferative effects, sirolimus has also been suggested to be a useful immunosuppressive agent in patients with a prior or current history of malignancy, such as HCC. Side effects include hyperlipidemia, peripheral edema, oral ulcers, and interstitial pneumonitis. Everolimus is a hydroxyethyl derivative of sirolimus that, when used in conjunction with low-dose tacrolimus, also provides successful protection against acute rejection, with decreased renal impairment compared to that associated with standard tacrolimus dosing. Everolimus and sirolimus share a similar adverse events profile; therefore, neither of these agents is approved for routine use in liver allograft recipients.

The most important principle of immunosuppression is that the ideal approach strikes a balance between immunosuppression and immunologic competence. In general, given sufficient immunosuppression, acute liver allograft rejection is nearly always reversible. On one hand, incompletely treated acute rejection predisposes to the development of chronic rejection, which can threaten graft survival. On the other hand, if the cumulative dose of immunosuppressive therapy is too large, the patient may succumb to opportunistic infection. In hepatitis C, pulse glucocorticoids or OKT3 use accelerate recurrent allograft hepatitis. Further complicating matters, acute rejection can be difficult to distinguish histologically from recurrent hepatitis C. Therefore, immunosuppressive drugs must be used judiciously, with strict attention to the infectious consequences of such therapy and careful confirmation of the diagnosis of acute rejection. In this vein, efforts have been made to minimize the use of glucocorticoids, a mainstay of immunosuppressive regimens, and steroid-free immunosuppression can be achieved in some instances. Patients who undergo liver transplantation for autoimmune diseases such as primary biliary cirrhosis, autoimmune hepatitis, and primary sclerosing cholangitis are less likely to achieve freedom from glucocorticoids.

POSTOPERATIVE COMPLICATIONS

Complications of liver transplantation can be divided into nonhepatic and hepatic categories (Tables 48-4 and 48-5). In addition, both immediate postoperative and late complications are encountered. As a rule, patients who undergo liver transplantation have been chronically ill for protracted periods and may be malnourished and wasted. The impact of such chronic illness and the multisystem failure that accompanies liver failure continue to require attention in the postoperative period. Because of the massive fluid losses and fluid shifts that occur during the operation, patients may remain fluid-overloaded during the immediate postoperative period, straining cardiovascular reserve; this effect can be amplified in the face of transient renal dysfunction and pulmonary capillary vascular permeability. Continuous monitoring of cardiovascular and pulmonary function, measures to maintain the integrity of the intravascular compartment and to treat extravascular volume overload, and scrupulous attention to potential sources and sites of infection are of paramount importance. Cardiovascular instability may also result from the electrolyte imbalance that may accompany reperfusion of the donor liver as well as from restoration of systemic vascular resistance following implantation. Pulmonary function may be compromised further by paralysis of the right hemidiaphragm associated with phrenic nerve injury. The hyperdynamic state with increased cardiac output that is characteristic of patients with liver failure reverses rapidly after successful liver transplantation.

TABLE 48-4

NONHEPATIC COMPLICATIONS OF LIVER TRANSPLANTATION

Fluid overload	
Cardiovascular instability	Arrhythmias Congestive heart failure Cardiomyopathy
Pulmonary compromise	Pneumonia Pulmonary capillary vascular permeability Fluid overload
Renal dysfunction	Prerenal azotemia Hypoperfusion injury (acute tubular necrosis) Drug nephrotoxicity ↓ Renal blood flow secondary to ↑ intraabdominal pressure
Hematologic	Anemia secondary to gastrointestinal and/or intraabdominal bleeding Hemolytic anemia, aplastic anemia Thrombocytopenia
Infection	Bacterial: early, common postoperative infections Fungal/parasitic: late, opportunistic infections Viral: late, opportunistic infections, recurrent hepatitis
Neuropsychiatric	Seizures Metabolic encephalopathy Depression Difficult psychosocial adjustment
Diseases of donor	Infectious Malignant
Malignancy	B cell lymphoma (posttransplantation lymphoproliferative disorders) De novo neoplasms (particularly squamous cell skin carcinoma)

TABLE 48-5

HEPATIC COMPLICATIONS OF LIVER TRANSPLANTATION

Hepatic Dysfunction Common after Major Surgery	
Prehepatic	Pigment load Hemolysis Blood collections (hematomas, abdominal collections)
Intrahepatic	
Early	Hepatotoxic drugs and anesthesia Hypoperfusion (hypotension, shock, sepsis) Benign postoperative cholestasis
Late	Transfusion-associated hepatitis Exacerbation of primary hepatic disease
Posthepatic	Biliary obstruction ↓ Renal clearance of conjugated bilirubin (renal dysfunction)
Hepatic Dysfunction Unique to Liver Transplantation	
Primary graft nonfunction	
Vascular compromise	Portal vein obstruction Hepatic artery thrombosis Anastomotic leak with intraabdominal bleeding
Bile duct disorder	Stenosis, obstruction, leak
Rejection	
Recurrent primary hepatic disease	

Other immediate management issues include renal dysfunction. Prerenal azotemia, acute kidney injury associated with hypoperfusion (acute tubular necrosis), and renal toxicity caused by antibiotics, tacrolimus, or cyclosporine are encountered frequently in the postoperative period, sometimes necessitating dialysis. Hemolytic-uremic syndrome can be associated with cyclosporine, tacrolimus, or OKT3. Occasionally, postoperative intraperitoneal bleeding may be sufficient to increase intraabdominal pressure, which, in turn, may reduce renal blood flow; this effect is rapidly reversible when abdominal distention is relieved by exploratory laparotomy to identify and ligate the bleeding site and to remove intraperitoneal clot.

Anemia may also result from acute upper gastrointestinal bleeding or from transient hemolytic anemia, which may be autoimmune, especially when blood group O livers are transplanted into blood group A or B recipients. This autoimmune hemolytic anemia is mediated by donor intrahepatic lymphocytes that recognize red blood cell A or B antigens on recipient erythrocytes. Transient in nature, this process resolves once the donor liver is repopulated by recipient bone marrow–derived lymphocytes; the hemolysis can be treated by transfusing blood group O red blood cells and/or by administering higher doses of glucocorticoids. Transient thrombocytopenia is also commonly encountered. Aplastic anemia, a late occurrence, is rare but has been reported in almost 30% of patients who underwent liver transplantation for acute, severe hepatitis of unknown cause.

Bacterial, fungal, or viral infections are common and may be life-threatening postoperatively. Early after transplant surgery, common postoperative infections predominate—pneumonia, wound infections, infected intraabdominal collections, urinary tract infections, and IV line infections—rather than opportunistic infections; these infections may involve the biliary tree and liver as well. Beyond the first postoperative month, the toll of immunosuppression becomes evident, and opportunistic infections—CMV, herpes viruses, fungal infections (*Aspergillus*, *Candida*, cryptococcal disease), mycobacterial infections, parasitic infections (*Pneumocystis*, *Toxoplasma*), bacterial infections (*Nocardia*, *Legionella*, *Listeria*)—predominate. Rarely, early infections represent those transmitted with the donor liver, either infections present in the donor or infections acquired during procurement processing. De novo viral hepatitis infections acquired from the donor organ or, almost unheard of now, from transfused blood products occur after typical incubation periods for these agents (well beyond the first month). Obviously, infections in an immunosuppressed host demand early recognition and prompt management; prophylactic antibiotic therapy is administered routinely in the immediate postoperative period. Use of sulfamethoxazole with trimethoprim reduces the incidence of postoperative *Pneumocystis carinii* pneumonia. Antiviral prophylaxis for CMV with ganciclovir should be administered in patients at high risk (e.g., when a CMV-seropositive donor organ is implanted into a CMV-seronegative recipient).

Neuropsychiatric complications include seizures (commonly associated with cyclosporine and tacrolimus toxicity), metabolic encephalopathy, depression, and difficult psychosocial adjustment. Rarely, diseases are transmitted by the allograft from the donor to the recipient. In addition to viral and bacterial infections, malignancies of donor origin have occurred. Posttransplantation lymphoproliferative disorders, especially B cell lymphoma, are a recognized complication associated with immunosuppressive drugs such as azathioprine, tacrolimus, and cyclosporine (see above). Epstein-Barr virus has been shown to play a contributory role in some of these tumors, which may regress when immunosuppressive therapy is reduced. De novo neoplasms appear at increased frequency after liver transplantation, particularly squamous cell carcinomas of the skin. Routine screening should be performed.

Long-term complications after liver transplantation attributable primarily to immunosuppressive medications include diabetes mellitus and osteoporosis (associated with glucocorticoids and calcineurin inhibitors) as well as hypertension, hyperlipidemia, and chronic renal insufficiency (associated with cyclosporine and tacrolimus). Monitoring and treating these disorders are routine components of posttransplantation care; in some cases, they respond to changes in immunosuppressive regimen, while in others, specific treatment of the disorder is introduced. Data from a large U.S. database showed that the prevalence of renal failure was 18% at year 5 and 25% at year 10 after liver transplantation. Similarly, the high frequency of diabetes, hypertension, hyperlipidemia, obesity, and the metabolic syndrome renders patients susceptible to cardiovascular disease after liver transplantation; although hepatic complications account for most of the mortality after liver transplantation, renal failure and cardiovascular disease are the other leading causes of late mortality after liver transplantation.

HEPATIC COMPLICATIONS

Hepatic dysfunction after liver transplantation is similar to the hepatic complications encountered after major abdominal and cardiothoracic surgery; however, in addition, hepatic complications include primary graft failure, vascular compromise, failure or stricture of the biliary anastomoses, and rejection. As in nontransplantation surgery, postoperative jaundice may result from prehepatic, intrahepatic, and posthepatic sources. *Prehepatic* sources represent the massive hemoglobin pigment load from transfusions, hemolysis, hematomas, ecchymoses, and other collections of blood. *Early intrahepatic* liver injury includes effects of hepatotoxic drugs and anesthesia; hypoperfusion injury associated with hypotension, sepsis, and shock; and benign postoperative cholestasis. *Late intrahepatic* sources of liver injury include exacerbation of primary disease. *Posthepatic* sources of hepatic dysfunction include biliary obstruction and reduced renal clearance of conjugated bilirubin. Hepatic complications unique to liver transplantation include primary graft failure associated with ischemic injury to the organ during harvesting; vascular compromise associated with thrombosis or stenosis of the portal vein or hepatic artery anastomoses; vascular anastomotic leak; stenosis, obstruction, or leakage of the anastomosed common bile duct; recurrence of primary hepatic disorder (see below); and rejection.

TRANSPLANT REJECTION

Despite the use of immunosuppressive drugs, rejection of the transplanted liver still occurs in a proportion of patients, beginning 1–2 weeks after surgery. Clinical signs suggesting rejection are fever, right upper quadrant pain, and reduced bile pigment and volume. Leukocytosis may occur, but the most reliable indicators are increases in serum bilirubin and aminotransferase levels. Because these tests lack specificity, distinguishing among rejection, biliary obstruction, primary graft nonfunction, vascular compromise, viral hepatitis, CMV infection, drug hepatotoxicity, and recurrent primary disease may be difficult. Radiographic visualization of the biliary tree and/or percutaneous liver biopsy often help to establish the correct diagnosis. Morphologic features of acute rejection include a mixed portal cellular infiltrate, bile duct injury, and/or endothelial inflammation ("endothelialitis"); some of these findings are reminiscent of graft-versus-host disease, primary biliary cirrhosis, or recurrent allograft hepatitis C. As soon as transplant rejection is suspected, treatment consists of IV methylprednisolone in repeated boluses; if this fails to abort rejection, many centers use thymoglobulin or OKT3. Caution should be exercised when managing acute rejection with pulse glucocorticoids or OKT3 in patients with HCV infection, because of the high risk of triggering recurrent allograft hepatitis C.

Chronic rejection is a relatively rare outcome that can follow repeated bouts of acute rejection or that occurs unrelated to preceding rejection episodes. Morphologically, chronic rejection is characterized by progressive cholestasis, focal parenchymal necrosis, mononuclear infiltration, vascular lesions (intimal fibrosis, subintimal foam cells, fibrinoid necrosis), and fibrosis. This process may be reflected as ductopenia—the vanishing bile duct syndrome, which is more common in patients undergoing liver transplantation for autoimmune liver disease. Reversibility of chronic rejection is limited; in patients with therapy-resistant chronic rejection, retransplantation has yielded encouraging results.

OUTCOME

SURVIVAL

The survival rate for patients undergoing liver transplantation has improved steadily since 1983. One-year survival rates have increased from ~70% in the early 1980s to 85–90% from 2003 to the present time. Currently, the 5-year survival rate exceeds 60%. An important observation is the relationship between clinical status before transplantation and outcome. For patients who undergo liver transplantation when their level of compensation is high (e.g., still working or only partially disabled), a 1-year survival rate of >85% is common. For those whose level of decompensation mandates continuous in-hospital care prior to transplantation, the 1-year survival rate is ~70%, whereas for those who are so decompensated that they require life support in an intensive care unit, the 1-year survival rate is ~50%. Since the adoption by UNOS in 2002 of the MELD system for organ allocation, posttransplantation survival has been found to be affected adversely for candidates with MELD scores >25, considered high disease severity. Thus, irrespective of allocation scheme, high disease severity before transplantation corresponds to diminished posttransplantation survival. Another important distinction in survival has been drawn between high- and low-risk patient categories. For patients who do not fit any "high-risk" designations, 1-year and 5-year survival rates of 85 and 80%, respectively, have been recorded. In contrast, among patients in high-risk categories—cancer, fulminant hepatitis, age >65, concurrent renal failure, respirator dependence, portal vein thrombosis, and history of a portacaval shunt or multiple right upper quadrant operations—survival statistics fall into the range of 60% at 1 year and 35% at 5 years. Survival after retransplantation for primary graft nonfunction is ~50%. Causes of failure of liver transplantation vary with time. Failures within the first 3 months result primarily from technical complications, postoperative infections, and hemorrhage. Transplant failures after the first 3 months are more likely to result from infection, rejection, or recurrent disease (such as malignancy or viral hepatitis).

RECURRENCE OF PRIMARY DISEASE

Features of autoimmune hepatitis, primary sclerosing cholangitis, and primary biliary cirrhosis overlap with those of rejection or posttransplantation bile duct injury. Whether autoimmune hepatitis and sclerosing cholangitis recur after liver transplantation is controversial; data supporting recurrent autoimmune hepatitis (in up to one-third of patients in some series) are more convincing than those supporting recurrent sclerosing cholangitis. Similarly, reports of recurrent primary biliary cirrhosis after liver transplantation have appeared; however, the histologic features of primary biliary cirrhosis and chronic rejection are virtually indistinguishable and occur as frequently in patients with primary biliary cirrhosis as in patients undergoing transplantation for other reasons. The presence of a florid inflammatory bile duct lesion is highly suggestive of the recurrence of primary biliary cirrhosis, but even this lesion can be observed in acute rejection. Hereditary disorders such as Wilson's disease and α_1-antitrypsin deficiency have not recurred after liver transplantation; however, recurrence of disordered iron metabolism has been observed in some patients with hemochromatosis. Hepatic vein thrombosis (Budd-Chiari syndrome) may recur; this can be minimized by treating underlying myeloproliferative disorders and by anticoagulation. Because cholangiocarcinoma recurs almost invariably, few centers now offer transplantation to such patients; however, a few highly selected patients with operatively confirmed stage I or II cholangiocarcinoma who undergo liver transplantation combined with neoadjuvant chemoradiation may experience excellent outcomes. In patients with intrahepatic HCC who meet criteria for transplantation, 1- and 5-year survivals are similar to those observed in patients undergoing liver transplantation for nonmalignant disease. Finally, metabolic disorders such as nonalcoholic steatohepatitis recur frequently, especially if the underlying metabolic predisposition is not altered. The metabolic syndrome occurs commonly after liver transplantation as a result of recurrent nonalcoholic fatty liver, immunosuppressive medications, and/or, in patients with hepatitis C related to the impact of HCV infection on insulin resistance, diabetes and fatty liver.

Hepatitis A can recur after transplantation for fulminant hepatitis A, but such acute reinfection has no serious clinical sequelae. In fulminant hepatitis B, recurrence is not the rule; however, in the absence of any prophylactic measures, hepatitis B usually recurs after transplantation for end-stage chronic hepatitis B. Before the introduction of prophylactic antiviral therapy, immunosuppressive therapy sufficient to prevent allograft rejection led inevitably to marked increases in hepatitis B viremia, regardless of pretransplantation levels. Overall graft and patient survival were poor, and some patients experienced a rapid recapitulation of severe injury—severe chronic hepatitis or even fulminant hepatitis—after transplantation. Also recognized in the era before availability of antiviral regimens was *fibrosing cholestatic hepatitis*, rapidly progressive liver injury associated with marked hyperbilirubinemia, substantial prolongation of the prothrombin time (both out of proportion to relatively modest elevations of aminotransferase activity), and rapidly progressive liver failure. This lesion has been suggested to represent a "choking off" of the hepatocyte by an overwhelming density of HBV proteins. Complications such as sepsis and pancreatitis were also observed more frequently in patients undergoing liver transplantation for hepatitis B prior to the introduction of antiviral therapy. The introduction of long-term prophylaxis with HBIg revolutionized liver transplantation for chronic hepatitis B. Preoperative hepatitis B vaccination, preoperative or postoperative interferon (IFN) therapy, or short-term (≤2 months) HBIg prophylaxis has not been shown to be effective, but a retrospective analysis of data from several hundred European patients followed for 3 years after transplantation has shown that long-term (≥6 months) prophylaxis with HBIg is associated with a lowering of the risk of HBV reinfection from ~75 to 35% and a reduction in mortality from ~50 to 20%.

As a result of long-term HBIg use following liver transplantation for chronic hepatitis B, similar improvements in outcome have been observed in the United States, with 1-year survival rates between 75% and 90%. Currently, with HBIg prophylaxis, the outcome of liver transplantation for chronic hepatitis B is indistinguishable from that for chronic liver disease unassociated with chronic hepatitis B; essentially, medical concerns regarding liver transplantation for chronic hepatitis B have been eliminated. Passive immunoprophylaxis with HBIg is begun during the anhepatic stage of surgery, repeated daily for the first 6 postoperative days, and then continued with infusions that are given either at regular intervals of 4–6 weeks or, alternatively, when anti-hepatitis B surface (HBs) levels fall below a threshold of 100 mIU/mL. The current approach in most centers is to continue HBIg indefinitely, which can add approximately $20,000 per year to the cost of care; some centers are evaluating regimens that shift to less frequent administration or to IM administration in the late posttransplantation period or, in low-risk patients, maintenance with antiviral therapy (see below) alone. Still, "breakthrough" HBV infection occasionally occurs.

Further improving the outcome of liver transplantation for chronic hepatitis B is the current availability of such antiviral drugs as lamivudine, adefovir, entecavir, and tenofovir disoproxil fumarate **(Chap. 41)**. When these drugs are administered to patients with decompensated liver disease, a proportion improve sufficiently to postpone imminent liver transplantation. In addition, antiviral therapy can be used to prevent recurrence of HBV infection when administered *prior to* transplantation; to treat hepatitis B that recurs *after* transplantation, including in patients who break through HBIg prophylaxis; and to reverse the course of otherwise fatal fibrosing cholestatic hepatitis. Clinical trials have shown that lamivudine antiviral therapy reduces the level of HBV replication substantially, sometimes even resulting in clearance of hepatitis B surface antigen (HBsAg); reduces alanine aminotransferase (ALT) levels; and improves histologic features of necrosis and inflammation. Long-term use of lamivudine is safe and effective, but after several months, a proportion of patients become resistant to lamivudine, resulting from YMDD (tyrosine-methionine-aspartate-aspartate) mutations in the HBV polymerase motif **(Chap. 41)**. In approximately one-half of such resistant patients, hepatic deterioration may ensue. Fortunately, adefovir and tenofovir disoproxil fumarate are available as well and can be used to treat lamivudine-associated YMDD variants, effectively "rescuing" patients experiencing hepatic decompensation after lamivudine breakthrough. Currently, most liver transplantation centers combine HBIg plus lamivudine, adefovir, entecavir, or tenofovir disoproxil fumarate. In low-risk patients with no detectable hepatitis B viremia at the time of transplantation, a number of clinical trials have suggested that antiviral prophylaxis can suffice, without HBIg or with a finite duration of HBIg, to prevent recurrent HBV infection of the allograft. Antiviral prophylactic approaches applied to patients undergoing liver transplantation for chronic hepatitis B are being used as well for patients without hepatitis B who receive organs from donors with antibody to hepatitis B core antigen (anti-HBc). Patients who undergo liver transplantation for chronic hepatitis B plus D are less likely to experience recurrent liver injury than patients undergoing liver transplantation for hepatitis B alone; still, such co-infected patients would also be offered standard post-transplantation prophylactic therapy for hepatitis B.

Accounting for up to 40% of all liver transplantation procedures, the most common indication for liver transplantation is end-stage liver disease resulting from chronic hepatitis C. Recurrence of HCV infection after liver transplantation can be documented in almost every patient. The clinical consequences of recurrent hepatitis C are limited during the first 5 years after transplantation. Nonetheless, despite the relative clinical benignity of recurrent hepatitis C in the early years after liver transplantation, and despite the negligible impact on patient survival during these early years, histologic studies have documented the presence of moderate to severe chronic hepatitis in more than one-half of all patients and cirrhosis in ~20% at 5 years. Allograft cirrhosis is even more common, occurring in up to two-thirds of patients at 5 years, if moderate hepatitis is detected in a 1-year liver biopsy. Not surprisingly, then, for patients undergoing liver transplantation for hepatitis C, allograft and patient survival are diminished substantially between 5 and 10 years after transplantation.

In a proportion of patients, even during the early posttransplantation period, recurrent hepatitis C may be sufficiently severe biochemically and histologically to merit antiviral therapy. Treatment with pegylated IFN can *suppress* HCV-associated liver injury but rarely leads to *sustained* benefit. Sustained virologic responses are the exception, and reduced tolerability is often dose-limiting. Preemptive combination antiviral therapy with pegylated IFN and the nucleoside analogue ribavirin immediately after transplantation does not appear to provide any advantage over therapy introduced after clinical hepatitis has occurred. Similarly, although IFN-based antiviral therapy is not recommended for patients with decompensated liver disease, some centers have experimented with pretransplantation antiviral therapy in an attempt to eradicate HCV replication prior to transplantation; preliminary results are promising, but IFN treatment of patients with end-stage liver disease can lead to worsening of hepatic decompensation, and HCV infection has recurred after transplantation in some of these recipients. Trials of hepatitis C immune globulin preparations to prevent recurrent hepatitis C after liver transplantation have not been successful. Similarly, a trial of a high-dose monoclonal antibody to the HCV E2 envelope glycoprotein delayed but did not prevent reappearance of viremia.

Although the current standard-of-care treatment of allograft hepatitis C is pegylated IFN and ribavirin, in a number of studies, the safety and efficacy of the addition of the approved HCV protease inhibitors telaprevir or boceprevir to pegylated IFN and ribavirin in genotype 1–infected patients with recurrent hepatitis C have been examined. Because of the profound inhibitory effects of the HCV protease inhibitors on the metabolism of the calcineurin inhibitors (increasing cyclosporine levels almost 5-fold and tacrolimus levels 70-fold), calcineurin inhibitor doses must be reduced to safe levels in these patients. In one multicenter study, treatment with a telaprevir- or boceprevir-based triple-drug regimen (with pegylated IFN and ribavirin) achieved rates of HCV clearance similar to those achieved in patients with chronic hepatitis C who had not undergone transplantation. Unfortunately, tolerability of these protease inhibitor–based regimens remains problematic in this population, particularly in persons with allograft cirrhosis, in whom the frequency of hepatic decompensation is increased. The approval of several new direct-acting antiviral (DAA) agents and of IFN-free DAA regimens against HCV will have a major impact on the management and outcome of both pretransplantation and posttransplantation HCV infection. Such therapeutic approaches (1) permit the clearance of viremia in a substantial proportion of decompensated cirrhotics, thereby preventing recurrent allograft infection and, possibly, even improving the clinical status of these patients, delaying or obviating the need for liver replacement; and (2) achieve sustained virologic responses in a much higher proportion of persons with allograft HCV infection, because of improvements in antiviral treatment efficacy and tolerability.

A small number of allograft recipients succumb to early HCV-associated liver injury, and a syndrome reminiscent of fibrosing cholestatic hepatitis (see above) has been observed rarely. Because patients with more episodes of rejection receive more immunosuppressive therapy, and because immunosuppressive therapy enhances HCV replication, patients with severe or multiple episodes of rejection are more likely to experience early recurrence of hepatitis C after transplantation. Both high viral levels and older donor age have been linked to recurrent HCV-induced liver disease and to earlier disease recurrence after transplantation.

Patients who undergo liver transplantation for end-stage alcoholic cirrhosis are at risk of resorting to drinking again after transplantation, a potential source of recurrent alcoholic liver injury. Currently, alcoholic liver disease is one of the more common indications for liver transplantation, accounting for 20–25% of all liver transplantation procedures, and most transplantation centers screen candidates carefully for predictors of continued abstinence. Recidivism is more likely in patients whose sobriety prior to transplantation was <6 months. For abstinent patients with alcoholic cirrhosis, liver transplantation can be undertaken successfully, with outcomes comparable to those for other categories of patients with chronic liver disease, when coordinated by a team approach that includes substance abuse counseling.

POSTTRANSPLANTATION QUALITY OF LIFE

Full rehabilitation is achieved in the majority of patients who survive the early postoperative months and escape chronic rejection or unmanageable infection. Psychosocial maladjustment interferes with medical compliance in a small number of patients, but most manage to adhere to immunosuppressive regimens, which must be continued indefinitely. In one study, 85% of patients who survived their transplant operations returned to gainful activities. In fact, some women have conceived and carried pregnancies to term after transplantation without demonstrable injury to their infants.

SECTION VIII

DISORDERS OF THE PANCREAS

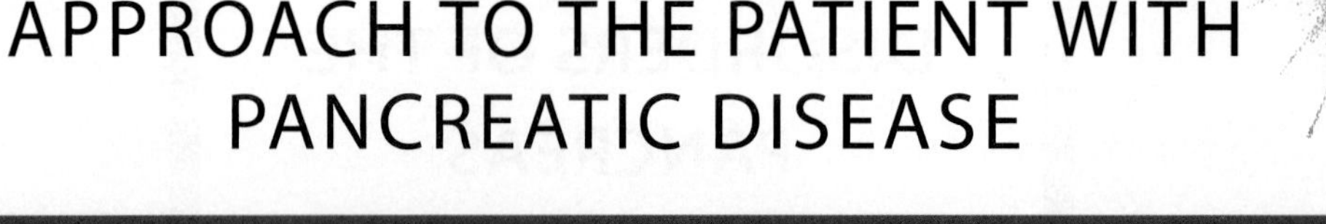

CHAPTER 49

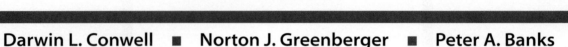

APPROACH TO THE PATIENT WITH PANCREATIC DISEASE

Darwin L. Conwell ■ Norton J. Greenberger ■ Peter A. Banks

GENERAL CONSIDERATIONS

As emphasized in **Chap. 50**, the etiologies as well as clinical manifestations of pancreatitis are quite varied. Although it is well-appreciated that pancreatitis is frequently secondary to biliary tract disease and alcohol abuse, it can also be caused by drugs, genetic mutations, trauma, and viral infections and is associated with metabolic and connective tissue disorders. In ~30% of patients with acute pancreatitis and 25–40% of patients with chronic pancreatitis, the etiology initially can be obscure.

The incidence of acute pancreatitis is about 5–35/100,000 new cases per year worldwide, with a mortality rate of about 3%. The incidence of chronic pancreatitis is about 4–8 new cases per 100,000 per year with a prevalence of 26–42 cases per 100,000. The number of patients admitted to the hospital who suffer with both acute and chronic pancreatitis in the United States is largely increasing and is now estimated to be 274,119 for acute pancreatitis and 19,724 for chronic pancreatitis. Acute pancreatitis is now the most common gastrointestinal diagnosis requiring hospitalization in the United States. Acute and chronic pancreatic disease costs an estimated 3 billion dollars annually in health care expenditures. These numbers may underestimate the true incidence and prevalence, because non–alcohol-induced pancreatitis has been largely ignored. At autopsy, the prevalence of chronic pancreatitis ranges from 0.04 to 5%.

The diagnosis of acute pancreatitis is generally clearly defined based on a combination of laboratory, imaging, and clinical symptoms. The diagnosis of chronic pancreatitis, especially in mild disease, is hampered by the relative inaccessibility of the pancreas to direct examination and the nonspecificity of the abdominal pain associated with chronic pancreatitis. Many patients with chronic pancreatitis do not have elevated blood amylase or lipase levels. Some patients with chronic pancreatitis develop signs and symptoms of pancreatic exocrine insufficiency, and thus, objective evidence for pancreatic disease can be demonstrated. However, there is a very large reservoir of pancreatic exocrine function. More than 90% of the pancreas must be damaged before maldigestion of fat and protein is manifested. Noninvasive, indirect tests of pancreatic exocrine function (fecal elastase) are much more likely to give abnormal results in patients with obvious advanced pancreatic disease (i.e., pancreatic calcification, steatorrhea, or diabetes mellitus) than in patients with occult disease. Invasive, direct tests of pancreatic secretory function (secretin tests) are the most sensitive and specific tests to detect early chronic pancreatic disease when imaging is equivocal or normal.

TESTS USEFUL IN THE DIAGNOSIS OF PANCREATIC DISEASE

Several tests have proved of value in the evaluation of pancreatic disease. Examples of specific tests and their usefulness in the diagnosis of acute and chronic pancreatitis are summarized in Table 49-1 and Fig. 49-1. At some institutions, pancreatic function tests are available and performed if the diagnosis of chronic pancreatic disease remains a possibility after noninvasive tests (ultrasound, computed tomography [CT], magnetic resonance cholangiopancreatography [MRCP]) or invasive tests (endoscopic retrograde cholangiopancreatography [ERCP], endoscopic ultrasonography [EUS]) have given normal or inconclusive results. In this regard, tests using *direct* stimulation of the pancreas with secretin are the most sensitive.

Pancreatic enzymes in body fluids

The serum amylase and lipase levels are widely used as screening tests for acute pancreatitis in the patient with

TABLE 49-1

TESTS USEFUL IN THE DIAGNOSIS OF ACUTE AND CHRONIC PANCREATITIS AND PANCREATIC TUMORS

TEST	PRINCIPLE	COMMENT
Pancreatic Enzymes in Body Fluids		
Serum lipase	Pancreatic inflammation leads to increased serum enzyme levels	Enzyme measurement of choice for diagnosis of acute pancreatitis
Amylase		
1. Serum	Pancreatic inflammation leads to increased serum enzyme levels	Simple; reliable if test results are three times the upper limit of normal
2. Urine	Renal clearance of amylase is increased in acute pancreatitis	Infrequently used
3. Ascitic fluid	Disruption of gland or main pancreatic duct leads to increased amylase concentration	Can help establish source of ascites; false positives occur with intestinal obstruction and perforated ulcer; can also measure lipase
4. Pleural fluid	Exudative pleural effusion with pancreatitis	False positives occur with carcinoma of the lung and esophageal perforation
Studies Pertaining to Pancreatic Structure		
Radiologic and radionuclide tests		
1. Plain film of the abdomen	Can be abnormal in acute and chronic pancreatitis	Infrequently used
2. Upper gastrointestinal x-rays		Infrequently used
3. Ultrasonography (US)	Can provide information on edema, inflammation, calcification, pseudocysts, and mass lesions	Simple, noninvasive; sequential studies quite feasible; useful in diagnosis of gallstones; pancreas visualization limited by interference from overlying bowel gas
4. Computed tomography (CT) scan	Permits detailed visualization of pancreas and surrounding structures, pancreatic fluid collection, pseudocyst; assessment of necrosis or interstitial disease	Useful in the diagnosis of pancreatic calcification, dilated pancreatic ducts, and pancreatic tumors; may not be able to distinguish between inflammatory and neoplastic mass lesions
5. Magnetic resonance cholangiopancreatography (MRCP)	Three-dimensional imaging has been used to produce very good images of the pancreatic-biliary ductal system by a noninvasive technique	Has replaced ERCP as a diagnostic test; noninvasive
6. Endoscopic ultrasonography (EUS)	High-frequency transducer used with EUS can produce very high-resolution images and depict changes in the pancreatic duct and parenchyma with great detail	Can be used to assess gallstones, chronic pancreatitis, and pancreatic carcinoma
7. Endoscopic retrograde cholangiopancreatography (ERCP)	Cannulation of pancreatic and common bile duct permits visualization of pancreatic-biliary ductal system	Primarily a therapeutic procedure; invasive
Pancreatic biopsy with US or CT guidance	Percutaneous aspiration biopsy of mass-forming lesions of the pancreas	High diagnostic yield; laparotomy avoided; can be done with EUS for the evaluation of chronic pancreatitis, autoimmune pancreatitis, and pancreatic carcinoma
Tests of Exocrine Pancreatic Function		
Direct stimulation of the pancreas with analysis of duodenal contents		
1. Secretin test	Secretin leads to increased output of pancreatic juice and HCO_3^-; pancreatic secretory response is related to the functional mass of pancreatic tissue	Sensitive enough to detect occult disease; involves duodenal intubation and fluoroscopic placement of gastroduodenal tube; poorly defined normal enzyme response; overlap in chronic pancreatitis; large secretory reserve capacity of the pancreas; currently done at only a few medical centers
2. Endoscopic secretin test	Replaces need for tube placement duodenum	Sensitive enough to detect occult disease; high negative predictive value; avoids intubation and fluoroscopy; requires sedation

(*continued*)

TABLE 49-1

TESTS USEFUL IN THE DIAGNOSIS OF ACUTE AND CHRONIC PANCREATITIS AND PANCREATIC TUMORS (*CONTINUED*)

TEST	PRINCIPLE	COMMENT
Measurement of intraluminal digestion products		
1. Quantitative stool fat determination	Lack of lipolytic enzymes brings about impaired fat digestion	Reliable reference standard for defining severity of malabsorption; does not distinguish between maldigestion and malabsorption
Measurement of pancreatic enzymes in feces		
1. Elastase	Pancreatic secretion of proteolytic enzymes; not degraded in intestine	Diagnostic accuracy best if value is <100 mg/g performed on a solid stool

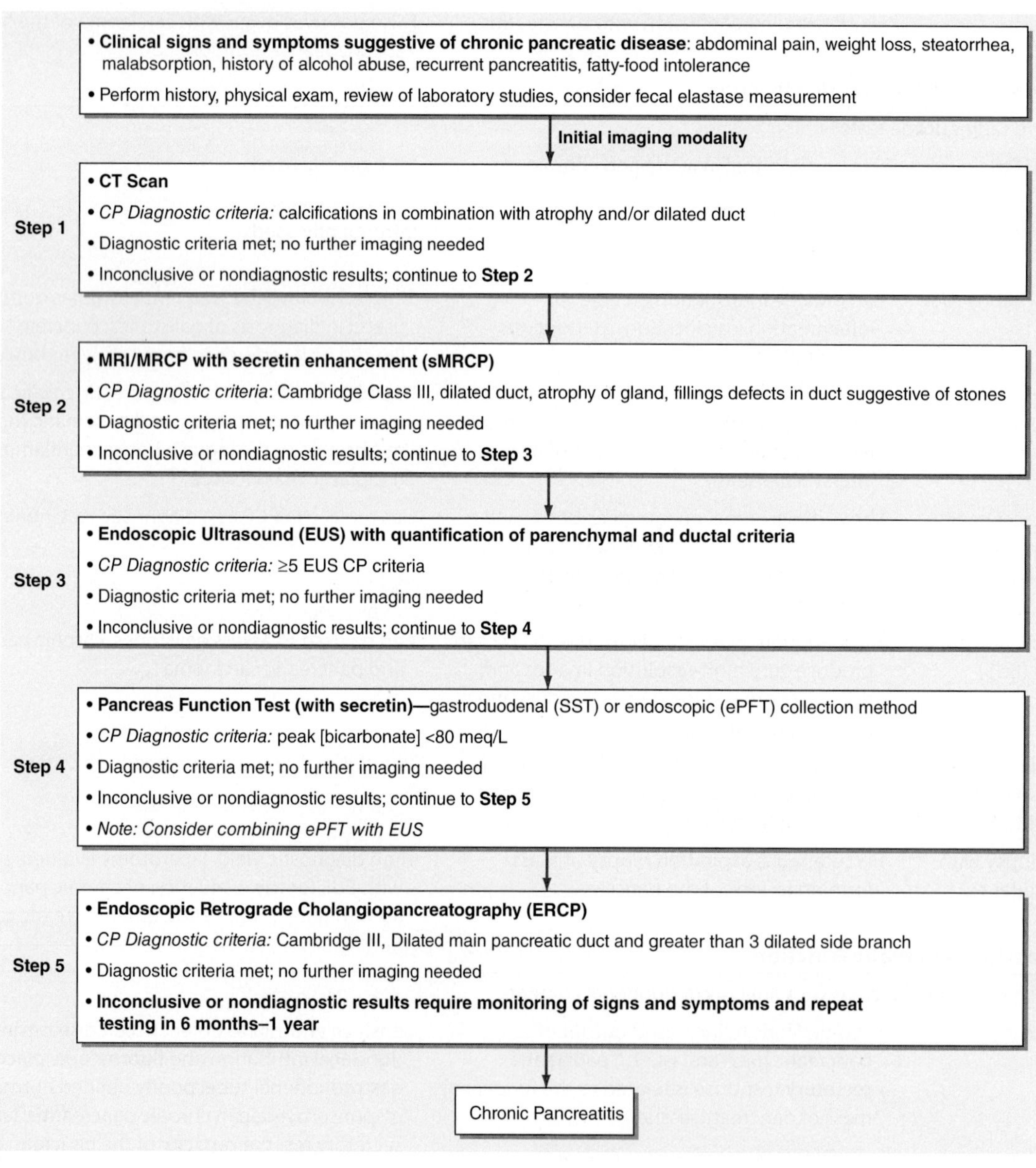

FIGURE 49-1

A stepwise diagnostic approach to the patient with suspected chronic pancreatitis (CP). Endoscopic ultrasonography (EUS) and magnetic resonance cholangiopancreatography (sMRCP/MRCP) are appropriate diagnostic alternatives to endoscopic retrograde cholangiopancreatography (ERCP). CT, computed tomography.

acute abdominal pain or back pain. Values greater than three times the upper limit of normal in combination with epigastric pain strongly suggest the diagnosis if gut perforation or infarction is excluded. In acute pancreatitis, the serum amylase and lipase are usually elevated within 24 h of onset and remain so for 3–7 days. Levels usually return to normal within 7 days unless there is pancreatic ductal disruption, ductal obstruction, or pseudocyst formation. Approximately 85% of patients with acute pancreatitis have a threefold or greater elevated serum lipase and amylase levels. The values may be normal if (1) there is a delay (of 2–5 days) before blood samples are obtained, (2) the underlying disorder is chronic pancreatitis rather than acute pancreatitis, or (3) hypertriglyceridemia is present. Patients with hypertriglyceridemia and proven pancreatitis have been found to have spuriously low levels of amylase and perhaps lipase activity. In the absence of objective evidence of pancreatitis by abdominal ultrasound, CT scan, MRCP, or EUS, mild to moderate elevations of amylase and/or lipase are not helpful in making a diagnosis of chronic pancreatitis.

The serum amylase can be elevated in other conditions (Table 49-2), in part because the enzyme is found in many organs. In addition to the pancreas and salivary glands, small quantities of amylase are found in the tissues of the fallopian tubes, lung, thyroid, and tonsils and can be produced by various tumors (carcinomas of the lung, esophagus, breast, and ovary). Isoamylase determinations do not accurately distinguish elevated blood amylase levels due to bona fide pancreatitis from elevated blood amylase levels due to a nonpancreatic source of amylase, especially when the blood amylase level is only moderately elevated. In patients with unexplained hyperamylasemia, measurement of macroamylase can avoid numerous tests in patients with this rare disorder.

Elevation of ascitic fluid amylase occurs in acute pancreatitis as well as in (1) ascites due to disruption of the main pancreatic duct or a leaking pseudocyst and (2) other abdominal disorders that simulate pancreatitis (e.g., intestinal obstruction, intestinal infarction, or perforated peptic ulcer). Elevation of pleural fluid amylase can occur in acute pancreatitis, chronic pancreatitis, carcinoma of the lung, and esophageal perforation. Lipase is the single best enzyme to measure for the diagnosis of acute pancreatitis. No single blood test is reliable for the diagnosis of acute pancreatitis in patients with renal failure. Pancreatic enzyme elevations are usually less than three times the upper limit of normal. Determining whether a patient with renal failure and abdominal pain has pancreatitis remains a difficult clinical problem. One study found that serum amylase levels were elevated in patients with renal dysfunction only when creatinine clearance was <0.8 mL/s (<50 mL/min). In such patients, the serum amylase level was invariably <500 IU/L in the absence of objective evidence of acute pancreatitis. In that study, serum lipase and trypsin levels paralleled serum amylase values. With these limitations in mind, the recommended screening test for acute pancreatitis in renal disease is serum lipase.

TABLE 49-2

CAUSES OF HYPERAMYLASEMIA AND HYPERAMYLASURIA

Pancreatic Disease

I. Pancreatitis
   A. Acute
   B. Chronic: ductal obstruction
   C. Complications of pancreatitis
      1. Pancreatic pseudocyst
      2. Ascites caused by pancreatic duct disruption
      3. Pancreatic necrosis
II. Pancreatic trauma
III. Pancreatic carcinoma

Nonpancreatic Disorders

I. Renal insufficiency
II. Salivary gland lesions
   A. Mumps
   B. Calculus
   C. Irradiation sialadenitis
   D. Maxillofacial surgery
III. "Tumor" hyperamylasemia
   A. Carcinoma of the lung, esophagus, breast, or ovary
IV. Macroamylasemia
V. Burns
VI. Diabetic ketoacidosis
VII. Pregnancy
VIII. Renal transplantation
IX. Cerebral trauma
X. Drugs: opiates

Other Abdominal Disorders

I. Biliary tract disease: cholecystitis, choledocholithiasis
II. Intraabdominal disease
   A. Perforated or penetrating peptic ulcer
   B. Intestinal obstruction or inflammation
   C. Ruptured ectopic pregnancy
   D. Peritonitis
   E. Aortic aneurysm
   F. Postoperative hyperamylasemia

Studies pertaining to pancreatic structure

Radiologic tests

Plain films of the abdomen, which once provided useful information in patients with acute and chronic pancreatitis, have been superseded by other more detailed imaging procedures (ultrasound, EUS, CT, MRCP).

Ultrasonography (US) can provide important information in patients with acute pancreatitis, chronic pancreatitis, pseudocysts, and pancreatic carcinoma. Echographic appearances can indicate the presence of edema, inflammation, and calcification (not obvious on plain films of the abdomen), as well as pseudocysts, mass lesions, and gallstones. In acute pancreatitis, the pancreas is characteristically enlarged. In pancreatic pseudocyst, the usual appearance is primarily that of smooth, round fluid collection. Pancreatic carcinoma distorts the usual landmarks, and mass lesions >3.0 cm are usually detected as localized, solid lesions. US is often the initial investigation for most patients with suspected pancreatic disease. However, obesity and excess small- and large-bowel gas can interfere with pancreatic imaging by US studies.

Computed tomography (CT) is the best imaging study for initial evaluation of a suspected pancreatic disorder and for the assessment of complications of acute and chronic pancreatitis. It is especially useful in the detection of pancreatic and peripancreatic acute fluid collections, fluid-containing lesions such as pseudocysts, walled-off necrosis, calcium deposits **(see Chap. 50, Figs. 50-1, 50-2, and 50-4)**, and pancreatic neoplasms. Acute pancreatitis is characterized by (1) enlargement of the pancreatic outline, (2) distortion of the pancreatic contour, and/or (3) a pancreatic fluid that has a different attenuation coefficient than normal pancreas. Oral, water-soluble contrast agents are used to opacify the stomach and duodenum during CT scans; this strategy permits more precise delineation of various organs as well as mass lesions. Dynamic CT (using rapid IV administration of contrast) is useful in estimating the extent of pancreatic necrosis and in predicting morbidity and mortality. CT provides clear images much more rapidly and essentially negates artifact caused by patient movement. If acute pancreatitis is confirmed with serology and physical examination findings, CT scan in the first 3 days is not recommended to avoid overuse and minimize costs.

Endoscopic ultrasonography (EUS) produces high-resolution images of the pancreatic parenchyma and pancreatic duct with a transducer fixed to an endoscope that can be directed onto the surface of the pancreas through the stomach or duodenum. EUS and MRCP have largely replaced ERCP for diagnostic purposes in many centers. EUS allows one to obtain information about the pancreatic duct as well as the parenchyma and has few procedure-related complications associated with it, in contrast to the 5–10% of post-ERCP pancreatitis observed. EUS is also helpful in detecting common bile duct stones in acute pancreatitis. Pancreatic masses can also be biopsied via EUS in cases with suspected pancreas cancer, and one can deliver nerve-blocking agents through EUS fine-needle injection in patients suffering from pancreatic pain from chronic pancreatitis or cancer. EUS has been studied as a diagnostic modality for chronic pancreatitis. Criteria for abnormalities on EUS in severe chronic pancreatic disease have been developed. There is general agreement that the presence of five or more of the nine criteria listed in Table 49-3 is highly predictive of chronic pancreatitis. Recent studies comparing EUS and ERCP to the secretin test in patients with unexplained abdominal pain suspected of having chronic pancreatitis show similar diagnostic accuracy in detecting early changes of chronic pancreatitis. The exact role of EUS versus CT, ERCP, or function testing in the early diagnosis of chronic pancreatitis has yet to be clearly defined.

TABLE 49-3

ENDOSCOPIC ULTRASONOGRAPHIC CRITERIA FOR CHRONIC PANCREATITIS (TOTAL CRITERIA = 9)

DUCTAL	PARENCHYMAL
Stones	Echogenic strands
Hyperechoic main duct margins	Echogenic foci
Main duct irregularity	Lobular contour
Main duct dilatation	Cyst
Visible side branches	

Magnetic resonance imaging (MRI) and *magnetic resonance cholangiopancreatography* (MRCP) are now being used to view the bile ducts, pancreatic duct, and the pancreas parenchyma in both acute pancreatitis and chronic pancreatitis. For diagnostic imaging in chronic pancreatitis, non-breath-holding and three-dimensional turbo spin-echo techniques are being used to produce superb MRCP images. The main pancreatic duct and common bile duct can be seen well, but there is still a question as to whether changes can be detected consistently in the secondary ducts. The secondary ducts are not visualized in a normal pancreas. Secretin-enhanced MRCP is currently under investigation but is emerging as a method to better evaluate ductal changes. In anteroposterior imaging, T2 imaging of fluid collections can differentiate necrotic debris from fluid in suspected walled-off necrosis, and T1 imaging can diagnose hemorrhage in suspected pseudoaneurysm rupture.

Both EUS and MRCP have largely replaced ERCP in the diagnostic evaluation of pancreatic disease. As these techniques become more refined, especially with the administration of secretin, they may well be the diagnostic tests of choice to evaluate the pancreatic duct. ERCP is still needed for treatment of bile duct and pancreatic duct lesions. ERCP is primarily of therapeutic value after CT, EUS, or MRCP has detected abnormalities requiring invasive endoscopic treatment. ERCP can also be helpful at clarification of equivocal findings discovered with other imaging techniques **(see Chap. 50, Fig. 50-1)**. Pancreatic carcinoma is characterized by stenosis or obstruction of either the pancreatic duct or the common bile duct; both ductal systems are often abnormal (double-duct sign). In chronic pancreatitis, ERCP abnormalities in the main pancreatic duct and side branches have been outlined by the Cambridge classification. The presence of ductal stenosis and irregularity can make it difficult to distinguish chronic pancreatitis from carcinoma. It is important to be aware that ERCP changes interpreted as indicating chronic pancreatitis actually may be due to the effects of aging on the pancreatic duct or sequelae of a recent attack of acute pancreatitis. Although aging may cause impressive ductal alterations, it does not affect the results of pancreatic function tests (i.e., the secretin test). Elevated serum amylase levels after ERCP have been reported in the majority of patients, and clinical pancreatitis in 5–10% of patients. Recent data suggest that pancreatic duct stenting and rectal indomethacin can decrease the incidence of ERCP-induced pancreatitis. ERCP should rarely be done for diagnostic purposes and should especially be avoided in high-risk patients.

Pancreatic biopsy with radiologic guidance

Percutaneous aspiration biopsy or a trucut biopsy of a pancreatic mass often distinguishes a pancreatic inflammatory mass from a pancreatic neoplasm.

TESTS OF EXOCRINE PANCREATIC FUNCTION

Pancreatic function tests (Table 49-1) can be divided into the following:

1. *Direct stimulation of the pancreas* by IV infusion of secretin followed by collection and measurement of duodenal contents

The secretin test, used to detect diffuse pancreatic disease, is based on the physiologic principle that the pancreatic secretory response is directly related to the functional mass of pancreatic tissue. In the standard assay, secretin is given IV in a dose of 0.2 mg/kg of synthetic human secretin as a bolus. Normal values for the standard secretin test are (1) volume output >2 mL/kg per hour, (2) bicarbonate (HCO_3^-) concentration >80 mmol/L, and (3) HCO_3^- output >10 mmol/L in 1 h. The most reproducible measurement, giving the highest level of discrimination between normal subjects and patients with chronic pancreatic exocrine insufficiency, appears to be the maximal bicarbonate concentration. A cutoff point below 80 mmol/L is considered abnormal and suggestive of abnormal secretory function that is most commonly observed in early chronic pancreatitis.

There may be a dissociation between the results of the secretin test and other tests of absorptive function. For example, patients with chronic pancreatitis often have abnormally low outputs of HCO_3^- after secretin but have normal fecal fat excretion. Thus the secretin test measures the secretory capacity of ductular epithelium, whereas fecal fat excretion indirectly reflects intraluminal lipolytic activity. Steatorrhea does not occur until intraluminal levels of lipase are markedly reduced, underscoring the fact that only small amounts of enzymes are necessary for intraluminal digestive activities. It must be emphasized that an abnormal secretin test result suggests only that chronic pancreatic damage is present.

2. *Measurement of fecal pancreatic enzymes* such as elastase

The amount of human elastase in stool reflects the pancreatic output of this proteolytic enzyme. Decreased elastase-1 activity (FE-1) in stool is an excellent test to detect severe pancreatic exocrine insufficiency (PEI) in patients with chronic pancreatitis and cystic fibrosis. FE-1 levels >200 mg/g are normal; levels of 100–200 mg/g are considered mild, and levels <100 mg/g are severe for PEI. Although the test is simple and noninvasive, it can give false-positive results and has a low sensitivity. Fecal levels <50 mg/g are definitive for PEI provided that the stool specimen is solid.

Tests useful in the diagnosis of exocrine pancreatic insufficiency and the differential diagnosis of malabsorption are also discussed in Chap. 50.

CHAPTER 50

ACUTE AND CHRONIC PANCREATITIS

Darwin L. Conwell ■ Peter A. Banks ■ Norton J. Greenberger

BIOCHEMISTRY AND PHYSIOLOGY OF PANCREATIC EXOCRINE SECRETION

GENERAL CONSIDERATIONS

The pancreas secretes 1500–3000 mL of isosmotic alkaline (pH >8) fluid per day containing about 20 enzymes. The pancreatic secretions provide the enzymes and bicarbonate needed to affect the major digestive activity of the gastrointestinal tract and provide an optimal pH for the function of these enzymes.

REGULATION OF PANCREATIC SECRETION

The exocrine pancreas is influenced by intimately interacting hormonal and neural systems. *Gastric acid* is the stimulus for the release of secretin from the duodenal mucosa (S cells), which stimulates the secretion of water and electrolytes from pancreatic ductal cells. Release of cholecystokinin (CCK) from the duodenal and proximal jejunal mucosa (Ito cells) is largely triggered by long-chain fatty acids, essential amino acids (tryptophan, phenylalanine, valine, methionine), and gastric acid itself. CCK evokes an enzyme-rich secretion from acinar cells in the pancreas. The *parasympathetic nervous system* (via the vagus nerve) exerts significant control over pancreatic secretion. Secretion evoked by secretin and CCK depends on permissive roles of vagal afferent and efferent pathways. This is particularly true for enzyme secretion, whereas water and bicarbonate secretions are heavily dependent on the hormonal effects of secretin and to a lesser extent CCK. Also, vagal stimulation affects the release of vasoactive intestinal peptide (VIP), a secretin agonist. Pancreatic exocrine secretion is also influenced by inhibitory neuropeptides such as somatostatin, pancreatic polypeptide, peptide YY, neuropeptide Y, enkephalin, pancreastatin, calcitonin gene–related peptides, glucagon, and galanin. Although pancreatic polypeptide and peptide YY may act primarily on nerves outside the pancreas, somatostatin acts at multiple sites. Nitric oxide (NO) is also an important neurotransmitter.

WATER AND ELECTROLYTE SECRETION

Bicarbonate is the ion of primary physiologic importance within pancreatic secretion. The ductal cells secrete bicarbonate predominantly derived from plasma (93%) more than from intracellular metabolism (7%). Bicarbonate enters the duct lumen through the sodium bicarbonate cotransporter with depolarization caused by chloride efflux through the cystic fibrosis transmembrane conductance regulator (CFTR). Secretin and VIP bind at the basolateral surface and cause an increase in secondary messenger intracellular cyclic AMP, and act on the apical surface of the ductal cells opening the CFTR in promoting secretion. CCK, acting as a neuromodulator, markedly potentiates the stimulatory effects of secretin. Acetylcholine also plays an important role in ductal cell secretion. Intraluminal bicarbonate secreted from the ductal cells helps neutralize gastric acid and creates the appropriate pH for the activity of pancreatic enzymes and bile salts on ingested food.

ENZYME SECRETION

The acinar cell is highly compartmentalized and is concerned with the secretion of pancreatic enzymes. Proteins synthesized by the rough endoplasmic reticulum are processed in the Golgi and then targeted to the appropriate site, whether that be zymogen granules, lysosomes, or other cell compartments. The zymogen granules migrate to the apical region of the acinar cell awaiting the appropriate neural or hormonal stimulatory response. The pancreas secretes amylolytic, lipolytic, and proteolytic enzymes into the duct lumen. *Amylolytic enzymes*, such as amylase, hydrolyze starch to oligosaccharides and to the disaccharide maltose. The *lipolytic enzymes* include lipase, phospholipase A_2, and cholesterol esterase. Bile salts inhibit lipase in isolation, but colipase, another constituent of pancreatic secretion, binds to lipase and prevents this inhibition. Bile salts activate phospholipase A and cholesterol esterase. *Proteolytic enzymes* include endopeptidases (trypsin, chymotrypsin), which act on internal peptide bonds of proteins and polypeptides; exopeptidases (carboxypeptidases, aminopeptidases), which act on the free carboxyl- and amino-terminal ends of peptides, respectively; and elastase. The proteolytic enzymes are secreted as inactive zymogen precursors. Ribonucleases (deoxyribonucleases, ribonuclease) are also secreted. *Enterokinase*, an enzyme found in the duodenal mucosa, cleaves the lysine-isoleucine bond of trypsinogen to form trypsin. Trypsin then activates the other proteolytic zymogens and phospholipase A_2 in a cascade phenomenon. All pancreatic enzymes have pH optima in the alkaline range. The nervous system initiates pancreatic enzyme secretion. The neurologic stimulation is cholinergic, involving extrinsic innervation by the vagus nerve and subsequent innervation by intrapancreatic cholinergic nerves. The stimulatory neurotransmitters are acetylcholine and gastrin-releasing peptides. These neurotransmitters activate calcium-dependent secondary messenger systems, resulting in the release of zymogens into the pancreas duct. VIP is present in intrapancreatic nerves and potentiates the effect of acetylcholine. In contrast to other species, there are no CCK receptors on acinar cells in humans. CCK in physiologic concentrations stimulates pancreatic secretion by stimulating afferent vagal and intrapancreatic nerves.

AUTOPROTECTION OF THE PANCREAS

Autodigestion of the pancreas is prevented by (1) the packaging of pancreatic proteases in precursor (proenzyme) form, (2) intracellular calcium homeostasis (low intracellular calcium in the cytosol of the acinar cell promotes the destruction of spontaneously activated trypsin), (3) acid-base balance, and (4) the synthesis of protective protease inhibitors (pancreatic secretory trypsin inhibitor [PSTI] or SPINK1), which can bind and inactivate about 20% of intracellular trypsin activity. Chymotrypsin C can also lyse and inactivate trypsin. These protease inhibitors are found in the acinar cell, the pancreatic secretions, and the α_1- and α_2-globulin fractions of plasma. Loss of any of these four protective mechanisms leads to premature enzyme activation, autodigestion, and acute pancreatitis.

ENTEROPANCREATIC AXIS AND FEEDBACK INHIBITION

Pancreatic enzyme secretion is controlled, at least in part, by a negative feedback mechanism induced by the presence of active serine proteases in the duodenum. To illustrate, perfusion of the duodenal lumen with phenylalanine (stimulates early digestion) causes a prompt increase in plasma CCK levels as well as increased secretion of chymotrypsin and other pancreatic enzymes. However, simultaneous perfusion with trypsin (stimulates late digestion) blunts both responses. Conversely, perfusion of the duodenal lumen with protease inhibitors actually leads to enzyme hypersecretion. The available evidence supports the concept that the duodenum contains a peptide called *CCK-releasing factor* (CCK-RF) that is involved in stimulating CCK release. It appears that serine proteases inhibit pancreatic secretion by inactivating a CCK-releasing peptide in the lumen of the small intestine. Thus, the integrative result of both bicarbonate and enzyme secretion depends on a feedback process for both bicarbonate and pancreatic enzymes. Acidification of the duodenum releases secretin, which stimulates vagal and other neural pathways to activate pancreatic duct cells, which secrete bicarbonate. This bicarbonate then neutralizes the duodenal acid, and the feedback loop is completed. Dietary proteins bind proteases, thereby leading to an increase in free CCK-RF. CCK is then released into the blood in physiologic concentrations, acting primarily through the neural pathways (vagal-vagal). This leads to acetylcholine-mediated pancreatic enzyme secretion. Proteases continue to be secreted from the pancreas until the protein within the duodenum is digested. At this point, pancreatic protease secretion is reduced to basic levels, thus completing this step in the feedback process.

ACUTE PANCREATITIS

GENERAL CONSIDERATIONS

Recent U.S. estimates from the National Inpatient Sample report that acute pancreatitis is the most common inpatient principal gastrointestinal diagnosis. The incidence of acute pancreatitis also varies in different countries and depends on cause (e.g., alcohol, gallstones, metabolic factors, drugs [Table 50-1]). The annual incidence ranges from 13–45/100,000 persons. Acute pancreatitis results in >250,000 hospitalizations per year. The median length of hospital stay is 4 days, with a median hospital cost of $6,096 and a mortality of 1%. The estimated cost annually approaches $2.6 billion. Hospitalization rates increase with age, are 88% higher among blacks, and are higher among males than females. The age-adjusted rate of hospital discharges with an acute pancreatitis diagnosis increased 62% between 1988 and 2004. From 2000 to 2009, the rate increased 30%. Thus, acute pancreatitis is increasing and is a significant burden on health care costs and resource utilization.

TABLE 50-1

CAUSES OF ACUTE PANCREATITIS
Common Causes
Gallstones (including microlithiasis)
Alcohol (acute and chronic alcoholism)
Hypertriglyceridemia
Endoscopic retrograde cholangiopancreatography (ERCP), especially after biliary manometry
Drugs (azathioprine, 6-mercaptopurine, sulfonamides, estrogens, tetracycline, valproic acid, anti-HIV medications, 5-aminosalicylic acid [5-ASA])
Trauma (especially blunt abdominal trauma)
Postoperative (abdominal and nonabdominal operations)
Uncommon Causes
Vascular causes and vasculitis (ischemic-hypoperfusion states after cardiac surgery)
Connective tissue disorders and thrombotic thrombocytopenic purpura (TTP)
Cancer of the pancreas
Hypercalcemia
Periampullary diverticulum
Pancreas divisum
Hereditary pancreatitis
Cystic fibrosis
Renal failure
Infections (mumps, coxsackievirus, cytomegalovirus, echovirus, parasites)
Autoimmune (e.g., type 1 and type 2)
Causes to Consider in Patients with Recurrent Bouts of Acute Pancreatitis Without an Obvious Etiology
Occult disease of the biliary tree or pancreatic ducts, especially microlithiasis, biliary sludge
Drugs
Alcohol abuse
Metabolic: Hypertriglyceridemia, hypercalcemia
Anatomic: Pancreas divisum
Pancreatic cancer
Intraductal papillary mucinous neoplasm (IPMN)
Hereditary pancreatitis
Cystic fibrosis
Autoimmune
Idiopathic

ETIOLOGY AND PATHOGENESIS

There are many causes of acute pancreatitis (Table 50-1), but the mechanisms by which these conditions trigger pancreatic inflammation have not been fully elucidated. Gallstones continue to be the leading cause of acute pancreatitis in most series (30–60%). The risk of acute pancreatitis in patients with at least one gallstone <5 mm in diameter is fourfold greater than that in patients with larger stones. Alcohol is the second most common cause, responsible for 15–30% of cases in the United States. The incidence of pancreatitis in alcoholics is surprisingly low (5/100,000), indicating that in addition to the amount of alcohol ingested, other factors affect a person's susceptibility to pancreatic injury such as cigarette smoking. Acute pancreatitis occurs in 5–10% of patients following endoscopic retrograde cholangiopancreatography (ERCP). Use of a prophylactic pancreatic duct stent and rectal nonsteroidal anti-inflammatory drugs (NSAIDs) has been shown to reduce pancreatitis after ERCP. Risk factors for post-ERCP pancreatitis include minor papilla sphincterotomy, sphincter of Oddi dysfunction, prior history of post-ERCP pancreatitis, age <60 years, >2 contrast injections into the pancreatic duct, and endoscopic trainee involvement.

Hypertriglyceridemia is the cause of acute pancreatitis in 1.3–3.8% of cases; serum triglyceride levels are usually >11.3 mmol/L (>1000 mg/dL). Most patients with hypertriglyceridemia, when subsequently examined, show evidence of an underlying derangement in lipid metabolism, probably unrelated to pancreatitis. Such patients are prone to recurrent episodes of pancreatitis. Any factor (e.g., drugs or alcohol) that causes an abrupt increase in serum triglycerides can precipitate a bout of acute pancreatitis. Patients with a deficiency of apolipoprotein CII have an increased incidence of pancreatitis; apolipoprotein CII activates lipoprotein lipase, which is important in clearing chylomicrons from the bloodstream. Patients with diabetes mellitus who have developed ketoacidosis and patients who are on certain medications such as oral contraceptives may also develop high triglyceride levels. Approximately 0.1–2% of cases of acute pancreatitis are drug related. Drugs cause pancreatitis either by a hypersensitivity reaction or by the generation of a toxic metabolite, although in some cases, it is not clear which of these mechanisms is operative (Table 50-1).

Pathologically, acute pancreatitis varies from *interstitial pancreatitis* (pancreas blood supply maintained), which is generally self-limited to *necrotizing pancreatitis* (pancreas blood supply interrupted), in which the extent of necrosis may correlate with the severity of the attack and its systemic complications. Autodigestion is a currently accepted pathogenic theory; according to this theory, pancreatitis results when proteolytic enzymes (e.g., trypsinogen, chymotrypsinogen, proelastase, and lipolytic enzymes such as phospholipase A_2) are activated in the pancreas acinar cell rather than in the intestinal lumen. A number of factors (e.g., endotoxins, exotoxins, viral infections, ischemia, oxidative stress, lysosomal calcium, and direct trauma) are believed to facilitate premature activation of trypsin. Activated proteolytic enzymes, especially trypsin, not only digest pancreatic and peripancreatic tissues but also can activate other enzymes, such as elastase and phospholipase A_2. Spontaneous activation of trypsin also can occur.

ACTIVATION OF PANCREATIC ENZYMES IN THE PATHOGENESIS OF ACUTE PANCREATITIS

Several recent studies have suggested that pancreatitis is a disease that evolves in three phases. The *initial phase* is characterized by intrapancreatic digestive enzyme activation and acinar cell injury. Trypsin activation appears to be mediated by lysosomal hydrolases such as cathepsin B that become colocalized with digestive enzymes in intracellular organelles; it is currently believed that acinar cell injury is the consequence of trypsin activation. The *second phase* of pancreatitis involves the activation, chemoattraction, and sequestration of leukocytes and macrophages in the pancreas, resulting in an enhanced intrapancreatic inflammatory reaction. Neutrophil depletion induced by prior administration of an antineutrophil serum has been shown to reduce the severity of experimentally induced pancreatitis. There is also evidence to support the concept that neutrophils can activate trypsinogen. Thus, intrapancreatic acinar cell activation of trypsinogen could be a two-step process (i.e., an early neutrophil-independent and a later neutrophil-dependent phase). The *third phase* of pancreatitis is due to the effects of activated proteolytic enzymes and cytokines, released by the inflamed pancreas, on distant organs. Activated proteolytic enzymes, especially trypsin, not only digest pancreatic and peripancreatic tissues but also activate other enzymes such as elastase and phospholipase A_2. The active enzymes and cytokines then digest cellular membranes and cause proteolysis, edema, interstitial hemorrhage, vascular damage, coagulation necrosis, fat necrosis, and parenchymal cell necrosis. Cellular injury and death result in the liberation of bradykinin peptides, vasoactive substances, and histamine that can produce vasodilation, increased vascular permeability, and edema with profound effects on many organs. The systemic inflammatory response syndrome (SIRS) and acute respiratory distress syndrome (ARDS), as well as multiorgan failure, may occur as a result of this cascade of local and distant effects.

A number of genetic factors can increase the susceptibility and/or modify the severity of pancreatic injury in acute pancreatitis, recurrent pancreatitis, and chronic pancreatitis. All of the major genetic susceptibility factors center on the control of trypsin activity within the pancreatic acinar cell, in part because they were identified as candidate genes linked to intrapancreatic trypsin control. Five genetic variants have been identified as being associated with susceptibility to pancreatitis. The genes that have been identified include (1) cationic trypsinogen gene (*PRSS1*), (2) pancreatic secretory trypsin inhibitor (*SPINK1*), (3) the cystic fibrosis transmembrane conductance regulator gene (*CFTR*), (4) the chymotrypsin C gene (*CTRC*), and (5) the calcium-sensing receptor (*CASR*). Investigations of other genetic variants are currently under way, and new genes will be added to this list in the future. Multiple medical, ethical, and psychological issues arise when these genes are discovered, and referral to genetic counselors is recommended.

APPROACH TO THE PATIENT: Abdominal Pain

Abdominal pain is the major symptom of acute pancreatitis. Pain may vary from a mild discomfort to severe, constant, and incapacitating distress. Characteristically, the pain, which is steady and boring in character, is located in the epigastrium and periumbilical region, and may radiate to the back, chest, flanks, and lower abdomen. Nausea, vomiting, and abdominal distention due to gastric and intestinal hypomotility and chemical peritonitis are also frequent complaints.

Physical examination frequently reveals a distressed and anxious patient. Low-grade fever, tachycardia, and hypotension are fairly common. Shock is not unusual and may result from (1) hypovolemia secondary to exudation of blood and plasma proteins into the retroperitoneal space; (2) increased formation and release of kinin peptides, which cause vasodilation and increased vascular permeability; and (3) systemic effects of proteolytic and lipolytic enzymes released into the circulation. Jaundice occurs infrequently; when present, it usually is due to edema of the head of the pancreas with compression of the intrapancreatic portion of the common bile duct or passage of a biliary stone or sludge. Erythematous skin nodules due to subcutaneous fat necrosis may rarely occur. In 10–20% of patients, there are pulmonary findings, including basilar rales, atelectasis, and pleural effusion, the latter most frequently left sided. Abdominal tenderness and muscle rigidity are present to a variable degree, but compared with the intense pain, these signs may be less impressive. Bowel sounds are usually diminished or absent. An enlarged pancreas from acute fluid collection, walled off necrosis, or a pseudocyst may be palpable in the upper abdomen later in the course of the disease (i.e., 4–6 weeks). A faint blue discoloration around the umbilicus (Cullen's sign) may occur as the result of hemoperitoneum, and a blue-red-purple or green-brown discoloration of the flanks (Turner's sign) reflects tissue catabolism of hemoglobin from severe necrotizing pancreatitis with hemorrhage.

LABORATORY DATA

Serum amylase and lipase values threefold or more above normal virtually clinch the diagnosis if gut perforation, ischemia, and infarction are excluded. Serum lipase is the preferred test. However, it should be noted that there is no correlation between the severity of pancreatitis and the degree of serum lipase and amylase elevations. After 3–7 days, even with continuing evidence of pancreatitis, total serum amylase values tend to return toward normal. However, pancreatic isoamylase and lipase levels may remain elevated for 7–14 days. It should be recognized that amylase elevations in serum and urine occur in many conditions other than pancreatitis **(see Chap. 49, Table 49-2)**. Importantly, patients with *acidemia* (arterial pH ≤7.32) may have spurious elevations in serum amylase. This finding explains why patients with diabetic ketoacidosis may have marked elevations in serum amylase without any other evidence of acute pancreatitis. Serum lipase activity increases in parallel with amylase activity and is more specific than amylase. A serum lipase measurement can be instrumental in differentiating a pancreatic or nonpancreatic cause for hyperamylasemia. *Leukocytosis* (15,000–20,000 leukocytes/μL) occurs frequently. Patients with more severe disease may show hemoconcentration with hematocrit values >44% and/or prerenal azotemia with a blood urea nitrogen (BUN) level >22 mg/dL resulting from loss of plasma into the retroperitoneal space and peritoneal cavity.

Hemoconcentration may be the harbinger of more severe disease (i.e., pancreatic necrosis), whereas azotemia is a significant risk factor for mortality. *Hyperglycemia* is common and is due to multiple factors, including decreased insulin release, increased glucagon release, and an increased output of adrenal glucocorticoids and catecholamines. *Hypocalcemia* occurs in ~25% of patients, and its pathogenesis is incompletely understood. Although earlier studies suggested that the response of the parathyroid gland to a decrease in serum calcium is impaired, subsequent observations have failed to confirm this phenomenon. Intraperitoneal saponification of calcium by fatty acids in areas of fat necrosis occurs occasionally, with large amounts (up to 6.0 g) dissolved or suspended in ascitic fluid. Such "soap formation" may also be significant in patients with pancreatitis, mild hypocalcemia, and little or no obvious ascites. *Hyperbilirubinemia* (serum bilirubin >68 mmoL or >4.0 mg/dL) occurs in ~10% of patients. However, jaundice is transient, and serum bilirubin levels return to normal in 4–7 days. Serum alkaline phosphatase and aspartate aminotransferase levels are also transiently elevated, and they parallel serum bilirubin values and may point to gallbladder-related disease or inflammation in the pancreatic head. *Hypertriglyceridemia* occurs in 5–10% of patients, and serum amylase levels in these individuals are often spuriously normal **(Chap. 49)**. Approximately 5–10% of patients have *hypoxemia* (arterial PO_2 ≤60 mmHg), which may herald the onset of ARDS. Finally, the electrocardiogram is occasionally abnormal in acute pancreatitis with ST-segment and T-wave abnormalities simulating myocardial ischemia.

An abdominal ultrasound is recommended in the emergency ward as the initial diagnostic imaging modality and is most useful to evaluate for gallstone disease and the pancreatic head.

The revised Atlanta criteria have clearly outlined the morphologic features of acute pancreatitis on computed tomography (CT) scan as follows: (1) interstitial pancreatitis, (2) necrotizing pancreatitis, (3) acute pancreatic fluid collection, (4) pancreatic pseudocyst, (5) acute necrotic collection (ANC), and (6) walled-off pancreatic necrosis (WON) **(Table 50-2 and Fig. 50-1)**. **Radiologic studies useful in the diagnosis of acute pancreatitis are discussed in Chap. 49 and listed in Table 49-1.**

DIAGNOSIS

Any severe acute pain in the abdomen or back should suggest the possibility of acute pancreatitis. The diagnosis is established by two of the following three criteria: (1) typical abdominal pain in the epigastrium that may radiate to the back, (2) threefold or greater elevation in serum lipase and/or amylase, and (3) confirmatory findings of acute pancreatitis on cross-sectional abdominal imaging. Patients also have associated nausea, emesis, fever, tachycardia, and abnormal findings on abdominal examination. Laboratory studies may reveal leukocytosis, hypocalcemia, and hyperglycemia. Although not required for diagnosis, markers of severity may include hemoconcentration (hematocrit >44%), admission azotemia (BUN >22 mg/dL), SIRS, and signs of organ failure **(Table 50-3)**.

The *differential diagnosis* should include the following disorders: (1) perforated viscus, especially peptic ulcer; (2) acute cholecystitis and biliary colic; (3) acute intestinal obstruction; (4) mesenteric vascular occlusion; (5) renal colic; (6) inferior myocardial infarction; (7) dissecting aortic aneurysm; (8) connective tissue disorders with vasculitis; (9) pneumonia; and (10) diabetic ketoacidosis. It may be difficult to differentiate acute cholecystitis from acute pancreatitis, because an elevated serum amylase may be found in both disorders. Pain of biliary tract origin is more right sided or epigastric than periumbilical or left upper quadrant and can be more severe; ileus is usually absent. Ultrasound is helpful in establishing the diagnosis of cholelithiasis and cholecystitis. Intestinal obstruction due to mechanical factors can be differentiated from pancreatitis by the history of crescendo-decrescendo pain, findings on abdominal examination, and CT of the abdomen showing changes characteristic of mechanical obstruction. Acute mesenteric vascular occlusion is usually suspected in elderly debilitated patients with brisk leukocytosis, abdominal distention, and bloody diarrhea, confirmed by CT or magnetic resonance angiography. Vasculitides secondary to systemic lupus erythematosus and polyarteritis nodosa may be confused

TABLE 50-2

REVISED ATLANTA DEFINITIONS OF MORPHOLOGIC FEATURES OF ACUTE PANCREATITIS

MORPHOLOGIC FEATURE	DEFINITION	COMPUTED TOMOGRAPHY CRITERIA
Interstitial pancreatitis	Acute inflammation of the pancreatic parenchyma and peripancreatic tissues, but without recognizable tissue necrosis	Pancreatic parenchyma enhancement by IV contrast agent No findings of peripancreatic necrosis
Necrotizing pancreatitis	Inflammation associated with pancreatic parenchymal necrosis and/or peripancreatic necrosis	Lack of pancreatic parenchymal enhancement by IV contrast agent and/or presence of findings of peripancreatic necrosis (see below—ANC and WON)
Acute pancreatic fluid collection	Peripancreatic fluid associated with interstitial edematous pancreatitis with no associated peripancreatic necrosis. This term applies only to areas of peripancreatic fluid seen within the first 4 weeks after onset of interstitial edematous pancreatitis and without the features of a pseudocyst.	Occurs in the setting of interstitial edematous pancreatitis Homogeneous collection with fluid density Confined by normal peripancreatic fascial planes No definable wall encapsulating the collection Adjacent to pancreas (no intrapancreatic extension)
Pancreatic pseudocyst	An encapsulated collection of fluid with a well-defined inflammatory wall usually outside the pancreas with minimal or no necrosis. This entity usually occurs >4 weeks after onset of interstitial edematous pancreatitis.	Well circumscribed, usually round or oval Homogeneous fluid density No nonliquid component Well-defined wall; that is, completely encapsulated Maturation usually requires >4 weeks after onset of acute pancreatitis; occurs after interstitial edematous pancreatitis
Acute necrotic collection (ANC)	A collection containing variable amounts of both fluid and necrosis associated with necrotizing pancreatitis; the necrosis can involve the pancreatic parenchyma and/or the peripancreatic tissues.	Occurs only in the setting of acute necrotizing pancreatitis Heterogeneous and nonliquid density of varying degrees in different locations (some appear homogeneous early in their course) No definable wall encapsulating the collection Location—intrapancreatic and/or extrapancreatic
Walled-off necrosis (WON)	A mature, encapsulated collection of pancreatic and/or peripancreatic necrosis that has developed a well-defined inflammatory wall. WON usually occurs >4 weeks after onset of necrotizing pancreatitis.	Heterogeneous with liquid and nonliquid density with varying degrees of loculations (some may appear homogeneous) Well-defined wall; that is, completely encapsulated Location—intrapancreatic and/or extrapancreatic Maturation usually requires 4 weeks after onset of acute necrotizing pancreatitis

Source: Modified from P Banks et al: *Gut* 62:102, 2013.

with pancreatitis, especially because pancreatitis may develop as a complication of these diseases. Diabetic ketoacidosis is often accompanied by abdominal pain and elevated total serum amylase levels, thus closely mimicking acute pancreatitis. However, the serum lipase level is not elevated in diabetic ketoacidosis.

CLINICAL COURSE, DEFINITIONS, AND CLASSIFICATIONS

The Revised Atlanta Classification (1) defines phases of acute pancreatitis, (2) defines severity of acute pancreatitis, and (3) clarifies imaging definitions as outlined below.

Phases of acute pancreatitis

Two phases of acute pancreatitis have been defined, early (<2 weeks) and late (>2 weeks), which primarily describes the hospital course of the disease. In the *early phase* of acute pancreatitis, which lasts 1–2 weeks, severity is defined by clinical parameters rather than morphologic findings. Most patients exhibit SIRS, and if this persists, patients are predisposed to organ failure. Three

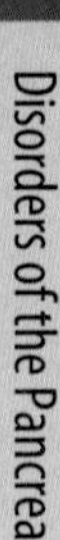

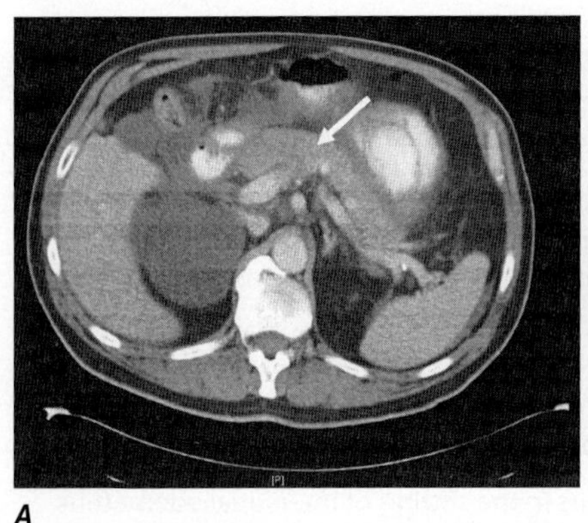

A

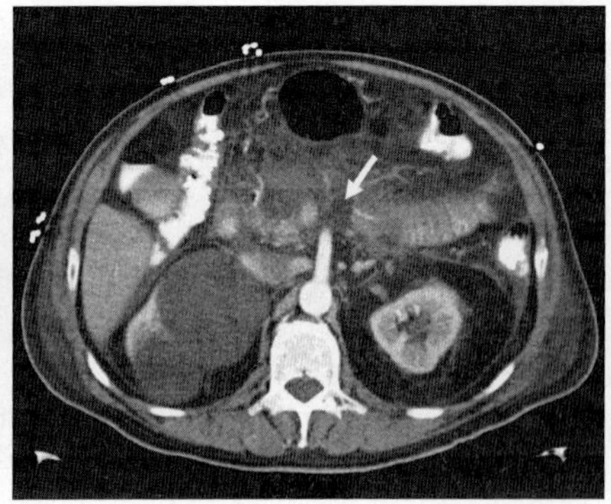

B

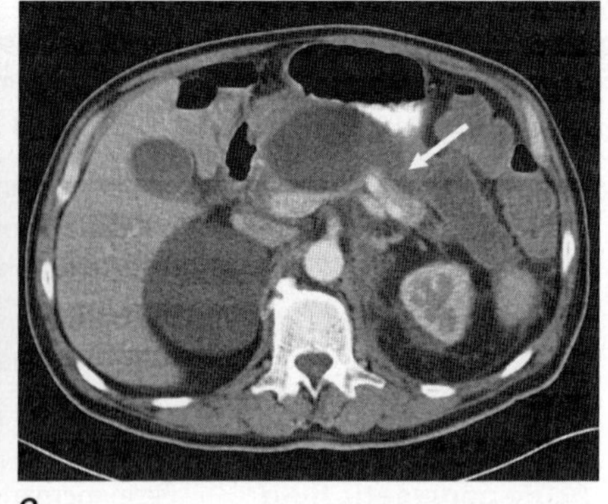

C

FIGURE 50-1

Acute pancreatitis: computed tomography (CT) evolution. ***A.*** Contrast-enhanced CT scan of the abdomen performed on admission for a patient with clinical and biochemical parameters suggestive of acute pancreatitis. Note the abnormal enhancement of the pancreatic parenchyma (*arrow*) suggestive of interstitial pancreatitis. ***B.*** Contrast-enhanced CT scan of the abdomen performed on the same patient 6 days later for persistent fever and systemic inflammatory response syndrome. The pancreas now demonstrates significant areas of nonenhancement consistent with development of necrosis, particularly in the body and neck region (*arrow*). Note that an early CT scan obtained within the first 48 h of hospitalization may underestimate or miss necrosis. **C.** Contrast-enhanced CT scan of the abdomen performed on the same patient 2 months after the initial episode of acute pancreatitis. CT now demonstrates evidence of a fluid collection consistent with walled-off pancreatic necrosis (*arrow*). *(Courtesy of Dr. KJ Mortele, Brigham and Women's Hospital; with permission.)*

TABLE 50-3

SEVERE ACUTE PANCREATITIS
Risk Factors for Severity
• Age >60 years
• Obesity, BMI >30
• Comorbid disease (Charlson Comorbidity Index)
Markers of Severity at Admission or within 24 h
• SIRS—defined by presence of 2 or more criteria:
• Core temperature <36° or >38°C
• Heart rate >90 beats/min
• Respirations >20/min or Pco_2 <32 mmHg
• White blood cell count >12,000/μL, <4000/μL, or 10% bands
• APACHE II
• Hemoconcentration (hematocrit >44%)
• Admission BUN (>22 mg/dL)
• BISAP Score
• (B) BUN >25 mg/dL
• (I) Impaired mental status
• (S) SIRS: ≥2 of 4 present
• (A) Age >60 years
• (P) Pleural effusion
• Organ failure (Modified Marshall Score)
• Cardiovascular: systolic BP <90 mmHg, heart rate >130 beats/min
• Pulmonary: Pao_2 <60 mmHg
• Renal: serum creatinine >2.0 mg%
Markers of Severity during Hospitalization
• Persistent organ failure
• Pancreatic necrosis

Abbreviations: APACHE II, Acute Physiology and Chronic Health Evaluation II; BMI, body mass index; BISAP, Bedside Index of Severity in Acute Pancreatitis; BP, blood pressure; BUN, blood urea nitrogen; SIRS, systemic inflammatory response syndrome.

organ systems should be assessed to define organ failure: respiratory, cardiovascular, and renal. Organ failure is defined as a score of 2 or more for one of these three organ systems using the modified Marshall scoring system. Persistent organ failure (>48 h) is the most important clinical finding in regard to severity of the acute pancreatitis episode. Organ failure that affects more than one organ is considered multisystem organ failure. CT imaging is usually not needed or recommended during the first 48 h of admission in acute pancreatitis.

The *late phase* is characterized by a protracted course of illness and may require imaging to evaluate for local complications. The important clinical parameter of severity, as in the early phase, is persistent organ failure. These patients may require supportive measures such as renal dialysis, ventilator support, or need for supplemental nutrition via the nasojejunal or parenteral route. The radiographic feature of greatest importance to recognize in this phase is the development of necrotizing pancreatitis on CT imaging. Necrosis generally prolongs hospitalization and, if infected, may require operative, endoscopic, or percutaneous intervention.

Severity of acute pancreatitis

Three severity classifications have also been defined: mild, moderately severe, and severe. *Mild acute pancreatitis* is without local complications or organ failure. Most patients with interstitial acute pancreatitis have mild pancreatitis. In mild acute pancreatitis, the disease is self-limited and subsides spontaneously, usually within 3–7 days after treatment is instituted. Oral intake can be resumed if the patient is hungry, has normal bowel function, and is without nausea and vomiting. Typically, a clear or full liquid diet has been recommended for the initial meal; however, a low-fat solid diet is a reasonable choice following recovery from mild acute pancreatitis.

Moderately severe acute pancreatitis is characterized by transient organ failure (resolves in <48 h) or local or systemic complications in the absence of persistent organ failure. These patients may or may not have necrosis, but may develop a local complication such as a fluid collection that requires a prolonged hospitalization greater than 1 week.

Severe acute pancreatitis is characterized by persistent organ failure (>48 h). Organ failure can be single or multiple. A CT scan or magnetic resonance imaging (MRI) should be obtained to assess for necrosis and/or complications. If a local complication is encountered, management is dictated by clinical symptoms, evidence of infection, maturity of fluid collection, and clinical stability of the patient. Prophylactic antibiotics are not recommended.

Imaging in acute pancreatitis

Two types of pancreatitis are recognized on imaging as *interstitial* or *necrotizing* based on pancreatic perfusion. CT imaging is best evaluated 3–5 days into hospitalization when patients are not responding to supportive care to look for local complications such as necrosis. Recent studies report the overutilization of CT imaging in acute pancreatitis and its inability to be better than clinical judgment in the early days of acute pancreatitis management. The revised criteria also outline the terminology for local complications and fluid collections along with a CT imaging template to guide reporting of findings. Local morphologic features are summarized in Table 50-1. *Interstitial pancreatitis* occurs in 90–95% of admissions for acute pancreatitis and is characterized by diffuse gland enlargement, homogenous contrast enhancement, and mild inflammatory changes or peripancreatic stranding. Symptoms generally resolve with a week of hospitalization. *Necrotizing pancreatitis* occurs in 5–10% of acute pancreatitis admissions and does not evolve until several days of hospitalization. It is characterized by lack of pancreatic parenchymal enhancement by intravenous contrast agent and/or presence of findings of peripancreatic necrosis. According to the revised Atlanta criteria, the natural history of pancreatic and peripancreatic necrosis is variable because it may remain solid or liquefy, remain sterile or become infected, and persist or disappear over time. CT identification of local complications, particularly necrosis, is critical in patients who are not responding to therapy because patients with infected and sterile necrosis are at greatest risk of mortality (Figs. 50-1*B*, 50-2, and 50-3). The median prevalence of organ failure is 54% in necrotizing pancreatitis. The prevalence of organ failure is perhaps slightly higher in infected versus sterile necrosis. With single-organ system failure, the mortality is 3–10% but increases to 47% with multisystem organ failure.

ACUTE PANCREATITIS MANAGEMENT

We will briefly describe the management of patients with acute pancreatitis from the time of diagnosis in the emergency ward to ongoing hospital admission and, finally, to time of discharge, highlighting salient features based on severity and complications. It is important to note that 85–90% of cases of acute pancreatitis are self-limited and subside spontaneously, usually within 3–7 days after initiation of treatment, and do not exhibit organ failure or local complications.

The management of acute pancreatitis begins in the emergency ward. After a diagnosis has been confirmed, aggressive fluid resuscitation is initiated, intravenous analgesics are administered, severity is assessed, and a search for etiologies that may impact acute care is begun. Patients who do not respond to aggressive fluid resuscitation in the emergency ward should be considered for admission to a step-down or intensive care unit for aggressive fluid resuscitation, hemodynamic monitoring, and management of necrosis or organ failure.

Fluid resuscitation and monitoring response to therapy

The most important treatment intervention for acute pancreatitis is safe, aggressive intravenous fluid resuscitation. The patient is made NPO to rest the pancreas and is given intravenous narcotic analgesics to control abdominal pain and supplemental oxygen (2 L) via nasal cannula.

Intravenous fluids of lactated Ringer's or normal saline are initially bolused at 15–20 cc/kg (1050–1400 mL), followed by 3 mg/kg per hour (200–250 mL/h), to maintain urine output >0.5 cc/kg per hour. Serial bedside evaluations are required every 6–8 h to assess vital signs, oxygen saturation, and change in physical examination. Lactated Ringer's solution has been shown to decrease systemic inflammation and may be a better crystalloid than normal saline. A *targeted resuscitation strategy* with measurement of hematocrit and BUN every 8–12 h is recommended to ensure adequacy of fluid resuscitation and monitor response to therapy, noting less aggressive resuscitation strategy may be needed in milder forms of pancreatitis. A rising BUN during hospitalization is not only associated with inadequate hydration but also higher in-hospital mortality.

A decrease in hematocrit and BUN during the first 12–24 h is strong evidence that sufficient fluids are being administered. Serial measurements and bedside

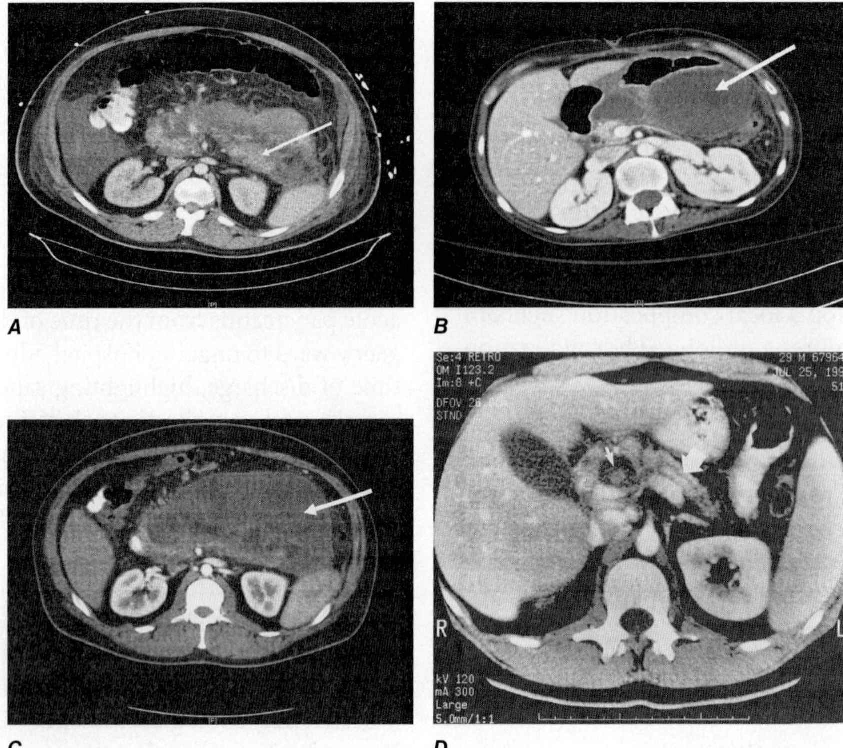

FIGURE 50-2

A. Acute necrotizing pancreatitis: computed tomography (CT) scan. Contrast-enhanced CT scan showing acute pancreatitis with necrosis. *Arrow* shows partially enhancing body/tail of pancreas surrounded by fluid with decreased enhancement in the neck/body of the pancreas. ***B.*** Acute fluid collection: CT scan. Contrast-enhanced CT scan showing fluid collection in the retroperitoneum (*arrow*) compressing the air-filled stomach arising from the pancreas in a patient with asparaginase-induced acute necrotizing pancreatitis. **C.** Walled-off pancreatic necrosis: CT scan. CT scan showing marked walled-off necrosis of the pancreas and peripancreatic area (*arrow*) in a patient with necrotizing pancreatitis. Addendum: In past years, both of these CT findings (Figs. 50-2*B* and 50-2*C*) would have been misinterpreted as pseudocysts. ***D.*** Spiral CT showing a pseudocyst (*small arrow*) with a pseudoaneurysm (*light area in pseudocyst*). Note the demonstration of the main pancreatic duct (*big arrow*), even though this duct is minimally dilated by endoscopic retrograde cholangiopancreatography. *(A, B, C, courtesy of Dr. KJ Mortele, Brigham and Women's Hospital; D, courtesy of Dr. PR Ros, Brigham and Women's Hospital; with permission.)*

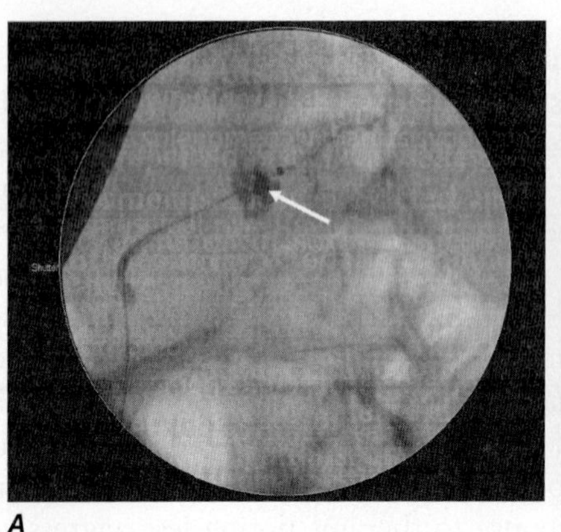

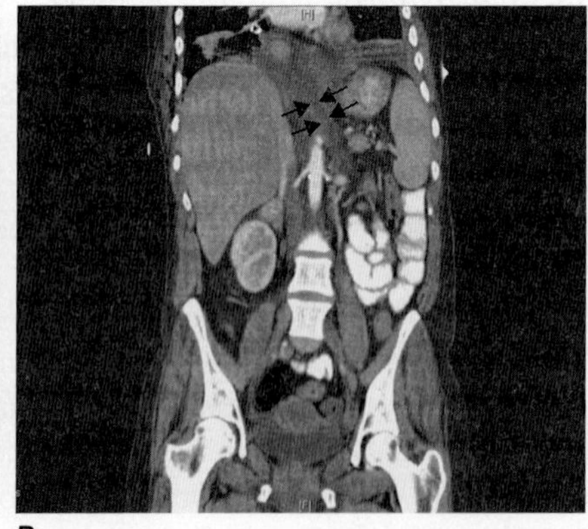

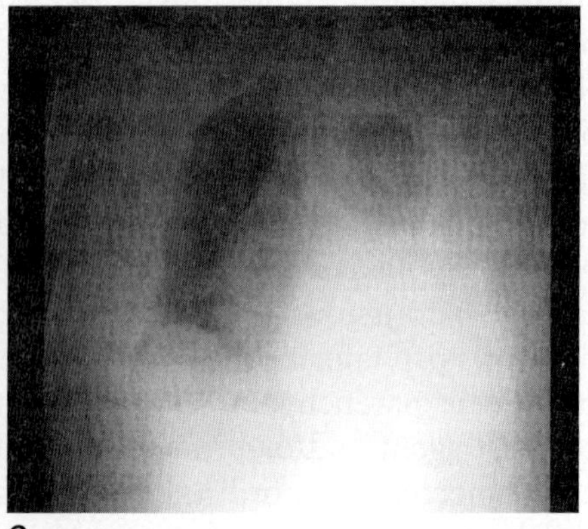

FIGURE 50-3

A. Pancreaticopleural fistula: pancreatic duct leak on endoscopic retrograde cholangiopancreatography. Pancreatic duct leak (*arrow*) demonstrated at the time of retrograde pancreatogram in a patient with acute exacerbation of alcohol-induced acute or chronic pancreatitis. ***B.*** Pancreaticopleural fistula: computed tomography (CT) scan. Contrast-enhanced CT scan (coronal view) with *arrows* showing fistula tract from pancreatic duct disruption in the pancreatic pleural fistula. **C.** Pancreaticopleural fistula: chest x-ray. Large pleural effusion in the left hemithorax from a disrupted pancreatic duct. Analysis of pleural fluid revealed elevated amylase concentration. *(Courtesy of Dr. KJ Mortele, Brigham and Women's Hospital; with permission.)*

assessment for fluid overload are continued, and fluid rates are maintained at the current rate. Adjustments in fluid resuscitation may be required in patients with cardiac, pulmonary, or renal disease. A rise in hematocrit or BUN during serial measurement should be treated with a repeat volume challenge with a 2-L crystalloid bolus followed by increasing the fluid rate by 1.5 mg/kg per hour. If the BUN or hematocrit fails to respond (i.e., remains elevated or does not decrease) to this bolus challenge and increase in fluid rate, consideration of transfer to an intensive care unit is strongly recommended for hemodynamic monitoring.

Assessment of severity and hospital triage

Severity of acute pancreatitis should be determined in the emergency ward to assist in patient triage to a regular hospital ward or step-down unit or direct admission to an intensive care unit. The Bedside Index of Severity in Acute Pancreatitis (BISAP) incorporates five clinical and laboratory parameters obtained within the first 24 h of hospitalization (Table 50-3)—BUN >25 mg/dL, impaired mental status (Glasgow coma score <15), SIRS, age >60 years, and pleural effusion on radiography—that can be useful in assessing severity. Presence of three or more of these factors was associated with substantially increased risk for in-hospital mortality among patients with acute pancreatitis. In addition, an elevated hematocrit >44% and admission BUN >22 mg/dL are also associated with more severe acute pancreatitis. Incorporating these indices with the overall patient response to initial fluid resuscitation in the emergency ward can be useful at triaging patients to the appropriate hospital acute care setting.

In general, patients with lower BISAP scores, hematocrits, and admission BUNs tend to respond to initial management and are triaged to a regular hospital ward for ongoing care. If SIRS is not present at 24 h, the patient is unlikely to develop organ failure or necrosis. Therefore, patients with persistent SIRS at 24 h or underlying comorbid illnesses (e.g., chronic obstructive pulmonary disease, congestive heart failure) should be considered for a step-down unit setting if available. Patients with higher BISAP scores and elevations in hematocrit and admission BUN that do not respond to initial fluid resuscitation and exhibit evidence of respiratory failure, hypotension, or organ failure should be considered for direct admission to an intensive care unit.

Special considerations based on etiology

A careful history, review of medications, selected laboratory studies (liver profile, serum triglycerides, serum calcium), and an abdominal ultrasound are recommended in the emergency ward to assess for etiologies that may impact acute management. An abdominal ultrasound is the initial imaging modality of choice and will evaluate the gallbladder and common duct and assess the pancreatic head.

Gallstone pancreatitis

Patients with evidence of ascending cholangitis (rising white blood cell count, increasing liver enzymes) should undergo ERCP within 24–48 h of admission. Patients with gallstone pancreatitis are at increased risk of recurrence, and consideration should be given to performing a cholecystectomy during the same admission or within 4–6 weeks of discharge. An alternative for patients who are not surgical candidates would be to perform an endoscopic biliary sphincterotomy before discharge.

Hypertriglyceridemia

Serum triglycerides >1000 mg/dL are associated with acute pancreatitis. Initial therapy may include insulin, heparin, or plasmapheresis. Outpatient therapies include control of diabetes if present, administration of lipid-lowering agents, weight loss, and avoidance of drugs that elevate lipid levels.

Other potential etiologies that may impact acute hospital care include *hypercalcemia*, *autoimmune pancreatitis*, *post-ERCP pancreatitis*, and *drug-induced pancreatitis*. Treatment of hyperparathyroidism or malignancy is effective at reducing serum calcium. Autoimmune pancreatitis is responsive to glucocorticoid administration. Pancreatic duct stenting and rectal indomethacin administration are effective at decreasing pancreatitis after ERCP. Drugs that cause pancreatitis should be discontinued. Multiple drugs have been implicated, but only about 30 have been challenged (Class 1A) and found to be causative.

Nutritional therapy

A low-fat solid diet can be administered to subjects with mild acute pancreatitis after the abdominal pain has resolved. Enteral nutrition should be considered 2–3 days after admission in subjects with more severe pancreatitis instead of total parenteral nutrition (TPN). Enteral feeding maintains gut barrier integrity, limits bacterial translocation, is less expensive, and has fewer complications than TPN. The choice of gastric versus nasojejunal enteral feeding is currently under investigation.

Management of local complications

Patients exhibiting signs of clinical deterioration despite aggressive fluid resuscitation and hemodynamic monitoring should be assessed for local complications, which may include necrosis, pseudocyst formation, pancreas duct disruption, peripancreatic vascular complications,

TABLE 50-4

COMPLICATIONS OF ACUTE PANCREATITIS

Local	
Necrosis	Pancreatic ascites
Sterile	Involvement of contiguous organs by necrotizing pancreatitis
Infected	Thrombosis of blood vessels (splenic vein, portal vein)
Walled-off necrosis	Pancreatic enteric fistula
Pancreatic fluid collections	Bowel infarction
Pancreatic pseudocyst	Obstructive jaundice
Disruption of main pancreatic duct or secondary branches	
Systemic	
Pulmonary	Renal
Pleural effusion	Oliguria (<300 mL/d)
Atelectasis	Azotemia
Mediastinal fluid	Renal artery and/or renal vein thrombosis
Pneumonitis	Acute tubular necrosis
Acute respiratory distress syndrome	Metabolic
Hypoxemia (unrecognized)	Hyperglycemia
Cardiovascular	Hypertriglyceridemia
Hypotension	Hypocalcemia
Hypovolemia	Encephalopathy
Nonspecific ST-T changes in electrocardiogram simulating myocardial infarction	Sudden blindness (Purtscher's retinopathy)
Pericardial effusion	Central nervous system
Hematologic	Psychosis
Disseminated intravascular coagulation	Fat emboli
Gastrointestinal hemorrhage	Fat necrosis
Peptic ulcer disease	Subcutaneous tissues (erythematous nodules)
Erosive gastritis	Bone
Hemorrhagic pancreatic necrosis with erosion into major blood vessels	Miscellaneous (mediastinum, pleura, nervous system)
Portal vein thrombosis, splenic vein thrombosis, variceal hemorrhage	

and extrapancreatic infections (Table 50-4). A multidisciplinary team approach is recommended including gastroenterology, surgery, interventional radiology, and intensive care specialists, and consideration should also be made for transfer to a pancreas center.

Necrosis

The management of necrosis requires a multidisciplinary team approach. Percutaneous aspiration of necrosis with Gram stain and culture should be performed if there are ongoing signs of possible pancreatic infection such as sustained leukocytosis, fever, or organ failure. There is currently no role for *prophylactic antibiotics* in necrotizing pancreatitis. It is reasonable to start broad-spectrum antibiotics in a patient who appears septic while awaiting the results of Gram stain and cultures. If cultures are negative, the antibiotics should be discontinued to minimize the risk of developing opportunistic or fungal superinfection. Repeated fine-needle aspiration and Gram stain with culture of pancreatic necrosis may be done every 5–7 days in the presence of persistent fever. Repeated CT or MRI imaging should also be considered with any change in clinical course to monitor for complications (e.g., thromboses, hemorrhage, abdominal compartment syndrome).

In general, *sterile necrosis* is most often managed conservatively unless complications arise. Once a diagnosis of *infected necrosis* is established and an organism identified, targeted antibiotics should be instituted. Pancreatic debridement (necrosectomy) should be considered for definitive management of *infected necrosis*, but clinical decisions are generally influenced by response to antibiotic treatment and overall clinical condition. Symptomatic local complications as outlined in the revised Atlanta criteria may require definitive therapy.

A step-up approach (percutaneous or endoscopic transgastric drainage followed, if necessary, by open necrosectomy) has been successfully reported by some pancreatic centers. One-third of the patients successfully treated with the step-up approach did not require major abdominal surgery. A recent randomized trial reported advantages to an initial endoscopic approach compared to an initial surgical necrosectomy approach in select patients requiring intervention for symptomatic WON. Taken together, a more conservative approach to the management of infected pancreatic necrosis has evolved over the years under the close supervision of a multidisciplinary team. If conservative therapy can be safely implemented for 4–6 weeks, to allow the pancreatic collections to resolve or "wall-off," surgical or endoscopic intervention is generally much safer and better tolerated by the patient.

Pseudocyst

The incidence of pseudocyst is low, and most acute collections resolve over time. Less than 10% of patients have persistent fluid collections after 6 weeks that would meet the definition of a pseudocyst. Only symptomatic collections should be drained with surgery or endoscopy or by percutaneous route.

Pancreatic duct disruption

Pancreatic duct disruption may present with symptoms of increasing abdominal pain or shortness of breath in the setting of an enlarging fluid collection. Diagnosis can be confirmed on magnetic resonance cholangiopancreatography (MRCP) or ERCP. Placement of a bridging pancreatic stent for at least 6 weeks is >90% effective at resolving the leak. Nonbridging stents are less effective.

Perivascular complications

Perivascular complications may include *splenic vein thrombosis* with gastric varices and pseudoaneurysms. *Gastric varices* bleed less than 5% of the time. Life-threatening bleeding from a ruptured *pseudoaneurysm* can be diagnosed and treated with mesenteric angiography and embolization.

Extrapancreatic infections

Hospital-acquired infections occur in up to 20% of patients with acute pancreatitis. Patients should be continually monitored for the development pneumonia, urinary tract infection, and line infection. Continued culturing of urine, monitoring of chest x-rays, and routine changing of intravenous lines are important during hospitalization.

Follow-up care

Hospitalizations for moderately severe and severe acute pancreatitis can last weeks to months and often involve a period of intensive care unit admission and outpatient rehabilitation or subacute nursing care. Follow-up evaluation should assess for development of diabetes, exocrine insufficiency, recurrent cholangitis, or development of infected fluid collections. As mentioned previously, cholecystectomy should be performed within 4–6 weeks of discharge if possible for patients with uncomplicated gallstone pancreatitis.

RECURRENT PANCREATITIS

Approximately 25% of patients who have had an attack of acute pancreatitis have a recurrence. The two most common etiologic factors are alcohol and cholelithiasis. In patients with recurrent pancreatitis without an obvious cause, the differential diagnosis should encompass occult biliary tract disease including microlithiasis, hypertriglyceridemia, drugs, pancreatic cancer, pancreas divisum, and cystic fibrosis (Table 50-1). In one series of 31 patients diagnosed initially as having idiopathic or recurrent acute pancreatitis, 23 were found to have occult gallstone disease. Thus, approximately two-thirds of patients with recurrent acute pancreatitis without an obvious cause actually have occult gallstone disease due to microlithiasis. Genetic defects as in hereditary pancreatitis and cystic fibrosis mutations can result in recurrent pancreatitis. Other diseases of the biliary tree and pancreatic ducts that can cause acute pancreatitis include choledochocele; ampullary tumors; pancreas divisum; and pancreatic duct stones, stricture, and tumor. Approximately 2–4% of patients with pancreatic carcinoma present with acute pancreatitis.

PANCREATITIS IN PATIENTS WITH AIDS

The incidence of acute pancreatitis is increased in patients with AIDS for two reasons: (1) the high incidence of infections involving the pancreas such as infections with cytomegalovirus, *Cryptosporidium*, and the *Mycobacterium avium* complex; and (2) the frequent use by patients with AIDS of medications such as didanosine, pentamidine, trimethoprim-sulfamethoxazole, and protease inhibitors. Incidence has been markedly reduced due to advances in therapy.

CHRONIC PANCREATITIS AND PANCREATIC EXOCRINE INSUFFICIENCY

PATHOPHYSIOLOGY

Chronic pancreatitis is a disease process characterized by irreversible damage to the pancreas as distinct from the reversible changes noted in acute pancreatitis (Table 50-4). The events that initiate and then perpetuate the inflammatory process in the pancreas are becoming more clearly understood. Irrespective of the mechanism of injury, it is becoming apparent that stellate cell activation that results in cytokine expression and production of extracellular matrix proteins cause acute and chronic inflammation and collagen deposition in the pancreas. Thus, the condition is defined by the presence of histologic abnormalities, including chronic inflammation, fibrosis, and progressive destruction of both exocrine and eventually endocrine tissue (atrophy). A number of etiologies have been associated with chronic pancreatitis resulting in the cardinal manifestations of the disease such as abdominal pain, steatorrhea, weight loss, and diabetes mellitus (Table 50-5).

Although alcohol has been believed to be the primary cause of chronic pancreatitis, other factors contribute to the disease because not all heavy consumers of alcohol develop pancreatic disease. There is also a strong association between smoking and chronic pancreatitis. Cigarette smoke leads to an increased susceptibility to pancreatic autodigestion and predisposes to dysregulation of duct cell CFTR function. Smoking is an independent, dose-dependent risk factor for chronic pancreatitis and recurrent acute pancreatitis. Both continued alcohol and smoking exposure are associated with pancreatic fibrosis, calcifications, and progression of disease

Recent characterization of pancreatic stellate cells (PSCs) has added insight into the underlying cellular responses behind development of chronic pancreatitis. Specifically, PSCs are believed to play a role in maintaining normal pancreatic architecture that can shift toward fibrogenesis in the case of chronic pancreatitis. The sentinel acute pancreatitis event (SAPE) hypothesis uniformly describes the events in the pathogenesis of chronic pancreatitis. It is believed that alcohol or additional stimuli lead to matrix metalloproteinase–mediated destruction of normal collagen in pancreatic

TABLE 50-5

CHRONIC PANCREATITIS AND PANCREATIC EXOCRINE INSUFFICIENCY: TIGAR-O CLASSIFICATION SYSTEM

Toxic-metabolic	Alcoholic
	Tobacco smoking
	Hypercalcemia
	Hyperlipidemia
	Chronic renal failure
	Medications—phenacetin abuse
	Toxins—organotin compounds (e.g., dibutylin dichloride, DBTC)
Idiopathic	Early onset
	Late onset
	Tropical
Genetic	Cationic trypsinogen (*PRSS1*)
	Cystic fibrosis transmembrane conductance regulator gene (*CFTR*)
	Calcium-sensing receptor (*CASR*)
	Chymotrypsin C gene (*CTRC*)
	Pancreatic secretory trypsin inhibitor gene (*SPINK1*)
Autoimmune	Type 1 autoimmune chronic pancreatitis
	IgG4 systemic
	Type 2 autoimmune chronic pancreatitis
Recurrent and severe acute pancreatitis	Postnecrotic (severe acute pancreatitis)
	Recurrent acute pancreatitis
	Vascular diseases/ischemia
	Radiation induced
Obstructive	Pancreas divisum
	Duct obstruction (e.g., tumor)
	Preampullary duodenal wall cysts
	Posttraumatic pancreatic duct scars

Abbreviations: DBTC, dibutylin dichloride; TIGAR-O, toxic-metabolic, idiopathic, genetic, autoimmune, recurrent and severe acute pancreatitis, obstructive.

parenchyma, which later allows for pancreatic remodeling. Proinflammatory cytokines, tumor necrosis factor α (TNF-α), interleukin 1 (IL-1), and interleukin 6 (IL-6), as well as oxidant complexes, are able to induce PSC activity with subsequent new collagen synthesis. In addition to being stimulated by cytokines, oxidants, or growth factors, PSCs also possess transforming growth factor β (TGF-β)–mediated self-activating autocrine pathways that may explain disease progression in chronic pancreatitis even after removal of noxious stimuli.

ETIOLOGIC CONSIDERATIONS

Among adults in the United States, alcoholism is the most common cause of clinically apparent chronic pancreatitis, whereas cystic fibrosis is the most frequent cause in children. As many as 25% of adults in the United States with chronic pancreatitis have the *idiopathic* form. Recent investigations have indicated that up to 15% of patients with idiopathic pancreatitis may have pancreatitis due to genetic defects (Table 50-5).

Whitcomb and associates studied several large families with hereditary chronic pancreatitis and were able to identify a genetic defect that affects the gene encoding for trypsinogen. Several additional defects of this gene have also been described. The defect prevents the destruction of prematurely activated trypsin and allows it to be resistant to the intracellular protective effect of trypsin inhibitor. It is hypothesized that this continual activation of digestive enzymes within the gland leads to acute injury and, finally, chronic pancreatitis. Since the initial discovery of the *PRSS1* mutation defect, other genetic diseases have been detected (Table 50-5).

Several other groups of investigators have documented mutations of *CFTR*. This gene functions as a cyclic AMP–regulated chloride channel. In patients with cystic fibrosis, the high concentration of macromolecules can block the pancreatic ducts. It must be appreciated, however, that there is a great deal of heterogeneity in relationship to the *CFTR* gene defect. More than 1000 putative mutations of the *CFTR* gene have been identified. Attempts to elucidate the relationship between the genotype and pancreatic manifestations have been hampered by the number of mutations. The ability to detect *CFTR* mutations has led to the recognition that the clinical spectrum of the disease is broader than previously thought. Two studies have clarified the association between mutations of the *CFTR* gene and another monosymptomatic form of cystic fibrosis (i.e., chronic pancreatitis). It is estimated that in patients with idiopathic pancreatitis, the frequency of a single *CFTR* mutation is 11 times the expected frequency and the frequency of two mutant alleles is 80 times the expected frequency. In these studies, the patients were adults when the diagnosis of pancreatitis was made; none had any clinical evidence of pulmonary disease, and sweat test results were not diagnostic of cystic fibrosis. The prevalence of such mutations is unclear, and further studies are certainly needed. In addition, the therapeutic and prognostic implication of these findings with respect to managing pancreatitis remains to be determined. Long-term follow-up of affected patients is needed. *CFTR* mutations are common in the general population. It is unclear whether the *CFTR* mutation alone can lead to pancreatitis as an autosomal recessive disease. A study evaluated 39 patients with idiopathic chronic pancreatitis to assess the risk associated with these mutations. Patients with two *CFTR* mutations (compound heterozygotes) demonstrated *CFTR* function at a level between that seen in typical cystic fibrosis and cystic fibrosis carriers and had a 40-fold increased risk of pancreatitis. The presence of an *N34S SPINK1* mutation increased the risk 20-fold. A combination of two *CFTR* mutations and an *N34S SPINK1* mutation increased the risk of pancreatitis 900-fold. Knowledge

TABLE 50-6

CLINICAL FEATURES OF AUTOIMMUNE PANCREATITIS (AIP)
• Mild symptoms, usually abdominal pain, but without frequent attacks of acute pancreatitis
• Diffuse swelling and enlargement of the pancreas
• Two-thirds of patients present with either obstructive jaundice or a "mass" in the head of the pancreas mimicking carcinoma
• Diffuse irregular narrowing of the pancreatic duct (MRCP or ERCP)
• Increased levels of serum gamma globulins, especially IgG4
• Presence of other autoantibodies (ANA), rheumatoid factor (RF)
• Can occur with other autoimmune diseases: Sjögren's syndrome, primary sclerosing cholangitis, ulcerative colitis, rheumatoid arthritis
• Extrapancreatic bile duct changes such as stricture of the common bile duct and intrahepatic ducts
• Pancreatic calcifications (rare)
• Pancreatic biopsies reveal extensive fibrosis and lymphoplasmacytic infiltration
• Glucocorticoids are effective in alleviating symptoms, decreasing size of the pancreas, and reversing histopathologic changes

Abbreviations: ERCP, endoscopic retrograde cholangiopancreatography; MRCP, magnetic resonance cholangiopancreatography.

of the genetic defects and downstream alterations in protein expression has led to the development of novel genetic therapy in cystic fibrosis children that potentiates the CFTR channel resulting in improvement in lung function, quality of life, and weight gain. Table 50-5 lists recognized causes of chronic pancreatitis and pancreatic exocrine insufficiency.

AUTOIMMUNE PANCREATITIS

Autoimmune pancreatitis (AIP) is an uncommon disorder of presumed autoimmune causation with characteristic laboratory, histologic, and morphologic findings (Table 50-6). In type 1 AIP, the pancreas is involved as part of an IgG4 systemic disease and meets HISORt criteria as defined below. The characteristic pancreatic histopathologic findings include lymphoplasmacytic infiltrate, storiform fibrosis, and abundant IgG4 cells. AIP type 2 is histologically confirmed idiopathic duct centric pancreatitis with granulocytic infiltration of the duct wall (termed GEL), but without IgG4 positive cells and systemic involvement. Although AIP was initially described as a primary pancreatic disorder, it is now recognized that it is associated with other disorders of presumed autoimmune etiology, and this has been termed IgG4 systemic disease. The clinical features include IgG4-associated cholangitis, rheumatoid arthritis, Sjögren's syndrome, ulcerative colitis, mediastinal fibrosis and adenopathy, autoimmune thyroiditis, tubulointerstitial nephritis, retroperitoneal fibrosis, chronic periaortitis, chronic sclerosing sialadenitis, and Mikulicz's disease. Mild symptoms, usually abdominal pain, and recurrent acute pancreatitis are unusual. Furthermore, AIP is not a common cause of idiopathic recurrent pancreatitis.

Weight loss and new onset of diabetes may also occur. An obstructive pattern on liver tests is common (i.e., disproportionately elevated serum alkaline phosphatase and minimally elevated serum aminotransferases). Elevated serum levels of IgG4 provide a marker for the disease, particularly in Western populations. Serum IgG4 normally accounts for only 5–6% of the total IgG4 in healthy patients but is elevated to values >280 mg/dL in those with AIP. CT scans reveal abnormalities in the majority of patients and include diffuse enlargement, focal enlargement, and a distinct enlargement at the head of the pancreas. ERCP or MRCP reveals strictures in the bile duct in more than one-third of patients with AIP; these may include common bile duct strictures, intrahepatic bile duct strictures, or proximal bile duct strictures, with accompanying narrowing of the pancreatic portion of the bile duct. This has been termed autoimmune IgG4 cholangitis. Characteristic histologic findings include extensive lymphoplasmacytic infiltrates with dense fibrosis around pancreatic ducts, as well as a lymphoplasmacytic infiltration, resulting in an obliterative phlebitis.

The Mayo Clinic HISORt criteria indicate that AIP can be diagnosed by the presence of at least two of the following: (1) *h*istology; (2) *i*maging; (3) *s*erology (elevated serum IgG4 levels); (4) *o*ther organ involvement; and (5) *r*esponse to glucocorticoid *t*herapy, with improvement in pancreatic and extrapancreatic manifestations.

Glucocorticoids have shown efficacy in alleviating symptoms, decreasing the size of the pancreas, and reversing histopathologic features in patients with AIP. Patients may respond dramatically to glucocorticoid therapy within a 2- to 4-week period. Prednisone is usually administered at an initial dose of 40 mg/d for 4 weeks followed by a taper of the daily dosage by 5 mg/wk based on monitoring of clinical parameters. Relief of symptoms, serial changes in abdominal imaging of the pancreas and bile ducts, decreased serum γ-globulin and IgG4 levels, and improvements in liver tests are parameters to follow. A poor response to glucocorticoids over a 2- to 4-week period should raise suspicion of pancreatic cancer or other forms of chronic pancreatitis. A recent multicenter international report reviewed 1064 patients with AIP. Clinical remission was achieved in 99% of type I and 92% of type II AIP patients with steroids. However, disease relapse occurred in 31% of type I and 9% of type II AIP patients. For treatment of disease relapse in type 1 AIP, glucocorticoids were successful in 201 of 295 (68%) patients, and azathioprine was successful in 52 of

58 patients (85%). A small number of patients responded favorably to 6-mercaptapurine, rituximab, cyclosporine, and cyclophosphamide. Types 1 and 2 AIP are highly responsive to initial glucocorticoid treatment. Relapse is common in type 1 patients, especially those with biliary tract strictures. Most relapses occur after glucocorticoids are discontinued. Patients with refractory symptoms and strictures generally require immunomodulator therapy as noted above. Appearance of interval cancers following a diagnosis of AIP is uncommon.

Clinical features of chronic pancreatitis

Patients with chronic pancreatitis seek medical attention predominantly because of two symptoms: abdominal pain or maldigestion and weight loss. The abdominal pain may be quite variable in location, severity, and frequency. The pain can be constant or intermittent with frequent pain-free intervals. Eating may exacerbate the pain, leading to a fear of eating with consequent weight loss. The spectrum of abdominal pain ranges from mild to quite severe, with narcotic dependence as a frequent consequence. Maldigestion is manifested as chronic diarrhea, steatorrhea, weight loss, and fatigue. Patients with chronic abdominal pain may or may not progress to maldigestion, and ~20% of patients will present with symptoms of maldigestion without a history of abdominal pain. Patients with chronic pancreatitis have significant morbidity and mortality and use appreciable amounts of societal resources. Despite steatorrhea, clinically apparent deficiencies of fat-soluble vitamins are surprisingly uncommon. Physical findings in these patients are usually unimpressive, so that there is a disparity between the severity of abdominal pain and the physical signs that usually consist of some mild tenderness.

The diagnosis of early or mild chronic pancreatitis can be challenging because there is no biomarker for the disease. In contrast to acute pancreatitis, the serum amylase and lipase levels are usually not strikingly elevated in chronic pancreatitis. Elevation of serum bilirubin and alkaline phosphatase may indicate cholestasis secondary to common bile duct stricture caused by chronic inflammation. Many patients have impaired glucose tolerance with elevated fasting blood glucose levels. The fecal elastase-1 and small-bowel biopsy are useful in the evaluation of patients with suspected pancreatic steatorrhea. The fecal elastase level will be abnormal and small-bowel histology will be normal in such patients. A decrease of fecal elastase level to <100 μg per gram of stool strongly suggests severe pancreatic exocrine insufficiency.

The radiographic evaluation of a patient with suspected chronic pancreatitis usually proceeds from a noninvasive to more invasive approach. Abdominal CT imaging (Fig. 50-4*A*, *B*) is the initial modality of choice, followed by MRI (Fig. 50-4*C*), endoscopic ultrasound, and pancreas function testing. In addition to

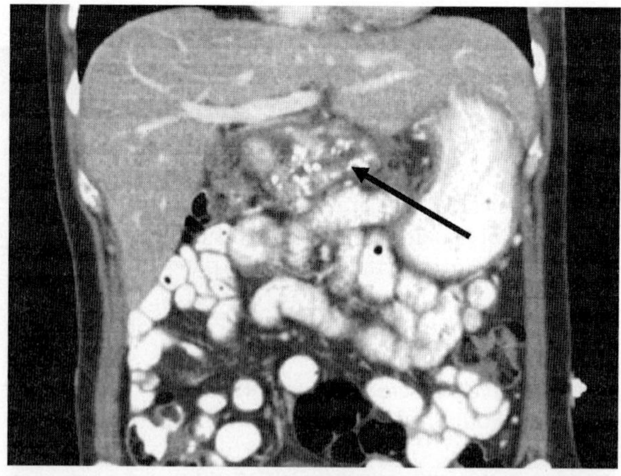

A

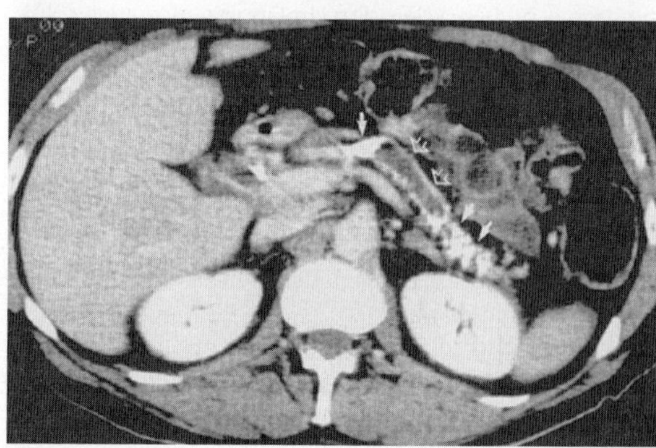

B

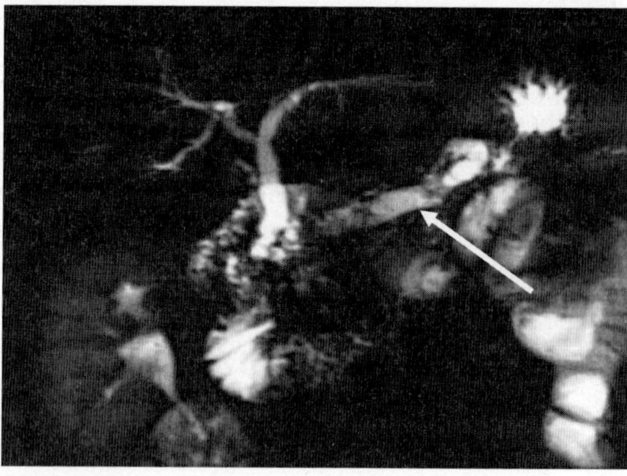

C

FIGURE 50-4

A. Chronic pancreatitis and pancreatic calculi: computed tomography (CT) scan. In this contrast-enhanced CT scan of the abdomen, there is evidence of an atrophic pancreas with multiple calcifications and stones in the parenchyma and dilated pancreatic duct (*arrow*). ***B.*** In this contrast-enhanced CT scan of the abdomen, there is evidence of an atrophic pancreas with multiple calcifications (*arrows*). Note the markedly dilated pancreatic duct seen in this section through the body and tail (*open arrows*). ***C.*** Chronic pancreatitis on magnetic resonance cholangiopancreatography (MRCP): dilated duct with filling defects. Gadolinium-enhanced magnetic resonance imaging/MRCP reveals a dilated pancreatic duct (*arrow*) in chronic pancreatitis with multiple filling defects suggestive of pancreatic duct calculi. *(A, C, courtesy of Dr. KJ Mortele, Brigham and Women's Hospital; with permission.)*

excluding a pseudocyst and pancreatic cancer, CT may show calcification, dilated ducts, or an atrophic pancreas. Although abdominal CT scanning and MRCP greatly aid in the diagnosis of pancreatic disease, the diagnostic test with the best sensitivity and specificity is the hormone stimulation test using secretin. The secretin test becomes abnormal when ≥60% of the pancreatic exocrine function has been lost. This usually correlates well with the onset of chronic abdominal pain. The role of endoscopic ultrasonography (EUS) in diagnosing early chronic pancreatitis is still being defined. A total of nine endosonographic features have been described in chronic pancreatitis. The presence of five or more features is considered diagnostic of chronic pancreatitis. EUS is not a sensitive enough test for detecting early chronic pancreatitis alone **(Chap. 49)** and may show positive features in patients who have dyspepsia or even normal aging individuals. Recent data suggest that EUS can be combined with endoscopic pancreatic function testing (EUS-ePFT) during a single endoscopy to screen for chronic pancreatitis in patients with chronic abdominal pain. Diffuse calcifications noted on plain film of the abdomen usually indicate significant damage to the pancreas and are pathognomic for chronic pancreatitis (Fig. 50-4*A*). Although alcohol is by far the most common cause of pancreatic calcification, such calcification may also be noted in hereditary pancreatitis, posttraumatic pancreatitis, hypercalcemic pancreatitis, idiopathic chronic pancreatitis, and tropical pancreatitis.

Complications of chronic pancreatitis

The complications of chronic pancreatitis are protean and are listed in Table 50-7. Although most patients have impaired glucose tolerance, diabetic ketoacidosis and diabetic coma are uncommon. Likewise, end-organ damage (retinopathy, neuropathy, nephropathy) is also uncommon. A nondiabetic retinopathy may be due to either vitamin A and/or zinc deficiency. Gastrointestinal bleeding may occur from peptic ulceration, gastritis, a pseudocyst eroding into the duodenum, arterial bleeding into the pancreatic duct (hemosuccus pancreaticus), or ruptured varices secondary to splenic vein thrombosis due to chronic inflammation of the tail of the pancreas. Jaundice, cholestasis, and biliary cirrhosis may occur from the chronic inflammatory reaction around the intrapancreatic portion of the common bile duct. Twenty years after the diagnosis of calcific chronic pancreatitis, the cumulative risk of pancreatic carcinoma is 4%. Patients with hereditary pancreatitis are at a 10-fold higher risk for pancreatic cancer.

TABLE 50-7

COMPLICATIONS OF CHRONIC PANCREATITIS	
Chronic abdominal pain	Jaundice
Narcotic addiction	Retinopathy
Diabetes mellitus/impaired glucose tolerance	Biliary stricture and/or biliary cirrhosis
Gastroparesis	Pseudocyst
Malabsorption/maldigestion	Metabolic bone disease
	Pancreatic cancer

TREATMENT Chronic Pancreatitis

STEATORRHEA The treatment of steatorrhea with pancreatic enzymes is straightforward even though complete correction of steatorrhea is unusual. Enzyme therapy usually brings diarrhea under control and restores absorption of fat to an acceptable level and affects weight gain. Thus, pancreatic enzyme replacement has been the cornerstone of therapy. In treating steatorrhea, it is important to use a potent pancreatic formulation that will deliver sufficient lipase into the duodenum to correct maldigestion and decrease steatorrhea. In an attempt to standardize the enzyme activity, potency, and bioavailability, the U.S. Food and Drug Administration (FDA) required that all pancreas enzyme drugs in the United States obtain a New Drug Application (NDA) by April 2008. Table 50-8 lists frequently used formulations, but availability will be based on compliance with the FDA mandate. Recent data suggest that dosages up to 80,000–100,000 units of lipase taken during the meal may be necessary to normalize nutritional parameters in malnourished chronic pancreatitis patients, and some may require acid suppression with proton pump inhibitors.

ABDOMINAL PAIN The management of pain in patients with chronic pancreatitis is problematic.

Recent meta-analyses have shown no consistent benefit of *enzyme therapy* at reducing pain in chronic pancreatitis. In some patients with idiopathic chronic pancreatitis, conventional non-enteric-coated enzyme preparations containing high concentrations of serine proteases may relieve mild abdominal pain or discomfort. The pain relief experienced by these patients actually may be due to improvements in the dyspepsia from maldigestion.

Gastroparesis is also quite common in patients with chronic pancreatitis. It is important to recognize and treat with prokinetic drugs because treatment with enzymes may fail simply because gastric dysmotility is interfering with the delivery of enzymes into the upper intestine. A recent prospective study reported that pregabalin can improve pain in chronic pancreatitis and lower pain medication requirement.

Endoscopic treatment of chronic pancreatitis pain may involve sphincterotomy, stenting, stone extraction, and drainage of a pancreatic pseudocyst. Therapy directed to the pancreatic duct would seem to be most appropriate in the setting of a dominant stricture, especially if a ductal stone has led to obstruction. The use of endoscopic stenting for patients

TABLE 50-8

FDA-APPROVED PANCREATIC ENZYME (PANCRELIPASE) PREPARATIONS

	ENZYME CONTENT/UNIT DOSE, U.S. PHARMACOPEIA UNITS		
PRODUCT	**LIPASE[a]**	**AMYLASE[a]**	**PROTEASE[a]**
Immediate-Release Capsule			
Non-enteric-coated			
Viokace 10,440	10,440	391,550	39,150
Viokace 20,880	20,880	78,300	78,300
Delayed-Release Capsules			
Enteric-coated mini-microspheres			
Creon 3000	3000	15,000	9500
Creon 6000	6000	30,000	19,000
Creon 12,000	12,000	60,000	38,000
Creon 24,000	24,000	120,000	76,000
Enteric-Coated Mini-Tablets			
Ultresa 13,800	13,800	27,600	27,600
Ultresa 20,700	20,700	41,400	41,400
Ultresa 23,000	23,000	46,000	46,000
Enteric-Coated Beads			
Zenpep 3000	3000	16,000	10,000
Zenpep 5000	5000	27,000	17,000
Zenpep 10,000	10,000	55,000	34,000
Zenpep 15,000	15,000	82,000	51,000
Zenpep 20,000	20,000	109,000	68,000
Zenpep 25,000	25,000	136,000	85,000
Enteric-Coated Micro-Tablets			
Pancreaze 4200	4200	17,500	10,000
Pancreaze 10,500	10,500	43,750	25,000
Pancreaze 16,800	16,800	70,000	40,000
Pancreaze 21,000	21,000	61,000	37,000
Bicarbonate-Buffered Enteric-Coated Microspheres			
Pertzye 8000	8000	30,250	28,750
Pertzye 16,000	16,000	60,500	57,500

[a]U.S. Pharmacopeia (USP) units per tablet or capsule

Note: The FDA has mandated all enzyme manufacturers to submit New Drug Applications (NDAs) for all pancreatic extract drug products after reviewing data that showed substantial variations among currently marketed products. Numerous manufacturers have investigations under way to seek FDA approval for the treatment of exocrine pancreatic insufficiency due to cystic fibrosis or other conditions under the new guidelines for this class of drugs (*www.fda.gov*).

with chronic pain, but without a dominant stricture, has not been subjected to any controlled trials. It is now appreciated that significant complications can occur from stenting (i.e., bleeding, cholangitis, stent migration, pancreatitis, and stent clogging). In patients with large-duct disease usually from alcohol-induced chronic pancreatitis, ductal decompression with *surgical therapy* has been the therapy of choice. Among such patients, 80% seem to obtain immediate relief; however, at the end of 3 years, one-half of the patients have recurrence of pain. Two randomized prospective trials comparing endoscopic to surgical therapy for chronic pancreatitis demonstrated that surgical therapy was superior to endoscopy at decreasing pain and improving quality of life in selected patients with dilated ducts and abdominal pain. This would suggest that chronic pancreatitis patients with dilated ducts and pain should be considered for surgical intervention. The role of preoperative stenting prior to surgery as a predictor of response has yet to be proven.

A Whipple procedure, total pancreatectomy, and autologous islet cell transplantation have been used in selected patients with chronic pancreatitis and abdominal pain refractory to conventional therapy. The patients who have benefited the most from total pancreatectomy have chronic pancreatitis without prior pancreatic surgery or evidence of islet cell insufficiency. The role of this procedure remains to be fully defined but may be an option in lieu of ductal decompression surgery or pancreatic resection in patients with intractable, painful small-duct disease, particularly as the standard surgical procedures tend to decrease islet cell yield. Celiac plexus block has not resulted in long-lasting pain relief.

HEREDITARY PANCREATITIS

Hereditary pancreatitis is a rare disease that is similar to chronic pancreatitis except for an early age of onset and evidence of hereditary factors. A genome-wide search using genetic linkage analysis identified the hereditary pancreatitis gene on chromosome 7. Mutations in ion codons 29 (exon 2) and 122 (exon 3) of the cationic trypsinogen gene cause autosomal dominant forms of hereditary pancreatitis. The codon 122 mutations lead to a substitution of the corresponding arginine with another amino acid, usually histidine. This substitution, when it occurs, eliminates a fail-safe trypsin self-destruction site necessary to eliminate trypsin that is prematurely activated within the acinar cell. These patients have recurring attacks of severe abdominal pain that may last from a few days to a few weeks. The serum amylase and lipase levels may be elevated during acute attacks but are usually normal. Patients frequently develop pancreatic calcification, diabetes mellitus, and steatorrhea; in addition, they have an increased incidence of pancreatic carcinoma, with the cumulative incidence being as high as 40% by age 70 years. A recent natural history study of hereditary pancreatitis in more than 200 patients from France reported that abdominal pain started in childhood at age 10 years, steatorrhea developed at age 29 years, diabetes at age 38 years, and pancreatic carcinoma at age 55 years. Such patients often require surgical ductal decompression for pain relief. Abdominal complaints in relatives of patients with hereditary pancreatitis should raise the question of pancreatic disease.

PSTI, or SPINK1, is a 56-amino-acid peptide that specifically inhibits trypsin by physically blocking its active site. SPINK1 acts as the first line of defense against prematurely activated trypsinogen in the acinar cell. Recently, it has been shown that the frequency of SPINK1 mutations in patients with idiopathic chronic pancreatitis is markedly increased, suggesting that these mutations may be associated with pancreatitis.

PANCREATIC ENDOCRINE TUMORS

Pancreatic endocrine tumors are discussed in Chap. 55.

OTHER CONDITIONS

ANNULAR PANCREAS

When the ventral pancreatic anlage fails to migrate correctly to make contact with the dorsal anlage, the result may be a ring of pancreatic tissue encircling the duodenum. Such an annular pancreas may cause intestinal obstruction in the neonate or the adult. Symptoms of postprandial fullness, epigastric pain, nausea, and vomiting may be present for years before the diagnosis is entertained. The radiographic findings are symmetric dilation of the proximal duodenum with bulging of the recesses on either side of the annular band, effacement but not destruction of the duodenal mucosa, accentuation of the findings in the right anterior oblique position, and lack of change on repeated examinations. The differential diagnosis should include duodenal webs, tumors of the pancreas or duodenum, postbulbar peptic ulcer, regional enteritis, and adhesions. Patients with annular pancreas have an increased incidence of pancreatitis and peptic ulcer. Because of these and other potential complications, the treatment is surgical even if the condition has been present for years. Retrocolic duodenojejeunostomy is the procedure of choice, although some surgeons advocate Billroth II gastrectomy, gastroenterostomy, and vagotomy.

PANCREAS DIVISUM

Pancreas divisum is present in 7–10% of the population and occurs when the embryologic ventral and dorsal pancreatic anlagen fail to fuse, so that pancreatic drainage is accomplished mainly through the accessory papilla. Pancreas divisum is the most common congenital anatomic variant of the human pancreas. Current evidence indicates that this anomaly does not predispose to the development of pancreatitis in the great majority of patients who harbor it. However, the combination of pancreas divisum and a small accessory orifice could result in dorsal duct obstruction. The challenge is to identify this subset of patients with dorsal duct pathology. Cannulation of the dorsal duct by ERCP is not as easily done as is cannulation of the ventral duct. Patients with pancreatitis and pancreas divisum demonstrated by MRCP or ERCP should be treated with conservative measures. In many of these patients, pancreatitis is idiopathic and unrelated to the pancreas divisum. Endoscopic or surgical intervention is indicated only if pancreatitis recurs and no other cause can be found. If marked dilation of the dorsal duct can be demonstrated, surgical ductal decompression should be performed. It should be stressed that the ERCP/MRCP appearance of pancreas divisum (i.e., a small-caliber ventral duct with an arborizing pattern) may be mistaken as representing an obstructed main pancreatic duct secondary to a mass lesion.

MACROAMYLASEMIA

In macroamylasemia, amylase circulates in the blood in a polymer form too large to be easily excreted by the kidney. Patients with this condition demonstrate an elevated serum amylase value and a low urinary amylase value. The presence of macroamylase can be documented by chromatography of the serum. The prevalence of macroamylasemia is 1.5% of the nonalcoholic general adult hospital population. Usually macroamylasemia is an incidental finding and is not related to disease of the pancreas or other organs. Macrolipasemia has now been documented in a few patients with cirrhosis or non-Hodgkin's lymphoma. In these patients, the pancreas appeared normal on ultrasound and CT examination. Lipase was shown to be complexed with immunoglobulin A. Thus, the possibility of *both* macroamylasemia and macrolipasemia should be considered in patients with elevated blood levels of these enzymes.

Acknowledgments

This chapter represents a revised version of chapters by Drs. Norton J. Greenberger, Phillip P. Toskes, and Bechien Wu that were in previous editions of Harrison's.

SECTION IX

NEOPLASTIC DISEASES OF THE GASTROINTESTINAL SYSTEM

CHAPTER 51

UPPER GASTROINTESTINAL TRACT CANCERS

Robert J. Mayer

Upper gastrointestinal cancers include malignancies arising in the esophagus, stomach, and small intestine.

ESOPHAGEAL CANCER

INCIDENCE AND ETIOLOGY

Cancer of the esophagus is an increasingly common and extremely lethal malignancy. The diagnosis was made in 18,170 Americans in 2014 and led to 15,450 deaths. Almost all esophageal cancers are either squamous cell carcinomas or adenocarcinomas; the two histologic subtypes have a similar clinical presentation but different causative factors.

Worldwide, squamous cell carcinoma is the more common cell type, having an incidence that rises strikingly in association with geographic location. It occurs frequently within a region extending from the southern shore of the Caspian Sea on the west to northern China on the east, encompassing parts of Iran, central Asia, Afghanistan, Siberia, and Mongolia. Familial increased risk has been observed in regions with high incidence, although gene associations are not yet defined. High-incidence "pockets" of the disease are also present in such disparate locations as Finland, Iceland, Curaçao, southeastern Africa, and northwestern France. In North America and western Europe, the disease is more common in blacks than whites and in males than females; it appears most often after age 50 and seems to be associated with a lower socioeconomic status. Such cancers generally arise in the cervical and thoracic portions of the esophagus.

A variety of causative factors have been implicated in the development of squamous cell cancers of the esophagus (Table 51-1). In the United States, the etiology of such cancers is primarily related to excess alcohol consumption and/or cigarette smoking. The relative risk increases with the amount of tobacco smoked or alcohol consumed, with these factors acting synergistically. The consumption of whiskey is linked to a higher incidence than the consumption of wine or beer. Squamous cell esophageal carcinoma has also been associated with the ingestion of nitrates, smoked opiates, and fungal toxins in pickled vegetables, as well as mucosal damage caused by such physical insults as long-term exposure to extremely hot tea, the ingestion of lye, radiation-induced strictures, and chronic achalasia. The presence of an esophageal web in association with glossitis and iron deficiency (i.e., Plummer-Vinson or Paterson-Kelly syndrome) and congenital hyperkeratosis and pitting of the palms and soles (i.e., tylosis palmaris et plantaris) have each been linked with squamous cell esophageal cancer, as have dietary deficiencies of molybdenum, zinc, selenium, and vitamin A. Patients with head and neck cancer are at increased risk of squamous cell cancer of the esophagus.

TABLE 51-1

SOME ETIOLOGIC FACTORS ASSOCIATED WITH SQUAMOUS CELL CANCER OF THE ESOPHAGUS
Excess alcohol consumption
Cigarette smoking
Other ingested carcinogens
Nitrates (converted to nitrites)
Smoked opiates
Fungal toxins in pickled vegetables
Mucosal damage from physical agents
Hot tea
Lye ingestion
Radiation-induced strictures
Chronic achalasia
Host susceptibility
Esophageal web with glossitis and iron deficiency (i.e., Plummer-Vinson or Paterson-Kelly syndrome)
Congenital hyperkeratosis and pitting of the palms and soles (i.e., tylosis palmaris et plantaris)
? Dietary deficiencies of selenium, molybdenum, zinc, and vitamin A

TABLE 51-2

SOME ETIOLOGIC FACTORS ASSOCIATED WITH ADENOCARCINOMA OF THE ESOPHAGUS
Chronic gastroesophageal reflux
Obesity
Barrett's esophagus
Male sex
Cigarette smoking

For unclear reasons, the incidence of squamous cell esophageal cancer has decreased somewhat in both the black and white populations in the United States over the past 40 years, whereas the rate of adenocarcinoma has risen sevenfold, particularly in white males (male-to-female ratio of 6:1). Whereas squamous cell cancers comprised the vast majority of esophageal cancers in the United States as recently as 40–50 years ago, more than 75% of esophageal tumors are now adenocarcinomas, with the incidence of this histologic subtype continuing to increase rapidly. Understanding the cause for this increase is the focus of current investigation.

Several strong etiologic associations have been observed to account for the development of adenocarcinoma of the esophagus (Table 51-2). Such tumors arise in the distal esophagus in association with chronic gastric reflux, often in the presence of Barrett's esophagus (replacement of the normal squamous epithelium of the distal esophagus by columnar mucosa), which occurs more commonly in obese individuals. Adenocarcinomas arise within dysplastic columnar epithelium in the distal esophagus. Even before frank neoplasia is detectable, aneuploidy and *p53* mutations are found in the dysplastic epithelium. These adenocarcinomas behave clinically like gastric adenocarcinomas, although they are not associated with *Helicobacter pylori* infections. Approximately 15% of esophageal adenocarcinomas overexpress the *HER2/neu* gene.

CLINICAL FEATURES

About 5% of esophageal cancers occur in the upper third of the esophagus (cervical esophagus), 20% in the middle third, and 75% in the lower third. Squamous cell carcinomas and adenocarcinomas cannot be distinguished radiographically or endoscopically.

Progressive dysphagia and weight loss of short duration are the initial symptoms in the vast majority of patients. Dysphagia initially occurs with solid foods and gradually progresses to include semisolids and liquids. By the time these symptoms develop, the disease is already very advanced, because difficulty in swallowing does not occur until >60% of the esophageal circumference is infiltrated with cancer. Dysphagia may be associated with pain on swallowing (odynophagia), pain radiating to the chest and/or back, regurgitation or vomiting, and aspiration pneumonia. The disease most commonly spreads to adjacent and supraclavicular lymph nodes, liver, lungs, pleura, and bone. Tracheoesophageal fistulas may develop, primarily in patients with upper and mid-esophageal tumors. As with other squamous cell carcinomas, hypercalcemia may occur in the absence of osseous metastases, probably from parathormone-related peptide secreted by tumor cells.

DIAGNOSIS

Attempts at endoscopic and cytologic screening for carcinoma in patients with Barrett's esophagus, while effective as a means of detecting high-grade dysplasia, have not yet been shown to reduce the likelihood of death from esophageal adenocarcinoma. Esophagoscopy should be performed in all patients suspected of having an esophageal abnormality, to both visualize and identify a tumor and also to obtain histopathologic confirmation of the diagnosis. Because the population of persons at risk for squamous cell carcinoma of the esophagus (i.e., smokers and drinkers) also has a high rate of cancers of the lung and the head and neck region, endoscopic inspection of the larynx, trachea, and bronchi should also be carried out. A thorough examination of the fundus of the stomach (by retroflexing the endoscope) is imperative as well. The extent of tumor spread to the mediastinum and para-aortic lymph nodes should be assessed by computed tomography (CT) scans of the chest and abdomen and by endoscopic ultrasound. Positron emission tomography scanning provides a useful assessment of the presence of distant metastatic disease, offering accurate information regarding spread to mediastinal lymph nodes, which can be helpful in defining radiation therapy fields. Such scans, when performed sequentially, appear to provide a means of making an early assessment of responsiveness to preoperative chemotherapy.

TREATMENT Esophageal Cancer

The prognosis for patients with esophageal carcinoma is poor. Approximately 10% of patients survive 5 years after the diagnosis; thus, management focuses on symptom control. Surgical resection of all gross tumor (i.e., total resection) is feasible in only 45% of cases, with residual tumor cells frequently present at the resection margins. Such esophagectomies have been associated with a postoperative mortality rate of approximately 5% due to anastomotic fistulas, subphrenic abscesses, and cardiopulmonary complications. Although debate regarding the comparative benefits of transthoracic versus transhiatal resections has continued, experienced thoracic surgeons are now favoring minimally invasive transthoracic esophagectomies. Endoscopic resections of superficial squamous cell cancers or adenocarcinomas are being examined but have not yet been shown to result in a similar likelihood of survival as observed with conventional surgical procedures. Similarly, the value of endoscopic ablation of dysplastic lesions in an area of Barrett's esophagus on reducing subsequent mortality from esophageal carcinoma is uncertain. Some experts have advocated fundoplication surgery (i.e., the removal of the gastroesophageal junction) as a means of cancer prevention in patients with Barrett's esophagus; again, objective data are not yet available to fully assess the risks versus benefits of this invasive procedure. About 20% of patients who survive a total surgical resection live for 5 years. The evaluation of chemotherapeutic agents in patients with esophageal carcinoma has been hampered by ambiguity in the definition of "response" and the debilitated physical condition of many treated individuals, particularly those with squamous cell cancers. Nonetheless, significant reductions in the size of measurable tumor masses have been reported in 15–25% of patients given single-agent treatment and in 30–60% of patients treated with drug combinations that include cisplatin. In the small subset of patients whose tumors overexpress the *HER2/neu* gene, the addition of the monoclonal antibody trastuzumab (Herceptin) appears to further enhance the likelihood of benefit, particularly in patients with gastroesophageal lesions. The use of the antiangiogenic agent bevacizumab (Avastin) seems to be of limited value in the setting of esophageal cancer. Combination chemotherapy and radiation therapy as the initial therapeutic approach, either alone or followed by an attempt at operative resection, seems to be beneficial. When administered along with radiation therapy, chemotherapy produces a better survival outcome than radiation therapy alone. The use of preoperative chemotherapy and radiation therapy followed by esophageal resection appears to prolong survival compared with surgery alone according to several randomized trials and a meta-analysis; some reports suggest that no additional benefit accrues when surgery is added if significant shrinkage of tumor has been achieved by the chemoradiation combination.

For the incurable, surgically unresectable patient with esophageal cancer, dysphagia, malnutrition, and the management of tracheoesophageal fistulas are major issues. Approaches to palliation include repeated endoscopic dilatation, the surgical placement of a gastrostomy or jejunostomy for hydration and feeding, endoscopic placement of an expansive metal stent to bypass the tumor, and radiation therapy.

TUMORS OF THE STOMACH

GASTRIC ADENOCARCINOMA

Incidence and epidemiology

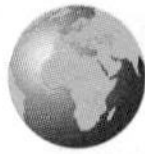

For unclear reasons, the incidence and mortality rates for gastric cancer have decreased in the United States during the past 80 years, although the disease remains the second most frequent cause of worldwide cancer-related death. The mortality rate from gastric cancer in the United States has dropped in men from 28 to 5.8 per 100,000 persons, whereas in women, the rate has decreased from 27 to 2.8 per 100,000. Nonetheless, in 2014, 22,220 new cases of stomach cancer were diagnosed in the United States, and 10,990 Americans died of the disease. Although the incidence of gastric cancer has decreased worldwide, it remains high in such disparate geographic regions as Japan, China, Chile, and Ireland.

The risk of gastric cancer is greater among lower socioeconomic classes. Migrants from high- to low-incidence nations maintain their susceptibility to gastric cancer, whereas the risk for their offspring approximates that of the new homeland. These findings suggest that an environmental exposure, probably beginning early in life, is related to the development of gastric cancer, with dietary carcinogens considered the most likely factor(s).

Pathology

About 85% of stomach cancers are adenocarcinomas, with 15% due to lymphomas, gastrointestinal stromal tumors (GISTs), and leiomyosarcomas. Gastric adenocarcinomas may be subdivided into two categories: a *diffuse type*, in which cell cohesion is absent, so that individual cells infiltrate and thicken the stomach wall without forming a discrete mass; and an *intestinal type*, characterized by cohesive neoplastic cells that form glandlike tubular structures. The diffuse carcinomas occur more often in younger patients, develop throughout the stomach (including the cardia), result in a loss of distensibility of the gastric wall (so-called *linitis plastica*, or "leather bottle" appearance), and carry a poorer prognosis. Diffuse cancers have defective intercellular adhesion, mainly as a consequence of loss of expression of E-cadherin. Intestinal-type lesions are frequently ulcerative, more commonly appear in the antrum and lesser curvature of the stomach, and are often preceded by a prolonged precancerous process, often initiated by *H. pylori* infection. Although the incidence of diffuse carcinomas is similar in most populations, the intestinal type tends to predominate in the high-risk geographic regions and is less likely to be found in areas where the frequency of gastric cancer is declining. Thus, different etiologic factor(s) are likely involved in these two subtypes. In the United States, ~30% of gastric cancers originate in the distal stomach, ~20% arise in the midportion of the stomach, and ~40% originate in the proximal third of the stomach. The remaining 10% involve the entire stomach.

Etiology

The long-term ingestion of high concentrations of nitrates found in dried, smoked, and salted foods

TABLE 51-3

NITRATE-CONVERTING BACTERIA AS A FACTOR IN THE CAUSATION OF GASTRIC CARCINOMA[a]
Exogenous sources of nitrate-converting bacteria:
Bacterially contaminated food (common in lower socioeconomic classes, who have a higher incidence of the disease; diminished by improved food preservation and refrigeration)
Helicobacter pylori infection
Endogenous factors favoring growth of nitrate-converting bacteria in the stomach:
Decreased gastric acidity
Prior gastric surgery (antrectomy) (15- to 20-year latency period)
Atrophic gastritis and/or pernicious anemia
? Prolonged exposure to histamine H_2-receptor antagonists

[a]Hypothesis: Dietary nitrates are converted to carcinogenic nitrites by bacteria.

appears to be associated with a higher risk. The nitrates are thought to be converted to carcinogenic nitrites by bacteria (Table 51-3). Such bacteria may be introduced exogenously through the ingestion of partially decayed foods, which are consumed in abundance worldwide by the lower socioeconomic classes. Bacteria such as *H. pylori* may also contribute to this effect by causing chronic inflammatory atrophic gastritis, loss of gastric acidity, and bacterial growth in the stomach. Although the risk for developing gastric cancer is thought to be sixfold higher in people infected with *H. pylori*, it remains uncertain whether eradicating the bacteria after infection has already occurred actually reduces this risk. Loss of acidity may occur when acid-producing cells of the gastric antrum have been removed surgically to control benign peptic ulcer disease or when achlorhydria, atrophic gastritis, and even pernicious anemia develop in the elderly. Serial endoscopic examinations of the stomach in patients with atrophic gastritis have documented replacement of the usual gastric mucosa by intestinal-type cells. This process of intestinal metaplasia may lead to cellular atypia and eventual neoplasia. Because the declining incidence of gastric cancer in the United States primarily reflects a decline in distal, ulcerating, intestinal-type lesions, it is conceivable that better food preservation and the availability of refrigeration for all socioeconomic classes have decreased the dietary ingestion of exogenous bacteria. *H. pylori* has not been associated with the diffuse, more proximal form of gastric carcinoma or with cancers arising at the gastroesophageal junction or in the distal esophagus. Approximately 10–15% of adenocarcinomas appearing in the proximal stomach, the gastroesophageal junction, and the distal esophagus overexpress the *HER2/neu* gene; individuals whose tumors demonstrate this overexpression benefit from treatment directed against this target (i.e., trastuzumab [Herceptin]).

Several additional etiologic factors have been associated with gastric carcinoma. Gastric ulcers and adenomatous polyps have occasionally been linked, but data on a cause-and-effect relationship are unconvincing. The inadequate clinical distinction between benign gastric ulcers and small ulcerating carcinomas may, in part, account for this presumed association. The presence of extreme hypertrophy of gastric rugal folds (i.e., Ménétrier's disease), giving the impression of polypoid lesions, has been associated with a striking frequency of malignant transformation; such hypertrophy, however, does not represent the presence of true adenomatous polyps. Individuals with blood group A have a higher incidence of gastric cancer than persons with blood group O; this observation may be related to differences in the mucous secretion, leading to altered mucosal protection from carcinogens. A germline mutation in the E-cadherin gene (*CDH1*), inherited in an autosomal dominant pattern and coding for a cell adhesion protein, has been linked to a high incidence of occult diffuse-type gastric cancers in young asymptomatic carriers. Duodenal ulcers are not associated with gastric cancer.

Clinical features

Gastric cancers, when superficial and surgically curable, usually produce no symptoms. As the tumor becomes more extensive, patients may complain of an insidious upper abdominal discomfort varying in intensity from a vague, postprandial fullness to a severe, steady pain. Anorexia, often with slight nausea, is very common but is not the usual presenting complaint. Weight loss may eventually be observed, and nausea and vomiting are particularly prominent in patients whose tumors involve the pylorus; dysphagia and early satiety may be the major symptoms caused by diffuse lesions originating in the cardia. There may be no early physical signs. A palpable abdominal mass indicates long-standing growth and predicts regional extension.

Gastric carcinomas spread by direct extension through the gastric wall to the perigastric tissues, occasionally adhering to adjacent organs such as the pancreas, colon, or liver. The disease also spreads via lymphatics or by seeding of peritoneal surfaces. Metastases to intraabdominal and supraclavicular lymph nodes occur frequently, as do metastatic nodules to the ovary (Krukenberg's tumor), periumbilical region ("Sister Mary Joseph node"), or peritoneal cul-de-sac (Blumer's shelf palpable on rectal or vaginal examination); malignant ascites may also develop. The liver is the most common site for hematogenous spread of tumor.

The presence of iron-deficiency anemia in men and of occult blood in the stool in both sexes mandates a search for an occult gastrointestinal tract lesion. A careful assessment is of particular importance in patients with atrophic gastritis or pernicious anemia. Unusual clinical features associated with gastric adenocarcinomas include migratory thrombophlebitis, microangiopathic hemolytic anemia, diffuse seborrheic keratoses (so-called Leser-Trélat sign), and acanthosis nigricans.

Diagnosis

The use of double-contrast radiographic examinations has been supplanted by esophagogastroscopy and CT scanning for the evaluation of patients with epigastric complaints.

Gastric ulcers identified at the time of such endoscopic procedure may appear benign but merit biopsy in order to exclude a malignancy. Malignant gastric ulcers must be recognized before they penetrate into surrounding tissues, because the rate of cure of early lesions limited to the mucosa or submucosa is >80%. Because gastric carcinomas are difficult to distinguish clinically or endoscopically from gastric lymphomas, endoscopic biopsies should be made as deeply as possible, due to the submucosal location of lymphoid tumors.

The staging system for gastric carcinoma is shown in Table 51-4.

TREATMENT Adenocarcinoma

Complete surgical removal of the tumor with resection of adjacent lymph nodes offers the only chance for cure. However, this is possible in less than a third of patients. A subtotal gastrectomy is the treatment of choice for patients with distal carcinomas, whereas total or near-total gastrectomies are required for more proximal tumors. The inclusion of extended lymph node dissection in these procedures appears to confer an added risk for complications without providing a meaningful enhancement in survival. The prognosis following complete surgical resection depends on the degree of tumor penetration into the stomach wall and is adversely influenced by regional lymph node involvement and vascular invasion, characteristics found in the vast majority of American patients. As a result, the probability of survival after 5 years for the 25–30% of patients able to undergo complete resection is ~20% for distal tumors and <10% for proximal tumors, with recurrences continuing for at least 8 years after surgery. In the absence of ascites or extensive hepatic or peritoneal metastases, even patients whose disease is believed to be incurable by surgery should be offered resection of the primary lesion. Reduction of tumor bulk is the best form of palliation and may enhance the probability of benefit from subsequent therapy. In high-incidence regions such as Japan and Korea, where the use of endoscopic screening programs has identified patients with superficial tumors, the use of laparoscopic gastrectomy has gained popularity. In the United

TABLE 51-4

STAGING SYSTEM FOR GASTRIC CARCINOMA

			DATA FROM ACS IN THE UNITED STATES	
STAGE	**TNM**	**FEATURES**	**NO. OF CASES, %**	**5-YEAR SURVIVAL, %**
0	$T_{is}N0M0$	Node negative; limited to mucosa	1	90
IA	T1N0M0	Node negative; invasion of lamina propria or submucosa	7	59
IB	T2N0M0 T1N1M0	Node negative; invasion of muscularis propria	10	44
II	T1N2M0 T2N1M0	Node positive; invasion beyond mucosa but within wall	17	29
		or		
	T3N0M0	Node negative; extension through wall		
IIIA	T2N2M0 T3N1-2M0	Node positive; invasion of muscularis propria or through wall	21	15
IIIB	T4N0-1M0	Node negative; adherence to surrounding tissue	14	9
IIIC	T4N2-3M0	>3 nodes positive; invasion of serosa or adjacent structures		
	T3N3M0	7 or more positive nodes; penetrates wall without invading serosa or adjacent structures		
IV	T4N2M0	Node positive; adherence to surrounding tissue	30	3
		or		
	T1-4N0-2-M1	Distant metastases		

Abbreviations: ACS, American Cancer Society; TNM, tumor, node, metastasis.

States and western Europe, the use of this less invasive surgical approach remains investigational.

Gastric adenocarcinoma is a relatively radioresistant tumor, and the adequate control of the primary tumor requires doses of external-beam irradiation that exceed the tolerance of surrounding structures, such as bowel mucosa and spinal cord. As a result, the major role of radiation therapy in patients has been palliation of pain. Radiation therapy alone after a complete resection does not prolong survival. In the setting of surgically unresectable disease limited to the epigastrium, patients treated with 3500–4000 cGy did not live longer than similar patients not receiving radiotherapy; however, survival was prolonged slightly when 5-fluorouracil (5-FU) plus leucovorin was given in combination with radiation therapy (3-year survival 50% vs 41% for radiation therapy alone). In this clinical setting, the 5-FU likely functions as a radiosensitizer.

The administration of combinations of cytotoxic drugs to patients with advanced gastric carcinoma has been associated with partial responses in 30–50% of cases; responders appear to benefit from treatment. Such drug combinations have generally included cisplatin combined with epirubicin or docetaxel and infusional 5-FU or capecitabine, or with irinotecan. Despite the encouraging response rates, complete remissions are uncommon, the partial responses are transient, and the overall impact of multidrug therapy on survival has been limited; the median survival time for patients treated in this manner remains less than 12 months. As with adenocarcinomas arising in the esophagus, the addition of bevacizumab (Avastin) to chemotherapy regimens in treating gastric cancer appears to provide limited benefit. However, preliminary results utilizing another antiangiogenic compound—ramucirumab (Cyranza)—in the treatment of gastric cancer are encouraging. The use of adjuvant chemotherapy alone following the complete resection of a gastric cancer has only minimally improved survival. However, combination chemotherapy administered before and after surgery (*perioperative treatment*) as well as postoperative chemotherapy combined with radiation therapy reduces the recurrence rate and prolongs survival.

PRIMARY GASTRIC LYMPHOMA

Primary lymphoma of the stomach is relatively uncommon, accounting for <15% of gastric malignancies and ~2% of all lymphomas. The stomach is, however, the most frequent extranodal site for lymphoma, and gastric lymphoma has increased in frequency during the past 35 years. The disease is difficult to distinguish clinically from gastric adenocarcinoma; both tumors are most often detected during the sixth decade of life; present with epigastric pain, early satiety, and generalized fatigue; and are usually characterized by ulcerations with a ragged, thickened mucosal pattern demonstrated by contrast radiographs or endoscopic appearance. The diagnosis of lymphoma of the stomach may occasionally be made through cytologic brushings of the gastric mucosa but usually requires a biopsy at gastroscopy or laparotomy. Failure of gastroscopic biopsies to detect lymphoma in a given case should not be interpreted as being conclusive, because superficial biopsies may miss the deeper lymphoid infiltrate. The macroscopic pathology of gastric lymphoma may also mimic adenocarcinoma, consisting of either a bulky ulcerated lesion localized in the corpus or antrum or a diffuse process spreading throughout the entire gastric submucosa and even extending into the duodenum. Microscopically, the vast majority of gastric lymphoid tumors are lymphomas of B-cell origin. Histologically, these tumors may range from well-differentiated, superficial processes (mucosa-associated lymphoid tissue [MALT]) to high-grade, large-cell lymphomas. Like gastric adenocarcinoma, infection with *H. pylori* increases the risk for gastric lymphoma in general and MALT lymphomas in particular. Large-cell lymphomas of the stomach spread initially to regional lymph nodes (often to Waldeyer's ring) and may then disseminate.

TREATMENT Primary Gastric Lymphoma

Primary gastric lymphoma is a far more treatable disease than adenocarcinoma of the stomach, a fact that underscores the need for making the correct diagnosis. Antibiotic treatment to eradicate *H. pylori* infection has led to regression of about 75% of gastric MALT lymphomas and should be considered before surgery, radiation therapy, or chemotherapy is undertaken in patients having such tumors. A lack of response to such antimicrobial treatment has been linked to a specific chromosomal abnormality, i.e., t(11;18). Responding patients should undergo periodic endoscopic surveillance because it remains unclear whether the neoplastic clone is eliminated or merely suppressed, although the response to antimicrobial treatment is quite durable. Subtotal gastrectomy, usually followed by combination chemotherapy, has led to 5-year survival rates of 40–60% in patients with localized high-grade lymphomas. The need for a major surgical procedure has been questioned, particularly in patients with preoperative radiographic evidence of nodal involvement, for whom chemotherapy (CHOP [cyclophosphamide, doxorubicin, vincristine, and prednisone]) plus rituximab is highly effective therapy. A role for radiation therapy is not defined because most recurrences develop at distant sites.

GASTRIC (NONLYMPHOID) SARCOMA

Leiomyosarcomas and GISTs make up 1–3% of gastric neoplasms. They most frequently involve the anterior and posterior walls of the gastric fundus and often ulcerate and bleed. Even those lesions that appear benign on histologic examination may behave in a malignant fashion. These tumors rarely invade adjacent viscera and characteristically do not metastasize to lymph nodes, but they may spread to the liver and lungs. The treatment of choice is surgical resection. Combination chemotherapy should be reserved for patients with metastatic disease. All such tumors should be analyzed for a mutation in the c-*kit* receptor. GISTs are unresponsive to conventional chemotherapy; yet ~50% of patients experience objective response and prolonged survival when treated with imatinib mesylate (Gleevec) (400–800 mg PO daily), a selective inhibitor of the c-*kit* tyrosine kinase. Many patients with GIST whose tumors have become refractory to imatinib subsequently benefit from sunitinib (Sutent) or regorafenib (Stivarga), other inhibitors of the c-*kit* tyrosine kinase.

TUMORS OF THE SMALL INTESTINE

Small-bowel tumors comprise <3% of gastrointestinal neoplasms. Because of their rarity and inaccessibility, a correct diagnosis is often delayed. Abdominal symptoms are usually vague and poorly defined, and conventional radiographic studies of the upper and lower intestinal tract often appear normal. Small-bowel tumors should be considered in the differential diagnosis in the following situations: (1) recurrent, unexplained episodes of crampy abdominal pain; (2) intermittent bouts of intestinal obstruction, especially in the absence of inflammatory bowel disease (IBD) or prior abdominal surgery; (3) intussusception in the adult; and (4) evidence of chronic intestinal bleeding in the presence of negative conventional and endoscopic examination. A careful small-bowel barium study should be considered in such a circumstance; the diagnostic accuracy may be improved by infusing barium through a nasogastric tube placed into the duodenum (enteroclysis). Alternatively, capsule endoscopic procedures have been used.

BENIGN TUMORS

The histology of benign small-bowel tumors is difficult to predict on clinical and radiologic grounds alone. The symptomatology of benign tumors is not distinctive, with pain, obstruction, and hemorrhage being the most frequent symptoms. These tumors are usually discovered during the fifth and sixth decades of life, more often in the distal rather than the proximal small intestine. The most common benign tumors are adenomas, leiomyomas, lipomas, and angiomas.

Adenomas

These tumors include those of the islet cells and Brunner's glands as well as polypoid adenomas. *Islet cell adenomas* are occasionally located outside the pancreas; the associated syndromes are discussed in **Chap. 55**. *Brunner's gland adenomas* are not truly neoplastic but represent a hypertrophy or hyperplasia of submucosal duodenal glands. These appear as small nodules in the duodenal mucosa that secrete a highly viscous alkaline mucus. Most often, this is an incidental radiographic finding not associated with any specific clinical disorder.

Polypoid adenomas

About 25% of benign small-bowel tumors are polypoid adenomas **(see Table 52-2)**. They may present as single polypoid lesions or, less commonly, as papillary villous adenomas. As in the colon, the sessile or papillary form of the tumor is sometimes associated with a coexisting carcinoma. Occasionally, patients with Gardner's syndrome develop premalignant adenomas in the small bowel; such lesions are generally in the duodenum. Multiple polypoid tumors may occur throughout the small bowel (and occasionally the stomach and colorectum) in the Peutz-Jeghers syndrome. The polyps are usually hamartomas (juvenile polyps) having a low potential for malignant degeneration. Mucocutaneous melanin deposits as well as tumors of the ovary, breast, pancreas, and endometrium are also associated with this autosomal dominant condition.

Leiomyomas

These neoplasms arise from smooth-muscle components of the intestine and are usually intramural, affecting the overlying mucosa. Ulceration of the mucosa may cause gastrointestinal hemorrhage of varying severity. Cramping or intermittent abdominal pain is frequently encountered.

Lipomas

These tumors occur with greatest frequency in the distal ileum and at the ileocecal valve. They have a characteristic radiolucent appearance and are usually intramural and asymptomatic, but on occasion cause bleeding.

Angiomas

While not true neoplasms, these lesions are important because they frequently cause intestinal bleeding. They may take the form of telangiectasia or hemangiomas. Multiple intestinal telangiectasias occur in a nonhereditary form confined to the gastrointestinal tract or as part of the hereditary Osler-Rendu-Weber syndrome. Vascular tumors may also take the form of isolated hemangiomas, most commonly in the jejunum.

Angiography, especially during bleeding, is the best procedure for evaluating these lesions.

MALIGNANT TUMORS

While rare, small-bowel malignancies occur in patients with long-standing regional enteritis and celiac sprue as well as in individuals with AIDS. Malignant tumors of the small bowel are frequently associated with fever, weight loss, anorexia, bleeding, and a palpable abdominal mass. After ampullary carcinomas (many of which arise from biliary or pancreatic ducts), the most frequently occurring small-bowel malignancies are adenocarcinomas, lymphomas, carcinoid tumors, and leiomyosarcomas.

ADENOCARCINOMAS

The most common primary cancers of the small bowel are adenocarcinomas, accounting for ~50% of malignant tumors. These cancers occur most often in the distal duodenum and proximal jejunum, where they tend to ulcerate and cause hemorrhage or obstruction. Radiologically, they may be confused with chronic duodenal ulcer disease or with Crohn's disease if the patient has long-standing regional enteritis. The diagnosis is best made by endoscopy and biopsy under direct vision. Surgical resection is the treatment of choice with suggested postoperative adjuvant chemotherapy options generally following treatment patterns used in the management of colon cancer.

LYMPHOMAS

Lymphoma in the small bowel may be primary or secondary. A diagnosis of a primary intestinal lymphoma requires histologic confirmation in a clinical setting in which palpable adenopathy and hepatosplenomegaly are absent and no evidence of lymphoma is seen on chest radiograph, CT scan, or peripheral blood smear or on bone marrow aspiration and biopsy. Symptoms referable to the small bowel are present, usually accompanied by an anatomically discernible lesion. Secondary lymphoma of the small bowel consists of involvement of the intestine by a lymphoid malignancy extending from involved retroperitoneal or mesenteric lymph nodes.

Primary intestinal lymphoma accounts for ~20% of malignancies of the small bowel. These neoplasms are non-Hodgkin's lymphomas; they usually have a diffuse, large-cell histology and are of T cell origin. Intestinal lymphoma involves the ileum, jejunum, and duodenum, in decreasing frequency—a pattern that mirrors the relative amount of normal lymphoid cells in these anatomic areas. The risk of small-bowel lymphoma is increased in patients with a prior history of malabsorptive conditions (e.g., celiac sprue), regional enteritis, and depressed immune function due to congenital immunodeficiency syndromes, prior organ transplantation, autoimmune disorders, or AIDS.

The development of localized or nodular masses that narrow the lumen results in periumbilical pain (made worse by eating) as well as weight loss, vomiting, and occasional intestinal obstruction. The diagnosis of small-bowel lymphoma may be suspected from the appearance on contrast radiographs of patterns such as infiltration and thickening of mucosal folds, mucosal nodules, areas of irregular ulceration, or stasis of contrast material. The diagnosis can be confirmed by surgical exploration and resection of involved segments. Intestinal lymphoma can occasionally be diagnosed by peroral intestinal mucosal biopsy, but because the disease mainly involves the lamina propria, full-thickness surgical biopsies are usually required.

Resection of the tumor constitutes the initial treatment modality. While postoperative radiation therapy has been given to some patients following a total resection, most authorities favor short-term (three cycles) systemic treatment with combination chemotherapy. The frequent presence of widespread intraabdominal disease at the time of diagnosis and the occasional multicentricity of the tumor often make a total resection impossible. The probability of sustained remission or cure is ~75% in patients with localized disease but is ~25% in individuals with unresectable lymphoma. In patients whose tumors are not resected, chemotherapy may lead to bowel perforation.

A unique form of small-bowel lymphoma, diffusely involving the entire intestine, was first described in oriental Jews and Arabs and is referred to as *immunoproliferative small intestinal disease* (IPSID), *Mediterranean lymphoma*, or *α heavy chain disease*. This is a B cell tumor. The typical presentation includes chronic diarrhea and steatorrhea associated with vomiting and abdominal cramps; clubbing of the digits may be observed. A curious feature in many patients with IPSID is the presence in the blood and intestinal secretions of an abnormal IgA that contains a shortened α heavy chain and is devoid of light chains. It is suspected that the abnormal α chains are produced by plasma cells infiltrating the small bowel. The clinical course of patients with IPSID is generally one of exacerbations and remissions, with death frequently resulting from either progressive malnutrition and wasting or the development of an aggressive lymphoma. The use of oral antibiotics such as tetracycline appears to be beneficial in the early phases of the disorder, suggesting a possible infectious etiology. Combination chemotherapy has been administered during later stages of the disease, with variable results. Results are better when antibiotics and chemotherapy are combined.

CARCINOID TUMORS

Carcinoid tumors arise from argentaffin cells of the crypts of Lieberkühn and are found from the distal duodenum to the ascending colon, areas embryologically derived from the midgut. More than 50% of intestinal carcinoids are found in the distal ileum, with most congregating close to the ileocecal valve. Most intestinal carcinoids are asymptomatic and of low malignant potential, but invasion and metastases may occur, leading to the carcinoid syndrome (**Chap. 55**).

LEIOMYOSARCOMAS

Leiomyosarcomas often are >5 cm in diameter and may be palpable on abdominal examination. Bleeding, obstruction, and perforation are common. Such tumors should be analyzed for the expression of mutant c-*kit* receptor (defining GIST), and in the presence of metastatic disease, justifying treatment with imatinib mesylate (Gleevec) or, in imatinib-refractory patients, sunitinib (Sutent) or regorafenib (Stivarga).

CHAPTER 52

LOWER GASTROINTESTINAL CANCERS

Robert J. Mayer

Lower gastrointestinal cancers include malignant tumors of the colon, rectum, and anus.

COLORECTAL CANCER

INCIDENCE

Cancer of the large bowel is second only to lung cancer as a cause of cancer death in the United States: 136,830 new cases occurred in 2014, and 50,310 deaths were due to colorectal cancer. The incidence rate has decreased significantly during the past 25 years, likely due to enhanced and more compliantly followed screening practices. Similarly, mortality rates in the United States have decreased by approximately 25%, resulting largely from earlier detection and improved treatment.

POLYPS AND MOLECULAR PATHOGENESIS

Most colorectal cancers, regardless of etiology, arise from adenomatous polyps. A polyp is a grossly visible protrusion from the mucosal surface and may be classified pathologically as a nonneoplastic hamartoma (e.g., *juvenile polyp*), a hyperplastic mucosal proliferation (*hyperplastic polyp*), or an adenomatous polyp. Only adenomas are clearly premalignant, and only a minority of adenomatous polyps evolve into cancer. Adenomatous polyps may be found in the colons of ~30% of middle-aged and ~50% of elderly people; however, <1% of polyps ever become malignant. Most polyps produce no symptoms and remain clinically undetected. Occult blood in the stool is found in <5% of patients with polyps.

A number of molecular changes are noted in adenomatous polyps and colorectal cancers that are thought to reflect a multistep process in the evolution of normal colonic mucosa to life-threatening invasive carcinoma. These developmental steps toward carcinogenesis include, but are not restricted to, point mutations in the K-*ras* protooncogene; hypomethylation of DNA, leading to gene activation; loss of DNA (*allelic loss*) at the site of a tumor-suppressor gene (the adenomatous polyposis coli [*APC*] gene) on the long arm of chromosome 5 (5q21); allelic loss at the site of a tumor-suppressor gene located on chromosome 18q (the deleted in colorectal cancer [*DCC*] gene); and allelic loss at chromosome 17p, associated with mutations in the *p53* tumor-suppressor gene. Thus, the altered proliferative pattern of the colonic mucosa, which results in progression to a polyp and then to carcinoma, may involve the mutational activation of an oncogene followed by and coupled with the loss of genes that normally suppress tumorigenesis. It remains uncertain whether the genetic aberrations always occur in a defined order. Based on this model, however, cancer is believed to develop only in those polyps in which most (if not all) of these mutational events take place.

Clinically, the probability of an adenomatous polyp becoming a cancer depends on the gross appearance of the lesion, its histologic features, and its size. Adenomatous polyps may be pedunculated (stalked) or sessile (flat-based). Invasive cancers develop more frequently in sessile polyps. Histologically, adenomatous polyps may be tubular, villous (i.e., papillary), or tubulovillous. Villous adenomas, most of which are sessile, become malignant more than three times as often as tubular adenomas. The likelihood that any polypoid lesion in the large bowel contains invasive cancer is related to the size of the polyp, being negligible (<2%) in lesions <1.5 cm, intermediate (2–10%) in lesions 1.5–2.5 cm, and substantial (10%) in lesions >2.5 cm in size.

Following the detection of an adenomatous polyp, the entire large bowel should be visualized endoscopically because synchronous lesions are noted in about one-third of cases. Colonoscopy should then be repeated periodically, even in the absence of a previously documented malignancy, because such patients have a 30–50% probability of developing another adenoma and are at a higher than average risk for developing a

TABLE 52-1

RISK FACTORS FOR THE DEVELOPMENT OF COLORECTAL CANCER
Diet: Animal fat
Hereditary syndromes
Polyposis coli
MYH-associated polyposis
Nonpolyposis syndrome (Lynch's syndrome)
Inflammatory bowel disease
Streptococcus bovis bacteremia
? Tobacco use

colorectal carcinoma. Adenomatous polyps are thought to require >5 years of growth before becoming clinically significant; colonoscopy need not be carried out more frequently than every 3 years for the vast majority of patients.

ETIOLOGY AND RISK FACTORS

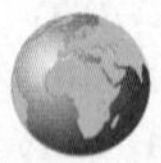

Risk factors for the development of colorectal cancer are listed in Table 52-1.

Diet

The etiology for most cases of large-bowel cancer appears to be related to environmental factors. The disease occurs more often in upper socioeconomic populations who live in urban areas. Mortality from colorectal cancer is directly correlated with per capita consumption of calories, meat protein, and dietary fat and oil as well as elevations in the serum cholesterol concentration and mortality from coronary artery disease. Geographic variations in incidence largely are unrelated to genetic differences, since migrant groups tend to assume the large-bowel cancer incidence rates of their adopted countries. Furthermore, population groups such as Mormons and Seventh Day Adventists, whose lifestyle and dietary habits differ somewhat from those of their neighbors, have significantly lower-than-expected incidence and mortality rates for colorectal cancer. The incidence of colorectal cancer has increased in Japan since that nation has adopted a more "Western" diet. At least three hypotheses have been proposed to explain the relationship to diet, none of which is fully satisfactory.

Animal fats

One hypothesis is that the ingestion of animal fats found in red meats and processed meat leads to an increased proportion of anaerobes in the gut microflora, resulting in the conversion of normal bile acids into carcinogens. This provocative hypothesis is supported by several reports of increased amounts of fecal anaerobes in the stools of patients with colorectal cancer. Diets high in animal (but not vegetable) fats are also associated with high serum cholesterol, which is also associated with enhanced risk for the development of colorectal adenomas and carcinomas.

Insulin resistance

The large number of calories in Western diets coupled with physical inactivity has been associated with a higher prevalence of obesity. Obese persons develop insulin resistance with increased circulating levels of insulin, leading to higher circulating concentrations of insulin-like growth factor type I (IGF-I). This growth factor appears to stimulate proliferation of the intestinal mucosa.

Fiber

Contrary to prior beliefs, the results of randomized trials and case-controlled studies have *failed* to show any value for dietary fiber or diets high in fruits and vegetables in preventing the recurrence of colorectal adenomas or the development of colorectal cancer.

The weight of epidemiologic evidence, however, implicates diet as being the major etiologic factor for colorectal cancer, particularly diets high in animal fat and in calories.

HEREDITARY FACTORS AND SYNDROMES

Up to 25% of patients with colorectal cancer have a family history of the disease, suggesting a hereditary predisposition. Inherited large-bowel cancers can be divided into two main groups: the well-studied but uncommon polyposis syndromes and the more common nonpolyposis syndromes (Table 52-2).

Polyposis coli

Polyposis coli (familial polyposis of the colon) is a rare condition characterized by the appearance of thousands of adenomatous polyps throughout the large bowel. It is transmitted as an autosomal dominant trait; the occasional patient with no family history probably developed the condition due to a spontaneous mutation. Polyposis coli is associated with a deletion in the long arm of chromosome 5 (including the *APC* gene) in both neoplastic (somatic mutation) and normal (germline mutation) cells. The loss of this genetic material (i.e., allelic loss) results in the absence of tumor-suppressor genes whose protein products would normally inhibit neoplastic growth. The presence of soft tissue and bony tumors, congenital hypertrophy of the retinal pigment epithelium, mesenteric desmoid tumors, and ampullary cancers in addition to the colonic polyps characterizes

TABLE 52-2

HEREDITABLE (AUTOSOMAL DOMINANT) GASTROINTESTINAL POLYPOSIS SYNDROMES

SYNDROME	DISTRIBUTION OF POLYPS	HISTOLOGIC TYPE	MALIGNANT POTENTIAL	ASSOCIATED LESIONS
Familial adenomatous polyposis	Large intestine	Adenoma	Common	None
Gardner's syndrome	Large and small intestines	Adenoma	Common	Osteomas, fibromas, lipomas, epidermoid cysts, ampullary cancers, congenital hypertrophy of retinal pigment epithelium
Turcot's syndrome	Large intestine	Adenoma	Common	Brain tumors
MYH-associated polyposis	Large intestine	Adenoma	Common	None
Nonpolyposis syndrome (Lynch's syndrome)	Large intestine (often proximal)	Adenoma	Common	Endometrial and ovarian tumors (most frequently) gastric, genitourinary, pancreatic, biliary cancers (less frequently)
Peutz-Jeghers syndrome	Small and large intestines, stomach	Hamartoma	Rare	Mucocutaneous pigmentation; tumors of the ovary, breast, pancreas, endometrium
Juvenile polyposis	Large and small intestines, stomach	Hamartoma, rarely progressing to adenoma	Rare	Various congenital abnormalities

a subset of polyposis coli known as *Gardner's syndrome*. The appearance of malignant tumors of the central nervous system accompanying polyposis coli defines *Turcot's syndrome*. The colonic polyps in all these conditions are rarely present before puberty but are generally evident in affected individuals by age 25. If the polyposis is not treated surgically, colorectal cancer will develop in almost all patients before age 40. Polyposis coli results from a defect in the colonic mucosa, leading to an abnormal proliferative pattern and impaired DNA repair mechanisms. Once the multiple polyps are detected, patients should undergo a total colectomy. Medical therapy with nonsteroidal anti-inflammatory drugs (NSAIDs) such as sulindac and selective cyclooxygenase-2 inhibitors such as celecoxib can decrease the number and size of polyps in patients with polyposis coli; however, this effect on polyps is only temporary, and the use of NSAIDs has not been shown to reduce the risk of cancer. Colectomy remains the primary therapy/prevention. The offspring of patients with polyposis coli, who often are prepubertal when the diagnosis is made in the parent, have a 50% risk for developing this premalignant disorder and should be carefully screened by annual flexible sigmoidoscopy until age 35. Proctosigmoidoscopy is a sufficient screening procedure because polyps tend to be evenly distributed from cecum to anus, making more invasive and expensive techniques such as colonoscopy or barium enema unnecessary. Testing for occult blood in the stool is an inadequate screening maneuver. If a causative germline *AP C* mutation has been identified in an affected family member, an alternative method for identifying carriers is testing DNA from peripheral blood mononuclear cells for the presence of the specific *APC* mutation. The detection of such a germline mutation can lead to a definitive diagnosis before the development of polyps.

MYH-associated polyposis

MYH-associated polyposis (MAP) is a rare autosomal recessive syndrome caused by a biallelic mutation in the *MUT4H* gene. This hereditary condition may have a variable clinical presentation, resembling polyposis coli or colorectal cancer occurring in younger individuals without polyposis. Screening and colectomy guidelines for this syndrome are less clear than for polyposis coli, but annual to biennial colonoscopic surveillance is generally recommended starting at age 25–30.

Hereditary nonpolyposis colon cancer

Hereditary nonpolyposis colon cancer (HNPCC), also known as *Lynch's syndrome*, is another autosomal dominant trait. It is characterized by the presence of three or more relatives with histologically documented colorectal cancer, one of whom is a first-degree relative of the other two; one or more cases of colorectal cancer diagnosed before age 50 in the family; and colorectal cancer involving at least two generations. In contrast to polyposis coli, HNPCC is associated with an unusually high frequency of cancer arising in the proximal large bowel. The median age for the appearance of an adenocarcinoma is <50 years, 10–15 years younger than the median age for the general population. Despite having a poorly differentiated, mucinous histologic appearance, the proximal colon tumors that characterize HNPCC have a better prognosis than sporadic tumors from patients of similar age. Families with HNPCC often include individuals with multiple primary cancers; the association of colorectal cancer with either ovarian or endometrial carcinomas is especially strong in women, and an increased appearance of gastric, small-bowel, genitourinary, pancreaticobiliary, and sebaceous skin tumors has been reported as well. It has been recommended that members of such families undergo annual or biennial colonoscopy beginning at age 25 years, with intermittent pelvic ultrasonography and endometrial biopsy for afflicted women; such a screening strategy has not yet been validated. HNPCC is associated with germline mutations of several genes, particularly *hMSH2* on chromosome 2 and *hMLH1* on chromosome 3. These mutations lead to errors in DNA replication and are thought to result in DNA instability because of defective repair of DNA mismatches resulting in abnormal cell growth and tumor development. Testing tumor cells through molecular analysis of DNA or immunohistochemical staining of paraffin-fixed tissue for "microsatellite instability" (sequence changes reflecting defective mismatch repair) in patients with colorectal cancer and a positive family history for colorectal or endometrial cancer may identify probands with HNPCC.

INFLAMMATORY BOWEL DISEASE

(Chap. 18) Large-bowel cancer is increased in incidence in patients with long-standing inflammatory bowel disease (IBD). Cancers develop more commonly in patients with ulcerative colitis than in those with granulomatous (i.e., Crohn's) colitis, but this impression may result in part from the occasional difficulty of differentiating these two conditions. The risk of colorectal cancer in a patient with IBD is relatively small during the initial 10 years of the disease, but then appears to increase at a rate of ~0.5–1% per year. Cancer may develop in 8–30% of patients after 25 years. The risk is higher in younger patients with pancolitis.

Cancer surveillance strategies in patients with IBD are unsatisfactory. Symptoms such as bloody diarrhea, abdominal cramping, and obstruction, which may signal the appearance of a tumor, are similar to the complaints caused by a flare-up of the underlying disease. In patients with a history of IBD lasting ≥15 years who continue to experience exacerbations, the surgical removal of the colon can significantly reduce the risk for cancer and also eliminate the target organ for the underlying chronic gastrointestinal disorder. The value of such surveillance techniques as colonoscopy with mucosal biopsies and brushings for less symptomatic individuals with chronic IBD is uncertain. The lack of uniformity regarding the pathologic criteria that characterize dysplasia and the absence of data that such surveillance reduces the development of lethal cancers have made this costly practice an area of controversy.

OTHER HIGH-RISK CONDITIONS

Streptococcus bovis bacteremia

For unknown reasons, individuals who develop endocarditis or septicemia from this fecal bacterium have a high incidence of occult colorectal tumors and, possibly, upper gastrointestinal cancers as well. Endoscopic or radiographic screening appears advisable.

Tobacco use

Cigarette smoking is linked to the development of colorectal adenomas, particularly after >35 years of tobacco use. No biologic explanation for this association has yet been proposed.

PRIMARY PREVENTION

Several orally administered compounds have been assessed as possible inhibitors of colon cancer. The most effective class of chemopreventive agents is aspirin and other NSAIDs, which are thought to suppress cell proliferation by inhibiting prostaglandin synthesis. Regular aspirin use reduces the risk of colon adenomas and carcinomas as well as death from large-bowel cancer; such use also appears to diminish the likelihood for developing additional premalignant adenomas following successful treatment for a prior colon carcinoma. This effect of aspirin on colon carcinogenesis increases with the duration and dosage of drug use. Oral folic acid supplements and oral calcium supplements appear to reduce the risk of adenomatous polyps and colorectal cancers in case-controlled studies. The value of vitamin D as a form of chemoprevention is under study. Antioxidant vitamins such as ascorbic acid, tocopherols, and β-carotene are ineffective at reducing the incidence of subsequent adenomas in patients who have undergone the removal of a colon adenoma. Estrogen replacement therapy has been associated with a reduction in the risk of colorectal cancer in women, conceivably by an effect on bile acid synthesis and composition or by decreasing synthesis of IGF-I.

SCREENING

The rationale for colorectal cancer screening programs is that the removal of adenomatous polyps will prevent colorectal cancer, and that earlier detection of localized, superficial cancers in asymptomatic individuals will increase the surgical cure rate. Such screening programs are particularly important for individuals with a family history of the disease in first-degree relatives. The relative risk for developing colorectal cancer increases to 1.75 in such individuals and may be even higher if the relative was afflicted before age 60. The prior use of proctosigmoidoscopy as a screening tool was based on the observation that 60% of early lesions are located in the rectosigmoid. For unexplained reasons, however, the proportion of large-bowel cancers arising in the rectum has been decreasing during the past several decades, with a corresponding increase in the proportion of cancers in the more proximal descending colon. As such, the potential for proctosigmoidoscopy to detect a sufficient number of occult neoplasms to make the procedure cost-effective has been questioned.

Screening strategies for colorectal cancer that have been examined during the past several decades are listed in Table 52-3.

Many programs directed at the early detection of colorectal cancers have focused on digital rectal examinations and fecal occult blood (i.e., stool guaiac) testing. The digital examination should be part of any routine physical evaluation in adults older than age 40 years, serving as a screening test for prostate cancer in men, a component of the pelvic examination in women, and an inexpensive maneuver for the detection of masses in the rectum. However, because of the proximal migration of colorectal tumors, its value as an overall screening modality for colorectal cancer has become limited. The development of the fecal occult blood test has greatly facilitated the detection of occult fecal blood. Unfortunately, even when performed optimally, the fecal occult blood test has major limitations as a screening technique. About 50% of patients with documented colorectal cancers have a negative fecal occult blood test, consistent with the intermittent bleeding pattern of these tumors. When random cohorts of asymptomatic persons have been tested, 2–4% have fecal occult blood-positive stools. Colorectal cancers have been found in <10% of these "test-positive" cases, with benign polyps being detected in an additional 20–30%. Thus, a colorectal neoplasm will not be found in most asymptomatic individuals with occult blood in their stool. Nonetheless, persons found to have fecal occult blood-positive stool routinely undergo further medical evaluation, including sigmoidoscopy and/or colonoscopy—procedures that are not only uncomfortable and expensive but also associated with a small risk for significant complications. The added cost of these studies would appear justifiable if the small number of patients found to have occult neoplasms because of fecal occult blood screening could be shown to have an improved prognosis and prolonged survival. Prospectively controlled trials have shown a statistically significant reduction in mortality rate from colorectal cancer for individuals undergoing annual stool guaiac screening. However, this benefit only emerged after >13 years of follow-up and was extremely expensive to achieve, because all positive tests (most of which were falsely positive) were followed by colonoscopy. Moreover, these colonoscopic examinations quite likely provided the opportunity for cancer prevention through the removal of potentially premalignant adenomatous polyps because the eventual development of cancer was reduced by 20% in the cohort undergoing annual screening.

TABLE 52-3

SCREENING STRATEGIES FOR COLORECTAL CANCER
Digital rectal examination
Stool testing
• Occult blood
• Fecal DNA
Imaging
• Contrast barium enema
• Virtual (i.e., computed tomography colonography)
Endoscopy
• Flexible sigmoidoscopy
• Colonoscopy

With the appreciation that the carcinogenic process leading to the progression of the normal bowel mucosa to an adenomatous polyp and then to a cancer is the result of a series of molecular changes, investigators have examined fecal DNA for evidence of mutations associated with such molecular changes as evidence of the occult presence of precancerous lesions or actual malignancies. Such a strategy has been tested in more than 4000 asymptomatic individuals whose stool was assessed for occult blood and for 21 possible mutations in fecal DNA; these study subjects also underwent colonoscopy. Although the fecal DNA strategy suggested the presence of more advanced adenomas and cancers than did the fecal occult blood testing approach, the overall sensitivity, using colonoscopic findings as the standard, was less than 50%, diminishing enthusiasm for further pursuit of the fecal DNA screening strategy.

The use of imaging studies to screen for colorectal cancers has also been explored. Air contrast barium enemas had been used to identify sources of occult blood in the stool prior to the advent of fiberoptic endoscopy; the cumbersome nature of the procedure and inconvenience to patients limited its widespread adoption. The introduction of computed tomography (CT) scanning led to the development of virtual (i.e., CT) colonography as an alternative to the growing use of endoscopic screening techniques. Virtual colonography was proposed as being equivalent in sensitivity to colonoscopy and being available in a more widespread manner because it did not require the same degree of operator expertise as fiberoptic endoscopy. However, virtual colonography requires the same cathartic preparation that has limited widespread acceptance of endoscopic colonoscopy, is diagnostic but not therapeutic (i.e., patients with suspicious findings must undergo a subsequent endoscopic procedure for polypectomy or biopsy), and, in the setting of general radiology practices, appears to be less sensitive as a screening technique when compared with endoscopic procedures.

With the appreciation of the inadequacy of fecal occult blood testing alone, concerns about the practicality of imaging approaches, and the wider adoption of endoscopic examinations by the primary care community, screening strategies in asymptomatic persons have changed. At present, both the American Cancer Society and the National Comprehensive Cancer Network suggest either fecal occult blood testing annually coupled with flexible sigmoidoscopy every 5 years or colonoscopy every 10 years beginning at age 50 in asymptomatic individuals with no personal or family history of polyps or colorectal cancer. The recommendation for the inclusion of flexible sigmoidoscopy is strongly supported by the recently published results of three randomized trials performed in the United States, the United Kingdom, and Italy, involving more than 350,000 individuals, which consistently showed that periodic (even single) sigmoidoscopic examinations, after more than a decade of median follow-up, lead to an approximate 21% reduction in the development of colorectal cancer and a more than 25% reduction in mortality from the malignant disease. Less than 20% of participants in these studies underwent a subsequent colonoscopy. In contrast to the cathartic preparation required before colonoscopic procedures, which is only performed by highly trained specialists, flexible sigmoidoscopy requires only an enema as preparation and can be accurately performed by nonspecialty physicians or physician-extenders. The randomized screening studies using flexible sigmoidoscopy led to the estimate that approximately 650 individuals needed to be screened to prevent one colorectal cancer death; this contrasts with the data for mammography where the number of women needing to be screened to prevent one breast cancer death is 2500, reinforcing the efficacy of endoscopic surveillance for colorectal cancer screening. Presumably the benefit from the sigmoidoscopic screening is the result of the identification and removal of adenomatous polyps; it is intriguing that this benefit has been achieved using a technique that leaves the proximal half of the large bowel unvisualized.

It remains to be seen whether surveillance colonoscopy, which has gained increasing popularity in the United States for colorectal cancer screening, will prove to be more effective than flexible sigmoidoscopy. Ongoing randomized trials being conducted in Europe are addressing this issue. Although flexible sigmoidoscopy only visualizes the distal half of the large bowel, leading to the assumption that colonoscopy represents a more informative approach, colonoscopy has been reported as being less accurate for screening the proximal rather than the distal colon, perhaps due to technical considerations but also possibly because of a greater frequency of serrated (i.e., "flat") polyps in the right colon, which are more difficult to identify. At present, colonoscopy performed every 10 years has been offered as an alternative to annual fecal occult blood testing with periodic (every 5 years) flexible sigmoidoscopy. Colonoscopy has been shown to be superior to double-contract barium enema and also to have a higher sensitivity for detecting villous or dysplastic adenomas or cancers than the strategy using occult fecal blood testing and flexible sigmoidoscopy. Whether colonoscopy performed every 10 years beginning at age 50 is medically superior and economically equivalent to flexible sigmoidoscopy remains to be determined.

CLINICAL FEATURES

Presenting symptoms

Symptoms vary with the anatomic location of the tumor. Because stool is relatively liquid as it passes through the ileocecal valve into the right colon, cancers arising in the cecum and ascending colon may become quite large without resulting in any obstructive symptoms or noticeable alterations in bowel habits. Lesions of the right colon commonly ulcerate, leading to chronic, insidious blood loss without a change in the appearance of the stool. Consequently, patients with tumors of the ascending colon often present with symptoms such as fatigue, palpitations, and even angina pectoris and are found to have a hypochromic, microcytic anemia indicative of iron deficiency. Because the cancers may bleed intermittently, a random fecal occult blood test may be negative. As a result, the unexplained presence of iron-deficiency anemia in any adult (with the possible exception of a premenopausal, multiparous woman) mandates a thorough endoscopic and/or radiographic visualization of the entire large bowel (Fig. 52-1).

Because stool becomes more formed as it passes into the transverse and descending colon, tumors arising there tend to impede the passage of stool, resulting in the development of abdominal cramping, occasional obstruction, and even perforation. Radiographs of the abdomen often reveal characteristic annular, constricting lesions ("apple-core" or "napkin-ring") (Fig. 52-2).

Cancers arising in the rectosigmoid are often associated with hematochezia, tenesmus, and narrowing of the caliber of stool; anemia is an infrequent finding.

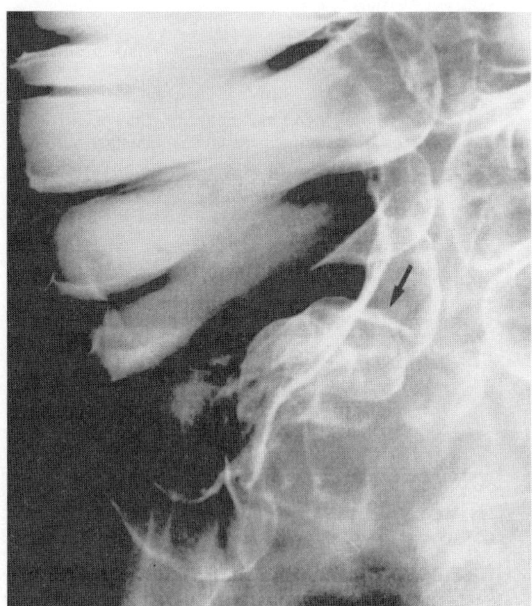

FIGURE 52-1
Double-contrast air-barium enema revealing a sessile tumor of the cecum in a patient with iron-deficiency anemia and guaiac-positive stool. The lesion at surgery was a stage II adenocarcinoma.

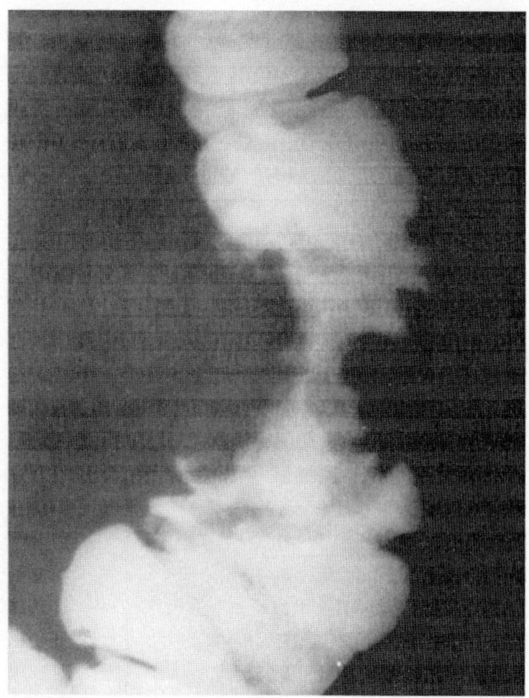

FIGURE 52-2
Annular, constricting adenocarcinoma of the descending colon. This radiographic appearance is referred to as an "apple-core" lesion and is always highly suggestive of malignancy.

While these symptoms may lead patients and their physicians to suspect the presence of hemorrhoids, the development of rectal bleeding and/or altered bowel habits demands a prompt digital rectal examination and proctosigmoidoscopy.

Staging, prognostic factors, and patterns of spread

The prognosis for individuals having colorectal cancer is related to the depth of tumor penetration into the bowel wall and the presence of both regional lymph node involvement and distant metastases. These variables are incorporated into the staging system introduced by Dukes and subsequently applied to a TNM classification method, in which T represents the depth of tumor penetration, N the presence of lymph node involvement, and M the presence or absence of distant metastases (Fig. 52-3). Superficial lesions that do not involve regional lymph nodes and do not penetrate through the submucosa (T1) or the muscularis (T2) are designated as *stage I* (T1–2N0M0) disease; tumors that penetrate through the muscularis but have not spread to lymph nodes are *stage II* disease (T3-4N0M0); regional lymph node involvement defines *stage III* (TXN1-2M0) disease; and metastatic spread to sites such as liver, lung, or bone indicates *stage IV* (TXNXM1) disease. Unless gross evidence of metastatic disease is present, disease stage cannot be determined accurately before surgical resection and pathologic analysis of the operative specimens. It is not clear whether the detection of nodal metastases by special immunohistochemical molecular techniques has the same prognostic implications as disease detected by routine light microscopy.

Most recurrences after a surgical resection of a large-bowel cancer occur within the first 4 years, making 5-year survival a fairly reliable indicator of cure. The likelihood for 5-year survival in patients with colorectal cancer is stage-related (Fig. 52-3). That likelihood has improved during the past several decades when similar surgical stages have been compared. The most plausible explanation for this improvement is more thorough intraoperative and pathologic staging. In particular, more exacting attention to pathologic detail has revealed that the prognosis following the resection of a colorectal cancer is not related merely to the presence or absence of regional lymph node involvement; rather, prognosis may be more precisely gauged by the number of involved lymph nodes (one to three lymph nodes ["N1"] vs four or more lymph nodes ["N2"]) and the number of nodes examined. A minimum of 12 sampled lymph nodes is thought necessary to accurately define tumor stage, and the more nodes examined, the better. Other predictors of a poor prognosis after a total surgical resection include tumor penetration through the bowel wall into pericolic fat, poorly differentiated histology, perforation and/or tumor adherence to adjacent organs (increasing the risk for an anatomically adjacent recurrence), and

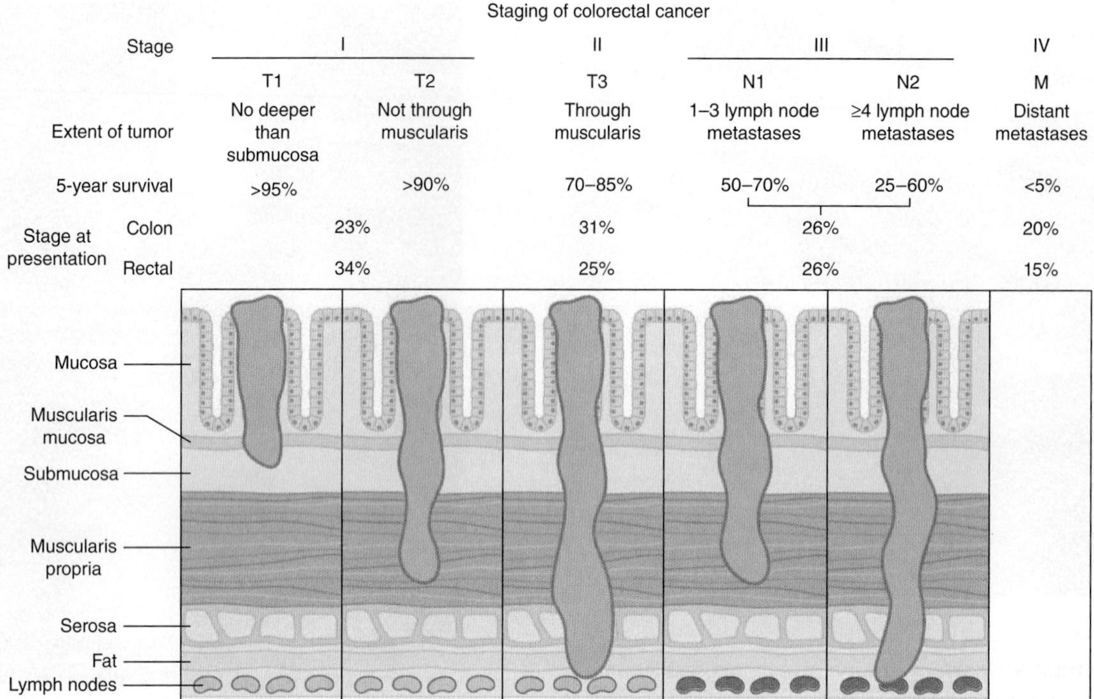

FIGURE 52-3

Staging and prognosis for patients with colorectal cancer.

TABLE 52-4

PREDICTORS OF POOR OUTCOME FOLLOWING TOTAL SURGICAL RESECTION OF COLORECTAL CANCER
Tumor spread to regional lymph nodes
Number of regional lymph nodes involved
Tumor penetration through the bowel wall
Poorly differentiated histology
Perforation
Tumor adherence to adjacent organs
Venous invasion
Preoperative elevation of CEA titer (>5 ng/mL)
Aneuploidy
Specific chromosomal deletion (e.g., mutation in the *b-raf* gene)

Abbreviation: CEA, carcinoembryonic antigen.

venous invasion by tumor (Table 52-4). Regardless of the clinicopathologic stage, a preoperative elevation of the plasma carcinoembryonic antigen (CEA) level predicts eventual tumor recurrence. The presence of aneuploidy and specific chromosomal deletions, such as a mutation in the *b-raf* gene in tumor cells, appears to predict for a higher risk for metastatic spread. Conversely, the detection of microsatellite instability in tumor tissue indicates a more favorable outcome. In contrast to most other cancers, the prognosis in colorectal cancer is not influenced by the size of the primary lesion when adjusted for nodal involvement and histologic differentiation.

Cancers of the large bowel generally spread to regional lymph nodes or to the liver via the portal venous circulation. The liver represents the most frequent visceral site of metastasis; it is the initial site of distant spread in one-third of recurring colorectal cancers and is involved in more than two-thirds of such patients at the time of death. In general, colorectal cancer rarely spreads to the lungs, supraclavicular lymph nodes, bone, or brain without prior spread to the liver. A major exception to this rule occurs in patients having primary tumors in the distal rectum, from which tumor cells may spread through the paravertebral venous plexus, escaping the portal venous system and thereby reaching the lungs or supraclavicular lymph nodes without hepatic involvement. The median survival after the detection of distant metastases has ranged in the past from 6–9 months (hepatomegaly, abnormal liver chemistries) to 24–30 months (small liver nodule initially identified by elevated CEA level and subsequent CT scan), but effective systemic therapy is significantly improving this prognosis.

Efforts to use gene expression profiles to identify patients at risk of recurrence or those particularly likely to benefit from adjuvant therapy have not yet yielded practice-changing results. Despite a burgeoning literature examining a host of prognostic factors, pathologic stage at diagnosis remains the best predictor of long-term prognosis. Patients with lymphovascular invasion and high preoperative CEA levels are likely to have a more aggressive clinical course.

TREATMENT Colorectal Cancer

Total resection of tumor is the optimal treatment when a malignant lesion is detected in the large bowel. An evaluation for the presence of metastatic disease, including a thorough physical examination, biochemical assessment of liver function, measurement of the plasma CEA level, and a CT scan of the chest, abdomen, and pelvis, should be performed before surgery. When possible, a colonoscopy of the entire large bowel should be performed to identify synchronous neoplasms and/or polyps. The detection of metastases should not preclude surgery in patients with tumor-related symptoms such as gastrointestinal bleeding or obstruction, but it often prompts the use of a less radical operative procedure. The necessity for a primary tumor resection in asymptomatic individuals with metastatic disease is an area of controversy. At the time of laparotomy, the entire peritoneal cavity should be examined, with thorough inspection of the liver, pelvis, and hemidiaphragm and careful palpation of the full length of the large bowel. Following recovery from a complete resection, patients should be observed carefully for 5 years by semiannual physical examinations and blood chemistry measurements. If a complete colonoscopy was not performed preoperatively, it should be carried out within the first several postoperative months. Some authorities favor measuring plasma CEA levels at 3-month intervals because of the sensitivity of this test as a marker for otherwise undetectable tumor recurrence. Subsequent endoscopic surveillance of the large bowel, probably at triennial intervals, is indicated, because patients who have been cured of one colorectal cancer have a 3–5% probability of developing an additional bowel cancer during their lifetime and a >15% risk for the development of adenomatous polyps. Anastomotic ("suture-line") recurrences are infrequent in colorectal cancer patients, provided the surgical resection margins are adequate and free of tumor. The value of periodic CT scans of the abdomen, assessing for an early, asymptomatic indication of tumor recurrence, is an area of uncertainty, with some experts recommending the test be performed annually for the first 3 postoperative years.

Radiation therapy to the pelvis is recommended for patients with rectal cancer because it reduces the 20–25% probability of regional recurrences following complete surgical resection of stage II or III tumors, especially if they have penetrated through the serosa. This alarmingly high rate of local disease recurrence is believed to be due to the fact that the contained anatomic space within the pelvis limits the extent of the resection and because the rich lymphatic network of the pelvic side wall immediately adjacent to the rectum facilitates the early spread of malignant cells into surgically inaccessible tissue. The use of sharp rather than blunt dissection of rectal cancers (*total mesorectal excision*) appears to reduce the likelihood of local disease recurrence to ~10%. Radiation therapy, either pre- or postoperatively, further reduces the likelihood of pelvic recurrences but does not appear to prolong survival. Combining radiation therapy with 5-fluorouracil (5-FU)-based chemotherapy, preferably prior to surgical resection, lowers local recurrence rates and improves overall survival. Preoperative radiotherapy is indicated for patients with large, potentially unresectable rectal cancers; such lesions may shrink enough to permit subsequent surgical removal. Radiation therapy is not effective as the primary treatment of colon cancer.

Systemic therapy for patients with colorectal cancer has become more effective. 5-FU remains the backbone of treatment for this disease. Partial responses are obtained in 15–20% of patients. The probability of tumor response appears to be somewhat greater for patients with liver metastases when chemotherapy is infused directly into the hepatic artery, but intraarterial treatment is costly and toxic and does not appear to appreciably prolong survival. The concomitant administration of folinic acid (leucovorin) improves the efficacy of 5-FU in patients with advanced colorectal cancer, presumably by enhancing the binding of 5-FU to its target enzyme, thymidylate synthase. A threefold improvement in the partial response rate is noted when folinic acid is combined with 5-FU; however, the effect on survival is marginal, and the optimal dose schedule remains to be defined. 5-FU is generally administered intravenously but may also be given orally in the form of capecitabine (Xeloda) with seemingly similar efficacy.

Irinotecan (CPT-11), a topoisomerase 1 inhibitor, prolongs survival when compared to supportive care in patients whose disease has progressed on 5-FU. Furthermore, the addition of irinotecan to 5-FU and leucovorin (LV) (e.g., FOLFIRI) improves response rates and survival of patients with metastatic disease. The *FOLFIRI regimen* is as follows: irinotecan, 180 mg/m^2 as a 90-min infusion on day 1; LV, 400 mg/m^2 as a 2-h infusion during irinotecan administration; immediately followed by 5-FU bolus, 400 mg/m^2, and 46-h continuous infusion of 2.4–3 g/m^2 every 2 weeks. Diarrhea is the major side effect from irinotecan. Oxaliplatin, a platinum analogue, also improves the response rate when added to 5-FU and LV (FOLFOX) as initial treatment of patients with metastatic disease. The *FOLFOX regimen* is as follows: 2-h infusion of LV (400 mg/m^2 per day) followed by a 5-FU bolus (400 mg/m^2 per day) and 22-h infusion (1200 mg/m^2) every 2 weeks, together with oxaliplatin, 85 mg/m^2 as a 2-h infusion on day 1. Oxaliplatin frequently causes a dose-dependent sensory neuropathy that often but not always resolves following the cessation of therapy. FOLFIRI and FOLFOX are equal in efficacy. In metastatic disease, these regimens may produce median survivals of 2 years.

Monoclonal antibodies are also effective in patients with advanced colorectal cancer. Cetuximab (Erbitux) and panitumumab (Vectibix) are directed against the epidermal growth factor receptor (EGFR), a transmembrane glycoprotein involved in signaling pathways affecting growth and proliferation of tumor cells. Both cetuximab and panitumumab, when given alone, have been shown to benefit a small proportion of previously treated patients, and cetuximab appears to have therapeutic synergy with such chemotherapeutic agents as irinotecan, even in patients previously resistant to this drug; this suggests that cetuximab can reverse cellular resistance to cytotoxic chemotherapy. The antibodies are not effective in the approximate 40% subset of colon tumors that contain mutated K-*ras*. The use of both cetuximab and panitumumab can lead to an acne-like rash, with the development and severity of the rash being correlated with the likelihood of antitumor efficacy. Inhibitors of the EGFR tyrosine kinase such as erlotinib (Tarceva) or sunitinib (Sutent) do not appear to be effective in colorectal cancer.

Bevacizumab (Avastin) is a monoclonal antibody directed against the vascular endothelial growth factor (VEGF) and is thought to act as an antiangiogenesis agent. The addition of bevacizumab to irinotecan-containing combinations and to FOLFOX initially appeared to significantly improve the outcome observed with chemotherapy alone, but subsequent studies have suggested a lesser degree of benefit. The use of bevacizumab can lead to hypertension, proteinuria, and an increased likelihood of thromboembolic events.

Patients with solitary hepatic metastases without clinical or radiographic evidence of additional tumor involvement should be considered for partial liver resection, because such procedures are associated with 5-year survival rates of 25–30% when performed on selected individuals by experienced surgeons.

The administration of 5-FU and LV for 6 months after resection of tumor in patients with stage III disease leads to a 40% decrease in recurrence rates and 30% improvement in survival. The likelihood of recurrence has been further reduced when oxaliplatin has been combined with 5-FU and LV (e.g., FOLFOX); unexpectedly, the addition of irinotecan to 5-FU and LV as well as the addition of either bevacizumab or cetuximab to FOLFOX did not significantly enhance outcome. Patients with stage II tumors do not appear to benefit appreciably from adjuvant therapy, with the use of such treatment generally restricted to those patients having biologic characteristics (e.g., perforated tumors, T4 lesions, lymphovascular invasion) that place them at higher likelihood for recurrence. The addition of oxaliplatin to adjuvant treatment for patients older than age 70 and those with stage II disease does not appear to provide any therapeutic benefit.

In rectal cancer, the delivery of preoperative or postoperative combined-modality therapy (5-FU plus radiation therapy) reduces the risk of recurrence and increases the chance of cure for patients with stage II and III tumors, with the preoperative approach being better tolerated. The 5-FU acts as a radiosensitizer when delivered together with radiation therapy. Life-extending adjuvant therapy is used in only about half of patients older than age 65 years. This age bias is unfortunate because the benefits and likely the tolerance of adjuvant therapy in patients age ≥65 years appear similar to those seen in younger individuals.

CANCERS OF THE ANUS

Cancers of the anus account for 1–2% of the malignant tumors of the large bowel. Most such lesions arise in the anal canal, the anatomic area extending from the anorectal ring to a zone approximately halfway between the pectinate (or dentate) line and the anal verge. Carcinomas arising proximal to the pectinate line (i.e., in the transitional zone between the glandular mucosa of the rectum and the squamous epithelium of the distal anus) are known as *basaloid*, *cuboidal*, or *cloacogenic* tumors; about one-third of anal cancers have this histologic pattern. Malignancies arising distal to the pectinate line have squamous histology, ulcerate more frequently, and constitute ~55% of anal cancers. The prognosis for patients with basaloid and squamous cell cancers of the anus is identical when corrected for tumor size and the presence or absence of nodal spread.

The development of anal cancer is associated with infection by human papillomavirus, the same organism etiologically linked to cervical cancer. The virus is sexually transmitted. The infection may lead to anal warts (condyloma acuminata), which may progress to anal intraepithelial neoplasia and on to squamous cell carcinoma. The risk for anal cancer is increased among homosexual males, presumably related to anal intercourse. Anal cancer risk is increased in both men and women with AIDS, possibly because their immunosuppressed state permits more severe papillomavirus infection. Vaccination against human papilloma viruses may reduce the eventual risk for anal cancer. Anal cancers occur most commonly in middle-aged persons and are more frequent in women than men. At diagnosis, patients may experience bleeding, pain, sensation of a perianal mass, and pruritus.

Radical surgery (abdominal-perineal resection with lymph node sampling and a permanent colostomy) was once the treatment of choice for this tumor type. The 5-year survival rate after such a procedure was 55–70% in the absence of spread to regional lymph nodes and <20% if nodal involvement was present. An alternative therapeutic approach combining external beam radiation therapy with concomitant chemotherapy (5-FU and mitomycin C) has resulted in biopsy-proven disappearance of all tumor in >80% of patients whose initial lesion was <3 cm in size. Tumor recurrences develop in <10% of these patients, meaning that ~70% of patients with anal cancers can be cured with nonoperative treatment and without the need for a colostomy. Surgery should be reserved for the minority of individuals who are found to have residual tumor after being managed initially with radiation therapy combined with chemotherapy.

CHAPTER 53

TUMORS OF THE LIVER AND BILIARY TREE

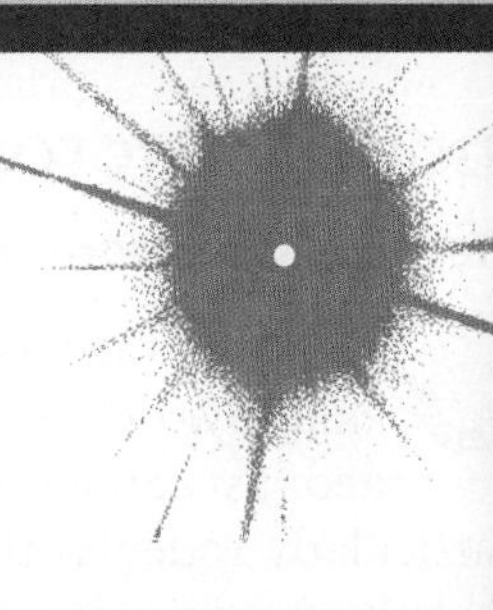

Brian I. Carr

HEPATOCELLULAR CARCINOMA

INCIDENCE

Hepatocellular carcinoma (HCC) is one of the most common malignancies worldwide. The annual global incidence is approximately 1 million cases, with a male-to-female ratio of approximately 4:1 (1:1 without cirrhosis to 9:1 in many high-incidence countries). The incidence rate equals the death rate. In the United States, approximately 22,000 new cases are diagnosed annually, with 18,000 deaths. The death rates in males in low-incidence countries such as the United States are 1.9 per 100,000 per year; in intermediate areas such as Austria and South Africa, they range from 5.1–20; and in high-incidence areas such as in the Orient (China and Korea), they are as high as 23.1–150 per 100,000 per year (Table 53-1). The incidence of HCC in the United States is approximately 3 per 100,000 persons, with significant gender, ethnic, and geographic variations. These numbers are rapidly increasing and may be an underestimate. Approximately 4 million chronic hepatitis C virus (HCV) carriers are in the United States alone. Approximately 10% of them, or 400,000, are likely to develop cirrhosis. Approximately 5%, or 20,000, of these patients may develop HCC annually. Add to this the two other common predisposing factors—hepatitis B virus (HBV) and chronic alcohol consumption—and 60,000 new HCC cases annually seem possible. Future advances in HCC survival will likely depend in part on immunization strategies for HBV (and HCV) and earlier diagnosis by screening of patients at risk of HCC development.

Current directions

With the U.S. HCV epidemic, HCC is increasing in most states, and obesity-associated liver disease (nonalcoholic steatohepatitis [NASH]) is increasingly recognized as a cause.

EPIDEMIOLOGY

There are two general types of epidemiologic studies of HCC—those of country-based incidence rates (Table 53-1) and those of migrants. Endemic hot spots occur in areas of China and sub-Saharan Africa, which are associated both with high endemic hepatitis B carrier rates as well as mycotoxin contamination of foodstuffs (aflatoxin B_1), stored grains, drinking water, and soil. Environmental factors are

TABLE 53-1

AGE-ADJUSTED INCIDENCE RATES FOR HEPATOCELLULAR CARCINOMA

	PERSONS PER 100,000 PER YEAR	
COUNTRY	**MALE**	**FEMALE**
Argentina	6.0	2.5
Brazil, Recife	9.2	8.3
Brazil, Sao Paulo	3.8	2.6
Mozambique	112.9	30.8
South Africa, Cape: Black	26.3	8.4
South Africa, Cape: White	1.2	0.6
Senegal	25.6	9.0
Nigeria	15.4	3.2
Gambia	33.1	12.6
Burma	25.5	8.8
Japan	7.2	2.2
Korea	13.8	3.2
China, Shanghai	34.4	11.6
India, Bombay	4.9	2.5
India, Madras	2.1	0.7
Great Britain	1.6	0.8
France	6.9	1.2
Italy, Varese	7.1	2.7
Norway	1.8	1.1
Spain, Navarra	7.9	4.7

important, for example, Japanese in Japan have a higher incidence than Japanese living in Hawaii, who in turn have a higher incidence than those living in California.

ETIOLOGIC FACTORS

Chemical carcinogens

Causative agents for HCC have been studied along two general lines. First are agents identified as carcinogenic in experimental animals (particularly rodents) that are thought to be present in the human environment (Table 53-2). Second is the association of HCC with various other clinical conditions. Probably the best-studied and most potent ubiquitous natural chemical carcinogen is a product of the *Aspergillus* fungus, called aflatoxin B_1. This mold and aflatoxin product can be found in a variety of stored grains in hot, humid places, where peanuts and rice are stored in unrefrigerated conditions. Aflatoxin contamination of foodstuffs correlates well with incidence rates in Africa and to some extent in China. In endemic areas of China, even farm animals such as ducks have HCC. The most potent carcinogens appear to be natural products of plants, fungi, and bacteria, such as bush trees containing pyrrolizidine alkaloids as well as tannic acid and safrole. Pollutants such as pesticides and insecticides are known rodent carcinogens.

Hepatitis

Both case-control and cohort studies have shown a strong association between chronic hepatitis B carrier rates and increased incidence of HCC. In Taiwanese male postal carriers who were hepatitis B surface antigen (HBsAg)-positive, a 98-fold greater risk for HCC was found compared to HBsAg-negative individuals. The incidence of HCC in Alaskan natives is markedly increased related to a high prevalence of HBV infection. HBV-based HCC may involve rounds of hepatic destruction with subsequent proliferation and not necessarily frank cirrhosis. The increase in Japanese HCC incidence rates in the last three decades is thought to be from hepatitis C. A large-scale World Health Organization (WHO)-sponsored intervention study is currently under way in Asia involving HBV vaccination of the newborn. HCC in African blacks is not associated with severe cirrhosis but is poorly differentiated and very aggressive. Despite uniform HBV carrier rates among the South African Bantu, there is a ninefold difference in HCC incidence between Mozambicans living along the coast and inland. These differences are attributed to the additional exposure to dietary aflatoxin B_1 and other carcinogenic mycotoxins. A typical interval between HCV-associated transfusion and subsequent HCC is approximately 30 years. HCV-associated HCC patients tend to have more frequent and advanced cirrhosis, but in HBV-associated HCC, only half the patients have cirrhosis, with the remainder having chronic active hepatitis (**Chap. 41**).

TABLE 53-2

FACTORS ASSOCIATED WITH AN INCREASED RISK OF DEVELOPING HEPATOCELLULAR CARCINOMA

COMMON	UNUSUAL
Cirrhosis from any cause	Primary biliary cirrhosis
Hepatitis B or C chronic infection	Hemochromatosis
	α_1 Antitrypsin deficiency
Ethanol chronic consumption	Glycogen storage diseases
NASH/NAFL	Citrullinemia
Aflatoxin B_1 or other mycotoxins	Porphyria cutanea tarda
	Hereditary tyrosinemia
	Wilson's disease

Abbreviations: NAFL, nonalcoholic fatty liver; NASH, nonalcoholic steatohepatitis.

Other etiologic conditions

The 75–85% association of HCC with underlying cirrhosis has long been recognized, more typically with macronodular cirrhosis in Southeast Asia, but also with micronodular cirrhosis (alcohol) in Europe and the United States (**Chap. 44**). It is still not clear whether cirrhosis itself is a predisposing factor to the development of HCC or whether the underlying causes of the cirrhosis are actually the carcinogenic factors. However, ~20% of U.S. patients with HCC do not have underlying cirrhosis. Several underlying conditions are associated with an increased risk for cirrhosis-associated HCC (Table 53-2), including hepatitis, alcohol, autoimmune chronic active hepatitis, cryptogenic cirrhosis, and NASH. A less common association is with primary biliary cirrhosis and several metabolic diseases including hemochromatosis, Wilson's disease, α_1 antitrypsin deficiency, tyrosinemia, porphyria cutanea tarda, glycogenesis types 1 and 3, citrullinemia, and orotic aciduria. The etiology of HCC in those 20% of patients who have no cirrhosis is currently unclear, and their HCC natural history is not well-defined.

Current directions

Many patients have multiple etiologies, and the interactions of HBV, HCV, alcohol, smoking, and aflatoxins are just beginning to be explored.

CLINICAL FEATURES

Symptoms

These include abdominal pain, weight loss, weakness, abdominal fullness and swelling, jaundice, and nausea (Table 53-3). Presenting signs and symptoms differ somewhat between high- and low-incidence areas. In high-risk areas, especially in South African blacks, the most common symptom is abdominal pain; by contrast, only 40–50% of Chinese and Japanese patients present with abdominal pain. Abdominal swelling may occur as a consequence of ascites due to the underlying chronic liver disease or may be due to a rapidly expanding tumor. Occasionally, central necrosis or acute hemorrhage into the peritoneal cavity leads to death. In countries with an active surveillance program, HCC tends to be identified at an earlier stage, when symptoms may be due only to the underlying disease. Jaundice is usually due to obstruction of the intrahepatic ducts from underlying liver disease. Hematemesis may occur due to esophageal varices from the underlying portal hypertension. Bone pain is seen in 3–12% of patients, but necropsies show pathologic bone metastases in ~20% of patients. However, 25% of patients may be asymptomatic.

TABLE 53-3

HEPATOCELLULAR CARCINOMA CLINICAL PRESENTATION (N = 547)

SYMPTOM	NO. OF PATIENTS (%)
No symptom	129 (24)
Abdominal pain	219 (40)
Other (workup of anemia and various diseases)	64 (12)
Routine physical exam finding, elevated LFTs	129 (24)
Weight loss	112 (20)
Appetite loss	59 (11)
Weakness/malaise	83 (15)
Jaundice	30 (5)
Routine CT scan screening of known cirrhosis	92 (17)
Cirrhosis symptoms (ankle swelling, abdominal bloating, increased girth, pruritus, GI bleed)	98 (18)
Diarrhea	7 (1)
Tumor rupture	1
Patient Characteristics	
Mean age (yr)	56 ± 13
Male:Female	3:1
Ethnicity	
White	72%
Middle Eastern	10%
Asian	13%
African American	5%
Cirrhosis	81%
No cirrhosis	19%
Tumor Characteristics	
Hepatic tumor numbers	
1	20%
2	25%
3 or more	65%
Portal vein invasion	75%
Unilobar	25%
Bilobar	75%

Abbreviations: CT, computed tomography; GI, gastrointestinal; LFT, liver function test.

Physical signs

Hepatomegaly is the most common physical sign, occurring in 50–90% of the patients. Abdominal bruits are noted in 6–25%, and ascites occurs in 30–60% of patients. Ascites should be examined by cytology. Splenomegaly is mainly due to portal hypertension. Weight loss and muscle wasting are common, particularly with rapidly growing or large tumors. Fever is found in 10–50% of patients, from unclear cause. The signs of chronic liver disease may often be present, including jaundice, dilated abdominal veins, palmar erythema, gynecomastia, testicular atrophy, and peripheral edema. Budd-Chiari syndrome can occur due to HCC invasion of the hepatic veins, with tense ascites and a large tender liver (**Chap. 44**).

Paraneoplastic syndromes

Most paraneoplastic syndromes in HCC are biochemical abnormalities without associated clinical consequences. They include hypoglycemia (also caused by end-stage liver failure), erythrocytosis, hypercalcemia, hypercholesterolemia, dysfibrinogenemia, carcinoid syndrome, increased thyroxin-binding globulin, changes in secondary sex characteristics (gynecomastia, testicular atrophy, and precocious puberty), and porphyria cutanea tarda. Mild hypoglycemia occurs in rapidly growing HCC as part of terminal illness, and profound hypoglycemia may occur, although the cause is unclear. Erythrocytosis occurs in 3–12% of patients and hypercholesterolemia in 10–40%. A high percentage of patients have thrombocytopenia associated with their fibrosis or leukopenia, resulting from portal hypertension, and not from cancer infiltration of bone marrow, as in other tumor types. Furthermore, large HCCs have normal or high platelet levels (thrombocytosis), as in ovarian and other gastrointestinal cancers, probably related to elevated interleukin 6 (IL-6) levels.

STAGING

Multiple clinical staging systems for HCC have been described. A widely used one has been the American Joint Committee on Cancer (AJCC) tumor-node-metastasis (TNM) classification. However, the Cancer of the Liver Italian Program (CLIP) system is now popular because it takes cirrhosis into account, based on the original Okuda system (Table 53-4). Patients with Okuda stage III disease have a dire prognosis because they usually cannot be curatively resected, and the condition of their liver typically precludes chemotherapy. Other staging systems have been proposed, and a consensus is needed. They are all based on combining the prognostic features of liver damage with those of tumor aggressiveness and include the Barcelona Clinic Liver Cancer (BCLC) system from Spain (Fig. 53-1), which is externally validated and incorporates baseline survival estimates; the Chinese University Prognostic Index (CUPI); the important and simple Japan Integrated Staging Score (JIS); and SLiDe, which stands for *s* tage, *li* ver damage, and *de* s-γ-carboxy prothrombin. CLIP and BCLC appear most popular in the West, whereas JIS is favored in Japan. Each system has its champions. The best prognosis is for stage I, solitary tumors less than 2 cm in diameter without vascular invasion. Adverse prognostic features include ascites, jaundice, vascular invasion, and elevated α fetoprotein (AFP). Vascular invasion in particular has profound effects on prognosis and may be microscopic or macroscopic (visible on computed tomography [CT] scans). Most large tumors have microscopic vascular invasion, so full staging can usually be made only after surgical resection. Stage III disease contains a mixture of lymph node–positive and–negative tumors. Stage III patients with positive lymph node disease have a poor prognosis, and few patients survive 1 year. The prognosis of stage IV is poor after either resection or transplantation, and 1-year survival is rare.

TABLE 53-4

CLIP AND OKUDA STAGING SYSTEMS FOR HEPATOCELLULAR CARCINOMA

CLIP CLASSIFICATION

	POINTS		
VARIABLES	**0**	**1**	**2**
i. Tumor number	Single	Multiple	–
Hepatic replacement by tumor (%)	<50	<50	>50
ii. Child-Pugh score	A	B	C
iii. α Fetoprotein level (ng/mL)	<400	≥400	–
iv. Portal vein thrombosis (CT)	No	Yes	–

CLIP stages (score = sum of points): CLIP 0, 0 points; CLIP 1, 1 point; CLIP 2, 2 points; CLIP 3, 3 points.

Okuda Classification

TUMOR EXTENT[a]		ASCITES		ALBUMIN (G/L)		BILIRUBIN (MG/DL)	
≥50%	<50	+	–	≤3	>3	≥ 3	<3
(+)	(–)	(+)	(–)	(+)	(–)	(+)	(–)

Okuda stages: stage 1, all (–); stage 2, 1 or 2 (+); stage 3, 3 or 4 (+).

[a]Extent of liver occupied by tumor.

Abbreviation: CLIP, Cancer of the Liver Italian Program.

New directions

Consensus is needed on staging. These systems will soon be refined or upended by proteomics.

APPROACH TO THE PATIENT: Hepatocellular Carcinoma

HISTORY AND PHYSICAL The history is important in evaluating putative predisposing factors, including a history of hepatitis or jaundice, blood transfusion, or use of intravenous drugs. A family history of HCC or hepatitis should be sought and a detailed social history taken to include job descriptions for industrial exposure to possible carcinogenic drugs as well as contraceptive hormones. Physical examination should include assessing stigmata of underlying liver disease such as jaundice, ascites, peripheral edema, spider nevi, palmar erythema, and weight loss. Evaluation of the abdomen for hepatic size, masses or ascites, hepatic nodularity and tenderness, and splenomegaly is needed, as is assessment of overall performance status and psychosocial evaluation.

SEROLOGIC ASSAYS AFP is a serum tumor marker for HCC; however, it is only increased in approximately one-half of U.S. patients. The lens culinaris agglutinin-reactive fraction of AFP (AFP-L3) assay is thought to be more specific. The other widely used assay is that for des-γ-carboxy prothrombin (DCP), a protein induced by vitamin K absence (PIVKA-2). This protein is increased in as many as 80% of HCC patients but may also be elevated in patients with vitamin K deficiency; it is always elevated after warfarin use. It may also predict for portal vein invasion. Both AFP-L3 and DCP are U.S. Food and Drug Administration (FDA) approved. Many other assays have been developed, such as glypican-3, but none have greater aggregate sensitivity and specificity. In a patient presenting with either a new hepatic mass or other indications of recent hepatic decompensation, carcinoembryonic antigen (CEA), vitamin B_{12}, AFP, ferritin, PIVKA-2, and antimitochondrial antibody should be measured, and standard liver function tests should be performed, including prothrombin time (PT), partial thromboplastin time (PTT), albumin, transaminases, γ-glutamyl transpeptidase, and alkaline phosphatase. γ-Glutamyl transpeptidase and alkaline phosphatase may

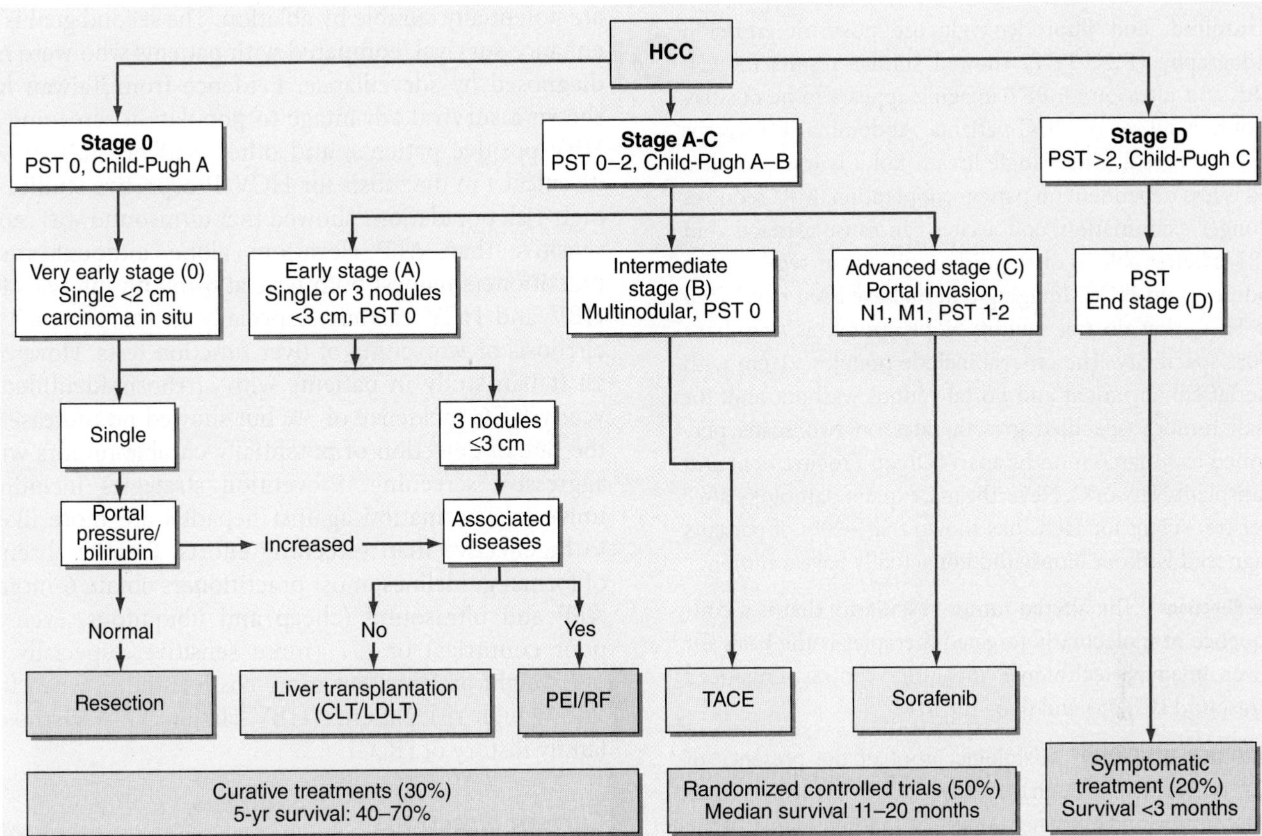

FIGURE 53-1

Barcelona Clinic Liver Cancer (BCLC) staging classification and treatment schedule. Patients with very early hepatocellular carcinoma (HCC) (stage 0) are optimal candidates for resection. Patients with early HCC (stage A) are candidates for radical therapy (resection, liver transplantation [LT], or local ablation via percutaneous ethanol injection [PEI] or radiofrequency [RF] ablation). Patients with intermediate HCC (stage B) benefit from transcatheter arterial chemoembolization (TACE). Patients with advanced HCC, defined as presence of macroscopic vascular invasion, extrahepatic spread, or cancer-related symptoms (Eastern Cooperative Oncology Group performance status 1 or 2) (stage C), benefit from sorafenib. Patients with end-stage disease (stage D) will receive symptomatic treatment. Treatment strategy will transition from one stage to another on treatment failure or contraindications for the procedures. CLT, cadaveric liver transplantation; LDLT, living donor liver transplantation; PST, Performance Status Test. *(Modified from JM Llovet et al: JNCI 100:698, 2008.)*

be particularly important in the 50% of HCC patients who have low AFP levels. Decreases in platelet count and white blood cell count may reflect portal hypertension and associated hypersplenism. Hepatitis A, B, and C serology should be measured. If HBV or HCV serology is positive, quantitative measurements of HBV DNA or HCV RNA are needed.

New directions Newer biomarkers are being evaluated, especially tissue- and serum-based genomics profiling. Newer plasma biomarkers include glypican-3, osteopontin, insulin-like growth factor I, and vascular endothelial growth factor. However, they are still in process of validation. Furthermore, the commercial availability of kits for isolating circulating tumor cells is permitting the molecular profiling of HCCs without the need for further tissue biopsy.

RADIOLOGY An ultrasound examination of the liver is an excellent screening tool. The two characteristic vascular abnormalities are hypervascularity of the tumor mass (neovascularization or abnormal tumor-feeding arterial vessels) and thrombosis by tumor invasion of otherwise normal portal veins. To determine tumor size and extent and the presence of portal vein invasion accurately, a helical/triphasic CT scan of the abdomen and pelvis, with fast-contrast bolus technique, should be performed to detect the vascular lesions typical of HCC. Portal vein invasion is normally detected as an obstruction and expansion of the vessel. A chest CT is used to exclude metastases. Magnetic resonance imaging (MRI) can also provide detailed information, especially with the newer contrast agents. Ethiodol (Lipiodol) is an ethiodized oil emulsion retained by liver tumors that can be delivered by hepatic artery injection (5–15 mL) for CT imaging 1 week later. For small tumors, Ethiodol injection is very helpful before biopsy because the histologic presence of the dye constitutes proof that the needle biopsied the mass under suspicion. A prospective comparison of triphasic CT, gadolinium-enhanced MRI, ultrasound, and fluorodeoxyglucose positron emission tomography (FDG-PET) showed similar results for CT, MRI, and ultrasound; PET imaging appears to be positive in only a subset of HCC patients. Abdominal CT versus MRI/CT uses a faster single breath-hold, is less complex, and is less dependent on patient cooperation. MRI requires a longer examination, and ascites can cause artifacts, but MRI is better able to distinguish dysplastic or regenerative nodules from HCC. Imaging criteria have been developed for HCC that do not require biopsy proof, as they have >90% specificity. The criteria include nodules >1 cm with arterial enhancement and portal venous washout and, for small tumors, specified growth rates on two scans performed less than 6 months apart (Organ Procurement and Transplant Network). Nevertheless, explant pathology after liver transplant for HCC has shown that ~20% of patients diagnosed without biopsy did not actually have a tumor.

New directions The altered tumor vascularity that is a consequence of molecularly targeted therapies is the basis for newer imaging techniques including contrast-enhanced ultrasound (CEUS) and dynamic MRI.

PATHOLOGIC DIAGNOSIS Histologic proof of the presence of HCC is obtained through a core liver biopsy of the liver mass under ultrasound guidance, as well as random biopsy of the underlying liver. Bleeding risk is increased compared to other cancers because (1) the tumors are hypervascular and (2) patients often have thrombocytopenia and decreased liver-dependent clotting factors. Bleeding risk is further increased in the presence of ascites. Tracking of tumor has an uncommon problem. Fine-needle aspirates can provide sufficient material for diagnosis of cancer, but core biopsies are preferred. Tissue architecture allows the distinction between HCC and adenocarcinoma. Laparoscopic approaches can also be used. For patients suspected of having portal vein involvement, a core biopsy of the portal vein may be performed safely. If positive, this is regarded as an exclusion criterion for transplantation for HCC.

New directions Immunohistochemistry has become mainstream. Prognostic subgroupings are being defined based on growth signaling pathway proteins and genotyping strategies, including a prognostically significant five-gene profile score. Furthermore, molecular profiling of the underlying liver has provided evidence for a "field-effect" of cirrhosis in generating recurrent or new HCCs after primary resection. In addition, characteristics of HCC stem cells have been identified and include EpCAM, CD44, and CD90 expression, which may form the basis of stem cell therapeutic targeting strategies.

SCREENING HIGH-RISK POPULATIONS

There are two goals of screening, both in patients at increased risk for developing HCC, such as those with cirrhosis. The first goal is to detect smaller tumors that are potentially curable by ablation. The second goal is to enhance survival, compared with patients who were not diagnosed by surveillance. Evidence from Taiwan has shown a survival advantage to population screening in HBV-positive patients, and other evidence has shown its efficacy in diagnosis for HCV. Prospective studies in high-risk populations showed that ultrasound was more sensitive than AFP elevations alone, although most practitioners request both tests at 6-month intervals for HBV and HCV carriers, especially in the presence of cirrhosis or worsening of liver function tests. However, an Italian study in patients with cirrhosis identified a yearly HCC incidence of 3% but showed no increase in the rate of detection of potentially curable tumors with aggressive screening. Prevention strategies including universal vaccination against hepatitis are more likely to be effective than screening efforts. Despite absence of formal guidelines, most practitioners obtain 6-month AFP and ultrasound (cheap and ubiquitous, even in poor countries) or CT (more sensitive, especially in overweight patients, but more costly) studies when following high-risk patients (HBV carriers, HCV cirrhosis, family history of HCC).

Current directions

Cost-benefit analysis is not yet convincing, even though screening is intuitively sound. However, studies from areas with high HBV carrier rates have shown a survival benefit for screening as a result of earlier stage at diagnosis. A definitive clinical trial on screening is unlikely, due to difficulties in obtaining informed consent for patients who are not to be screened. γ-Glutamyl transpeptidase appears useful for detecting small tumors.

PREVENTION

Prevention strategies can only be planned when the causes of a cancer are known or strongly suspected. This is true of few human cancers, with significant exceptions being smoking and lung cancer, papilloma virus and cancer of the cervix uteri, and cirrhosis of any cause or dietary contamination by aflatoxin B_1 for HCC. Aflatoxin B_1 is one of the most potent known chemical carcinogens and is a product of the *Aspergillus* mold that grows on peanuts and rice when stored in hot and humid climates. The obvious strategy is to refrigerate these foodstuffs when stored and to conduct surveillance programs for elevated aflatoxin B_1 levels, as happens in the United States, but not usually in Asia. HBV is commonly transmitted from mother to fetus in Asia (except Japan), and neonatal HBV vaccination programs have resulted in a big decrease in adolescent HBV and, thus, in predicted HCC rates. There are millions of HBV and HCV carriers (4 million with HCV in the United States) who are already infected. Nucleoside analogue–based chemoprevention (entecavir) of HBV-mediated HCC in Japan resulted in a fivefold decrease in HCC incidence over 5 years in cirrhotic but not in noncirrhotic HBV patients. More powerful and effective HCV therapies promise the possibility of prevention of HCV-based HCC in the future.

TREATMENT Hepatocellular Carcinoma

Most HCC patients have two liver diseases, cirrhosis and HCC, each of which is an independent cause of death. The presence of cirrhosis usually places constraints on resection surgery, ablative therapies, and chemotherapy. Thus patient assessment and treatment planning have to take the severity of the nonmalignant liver disease into account. The clinical management choices for HCC can be complex (Fig. 53-2, Tables 53-5 and 53-6). The natural history of HCC is highly variable. Patients presenting with advanced tumors (vascular invasion, symptoms, extrahepatic spread) have a median survival of ~4 months, with or without treatment. Treatment results from the literature are difficult to interpret. Survival is not always a measure of the efficacy of therapy because of the adverse effects on survival of the underlying liver disease. A multidisciplinary team, including a hepatologist, interventional radiologist, surgical oncologist, resection surgeon, transplant surgeon, and medical oncologist, is important for the comprehensive management of HCC patients.

TNM STAGES I AND II HCC Early-stage tumors are successfully treated using various techniques, including surgical resection, local ablation (thermal, radiofrequency [RFA], or microwave ablation (MWA]), and local injection therapies (Table 53-6). Because the majority of patients with HCC suffer from a field defect in the cirrhotic liver, they are at risk for subsequent multiple primary liver tumors. Many will also have significant underlying liver disease and may not tolerate major surgical loss of hepatic parenchyma, and they may be eligible for orthotopic liver transplant (OLTX). Living related donor transplants have increased in popularity, resulting in absence of waiting for a transplant. An important principle in treating early-stage HCC in the nontransplant setting is to use liver-sparing treatments and to focus on treatment of both the tumor and the cirrhosis.

Surgical Excision The risk of major hepatectomy is high (5–10% mortality rate) due to the underlying liver disease and the potential for liver failure, but acceptable in selected cases and highly dependent on surgical experience. The risk is lower in high-volume centers. Preoperative portal vein occlusion can sometimes be performed to cause atrophy of the HCC-involved lobe and compensatory hypertrophy of the noninvolved liver, permitting safer resection.

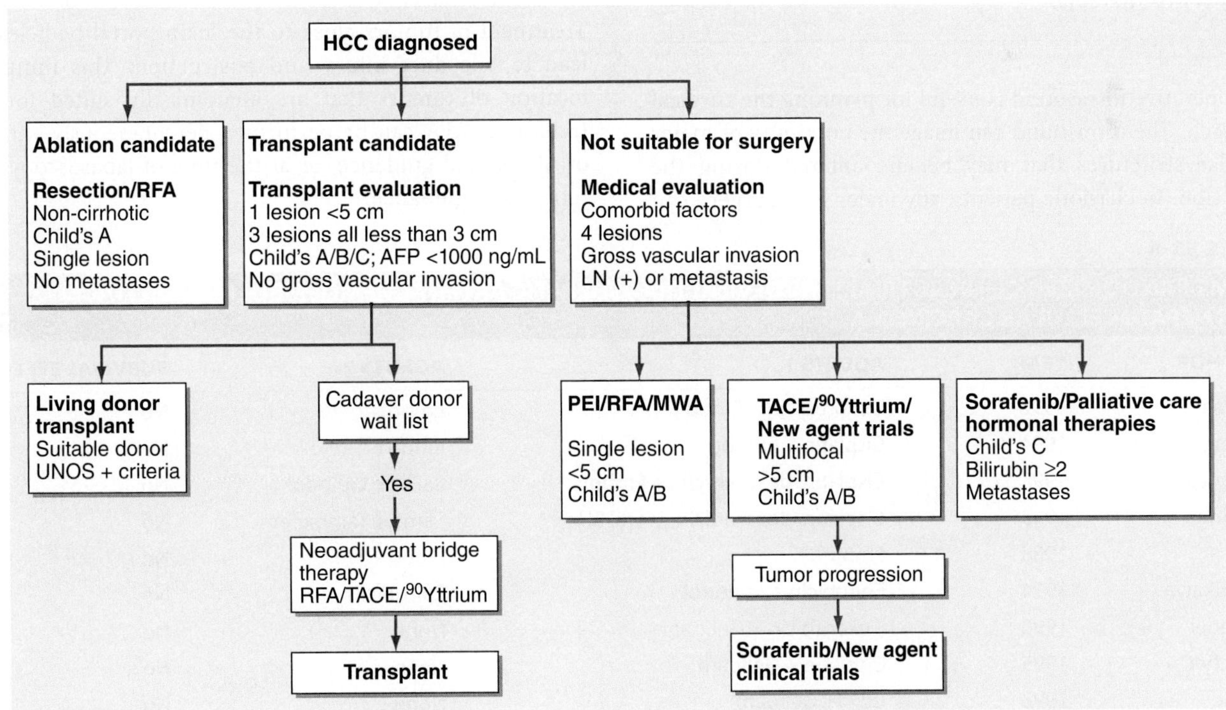

FIGURE 53-2

Hepatocellular carcinoma (HCC) treatment algorithm. The initial clinical evaluation is aimed at assessing the extent of the tumor and the underlying functional compromise of the liver by cirrhosis. Patients are classified as having resectable disease or unresectable disease or as being candidates for transplantation. AFP, α fetoprotein; LN, lymph node; MWA, microwave ablation; OLTX, orthotopic liver transplantation; PEI, percutaneous ethanol injection; RFA, radiofrequency ablation; TACE, transcatheter arterial chemoembolization; UNOS, United Network for Organ Sharing. Child's A/B/C refers to the Child-Pugh classification of liver failure.

TABLE 53-5

TREATMENT OPTIONS FOR HEPATOCELLULAR CARCINOMA
Surgery
Resection
Liver transplantation
Local Ablative Therapies
Radiofrequency ablation (RFA)
Microwave ablation (MWA)
Cryosurgery
Percutaneous ethanol injection (PEI)
Regional Therapies: Hepatic Artery Transcatheter Treatments
Transarterial chemotherapy
Transarterial embolization
Transarterial chemoembolization
Transarterial drug-eluting beads
Transarterial radiotherapies:
^{90}Yttrium microspheres
^{131}Iodine– Ethiodol
Proton beam radiation
Conformal External-Beam Radiation and Intensity-Modulated Radiation Therapy
Systemic therapies
Molecularly targeted therapies (sorafenib, etc.)
Chemotherapy
Immunotherapy
Hormonal therapy + growth control
Supportive Therapies

Intraoperative ultrasound is useful for planning the surgical approach. The ultrasound can image the proximity of major vascular structures that may be encountered during the dissection. In cirrhotic patients, any major liver surgery can result in liver failure. The Child-Pugh classification of liver failure is still a reliable prognosticator for tolerance of hepatic surgery, and only Child A patients should be considered for surgical resection. Child B and C patients with stages I and II HCC should be referred for OLTX if appropriate, as well as patients with ascites or a recent history of variceal bleeding. Although open surgical excision is the most reliable, the patient may be better served with a laparoscopic approach to resection, using RFA, MWA, or percutaneous ethanol injection (PEI). No adequate comparisons of these different techniques have been undertaken, and the choice of treatment is usually based on physician skill. However, RFA has been shown to be superior to PEI in necrosis induction for tumors <3 cm in diameter and is thought to be equivalent to open resection and, thus, is the treatment of first choice for these small tumors. As tumors get larger than 3 cm, especially ≥5 cm, the effectiveness of RFA-induced necrosis diminishes. The combination of transcatheter arterial chemoembolization (TACE) with RFA has shown superior results to TACE alone in a prospective, randomized trial. Although vascular invasion is a preeminent negative prognostic factor, microvascular invasion in small tumors appears not to be a negative factor.

Local ablation strategies RFA uses heat to ablate tumors. The maximum size of the probe arrays allows for a 7-cm zone of necrosis, which would be adequate for a 3- to 4-cm tumor. The heat reliably kills cells within the zone of necrosis. Treatment of tumors close to the main portal pedicles can lead to bile duct injury and obstruction. This limits the location of tumors that are anatomically suited for this technique. RFA can be performed percutaneously with CT or ultrasound guidance, or at the time of laparoscopy with ultrasound guidance.

TABLE 53-6

SOME RANDOMIZED CLINICAL TRIALS INVOLVING TRANSHEPATIC ARTERY CHEMOEMBOLIZATION (TACE) FOR HEPATOCELLULAR CARCINOMA

AUTHOR	YEAR	AGENTS 1	AGENTS 2	SURVIVAL EFFECT
Kawaii	1992	Doxorubicin + Embo	Embo	No
Chang	1994	Cisplatin + Embo	Embo	No
Hatanaka	1995	Cisplatin, doxorubicin, + Embo	Same + Lipiodol	No
Uchino	1993	Cisplatin, doxorubicin, + oral FU	Same + Tamoxifen	No
Lin	1988	Embo	Embo + IV FU	No
Yoshikawa	1994	Epirubicin + Ethiodol	Epirubicin	No
Pelletier	1990	Doxorubicin + Gelfoam	None	No
Trinchet	1995	Cisplatin + Gelfoam	None	No
Bruix	1998	Coils + Gelfoam	None	No
Pelletier	1998	Cisplatin + Ethiodol	None	No
Trinchet	1995	Cisplatin + Gelfoam	None	No
Lo	2002	Cisplatin + Ethiodol	None	Yes
Llovet	2002	Doxorubicin + Ethiodol	None	Yes

Abbreviations: Embo, embolization; FU, 5-fluorouracil.

Local injection therapy Numerous agents have been used for local injection into tumors, most commonly ethanol (PEI). The relatively soft HCC within the hard background cirrhotic liver allows for injection of large volumes of ethanol into the tumor without diffusion into the hepatic parenchyma or leakage out of the liver. PEI causes direct destruction of cancer cells, but it is not selective for cancer and will destroy normal cells in the vicinity. However, it usually requires multiple injections (average three), in contrast to one for RFA. The maximum size of tumor reliably treated is 3 cm, even with multiple injections.

Current directions Resection and RFA each obtain similar results. However, a distinction has been made between the causes and prevention strategies needed to prevent early versus late tumor recurrences after resection. Early recurrence has been linked to tumor invasion factors, especially microvascular tumor invasion with elevated transaminases, whereas late recurrence has been associated with cirrhosis and virus hepatitis factors and, thus, the development of new tumors. See the section on virus-directed adjuvant therapy below.

Liver transplantation (OLTX) A viable option for stages I and II tumors in the setting of cirrhosis is OLTX, with survival approaching that for noncancer cases. OLTX for patients with a single lesion ≤5 cm or three or fewer nodules, each ≤3 cm (Milan criteria), resulted in excellent tumor-free survival (≥70% at 5 years). For advanced HCC, OLTX has been abandoned due to high tumor recurrence rates. Priority scoring for OLTX previously led to HCC patients waiting too long for their OLTX, resulting in some tumors becoming too advanced during the patient's wait for a donated liver. A variety of therapies were used as a "bridge" to OLTX, including RFA, TACE, and hepatic arterial ^{90}Y-radioembolization. These pretransplant treatments allow patients to remain on the waiting list longer, giving them greater opportunities to be transplanted, because they can stabilize the tumor and prevent it from growing in the months until a donor liver becomes available. What remains unclear, however, is whether this translates into prolonged survival after transplant. Further, it is not known whether patients who have had their tumor(s) treated preoperatively follow the recurrence pattern predicted by their tumor status at the time of transplant (i.e., post–local ablative therapy), or if they follow the course set by their tumor parameters present before such treatment. The United Network for Organ Sharing (UNOS) point system for priority scoring of OLTX recipients now includes additional points for patients with HCC. The success of living related donor liver transplantation programs has also led to patients receiving transplantation earlier for HCC and often with greater than minimal tumors.

Current directions Expanded criteria for larger HCCs beyond the Milan criteria (one lesion <5 cm or three lesions, each <3 cm), such as the University of California, San Francisco (UCSF) criteria (single lesion ≤6.5 cm or two lesions ≤4.5 cm with a total diameter ≤8 cm; 1- and 5-year survival rates of 90 and 75%, respectively), are being increasingly accepted by various UNOS areas for OLTX with satisfactory longer-term survival comparable to Milan criteria results. Furthermore, downstaging of HCCs that are too large for the Milan criteria by medical therapy (TACE) is increasingly recognized as acceptable treatment before OLTX with equivalent outcomes to patients who originally were within Milan criteria. Within-criteria patients with AFP levels >1000 ng/mL have exceptionally high post-OLTX recurrence rates. Also, the use of "salvage" OLTX after recurrent HCC after resection has produced conflicting outcomes. Shortages of organs combined with advances in resection safety have led to increasing use of resection for patients with good liver function.

Adjuvant therapy The role of adjuvant chemotherapy for patients after resection or OLTX remains unclear. Both adjuvant and neoadjuvant approaches have been studied, but no clear advantage in disease-free or overall survival has been found. However, a meta-analysis of several trials revealed a significant improvement in disease-free and overall survival. Although analysis of postoperative adjuvant systemic chemotherapy trials demonstrated no disease-free or overall survival advantage, single studies of TACE and neoadjuvant ^{131}I-Ethiodol showed enhanced survival after resection.

Antiviral therapy, instead of anticancer therapy, has been successful in decreasing postresection tumor recurrences in the postresection adjuvant setting. Nucleoside analogues in HBV-based HCC and peg-interferon plus ribavirin for HCV-based HCC have both been effective in reducing recurrence rates.

Current directions A large adjuvant trial examining resection and transplantation, with or without sorafenib (see below) is in progress. The success of viral therapies in decreasing HCC recurrence after resection is part of a broader focus on the tumor microenvironment (stroma, blood vessels, inflammatory cells, and cytokines) as mediators of HCC progression and as targets for new therapies.

TNM STAGES III AND IV HCC Fewer surgical options exist for stage III tumors involving major vascular structures. In patients without cirrhosis, a major hepatectomy is feasible, although prognosis is poor. Patients with Child A cirrhosis may be resected, but a lobectomy is associated with significant morbidity and mortality rates, and long-term prognosis is poor. Nevertheless, a small percentage of patients will achieve long-term survival, justifying an attempt at resection when feasible. Because of the advanced nature of these tumors, even successful resection can be followed by rapid recurrence. These patients are not considered candidates for transplantation because of the high tumor recurrence rates, unless their tumors can first be downstaged with neoadjuvant therapy. Decreasing the size of the primary tumor allows for less surgery, and the delay in surgery allows for extrahepatic disease to manifest on imaging studies and avoid unhelpful OLTX. The prognosis is poor for stage IV tumors, and no surgical treatment is recommended.

Systemic chemotherapy A large number of controlled and uncontrolled clinical studies have been performed with most of the major classes of cancer chemotherapy. No single agent or combination of agents given systemically reproducibly leads to even a 25% response rate or has any effect on survival.

Regional chemotherapy In contrast to the dismal results of systemic chemotherapy, a variety of agents given via the hepatic artery have activity for HCC confined to the liver (Table 53-6). Two randomized controlled trials have shown a survival advantage for TACE in a selected subset of patients. One used doxorubicin, and the other used cisplatin. Despite the fact that increased hepatic extraction of chemotherapy has been shown for very few drugs, some drugs such as cisplatin, doxorubicin, mitomycin C, and possibly neocarzinostatin, produce substantial objective responses when administered regionally. Few data are available on continuous hepatic arterial infusion for HCC, although pilot studies with cisplatin have shown encouraging responses. Because the reports have not usually stratified responses or survival based on TNM staging, it is difficult to know long-term prognosis in relation to tumor extent. Most of the studies on regional hepatic arterial chemotherapy also use an embolizing agent such as Ethiodol, gelatin sponge particles (Gelfoam), starch (Spherex), or microspheres. Two products are composed of microspheres of defined size ranges—Embospheres (Biospheres) and Contour SE—using particles of 40–120, 100–300, 300–500, and 500–1000 μm in size. The optimal diameter of the particles for TACE has yet to be defined. Consistently higher objective response rates are reported for arterial administration of drugs together with some form of hepatic artery occlusion compared with any form of systemic chemotherapy to date. The widespread use of some form of embolization in addition to chemotherapy has added to its toxicities. These include a frequent but transient fever, abdominal pain, and anorexia (all in >60% of patients). In addition, >20% of patients have increased ascites or transient elevation of transaminases. Cystic artery spasm and cholecystitis are also not uncommon. However, higher responses have also been obtained. The hepatic toxicities associated with embolization may be ameliorated by the use of degradable starch microspheres, with 50–60% response rates. Two randomized studies of TACE versus placebo showed a survival advantage for treatment (Table 53-6). In addition, it is not clear that formal oncologic CT response criteria are adequate for HCC. A loss of vascularity on CT without size change may be an index of loss of viability and thus of response to TACE. A major problem that TACE trials have had in showing a survival advantage is that many HCC patients die of their underlying cirrhosis, not the tumor. Nevertheless, two randomized controlled trials, one using doxorubicin and the other using cisplatin, showed a survival advantage for TACE versus placebo (Table 53-6). However, improving quality of life is a legitimate goal of regional therapy. Drug-eluting beads using doxorubicin (DEB-TACE) have been claimed to produce equivalent survival with less toxicity, but this strategy has not been tested in a randomized trial.

Kinase inhibitors A survival advantage has been observed for the oral multikinase inhibitor, sorafenib (Nexavar), versus placebo in two randomized trials. It targets both the Raf mitogenic pathway and the vascular endothelial growth factor receptor (VEGFR) endothelial vasculogenesis pathway. However, tumor responses were negligible, and the survival in the treatment arm in Asians was less than the placebo arm in the Western trial (Table 53-7). Sorafenib has considerable toxicity, with 30–40% of patients requiring "drug holidays," dose reductions, or cessation of therapy. The most common toxicities include fatigue, hypertension, diarrhea, mucositis, and skin changes, such as the painful hand-foot syndrome, hair loss, and itching, each in 20–40% of patients. Several "look-alike" new agents that also target angiogenesis have either proved to be inferior or more toxic. These include sunitinib, brivanib, linifanib, everolimus, and bevacizumab (Table 53-8). The idea of angiogenesis alone as a major HCC therapeutic target may need revision.

TABLE 53-7

TARGETED THERAPIES IN HEPATOCELLULAR CARCINOMA: TRIALS

PHASE III	TARGET	SURVIVAL (MO)
Sorafenib vs placebo	Raf, VEGFR, PDGFR	10.7 vs 7.9
Sorafenib vs placebo (Asians)	Raf, VEGFR, PDGFR	6.5 vs 4.2

Abbreviations: PDGFR, platelet-derived growth factor receptor; Raf, rapidly accelerated fibrosarcoma; VEGFR vascular endothelial growth factor receptor.

New therapies Although prolonged survival has been reported in phase II trials using newer agents, such as bevacizumab plus erlotinib, the data from a phase III trial were disappointing. Several forms of *radiation therapy* have been used in the treatment of HCC, including external-beam radiation and conformal radiation therapy. Radiation hepatitis remains a dose-limiting problem. The pure beta emitter ^{90}Yttrium attached to either glass (TheraSphere) or resin (SIR-Spheres) microspheres injected into a major branch hepatic artery has been assessed in phase II trials of HCC and has encouraging tumor control and survival effects with minimal toxicities. Randomized phase III trials comparing it to TACE have yet

TABLE 53-8

PROMISING TARGETED THERAPIES THAT FAILED THEIR CLINICAL TRIAL GOALS
Sunitinib
Brivanib
Linifanib
Everolimus
Erlotinib
ThermaDox
Oncolytic virus JX-594
Bevacizumab
Bevacizumab plus erlotinib vs sorafenib
Sorafenib plus erlotinib vs sorafenib

to be completed. The main attractiveness of ^{90}Yttrium therapy is its safety in the presence of major branch portal vein thrombosis, where TACE is dangerous or contraindicated. Furthermore, external-beam radiation has been reported to be safe and useful in the control of major branch portal or hepatic vein invasion (thrombosis) by tumors. The studies have all been small. Vitamin K has been assessed in clinical trials at high dosage for its HCC-inhibitory actions. This idea is based on the characteristic biochemical defect in HCC of elevated plasma levels of immature prothrombin (DCP or PIVKA-2), due to a defect in the activity of prothrombin carboxylase, a vitamin K–dependent enzyme. Two vitamin K randomized controlled trials from Japan show decreased tumor occurrence, but a major phase III trial aimed at limiting postresection recurrence was not successful.

Current directions A number of new kinase inhibitors are being evaluated for HCC (Tables 53-9 and 53-10). These include the biologicals, such as Raf kinase and vascular endothelial growth factor (VEGF) inhibitors, and agents that target various steps of the cell growth pathway. Current hopes focus particularly on the Met pathway inhibitors such as tivantinib and several IGF receptor antagonists. ^{90}Yttrium looks promising and without chemotherapy toxicities. It is particularly attractive because, unlike TACE, it seems safe in the presence of portal vein thrombosis, a pathognomonic feature of HCC aggressiveness. The bottleneck of liver donors for OLTX is at last widening with increasing use of living donors, and criteria for OLTX for larger HCCs are slowly expanding. Patient participation in clinical trials assessing new therapies is encouraged (www.clinicaltrials.gov).

TABLE 53-9

NEW TARGETED AGENTS AND THEIR TARGETS IN CURRENT CLINICAL TRIALS

TARGETS	INHIBITORS
EGF receptor	Erlotinib Gefitinib Cetuximab Panitumumab
cMET	Tivantinib (ARQ197) EMD1204831 Cabozantinib
VEGF receptor	Bevacizumab Regorafenib Brivanib Cediranib Sunitinib
FGF1 receptor	AEW54 R1507 (MAb) Linsitinib (OSI-906) Brivanib
TRAIL-R1 (proapoptosis)	Mapatumumab
PDGF receptor	Sorafenib Dovitinib Linifanib
IGF-I receptor	IMC-A12 B11B022 Cixutumumab
Ubiquitin-proteasome	Bortezomib

Abbreviations: EGF, epidermal growth factor; FGF1, fibroblast growth factor 1; IGF-I, insulin-like growth factor I; PDGF, platelet-derived growth factor; VEGF, vascular endothelial growth factor.

TABLE 53-10

SOME NOVEL MEDICAL TREATMENTS FOR HEPATOCELLULAR CARCINOMA
EGF receptor antagonists: erlotinib, gefitinib, lapatinib, cetuximab, brivanib
Multikinase antagonists: sorafenib, sunitinib
VEGF antagonist: bevacizumab
VEGFR antagonist: ABT-869 (linifanib)
mTOR antagonists: sirolimus, temsirolimus, everolimus
Proteasome inhibitors: bortezomib
Vitamin K
^{131}I–Ethiodol (lipiodol)
^{131}I–Ferritin
^{90}Yttrium microspheres (TheraSphere, SIR-Spheres)
^{166}Holmium, ^{188}Rhenium
Three-dimensional conformal radiation
Proton beam high-dose radiotherapy
Gamma knife, CyberKnife
New targets: inhibitors of cyclin dependent kinases (Cdk), TRAIL induction caspases, and stem cells

Abbreviations: EGF, epidermal growth factor; mTOR, mammalian target of rapamycin; VEGF, vascular endothelial growth factor; VEGFR, vascular endothelial growth factor receptor.

The main effort now is the evaluation of combinations of the compounds listed in Tables 53-7, 53-8, and 53-9 that target different pathways, as well as the combination of any of these targeted therapies, but especially sorafenib, with TACE or ^{90}Yttrium radioembolization. Combining TACE with sorafenib appears to be safe in phase II studies with promising survival data, but randomized studies are still in progress. The same is true for intra-arterial ^{90}Yttrium plus sorafenib as therapy for HCC and as bridge to transplant therapy.

SIGNIFICANCE AND EVALUATION OF RESPONSES TO NONSURGICAL THERAPIES

Tumor growth or spread is considered a poor prognostic sign and evidence of treatment failure. By contrast, patients receiving chemotherapy are judged to have a response if there is shrinkage of tumor size. Lack of response/size decrease has been thought of as treatment failure. Three considerations in HCC management have completely changed the views concerning nonshrinkage after therapy. First, the correlation between response to chemotherapy and survival is poor in various tumors; in some tumors, such as ovarian cancer and small-cell lung cancer, substantial tumor shrinkage on chemotherapy is followed by rapid tumor regrowth. Second, the Sorafenib HCC Assessment Randomized Protocol (SHARP) phase III trial of sorafenib versus placebo for unresectable HCC showed that survival could be significantly enhanced in the treatment arm with only 2% of the patients having tumor response but 70% of patients having disease stabilization. This observation has led to a reconsideration of the usefulness of response and the significance of disease stability. Third, HCC is a typically highly vascular tumor, and the vascularity is considered to be a measure of tumor viability. As a result, the Response Evaluation Criteria in Solid Tumors (RECIST) have been modified to mRECIST, which requires measurement of vascular/viable tumor on the CT or MRI scan. A partial response is defined as a 30% decrease in the sum of diameters of viable (arterially enhancing) target tumors. The need for semiquantitation of tumor vascularity on scans has led to the introduction of diffusion-weighted MRI imaging. Tissue-specific imaging agents such as gadoxetic acid (Primovist or Eovist) and the move to functional and genetic imaging mark a shift in approaches. Furthermore, plasma AFP response may be a biologic marker of radiologic response.

TREATMENT SUMMARY

Long-term survival is associated with resection or ablation or transplantation, all of which can yield >70% 5-year survival. Liver transplant is the only therapy that can treat the tumor and the underlying liver disease simultaneously and may be the most important advance in HCC therapy in 50 years. Unfortunately, it benefits only patients with limited size tumors without macrovascular portal vein invasion. Untreated patients with multinodular asymptomatic tumors without vascular invasion or extrahepatic spread have a median survival of approximately 16 months. Chemoembolization (TACE) improves their median survival to 19–20 months and is considered standard therapy for these patients, who represent the majority of HCC patients, although ^{90}Yttrium therapy may provide similar results with less toxicity. Patients with advanced-stage disease, vascular invasion, or metastases have a median survival of around 6 months. Among this group, outcomes may vary according to their underlying liver disease. It is this group at which kinase inhibitors are directed.

SUMMARY

The most common modes of patient presentation

1. A patient with known history of hepatitis, jaundice, or cirrhosis, with an abnormality on ultrasound or CT scan, or rising AFP or DCP (PIVKA-2) (Table 53-5)
2. A patient with an abnormal liver function test as part of a routine examination
3. Radiologic workup for liver transplant for cirrhosis
4. Symptoms of HCC including cachexia, abdominal pain, or fever

History and physical examination

1. Clinical jaundice, asthenia, itching (scratches), tremors, or disorientation
2. Hepatomegaly, splenomegaly, ascites, peripheral edema, skin signs of liver failure

Clinical evaluation

1. Blood tests: full blood count (splenomegaly), liver function tests, ammonia levels, electrolytes, AFP and DCP (PIVKA-2), Ca^{2+} and Mg^{2+}; hepatitis B, C, and D serology (and quantitative HBV DNA or HCV RNA, if either is positive); neurotensin (specific for fibrolamellar HCC)
2. Triphasic dynamic helical (spiral) CT scan of liver (if inadequate, then follow with an MRI); chest CT scan; upper and lower gastrointestinal endoscopy (for varices, bleeding, ulcers); and brain scan (only if symptoms suggest)
3. Core biopsy: of the tumor and separate biopsy of the underlying liver

Therapy

1. HCC <2 cm: RFA, PEI, or resection (Tables 53-5 and 53-6)
2. HCC >2 cm, no vascular invasion: liver resection, RFA, or OLTX
3. Multiple unilobar tumors or tumor with vascular invasion: TACE or sorafenib
4. Bilobar tumors, no vascular invasion: TACE with OLTX for patients with tumor response
5. Extrahepatic HCC or elevated bilirubin: sorafenib or bevacizumab plus erlotinib (combination agent trials are in progress)

OTHER PRIMARY LIVER TUMORS

FIBROLAMELLAR HCC (FL-HCC)

This rarer variant of HCC has a quite different biology than adult-type HCC. None of the known HCC causative factors seem important here. It is typically a disease of younger adults, often teenagers and predominantly females. It is AFP-negative, but patients typically have elevated blood neurotensin levels, normal liver function tests, and no cirrhosis. Radiology is similar for

HCC, except that characteristic adult-type portal vein invasion is less common. Although it is often multifocal in the liver, and therefore not resectable, metastases are common, especially to lungs and locoregional lymph nodes, but survival is often much better than with adult-type HCC. Resectable tumors are associated with 5-year survival ≥50%. Patients often present with a huge liver or unexplained weight loss, fever, or elevated liver function tests on routine evaluations. These huge masses suggest quite slow growth for many tumors. Surgical resection is the best management option, even for metastases, as these tumors respond much less well to chemotherapy than adult-type HCC. Although several series of OLTX for FL-HCC have been reported, the patients seem to die from tumor recurrences, with a 2- to 5-year lag compared with OLTX for adult-type HCC. Anecdotal responses to gemcitabine plus cisplatin-TACE are reported.

Epithelioid hemangioendothelioma (EHE)

This rare vascular tumor of adults is also usually multifocal and can also be associated with prolonged survival, even in the presence of metastases, which are commonly in the lung. There is usually no underlying cirrhosis. Histologically, these tumors are usually of borderline malignancy and express factor VIII, confirming their endothelial origin. OLTX may produce prolonged survival.

Cholangiocarcinoma (CCC)

CCC typically refers to mucin-producing adenocarcinomas (different from HCC) that arise from the biliary tract and have features of cholangiocyte differentiation. They are grouped by their anatomic site of origin, as intrahepatic (IHC), perihilar (central, ~65% of CCCs), and peripheral (or distal, ~30% of CCCs). IHC is the second most common primary liver tumor. Depending on the site of origin, they have different features and require different treatments. They arise on the basis of cirrhosis less frequently than HCC, but may complicate primary biliary cirrhosis. However, cirrhosis and both primary biliary cirrhosis and HCV predispose to IHC. Nodular tumors arising at the bifurcation of the common bile duct are called *Klatskin* tumors and are often associated with a collapsed gallbladder, a finding that mandates visualization of the entire biliary tree. The approach to management of central and peripheral CCC is quite different. Incidence is increasing. Although most CCCs have no obvious cause (etiology unknown), a number of predisposing factors have been identified. Predisposing diseases include primary sclerosing cholangitis (10–20% of primary sclerosing cholangitis [PSC] patients), an autoimmune disease, and liver fluke in Asians, especially *Opisthorchis viverrini* and *Clonorchis sinensis.* CCC seems also to be associated with any cause of chronic biliary inflammation and injury, with alcoholic liver disease, choledocholithiasis, choledochal cysts (10%), and Caroli's disease (a rare inherited form of bile duct ectasia). CCC most typically presents as painless jaundice, often with pruritus or weight loss. Diagnosis is made by biopsy, percutaneously for peripheral liver lesions, or more commonly via endoscopic retrograde cholangiopancreatography (ERCP) under direct vision for central lesions. The tumors often stain positively for cytokeratins 7, 8, and 19 and negatively for cytokeratin 20. However, histology alone cannot usually distinguish CCC from metastases from colon or pancreas primary tumors. Serologic tumor markers appear to be nonspecific, but CEA, CA 19-9, and CA-125 are often elevated in CCC patients and are useful for following response to therapy. Radiologic evaluation typically starts with ultrasound, which is very useful in visualizing dilated bile ducts, and then proceeds with either MRI or magnetic resonance cholangiopancreatography (MRCP) or helical CT scans. Invasive cholangiopancreatography (ERCP) is then needed to define the biliary tree and obtain a biopsy or is needed therapeutically to decompress an obstructed biliary tree with internal stent placement. If that fails, then percutaneous biliary drainage will be needed, with the biliary drainage flowing into an external bag. Central tumors often invade the porta hepatis, and locoregional lymph node involvement by tumor is frequent. Incidence has been increasing in recent decades; few patients survive 5 years. The usual treatment is surgical, but combination systemic chemotherapy may be effective. After complete surgical resection for IHC, 5-year survival is 25–30%. Combination radiation therapy with liver transplant has produced a 5-year recurrence-free survival rate of 65%.

TREATMENT Cholangiocarcinoma

Hilar CCC is resectable in ~30% of patients and usually involves bile duct resection and lymphadenectomy for prognostication. Typical survival is approximately 24 months, with recurrences being mainly in the operative bed but with ~30% in the lungs and liver. Distal CCC, which involves the main ducts, is normally treated by resection of the extrahepatic bile ducts, often with pancreaticoduodenectomy. Survival is similar. Due to the high rates of locoregional recurrences or positive surgical margins, many patients receive postoperative adjuvant radiotherapy. Its effect on survival has not been assessed. Intraluminal brachyradiotherapy has also shown some promise. However, photodynamic therapy enhanced survival in one study. In this technique, sodium porfimer is injected intravenously and then subjected to intraluminal red light laser photoactivation. OLTX has been assessed for treatment of unresectable

CCC. Five-year survival was ~20%, so enthusiasm waned. However, neoadjuvant radiotherapy with sensitizing chemotherapy has shown better survival rates for CCC treated by OLTX and is currently used by UNOS for perihilar CCC <3 cm with neither intrahepatic or extrahepatic metastases. A 12-center data collection study of 287 patients with perihilar CCC confirmed the benefit of this approach in a subset of patients, with a 53% 5-year survival rate but with 10% patient dropout before transplantation. The patients had neoadjuvant external radiation with radiosensitizing therapy. Patients with tumors >3 cm had significantly shorter survival. Multiple chemotherapeutic agents have been assessed for activity and survival in unresectable CCC. Most have been inactive. However, both systemic and hepatic arterial gemcitabine have shown promising results. The combination of cisplatin plus gemcitabine has produced a survival advantage compared with gemcitabine alone in a 410-patient randomized controlled phase III trial for patients with locally advanced or metastatic CCC and is now considered standard therapy for unresectable CCC. Median overall survival in the combination arm was 11.7 months versus 8.1 months for gemcitabine alone. Significant responses were seen mainly in patients with IHC and gallbladder cancer. However, neither surgery for lymph node–positive disease nor regional chemotherapy in nonsurgical patients has shown any survival advantage thus far. Several case series have shown safety and some responses for hepatic arterial chemotherapy with gemcitabine, drug-eluting beads, and ^{90}Yttrium microspheres, but no convincing clinical trials are available. Clinical trials are under way with targeted therapies. Bevacizumab plus erlotinib gave a 10% partial response rate with median overall survival of 9.9 months. A sorafenib trial yielded an overall survival of 4.4 months, but 50% of the patients had received previous chemotherapy. Patients with unresectable tumors should be treated in clinical trials.

GALLBLADDER CANCER

Gallbladder (GB) cancer has an even worse prognosis than CCC, with a typical survival of ~6 months or less. Women are affected much more commonly than men (4:1), unlike HCC or CCC, and GB cancer occurs more frequently than CCC. Most patients have a history of antecedent gallstones, but very few patients with gallstones develop GB cancer (~0.2%). GB cancer presents similarly to CCC and is often diagnosed unexpectedly during gallstone or cholecystitis surgery. Presentation is typically that of chronic cholecystitis, chronic right upper quadrant pain, and weight loss. Useful but nonspecific serum markers include CEA and CA 19-9. CT scans or MRCP typically reveal a GB mass. The mainstay of treatment is surgical, either simple or radical cholecystectomy for stage I or II disease, respectively. Survival rates are near 100% at 5 years for stage I, and range from 60–90% at 5 years for stage II. More advanced GB cancer has worse survival, and many patients are unresectable. Adjuvant radiotherapy, used in the presence of local lymph node disease, has not been shown to enhance survival. Chemotherapy is not useful in advanced or metastatic GB cancer.

CARCINOMA OF THE AMPULLA OF VATER

This tumor arises within 2 cm of the distal end of the common bile duct and is mainly (90%) an adenocarcinoma. Locoregional lymph nodes are commonly involved (50%), and the liver is the most frequent site for metastases. The most common clinical presentation is jaundice, and many patients also have pruritus, weight loss, and epigastric pain. Initial evaluation is performed with an abdominal ultrasound to assess vascular involvement, biliary dilation, and liver lesions. This is followed by a CT scan or MRI and especially MRCP. The most effective therapy is resection by pylorus-sparing pancreaticoduodenectomy, an aggressive procedure resulting in better survival rates than with local resection. Survival rates are ~25% at 5 years in operable patients with involved lymph nodes and ~50% in patients without involved nodes. Unlike CCC, approximately 80% of patients are thought to be resectable at diagnosis. Adjuvant chemotherapy or radiotherapy has not been shown to enhance survival. For metastatic tumors, chemotherapy is currently experimental.

TUMORS METASTATIC TO THE LIVER

These are predominantly from colon, pancreas, and breast primary tumors but can originate from any organ primary. Ocular melanomas are prone to liver metastasis. Tumor spread to the liver normally carries a poor prognosis for that tumor type. Colorectal and breast hepatic metastases were previously treated with continuous hepatic arterial infusion chemotherapy. However, more effective systemic drugs for each of these two cancers, especially the addition of oxaliplatin to colorectal cancer regimens, have reduced the use of hepatic artery infusion therapy. In a large randomized study of systemic versus infusional plus systemic chemotherapy for resected colorectal metastases to the liver, the patients receiving infusional therapy had no survival advantage, mainly due to extrahepatic tumor spread. ^{90}Yttrium resin beads are approved in the United States for treatment of colorectal hepatic metastases. The role of this modality, either alone or in combination with chemotherapy, is being evaluated in many centers. Palliation may be obtained from chemoembolization, PEI, or RFA.

BENIGN LIVER TUMORS

Three common benign tumors occur and all are found predominantly in women. They are *hemangiomas, adenomas,* and *focal nodular hyperplasia* (FNH). FNH is typically benign, and usually no treatment is needed. Hemangiomas are the most common and are entirely benign. Treatment is unnecessary unless their expansion causes symptoms. Adenomas are associated with contraceptive hormone use. They can cause pain and can bleed or rupture, causing acute problems. Their main interest for the physician is a low potential for malignant change and a 30% risk of bleeding. For this reason, considerable effort has gone into differentiating these three entities radiologically. On discovery of a liver mass, patients are usually advised to stop taking sex steroids, because adenoma regression may then occasionally occur. Adenomas can often be large masses ranging from 8–15 cm. Due to their size and definite, but low, malignant potential and potential for bleeding, adenomas are typically resected. The most useful diagnostic differentiating tool is a triphasic CT scan performed with HCC fast bolus protocol for arterial-phase imaging, together with subsequent delayed venous-phase imaging. Adenomas usually do not appear on the basis of cirrhosis, although both adenomas and HCCs are intensely vascular on the CT arterial phase and both can exhibit hemorrhage (40% of adenomas). However, adenomas have smooth, well-defined edges, and enhance homogeneously, especially in the portal venous phase on delayed images, when HCCs no longer enhance. FNHs exhibit a characteristic central scar that is hypovascular on the arterial-phase and hypervascular on the delayed-phase CT images. MRI is even more sensitive in depicting the characteristic central scar of FNH.

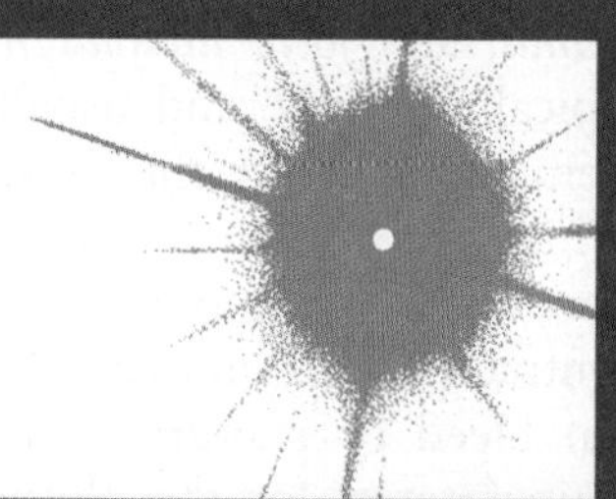

CHAPTER 54

PANCREATIC CANCER

Elizabeth Smyth ■ David Cunningham

Pancreatic cancer is the fourth leading cause of cancer death in the United States and is associated with a poor prognosis. Endocrine tumors affecting the pancreas are discussed in **Chap. 55**. Infiltrating ductal adenocarcinomas, the subject of this Chapter, account for the vast majority of cases and arise most frequently in the head of pancreas. At the time of diagnosis, 85–90% of patients have inoperable or metastatic disease, which is reflected in the 5-year survival rate of only 6% for all stages combined. An improved 5-year survival of up to 24% may be achieved when the tumor is detected at an early stage and when complete surgical resection is accomplished.

EPIDEMIOLOGY

Pancreatic cancer represents 3% of all newly diagnosed malignancies in the United States. The most common age group at diagnosis is 65–84 years for both sexes. Pancreatic cancer was estimated to have been diagnosed in approximately 45,220 patients and accounted for approximately 38,460 deaths in 2013. Although survival rates have almost doubled over the past 35 years for this disease, overall survival remains low.

GLOBAL CONSIDERATIONS

An estimated 278,684 cases of pancreatic cancer occur annually worldwide (the thirteenth most common cancer globally), with up to 60% of these cases diagnosed in more developed countries. It remains the eighth most common cause of cancer death in men and the ninth most common in women. The incidence is highest in the United States and western Europe and lowest in parts of Africa and South Central Asia. However, increasing rates of obesity, diabetes, and tobacco use in addition to access to diagnostic radiology in the developing world are likely to increase incidence rates in these countries. In this situation, consideration of the cost implications of adoption of current treatment paradigms in resource-constrained environments will be necessary. Primary prevention such as limiting tobacco use and avoiding obesity may be more cost effective than improvements in treatment of preexisting disease.

RISK FACTORS

Cigarette smoking may be the cause of up to 20–25% of all pancreatic cancers and is the most common environmental risk factor for this disease. A longstanding history of type 1 or type 2 diabetes also appears to be a risk factor; however, diabetes may also occur in association with pancreatic cancer, possibly confounding this interpretation. Other risk factors may include obesity, chronic pancreatitis, and ABO blood group status. Alcohol does not appear to be a risk factor unless excess consumption gives rise to chronic pancreatitis.

GENETIC AND MOLECULAR CONSIDERATIONS

Pancreatic cancer is associated with a number of well-defined molecular hallmarks. The four genes most commonly mutated or inactivated in pancreatic cancer are *KRAS* (predominantly codon 12, in 60–75% of pancreatic cancers), the tumor-suppressor genes *p16* (deleted in 95% of tumors), *p53* (inactivated or mutated in 50–70% of tumors), and *SMAD4* (deleted in 55% of tumors). The pancreatic cancer precursor lesion pancreatic intraepithelial neoplasia (PanIN) acquires these genetic abnormalities in a progressive manner associated with increasing dysplasia; initial *KRAS* mutations are followed by *p16* loss and finally *p53* and *SMAD4* alterations. *SMAD4* gene inactivation is associated with a pattern of widespread metastatic disease in advanced-stage patients and poorer survival in patients with surgically resected pancreatic adenocarcinoma.

Up to 16% of pancreatic cancers may be inherited. Germline mutations in the following genes are associated with a significantly increased risk of pancreatic cancer and other cancers: (1) *STK11* gene (Peutz-Jeghers syndrome), which carries a 132-fold increased lifetime risk of pancreatic cancer above the general population; (2) *BRCA2* (increased risk of breast, ovarian, and pancreatic cancer); (3) *p16/CDKN2A* (familial atypical multiple mole melanoma), which carries an increased risk of melanoma and pancreatic cancer; (4) *PALB2*, which confers an increased risk of breast and pancreatic cancer; (5) *hMLH1* and *MSH2* (Lynch syndrome), which carries an increased risk of colon and pancreatic cancer; and (6) *ATM* (ataxia-telangiectasia), which carries an increased risk of breast cancer, lymphoma, and pancreatic cancer. Familial pancreatitis and an increased risk of pancreatic cancer are associated with mutations of the *PRSS1* (serine protease 1) gene. However, for most familial pancreatic syndromes, the underlying genetic cause remains unexplained. The absolute number of affected first-degree relatives is also correlated with increased cancer risk, and patients with at least two first-degree relatives with pancreatic cancer should be considered to have familial pancreatic cancer until proven otherwise.

The desmoplastic stroma surrounding pancreatic adenocarcinoma functions as a mechanical barrier to chemotherapy and secretes compounds essential for tumor progression and metastasis. Key mediators of these functions include the activated pancreatic stellate cell and the glycoprotein SPARC (secreted protein acidic and rich in cysteine), which is expressed in 80% of pancreatic ductal adenocarcinomas. Targeting this extracellular environment has become increasingly important in the treatment of advanced disease.

SCREENING AND PRECURSOR LESIONS

Screening is not routinely recommended because the incidence of pancreatic cancer in the general population is low (lifetime risk 1.3%), putative tumor markers such as carbohydrate antigen 19-9 (CA19-9) and carcinoembryonic antigen (CEA) have insufficient sensitivity, and computed tomography (CT) has inadequate resolution to detect pancreatic dysplasia. Endoscopic ultrasound (EUS) is a more promising screening tool, and preclinical efforts are focused on identifying biomarkers that may detect pancreatic cancer at an early stage. Consensus practice recommendations based largely on expert opinion have chosen a threshold of greater than five-fold increased risk for developing pancreatic cancer to select individuals who may benefit from screening. This includes people with two or more first-degree relatives with pancreatic cancer, patients with Peutz-Jeghers syndrome, and *BRCA* 2, *p16*, and hereditary nonpolyposis colorectal cancer (HNPCC) mutation carriers with one or more affected first-degree relatives.

PanIN represents a spectrum of small (<5 mm) neoplastic but noninvasive precursor lesions of the pancreatic ductal epithelium demonstrating mild, moderate, or severe dysplasia (PanIN 1–3, respectively); however, not all PanIN lesions will progress to frank invasive malignancy. Cystic pancreatic tumors such as intraductal mucinous papillary neoplasms (IPMNs) and mucinous cystic neoplasms (MCNs) are increasingly detected radiologically and are frequently asymptomatic. Main duct IPMNs are more likely to occur in older persons and have higher malignant potential than branched duct IPMNs (invasive cancer in 45% vs 18% of resected lesions, respectively). In contrast, MCNs are solitary lesions of the distal pancreas that do not communicate with the duct system. MCNs have an almost exclusive female distribution (95%). The rate of invasive cancer in resected MCNs is lower (<18%) with increased rates associated with larger tumors or the presence of nodules.

CLINICAL FEATURES

Clinical presentation

Obstructive jaundice occurs frequently when the cancer is located in the head of the pancreas. This may be accompanied by symptoms of abdominal discomfort, pruritus, lethargy, and weight loss. Less common presenting features include epigastric pain, backache, new-onset diabetes mellitus, and acute pancreatitis caused by pressure effects on the pancreatic duct. Nausea and vomiting, resulting from gastroduodenal obstruction, may also be a symptom of this disease.

Physical signs

Patients can present with jaundice and cachexia, and scratch marks may be present. Of patients with operable tumors, 25% have a palpable gallbladder (Courvoisier's sign). Physical signs related to the development of distant metastases include hepatomegaly, ascites, left supraclavicular lymphadenopathy (Virchow's node), and periumbilical nodules (Sister Mary Joseph's nodes).

DIAGNOSIS

Diagnostic imaging

Patients who present with clinical features suggestive of pancreatic cancer undergo imaging to confirm the presence of a tumor and to establish whether the mass is likely to be inflammatory or malignant in nature. Other imaging objectives include the local and distant staging of the tumor, which will determine resectability and

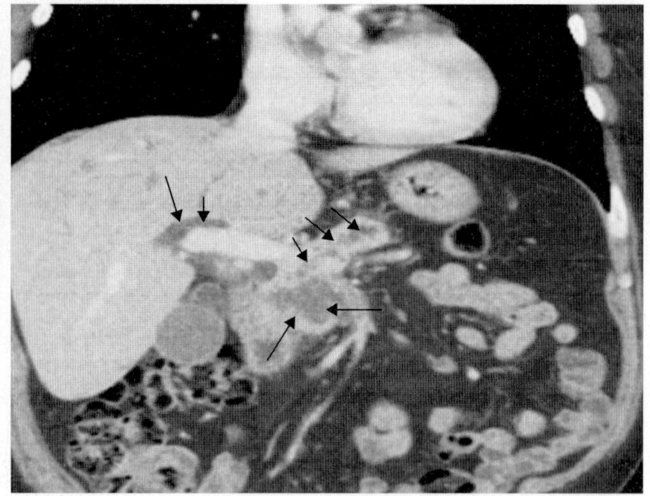

FIGURE 54-1
Coronal computed tomography showing pancreatic cancer and dilated intrahepatic and pancreatic ducts (*arrows*).

provide prognostic information. Dual-phase, contrast-enhanced spiral CT is the imaging modality of choice (Fig. 54-1). It provides accurate visualization of surrounding viscera, vessels, and lymph nodes, thus determining tumor resectability. Intestinal infiltration and liver and lung metastases are also reliably depicted on CT. There is no advantage of magnetic resonance imaging (MRI) over CT in predicting tumor resectability, but selected cases may benefit from MRI to characterize the nature of small indeterminate liver lesions and to evaluate the cause of biliary dilatation when no obvious mass is seen on CT. Endoscopic retrograde cholangiopancreatography (ERCP) is useful for revealing small pancreatic lesions, identifying stricture or obstruction in pancreatic or common bile ducts, and facilitating stent placement; however, it is associated with a risk of pancreatitis (Fig. 54-2). Magnetic resonance cholangiopancreatography (MRCP) is a noninvasive method for accurately depicting the level and degree of bile and pancreatic duct dilatation. EUS is highly sensitive in detecting lesions less than 3 cm in size (more sensitive than CT for lesions <2 cm) and is useful as a local staging tool for assessing vascular invasion and lymph node involvement. Fluorodeoxyglucose positron emission tomography (FDG-PET) should be considered before surgery or radical chemoradiotherapy (CRT), because it is superior to conventional imaging in detecting distant metastases.

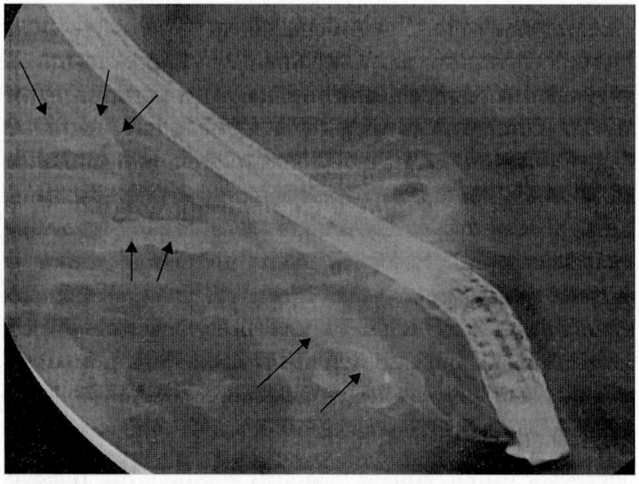

FIGURE 54-2
Endoscopic retrograde cholangiopancreatography showing contrast in dilated pancreatic duct (*arrows*).

TISSUE DIAGNOSIS AND CYTOLOGY

Preoperative confirmation of malignancy is not always necessary in patients with radiologic appearances consistent with operable pancreatic cancer. However, EUS-guided fine-needle aspiration is the technique of choice when there is any doubt, and also for use in patients who require neoadjuvant treatment. It has an accuracy of approximately 90% and has a smaller risk of intraperitoneal dissemination compared with the percutaneous route. Percutaneous biopsy of the pancreatic primary or liver metastases is only acceptable in patients with inoperable or metastatic disease. ERCP is a useful method for obtaining ductal brushings, but the sensitivity of ERCP for diagnosis ranges from 35 to 70%.

Serum markers

Tumor-associated CA19-9 is elevated in approximately 70–80% of patients with pancreatic carcinoma but is not recommended as a routine diagnostic or screening test because its sensitivity and specificity are inadequate for accurate diagnosis. Preoperative CA19-9 levels correlate with tumor stage, and postresection CA19-9 level has prognostic value. It is an indicator of asymptomatic recurrence in patients with completely resected tumors and is used as a biomarker of response in patients with advanced disease undergoing chemotherapy. A number of studies have established a high pretreatment CA19-9 level as an independent prognostic factor.

STAGING

The American Joint Committee on Cancer (AJCC) tumor-node-metastasis (TNM) staging of pancreatic cancer takes into account the location and size of the tumor, the involvement of lymph nodes, and distant metastasis. This information is then combined to assign a stage (Fig. 54-3). From a practical standpoint, patients are grouped according to whether the cancer is resectable, locally advanced (unresectable, but without distant spread), or metastatic.

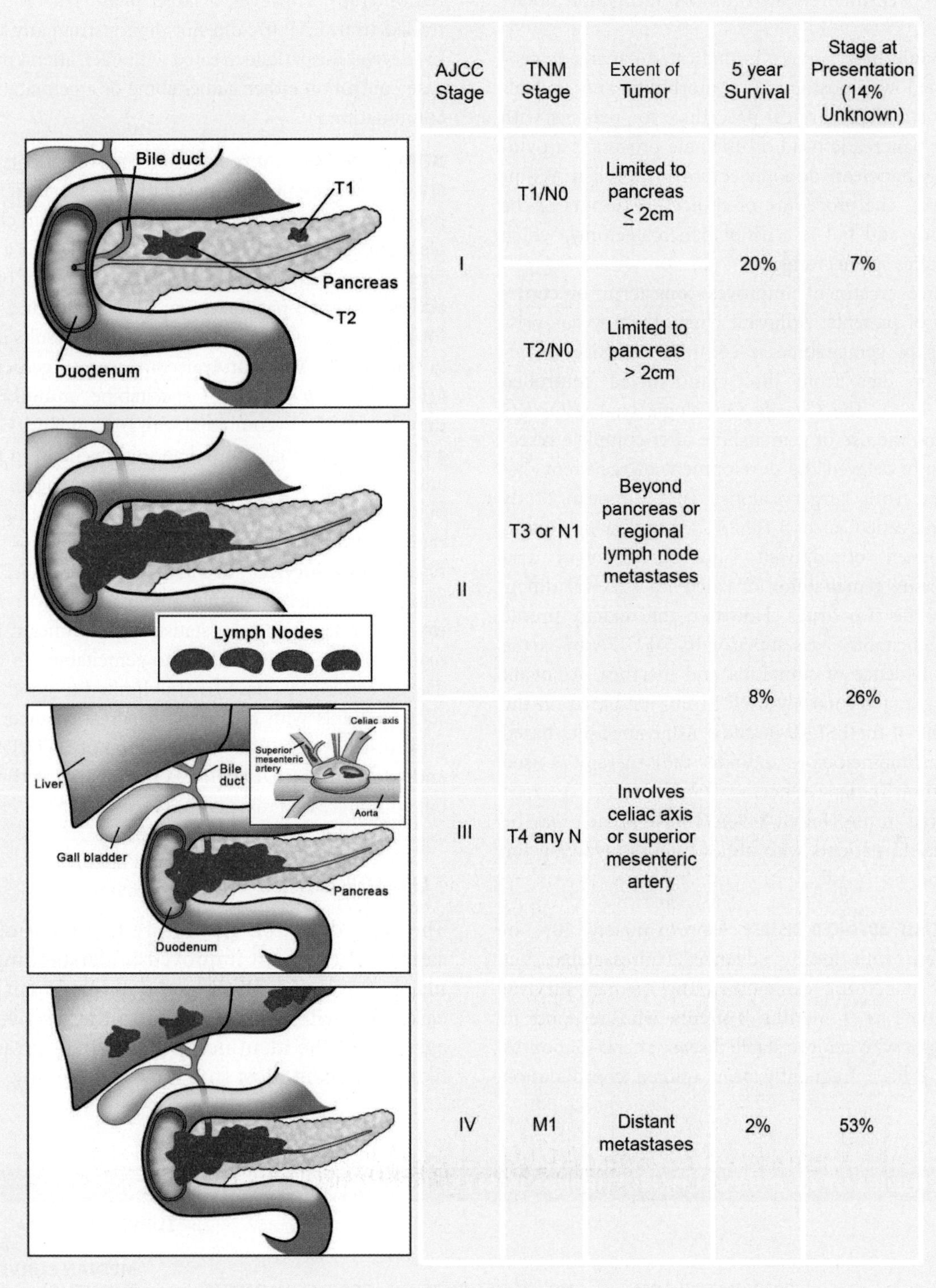

AJCC Stage	TNM Stage	Extent of Tumor	5 year Survival	Stage at Presentation (14% Unknown)
I	T1/N0	Limited to pancreas ≤ 2cm	20%	7%
	T2/N0	Limited to pancreas > 2cm		
II	T3 or N1	Beyond pancreas or regional lymph node metastases	8%	26%
III	T4 any N	Involves celiac axis or superior mesenteric artery		
IV	M1	Distant metastases	2%	53%

FIGURE 54-3

Staging of pancreatic cancer, and survival according to stage. AJCC, American Joint Committee on Cancer. *(Illustration by Stephen Millward.)*

TREATMENT Pancreatic Cancer

RESECTABLE DISEASE Approximately 10% of patients present with localized nonmetastatic disease that is potentially suitable for surgical resection. Approximately 30% of patients have R1 resection (microscopic residual disease) following surgery. Those who undergo R0 resection (no microscopic or macroscopic residual tumor) and who receive adjuvant treatment have the best chance of cure, with an estimated median survival of 20–23 months and a 5-year survival of approximately 20%. Outcomes are more favorable in patients with small (<3 cm), well-differentiated tumors and lymph node–negative disease.

Patients should have surgery in dedicated pancreatic centers that have lower postoperative morbidity and mortality rates. The standard surgical procedure for patients with tumors of the pancreatic head or uncinate process is a pylorus-preserving pancreaticoduodenectomy (modified Whipple's procedure). The procedure of choice for tumors of the pancreatic body and tail is a distal pancreatectomy, which routinely includes splenectomy.

Postoperative treatment improves long-term outcomes in this group of patients. Adjuvant chemotherapy comprising six cycles of gemcitabine is common practice worldwide based on data from three randomized controlled trials (Table 54-1). The Charité Onkologie trial (CONKO 001) found that the use of gemcitabine after complete resection significantly delayed the development of recurrent disease compared with surgery alone. The European Study Group for Pancreatic Cancer 3 (ESPAC-3) trial, which investigated the benefit of adjuvant 5-fluorouracil/folinic acid (5-FU/FA) versus gemcitabine, revealed no survival difference between the two drugs. However, the toxicity profile of adjuvant gemcitabine was superior to 5-FU/FA by virtue of its lower incidence of stomatitis and diarrhea. Adjuvant radiotherapy is not commonly used in Europe based on the negative results of the ESPAC-1 study. Adjuvant 5-FU-based CRT with gemcitabine before and after radiotherapy as used in the Radiation Therapy Oncology Group (RTOG) 97-04 trial is preferred in the United States. This approach may be most beneficial in patients with bulky tumors involving the pancreatic head.

INOPERABLE LOCALLY ADVANCED DISEASE Approximately 30% of patients present with locally advanced, unresectable, but nonmetastatic pancreatic carcinoma. The median survival with gemcitabine is 9 months. Patients who respond to chemotherapy or who achieve stable disease after 3–6 months of gemcitabine have frequently been offered consolidation radiotherapy. However, a large, phase III, randomized controlled trial, LAP-07, did not demonstrate any improvement in survival for patients treated with CRT after 4 months of disease control on either gemcitabine or a gemcitabine/erlotinib combination.

METASTATIC DISEASE Approximately 60% of patients with pancreatic cancer present with metastatic disease. Patients with poor performance status do not usually benefit from chemotherapy. Gemcitabine was the standard treatment with a median survival of 6 months and a 1-year survival rate of only 20%. The addition of nab-paclitaxel (an albumin bound nanoparticle formulation of paclitaxel) to gemcitabine results in significantly improved 1-year survival compared to gemcitabine alone (35% vs 22%, $p < 0.001$). Capecitabine, an oral fluoropyrimidine, has also been combined with gemcitabine (GEM-CAP) in a phase III trial that showed an improvement in response rate and progression-free survival over single-agent gemcitabine, but no overall survival benefit. However, pooling of two other randomized controlled trials with this trial in a meta-analysis resulted in a survival advantage with GEM-CAP. Addition of erlotinib, a small-molecule epidermal growth factor receptor inhibitor, produced a statistically significant but clinically marginal benefit when added to gemcitabine in the advanced disease setting. A phase III trial limited to good performance status patients with metastatic pancreatic cancer showed improved survival with the combination of 5-FU/FA, irinotecan, and oxaliplatin (FOLFIRINOX) compared with gemcitabine, but with increased toxicity (Table 54-2).

FUTURE DIRECTIONS

The early detection and future treatment of pancreatic cancer relies on an improved understanding of molecular pathways involved in the development of this disease. This will ultimately lead to the discovery of novel agents and the identification of patient groups who are likely to benefit most from targeted therapy.

TABLE 54-1

PHASE III STUDIES OF ADJUVANT CHEMOTHERAPY IN RESECTED PANCREATIC CANCER

			SURVIVAL	
STUDY	COMPARATOR ARM	NO. OF PATIENTS	PFS/DFS (MONTHS)	MEDIAN SURVIVAL (MONTHS)
ESPAC-1, Neoptolemos et al: N Engl J Med 350:1200, 2004	Chemotherapy (folinic acid + bolus 5-FU) vs no chemotherapy	289	PFS 15.3 vs 9.4. ($p = .02$)	20.1 vs 15.5 (HR 0.71; 95% CI 0.55–0.92; $p = .009$)
CONKO 001, Oettle et al: JAMA 297:267, 2007	Gemcitabine vs observation	368	Median DFS 13.4 vs 6.9 ($p < .001$)	22.1 vs 20.2 ($p = .06$)
ESPAC-3, Neoptolemos et al: JAMA 304:1073, 2010	5-FU/LV vs gemcitabine	1088		23 vs 23.6 (HR 0.94; 95% CI 0.81–1.08, $p = .39$)

Abbreviations: CI, confidence interval; CONKO, Charité Onkologie; DFS, disease-free survival; ESPAC, European Study Group for Pancreatic Cancer; 5-FU, 5-fluorouracil; HR, hazard ratio; LV, leucovorin; PFS, progression-free survival.

TABLE 54-2

SELECTED PHASE III STUDIES EVALUATING CHEMOTHERAPY TREATMENT IN ADVANCED PANCREATIC CANCER

			SURVIVAL	
STUDY	**COMPARATOR ARM**	**NO. OF PATIENTS**	**PFS (MONTHS)**	**MEDIAN SURVIVAL (MONTHS)**
Moore et al: J Clin Oncol 26:1960, 2007	Gemcitabine vs gemcitabine + erlotinib	569	3.55 vs 3.75 (HR 0.77; 95% CI 0.64–0.92; $p = .004$)	5.91 vs 6.24 (HR 0.82; 95% CI 0.69–0.99; $p = .038$)
Cunningham et al: J Clin Oncol 27:5513, 2009	Gemcitabine vs gemcitabine + capecitabine (GEM-CAP)	533	3.8 vs 5.3 (HR 0.78; 95% CI 0.66–0.93; $p = .004$)	6.2 vs 7.1 (HR 0.86; 95% CI 0.72–1.02; $p = .08$)
Von Hoff et al: N Engl J Med 369:1691, 2013	Gemcitabine vs gemcitabine + nab-paclitaxel	861	3.7 vs 5.5 (HR 0.69; 95% CI 0.58–0.82; $p < .001$)	6.7 vs 8.5 (HR 0.72; 95% CI 0.62–0.83; $p < .001$)
Conroy et al: N Engl J Med 364:1817, 2011	Gemcitabine vs FOLFIRINOX	342	3.3 vs 6.4 (HR 0.47; 95% CI 0.37–0.59; $p < .001$)	6.8 vs 11.1 (HR 0.57; 95% CI 0.45–0.73; $p < .001$)

ACKNOWLEDGMENT

Dr. Irene Chong is acknowledged for her work on this chapter in the 18th edition of Harrison's Principles of Internal Medicine.

CHAPTER 55

ENDOCRINE TUMORS OF THE GASTROINTESTINAL TRACT AND PANCREAS

Robert T. Jensen

GENERAL FEATURES OF GASTROINTESTINAL NEUROENDOCRINE TUMORS

Gastrointestinal (GI) neuroendocrine tumors (NETs) are tumors derived from the diffuse neuroendocrine system of the GI tract; that system is composed of amine- and acid-producing cells with different hormonal profiles, depending on the site of origin. The tumors historically are divided into GI-NETs (in the GI tract) (also frequently called *carcinoid tumors*) and pancreatic neuroendocrine tumors (pNETs), although newer pathologic classifications have proposed that they all be classified as GI-NETs. The term *GI-NET* has been proposed to replace the term *carcinoid*; however, the term *carcinoid* is widely used, and many are not familiar with this change. Accordingly, this chapter will use the term *GI-NETs* (carcinoids). These tumors originally were classified as APUDomas (for *a*mine *p*recursor *u*ptake and *d*ecarboxylation), as were pheochromocytomas, melanomas, and medullary thyroid carcinomas, because they share certain cytochemical features as well as various pathologic, biologic, and molecular features (Table 55-1). It was originally proposed that APUDomas had a similar embryonic origin from neural crest cells, but it is now known the peptide-secreting cells are not of neuroectodermal origin. Nevertheless, the concept of APUDomas is useful because these tumors have important similarities as well as some differences (Table 55-1). In this section, the areas of similarity between pNETs and GI-NETs (carcinoids) will be discussed together, and areas in which there are important differences will be discussed separately.

CLASSIFICATION/PATHOLOGY/TUMOR BIOLOGY OF NETS

NETs generally are composed of monotonous sheets of small round cells with uniform nuclei, and mitoses are uncommon. They can be identified tentatively on routine histology; however, these tumors are now recognized principally by their histologic staining patterns due to shared cellular proteins. Historically, silver staining was used, and tumors were classified as showing an argentaffin reaction if they took up and reduced silver or as being argyrophilic if they did not reduce it. Currently, immunocytochemical localization of chromogranins (A, B, C), neuron-specific enolase, and synaptophysin, which are all neuroendocrine cell markers, is used (Table 55-1). Chromogranin A is the most widely used.

Ultrastructurally, these tumors possess electron-dense neurosecretory granules and frequently contain small clear vesicles that correspond to synaptic vesicles of neurons. NETs synthesize numerous peptides, growth factors, and bioactive amines that may be ectopically secreted, giving rise to a specific clinical syndrome (Table 55-2). The diagnosis of the specific syndrome requires the clinical features of the disease (Table 55-2) and cannot be made from the immunocytochemistry results alone. The presence or absence of a specific clinical syndrome also cannot be predicted from the immunocytochemistry alone (Table 55-1). Furthermore, pathologists cannot distinguish between benign and malignant NETs unless metastasis or invasion is present.

GI-NETs (carcinoids) frequently are classified according to their anatomic area of origin (i.e., foregut, midgut, hindgut) because tumors with similar areas of origin share functional manifestations, histochemistry, and secretory products (Table 55-3). Foregut tumors generally have a low serotonin (5-HT) content; are argentaffin-negative but argyrophilic; occasionally secrete adrenocorticotropic hormone (ACTH) or 5-hydroxytryptophan (5-HTP), causing an atypical carcinoid syndrome (Fig. 55-1); are often multihormonal; and may metastasize to bone. They uncommonly produce a clinical syndrome due to the secreted products. Midgut carcinoids are argentaffin-positive, have a high

TABLE 55-1

GENERAL CHARACTERISTICS OF GASTROINTESTINAL NEUROENDOCRINE TUMORS (GI-NETs [CARCINOIDS], PANCREATIC NEUROENDOCRINE TUMORS [pNETs])
A. Share general neuroendocrine cell markers (identification used for diagnosis) 1. Chromogranins (A, B, C) are acidic monomeric soluble proteins found in the large secretory granules. Chromogranin A is the most widely used. 2. Neuron-specific enolase (NSE) is the γ-γ dimer of the enzyme enolase and is a cytosolic marker of neuroendocrine differentiation. 3. Synaptophysin is an integral membrane glycoprotein of 38,000 molecular weight found in small vesicles of neurons and neuroendocrine tumors.
B. Pathologic similarities 1. All are APUDomas showing *a*mine *p*recursor *u*ptake and *d*ecarboxylation. 2. Ultrastructurally, they have dense-core secretory granules (>80 nm). 3. Histologically, they generally appear similar with few mitoses and uniform nuclei. 4. Frequently synthesize multiple peptides/amines, which can be detected immunocytochemically but may not be secreted. 5. Presence or absence of clinical syndrome or type cannot be predicted by immunocytochemical studies. 6. Histologic classifications (grading, TNM classification) have prognostic significance. Only invasion or metastases establish malignancy.
C. Similarities of biologic behavior 1. Generally slow growing, but some are aggressive. 2. Most are well-differentiated tumors having low proliferative indices. 3. Secrete biologically active peptides/amines, which can cause clinical symptoms. 4. Generally have high densities of somatostatin receptors, which are used for both localization and treatment. 5. Most (>70%) secrete chromogranin A, which is frequently used as a tumor marker.
D. Similarities/differences in molecular abnormalities 1. Similarities a. Uncommon—mutations in common oncogenes (*ras, jun, fos,* etc). b. Uncommon—mutations in common tumor-suppressor genes (*p53*, retinoblastoma). c. Alterations at MEN 1 locus (11q13) (frequently foregut, less commonly mid/hindgut NETs) and $p16^{INK4a}$ (9p21) occur in a proportion (10–45%). d. Methylation of various genes occurs in 40–87% (*ras*-associated domain family I, p14, p16, O^6-methylguanine methyltransferases, retinoic acid receptor β). 2. Differences a. pNETs—loss of 1p (21%), 3p (8–47%), 3q (8–41%), 11q (21–62%), 6q (18–68%), Y (45%). Gains at 17q (10–55%), 7q (16–68%), 4q (33%), 18 (up to 45%). b. GI-NETs (carcinoids)—loss of 18q (38–88%), >18p (33–43%), >9p, 16q21 (21–23%). Gains at 17q, 19p (57%), 4q (33%), 14q (20%), 5 (up to 36%). c. pNETs: *ATRX/DAXX* mutations in 43%, MEN 1 mutations in 44%, mTor mutations (14%); uncommon in midgut GI-NETs (0–2%).

Abbreviations: *ATRX,* alpha-thalassemia X-lined mental retardation protein; *DAXX*, death domain associated protein; *MEN 1*, multiple endocrine neoplasia type 1; TNM, tumor, node, metastasis.

serotonin content, most frequently cause the typical carcinoid syndrome when they metastasize (Table 55-3, Fig. 55-1), release serotonin and tachykinins (substance P, neuropeptide K, substance K), rarely secrete 5-HTP or ACTH, and less commonly metastasize to bone. Hindgut carcinoids (rectum, transverse and descending colon) are argentaffin-negative, are often argyrophilic, rarely contain serotonin or cause the carcinoid syndrome (Fig. 55-1, Table 55-3), rarely secrete 5-HTP or ACTH, contain numerous peptides, and may metastasize to bone.

pNETs can be classified into nine well-established specific functional syndromes (Table 55-2), six additional very rare specific functional syndromes (less than five cases described), five possible specific functional syndromes (pNETs secreting calcitonin, neurotensin, pancreatic polypeptide, ghrelin) (Table 55-2), and nonfunctional pNETs. Other functional hormonal syndromes due to nonpancreatic tumors (usually intraabdominal in location) have been described only rarely and are not included in (Table 55-2). These include secretion by intestinal and ovarian tumors of peptide tyrosine tyrosine (PYY), which results in altered motility and constipation, and ovarian tumors secreting renin or aldosterone causing alterations in blood pressure or somatostatin causing diabetes or reactive hypoglycemia. Each of the functional syndromes listed in Table 55-2 is associated with symptoms due to the specific hormone released. In contrast, nonfunctional pNETs release no products that cause a specific clinical syndrome. "Nonfunctional" is a misnomer in the strict sense because those tumors frequently ectopically secrete a number of peptides (pancreatic polypeptide [PP], chromogranin A, ghrelin, neurotensin, α subunits

TABLE 55-2

GASTROINTESTINAL NEUROENDOCRINE TUMOR SYNDROMES

NAME	BIOLOGICALLY ACTIVE PEPTIDE(S) SECRETED	INCIDENCE (NEW CASES/10^6 POPULATION/ YEAR)	TUMOR LOCATION	MALIGNANT, %	ASSOCIATED WITH MEN 1, %	MAIN SYMPTOMS/ SIGNS
I. Established Specific Functional Syndromes						
A. Carcinoid syndrome due to GI-NET						
Carcinoid syndrome	Serotonin, possibly tachykinins, motilin, prostaglandins	0.5–2	Midgut (75–87%) Foregut (2–33%) Hindgut (1–8%) Unknown (2–15%)	95–100	Rare	Diarrhea (32–84%) Flushing (63–75%) Pain (10–34%) Asthma (4–18%) Heart disease (11–41%)
B. Well-established functional pNET syndromes						
Zollinger-Ellison syndrome	Gastrin	0.5–1.5	Duodenum (70%) Pancreas (25%) Other sites (5%)	60–90	20–25	Pain (79–100%) Diarrhea (30–75%) Esophageal symptoms (31–56%)
Insulinoma	Insulin	1–2	Pancreas (>99%)	<10	4–5	Hypoglycemic symptoms (100%)
VIPoma (Verner-Morrison syndrome, pancreatic cholera, WDHA)	Vasoactive intestinal peptide	0.05–0.2	Pancreas (90%, adult) Other (10%, neural, adrenal, periganglionic)	40–70	6	Diarrhea (90–100%) Hypokalemia (80–100%) Dehydration (83%)
Glucagonoma	Glucagon	0.01–0.1	Pancreas (100%)	50–80	1–20	Rash (67–90%) Glucose intolerance (38–87%) Weight loss (66–96%)
Somatostatinoma	Somatostatin	Rare	Pancreas (55%) Duodenum/jejunum (44%)	>70	45	Diabetes mellitus (63–90%) Cholelithiasis (65–90%) Diarrhea (35–90%)
GRFoma	Growth hormone–releasing hormone	Unknown	Pancreas (30%) Lung (54%) Jejunum (7%) Other (13%)	>60	16	Acromegaly (100%)
ACTHoma	ACTH	Rare	Pancreas (4–16% all ectopic Cushing's)	>95	Rare	Cushing's syndrome (100%)
pNET causing carcinoid syndrome	Serotonin, ?tachykinins	Rare (43 cases)	Pancreas (<1% all carcinoids)	60–88	Rare	Same as carcinoid syndrome above
pNET causing hypercalcemia	PTHrP Others unknown	Rare	Pancreas (rare cause of hypercalcemia)	84	Rare	Abdominal pain due to hepatic metastases
II. Rare Specific Functional Syndromes						
pNET secreting renin	Renin	Rare	Pancreas	Unknown	No	Hypertension
pNET secreting luteinizing hormone	Luteinizing hormone	Rare	Pancreas	Unknown	No	Anovulation, virilization (female); reduced libido (male)
pNET secreting erythropoietin	Erythropoietin	Rare	Pancreas	100	No	Polycythemia

(*continued*)

TABLE 55-2

GASTROINTESTINAL NEUROENDOCRINE TUMOR SYNDROMES (*CONTINUED*)

NAME	BIOLOGICALLY ACTIVE PEPTIDE(S) SECRETED	INCIDENCE (NEW CASES/10^6 POPULATION/ YEAR)	TUMOR LOCATION	MALIGNANT, %	ASSOCIATED WITH MEN 1, %	MAIN SYMPTOMS/ SIGNS
pNET secreting IGF-II	Insulin-like growth factor II	Rare	Pancreas	Unknown	No	Hypoglycemia
pNET secreting GLP-1	Glucagon-like peptide-1	Rare	Pancreas	Unknown	No	Hypoglycemia, diabetes
pNET secreting enteroglucagon	Enteroglucagon	Rare	Pancreas, small intestine	Unknown	Rare	Small intestinal hypertrophy, intestinal stasis, malabsorption
III. Possible Specific Functional pNET Syndromes						
pNET secreting calcitonin	Calcitonin	Rare	Pancreas (rare cause of hyper-calcitonemia)	>80	16	Diarrhea (50%)
pNET secreting neurotensin	Neurotensin	Rare	Pancreas (100%)	Unknown	No	Motility disturbances, vascular symptoms
pNET secreting pancreatic polypeptide (PPoma)	Pancreatic polypeptide	1–2	Pancreas	>60	18–44	Watery diarrhea
pNET secreting ghrelin	Ghrelin	Rare	Pancreas	Unknown	No	Effects on appetite, body weight
IV. Non Functional Syndrome pNET						
PPoma/ nonfunctional[a]	None	1–2	Pancreas (100%)	>60	18–44	Weight loss (30–90%) Abdominal mass (10–30%) Pain (30–95%)

Abbreviations: ACTH, adrenocorticotropic hormone; GRFoma, growth hormone–releasing factor secreting pancreatic endocrine tumor; IGF-II, insulin-like growth factor II; MEN, multiple endocrine neoplasia; pNET, pancreatic neuroendocrine tumor; PPoma, tumor secreting pancreatic polypeptide; PTHrP, parathyroid hormone–related peptide; VIPoma, tumor secreting vasoactive intestinal peptide; WDHA, *w*atery *d*iarrhea, *h*ypokalemia, and *a*chlorhydria syndrome.

[a]Pancreatic polypeptide–secreting tumors (PPomas) are listed in two places because most authorities classify these as not associated with a specific hormonal syndrome (nonfunctional); however, rare cases of watery diarrhea proposed to be due to PPomas have been reported.

of human chorionic gonadotropin, and neuron-specific enolase); however, they cause no specific clinical syndrome. The symptoms caused by nonfunctional pNETs are entirely due to the tumor per se. pNETs frequently ectopically secrete PP (60–85%), neurotensin (30–67%), calcitonin (30–42%), and to a lesser degree, ghrelin (5–65%). Whereas a few studies have proposed their secretion can cause a specific functional syndrome, most studies support the conclusion that their ectopic secretion is not associated with a specific clinical syndrome, and thus they are listed in Table 55-2 as possible clinical syndromes. Because a large proportion of nonfunctional pNETs (60–90%) secrete PP, these tumors are often referred to as PPomas (Table 55-2).

GI-NETs (carcinoids) can occur in almost any GI tissue (Table 55-3); however, at present, most (70%) have their origin in one of three sites: bronchus, jejunoileum, or colon/rectum. In the past, GI-NET (carcinoids) most frequently were reported in the appendix (i.e., 40%); however, the bronchus/lung, rectum, and small intestine are now the most common sites. Overall, the GI tract is the most common site for these tumors, accounting for 64%, with the respiratory tract a distant second at 28%. Both race and sex can affect the frequency as well as the distribution of GI-NETs (carcinoids). African Americans have a higher incidence of carcinoids. Race is particularly important for rectal carcinoids, which are found in 41% of Asians/Pacific

TABLE 55-3

GI-NET (CARCINOID) LOCATION, FREQUENCY OF METASTASES, AND ASSOCIATION WITH THE CARCINOID SYNDROME

	LOCATION (% OF TOTAL)	INCIDENCE OF METASTASES	INCIDENCE OF CARCINOID SYNDROME
Foregut			
Esophagus	<0.1	—	—
Stomach	4.6	10	9.5
Duodenum	2.0	—	3.4
Pancreas	0.7	71.9	20
Gallbladder	0.3	17.8	5
Bronchus, lung, trachea	27.9	5.7	13
Midgut			
Jejunum	1.8	{58.4	9
Ileum	14.9		9
Meckel's diverticulum	0.5	—	13
Appendix	4.8	38.8	<1
Colon	8.6	51	5
Liver	0.4	32.	—
Ovary	1.0	2 32	50
Testis	<0.1	—	50
Hindgut			
Rectum	13.6	3.9	—

Abbreviation: GI-NET, gastrointestinal neuroendocrine tumor.
Source: Location is from the PAN-SEER data (1973–1999), and incidence of metastases is from the SEER data (1992–1999), reported by IM Modlin et al: Cancer 97:934, 2003. Incidence of carcinoid syndrome is from 4349 cases studied from 1950–1971, reported by JD Godwin: Cancer 36:560, 1975.

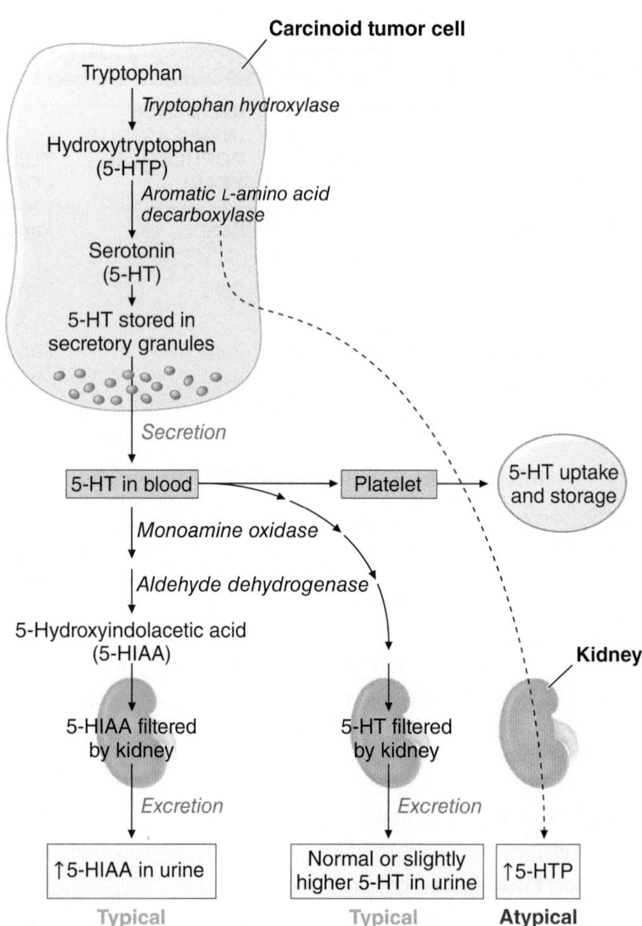

FIGURE 55-1
Synthesis, secretion, and metabolism of serotonin (5-HT) in patients with typical and atypical carcinoid syndromes. 5-HIAA, 5-hydroxyindolacetic acid.

Islanders with NETs compared to 32% of American Indians/Alaskan natives, 26% of African Americans, and 12% of white Americans. Females have a lower incidence of small intestinal and pancreatic carcinoids.

The term *pancreatic neuroendocrine* or *endocrine tumor*, although widely used and therefore retained here, is also a misnomer, strictly speaking, because these tumors can occur either almost entirely in the pancreas (insulinomas, glucagonomas, nonfunctional pNETs, pNETs causing hypercalcemia) or at both pancreatic and extrapancreatic sites (gastrinomas, VIPomas [vasoactive intestinal peptide], somatostatinomas, GRFomas [growth hormone–releasing factor]). pNETs are also called islet cell tumors; however, the use of this term is discouraged because it is not established that they originate from the islets, and many can occur at extrapancreatic sites.

Whereas the classification of GI neuroendocrine tumors into foregut, midgut, or hindgut is widely used and generally useful because the NETs within these areas have many similarities, they also have marked differences, particularly in biologic behavior, and it has not proved useful for prognostic purposes. More general classifications have been developed that allow NETs with similar features in different locations to be compared, have proven prognostic value, and are widely used. New classification systems have been developed for both GI-NETs (carcinoids) and pNETs by the World Health Organization (WHO), European Neuroendocrine Tumor Society (ENETS), and the American Joint Committee on Cancer/International Union Against Cancer (AJCC/UICC). Although there are some differences between these different classification systems, each uses similar information, and it is now recommended that the basic data underlying the classification be included in all standard pathology reports. These classification systems divide NETs from all sites into those that are well differentiated (low grade [G1] or intermediate grade [G2]) and those that are poorly differentiated (high grade [G3] divided into either small-cell carcinoma or large-cell neuroendocrine carcinoma). In these classification systems, both pNETs and GI-NETs (carcinoids) are classified as neuroendocrine tumors, and the old term of carcinoid is equivalent to well-differentiated

TABLE 55-4

COMPARISON OF THE CRITERIA FOR THE TUMOR CATEGORY IN THE ENETS AND SEVENTH EDITION AJCC TNM CLASSIFICATIONS OF PANCREATIC AND APPENDICEAL NETs

	ENETS TNM	AJCC/UICC TNM
pNETs		
T1	Confined to pancreas, <2 cm	Confined to pancreas, <2 cm
T2	Confined to pancreas, 2–4 cm	Confined to pancreas, >2 cm
T3	Confined to pancreas, >4 cm, or invasion of duodenum or bile duct	Peripancreatic spread, but without major vascular invasion (truncus coeliacus, superior mesenteric artery)
T4	Invasion of adjacent organs or major vessels	Major vascular invasion
Appendiceal NETs		
T1	≤1 cm; invasion of muscularis propria	T1a, ≤1 cm; T1b, >1–2 cm
T2	≤2 cm and <3 mm invasion of subserosa/mesoappendix	>2–4 cm or invasion of cecum
T3	>2 cm or >3 mm invasion of subserosa/mesoappendix	>4 cm or invasion of ileum
T4	Invasion of peritoneum/other organs	Invasion of peritoneum/other organs

Abbreviations: AJCC, American Joint Committee on Cancer; ENETS, European Neuroendocrine Tumor Society; NET, neuroendocrine tumor; pNET, pancreatic neuroendocrine tumor; TNM, tumor, node, metastasis; UICC, International Union Against Cancer.
Source: Modified from DS Klimstra: Semin Oncol 40:23, 2013 and G Kloppel et al: Virchow Arch 456:595, 2010.

neuroendocrine tumors of the GI tract. These classification systems are based on not only the differentiation of the NET, but also a grading system assessing proliferative indices (Ki-67 and the mitotic count). NETs are considered low grade (ENETS G1) if the Ki-67 is <3% and the mitotic count is <2 mitoses/high-power field (HPF), intermediate grade (ENETS G2) if the Ki-67 is 3–20% and the mitotic count is 2–20 mitoses/HPF, and high grade (ENETS G3) if the Ki-67 is >20% and the mitotic count is >20 mitoses/HPF. In addition to the grading system, a TNM classification has been proposed that is based on the level of tumor invasion, tumor size, and tumor extent (see Table 55-4 for an example with pNETs and appendiceal GI-NETs [carcinoids]). Because of the proven prognostic value of these classification and grading systems, as well as the fact that NETs with different classifications/grades respond differently to treatments, the systems are now essential for the management of all NETs.

In addition to these classification/grading systems, a number of other factors have been identified that provide important prognostic information that can guide treatment (Table 55-5).

The exact incidence of GI-NETs (carcinoids) or pNETs varies according to whether only symptomatic tumors or all tumors are considered. The incidence of clinically significant carcinoids is 7–13 cases/million population per year, whereas any malignant carcinoids at autopsy are reported in 21–84 cases/million population per year. The incidence of GI-NETs (carcinoids) is approximately 25–50 cases per million in the United States, which makes them less common than adenocarcinomas of the GI tract. However, their incidence has increased sixfold in the last 30 years. In an analysis of 35,825 GI-NETs (carcinoids) (2004) from the U.S. Surveillance, Epidemiology, and End Results (SEER) database, their incidence was 5.25/100,000 per year, and the 29-year prevalence was 35/100,000. Clinically significant pNETs have a prevalence of 10 cases/million population, with insulinomas, gastrinomas, and nonfunctional pNETs having an incidence of 0.5–2 cases/million population per year (Table 55-2). pNETs account for 1–10% of all tumors arising in the pancreas and 1.3% of tumors in the SEER database, which consists primarily of malignant tumors. VIPomas are 2–8 times less common, glucagonomas are 17–30 times less common, and somatostatinomas are the least common. In autopsy studies, 0.5–1.5% of all cases have a pNET; however, in less than 1 in 1000 cases was a functional tumor thought to occur.

Both GI-NETs (carcinoids) and pNETs commonly show malignant behavior (Tables 55-2 and 55-3). With pNETs, except for insulinomas in which <10% are malignant, 50–100% in different series are malignant. With GI-NETs (carcinoids), the percentage showing malignant behavior varies in different locations (Table 55-3). For the three most common sites of occurrence, the incidence of metastases varies greatly from the jejunoileum (58%), lung/bronchus (6%), and rectum (4%) (Table 55-3). With both GI-NETs (carcinoids) and pNETs, a number of factors (Table 55-5) are important prognostic factors in determining survival and the aggressiveness of the tumor. Patients with pNETs (excluding insulinomas) generally have a poorer prognosis than do patients with GI-NETs (carcinoids).

TABLE 55-5

PROGNOSTIC FACTORS IN NEUROENDOCRINE TUMORS

I. Both GI-NETs (carcinoids) and pNETs

- Symptomatic presentation (p <.05)
- Presence of liver metastases (p <.001)
- Extent of liver metastases (p <.001)
- Presence of lymph node metastases (p <.001)
- Development of bone or extrahepatic metastases (p <.01)
- Depth of invasion (p <.001)
- Rapid rate of tumor growth
- Elevated serum alkaline phosphatase levels (p = .003)
- Primary tumor site (p <.001)
- Primary tumor size (p <.005)
- High serum chromogranin A level (p <.01)
- Presence of one or more circulating tumor cells (p <.001)
- Various histologic features
  - Tumor differentiation (p <.001)
  - High growth indices (high Ki-67 index, PCNA expression)
  - High mitotic counts (p <.001)
  - Necrosis present
  - Presence of cytokeratin 19 (p <.02)
  - Vascular or perineural invasion
  - Vessel density (low microvessel density, increased lymphatic density)
  - High CD10 metalloproteinase expression (in series with all grades of NETs)
  - Flow cytometric features (i.e., aneuploidy)
  - High VEGF expression (in low-grade or well-differentiated NETs only)
- WHO, ENETS, AJCC/UICC, and grading classification
- Presence of a pNET rather than GI-NET associated with poorer prognosis (p = .0001)
- Older age (p <.01)

II. GI-NETs (Carcinoids)

- Location of primary: appendix < lung, rectum < small intestine < pancreas
- Presence of carcinoid syndrome
- Laboratory results (urinary 5-HIAA levels [p <.01], plasma neuropeptide K [p <.05], serum chromogranin A [p <.01])
- Presence of a second malignancy
- Male sex (p <.001)
- Molecular findings (TGF-α expression [p <.05], chr 16q LOH or gain chr 4p [p <.05])
- WHO, ENETS, AJCC/UICC, and grading classification
- Molecular findings (gain in chr 14, loss of 3p13 [ileal carcinoid], upregulation of Hoxc6)

III. pNETs

- Location of primary: duodenal (gastrinoma) better than pancreatic
- Ha-*ras* oncogene or p53 overexpression
- Female gender
- MEN 1 syndrome absent
- Presence of nonfunctional tumor (some studies, not all)
- WHO, ENETS, AJCC/UICC, and grading classification
- Various histologic features: IHC positivity for c-KIT, low cyclin B1 expression (p <.01), loss of PTEN or of tuberous sclerosis-2 IHC, expression of fibroblast growth factor-13
- Laboratory findings (increased chromogranin A in some studies; gastrinomas—increased gastrin level)
- Molecular findings (increased HER2/*neu* expression [p = .032], chr 1q, 3p, 3q, or 6q LOH [p = .0004], EGF receptor overexpression [p = .034], gains in chr 7q, 17q, 17p, 20q; alterations in the VHL gene [deletion, methylation]; presence of FGFR4-G388R single-nucleotide polymorphism)

Abbreviations: 5-HIAA, 5-hydroxyindoleacetic acid; AJCC, American Joint Committee on Cancer; chr, chromosome; EGF, epidermal growth factor; FGFR, fibroblast growth factor receptor; GI-NET, gastrointestinal neuroendocrine tumor; IHC, immunohistochemistry; Ki-67, proliferation-associated nuclear antigen recognized by Ki-67 monoclonal antibody; LOH, loss of heterozygosity; MEN, multiple endocrine neoplasia; NET, neuroendocrine tumors; PCNA, proliferating cell nuclear antigen; pNET, pancreatic neuroendocrine tumor; PTEN, phosphatase and tensin homologue deleted from chromosome 10; TGF-α, transforming growth factor α; TNM, tumor, node, metastasis; UICC, International Union Against Cancer; VEGF, vascular endothelial growth factor; WHO, World Health Organization.

The presence of liver metastases is the single most important prognostic factor in single and multivariate analyses for both GI-NETs (carcinoids) and pNETs. Particularly important in the development of liver metastases is the size of the primary tumor. For example, with small intestinal carcinoids, which are the most common cause of the carcinoid syndrome due to metastatic disease in the liver (Table 55-2), metastases occur in 15–25% if the tumor is <1 cm in diameter, 58–80% if it is 1–2 cm in diameter, and >75% if it is >2 cm in diameter. Similar data exist for gastrinomas and other pNETs; the size of the primary tumor is an independent predictor of the development of liver metastases. The presence of lymph node metastases or extrahepatic metastases; the depth of invasion; the rapid rate of growth; various histologic features (differentiation, mitotic rates, growth indices, vessel density, vascular endothelial growth factor [VEGF], and CD10 metalloproteinase expression); necrosis; presence of cytokeratin; elevated serum alkaline phosphatase levels; older age; presence of circulating tumor cells; and flow cytometric results, such as the presence of aneuploidy, are all important prognostic factors for the development of metastatic disease (Table 55-5). For patients with GI-NETs (carcinoids), additional associations with a worse prognosis include the development of the carcinoid syndrome (especially the development of carcinoid heart disease), male sex, the presence of a symptomatic tumor or greater increases in a number of tumor markers (5-hydroxyindolacetic acid [5-HIAA], neuropeptide K, chromogranin A), and the presence of various molecular features. With pNETs or gastrinomas, a

TABLE 55-6

GENETIC SYNDROMES ASSOCIATED WITH AN INCREASED INCIDENCE OF NEUROENDOCRINE TUMORS (NETs) (GI-NETs [CARCINOIDS] OR pNETs)

SYNDROME	LOCATION OF GENE MUTATION AND GENE PRODUCT	NETS SEEN/FREQUENCY
Multiple endocrine neoplasia type 1 (MEN 1)	11q13 (encodes 610-amino-acid protein, menin)	80–100% develop pNETs (microscopic), 20–80% (clinical): (nonfunctional > gastrinoma > insulinoma) GI-NETs (Carcinoids): gastric (13–30%), bronchial/thymic (8%)
von Hippel–Lindau disease	3q25 (encodes 213-amino-acid protein)	12–17% develop pNETs (almost always nonfunctional)
von Recklinghausen's disease (neurofibromatosis 1 [NF-1])	17q11.2 (encodes 2485-amino-acid protein, neurofibromin)	0–10% develop pNETs, primarily duodenal somatostatinomas (usually nonfunctional) Rarely insulinoma, gastrinoma
Tuberous sclerosis	9q34 (TSCI) (encodes 1164-amino-acid protein, hamartin), 16p13 (TSC2) (encodes 1807-amino-acid protein, tuberin)	Uncommonly develop pNETs (nonfunctional and functional [insulinoma, gastrinoma])

Abbreviations: GI, gastrointestinal; PNETs, pancreatic neuroendocrine tumors.

worse prognosis is associated with female sex, overexpression of the Ha-*ras* oncogene or p53, the absence of multiple endocrine neoplasia type 1 (MEN 1), higher levels of various tumor markers (i.e., chromogranin A, gastrin), and presence of various histologic features (immunohistochemistry for c-KIT, low cyclin B1, loss of PTEN/TSC-2, expression of fibroblast growth factor-13) and various molecular features (Table 55-5). The TNM classification systems and the grading systems (G1–G3) have important prognostic value.

A number of diseases due to various genetic disorders are associated with an increased incidence of NETs (Table 55-6). Each one is caused by a loss of a possible tumor-suppressor gene. The most important is MEN 1, which is an autosomal dominant disorder due to a defect in a 10-exon gene on 11q13, which encodes for a 610-amino-acid nuclear protein, menin. Patients with MEN 1 develop hyperparathyroidism due to parathyroid hyperplasia in 95–100% of cases, pNETs in 80–100%, pituitary adenomas in 54–80%, adrenal adenomas in 27–36%, bronchial carcinoids in 8%, thymic carcinoids in 8%, gastric carcinoids in 13–30% of patients with Zollinger-Ellison syndrome, skin tumors (angiofibromas [88%], collagenomas [72%]), central nervous system (CNS) tumors (meningiomas [<8%]), and smooth-muscle tumors (leiomyomas, leiomyosarcomas [1–7%]). Among patients with MEN 1, 80–100% develop nonfunctional pNETs (most are microscopic with 0–13% large/symptomatic), and functional pNETs occur in 20–80% in different series, with a mean of 54% developing Zollinger-Ellison syndrome, 18% insulinomas, 3% glucagonomas, 3% VIPomas, and <1% GRFomas or somatostatinomas. MEN 1 is present in 20–25% of all patients with Zollinger-Ellison syndrome, 4% of patients with insulinomas, and a low percentage (<5%) of patients with other pNETs.

Three phacomatoses associated with NETs are von Hippel–Lindau disease (VHL), von Recklinghausen's disease (neurofibromatosis type 1 [NF-1]), and tuberous sclerosis (Bourneville's disease) (Table 55-6). VHL is an autosomal dominant disorder due to defects on chromosome 3p25, which encodes for a 213-amino-acid protein that interacts with the elongin family of proteins as a transcriptional regulator. In addition to cerebellar hemangioblastomas, renal cancer, and pheochromocytomas, 10–17% develop a pNET. Most are nonfunctional, although insulinomas and VIPomas have been reported. Patients with NF-1 (von Recklinghausen's disease) have defects in a gene on chromosome 17q11.2 that encodes for a 2845-amino-acid protein, neurofibromin, which functions in normal cells as a suppressor of the *ras* signaling cascade. Up to 10% of these patients develop an upper GI-NET (carcinoid), characteristically in the periampullary region (54%). Many are classified as somatostatinomas because they contain somatostatin immunocytochemically; however, they uncommonly secrete somatostatin and rarely produce a clinical somatostatinoma syndrome. NF-1 has rarely been associated with insulinomas and Zollinger-Ellison syndrome. NF-1 accounts for 48% of all duodenal somatostastinomas and 23% of all ampullary GI-NETs (carcinoids). Tuberous sclerosis is caused by mutations that alter either the 1164-amino-acid protein hamartin (TSC1) or the 1807-amino-acid protein tuberin (TSC2). Both hamartin and tuberin interact in a pathway related to phosphatidylinositol 3-kinases and mammalian target of rapamycin (mTOR) signaling cascades. A few cases including nonfunctional and functional pNETs (insulinomas and gastrinomas) have been reported in these patients (Table 55-6). Mahvash disease is associated with the development of α-cell hyperplasia, hyperglucagonemia, and the development of NF pNETs and is due to a homozygous P86S mutation of the human glucagon receptor.

Mutations in common oncogenes (*ras, myc, fos, src, jun*) or common tumor-suppressor genes (*p53*, retinoblastoma susceptibility gene) are not commonly found in either pNETs or GI-NETs (carcinoids) (Table 5-1). However, frequent (70%) gene amplifications in *MDM2, MDM4,* and *WIPI* inactivating the p53 pathway are noted in well-differentiated pNETs, and the retinoblastoma pathway is altered in the majority of pNETs. In addition to these genes, additional alterations that may be important in their pathogenesis include changes in the *MEN1* gene, *p16/MTS1* tumor-suppressor gene, and *DPC4/Smad4* gene; amplification of the HER-2/*neu* protooncogene; alterations in transcription factors (Hoxc6 [GI carcinoids]), growth factors, and their receptors; methylation of a number of genes that probably results in their inactivation; and deletions of unknown tumor-suppressor genes as well as gains in other unknown genes (Table 55-1). The clinical antitumor activity of everolimus, an mTOR inhibitor, and sunitinib, a tyrosine kinase inhibitor (PDGFR, VEGFR1, VEGFR2, c-KIT, FLT-3), support the importance of the mTOR-AKT pathway and tyrosine kinase receptors in mediating growth of malignant NETs (especially pNETs). The importance of the mTOR pathway in pNET growth is further supported by the finding that a single-nucleotide polymorphism (FGFR4-G388R, in fibroblast growth factor receptor 4) affects selectivity to the mTOR inhibitor and can result in significantly higher risk of advanced pNET stage and liver metastases (Table 55-5). Comparative genomic hybridization, genome-wide allelotyping studies, and genome-wide single-nucleotide polymorphism analyses have shown that chromosomal losses and gains are common in pNETs and GI-NETs (carcinoids), but they differ between these two NETs, and some have prognostic significance (Table 55-5). Mutations in the *MEN1* gene are probably particularly important. Loss of heterozygosity at the MEN 1 locus on chromosome 11q13 is noted in 93% of sporadic pNETs (i.e., in patients without MEN 1) and in 26–75% of sporadic GI-NETs (carcinoids). Mutations in the *MEN1* gene are reported in 31–34% of sporadic gastrinomas. Exomic sequencing of sporadic pNETs found that the most frequently altered gene was *MEN1*, occurring in 44% of patients, followed by mutations in 43% of patients in genes encoding for two subunits of a transcription/chromatin remodeling complex consisting of DAXX (death-domain-associated protein) and ATRX (α-thalassemia/mental retardation syndrome X-linked) and in 15% of patients in the mTOR pathway. The presence of a number of these molecular alterations in pNETs or GI-NETs (carcinoids) correlates with tumor growth, tumor size, and disease extent or invasiveness and may have prognostic significance (Table 55-5).

GI-NETs (CARCINOIDS) AND CARCINOID SYNDROME

CHARACTERISTICS OF THE MOST COMMON GI-NETs (CARCINOIDS)

Appendiceal nets (carcinoids)

Appendiceal NETs (carcinoids) occur in 1 in every 200–300 appendectomies, usually in the appendiceal tip, have an incidence of 0.15/100,000 per year, comprise 2–5% of all GI-NETs (carcinoids), and comprise 32–80% of all appendiceal tumors. Most (i.e., >90%) are <1 cm in diameter without metastases in older studies, but more recently, 2–35% have had metastases (Table 55-3). In the SEER data of 1570 appendiceal carcinoids, 62% were localized, 27% had regional metastases, and 8% had distant metastases. The risk of metastases increases with size, with those <1 cm having a 0 to <10% risk of metastases and those >2 cm having a 25–44% risk. Besides tumor size, other important prognostic factors for metastases include basal location, invasion of mesoappendix, poor differentiation, advanced stage or WHO/ENETS classification, older age, and positive resection margins. The 5-year survival is 88–100% for patients with localized disease, 78–100% for patients with regional involvement, and 12–28% for patients with distal metastases. In patients with tumors <1 cm in diameter, the 5-year survival is 95–100%, whereas it is 29% if tumors are >2 cm in diameter. Most tumors are well-differentiated G1 tumors (87%) (Table 55-4), with the remainder primarily well-differentiated G2 tumors (13%); poorly differentiated G3 tumors are uncommon (<1%). Their percentage of the total number of carcinoids decreased from 43.9% (1950–1969) to 2.4% (1992–1999). Appendiceal goblet cell (GC) NETs (carcinoids)/carcinomas are a rare subtype (<5%) that are mixed adeno-neuroendocrine carcinomas. They are malignant and are thought to comprise a distinct entity; they frequently present with advanced disease and are recommended to be treated as adenocarcinomas, not carcinoid tumors.

SMALL INTESTINAL NETs (CARCINOIDS)

Small intestinal (SI) NETs (carcinoids) have a reported incidence of 0.67/100,000 in the United States, 0.32/100,000 in England, and 1.12/100,000 in Sweden and comprise >50% of all SI tumors. There is a male predominance (1.5:1), and race affects frequency, with a lower frequency in Asians and greater frequency in

African Americans. The mean age of presentation is 52–63 years, with a wide range (1–93 years). Familial SI carcinoid families exist but are very uncommon. These are frequently multiple; 9–18% occur in the jejunum, 70–80% are present in the ileum, and 70% occur within 6 cm (2.4 in.) of the ileocecal valve. Forty percent are <1 cm in diameter, 32% are 1–2 cm, and 29% are >2 cm. They are characteristically well differentiated; however, they are generally invasive, with 1.2% being intramucosal in location, 27% penetrating the submucosa, and 20% invading the muscularis propria. Metastases occur in a mean of 47–58% (range 20–100%). Liver metastases occur in 38%, to lymph nodes in 37% and more distant in 20–25%. They characteristically cause a marked fibrotic reaction, which can lead to intestinal obstruction. Tumor size is an important variable in the frequency of metastases. However, even small NETs (carcinoids) of the small intestine (<1 cm) have metastases in 15–25% of cases, whereas the proportion increases to 58–100% for tumors 1–2 cm in diameter. Carcinoids also occur in the duodenum, with 31% having metastases. Duodenal tumors <1 cm virtually never metastasize, whereas 33% of those >2 cm had metastases. SI NETs (carcinoids) are the most common cause (60–87%) of the carcinoid syndrome and are discussed in a later section (Table 55-7). Important prognostic factors are listed in (Table 55-5), and particularly important are the tumor extent, proliferative index by grading, and stage (Table 55-4). The overall survival at 5 years is 55–75%; however, it varies markedly with disease extent, being 65–90% with localized disease, 66–72% with regional involvement, and 36–43% with distant disease.

TABLE 55-7

CLINICAL CHARACTERISTICS IN PATIENTS WITH CARCINOID SYNDROME

	PERCENTAGE (RANGE)	
	AT PRESENTATION	DURING COURSE OF DISEASE
Symptoms/signs		
Diarrhea	32–93%	68–100%
Flushing	23–100%	45–96%
Pain	10%	34%
Asthma/wheezing	4–14%	3–18%
Pellagra	0–7%	0–5%
None	12%	22%
Carcinoid heart disease present	11–40%	14–41%
Demographics		
Male	46–59%	46–61%
Age		
Mean	57 yrs	59.2 yrs
Range	25–79 yrs	18–91 yrs
Tumor location		
Foregut	5–14%	0–33%
Midgut	57–87%	60–100%
Hindgut	1–7%	0–8%
Unknown	2–21%	0–26%

Rectal NETs (carcinoids)

Rectal NETs (carcinoids) comprise 27% of all GI-NETs (carcinoids) and 16% of all NETs and are increasing in frequency. In the U.S. SEER data, they currently have an incidence of 0.86/100,000 per year (up from 0.2/100,000 per year in 1973) and represent 1–2% of all rectal tumors. They are found in approximately 1 in every 1500/2500 proctoscopies/colonoscopies or 0.05–0.07% of individuals undergoing these procedures. Nearly all occur between 4 and 13 cm above the dentate line. Most are small, with 66–80% being <1 cm in diameter, and rarely metastasize (5%). Tumors between 1 and 2 cm can metastasize in 5–30%, and those >2 cm, which are uncommon, in >70%. Most invade only to the submucosa (75%), with 2.1% confined to the mucosa, 10% to the muscular layer, and 5% to adjacent structures. Histologically, most are well differentiated (98%) with 72% ENETS/WHO grade G1 and 28% grade G2 (Table 55-4). Overall survival is 88%; however, it is very much dependent of the stage, with 5-year survival of 91% for localized disease, 36–49% for regional disease, and 20–32% for distant disease. Risk factors are listed in Table 55-5 and particularly include tumor size, depth of invasion, presence of metastases, differentiation, and recent TNM classification and grade.

Bronchial NETs (carcinoids)

Bronchial NETs (carcinoids) comprise 25–33% of all well-differentiated NETs and 90% of all the poorly differentiated NETs found, likely due to a strong association with smoking. Their incidence ranges from 0.2 to 2/100,000 per year in the United States and European countries and is increasing at a rate of 6% per year. They are slightly more frequent in females and in whites compared with those of Hispanic/Asian/African descent, and are most commonly seen in the sixth decade of life, with a younger age of presentation for typical carcinoids (45 years) compared to atypical carcinoids (55 years).

A number of different classifications of bronchial GI-NETs (carcinoids) have been proposed. In some studies, they are classified into four categories: typical carcinoid (also called bronchial carcinoid tumor, Kulchitsky cell carcinoma I [KCC-I]), atypical carcinoid (also called well-differentiated neuroendocrine carcinoma [KC-II]), intermediate small-cell neuroendocrine carcinoma, and small-cell neuroendocarcinoma (KC-III). Another proposed classification includes three categories of lung NETs: benign or low-grade malignant (typical carcinoid), low-grade malignant (atypical carcinoid), and high-grade malignant (poorly differentiated carcinoma of the large-cell or small-cell type). The WHO classification includes four general categories: typical carcinoid, atypical carcinoid, large-cell neuroendocrine carcinoma, and small-cell carcinoma. The ratio of typical to atypical carcinoids is 8–10:1, with the typical carcinoids comprising 1–2% of lung tumors, atypical 0.1–0.2%, large-cell neuroendocrine tumors 0.3%, and small-cell lung cancer 9.8% of all lung tumors. These different categories of lung NETs have different prognoses, varying from excellent for typical carcinoid to poor for small-cell neuroendocrine carcinomas. The occurrence of large-cell and small-cell lung carcinoids, but not typical or atypical lung carcinoids, is related to tobacco use. The 5-year survival is very much influenced by the classification of the tumor, with survival of 92–100% for patients with a typical carcinoid, 61–88% with an atypical carcinoid, 13–57% with a large-cell neuroendocrine tumor, and 5% with a small-cell lung cancer.

Gastric NET (carcinoids)

Gastric NETs (carcinoids) account for 3 of every 1000 gastric neoplasms and 1.3–2% of all carcinoids, and their relative frequency has increased three- to fourfold over the last five decades (2.2% in 1950 to 9.6% in 2000–2007, SEER data). At present, it is unclear whether this increase is due to better detection with the increased use of upper GI endoscopy or to a true increase in incidence. Gastric NETs (carcinoids) are classified into three different categories, and this has important implications for pathogenesis, prognosis, and treatment. Each originates from gastric enterochromaffin-like (ECL) cells, one of the six types of gastric neuroendocrine cells, in the gastric mucosa. Two subtypes are associated with hypergastrinemic states, either chronic atrophic gastritis (type I) (80% of all gastric NETs [carcinoids]) or Zollinger-Ellison syndrome, which is almost always a part of the MEN 1 syndrome (type II) (6% of all cases). These tumors generally pursue a benign course, with type I uncommonly (<10%) associated with metastases, whereas type II tumors are slightly more aggressive, with 10–30% associated with metastases. They are usually multiple, small, and infiltrate only to the submucosa. The third subtype of gastric NETs (carcinoids) (type III) (sporadic) occurs without hypergastrinemia (14–25% of all gastric carcinoids) and has an aggressive course, with 54–66% developing metastases. Sporadic carcinoids are usually single, large tumors; 50% have atypical histology, and they can be a cause of the carcinoid syndrome. Five-year survival is 99–100% in patients with type I, 60–90% in patients with type II, and 50% in patients with type III gastric NETs (carcinoids).

CLINICAL PRESENTATION OF NETs (CARCINOIDS)

Gi/lung NET (carcinoid) without the carcinoid syndrome

The age of patients at diagnosis ranges from 10 to 93 years, with a mean age of 63 years for the small intestine and 66 years for the rectum. The presentation is diverse and is related to the site of origin and the extent of malignant spread. In the appendix, NETs (carcinoids) usually are found incidentally during surgery for suspected appendicitis. SI NETs (carcinoids) in the jejunoileum present with periodic abdominal pain (51%), intestinal obstruction with ileus/invagination (31%), an abdominal tumor (17%), or GI bleeding (11%). Because of the vagueness of the symptoms, the diagnosis usually is delayed approximately 2 years from onset of the symptoms, with a range up to 20 years. Duodenal, gastric, and rectal NETs (carcinoids) are most frequently found by chance at endoscopy. The most common symptoms of rectal carcinoids are melena/bleeding (39%), constipation (17%), and diarrhea (12%). Bronchial NETs (carcinoids) frequently are discovered as a lesion on a chest radiograph, and 31% of the patients are asymptomatic. Thymic NETs (carcinoids) present as anterior mediastinal masses, usually on chest radiograph or computed tomography (CT) scan. Ovarian and testicular NETs (carcinoids) usually present as masses discovered on physical examination or ultrasound. Metastatic NETs (carcinoids) in the liver frequently presents as hepatomegaly in a patient who may have minimal symptoms and nearly normal liver function test results.

GI-NETs (CARCINOIDS) WITH SYSTEMIC SYMPTOMS DUE TO SECRETED PRODUCTS

GI/lung NETs (carcinoids) immunocytochemically can contain numerous GI peptides: gastrin, insulin, somatostatin, motilin, neurotensin, tachykinins (substance K, substance P, neuropeptide K), glucagon, gastrin-releasing peptide, vasoactive intestinal peptide (VIP), PP, ghrelin, other biologically active peptides (ACTH, calcitonin, growth hormone), prostaglandins, and bioactive amines (serotonin). These substances may or may not be released in sufficient amounts to cause symptoms. In various studies of patients with GI-NETs (carcinoids), elevated serum levels of PP were found in 43%, motilin in 14%, gastrin in 15%, and VIP in 6%. Foregut NETs (carcinoids) are more likely to produce various GI peptides than are midgut NETs (carcinoids). Ectopic ACTH production causing Cushing's syndrome is seen increasingly with foregut carcinoids (respiratory tract primarily) and, in some series, has been the most common cause of the ectopic ACTH syndrome, accounting for 64% of all cases. Acromegaly due to growth hormone–releasing factor release occurs with foregut NETs (carcinoids), as does the somatostatinoma syndrome, but rarely occurs with duodenal NETs (carcinoids). The most common systemic syndrome with GI-NETs (carcinoids) is the carcinoid syndrome, which is discussed in detail in the next section.

CARCINOID SYNDROME

Clinical features

The cardinal features from a number of series at presentation as well as during the disease course are shown in Table 55-7. Flushing and diarrhea are the two most common symptoms, occurring in a mean of 69–70% of patients initially and in up to 78% of patients during the course of the disease. The characteristic flush is of sudden onset; it is a deep red or violaceous erythema of the upper body, especially the neck and face, often associated with a feeling of warmth and occasionally associated with pruritus, lacrimation, diarrhea, or facial edema. Flushes may be precipitated by stress; alcohol; exercise; certain foods, such as cheese; or certain agents, such as catecholamines, pentagastrin, and serotonin reuptake inhibitors. Flushing episodes may be brief, lasting 2–5 min, especially initially, or may last hours, especially later in the disease course. Flushing usually is associated with metastatic midgut NETs (carcinoids) but can also occur with foregut NETs (carcinoids). With bronchial NETs (carcinoids), the flushes frequently are prolonged for hours to days, reddish in color, and associated with salivation, lacrimation, diaphoresis, diarrhea, and hypotension. The flush associated with gastric NETs (carcinoids) can also be reddish in color, but with a patchy distribution over the face and neck, although the classic flush seen with midgut NETs (carcinoids) can also be seen with gastric NETs (carcinoids). It may be provoked by food and have accompanying pruritus.

Diarrhea usually occurs with flushing (85% of cases). The diarrhea usually is described as watery, with 60% of patients having <1 L/d of diarrhea. Steatorrhea is present in 67%, and in 46%, it is >15 g/d (normal <7 g). Abdominal pain may be present with the diarrhea or independently in 10–34% of cases.

Cardiac manifestations occur initially in 11–40% (mean 26%) of patients with carcinoid syndrome and in 14–41% (mean 30%) at some time in the disease course. The cardiac disease is due to the formation of fibrotic plaques (composed of smooth-muscle cells, myofibroblasts, and elastic tissue) involving the endocardium, primarily on the right side, although lesions on the left side also occur occasionally, especially if a patent foramen ovale exists. The dense fibrous deposits are most commonly on the ventricular aspect of the tricuspid valve and less commonly on the pulmonary valve cusps. They can result in constriction of the valves, and pulmonic stenosis is usually predominant, whereas the tricuspid valve is often fixed open, resulting in regurgitation predominating. Overall, in patients with carcinoid heart disease, 90–100% have tricuspid insufficiency, 43–59% have tricuspid stenosis, 50–81% have pulmonary insufficiency, 25–59% have pulmonary stenosis, and 11% (0–25%) left-side lesions. Up to 80% of patients with cardiac lesions develop heart failure. Lesions on the left side are much less extensive, occur in 30% at autopsy, and most frequently affect the mitral valve. Up to 80% of patients with cardiac lesions have evidence of heart failure. At diagnosis in various series, 27–43% of patients are in New York Heart Association class I, 30–40% are in class II, 13–31% are in class III, and 3–12% are in class IV. At present, carcinoid heart disease is reported to be decreasing in frequency and severity, with mean occurrence in 20% of patients and occurrence in as few as 3–4% in some reports. Whether this decrease is due to the widespread use of somatostatin analogues, which control the release of bioactive agents thought involved in mediating the heart disease, is unclear.

Other clinical manifestations include wheezing or asthma-like symptoms (8–18%), pellagra-like skin lesions (2–25%), and impaired cognitive function. A variety of noncardiac problems due to increased fibrous tissue have been reported, including retroperitoneal fibrosis causing urethral obstruction, Peyronie's disease of the penis, intraabdominal fibrosis, and occlusion of the mesenteric arteries or veins.

Pathobiology

Carcinoid syndrome occurred in 8% of 8876 patients with GI-NETs (carcinoids), with a rate of 1.7–18.4% in different studies. It occurs only when sufficient concentrations of products secreted by the tumor reach the systemic circulation. In 91–100% of cases, this occurs after distant metastases to the liver. Rarely, primary GI-NETs (carcinoids) with nodal metastases with extensive retroperitoneal invasion, pNETs (carcinoids) with retroperitoneal lymph nodes, or NETs (carcinoids) of the lung or ovary with direct access to the systemic circulation can cause the carcinoid syndrome without hepatic metastases. All GI-NETs (carcinoids) do not have the same propensity to metastasize and cause the carcinoid syndrome (Table 55-3). Midgut NETs (carcinoids) account for 57–67% of cases of carcinoid syndrome, foregut NETs (carcinoids) for 0–33%, hindgut for 0–8%, and an unknown primary location for 2–26% (Tables 55-3 and 55-7).

One of the main secretory products of GI-NETs (carcinoids) involved in the carcinoid syndrome is serotonin (5-HT) (Fig. 55-1), which is synthesized from tryptophan. Up to 50% of dietary tryptophan can be used in this synthetic pathway by tumor cells, and this can result in inadequate supplies for conversion to niacin; hence, some patients (2.5%) develop pellagra-like lesions. Serotonin has numerous biologic effects, including stimulating intestinal secretion with inhibition of absorption, stimulating increases in intestinal motility, and stimulating fibrogenesis. In various studies, 56–88% of all GI-NETs (carcinoids) were associated with serotonin overproduction; however, 12–26% of the patients did not have the carcinoid syndrome. In one study, platelet serotonin was elevated in 96% of patients with midgut NETs (carcinoids), 43% with foregut tumors, and 0% with hindgut tumors. In 90–100% of patients with the carcinoid syndrome, there is evidence of serotonin overproduction. Serotonin is thought to be predominantly responsible for the diarrhea. Patients with the carcinoid syndrome have increased colonic motility with a shortened transit time and possibly a secretory/absorptive alteration that is compatible with the known actions of serotonin in the gut mediated primarily through 5-HT_3 and, to a lesser degree, 5-HT_4 receptors. Serotonin receptor antagonists (especially 5-HT_3 antagonists) relieve the diarrhea in many, but not all, patients. A tryptophan 5-hydroxylase inhibitor, LX-1031, which inhibits serotonin synthesis in peripheral tissues, is reported to cause a 44% decrease in bowel movement frequency and a 20% improvement in stool form in patients with the carcinoid syndrome. Additional studies suggest that tachykinins may be important mediators of diarrhea in some patients. In one study, plasma tachykinin levels correlated with symptoms of diarrhea. Serotonin does not appear to be involved in the flushing because serotonin receptor antagonists do not relieve flushing. In patients with gastric carcinoids, the characteristic red, patchy pruritic flush is thought due to histamine release because H_1 and H_2 receptor antagonists can prevent it. Numerous studies have shown that tachykinins (substance P, neuropeptide K) are stored in GI-NETs (carcinoids) and released during flushing. However, some studies have demonstrated that octreotide can relieve the flushing induced by pentagastrin in these patients without altering the stimulated increase in plasma substance P, suggesting that other mediators must be involved in the flushing. A correlation between plasma tachykinin levels (but not substance P levels) and flushing has been reported. Prostaglandin release could be involved in mediating either the diarrhea or flush, but conflicting data exist. Both histamine and serotonin may be responsible for the wheezing as well as the fibrotic reactions involving the heart, causing Peyronie's disease and intraabdominal fibrosis.

The exact mechanism of the heart disease remains unclear, although increasing evidence supports a central role for serotonin. Patients with heart disease have higher plasma levels of neurokinin A, substance P, plasma atrial natriuretic peptide (ANP), pro-brain natriuretic peptide, chromogranin A, and activin A as well as higher urinary 5-HIAA excretion.

The valvular heart disease caused by the appetite-suppressant drug dexfenfluramine is histologically indistinguishable from that observed in carcinoid disease. Furthermore, ergot-containing dopamine receptor agonists used for Parkinson's disease (pergolide, cabergoline) cause valvular heart disease that closely resembles that seen in the carcinoid syndrome. Furthermore, in animal studies, the formation of valvular plaques/fibrosis occurs after prolonged treatment with serotonin as well as in animals with a deficiency of the 5-HIAA transporter gene, which results in an inability to inactivate serotonin. Metabolites of fenfluramine, as well as the dopamine receptor agonists, have high affinity for serotonin receptor subtype 5-HT_{2B} receptors, whose activation is known to cause fibroblast mitogenesis. Serotonin receptor subtypes 5-$HT_{1B,1D,2A,2B}$ normally are expressed in human heart valve interstitial cells. High levels of 5-HT_{2B} receptors are known to occur in heart valves and occur in cardiac fibroblasts and cardiomyocytes. Studies of cultured interstitial cells from human cardiac valves have demonstrated that these valvulopathic drugs induce mitogenesis by activating 5-HT_{2B} receptors and stimulating upregulation of transforming growth factor β and collagen biosynthesis. These observations support the conclusion that serotonin overproduction by GI-NETs (carcinoids) is important in mediating the valvular changes, possibly by activating 5-HT_{2B} receptors in the endocardium. Both the magnitude of serotonin overproduction and prior chemotherapy are important predictors of progression of the heart disease, whereas patients with high plasma levels of ANP have a worse prognosis. Plasma connective tissue growth factor levels are elevated in many fibrotic conditions; elevated levels occur in patients with carcinoid heart disease and correlate with the presence of right ventricular dysfunction and the extent of valvular regurgitation in patients with GI-NETs (carcinoids).

Patients may develop either a typical or, rarely, an atypical carcinoid syndrome (Fig. 55-1). In patients with the typical form, which characteristically is caused by midgut NETs (carcinoids), the conversion of tryptophan to 5-HTP is the rate-limiting step (Fig. 55-1). Once 5-HTP is formed, it is rapidly converted to 5-HT and stored in secretory granules of the tumor or in platelets. A small amount remains in plasma and is converted to 5-HIAA, which appears in large amounts in the urine. These patients have an expanded serotonin pool size, increased blood and platelet serotonin, and increased urinary 5-HIAA. Some GI-NETs (carcinoids) cause an atypical carcinoid syndrome that is thought to be due to a deficiency in the enzyme dopa decarboxylase; thus, 5-HTP cannot be converted to 5-HT (serotonin), and 5-HTP is secreted into the bloodstream (Fig. 55-1). In these patients, plasma serotonin levels are normal but urinary levels may be increased because some 5-HTP is converted to 5-HT in the kidney. Characteristically, urinary 5-HTP and 5-HT are increased, but urinary 5-HIAA levels are only slightly elevated. Foregut carcinoids are the most likely to cause an atypical carcinoid syndrome; however, they also can cause a typical carcinoid syndrome.

One of the most immediate life-threatening complications of the carcinoid syndrome is the development of a carcinoid crisis. This is more common in patients who have intense symptoms or have greatly increased urinary 5-HIAA levels (i.e., >200 mg/d). The crisis may occur spontaneously; however, it is usually provoked by procedures such as anesthesia, chemotherapy, surgery, biopsy, endoscopy, or radiologic examinations such as during biopsies, hepatic artery embolization, and vessel catheterization. It can be provoked by stress or procedures as mild as repeated palpation of the tumor during physical examination. Patients develop intense flushing, diarrhea, abdominal pain, cardiac abnormalities including tachycardia, hypertension, or hypotension, and confusion or stupor. If not adequately treated, this can be a terminal event.

DIAGNOSIS OF THE CARCINOID SYNDROME AND GI-NETs (CARCINOIDS)

The diagnosis of carcinoid syndrome relies on measurement of urinary or plasma serotonin or its metabolites in the urine. The measurement of 5-HIAA is used most frequently. False-positive elevations may occur if the patient is eating serotonin-rich foods such as bananas, pineapples, walnuts, pecans, avocados, or hickory nuts or is taking certain medications (cough syrup containing guaifenesin, acetaminophen, salicylates, serotonin reuptake inhibitors, or L-dopa). The normal range for daily urinary 5-HIAA excretion is 2–8 mg/d. Serotonin overproduction was noted in 92% of patients with carcinoid syndrome in one study, and in another study, 5-HIAA had 73% sensitivity and 100% specificity for carcinoid syndrome. Serotonin overproduction is *not* synonymous with the presence of clinical carcinoid syndrome because 12–26% of patients with serotonin overproduction do not have clinical evidence of the carcinoid syndrome.

Most physicians use only the urinary 5-HIAA excretion rate; however, plasma and platelet serotonin levels, if available, may provide additional information. Platelet serotonin levels are more sensitive than urinary 5-HIAA but are not generally available. A single plasma 5-HIAA determination was found to correlate with the 24-h urinary values, raising the possibility that this could replace the standard urinary collection because of its greater convenience and avoidance of incomplete or improper collections. Because patients with foregut NETs (carcinoids) may produce an atypical carcinoid syndrome, if this syndrome is suspected and the urinary 5-HIAA is minimally elevated or normal, other urinary metabolites of tryptophan, such as 5-HTP and 5-HT, should be measured (Fig. 55-1).

Flushing occurs in a number of other diseases, including systemic mastocytosis, chronic myeloid leukemia with increased histamine release, menopause, reactions to alcohol or glutamate, and side effects of chlorpropamide, calcium channel blockers, and nicotinic acid. None of these conditions cause increased urinary 5-HIAA.

The diagnosis of carcinoid tumor can be suggested by the carcinoid syndrome, recurrent abdominal symptoms in a healthy-appearing individual, or the discovery of hepatomegaly or hepatic metastases associated with minimal symptoms. Ileal NETs (carcinoids), which make up 25% of all clinically detected carcinoids, should be suspected in patients with bowel obstruction, abdominal pain, flushing, or diarrhea.

Serum chromogranin A levels are elevated in 56–100% of patients with GI-NETs (carcinoids), and the level correlates with tumor bulk. Serum chromogranin A levels are not specific for GI-NETs (carcinoids) because they are also elevated in patients with pNETs and other NETs. Furthermore, a major problem is caused by potent acid antisecretory drugs such as proton pump inhibitors (omeprazole and related drugs) because they almost invariably cause elevation of plasma chromogranin A levels; the elevation occurs rapidly (3–5 days) with continued use, and the elevated levels overlap with the levels seen in many patients with NETs. Plasma neuron-specific enolase levels are also used as a marker of GI-NETs (carcinoids) but are less sensitive than chromogranin A, being increased in only 17–47% of patients. Newer markers have been proposed including pancreastatin (a chromogranin A breakdown product) and activin A. The former is not affected by proton pump inhibitors; however, its sensitivity and specificity are not established. Plasma activin elevations are reported to correlate with the presence of cardiac disease with a sensitivity of 87% and specificity of 57%.

TREATMENT Carcinoid Syndrome and Nonmetastatic Gastrointestinal Neuroendocrine Tumors (Carcinoids)

CARCINOID SYNDROME Treatment includes avoiding conditions that precipitate flushing, dietary supplementation with nicotinamide, treatment of heart failure with diuretics, treatment of wheezing with oral bronchodilators, and control of the diarrhea with antidiarrheal agents such as loperamide and diphenoxylate. If patients still have symptoms, serotonin receptor antagonists or somatostatin analogues (Fig. 55-2) are the drugs of choice.

There are 14 subclasses of serotonin receptors, and antagonists for many are not available. The 5-HT_1 and 5-HT_2 receptor antagonists methysergide, cyproheptadine, and ketanserin have all been used to control the diarrhea

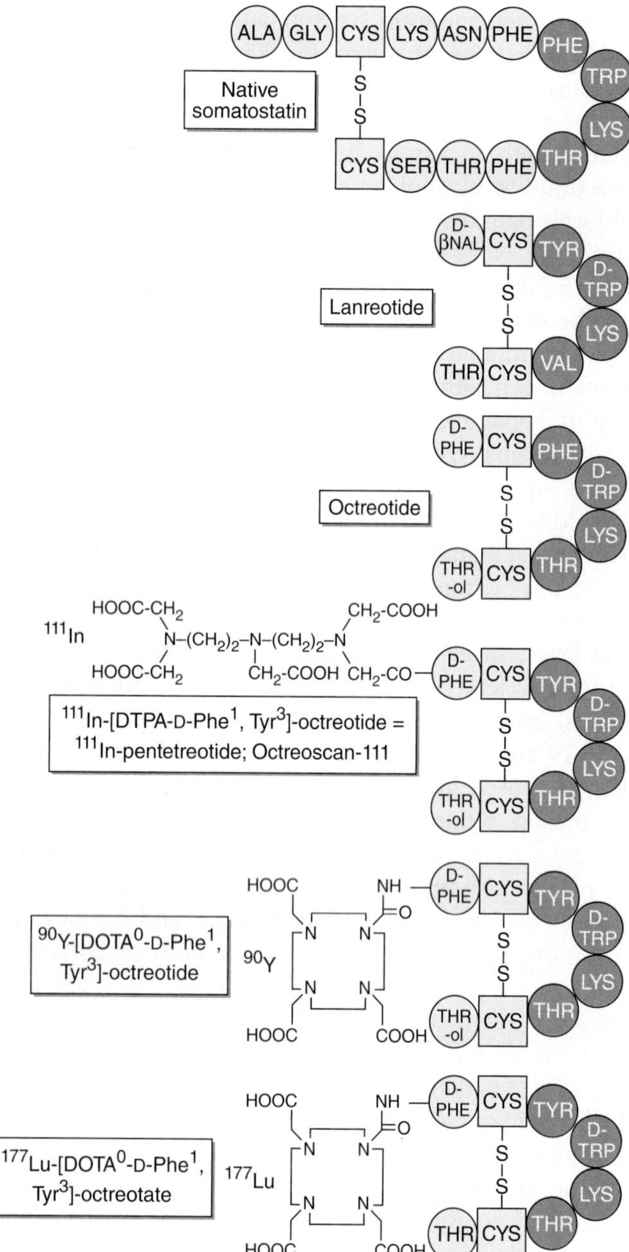

FIGURE 55-2

Structure of somatostatin and synthetic analogues used for diagnostic or therapeutic indications.

but usually do not decrease flushing. The use of methysergide is limited because it can cause or enhance retroperitoneal fibrosis. Ketanserin diminishes diarrhea in 30–100% of patients. 5-HT_3 receptor antagonists (ondansetron, tropisetron, alosetron) can control diarrhea and nausea in up to 100% of patients and occasionally ameliorate the flushing. A combination of histamine H_1 and H_2 receptor antagonists (i.e., diphenhydramine and cimetidine or ranitidine) may control flushing in patients with foregut carcinoids. The tryptophan 5-hydoxylase inhibitor telotristat etiprate decreased bowel frequency in 44% and improved stool consistency in 20%.

Synthetic analogues of somatostatin (octreotide, lanreotide) are now the most widely used agents to control the symptoms of patients with carcinoid syndrome (Fig. 55-2). These drugs are effective at relieving symptoms and decreasing urinary 5-HIAA levels in patients with this syndrome. Octreotide-LAR and lanreotide-SR/autogel (Somatuline) (sustained-release formulations allowing monthly injections) control symptoms in 74% and 68% of patients, respectively, with carcinoid syndrome and show a biochemical response in 51% and 64%, respectively. Patients with mild to moderate symptoms usually are treated initially with octreotide 100 μg SC every 8 h and then begun on the long-acting monthly depot forms (octreotide-LAR or lanreotide-autogel). Forty percent of patients escape control after a median time of 4 months, and the depot dosage may have to be increased as well as supplemented with the shorter-acting formulation, SC octreotide. Pasireotide (SOM230) is a somatostatin analogue with broader selectivity (high-affinity somatostatin receptors [sst_1, sst_2, sst_3, sst_5]) than octreotide/lanreotide (sst_2, sst_5). In a phase II study of patients with refractory carcinoid syndrome, pasireotide controlled symptoms in 27%.

Carcinoid heart disease is associated with a decreased mean survival (3.8 years), and therefore, it should be sought for and carefully assessed in all patients with carcinoid syndrome. Transthoracic echocardiography remains a key element in establishing the diagnosis of carcinoid heart disease and determining the extent and type of cardiac abnormalities. Treatment with diuretics and somatostatin analogues can reduce the negative hemodynamic effects and secondary heart failure. It remains unclear whether long-term treatment with these drugs will decrease the progression of carcinoid heart disease. Balloon valvuloplasty for stenotic valves or cardiac valve surgery may be required.

In patients with carcinoid crises, somatostatin analogues are effective at both treating the condition and preventing their development during known precipitating events such as surgery, anesthesia, chemotherapy, and stress. It is recommended that octreotide 150–250 μg SC every 6 to 8 h be used 24–48 h before anesthesia and then continued throughout the procedure.

Currently, sustained-release preparations of both octreotide (octreotide-LAR [long-acting release], 10, 20, 30 mg) and lanreotide (lanreotide-PR [prolonged release, lanreotide-autogel], 60, 90, 120 mg) are available and widely used because their use greatly facilitates long-term treatment. Octreotide-LAR (30 mg/month) gives a plasma level ≥1 ng/mL for 25 days, whereas this requires three to six injections a day of the non-sustained-release form. Lanreotide-autogel (Somatuline) is given every 4–6 weeks.

Short-term side effects occur in up to one-half of patients. Pain at the injection site and side effects related to the GI tract (59% discomfort, 15% nausea, diarrhea) are the most common. They are usually short-lived and do not interrupt treatment. Important long-term side effects include gallstone formation, steatorrhea, and deterioration in glucose tolerance. The overall incidence of gallstones/biliary sludge in one study was 52%, with 7% having symptomatic disease that required surgical treatment.

Interferon α is reported to be effective in controlling symptoms of the carcinoid syndrome either alone or combined with hepatic artery embolization. With interferon α alone, the clinical response rate is 30–70%, and with interferon α with hepatic artery embolization, diarrhea was controlled for 1 year in 43% and flushing was controlled in 86%. Side effects develop in almost all patients, with the most frequent being a flu-like syndrome (80–100%), followed by anorexia and fatigue, even though these frequently improve with continued treatment. Other more severe side effects include bone marrow toxicity, hepatotoxicity, autoimmune disorders, and rarely CNS side effects (depression, mental disorders, visual problems).

Hepatic artery embolization alone or with chemotherapy (chemoembolization) has been used to control the symptoms of carcinoid syndrome. Embolization alone is reported to control symptoms in up to 76% of patients, and chemoembolization (5-fluorouracil, doxorubicin, cisplatin, mitomycin) controls symptoms in 60–75% of patients. Hepatic artery embolization can have major side effects, including nausea, vomiting, pain, and fever. In two studies, 5–7% of patients died from complications of hepatic artery occlusion.

Other drugs have been used successfully in small numbers of patients to control the symptoms of carcinoid syndrome. Parachlorophenylanine can inhibit tryptophan hydroxylase and therefore the conversion of tryptophan to 5-HTP. However, its severe side effects, including psychiatric disturbances, make it intolerable for long-term use. α-Methyldopa inhibits the conversion of 5-HTP to 5-HT, but its effects are only partial.

Peptide radioreceptor therapy (using radiotherapy with radiolabeled somatostatin analogues), the use of radiolabeled microspheres, and other methods for treatment of advanced metastatic disease may facilitate control of the carcinoid syndrome and are discussed in a later section dealing with treatment of advanced disease.

GI-NETs (CARCINOIDS) (NONMETASTATIC) Surgery is the only potentially curative therapy. Because with most GI-NETs (carcinoids), the probability of metastatic disease increases with increasing size, the extent of surgical resection is determined accordingly. With appendiceal NETs (carcinoids) <1 cm, simple appendectomy was curative in 103 patients followed for up to 35 years. With rectal NETs (carcinoids) <1 cm, local resection is curative. With SI NETs (carcinoids) <1 cm, there is not complete agreement. Because 15–69% of SI NETs (carcinoids) this size have metastases in different studies, some recommend a wide resection with en bloc resection of the adjacent lymph-bearing mesentery. If the tumor is >2 cm for rectal, appendiceal, or SI NETs (carcinoids), a full cancer operation should be done. This includes a right hemicolectomy for appendiceal NETs (carcinoids), an abdominoperineal resection or low anterior resection for rectal NETs (carcinoids), and an en bloc resection of adjacent lymph nodes for SI NETs (carcinoids). For appendiceal NETs (carcinoids) 1–2 cm in diameter, a simple appendectomy is proposed by some, whereas others favor a formal right hemicolectomy. For 1–2 cm rectal NETs (carcinoids), it is recommended that a wide, local, full-thickness excision be performed.

With type I or II gastric NETs (carcinoids), which are usually <1 cm, endoscopic removal is recommended. In type I or II gastric carcinoids, if the tumor is >2 cm or if there is local invasion, some recommend total gastrectomy, whereas others recommend antrectomy in type I to reduce the hypergastrinemia, which has led to regression of the carcinoids in a number of studies. For types I and II gastric NETs (carcinoids) of 1–2 cm, there is no agreement, with some recommending endoscopic treatment followed by chronic somatostatin treatment and careful follow-up and others recommending surgical treatment. With type III gastric NETs (carcinoids) >2 cm, excision and regional lymph node clearance are recommended. Most tumors <1 cm are treated endoscopically.

Resection of isolated or limited hepatic metastases may be beneficial and will be discussed in a later section on treatment of advanced disease.

PANCREATIC NEUROENDOCRINE TUMORS

Functional pNETs usually present clinically with symptoms due to the hormone-excess state (Table 55-2). Only late in the course of the disease does the tumor per se cause prominent symptoms such as abdominal pain. In contrast, all the symptoms due to nonfunctional pNETs are due to the tumor per se. The overall result of this is that some functional pNETs may present with severe symptoms with a small or undetectable primary tumor, whereas nonfunctional tumors usually present late in the disease course with large tumors, which are frequently metastatic. The mean delay between onset of continuous symptoms and diagnosis of a functional pNET syndrome is 4–7 years. Therefore, the diagnoses frequently are missed for extended periods.

TREATMENT Pancreatic Neuroendocrine Tumor (General Points)

Treatment of pNETs requires two different strategies. First, treatment must be directed at the hormone-excess state such as the gastric acid hypersecretion in gastrinomas or the hypoglycemia in insulinomas. Ectopic hormone secretion usually causes the presenting symptoms and can cause life-threatening complications. Second, with all the tumors except insulinomas, >50% are malignant (Table 55-2); therefore, treatment must also be directed against the tumor per se. Because in many patients these tumors are not surgically curable due to the presence of advanced disease at diagnosis, surgical resection for cure, which addresses both treatment aspects, is often not possible.

GASTRINOMA (ZOLLINGER-ELLISON SYNDROME)

A gastrinoma is an NET that secretes gastrin; the resultant hypergastrinemia causes gastric acid hypersecretion (Zollinger-Ellison syndrome [ZES]). The chronic hypergastrinemia results in marked gastric acid hypersecretion and growth of the gastric mucosa with increased numbers of parietal cells and proliferation of gastric ECL cells. The gastric acid hypersecretion characteristically causes peptic ulcer disease (PUD), often refractory and severe, as well as diarrhea. The most common presenting symptoms are abdominal pain (70-100%), diarrhea (37-73%), and gastroesophageal reflux disease (GERD) (30-35%); 10-20% of patients have diarrhea only. Although peptic ulcers may occur in unusual locations, most patients have a typical duodenal ulcer. Important observations that should suggest this diagnosis include PUD with diarrhea; PUD in an unusual location or with multiple ulcers; PUD refractory to treatment or persistent; PUD associated with prominent gastric folds; PUD associated with findings suggestive of MEN 1 (endocrinopathy, family history of ulcer or endocrinopathy, nephrolithiases); and PUD without *Helicobacter pylori* present. *H. pylori* is present in >90% of idiopathic peptic ulcers but is present in <50% of patients with gastrinomas. Chronic unexplained diarrhea also should suggest ZES.

Approximately 20-25% of patients with ZES have MEN 1 (MEN1/ZES), and in most cases, hyperparathyroidism is present before the ZES develops. These patients are treated differently from those without MEN 1 (sporadic ZES); therefore, MEN 1 should be sought in all patients with ZES by family history and by measuring plasma ionized calcium and prolactin levels and plasma hormone levels (parathormone, growth hormone).

Most gastrinomas (50–90%) in sporadic ZES are present in the duodenum, followed by the pancreas (10–40%) and other intraabdominal sites (mesentery, lymph nodes, biliary tract, liver, stomach, ovary). Rarely, the tumor may involve extraabdominal sites (heart, lung cancer). In MEN 1/ZES the gastrinomas are also usually in the duodenum (70–90%), followed by the pancreas (10–30%), and are almost always multiple. About 60–90% of gastrinomas are malignant (Table 55-2) with metastatic spread to lymph nodes and liver. Distant metastases to bone occur in 12–30% of patients with liver metastases.

Diagnosis

The diagnosis of ZES requires the demonstration of inappropriate fasting hypergastrinemia, usually by demonstrating hypergastrinemia occurring with an increased basal gastric acid output (BAO) (hyperchlorhydria). More than 98% of patients with ZES have fasting hypergastrinemia, although in 40–60% the level may be elevated less than tenfold. Therefore, when the diagnosis is suspected, a fasting gastrin is usually the initial test performed. It is important to remember that potent gastric acid suppressant drugs such as proton pump inhibitors (PPIs) (omeprazole, esomeprazole, pantoprazole, lansoprazole, rabeprazole) can suppress acid secretion sufficiently to cause hypergastrinemia; because of their prolonged duration of action, these drugs have to be tapered or frequently discontinued for a week before the gastrin determination. Withdrawal of PPIs should be performed carefully because PUD complications can rapidly develop in some patients and is best done in consultation with GI units with experience in this area. The widespread use of PPIs can confound the diagnosis of ZES by raising a false-positive diagnosis by causing hypergastrinemia in a patient being treated with idiopathic PUD (without ZES) and lead to a false-negative diagnosis because at routine doses used to treat patients with idiopathic PUD, PPIs control symptoms in most ZES patients and thus mask the diagnosis. If ZES is suspected and the gastrin level is elevated, it is important to show that it is increased when gastric pH is ≤2.0 because physiologically hypergastrinemia secondary to achlorhydria (atrophic gastritis, pernicious anemia) is one of the most common causes of hypergastrinemia. Nearly all ZES patients have a fasting pH ≤2 when off antisecretory drugs. If the fasting gastrin is >1000 pg/mL (increased tenfold) and the pH is ≤2.0, which occurs in 40–60% of patients with ZES, the diagnosis of ZES is established after the possibility of retained antrum syndrome has been ruled out by history. In patients with hypergastrinemia with fasting gastrins <1000 pg/mL (<10-fold increased) and gastric pH ≤2.0, other conditions, such as *H. pylori* infections, antral G-cell hyperplasia/hyperfunction, gastric outlet obstruction, and, rarely, renal failure, can masquerade as ZES. To establish the diagnosis in this group, a determination of BAO and a secretin provocative test should be done. In patients with ZES without previous gastric acid–reducing surgery, the BAO is usually (>90%) elevated (i.e., >15 mEq/h). The secretin provocative test is usually positive, with the criterion of a >120-pg/mL increase over the basal level having the highest sensitivity (94%) and specificity (100%). Unfortunately the diagnosis of ZES is becoming increasing more difficult. This is due not only to the widespread use of PPIs (leading to false-positive results as well as masking ZES presentation), but also recent studies demonstrate than many of the commercial gastrin kits that are used by most laboratories to measure fasting serum gastrin levels are not reliable. In one study, 7 of the 12 tested commercial gastrin kits inaccurately assessed the true serum concentration of gastrin primarily because the antibodies used had inappropriate specificity for the different circulating forms of gastrin and were not adequately validated. Both underestimation and overestimation of fasting serum gastrin levels occurred using these commercial kits. To circumvent this problem, it is either necessary to use one of the five reliable kits identified or, alternatively, to refer the patient to a center with expertise in making the diagnosis in your area, or if this is not possible, to contact such a center and use the gastrin assay they recommend. An accurate gastrin assay is essential for accurate measurement of fasting serum gastrin level as well as for assessing gastrin levels during the secretin provocative test, and thus, the diagnosis of ZES cannot reliably be made without one.

TREATMENT Zollinger-Ellison Syndrome

Gastric acid hypersecretion in patients with ZES can be controlled in almost every case by oral gastric antisecretory drugs. Because of their long duration of action and potency, which allows dosing once or twice a day, the PPIs (H^+, K^+-ATPase inhibitors) are the drugs of choice. Histamine H_2-receptor antagonists are also effective, although more frequent dosing (q 4–8 h) and high doses are required. In patients with MEN 1/ZES with hyperparathyroidism, correction of the hyperparathyroidism increases the sensitivity to gastric antisecretory drugs and decreases the basal acid output. Long-term treatment with PPIs (>15 years) has proved to be safe and effective, without development of tachyphylaxis. Although patients with ZES, especially those with MEN 1/ZES, more frequently develop gastric NETs (carcinoids), no data suggest that the long-term use of PPIs increases this risk in these patients. With long-term PPI use in ZES patients, vitamin B_{12} deficiency can develop; thus, vitamin B_{12} levels should be assessed during follow-up. Epidemiologic studies suggest that long-term PPI use may be associated with an increased incidence of bone fractures; however, at present, there is no such report in ZES patients.

With the increased ability to control acid hypersecretion, more than 50% of patients who are not cured (>60% of patients) will die from tumor-related causes. At presentation, careful imaging studies are essential to localize the extent of the tumor to determine the appropriate treatment. A third of patients present with hepatic metastases, and in <15% of those patients, the disease is limited, so that surgical resection may be possible. Surgical short-term cure is possible in 60% of all patients without MEN 1/ZES or liver metastases (40% of all patients) and in 30% of patients long term. In patients with MEN 1/ZES, long-term surgical cure is rare because the tumors are multiple, frequently with lymph node metastases. Surgical studies demonstrate that successful resection of the gastrinoma not only decreases the chances of developing liver metastases but also increases the disease-related survival rate. Therefore, all patients with gastrinomas without MEN 1/ZES or a medical condition that limits life expectancy should undergo surgery by a surgeon experienced in the treatment of these disorders.

INSULINOMAS

An insulinoma is an NET of the pancreas that is thought to be derived from beta cells that ectopically secrete insulin, which results in hypoglycemia. The average age of occurrence is 40–50 years old. The most common clinical symptoms are due to the effect of the hypoglycemia on the CNS (neuroglycemic symptoms) and include confusion, headache, disorientation, visual difficulties, irrational behavior, and even coma. Also, most patients have symptoms due to excess catecholamine release secondary to the hypoglycemia, including sweating, tremor, and palpitations. Characteristically, these attacks are associated with fasting.

Insulinomas are generally small (>90% are <2 cm) and usually not multiple (90%); only 5–15% are malignant, and they almost invariably occur only in the pancreas, distributed equally in the pancreatic head, body, and tail.

Insulinomas should be suspected in all patients with hypoglycemia, especially when there is a history suggesting that attacks are provoked by fasting, or with a family history of MEN 1. Insulin is synthesized as proinsulin, which consists of a 21-amino-acid α chain and a 30-amino-acid β chain connected by a 33-amino-acid connecting peptide (C peptide). In insulinomas, in addition to elevated plasma insulin levels, elevated plasma proinsulin levels are found, and C-peptide levels are elevated.

Diagnosis

The diagnosis of insulinoma requires the demonstration of an elevated plasma insulin level at the time of hypoglycemia. A number of other conditions may cause fasting hypoglycemia, such as the inadvertent or surreptitious use of insulin or oral hypoglycemic agents, severe liver disease, alcoholism, poor nutrition, and other extrapancreatic tumors. Furthermore, postprandial hypoglycemia can be caused by a number of conditions that confuse the diagnosis of insulinoma. Particularly important here is the increased occurrence of hypoglycemia after gastric bypass surgery for obesity, which is now widely performed. A new entity, insulinomatosis, was described that can cause hypoglycemia and mimic insulinomas. It occurs in 10% of patients with persistent hyperinsulinemic hypoglycemia and is characterized by the occurrence of multiple macro-/microadenomas expressing insulin, and it is not clear how to distinguish this entity from insulinoma preoperatively. The most reliable test to diagnose insulinoma is a fast up to 72 h with serum glucose, C-peptide, proinsulin, and insulin measurements every 4–8 h. If at any point the patient becomes symptomatic or glucose levels are persistently below <2.2 mmol/L (40 mg/dL), the test should be terminated, and repeat samples for the above studies should be obtained before glucose is given. Some 70–80% of patients will develop hypoglycemia during the first 24 h, and 98% by 48 h. In nonobese normal subjects, serum insulin levels should decrease to <43 pmol/L (<6 μU/mL) when blood glucose decreases to <2.2 mmol/L (<40 mg/dL) and the ratio of insulin to glucose is <0.3 (in mg/dL). In addition to having an insulin level >6 μU/mL when blood glucose is <40 mg/dL, some investigators also require an elevated C-peptide and serum proinsulin level, an insulin/glucose ratio >0.3, and a decreased plasma β-hydroxybutyrate level for the diagnosis of insulinomas. Surreptitious use of insulin or hypoglycemic agents may be difficult to distinguish from insulinomas. The combination of proinsulin levels (normal in exogenous insulin/hypoglycemic agent users), C-peptide levels (low in exogenous insulin users), antibodies to insulin (positive in exogenous insulin users), and measurement of sulfonylurea levels in serum or plasma will allow the correct diagnosis to be made. The diagnosis of insulinoma has been complicated by the introduction of specific insulin assays that do not also interact with proinsulin, as do many of the older radioimmunoassays (RIAs), and therefore give lower plasma insulin levels. The increased use of these specific insulin assays has resulted in increased numbers of patients with insulinomas having lower plasma insulin values (<6 μU/mL) than levels proposed to be characteristic of insulinomas by RIA. In these patients, the assessment of proinsulin and C-peptide levels at the time of hypoglycemia is particularly helpful for establishing the correct diagnosis. An elevated proinsulin level when the fasting glucose level is <45 mg/dL is sensitive and specific.

TREATMENT Insulinomas

Only 5–15% of insulinomas are malignant; therefore, after appropriate imaging (see below), surgery should be performed. In different studies, 75–100% of patients are cured by surgery. Before surgery, the hypoglycemia can be controlled by frequent small meals and the use of diazoxide (150–800 mg/d). Diazoxide is a benzothiadiazide whose hyperglycemic effect is attributed to inhibition of insulin release. Its side effects are sodium retention and GI symptoms such as nausea. Approximately 50–60% of patients respond to diazoxide. Other agents effective in some patients to control the hypoglycemia include verapamil and diphenylhydantoin. Long-acting somatostatin analogues such as octreotide and lanreotide are acutely effective in 40% of patients. However, octreotide must be used with care because it inhibits growth hormone secretion and can alter plasma glucagon levels; therefore, in some patients, it can worsen the hypoglycemia.

For the 5–15% of patients with malignant insulinomas, these drugs or somatostatin analogues are used initially. In a small number of patients with insulinomas, some with malignant tumors, mammalian target of rapamycin (mTOR) inhibitors (everolimus, rapamycin) are reported to control the hypoglycemia. If they are not effective, various antitumor treatments such as hepatic arterial embolization, chemoembolization, chemotherapy, and peptide receptor radiotherapy have been used (see below).

Insulinomas, which are usually benign (>90%) and intrapancreatic in location, are increasingly resected using a laparoscopic approach, which has lower morbidity rates. This approach requires that the insulinoma be localized on preoperative imaging studies.

GLUCAGONOMAS

A glucagonoma is NET of the pancreas that secretes excessive amounts of glucagon, which causes a distinct syndrome characterized by dermatitis, glucose intolerance or diabetes, and weight loss. Glucagonomas principally occur between 45 and 70 years of age. The tumor is clinically heralded by a characteristic dermatitis (migratory necrolytic erythema) (67–90%), accompanied by glucose intolerance (40–90%), weight loss (66–96%), anemia (33–85%), diarrhea (15–29%), and thromboembolism (11–24%). The characteristic rash usually starts as an annular erythema at intertriginous and periorificial sites, especially in the groin or buttock. It subsequently becomes raised, and bullae form; when the bullae rupture, eroded areas form. The lesions can wax and wane. The development of a similar rash in patients receiving glucagon therapy suggests that the rash is a direct effect of the hyperglucagonemia. A characteristic laboratory finding is hypoaminoacidemia, which occurs in 26–100% of patients.

Glucagonomas are generally large tumors at diagnosis (5–10 cm). Some 50–80% occur in the pancreatic tail. From 50 to 82% have evidence of metastatic spread at presentation, usually to the liver. Glucagonomas are rarely extrapancreatic and usually occur singly.

Two new entities have been described that can also cause hyperglucagonemia and may mimic glucagonomas. Mahvah disease is due to a homozygous P86S mutation of the human glucagon receptor. It is associated with the development of α-cell hyperplasia, hyperglucagonemia, and the development of nonfunctioning pNETs. A second disease called *glucagon cell adenomatosis* can mimic glucagonoma syndrome clinically and is characterized by the presence of hyperplastic islets staining positive for glucagon instead of a single glucagonoma.

Diagnosis

The diagnosis is confirmed by demonstrating an increased plasma glucagon level. Characteristically, plasma glucagon levels exceed 1000 pg/mL (normal is <150 pg/mL) in 90%; 7% are between 500 and 1000 pg/mL, and 3% are <500 pg/mL. A trend toward lower levels at diagnosis has been noted in the last decade. A plasma glucagon level >1000 pg/mL is considered diagnostic of glucagonoma. Other diseases causing increased plasma glucagon levels include cirrhosis, diabetic ketoacidosis, celiac disease, renal insufficiency, acute pancreatitis, hypercorticism, hepatic insufficiency, severe stress, and prolonged fasting or familial hyperglucagonemia, as well as danazol treatment. With the exception of cirrhosis, these disorders do not increase plasma glucagon >500 pg/mL.

Necrolytic migratory erythema is not pathognomonic for glucagonoma and occurs in myeloproliferative disorders, hepatitis B infection, malnutrition, short-bowel syndrome, inflammatory bowel disease, zinc deficiency, and malabsorption disorders.

TREATMENT Glucagonomas

In 50–80% of patients, hepatic metastases are present, and so curative surgical resection is not possible. Surgical debulking in patients with advanced disease or other antitumor treatments may be beneficial (see below). Long-acting somatostatin analogues such as octreotide and lanreotide improve the skin rash in 75% of patients and may improve the weight loss, pain, and diarrhea, but usually do not improve the glucose intolerance.

SOMATOSTATINOMA SYNDROME

The somatostatinoma syndrome is due to an NET that secretes excessive amounts of somatostatin, which causes a distinct syndrome characterized by diabetes mellitus, gallbladder disease, diarrhea, and steatorrhea. There is no general distinction in the literature between a tumor that contains somatostatin-like immunoreactivity (somatostatinoma) and does (11–45%) or does not (55–90%) produce a clinical syndrome (somatostatinoma syndrome) by secreting somatostatin. In a review of 173 cases of somatostatinomas, only 11% were associated with the somatostatinoma syndrome. The mean age is 51 years. Somatostatinomas occur primarily in the pancreas and small intestine, and the frequency of the symptoms and occurrence of the somatostatinoma syndrome differ in each. Each of the usual symptoms is more common in pancreatic than in intestinal somatostatinomas: diabetes mellitus (95% vs 21%), gallbladder disease (94% vs 43%), diarrhea (92% vs 38%), steatorrhea (83% vs 12%), hypochlorhydria (86% vs 12%), and weight loss (90% vs 69%). The somatostatinoma syndrome occurs in 30–90% of pancreatic and 0–5% of SI somatostatinomas. In various series, 43% of all duodenal NETs contain somatostatin; however, the somatostatinoma syndrome is rarely present (<2%). Somatostatinomas occur in the pancreas in 56–74% of cases, with the primary location being the pancreatic head. The tumors are usually solitary (90%) and large (mean size 4.5 cm). Liver metastases are common, being present in 69–84% of patients. Somatostatinomas are rare in patients with MEN 1, occurring in only 0.65%.

Somatostatin is a tetradecapeptide that is widely distributed in the CNS and GI tract, where it functions as a neurotransmitter or has paracrine and autocrine actions. It is a potent inhibitor of many processes, including release of almost all hormones, acid secretion, intestinal and pancreatic secretion, and intestinal absorption. Most of the clinical manifestations are directly related to these inhibitory actions.

Diagnosis

In most cases, somatostatinomas have been found by accident either at the time of cholecystectomy or during endoscopy. The presence of psammoma bodies in a duodenal tumor should particularly raise suspicion. Duodenal somatostatin-containing tumors are increasingly associated with von Recklinghausen's disease (NF-1) (Table 55-6). Most of these tumors (>98%) do not cause the somatostatinoma syndrome. The diagnosis of the somatostatinoma syndrome requires the demonstration of elevated plasma somatostatin levels.

TREATMENT Somatostatinomas

Pancreatic tumors are frequently (70–92%) metastatic at presentation, whereas 30–69% of SI somatostatinomas have metastases. Surgery is the treatment of choice for those without widespread hepatic metastases. Symptoms in patients with the somatostatinoma syndrome are also improved by octreotide treatment.

VIPOMAS

VIPomas are NETs that secrete excessive amounts of vasoactive intestinal peptide (VIP), which causes a distinct syndrome characterized by large-volume diarrhea, hypokalemia, and dehydration. This syndrome also is called Verner-Morrison syndrome, pancreatic cholera, and WDHA syndrome for *w*atery *d*iarrhea, *h*ypokalemia, and *a*chlorhydria, which some patients develop. The mean age of patients with this syndrome is 49 years; however, it can occur in children, and when it does, it is usually caused by a ganglioneuroma or ganglioneuroblastoma.

The principal symptoms are large-volume diarrhea (100%) severe enough to cause hypokalemia (80–100%), dehydration (83%), hypochlorhydria (54–76%), and flushing (20%). The diarrhea is secretory in nature, persisting during fasting, and is almost always >1 L/d and in 70% is >3 L/d. In a number of studies, the diarrhea was intermittent initially in up to half the patients. Most patients do not have accompanying steatorrhea (16%), and the increased stool volume is due to increased excretion of sodium and potassium, which, with the anions, accounts for the osmolality of the stool. Patients frequently have hyperglycemia (25–50%) and hypercalcemia (25–50%).

VIP is a 28-amino-acid peptide that is an important neurotransmitter, ubiquitously present in the CNS and GI tract. Its known actions include stimulation of SI chloride secretion as well as effects on smooth-muscle contractility, inhibition of acid secretion, and vasodilatory effects, which explain most features of the clinical syndrome.

In adults, 80–90% of VIPomas are pancreatic in location, with the rest due to VIP-secreting pheochromocytomas, intestinal carcinoids, and rarely ganglioneuromas. These tumors are usually solitary, 50–75% are in the pancreatic tail, and 37–68% have hepatic metastases at diagnosis. In children <10 years old, the syndrome is usually due to ganglioneuromas or ganglioblastomas and is less often malignant (10%).

Diagnosis

The diagnosis requires the demonstration of an elevated plasma VIP level and the presence of large-volume diarrhea. A stool volume <700 mL/d is proposed to exclude the diagnosis of VIPoma. When the patient fasts, a number of diseases can be excluded that can cause marked diarrhea because the high volume of diarrhea is not sustained during the fast. Other diseases that can produce a secretory large-volume diarrhea include gastrinomas, chronic laxative abuse, carcinoid syndrome, systemic mastocytosis, rarely medullary thyroid cancer, diabetic diarrhea, sprue, and AIDS. Among these conditions, only VIPomas caused a marked increase in plasma VIP. Chronic surreptitious use of laxatives/diuretics can be particularly difficult to detect clinically. Hence, in a patient with unexplained chronic diarrhea, screens for laxatives should be performed; they will detect many, but not all, laxative abusers. Elevated plasma levels of VIP should not be the only basis of the diagnosis of VIPomas because they can occur with some diarrheal states including inflammatory bowel disease, post small bowel resection, and radiation enteritis. Furthermore, nesidioblastosis can mimic VIPomas by causing elevated plasma VIP levels, diarrhea, and even false-positive location in the pancreatic region on somatostatin receptor scintigraphy.

TREATMENT VIPomas

The most important initial treatment in these patients is to correct their dehydration, hypokalemia, and electrolyte losses with fluid and electrolyte replacement. These patients may require 5 L/d of fluid and >350 mEq/d of potassium. Because 37–68% of adults with VIPomas have metastatic disease in the liver at presentation, a significant number of patients cannot be cured surgically. In these patients, long-acting somatostatin analogues such as octreotide and lanreotide are the drugs of choice.

Octreotide/lanreotide will control the diarrhea short- and long-term in 75–100% of patients. In nonresponsive patients, the combination of glucocorticoids and octreotide/lanreotide has proved helpful in a small number of patients. Other drugs reported to be helpful in small numbers of patients include prednisone (60–100 mg/d), clonidine, indomethacin, phenothiazines, loperamide, lidamidine, lithium, propranolol, and metoclopramide. Treatment of advanced disease with cytoreductive surgery, embolization, chemoembolization, chemotherapy, radiotherapy, radiofrequency ablation, and peptide receptor radiotherapy may be helpful (see below).

NONFUNCTIONAL PANCREATIC NEUROENDOCRINE TUMORS (NF-pNETs)

NF-pNETs are NETs that originate in the pancreas and either secrete no products or their products do not cause a specific clinical syndrome. Their symptoms are due entirely to the tumor per se. NF-pNETs secrete chromogranin A (90–100%), chromogranin B (90–100%), α-HCG (human chorionic gonadotropin) (40%), neuron-specific enolase (31%), and β-HCG (20%), and because 40–90% secrete PP, they are also often called PPomas. Because the symptoms are due to the tumor mass, patients with NF-pNETs usually present late in the disease course with invasive tumors and hepatic metastases (64–92%), and the tumors are usually large (72% >5 cm). NF-pNETs are usually solitary except in patients with MEN 1, in which case they are multiple. They occur primarily in the pancreatic head. Even though these tumors do not cause a functional syndrome, immunocytochemical studies show that they synthesize numerous peptides and cannot be distinguished from functional pNETs by immunocytochemistry. In MEN 1, 80–100% of patients have microscopic NF-pNETs, but they become large or symptomatic in a minority (0–13%) of cases. In VHL, 12–17% develop NF-pNETs, and in 4%, they are ≥3 cm in diameter.

The most common symptoms are abdominal pain (30–80%), jaundice (20–35%), and weight loss, fatigue, or bleeding; 10–35% are found incidentally. The average time from the beginning of symptoms to diagnosis is 5 years.

Diagnosis

The diagnosis is established by histologic confirmation in a patient without either the clinical symptoms or the elevated plasma hormone levels of one of the established syndromes. The principal difficulty in diagnosis is to distinguish an NF-pNET from a nonendocrine pancreatic tumor, which is more common, as well as from a functional pNET. Even though chromogranin A levels are elevated in almost every patient, this is not specific for this disease as it can be found in functional pNETs, GI-NETs (carcinoids), and other neuroendocrine disorders. Plasma PP elevations should strongly suggest the diagnosis in a patient with a pancreatic mass because it is usually normal in patients with pancreatic adenocarcinomas. Elevated plasma PP is not diagnostic of this tumor because it is elevated in a number of other conditions, such as chronic renal failure, old age, inflammatory conditions, alcohol abuse, pancreatitis, hypoglycemia, postprandially, and diabetes. A positive somatostatin receptor scan in a patient with a pancreatic mass should suggest the presence of pNET/NF-pNET rather than a nonendocrine tumor.

TREATMENT Nonfunctional Pancreatic Neuroendocrine Tumors (NF-pNETs)

Overall survival in patients with sporadic NF-pNET is 30–63% at 5 years, with a median survival of 6 years. Unfortunately, surgical curative resection can be considered only in a minority of these patients because 64–92% present with diffuse metastatic disease. Treatment needs to be directed against the tumor per se using the various modalities discussed below for advanced disease. The treatment of NF-pNETs in either MEN 1 patients or patients with VHL is controversial. Most recommend surgical resection for any tumor >2–3 cm in diameter; however, there is no consensus on smaller NF-pNETs in these inherited disorders, with most recommending careful surveillance of these patients. The treatment of small sporadic, asymptomatic NF-pNETs (≤2 cm) is also controversial. Most of these are low- or intermediate-grade lesions, and <7% are malignant. Some advocate a nonoperative approach with careful, regular follow-up, whereas other recommend an operative approach with specially consideration for a laparoscopic surgical approach.

GRFOMAS

GRFomas are NETs that secrete excessive amounts of growth hormone–releasing factor (GRF) that cause acromegaly. GRF is a 44-amino-acid peptide, and 25–44% of pNETs have GRF immunoreactivity, although it is uncommonly secreted. GRFomas are lung tumors in 47–54% of cases, pNETs in 29–30%, and SI carcinoids in 8–10%; up to 12% occur at other sites. Patients have a mean age of 38 years, and the symptoms usually are due to either acromegaly or the tumor per se. The acromegaly caused by GRFomas is indistinguishable from classic acromegaly. The pancreatic tumors are usually large (>6 cm), and liver metastases are present in 39%. They should be suspected in any patient with acromegaly and an abdominal tumor, a patient with MEN 1 with acromegaly, or a patient without a pituitary adenoma with acromegaly or associated with hyperprolactinemia, which occurs in 70% of GRFomas. GRFomas are an uncommon cause of acromegaly. GRFomas occur in <1% of MEN 1 patients. The diagnosis is established by performing plasma assays for GRF and growth hormone. Most GRFomas have a plasma GRF level >300 pg/mL (normal <5 pg/mL men, <10 pg/mL women). Patients with GRFomas also have increased plasma levels of insulin-like growth factor type I (IGF-I) similar to those in classic acromegaly. Surgery is the treatment of choice if diffuse metastases are not present. Long-acting somatostatin analogues such as octreotide and lanreotide are the agents of choice, with 75–100% of patients responding.

OTHER RARE PANCREATIC NEUROENDOCRINE TUMOR SYNDROMES

Cushing's syndrome (ACTHoma) due to a pNET occurs in 4–16% of all ectopic Cushing's syndrome cases. It occurs in 5% of cases of sporadic gastrinomas, almost invariably in patients with hepatic metastases, and is an independent poor prognostic factor. Paraneoplastic hypercalcemia due to pNETs releasing parathyroid hormone–related peptide (PTHrP), a PTH-like material, or unknown factor, is rarely reported. The tumors are usually large, and liver metastases are usually present. Most (88%) appear to be due to release of PTHrP. pNETs occasionally can cause the carcinoid syndrome. A number of very rare pNET syndromes involving a few cases (less than five) have been described; these include a renin-producing pNET in a patient presenting with hypertension; pNETs secreting luteinizing hormone, resulting in masculinization or decreased libido; a pNET secreting erythropoietin, resulting in polycythemia; pNETs secreting IGF-II, causing hypoglycemia; and pNETs secreting enteroglucagon, causing small intestinal hypertrophy, colonic/SI stasis, and malabsorption (Table 55-2). A number of other possible functional pNETs have been proposed, but most authorities classify these as unclear or as a nonfunctional pNET because in each case numerous patients have been described with similar plasma hormone elevations that do not cause any symptoms. These include pNETs secreting calcitonin, neurotensin (neurotensinoma), PP (PPoma), and ghrelin (Table 55-2).

TUMOR LOCALIZATION

Localization of the primary tumor and knowledge of the extent of the disease are essential to the proper management of all GI-NETs (carcinoids) and pNETs. Without proper localization studies, it is not possible to determine whether the patient is a candidate for surgical resection (curative or cytoreductive) or requires antitumor treatment, to determine whether the patient is responding to antitumor therapies, or to appropriately classify/stage the patient's disease to assess prognosis.

Numerous tumor localization methods are used in both types of NETs, including cross-sectional imaging studies (CT, magnetic resonance imaging [MRI], transabdominal ultrasound), selective angiography, somatostatin receptor scintigraphy (SRS), and positron emission tomography. In pNETs, endoscopic ultrasound (EUS) and functional localization by measuring venous hormonal gradients are also reported to be useful. Bronchial carcinoids are usually detected by standard chest radiography and assessed by CT. Rectal, duodenal, colonic, and gastric carcinoids are usually detected by GI endoscopy. Because of their wide availability, CT and MRI are generally initially used to determine the location of the primary NETs and the extent of disease. NETs are hypervascular tumors, and with both MRI and CT, contrast enhancement is essential for maximal sensitivity, and it is recommended that generally triple-phase scanning be used. The ability of cross-sectional imaging and, to a lesser extent, SRS to detect NETs is a function of NET size. With CT and MRI, <10% of tumors <1 cm in diameter are detected, 30–40% of tumors 1–3 cm are detected, and >50% of tumors >3 cm are detected. Many primary GI-NETs (carcinoids) are small, as are insulinomas and duodenal gastrinomas, and are frequently not detected by cross-sectional imaging, whereas most other pNETs present late in the course of their disease and are large (>4 cm). Selective angiography is more sensitive, localizing 60–90% of all NETs; however, it is now used infrequently. For detecting liver metastases, CT and MRI are more sensitive than ultrasound, and with recent improvements, 5–25% of patients with liver metastases will be missed by CT and/or MRI.

pNETs, as well as GI-NETs (carcinoids), frequently (>80%) overexpress high-affinity somatostatin receptors in both the primary tumors and the metastases. Of the five types of somatostatin receptors (sst_{1-5}), radiolabeled octreotide binds with high affinity to sst_2 and sst_5, has a lower affinity for sst_3, and has a very low affinity for sst_1 and sst_4. Between 80 and 100% of GI-NETs (carcinoids) and pNETs possess sst_2, and many also have the other four sst subtypes. Interaction with these receptors can be used to treat these tumors as well as to localize NETs by using radiolabeled somatostatin analogues (SRS). In the United States, [^{111}In-DTPA-D-Phe^1]octreotide (octreoscan) is generally used with gamma camera detection using single-photon emission computed tomography (SPECT) imaging. Numerous studies, primarily in Europe, using gallium-68-labeled somatostatin analogues and positron emission tomography (PET) detection, demonstrate even greater sensitivity than with SRS with ^{111}In-labeled somatostatin analogues. Although not yet approved in the United States, there are a number of centers starting to use this approach. Because of its sensitivity and ability to localize tumor throughout the body, SRS is the initial imaging modality of choice for localizing both the primary tumor and metastatic NETs. SRS localizes tumor in 73–95% of patients with GI-NETs (carcinoids) and in 56–100% of patients with pNETs, except insulinomas. Insulinomas are usually small and have low densities of sst receptors, resulting in SRS being positive in only 12–50% of patients with insulinomas. SRS identifies >90–95% of patients with liver metastases due to NETs. Figure 55-3 shows an example of the increased sensitivity of SRS in a patient with a GI-NET (carcinoid) tumor. The CT scan showed a single liver metastasis, whereas the SRS demonstrated three metastases in the liver in multiple locations. Occasional false-positive responses with SRS can occur (12% in one study) because numerous other normal tissues as well as diseases can have high densities of sst receptors, including granulomas (sarcoid, tuberculosis, etc.), thyroid

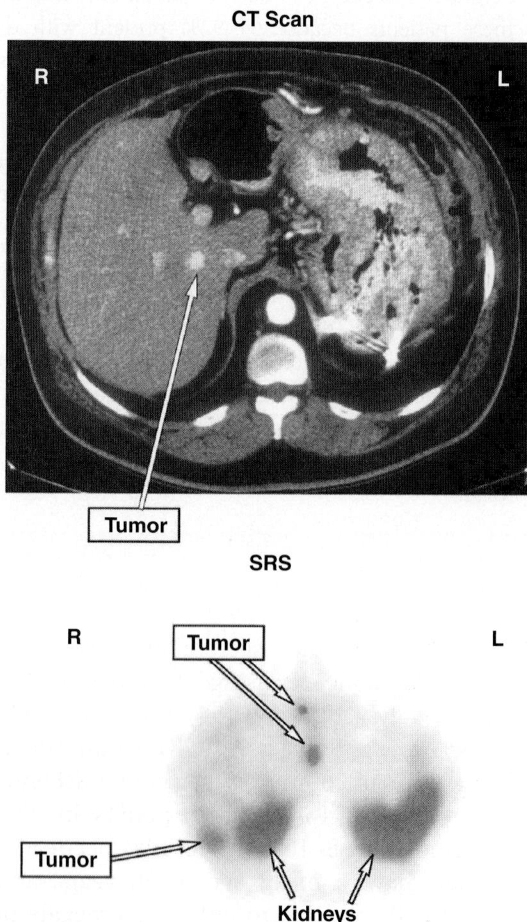

FIGURE 55-3
Ability of computed tomography (CT) scanning (*top*) or somatostatin receptor scintigraphy (SRS) (*bottom*) to localize metastatic carcinoid in the liver.

diseases (goiter, thyroiditis), and activated lymphocytes (lymphomas, wound infections). If liver metastases are identified by SRS, to plan the proper treatment, either a CT or an MRI (with contrast enhancement) is recommended to assess the size and exact location of the metastases because SRS does not provide information on tumor size. For pNETs in the pancreas, EUS is highly sensitive, localizing 77–100% of insulinomas, which occur almost exclusively within the pancreas. Endoscopic ultrasound is less sensitive for extrapancreatic tumors. It is increasingly used in patients with MEN 1, and to a lesser extent VHL, to detect small pNETs not seen with other modalities or for serial pNET assessments to determine size changes or rapid growth in patients in whom surgery is deferred. EUS with cytologic evaluation also is used frequently to distinguish an NF-pNET from a pancreatic adenocarcinoma or another nonendocrine pancreatic tumor. Not infrequently patients present with liver metastases due to an NET and the primary site is unclear. Occult small intestinal NETs (carcinoids) are increasingly detected by double-balloon enteroscopy or capsule endoscopy.

Insulinomas frequently overexpress receptors for glucagon-like peptide-1 (GLP-1), and radiolabeled GLP-1 analogues have been developed that can detect occult insulinomas not localized by other imaging modalities. Functional localization by measuring hormonal gradients is now uncommonly used with gastrinomas (after intra-arterial secretin injections) but is still frequently used in insulinoma patients in whom other imaging studies are negative (assessing hepatic vein insulin concentrations post-intra-arterial calcium injections). Functional localization measuring hormone gradients in insulinomas or gastrin gradients in gastrinoma is a sensitive method, being positive in 80–100% of patients. The intra-arterial calcium test may also allow differentiation of the cause of the hypoglycemia and indicate whether it is due to an insulinoma or a nesidioblastosis. The latter entity is becoming increasingly important because hypoglycemia after gastric bypass surgery for obesity is increasing in frequency, and it is primarily due to nesidioblastosis, although it can occasionally be due to an insulinoma.

PET and use of hybrid scanners such as CT and SRS may have increased sensitivity. PET scanning with ^{18}F-fluoro-DOPA in patients with carcinoids or with ^{11}C-5-HTP in patients with pNETs or GI-NETs (carcinoids) has greater sensitivity than cross-sectional imaging studies and may be used increasingly in the future. PET scanning for GI-NETs is not currently approved in the United States.

TREATMENT Advanced Disease (Diffuse Metastatic Disease)

The single most important prognostic factor for survival is the presence of liver metastases (Fig. 55-4). For patients with foregut carcinoids without hepatic metastases, the 5-year survival in one study was 95%, and with distant metastases, it was 20% (Fig. 55-4). With gastrinomas, the 5-year survival without liver metastases is 98%; with limited metastases in one hepatic lobe, it is 78%; and with diffuse metastases, 16% (Fig. 55-4). In a large study of 156 patients (67 pNETs, rest carcinoids), the overall 5-year survival rate was 77%; it was 96% without liver metastases, 73% with liver metastases, and 50% with distant disease. Another very important prognostic factor is whether the NET is well-differentiated (G1/G2) or poorly differentiated (<1% of all NETs) (G3). Well-differentiated NETs have a 5-year survival of 50–80%, whereas poorly differentiated NETs have a 5-year survival of only 0–15%.

Therefore, treatment for advanced metastatic disease is an important challenge. A number of different modalities are reported to be effective, including cytoreductive surgery (surgically or by radiofrequency ablation [RFA]), treatment with chemotherapy, somatostatin analogues, interferon α, hepatic embolization alone or with chemotherapy (chemoembolization), molecular targeted therapy, radiotherapy with radiolabeled beads/microspheres, peptide radioreceptor therapy (PRRT), and liver transplantation.

SPECIFIC ANTITUMOR TREATMENTS Cytoreductive surgery is considered if either all of the visible metastatic disease or at last 90% is thought resectable; however, unfortunately, this is possible in only the 9–22% of patients who present with limited hepatic metastases. Although no randomized studies have proven that it extends life, results from a number of studies suggest that it may increase survival; therefore, it is recommended, if possible. RFA can be applied to NET liver metastases if they are limited in number (usually less than five) and size (usually <3.5 cm in diameter). It can be used at the time of surgery (either general or laparoscopic) or using radiologic guidance.

Response rates are >80%, the responses can last up to 3 years, the morbidity rate is low, and this procedure may be particularly helpful in patients with functional pNETs that are difficult to control medically. Although RFA has not been established in a controlled trial, both the European and North American Neuroendocrine Tumor Society guidelines (ENETS, NANETS) state it can be an effective antitumor treatment for both refractory functional syndromes and for palliative treatment.

Chemotherapy plays a different role in the treatment of patients with pNETs and GI-NETs (carcinoids). Chemotherapy continues to be widely used in the treatment of patients with advanced pNETs with moderate success (response rates 20–70%); however, in general, its results in patients with metastatic GI-NETs (carcinoids) has been disappointing, with response rates of 0–30% with various two- and three-drug combinations, and thus, it is infrequently used in these patients. An important distinction in patients with pNETs is whether the tumor is well differentiated (G1/G2) or poorly differentiated (G3). The chemotherapeutic approach is different for these two groups. The current regimen of choice for

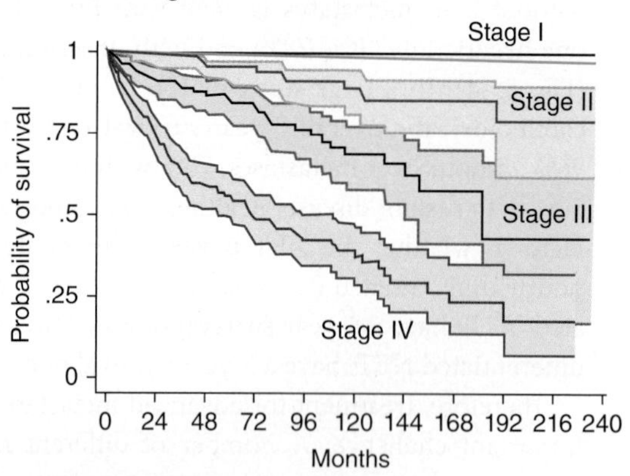

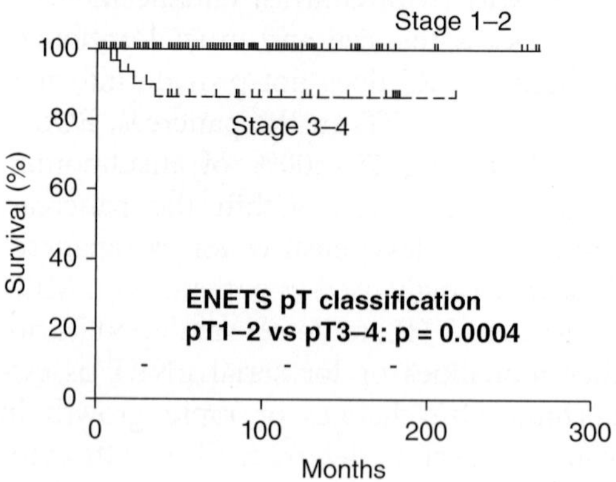

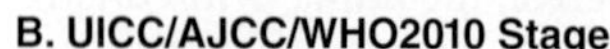

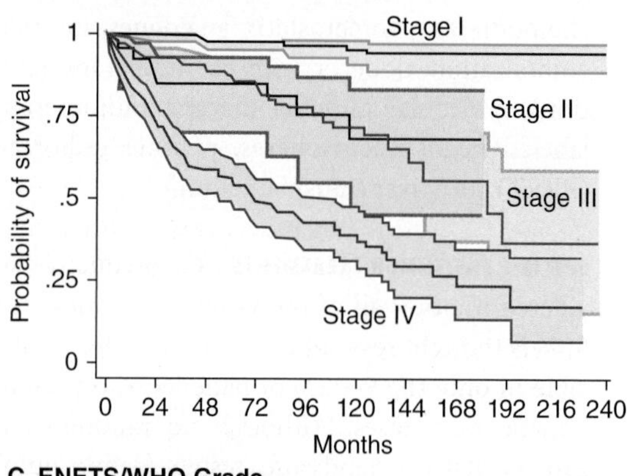

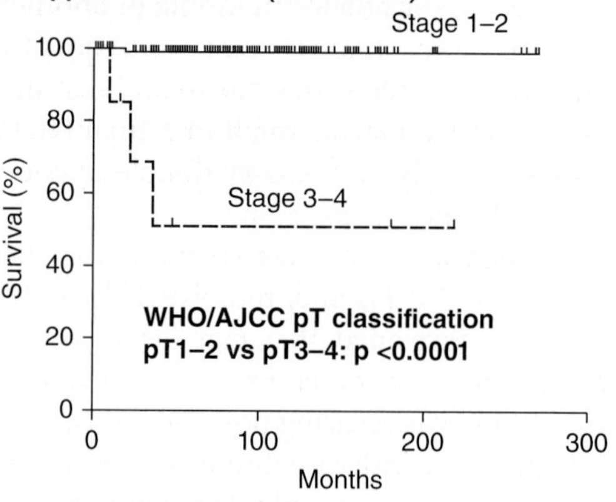

C. ENETS/WHO Grade

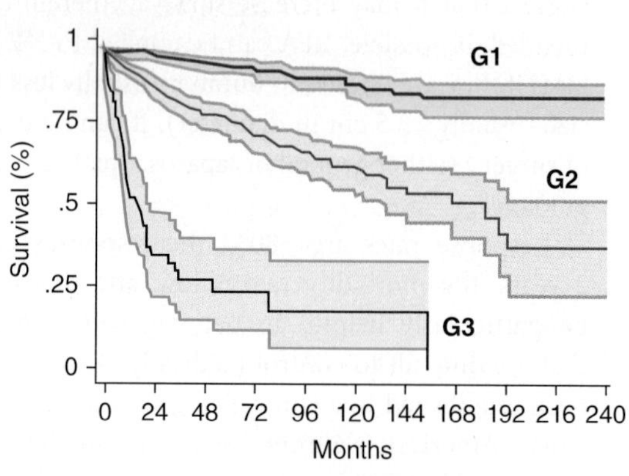

F. Midgut NETs (Carcinoids)

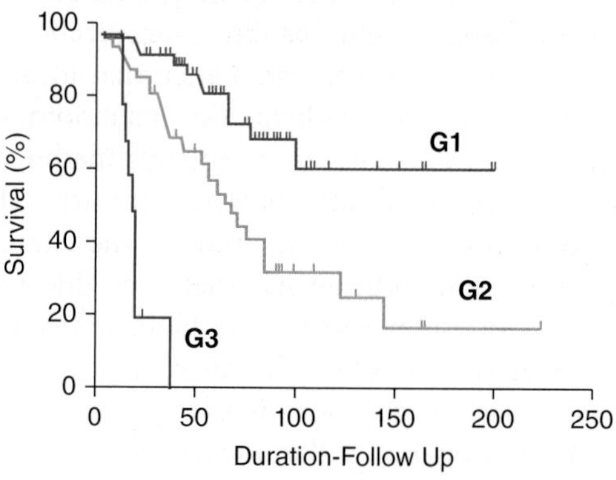

FIGURE 55-4

Survival (Kaplan-Meier plots) of patients with pancreatic neuroendocrine tumors (pNETs; n = 1072) (*A–C*) or gastrointestinal neuroendocrine tumors (GI-NETs; carcinoids) (appendix, n = 138; midgut, n = 238) (*D–F*) stratified according to recent proposed classification and grading systems. *(Panels A–C are drawn from data in G Rindi et al: J Natl Cancer Inst 104:764, 2012; panels D and E are drawn from data in M Volante et al: Am J Surg Pathol 37:606, 2013; and panel F is drawn from data in MS Khan: Br J Cancer 108:1838, 2013.)*

patients with well-differentiated pNETs is the combination of streptozotocin and doxorubicin with or without 5-fluorouracil. Streptozotocin is a glucosamine nitrourea compound originally found to have cytotoxic effects on pancreatic islets, and later in studies with doxorubicin with or without 5-fluorouracil, it produced response rates of 20–45% in advanced pNETs. Streptozotocin causes considerable morbidity, with 70–100% of patients developing side effects (most prominent being nausea/vomiting in 60–100% or leukopenia/thrombocytopenia) and 15–40% of patients developing some degree of renal dysfunction (proteinuria in 40–50%, decreased creatine clearance). The combination of temozolomide (TMZ) with capecitabine produces partial response rates as high as 70% in patients with advance pNETs and a 2-year survival of 92%. The use of TMZ or another alkylating agent in advanced pNETs is supported by studies that show low levels of the DNA repair enzyme O^6-methylguanine DNA methyltransferase in pNETs, but not in GI-NETs (carcinoids), which increases the sensitivity of pNETs to TMZ. In poorly differentiated NETs (G3), chemotherapy with a cisplatin-based regimen with etoposide or other agents (vincristine, paclitaxel) is the recommended treatment, with response rates of 40–70%; however, responses are generally short-lived (<12 months). This chemotherapy regimen can be associated with significant toxicity including GI toxicities (nausea, vomiting), myelosuppression, and renal toxicity.

In addition to the effectiveness in controlling the functional hormonal state, long-acting somatostatin analogues such as octreotide and lanreotide are increasingly used for their antiproliferative effects. Whereas somatostatin analogues rarely decrease tumor size (i.e., 0–17%), these drugs have tumoristatic effects, stopping additional growth in 26–95% of patients with NETs. In a randomized, double-blind study in patients with metastatic midgut carcinoids (PROMID study) octreotide-LAR demonstrated a marked lengthening of time to progression (14.3 vs 6 months, $p = .000072$). This improvement was seen in patients with limited liver involvement. This study did not assess whether such treatment will extend survival. A double-blind, randomized, placebo-controlled, phase III study in patients with well-differentiated, metastatic, inoperable pNETs (45%) or GI-NETs (carcinoids) (55%) (CLARINET study) showed that monthly treatment with lanreotide-autogel reduced tumor progression or death by 53%. Somatostatin analogues can induce apoptosis in GI-NETs (carcinoids), which probably contributes to their tumoristatic effects. Treatment with somatostatin analogues is generally well-tolerated, with most side effects being mild and uncommonly leading to stopping the drug. Potential long-term side effects include diabetes/glucose intolerance, steatorrhea, and the development of gallbladder sludge/gallstones (10–80%), although only 1% of patients develop symptomatic gallbladder disease. Because of these phase III studies, somatostatin analogues are generally recommended as first-line treatment for patients with well-differentiated metastatic NETs.

Interferon α, similar to somatostatin analogues, is effective at controlling the hormonal excess symptoms of NETs and has antiproliferative effects in NETs, which primarily result in disease stabilization (30–80%), with a decrease in tumor size in <15% of patients. Interferon can inhibit DNA synthesis, block cell cycle progression in the G_1 phase, inhibit protein synthesis, inhibit angiogenesis, and induce apoptosis. Interferon α treatment results in side effects in the majority of patients, with the most frequent being a flu-like syndrome (80–100%), anorexia with weight loss, and fatigue. These side effects frequently decrease in severity with continued treatment. In addition, patients become accommodated to the symptoms. More serious side effects include hepatotoxicity (31%), hyperlipidemia (31%), bone marrow toxicity, thyroid disease (19%), and rarely CNS side effects (depression, mental/visual disorders). ENETS 2012 guidelines conclude that in patients with well-differentiated NETs that are slowly progressive, interferon α treatment should be considered if the tumor is somatostatin receptor negative or if somatostatin treatment fails.

Selective internal radiation therapy (SIRT) using yttrium-90 (^{90}Y) glass or resin microspheres is a relatively newer approach being evaluated in patients with unresectable NET liver metastases, with approximately 500 NET patients treated. The treatment requires careful evaluation for vascular shunting before treatment and a pretreatment angiogram to evaluate placement of the catheter and is generally is reserved for patients without extrahepatic metastatic disease and with adequate hepatic reserve. One of two types of ^{90}Y microspheres are used: either microspheres with a 20- to 60-μm diameter and 50 Bq/sphere (SIR-Spheres) or glass microspheres (TheraSpheres) with a 20- to 30-μm diameter and 2500 Bq/sphere. The ^{90}Y-microspheres are delivered to the liver by intra-arterial injection from percutaneously placed catheters. In four studies involving metastatic NETs, the response rate varied from 50–61% (partial or complete), tumor stabilization occurred in 22–41%, 60–100% had symptomatic improvement, and overall survival varied from 25–70 months. Side effects include postembolization syndrome (pain, fever, nausea/vomiting [frequent]), which is usually mild, although grade 2 (43%) or grade 3 (1%) symptoms can occur; radiation-induced liver disease (<1%); and radiation pneumonitis (<1%). Contraindications to use include excess shunting to the GI tract or lung, inability to isolate the liver arterial supply, and inadequate liver reserve. Because of the limited data available in the ENETS 2012 guidelines, treatment with SIRTs is considered experimental.

Molecular targeted medical treatment with either an mTOR inhibitor (everolimus) or a tyrosine kinase inhibitor (sunitinib) is now approved treatment in the United States and Europe for patients with metastatic unresectable pNET, each supported by a phase III, double-blind, prospective, placebo-controlled trial. mTOR is a serine-threonine kinase that plays an important role in proliferation, cell growth, and apoptosis in both normal and neoplastic cells. Activation of the mTOR cascade is important in mediating NET cell growth, especially in pNETs. A number of mTOR inhibitors have shown promising antitumor activity in NETs including everolimus and temsirolimus, with the former undergoing a phase III trial (RADIANT-3) involving 410 patients with advance progressive pNETs. Everolimus caused significant improvement in progression-free survival (11 vs 4.6 months, $p < .001$) and increased by a factor of 3.7 the proportion of patients progression-free at 18 months (37% vs 9%). Everolimus treatment was associated with frequent side effects, causing a twofold increase in adverse events, with the most frequent being grade 1 or 2. Grade 3 or 4 side effects included hematologic, GI (diarrhea), stomatitis, or hypoglycemia occurring in 3–7% of patients. Most grade 3 or 4 side effects were controlled by dose reduction or drug interruption.

The ENETS 2012 guidelines conclude that everolimus, similar to sunitinib (below), should be considered as a first-line treatment in selected cases of well-differentiated pNETs that are unresectable. NETs, like other normal and neoplastic cells, frequently possess multiple types of the 20 different tyrosine kinase (TK) receptors that are known and mediate the action of different growth factors. Numerous studies demonstrate that TK receptors in normal and neoplastic tissues as well as NETs are especially important in mediating cell growth, angiogenesis, differentiation, and apoptosis. Whereas a number of TK inhibitors show antiproliferative activity in NETs only sunitinib has undergone a phase III controlled trial. Sunitinib is an orally active small-molecule inhibitor of TK receptors (PDGFRs, VEGFR-1, VEGFR-2, c-KIT, FLT-3). In a phase III study in which 171 patients with progressive, metastatic, nonresectable pNETs were treated with sunitinib (37.5 mg/d) or placebo, sunitinib treatment caused a doubling of progression-free survival (11.4 vs 4.5 months, $p < .001$), an increase in objective tumor response rate (9% vs 0%, $p = .007$), and an increase in overall survival. Sunitinib treatment was associated with an overall threefold increase in side effects, although most were grade 1 or 2. The most frequent grade 3 or 4 side effects were neutropenia (12%) and hypertension (9.6%), which were controlled by dose reduction or temporary interruption. There is no consensus regarding the order of sunitinib or everolimus use in patients with advanced, well-differentiated, progressive pNETs.

PRRT for NETs involves treatment with radiolabeled somatostatin analogues. The success of this approach is based on the finding that somatostatin receptors (sst) are overexpressed or ectopically expressed by 60–100% of all NETs, which allows the targeting of cytotoxic, radiolabeled somatostatin receptor ligands.

Three different radionuclides are being used. High doses of [^{111}In-DTPA-D-Phe^{1}]octreotide, which emits γ-rays, internal conversion, and Auger electrons; ^{90}yttrium, which emits high-energy β-particles coupled by a DOTA chelating group to octreotide or octreotate; and ^{177}lutetium-coupled analogues, which emit both, are all in clinical studies. At present, the ^{177}lutetium-coupled analogues are the most widely used. ^{111}Indium-, ^{90}yttrium-, and ^{177}lutetium-labeled compounds caused tumor stabilization in 41–81%, 44–88%, and 23–40%, respectively, and a decrease in tumor size in 8–30%, 6–37%, and 38%, respectively, of patients with advanced metastatic NETs. In one large study involving 504 patients with malignant NETs, ^{177}lutetium-labeled analogues produced a reduction of tumor size of >50% in 30% of patients (2% complete) and tumor stabilization in 51% of patients. An effect on survival has not been established. At present, PRRT is not approved for use in either the United States or Europe, but because of the above promising results, a large phase III study is now being conducted in both the United States and Europe. The ENETS 2012, NANETS 2010, Nordic 2010, and European Society for Medical Oncology (ESMO) guidelines list PRRT as an experimental or investigational treatment at present.

The use of liver transplantation has been abandoned for treatment of most metastatic tumors to the liver. However, for metastatic NETs, it is still a consideration. Among 213 European patients with NETs (50% functional NETs) who had liver transplantation from 1982 to 2009, the overall 5-year survival was 52% and disease free-survival was 30%. In various studies, the postoperative mortality rate is 10–14%. These results are similar to the United Network for Organ Sharing data in the United States in which 150 NET patients had liver transplants and the 5-year survival was 49%. In various studies, important prognostic factors for a poor outcome include a major resection performed in addition at the time of the liver transplant; poor tumor differentiation; hepatomegaly; age >45 years; a primary NET in the duodenum or pancreas; the presence of extrahepatic metastatic disease or extensive liver involvement (>50%); Ki-67 proliferative index >10%; and abnormal E-cadherin staining. The ENETS 2012 guidelines conclude that liver transplantation should be viewed as providing palliative care, with cure an exception, and recommend it be reserved for patients with life-threatening hormonal disturbances refractory to other treatments or for selected patients with a nonfunctional tumor with diffuse liver metastatic disease refractory to all other treatments.

SECTION X

NUTRITION

CHAPTER 56

NUTRIENT REQUIREMENTS AND DIETARY ASSESSMENT

Johanna Dwyer

Nutrients are substances that are not synthesized in sufficient amounts in the body and therefore must be supplied by the diet. Nutrient requirements for groups of healthy persons have been determined experimentally. The absence of essential nutrients leads to growth impairment, organ dysfunction, and failure to maintain nitrogen balance or adequate status of other nutrients. For good health, we require energy-providing nutrients (protein, fat, and carbohydrate), vitamins, minerals, and water. Requirements for organic nutrients include 9 essential amino acids, several fatty acids, glucose, 4 fat-soluble vitamins, 10 water-soluble vitamins, dietary fiber, and choline. Several inorganic substances, including 4 minerals, 7 trace minerals, 3 electrolytes, and the ultratrace elements, must also be supplied by diet.

The amounts of the essential nutrients that are required by individuals differ by age and physiologic state. Conditionally essential nutrients are not required in the diet but must be supplied to individuals who do not synthesize them in adequate amounts, such as those with genetic defects, those with pathologic conditions such as infection or trauma with nutritional implications, and developmentally immature infants. For example, inositol, taurine, arginine, and glutamine may be needed by premature infants. Many other organic and inorganic compounds that are present in foods, such as pesticides and lead, also have health effects.

ESSENTIAL NUTRIENT REQUIREMENTS

Energy

For weight to remain stable, energy intake must match energy output. The major components of energy output are resting energy expenditure (REE) and physical activity; minor components include the energy cost of metabolizing food (thermic effect of food, or specific dynamic action) and shivering thermogenesis (e.g., cold-induced thermogenesis). The average energy intake is ~2600 kcal/d for American men and ~1800 kcal/d for American women, though these estimates vary with body size and activity level. Formulas for roughly estimating REE are useful in assessing the energy needs of an individual whose weight is stable. Thus, for males, REE = 900 + 10m, and for females, REE = 700 + 7m, where is m mass in kilograms. The calculated REE is then adjusted for physical activity level by multiplying by 1.2 for sedentary, 1.4 for moderately active, or 1.8 for very active individuals. The final figure, the estimated energy requirement (EER), provides an approximation of total caloric needs in a state of energy balance for a person of a certain age, sex, weight, height, and physical activity level. **For further discussion of energy balance in health and disease, see Chap. 58.**

Protein

Dietary protein consists of both essential and nonessential amino acids that are required for protein synthesis. The nine essential amino acids are histidine, isoleucine, leucine, lysine, methionine/cystine, phenylalanine/tyrosine, threonine, tryptophan, and valine. Certain amino acids, such as alanine, can also be used for energy and gluconeogenesis. When energy intake is inadequate, protein intake must be increased, because ingested amino acids are diverted into pathways of glucose synthesis and oxidation. In extreme energy deprivation, protein-calorie malnutrition may ensue **(Chap. 58)**.

For adults, the recommended dietary allowance (RDA) for protein is ~0.6 g/kg desirable body mass per day, assuming that energy needs are met and that the protein is of relatively high biologic value. Current recommendations for a healthy diet call for at least 10–14% of calories from protein. Most American diets provide at least those amounts. Biologic value tends to be highest for animal proteins, followed by proteins from legumes (beans), cereals (rice, wheat, corn), and roots. Combinations of plant proteins that complement one another in biologic value or combinations of animal and plant proteins can increase biologic value and lower total protein requirements. In healthy people with adequate diets, the timing of protein intake over the course of the day has little effect.

Protein needs increase during growth, pregnancy, lactation, and rehabilitation after injury or malnutrition. Tolerance to dietary protein is decreased in renal insufficiency (with consequent uremia) and in liver failure. Normal protein intake can precipitate encephalopathy in patients with cirrhosis of the liver.

Fat and carbohydrate

Fats are a concentrated source of energy and constitute, on average, 34% of calories in U.S. diets. However, for optimal health, fat intake should total no more than 30% of calories. Saturated fat and trans fat should be limited to <10% of calories and polyunsaturated fats to <10% of calories, with monounsaturated fats accounting for the remainder of fat intake. At least 45–55% of total calories should be derived from carbohydrates. The brain requires ~100 g of glucose per day for fuel; other tissues use about 50 g/d. Some tissues (e.g., brain and red blood cells) rely on glucose supplied either exogenously or from muscle proteolysis. Over time, adaptations in carbohydrate needs are possible during hypocaloric states. Like fat (9 kcal/g), carbohydrate (4 kcal/g), and protein (4 kcal/g), alcohol (ethanol) provides energy (7 kcal/g). However, it is not a nutrient.

Water

For adults, 1–1.5 mL of water per kilocalorie of energy expenditure is sufficient under usual conditions to allow for normal variations in physical activity, sweating, and solute load of the diet. Water losses include 50–100 mL/d in the feces; 500–1000 mL/d by evaporation or exhalation; and, depending on the renal solute load, ≥1000 mL/d in the urine. If external losses increase, intakes must increase accordingly to avoid underhydration. Fever increases water losses by ~200 mL/d per °C; diarrheal losses vary but may be as great as 5 L/d in severe diarrhea. Heavy sweating, vigorous exercise, and vomiting also increase water losses. When renal function is normal and solute intakes are adequate, the kidneys can adjust to increased water intake by excreting up to 18 L of excess water per day. However, obligatory urine outputs can compromise hydration status when there is inadequate water intake or when losses increase in disease or kidney damage.

Infants have high requirements for water because of their large ratio of surface area to volume, their inability to communicate their thirst, and the limited capacity of the immature kidney to handle high renal solute loads. Increased water needs during pregnancy are ~30 mL/d. During lactation, milk production increases daily water requirements so that ~1000 mL of additional water is needed, or 1 mL for each milliliter of milk produced. Special attention must be paid to the water needs of the elderly, who have reduced total body water and blunted thirst sensation and are more likely to be taking medications such as diuretics.

Other nutrients

See Chap. 57 for detailed descriptions of vitamins and trace minerals.

DIETARY REFERENCE INTAKES AND RECOMMENDED DIETARY ALLOWANCES

Fortunately, human life and well-being can be maintained within a fairly wide range for most nutrients. However, the capacity for adaptation is not infinite—too much, as well as too little, intake of a nutrient can have adverse effects or alter the health benefits conferred by another nutrient. Therefore, benchmark recommendations regarding nutrient intakes have been developed to guide clinical practice. These quantitative estimates of nutrient intakes are collectively referred to as the *dietary reference intakes* (DRIs). The DRIs have supplanted the RDAs—the single reference values used in the United States until the early 1990s. DRIs include the *estimated average requirement* (EAR) for nutrients as well as other reference values used for dietary planning for individuals: the RDA, the *adequate intake* (AI), and the tolerable *upper level* (UL). The DRIs also include acceptable macronutrient distribution ranges (AMDRs) for protein, fat, and carbohydrate. The current DRIs for vitamins and elements are provided in Tables 56-1 and 56-2, respectively. Table 56-3 provides DRIs for water and macronutrients. **EERs are discussed in Chap. 58 on energy balance in health and disease.**

Estimated average requirement

When florid manifestations of the classic dietary-deficiency diseases such as rickets (deficiency of vitamin D and calcium), scurvy (deficiency of vitamin C), xerophthalmia (deficiency of vitamin A), and protein-calorie malnutrition were common, nutrient adequacy was inferred from the absence of their clinical signs. Later, biochemical and other changes were found to be evident long before the deficiency became clinically apparent. Consequently, criteria of adequacy are now based on biologic markers when they are available. Priority is given to sensitive biochemical, physiologic, or behavioral tests that reflect early changes in regulatory

TABLE 56-1

DIETARY REFERENCE INTAKES (DRIs): RECOMMENDED DIETARY ALLOWANCES AND ADEQUATE INTAKES FOR VITAMINS

LIFE-STAGE GROUP	VITA-MIN A (μg/d)[a]	VITAMIN C (mg/d)	VITAMIN D (μg/d)[b,c]	VITAMIN E (mg/d)[d]	VITAMIN K (μg/d)	THIAMIN (mg/d)	RIBOFLAVIN (mg/d)	NIACIN (mg/d)[e]	VITAMIN B_6 (mg/d)	FOLATE (μg/d)[f]	VITAMIN B_{12} (μg/d)	PANTOT-HENIC ACID (mg/d)	BIOTIN (μg/d)	CHOLINE (mg/d)[g]
Infants														
Birth to 6 mo	400*	40*	10	4*	2.0*	0.2*	0.3*	2*	0.1*	65*	0.4*	1.7*	5*	125*
6–12 mo	500*	50*	10	5*	2.5*	0.3*	0.4*	4*	0.3*	80*	0.5*	1.8*	6*	150*
Children														
1–3 y	**300**	**15**	**15**	**6**	30*	**0.5**	**0.5**	**6**	**0.5**	**150**	**0.9**	2*	8*	200*
4–8 y	**400**	**25**	**15**	**7**	55*	**0.6**	**0.6**	**8**	**0.6**	**200**	**1.2**	3*	12*	250*
Males														
9–13 y	**600**	**45**	**15**	**11**	60*	**0.9**	**0.9**	**12**	**1.0**	**300**	**1.8**	4*	20*	375*
14–18 y	**900**	**75**	**15**	**15**	75*	**1.2**	**1.3**	**16**	**1.3**	**400**	**2.4**	5*	25*	550*
19–30 y	**900**	**90**	**15**	**15**	120*	**1.2**	**1.3**	**16**	**1.3**	**400**	**2.4**	5*	30*	550*
31–50 y	**900**	**90**	**15**	**15**	120*	**1.2**	**1.3**	**16**	**1.3**	**400**	**2.4**	5*	30*	550*
51–70 y	**900**	**90**	**15**	**15**	120*	**1.2**	**1.3**	**16**	**1.7**	**400**	**2.4**[h]	5*	30*	550*
>70 y	**900**	**90**	**20**	**15**	120*	**1.2**	**1.3**	**16**	**1.7**	**400**	**2.4**[h]	5*	30*	550*
Females														
9–13 y	**600**	**45**	**15**	**11**	60*	**0.9**	**0.9**	**12**	**1.0**	**300**	**1.8**	4*	20*	375*
14–18 y	**700**	**65**	**15**	**15**	75*	**1.0**	**1.0**	**14**	**1.2**	**400**[i]	**2.4**	5*	25*	400*
19–30 y	**700**	**75**	**15**	**15**	90*	**1.1**	**1.1**	**14**	**1.3**	**400**[i]	**2.4**	5*	30*	425*
31–50 y	**700**	**75**	**15**	**15**	90*	**1.1**	**1.1**	**14**	**1.3**	**400**[i]	**2.4**	5*	30*	425*
51–70 y	**700**	**75**	**15**	**15**	90*	**1.1**	**1.1**	**14**	**1.5**	**400**	**2.4**[h]	5*	30*	425*
>70 y	**700**	**75**	**20**	**15**	90*	**1.1**	**1.1**	**14**	**1.5**	**400**	**2.4**[h]	5*	30*	425*
Pregnant women														
14–18 y	**750**	**80**	**15**	**15**	75*	**1.4**	**1.4**	**18**	**1.9**	**600**[j]	**2.6**	6*	30*	450*
19–30 y	**770**	**85**	**15**	**15**	90*	**1.4**	**1.4**	**18**	**1.9**	**600**[j]	**2.6**	6*	30*	450*
31–50 y	**770**	**85**	**15**	**15**	90*	**1.4**	**1.4**	**18**	**1.9**	**600**[j]	**2.6**	6*	30*	450*

(continued)

TABLE 56-1

DIETARY REFERENCE INTAKES (DRIs): RECOMMENDED DIETARY ALLOWANCES AND ADEQUATE INTAKES FOR VITAMINS (*CONTINUED*)

LIFE-STAGE GROUP	VITA-MIN A (μg/d)[a]	VITAMIN C (mg/d)	VITAMIN D (μg/d)[b,c]	VITAMIN E (mg/d)[d]	VITAMIN K (μg/d)	THIAMIN (mg/d)	RIBOFLAVIN (mg/d)	NIACIN (mg/d)[e]	VITAMIN B_6 (mg/d)	FOLATE (μg/d)[f]	VITAMIN B_{12} (μg/d)	PANTOT-HENIC ACID (mg/d)	BIOTIN (μg/d)	CHOLINE (mg/d)[g]
Lactating women														
14–18 y	**1200**	**115**	**15**	**19**	75*	**1.4**	**1.6**	**17**	**2.0**	**500**	**2.8**	7*	35*	550*
19–30 y	**1300**	**120**	**15**	**19**	90*	**1.4**	**1.6**	**17**	**2.0**	**500**	**2.8**	7*	35*	550*
31–50 y	**1300**	**120**	**15**	**19**	90*	**1.4**	**1.6**	**17**	**2.0**	**500**	**2.8**	7*	35*	550*

Note: This table (taken from the DRI reports; see www.nap.edu) presents recommended dietary allowances (RDAs) in **bold type** and adequate intakes (AIs) in ordinary type followed by an asterisk (*). An RDA is the average daily dietary intake level sufficient to meet the nutrient requirements of nearly all healthy individuals (97–98%) in a group. The RDA is calculated from an estimated average requirement (EAR). If sufficient scientific evidence is not available to establish an EAR and thus to calculate an RDA, an AI is usually developed. For healthy breast-fed infants, an AI is the mean intake. The AI for other life-stage and sex-specific groups is believed to cover the needs of all healthy individuals in those groups, but lack of data or uncertainty in the data makes it impossible to specify with confidence the percentage of individuals covered by this intake.

[a]As retinol activity equivalents (RAEs). 1 RAE = 1 μg retinol, 12 μg β-carotene, 24 μg α-carotene, or 24 μg β-cryptoxanthin. The RAE for dietary provitamin A carotenoids is twofold greater than the retinol equivalent (RE), whereas the RAE for preformed vitamin A is the same as the RE.

[b]As cholecalciferol. 1 μg cholecalciferol = 40 IU vitamin D.

[c]Under the assumption of minimal sunlight.

[d]As α-tocopherol. α-Tocopherol includes RRR-α-tocopherol, the only form of α-tocopherol that occurs naturally in foods, and the *2R*-stereoisomeric forms of α-tocopherol (RRR-, RSR-, RRS-, and RSS-α-tocopherol) that occur in fortified foods and supplements. It does not include the 2S-stereoisomeric forms of α-tocopherol (SRR-, SSR-, SRS-, and SSS-α-tocopherol) also found in fortified foods and supplements.

[e]As niacin equivalents (NEs). 1 mg of niacin = 60 mg of tryptophan; 0–6 months = preformed niacin (not NE).

[f]As dietary folate equivalents (DFEs). 1 DFE = 1 μg food folate = 0.6 μg of folic acid from fortified food or as a supplement consumed with food = 0.5 μg of a supplement taken on an empty stomach.

[g]Although AIs have been set for choline, there are few data to assess whether a dietary supply of choline is needed at all stages of the life cycle, and it may be that the choline requirement can be met by endogenous synthesis at some of these stages.

[h]Because 10–30% of older people may malabsorb food-bound B12, it is advisable for those >50 years of age to meet their RDA mainly by consuming foods fortified with B_{12} or a supplement containing B_{12}.

[i]In view of evidence linking inadequate folate intake with neural tube defects in the fetus, it is recommended that all women capable of becoming pregnant consume 400 μg of folate from supplements or fortified foods in addition to intake of food folate from a varied diet.

[j]It is assumed that women will continue consuming 400 μg from supplements or fortified food until their pregnancy is confirmed and they enter prenatal care, which ordinarily occurs after the end of the periconceptional period—the critical time for formation of the neural tube.

Source: Food and Nutrition Board, Institute of Medicine, National Academies (http://www.iom.edu/Activities/Nutrition/SummaryDRIs/DRI-Tables.aspx).

TABLE 56-2

DIETARY REFERENCE INTAKES (DRIs): RECOMMENDED DIETARY ALLOWANCES AND ADEQUATE INTAKES FOR ELEMENTS

LIFE-STAGE GROUP	CALCIUM (mg/d)	CHROMIUM (µg/d)	COPPER (µg/d)	FLUORIDE (mg/d)	IODINE (µg/d)	IRON (mg/d)	MAG-NESIUM (mg/d)	MAN-GANESE (mg/d)	MOLY-BDENUM (µg/d)	PHOS-PHORUS (mg/d)	SELENIUM (µg/d)	ZINC (mg/d)	POT-ASSIUM (g/d)	SODIUM (g/d)	CHLORIDE (g/d)
Infants															
Birth to 6 mo	200*	0.2*	200*	0.01*	110*	0.27*	30*	0.003*	2*	100*	15*	2*	0.4*	0.12*	0.18*
6–12 mo	260*	5.5*	220*	0.5*	130*	**11**	75*	0.6*	3*	275*	20*	**3**	0.7*	0.37*	0.57*
Children															
1–3 y	**700**	11*	**340**	0.7*	**90**	**7**	**80**	1.2*	**17**	**460**	**20**	**3**	3.0*	1.0*	1.5*
4–8 y	**1000**	15*	**440**	1*	**90**	**10**	**130**	1.5*	**22**	**500**	**30**	**5**	3.8*	1.2*	1.9*
Males															
9–13 y	**1300**	25*	**700**	2*	**120**	**8**	**240**	1.9*	**34**	**1250**	**40**	**8**	4.5*	1.5*	2.3*
14–18 y	**1300**	35*	**890**	3*	**150**	**11**	**410**	2.2*	**43**	**1250**	**55**	**11**	4.7*	1.5*	2.3*
19–30 y	**1000**	35*	**900**	4*	**150**	**8**	**400**	2.3*	**45**	**700**	**55**	**11**	4.7*	1.5*	2.3*
31–50 y	**1000**	35*	**900**	4*	**150**	**8**	**420**	2.3*	**45**	**700**	**55**	**11**	4.7*	1.5*	2.3*
51–70 y	**1000**	30*	**900**	4*	**150**	**8**	**420**	2.3*	**45**	**700**	**55**	**11**	4.7*	1.3*	2.0*
>70 y	**1200**	30*	**900**	4*	**150**	**8**	**420**	2.3*	**45**	**700**	**55**	**11**	4.7*	1.2*	1.8*
Females															
9–13 y	**1300**	21*	**700**	2*	**120**	**8**	**240**	1.6*	**34**	**1250**	**40**	**8**	4.5*	1.5*	2.3*
14–18 y	**1300**	24*	**890**	3*	**150**	**15**	**360**	1.6*	**43**	**1250**	**55**	**9**	4.7*	1.5*	2.3*
19–30 y	**1000**	25*	**900**	3*	**150**	**18**	**310**	1.8*	**45**	**700**	**55**	**8**	4.7*	1.5*	2.3*
31–50 y	**1000**	25*	**900**	3*	**150**	**18**	320	1.8*	**45**	**700**	**55**	**8**	4.7*	1.5*	2.3*
51–70 y	**1200**	20*	**900**	3*	**150**	**8**	**320**	1.8*	**45**	**700**	**55**	**8**	4.7*	1.3*	2.0*
>70 y	**1200**	20*	**900**	3*	**150**	**8**	**320**	1.8*	**45**	**700**	**55**	**8**	4.7*	1.2*	1.8*
Pregnant women															
14–18 y	**1300**	29*	**1000**	3*	**220**	**27**	**400**	2.0*	**50**	**1250**	**60**	**12**	4.7*	1.5*	2.3*
19–30 y	**1000**	30*	**1000**	3*	**220**	**27**	**350**	2.0*	**50**	**700**	**60**	**11**	4.7*	1.5*	2.3*
31–50 y	**1000**	30*	**1000**	3*	**220**	**27**	**360**	2.0*	**50**	**700**	**60**	**11**	4.7*	1.5*	2.3*

(*continued*)

TABLE 56-2

DIETARY REFERENCE INTAKES (DRIs): RECOMMENDED DIETARY ALLOWANCES AND ADEQUATE INTAKES FOR ELEMENTS *(CONTINUED)*

LIFE-STAGE GROUP	CALCIUM (mg/d)	CHROMIUM (μg/d)	COPPER (μg/d)	FLUORIDE (mg/d)	IODINE (μg/d)	IRON (mg/d)	MAG-NESIUM (mg/d)	MAN-GANESE (mg/d)	MOLY-BDENUM (μg/d)	PHOS-PHORUS (mg/d)	SELENIUM (μg/d)	ZINC (mg/d)	POT-ASSIUM (g/d)	SODIUM (g/d)	CHLORIDE (g/d)
Lactating women															
14–18 y	**1300**	44*	**1300**	3*	**290**	**10**	**360**	2.6*	**50**	**1250**	**70**	**13**	5.1*	1.5*	2.3*
19–30 y	**1000**	45*	**1300**	3*	**290**	**9**	**310**	2.6*	**50**	**700**	**70**	**12**	5.1*	1.5*	2.3*
31–50 y	**1000**	45*	**1300**	3*	**290**	**9**	**320**	2.6*	**50**	**700**	**70**	**12**	5.1*	1.5*	2.3*

Note: This table (taken from the DRI reports; see *www.nap.edu*) presents recommended dietary allowances (RDAs) in **bold type** and adequate intakes (AIs) in ordinary type followed by an asterisk (*). An RDA is the average daily dietary intake level sufficient to meet the nutrient requirements of nearly all healthy individuals (97–98%) in a group. The RDA is calculated from an estimated average requirement (EAR). If sufficient scientific evidence is not available to establish an EAR and thus to calculate an RDA, an AI is usually developed. For healthy breast-fed infants, an AI is the mean intake. The AI for other life-stage and sex-specific groups is believed to cover the needs of all healthy individuals in those groups, but lack of data or uncertainty in the data makes it impossible to specify with confidence the percentage of individuals covered by this intake.

Sources: Food and Nutrition Board, Institute of Medicine, National Academies (*http://www.iom.edu/Activities/Nutrition/SummaryDRIs/DRI-Tables.aspx*), based on: Dietary Reference Intakes for Calcium, Phosphorus, Magnesium, Vitamin D, and Fluoride (1997); Dietary Reference Intakes for Thiamin, Riboflavin, Niacin, Vitamin B_6, Folate, Vitamin B_{12}, Pantothenic Acid, Biotin, and Choline (1998); Dietary Reference Intakes for Vitamin C, Vitamin E, Selenium, and Carotenoids (2000); and Dietary Reference Intakes for Vitamin A, Vitamin K, Arsenic, Boron, Chromium, Copper, Iodine, Iron, Manganese, Molybdenum, Nickel, Silicon, Vanadium, and Zinc (2001); Dietary Reference Intakes for Water, Potassium, Sodium, Chloride, and Sulfate (2005); and Dietary Reference Intakes for Calcium and Vitamin D (2011). These reports can be accessed via www.nap.edu.

TABLE 56-3

DIETARY REFERENCE INTAKES (DRIs): RECOMMENDED DIETARY ALLOWANCES AND ADEQUATE INTAKES FOR TOTAL WATER AND MACRONUTRIENTS

LIFE-STAGE GROUP	TOTAL WATER[a] (L/d)	CARBOHYDRATE (g/d)	TOTAL FIBER (g/d)	FAT (g/d)	LINOLEIC ACID (g/d)	α-LINOLENIC ACID (g/d)	PROTEIN[b] (g/d)
Infants							
Birth to 6 mo	0.7*	60*	ND[c]	31*	4.4*	0.5*	9.1*
6–12 mo	0.8*	95*	ND	30*	4.6*	0.5*	**11.0**
Children							
1–3 y	1.3*	**130**	19*	ND	7*	0.7*	**13**
4–8 y	1.7*	**130**	25*	ND	10*	0.9*	**19**
Males							
9–13 y	2.4*	**130**	31*	ND	12*	1.2*	**34**
14–18 y	3.3*	**130**	38*	ND	16*	1.6*	**52**
19–30 y	3.7*	**130**	38*	ND	17*	1.6*	**56**
31–50 y	3.7*	**130**	38*	ND	17*	1.6*	**56**
51–70 y	3.7*	**130**	30*	ND	14*	1.6*	**56**
>70 y	3.7*	**130**	30*	ND	14*	1.6*	**56**
Females							
9–13 y	2.1*	**130**	26*	ND	10*	1.0*	**34**
14–18 y	2.3*	**130**	26*	ND	11*	1.1*	**46**
19–30 y	2.7*	**130**	25*	ND	12*	1.1*	**46**
31–50 y	2.7*	**130**	25*	ND	12*	1.1*	**46**
51–70 y	2.7*	**130**	21*	ND	11*	1.1*	**46**
>70 y	2.7*	**130**	21*	ND	11*	1.1*	**46**
Pregnant women							
14–18 y	3.0*	**175**	28*	ND	13*	1.4*	**71**
19–30 y	3.0*	**175**	28*	ND	13*	1.4*	**71**
31–50 y	3.0*	**175**	28*	ND	13*	1.4*	**71**
Lactating women							
14–18	3.8*	**210**	29*	ND	13*	1.3*	**71**
19–30 y	3.8*	**210**	29*	ND	13*	1.3*	**71**
31–50 y	3.8*	**210**	29*	ND	13*	1.3*	**71**

Note: This table (taken from the DRI reports; see www.nap.edu) presents recommended dietary allowances (RDAs) in **bold type** and adequate intakes (AIs) in ordinary type followed by an asterisk (*). An RDA is the average daily dietary intake level sufficient to meet the nutrient requirements of nearly all healthy individuals (97–98%) in a group. The RDA is calculated from an estimated average requirement (EAR). If sufficient scientific evidence is not available to establish an EAR and thus to calculate an RDA, an AI is usually developed. For healthy breast-fed infants, an AI is the mean intake. The AI for other life-stage and sex-specific groups is believed to cover the needs of all healthy individuals in those groups, but lack of data or uncertainty in the data make it impossible to specify with confidence the percentage of individuals covered by this intake.

[a]Total water includes all water contained in food, beverages, and drinking water.

[b]Based on grams of protein per kilogram of body weight for the reference body weight (e.g., for adults: 0.8 g/kg body weight for the reference body weight).

[c]Not determined.

Source: Food and Nutrition Board, Institute of Medicine, National Academies (*http://www.iom.edu/Activities/Nutrition/SummaryDRIs/DRI-Tables.aspx*), based on: Dietary Reference Intakes for Energy, Carbohydrate, Fiber, Fat, Fatty Acids, Cholesterol, Protein, and Amino Acids (2002/2005) and Dietary Reference Intakes for Water, Potassium, Sodium, Chloride, and Sulfate (2005). These reports can be accessed via *www.nap.edu*.

processes; maintenance of body stores of nutrients; or, if available, the amount of a nutrient that minimizes the risk of chronic degenerative disease. Current efforts focus on this last variable, but relevant markers often are not available.

The EAR is the amount of a nutrient estimated to be adequate for half of the healthy individuals of a specific age and sex. The types of evidence and criteria used to establish nutrient requirements vary by nutrient, age, and physiologic group. The EAR is not an effective estimate of nutrient adequacy in individuals because it is a median requirement for a group; 50% of individuals in a group fall below the requirement and 50% fall above it. Thus, a person with a usual intake at the EAR has a 50% risk of inadequate intake. For these reasons, other standards, described below, are more useful for clinical purposes.

Recommended dietary allowances

The RDA is the average daily dietary intake level that meets the nutrient requirements of nearly all healthy persons of a specific sex, age, life stage, or physiologic condition (e.g., pregnancy or lactation). The RDA, which is the nutrient-intake goal for planning diets of individuals, is defined statistically as two standard deviations above the EAR to ensure that the needs of any given individual are met. The online tool at *http://fnic.nal.usda.gov/interactiveDRI/* allows health professionals to calculate individualized daily nutrient recommendations for dietary planning based on the DRIs for persons of a given age, sex, and weight. The RDAs are used to formulate food guides such as the U.S. Department of Agriculture (USDA) MyPlate Food Guide for individuals (*www.supertracker.usda.gov/default.aspx*), to create food-exchange lists for therapeutic diet planning, and as a standard for describing the nutritional content of foods and nutrient-containing dietary supplements.

The risk of dietary inadequacy increases as intake falls below the RDA. However, the RDA is an overly generous criterion for evaluating nutrient adequacy. For example, by definition, the RDA exceeds the actual requirements of all but ~2–3% of the population. Therefore, many people whose intake falls below the RDA may still be getting enough of the nutrient. On food labels, the nutrient content in a food is stated by weight or as a percent of the daily value (DV), a variant of the RDA used on the nutrition facts panel that, for an adult, represents the highest RDA for an adult consuming 2000 kcal.

Adequate intake

It is not possible to set an RDA for some nutrients that do not have an established EAR. In this circumstance, the AI is based on observed or experimentally determined approximations of nutrient intakes in healthy people. In the DRIs, AIs rather than RDAs are proposed for nutrients consumed by infants (up to age 1 year) as well as for chromium, fluoride, manganese, sodium, potassium, pantothenic acid, biotin, choline, and water consumed by persons of all ages. Vitamin D and calcium recommendations were recently revised, and more precise estimates are now available.

Tolerable upper levels of nutrient intake

Healthy individuals derive no established benefit from consuming nutrient levels above the RDA or AI. In fact, excessive nutrient intake can disturb body functions and cause acute, progressive, or permanent disabilities. The tolerable UL is the highest level of chronic nutrient intake (usually daily) that is unlikely to pose a risk of adverse health effects for most of the population. Data on the adverse effects of large amounts of many nutrients are unavailable or too limited to establish a UL. Therefore, the lack of a UL does *not* mean that the risk of adverse effects from high intake is nonexistent. Nutrients in commonly eaten foods rarely exceed the UL. However, highly fortified foods and dietary supplements provide more concentrated amounts of nutrients per serving and thus pose a potential risk of toxicity. Nutrient supplements are labeled with supplement facts that express the amount of nutrient in absolute units or as the percentage of the DV provided per recommended serving size. Total nutrient consumption, including that in foods, supplements, and over-the-counter medications (e.g., antacids), should not exceed RDA levels.

Acceptable macronutrient distribution ranges

The AMDRs are not experimentally determined but are rough ranges for energy-providing macronutrient intakes (protein, carbohydrate, and fat) that the Institute of Medicine's Food and Nutrition Board considers to be healthful. These ranges are 10–35% of calories for protein, 20–35% of calories for fat, and 45–65% of calories for carbohydrate. Alcohol, which also provides energy, is not a nutrient; therefore, no recommendations are not provided.

FACTORS ALTERING NUTRIENT NEEDS

The DRIs are affected by age, sex, rate of growth, pregnancy, lactation, physical activity level, concomitant diseases, drugs, and dietary composition. If requirements for nutrient sufficiency are close to levels indicating excess of a nutrient, dietary planning is difficult.

Physiologic factors

Growth, strenuous physical activity, pregnancy, and lactation all increase needs for energy and several essential nutrients. Energy needs rise during pregnancy due to the demands of fetal growth and during lactation because of the increased energy required for milk production. Energy needs decrease with loss of lean body mass, the major determinant of REE. Because lean tissue, physical activity, and health often decline with age, energy needs of older persons, especially those over 70, tend to be lower than those of younger persons.

Dietary composition

Dietary composition affects the biologic availability and use of nutrients. For example, the absorption of iron may be impaired by large amounts of calcium or lead; likewise, non-heme iron uptake may be impaired by a lack of ascorbic acid and amino acids in the meal. Protein use by the body may be decreased when essential amino acids are not present in sufficient amounts—a rare scenario in U.S. diets. Animal foods, such as milk, eggs, and meat, have high biologic values, with most of the needed amino acids present in adequate amounts. Plant proteins in corn (maize), soy, rice, and wheat have lower biologic values and must be combined with other plant or animal proteins or fortified with the amino acids that are deficient to achieve optimal use by the body.

Route of intake

The RDAs apply only to oral intakes. When nutrients are administered parenterally, similar values can sometimes be used for amino acids, glucose (carbohydrate), fats, sodium, chloride, potassium, and most vitamins because their intestinal absorption rate is nearly 100%. However, the oral bioavailability of most mineral elements may be only half that obtained by parenteral administration. For some nutrients that are not readily stored in the body or that cannot be stored in large amounts, timing of administration may also be important. For example, amino acids cannot be used for protein synthesis if they are not supplied together; instead, they will be used for energy production, although in healthy individuals eating adequate diets, the distribution of protein intake over the course of the day has little effect on health.

Disease

Dietary deficiency diseases include protein-calorie malnutrition, iron-deficiency anemia, goiter (due to iodine deficiency), rickets and osteomalacia (vitamin D deficiency), and xeropthalmia (vitamin A deficiency), megaloblastic anemia (vitamin B_{12} or folic acid deficiency), scurvy (vitamin C/ascorbic acid deficiency), beriberi (thiamin deficiency), and pellagra (niacin and tryptophan deficiency) **(Chaps. 57 and 58)**. Each deficiency disease is characterized by imbalances at the cellular level between the supply of nutrients or energy and the body's nutritional needs for growth, maintenance, and other functions. Imbalances and excesses in nutrient intakes are recognized as risk factors for certain chronic degenerative diseases, such as saturated fat and cholesterol in coronary artery disease; sodium in hypertension; obesity in hormone-dependent endometrial and breast cancers; and ethanol in alcoholism. Because the etiology and pathogenesis of these disorders are multifactorial, diet is only one of many risk factors. Osteoporosis, for example, is associated with calcium deficiency, sometimes secondary to vitamin D deficiency, as well as with risk factors related to environment (e.g., smoking, sedentary lifestyle), physiology (e.g., estrogen deficiency), genetic determinants (e.g., defects in collagen metabolism), and drug use (chronic steroid and aromatase inhibitors).

DIETARY ASSESSMENT

In clinical situations, nutritional assessment is an iterative process that involves: (1) screening for malnutrition, (2) assessing the diet and other data to establish either the absence or the presence of malnutrition and its possible causes, (3) planning and implementing the most appropriate nutritional therapy, and (4) reassessing intakes to make sure that they have been consumed. Some disease states affect the bioavailability, requirements, use, or excretion of specific nutrients. In these circumstances, specific measurements of various nutrients or their biomarkers may be required to ensure adequate replacement **(Chap. 57)**.

Most health care facilities have nutrition-screening processes in place for identifying possible malnutrition after hospital admission. Nutritional screening is required by the Joint Commission, which accredits and certifies health care organizations in the United States. However, there are no universally recognized or validated standards. The factors that are usually assessed include abnormal weight for height or body mass index (e.g., BMI <19 or >25); reported weight change (involuntary loss or gain of >5 kg in the past 6 months) **(Chap. 10)**; diagnoses with known nutritional implications (e.g., metabolic disease, any disease affecting the gastrointestinal tract, alcoholism); present therapeutic dietary prescription; chronic poor appetite; presence of chewing and swallowing problems or major food intolerances; need for assistance with preparing or shopping for food, eating, or other aspects of self-care; and social isolation. The nutritional status of hospitalized patients should be reassessed periodically—at least once every week.

A more complete dietary assessment is indicated for patients who exhibit a high risk of or frank malnutrition on nutritional screening. The type of assessment varies with the clinical setting, the severity of the patient's illness, and the stability of the patient's condition.

Acute-care settings

In acute-care settings, anorexia, various other diseases, test procedures, and medications can compromise dietary intake. Under such circumstances, the goal is to identify and avoid inadequate intake and to assure appropriate alimentation. Dietary assessment focuses on what patients are currently eating, whether or not they are able and willing to eat, and whether or not they experience any problems with eating. Dietary intake assessment is based on information from observed intakes; medical records; history; clinical examination; and anthropometric, biochemical, and functional status evaluations. The objective is to gather enough information to establish the likelihood of malnutrition due to poor dietary intake or other causes in order to assess whether nutritional therapy is indicated **(Chap. 59)**.

Simple observations may suffice to suggest inadequate oral intake. These include dietitians' and nurses' notes; observation of a patient's frequent refusal to eat or the amount of food eaten on trays; the frequent performance of tests and procedures that are likely to cause meals to be skipped; adherence to nutritionally inadequate diet orders (e.g., clear liquids or full liquids) for more than a few days; the occurrence of fever, gastrointestinal distress, vomiting, diarrhea, or a comatose state; and the presence of diseases or use of treatments that involve any part of the alimentary tract. Acutely ill patients with diet-related diseases such as diabetes need assessment because an inappropriate diet may exacerbate these conditions and adversely affect other therapies. Abnormal biochemical values (serum albumin levels <35 g/L [<3.5 mg/dL]; serum cholesterol levels <3.9 mmol/L [<150 mg/dL]) are nonspecific but may indicate a need for further nutritional assessment.

Most therapeutic diets offered in hospitals are calculated to meet individual nutrient requirements and the RDA *if they are eaten*. Exceptions include clear liquids, some full-liquid diets, and test diets (such as those adhered to in preparation for gastrointestinal procedures), which are inadequate for several nutrients and should not be used, if possible, for more than 24 h. However, because as much as half of the food served to hospitalized patients is not eaten, it cannot be assumed that the intakes of hospitalized patients are adequate. Dietary assessment should compare how much and what kinds of food the patient has consumed with the diet that has been provided. Major deviations in intakes of energy, protein, fluids, or other nutrients of special concern for the patient's illness should be noted and corrected.

Nutritional monitoring is especially important for patients who are very ill and who have extended lengths of hospital stay. Patients who are fed by enteral and parenteral routes also require special nutritional assessment and monitoring by physicians and/or dietitians with certification in nutritional support **(Chap. 59)**.

Ambulatory settings

The aim of dietary assessment in the outpatient setting is to determine whether or not the patient's usual diet is a health risk in itself or if it contributes to existing chronic disease-related problems. Dietary assessment also provides the basis for planning a diet that fulfills therapeutic goals while ensuring patient adherence. The outpatient dietary assessment should review the adequacy of present and usual food intakes, including vitamin and mineral supplements, oral nutritional supplements, medical foods, other dietary supplements, medications, and alcohol, because all of these may affect the patient's nutritional status. The assessment should focus on the dietary constituents that are most likely to be involved or compromised by a specific diagnosis as well as on any comorbidities that are present. More than one day's intake should be reviewed to provide a better representation of the usual diet.

There are many ways to assess the adequacy of a patient's habitual diet. These include use of a food guide, a food-exchange list, a diet history, or a food-frequency questionnaire. A commonly used food guide for healthy persons is the USDA's Choose My Plate, which is useful as a rough guide for avoiding inadequate intakes of essential nutrients as well as likely excesses in the amounts of fat (especially saturated and trans fats), sodium, sugar, and alcohol consumed (Table 56-4). The Choose My Plate graphic emphasizes a balance between calories and nutritional needs, encouraging increased intake of fruits and vegetables, whole grains, and low-fat milk in conjunction with reduced intake of sodium and high-calorie sugary drinks. The Web version of the guide provides a calculator that tailors the number of servings suggested for healthy patients of different weights, sexes, ages, and life-cycle stages to help them to meet their needs while avoiding excess *(http://www.supertracker.usda.gov/default.aspx and www.ChooseMyPlate.gov)*. Patients who follow ethnic or unusual dietary patterns may need extra instruction on how foods should be categorized and on the appropriate portion sizes that constitute a serving. The process of reviewing the guide with patients helps them transition to healthier dietary patterns and identifies food groups eaten in excess of recommendations or in insufficient quantities. For persons on therapeutic diets, assessment against food-exchange lists may be useful. These include, for example, American Diabetes Association food-exchange lists for diabetes and the Academy of Nutrition and Dietetics food-exchange lists for renal disease.

NUTRITIONAL STATUS ASSESSMENT

Full nutritional status assessment is reserved for seriously ill patients and those at very high nutritional risk when the cause of malnutrition is still uncertain after the initial clinical evaluation and dietary assessment. It involves multiple dimensions, including documentation of dietary intake, anthropometric measurements, biochemical measurements of blood and urine, clinical examination, health history elicitation, and functional status evaluation. Therapeutic dietary prescriptions and menu plans for most diseases are available from most hospitals and from the Academy of Nutrition and Dietetics. **For further discussion of nutritional assessment, see Chap. 58.**

GLOBAL CONSIDERATIONS

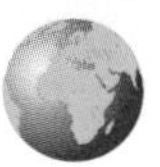

The DRIs (e.g., the EAR, the UL, and energy needs) are estimates of physiologic requirements based on experimental evidence. Assuming that

TABLE 56-4

CHOOSE MY PLATE: A GUIDE TO INDIVIDUALIZED DIETARY PLANNING

DIETARY FACTOR, UNIT OF MEASURE (ADVICE)	EXAMPLES OF STANDARD PORTION SIZES AT INDICATED ENERGY LEVEL		
	LOWER: 1600 kcal	MODERATE: 2200 kcal	HIGHER: 2800 kcal
Fruits, cups (Focus on fruits.)	1.5	2	2.5
Vegetables, cups (Vary vegetables.)	2	3	3.5
Grains, oz eq (Make at least half of grains whole.)[a]	5	7	10
Protein foods, oz eq (Go lean with protein.)[b]	5	6	7
Dairy, cups or oz[c] (Choose calcium-rich foods.)	3	3	3
"Empty" calories, kcal[d]	120	260	400
Sodium, mg	<2300 at all energy levels		
Physical activity, min	At least 150 min vigorous physical activity per week at all energy levels		

Note: Oils (formerly listed with portions of 5, 6, and 8 teaspoons for the lower, moderate, and higher energy levels, respectively) are no longer singled out in Choose My Plate, but rather are included in the empty calories/added sugar category with SOFAS (calories from solid fats and added sugars). The limit is the remaining number of calories in each food pattern above after intake of the recommended amounts of the nutrient-dense foods.

[a]For example, 1 serving equals 1 slice bread, 1 cup ready-to-eat cereal, or 0.5 cup cooked rice, pasta, or cooked cereal.

[b]For example, 1 serving equals 1 oz lean meat, poultry, or fish; 1 egg; 1 tablespoon peanut butter; 0.25 cup cooked dry beans; or 0.5 oz nuts or seeds.

[c]For example, 1 serving equals 1 cup milk or yogurt, 1.5 oz natural cheese, or 2 oz processed cheese.

[d]Formerly called "discretionary calorie allowance." Portions are calculated as the number of calories remaining after all of the above allotments are accounted for.

Abbreviation: oz eq, ounce equivalent.

Source: Data from U.S. Department of Agriculture *(http://www.Choosemyplate.gov)*.

appropriate adjustments are made for age, sex, body size, and physical activity level, these estimates should be applicable to individuals in most parts of the world. However, the AIs are based on customary and adequate intakes in U.S. and Canadian populations, which appear to be compatible with good health, rather than on a large body of direct experimental evidence. Similarly, the AMDRs represent expert opinion regarding the approximate intakes of energy-providing nutrients that are healthful in these North American populations. Thus these measures should be used with caution in other settings. Nutrient-based standards like the DRIs have also been developed by the World Health Organization/Food and Agricultural Organization of the United Nations and are available on the Web (*http://www.who.int/nutrition/topics/nutrecomm/en/index.html*). The European Food Safety Authority (EFSA) Panel on Dietetic Products, Nutrition and Allergies periodically publishes its recommendations in the EFSA *Journal.* Other countries have promulgated similar recommendations. The different standards have many similarities in their basic concepts, definitions, and nutrient recommendation levels, but there are some differences from the DRIs as a result of the functional criteria chosen, environmental differences, the timeliness of the evidence reviewed, and expert judgment.

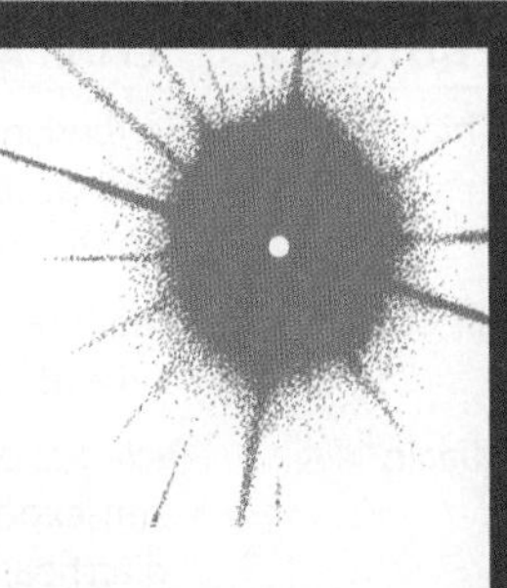

CHAPTER 57

VITAMIN AND TRACE MINERAL DEFICIENCY AND EXCESS

Robert M. Russell ■ Paolo M. Suter

Vitamins are required constituents of the human diet since they are synthesized inadequately or not at all in the human body. Only small amounts of these substances are needed to carry out essential biochemical reactions (e.g., by acting as coenzymes or prosthetic groups). Overt vitamin or trace mineral deficiencies are rare in Western countries because of a plentiful, varied, and inexpensive food supply; food fortification; and use of supplements. However, multiple nutrient deficiencies may appear together in persons who are chronically ill or alcoholic. After gastric bypass surgery, patients are at high risk for multiple nutrient deficiencies. Moreover, subclinical vitamin and trace mineral deficiencies, as diagnosed by laboratory testing, are quite common in the normal population, especially in the geriatric age group. Conversely, because of the widespread use of nutrient supplements, nutrient toxicities are gaining pathophysiologic and clinical importance.

Victims of famine, emergency-affected and displaced populations, and refugees are at increased risk for protein-energy malnutrition and classic micronutrient deficiencies (vitamin A, iron, iodine) as well as for overt deficiencies in thiamine (beriberi), riboflavin, vitamin C (scurvy), and niacin (pellagra).

Body stores of vitamins and minerals vary tremendously. For example, stores of vitamin B_{12} and vitamin A are large, and an adult may not become deficient until ≥1 year after beginning to eat a deficient diet. However, folate and thiamine may become depleted within weeks among those eating a deficient diet. Therapeutic modalities can deplete essential nutrients from the body; for example, hemodialysis removes water-soluble vitamins, which must be replaced by supplementation.

Vitamins and trace minerals play several roles in diseases: (1) Deficiencies of vitamins and minerals may be caused by disease states such as malabsorption. (2) Either deficiency or excess of vitamins and minerals can cause disease in and of itself (e.g., vitamin A intoxication and liver disease). (3) Vitamins and minerals in high doses may be used as drugs (e.g., niacin for hypercholesterolemia). Since they are covered elsewhere, the hematologic-related vitamins and minerals either are not considered or are considered only briefly in this chapter, as are the bone-related vitamins and minerals (vitamin D, calcium, phosphorus, magnesium).

VITAMINS

See also Table 57-1 and Fig. 57-1.

THIAMINE (VITAMIN B_1)

Thiamine was the first B vitamin to be identified and therefore is referred to as vitamin B_1. Thiamine functions in the decarboxylation of α-ketoacids (e.g., pyruvate α-ketoglutarate) and branched-chain amino acids and thus is essential for energy generation. In addition, thiamine pyrophosphate acts as a coenzyme for a transketolase reaction that mediates the conversion of hexose and pentose phosphates. It has been postulated that thiamine plays a role in peripheral nerve conduction, although the exact chemical reactions underlying this function are not known.

Food sources

The median intake of thiamine in the United States from food alone is 2 mg/d. Primary food sources for thiamine include yeast, organ meat, pork, legumes, beef, whole grains, and nuts. Milled rice and grains contain little thiamine. Thiamine deficiency is therefore more common in cultures that rely heavily on a rice-based diet. Tea, coffee (regular and decaffeinated), raw fish, and shellfish contain thiaminases, which can destroy the

TABLE 57-1

PRINCIPAL CLINICAL FINDINGS OF VITAMIN MALNUTRITION

NUTRIENT	CLINICAL FINDING	DIETARY LEVEL PER DAY ASSOCIATED WITH OVERT DEFICIENCY IN ADULTS	CONTRIBUTING FACTORS TO DEFICIENCY
Thiamine	Beriberi: neuropathy, muscle weakness and wasting, cardiomegaly, edema, ophthalmoplegia, confabulation	<0.3 mg/1000 kcal	Alcoholism, chronic diuretic use, hyperemesis, thiaminases in food
Riboflavin	Magenta tongue, angular stomatitis, seborrhea, cheilosis	<0.6 mg	Alcoholism
Niacin	Pellagra: pigmented rash of sun-exposed areas, bright red tongue, diarrhea, apathy, memory loss, disorientation	<9.0 niacin equivalents	Alcoholism, vitamin B_6 deficiency, riboflavin deficiency, tryptophan deficiency
Vitamin B_6	Seborrhea, glossitis, convulsions, neuropathy, depression, confusion, microcytic anemia	<0.2 mg	Alcoholism, isoniazid
Folate	Megaloblastic anemia, atrophic glossitis, depression, ↑ homocysteine	<100 μg/d	Alcoholism, sulfasalazine, pyrimethamine, triamterene
Vitamin B_{12}	Megaloblastic anemia, loss of vibratory and position sense, abnormal gait, dementia, impotence, loss of bladder and bowel control, ↑ homocysteine, ↑ methylmalonic acid	<1.0 μg/d	Gastric atrophy (pernicious anemia), terminal ileal disease, strict vegetarianism, acid-reducing drugs (e.g., H_2 blockers), metformin
Vitamin C	Scurvy: petechiae, ecchymosis, coiled hairs, inflamed and bleeding gums, joint effusion, poor wound healing, fatigue	<10 mg/d	Smoking, alcoholism
Vitamin A	Xerophthalmia, night blindness, Bitot's spots, follicular hyperkeratosis, impaired embryonic development, immune dysfunction	<300 μg/d	Fat malabsorption, infection, measles, alcoholism, protein-energy malnutrition
Vitamin D	Rickets: skeletal deformation, rachitic rosary, bowed legs; osteomalacia	<2.0 μg/d	Aging, lack of sunlight exposure, fat malabsorption, deeply pigmented skin
Vitamin E	Peripheral neuropathy, spinocerebellar ataxia, skeletal muscle atrophy, retinopathy	Not described unless underlying contributing factor is present	Occurs only with fat malabsorption or genetic abnormalities of vitamin E metabolism/transport
Vitamin K	Elevated prothrombin time, bleeding	<10 μg/d	Fat malabsorption, liver disease, antibiotic use

vitamin. Thus, drinking large amounts of tea or coffee can theoretically lower thiamine body stores.

Deficiency

Most dietary deficiency of thiamine worldwide is the result of poor dietary intake. In Western countries, the primary causes of thiamine deficiency are alcoholism and chronic illnesses such as cancer. Alcohol interferes directly with the absorption of thiamine and with the synthesis of thiamine pyrophosphate, and it increases urinary excretion. Thiamine should always be replenished when a patient with alcoholism is being refed, as carbohydrate repletion without adequate thiamine can precipitate acute thiamine deficiency with lactic acidosis. Other at-risk populations are women with prolonged hyperemesis gravidarum and anorexia, patients with overall poor nutritional status who are receiving parenteral glucose, patients who have had bariatric bypass surgery (*bariatric Wernicke*), and patients receiving chronic diuretic therapy (e.g., in hypertension or heart failure) due to increased urinary thiamine losses. Maternal thiamine deficiency can lead to infantile beriberi in breast-fed children. Thiamine deficiency could be an underlying factor in motor vehicle accidents and could be overlooked in the setting of head injury.

Thiamine deficiency in its early stage induces anorexia and nonspecific symptoms (e.g., irritability, decrease in short-term memory). Prolonged thiamine

Vitamin	Active derivative or cofactor form	Principal function
Thiamine (B_1) 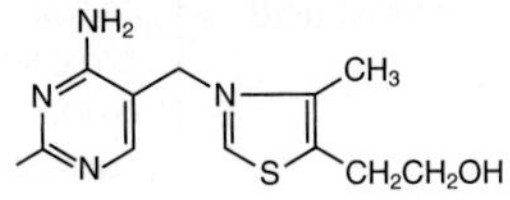	Thiamine pyrophosphate	Coenzyme for cleavage of carbon-carbon bonds; amino acid and carbohydrate metabolism
Riboflavin (B_2) 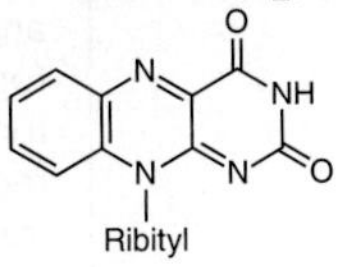	Flavin mononucleotide (FMN) and flavin adenine dinucleotide (FAD)	Cofactor for oxidation, reduction reactions, and covalently attached prosthetic groups for some enzymes
Niacin 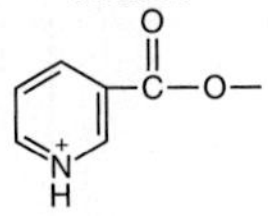	Nicotinamide adenine dinucleotide phosphate (NADP) and nicotinamide adenine dinucleotide (NAD)	Coenzymes for oxidation and reduction reactions
Vitamin B_6 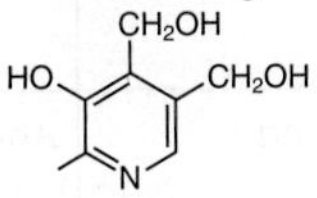	Pyridoxal phosphate	Cofactor for enzymes of amino acid metabolism
Folate 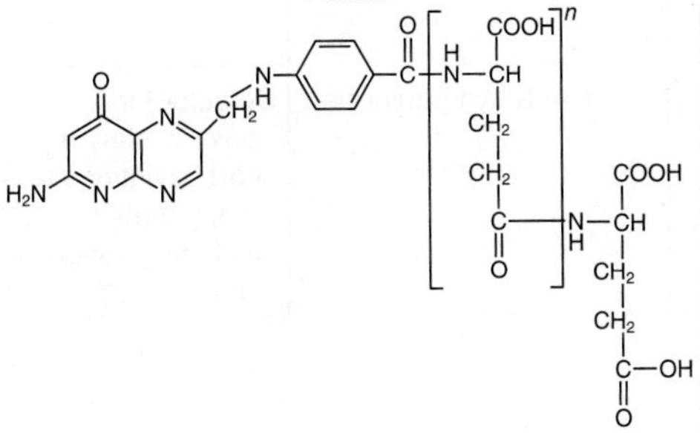	Polyglutamate forms of (5, 6, 7, 8) tetrahydrofolate with carbon unit attachments	Coenzyme for one carbon transfer in nucleic acid and amino acid metabolism
Vitamin B_{12} 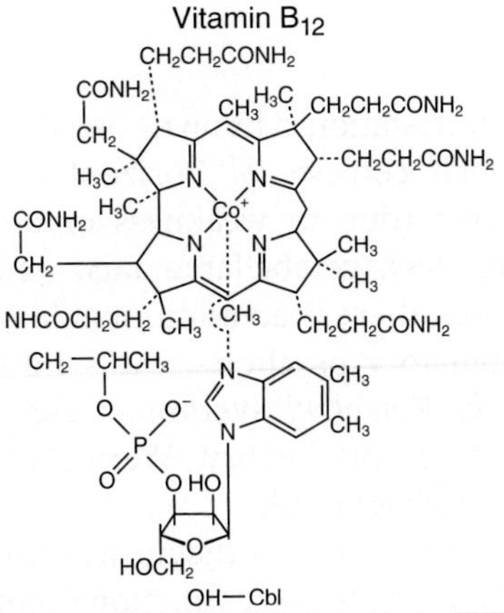	Methylcobalamine Adenosylcobalamin	Coenzyme for methionine synthase and L-methylmalonyl-CoA mutase

FIGURE 57-1
Structures and principal functions of vitamins associated with human disorders.

Vitamin	Active derivative or cofactor form	Principal function
Vitamin C 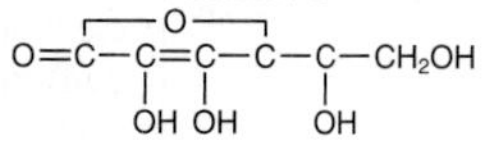 O=C—C=C—C—C—CH$_2$OH (ring via O) OH OH OH	Ascorbic acid and dehydroascorbic acid	Participation as a redox ion in many biologic oxidation and hydrogen transfer reactions
Vitamin A 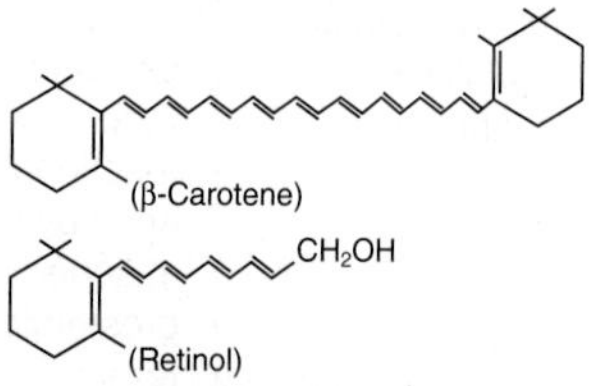 (β-Carotene) CH$_2$OH (Retinol)	Retinol, retinaldehyde, and retinoic acid	Formation of rhodopsin (vision) and glycoproteins (epithelial cell function); also regulates gene transcription
Vitamin D 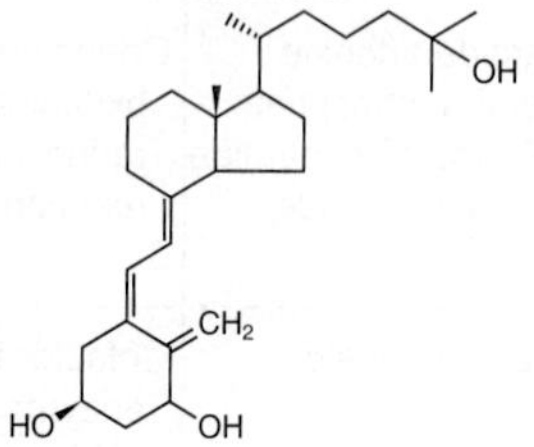 OH CH$_2$ HO OH	1,25-Dihydroxyvitamin D	Maintenance of blood calcium and phosphorus levels; antiproliferative hormone
Vitamin E 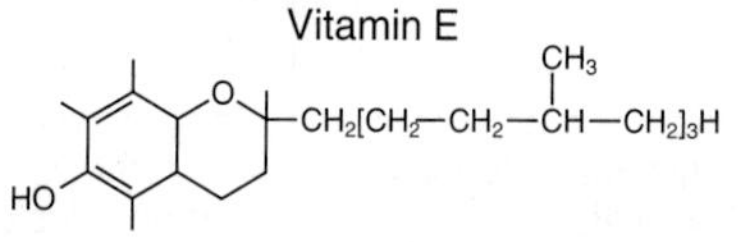 CH$_3$ O —CH$_2$[CH$_2$—CH$_2$—CH—CH$_2$]$_3$H HO	Tocopherols and tocotrienols	Antioxidants
Vitamin K 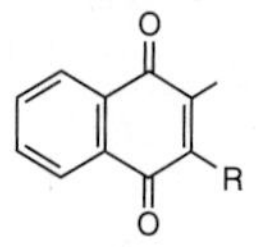 O R O	Vitamin K hydroquinone	Cofactor for posttranslation carboxylation of many proteins including essential clotting factors

FIGURE 57-1
(Continued)

deficiency causes *beriberi*, which is classically categorized as wet or dry although there is considerable overlap between the two categories. In either form of beriberi, patients may complain of pain and paresthesia. *Wet beriberi* presents primarily with cardiovascular symptoms that are due to impaired myocardial energy metabolism and dysautonomia; it can occur after 3 months of a thiamine-deficient diet. Patients present with an enlarged heart, tachycardia, high-output congestive heart failure, peripheral edema, and peripheral neuritis. Patients with *dry beriberi* present with a symmetric peripheral neuropathy of the motor and sensory systems, with diminished reflexes. The neuropathy affects the legs most markedly, and patients have difficulty rising from a squatting position.

Alcoholic patients with chronic thiamine deficiency also may have central nervous system (CNS) manifestations known as *Wernicke's encephalopathy*, which consists of horizontal nystagmus, ophthalmoplegia (due to weakness of one or more extraocular muscles), cerebellar ataxia, and mental impairment . When there is an additional loss of memory and a confabulatory psychosis, the syndrome is known as *Wernicke-Korsakoff syndrome*. Despite the typical clinical picture and history, Wernicke-Korsakoff syndrome is underdiagnosed.

The laboratory diagnosis of thiamine deficiency usually is made by a functional enzymatic assay of transketolase activity measured before and after the addition of thiamine pyrophosphate. A >25% stimulation in response to the addition of thiamine pyrophosphate (i.e., an activity coefficient of 1.25) is interpreted as abnormal. Thiamine or the phosphorylated esters of thiamine in serum or blood also can be measured by high-performance liquid chromatography to detect deficiency.

TREATMENT Thiamine Deficiency

In acute thiamine deficiency with either cardiovascular or neurologic signs, 200 mg of thiamine three times daily should be given intravenously until there is no further improvement in acute symptoms; oral thiamine (10 mg/d) should subsequently be given until recovery is complete. Cardiovascular and ophthalmoplegic improvement occurs within 24 h. Other manifestations gradually clear, although psychosis in Wernicke-Korsakoff syndrome may be permanent or may persist for several months. Other nutrient deficiencies should be corrected concomitantly.

Toxicity

Although anaphylaxis has been reported after high intravenous doses of thiamine, no adverse effects have been recorded from either food or supplements at high doses. Thiamine supplements may be bought over the counter in doses of up to 50 mg/d.

RIBOFLAVIN (VITAMIN B_2)

Riboflavin is important for the metabolism of fat, carbohydrate, and protein, acting as a respiratory coenzyme and an electron donor. Enzymes that contain flavin adenine dinucleotide (FAD) or flavin mononucleotide (FMN) as prosthetic groups are known as *flavoenzymes* (e.g., succinic acid dehydrogenase, monoamine oxidase, glutathione reductase). FAD is a cofactor for methyltetrahydrofolate reductase and therefore modulates homocysteine metabolism. The vitamin also plays a role in drug and steroid metabolism, including detoxification reactions.

Although much is known about the chemical and enzymatic reactions of riboflavin, the clinical manifestations of riboflavin deficiency are nonspecific and are similar to those of other deficiencies of B vitamins. Riboflavin deficiency is manifested principally by lesions of the mucocutaneous surfaces of the mouth and skin. In addition, corneal vascularization, anemia, and personality changes have been described with riboflavin deficiency.

Deficiency and excess

Riboflavin deficiency almost always is due to dietary deficiency. Milk, other dairy products, and enriched breads and cereals are the most important dietary sources of riboflavin in the United States, although lean meat, fish, eggs, broccoli, and legumes are also good sources. Riboflavin is extremely sensitive to light, and milk should be stored in containers that protect against photodegradation. Laboratory diagnosis of riboflavin deficiency can be made by determination of red blood cell or urinary riboflavin concentrations or by measurement of erythrocyte glutathione reductase activity, with and without added FAD. Because the capacity of the gastrointestinal tract to absorb riboflavin is limited (~20 mg after one oral dose), riboflavin toxicity has not been described.

NIACIN (VITAMIN B_3)

The term *niacin* refers to nicotinic acid and nicotinamide and their biologically active derivatives. Nicotinic acid and nicotinamide serve as precursors of two coenzymes, nicotinamide adenine dinucleotide (NAD) and NAD phosphate (NADP), which are important in numerous oxidation and reduction reactions in the body. In addition, NAD and NADP are active in adenine diphosphate–ribose transfer reactions involved in DNA repair and calcium mobilization.

Metabolism and requirements

Nicotinic acid and nicotinamide are absorbed well from the stomach and small intestine. The bioavailability of niacin from beans, milk, meat, and eggs is high; bioavailability from cereal grains is lower. Since flour is enriched with "free" niacin (i.e., the non-coenzyme form), bioavailability is excellent. Median intakes of niacin in the United States considerably exceed the recommended dietary allowance (RDA).

The amino acid tryptophan can be converted to niacin with an efficiency of 60:1 by weight. Thus, the RDA for niacin is expressed in niacin equivalents. A lower-level conversion of tryptophan to niacin occurs in vitamin B_6 and/or riboflavin deficiencies and in the presence of isoniazid. The urinary excretion products of niacin include 2-pyridone and 2-methyl nicotinamide, measurements of which are used in the diagnosis of niacin deficiency.

Deficiency

Niacin deficiency causes *pellagra*, which is found mostly among people eating corn-based diets in parts of China, Africa, and India. Pellagra in North America is found mainly among alcoholics; among patients with congenital defects of intestinal and kidney absorption of tryptophan (Hartnup disease); and among patients with carcinoid syndrome, in which there is increased conversion of tryptophan to serotonin. The antituberculosis drug isoniazid is a structural analog of niacin and can precipitate pellagra. In the setting of famine or population displacement, pellagra results from the absolute lack of niacin but also from the deficiency of micronutrients required for the conversion of tryptophan to niacin (e.g., iron, riboflavin, and pyridoxine).

The early symptoms of pellagra include loss of appetite, generalized weakness and irritability, abdominal pain, and vomiting. Bright red glossitis then ensues and is followed by a characteristic skin rash that is pigmented and scaling, particularly in skin areas exposed to sunlight. This rash is known as *Casal's necklace* because it forms a ring around the neck; it is seen in advanced cases. Vaginitis and esophagitis also may occur. Diarrhea (due in part to proctitis and in part to malabsorption), depression, seizures, and dementia are also part of the pellagra syndrome. The primary manifestations of this syndrome are sometimes referred to as "the four *D's*": *d*ermatitis, *d*iarrhea, and *d*ementia leading to *d*eath.

TREATMENT Pellagra

Treatment of pellagra consists of oral supplementation with 100–200 mg of nicotinamide or nicotinic acid three times daily for 5 days. High doses of nicotinic acid (2 g/d in a time-release form) are used for the treatment of elevated cholesterol and triglyceride levels and/or low high-density lipoprotein cholesterol levels.

Toxicity

Prostaglandin-mediated flushing due to binding of the vitamin to a G protein–coupled receptor has been observed at daily nicotinic acid doses as low as 30 mg taken as a supplement or as therapy for dyslipidemia. There is no evidence of toxicity from niacin that is derived from food sources. Flushing always starts in the face and may be accompanied by skin dryness, itching, paresthesia, and headache. Pharmaceutical preparations of nicotinic acid combined with laropiprant, a selective prostaglandin D_2 receptor 1 antagonist, or premedication with aspirin may alleviate these symptoms. Flushing is subject to tachyphylaxis and often improves with time. Nausea, vomiting, and abdominal pain also occur at similar doses of niacin. Hepatic toxicity is the most serious toxic reaction caused by sustained-release niacin and may present as jaundice with elevated aspartate aminotransferase (AST) and alanine aminotransferase (ALT) levels. A few cases of fulminant hepatitis requiring liver transplantation have been reported at doses of 3–9 g/d. Other toxic reactions include glucose intolerance, hyperuricemia, macular edema, and macular cysts. The combination of nicotinic acid preparations for dyslipidemia with 3-hydroxy-3-methylglutaryl coenzyme A (HMG-CoA) reductase inhibitors may increase the risk of rhabdomyolysis. The upper limit for daily niacin intake has been set at 35 mg. However, this upper limit does not pertain to the therapeutic use of niacin.

PYRIDOXINE (VITAMIN B_6)

Vitamin B_6 refers to a family of compounds that includes pyridoxine, pyridoxal, pyridoxamine, and their 5′-phosphate derivatives. 5′-Pyridoxal phosphate (PLP) is a cofactor for more than 100 enzymes involved in amino acid metabolism. Vitamin B_6 also is involved in heme and neurotransmitter synthesis and in the metabolism of glycogen, lipids, steroids, sphingoid bases, and several vitamins, including the conversion of tryptophan to niacin.

Dietary sources

Plants contain vitamin B_6 in the form of pyridoxine, whereas animal tissues contain PLP and pyridoxamine phosphate. The vitamin B_6 contained in plants is less bioavailable than that in animal tissues. Rich food sources of vitamin B_6 include legumes, nuts, wheat bran, and meat, although it is present in all food groups.

Deficiency

Symptoms of vitamin B_6 deficiency include epithelial changes, as seen frequently with other B vitamin deficiencies. In addition, severe vitamin B_6 deficiency can lead to peripheral neuropathy, abnormal electroencephalograms, and personality changes that include depression and confusion. In infants, diarrhea, seizures, and anemia have been reported. Microcytic hypochromic anemia is due to diminished hemoglobin synthesis, since the first enzyme involved in heme biosynthesis (aminolevulinate synthase) requires PLP as a cofactor. In some case reports, platelet dysfunction has been reported. Since vitamin B_6 is necessary for the conversion of homocysteine to cystathionine, it is possible that chronic low-grade vitamin B_6 deficiency may result in hyperhomocysteinemia and increased risk of cardiovascular disease. Independent of homocysteine, low levels of circulating vitamin B_6 have been associated with inflammation and elevated levels of C-reactive protein.

Certain medications, such as isoniazid, L-dopa, penicillamine, and cycloserine, interact with PLP due to a reaction with carbonyl groups. Pyridoxine should be given concurrently with isoniazid to avoid neuropathy. The increased ratio of AST to ALT seen in alcoholic liver disease reflects the relative vitamin B_6 dependence of ALT. Vitamin B_6 dependency syndromes that require pharmacologic doses of vitamin B_6 are rare; they include cystathionine β-synthase deficiency, pyridoxine-responsive (primarily sideroblastic) anemias, and gyrate atrophy with chorioretinal degeneration due to decreased activity of the mitochondrial enzyme ornithine aminotransferase. In these situations, 100–200 mg/d of oral vitamin B_6 is required for treatment.

High doses of vitamin B_6 have been used to treat carpal tunnel syndrome, premenstrual syndrome, schizophrenia, autism, and diabetic neuropathy but have not been found to be effective.

The laboratory diagnosis of vitamin B_6 deficiency is generally based on low plasma PLP values (<20 nmol/L). Vitamin B_6 deficiency is treated with 50 mg/d; higher doses of 100–200 mg/d are given if the deficiency is related to medication use. Vitamin B_6 should not be given with l-dopa, since the vitamin interferes with the action of this drug.

Toxicity

The safe upper limit for vitamin B_6 has been set at 100 mg/d, although no adverse effects have been associated with high intakes of vitamin B_6 from food sources only. When toxicity occurs, it causes severe sensory neuropathy, leaving patients unable to walk. Some cases of photosensitivity and dermatitis have been reported.

FOLATE (VITAMIN B_{12})

VITAMIN C

Both ascorbic acid and its oxidized product dehydroascorbic acid are biologically active. Actions of vitamin C include antioxidant activity, promotion of nonheme iron absorption, carnitine biosynthesis, conversion of dopamine to norepinephrine, and synthesis of many peptide hormones. Vitamin C is also important for connective tissue metabolism and cross-linking (proline hydroxylation), and it is a component of many drug-metabolizing enzyme systems, particularly the mixed-function oxidase systems.

Absorption and dietary sources

Vitamin C is almost completely absorbed if <100 mg is administered in a single dose; however, only 50% or less is absorbed at doses >1 g. Enhanced degradation and fecal and urinary excretion of vitamin C occur at higher intake levels.

Good dietary sources of vitamin C include citrus fruits, green vegetables (especially broccoli), tomatoes, and potatoes. Consumption of five servings of fruits and vegetables a day provides vitamin C in excess of the RDA of 90 mg/d for men and 75 mg/d for women. In addition, ~40% of the U.S. population consumes vitamin C as a dietary supplement in which "natural forms" of the vitamin are no more bioavailable than synthetic forms. Smoking, hemodialysis, pregnancy, and stress (e.g., infection, trauma) appear to increase vitamin C requirements.

Deficiency

Vitamin C deficiency causes scurvy. In the United States, this condition is seen primarily among the poor and the elderly, in alcoholics who consume <10 mg/d of vitamin C, and in individuals consuming macrobiotic diets. Vitamin C deficiency also can occur in young adults who eat severely unbalanced diets. In addition to generalized fatigue, symptoms of scurvy primarily reflect impaired formation of mature connective tissue and include bleeding into the skin (petechiae, ecchymoses, perifollicular hemorrhages); inflamed and bleeding gums; and manifestations of bleeding into joints, the peritoneal cavity, the pericardium, and the adrenal glands. In children, vitamin C deficiency may cause impaired bone growth. Laboratory diagnosis of vitamin C deficiency is based on low plasma or leukocyte levels.

Administration of vitamin C (200 mg/d) improves the symptoms of scurvy within several days. High-dose vitamin C supplementation (e.g., 1–2 g/d) may slightly decrease the symptoms and duration of upper respiratory tract infections. Vitamin C supplementation has also been reported to be useful in Chédiak-Higashi syndrome and osteogenesis imperfecta. Diets high in vitamin C have been claimed to lower the incidence of certain cancers, particularly esophageal and gastric cancers. If proved, this effect may be due to the fact that vitamin C can prevent the conversion of nitrites and secondary amines to carcinogenic nitrosamines. However, an intervention study from China did not show vitamin C to be protective. A potential role for parenteral ascorbic acid in the treatment of advanced cancers has been suggested.

Toxicity

Taking >2 g of vitamin C in a single dose may result in abdominal pain, diarrhea, and nausea. Since vitamin C may be metabolized to oxalate, it is feared that chronic high-dose vitamin C supplementation could result in an increased prevalence of kidney stones. However, except in patients with preexisting renal disease, this association has not been borne out in several trials. Nevertheless, it is reasonable to advise patients with a history of kidney stones not to take large doses of vitamin C. There is also an unproven but possible risk that chronic high doses of vitamin C could promote iron overload and iron toxicity. High doses of vitamin C can induce hemolysis in patients with glucose-6-phosphate dehydrogenase deficiency, and doses >1 g/d can cause false-negative guaiac reactions and interfere with tests for urinary glucose. High doses may interfere with the activity of certain drugs (e.g., bortezomib in myeloma patients).

BIOTIN

Biotin is a water-soluble vitamin that plays a role in gene expression, gluconeogenesis, and fatty acid synthesis and serves as a CO_2 carrier on the surface of both cytosolic and mitochondrial carboxylase enzymes. The vitamin also functions in the catabolism of specific amino acids (e.g., leucine) and in gene regulation by histone biotinylation. Excellent food sources of biotin include organ meat such as liver or kidney, soy and other beans, yeast, and egg yolks; however, egg white contains the protein avidin, which strongly binds the vitamin and reduces its bioavailability.

Biotin deficiency due to low dietary intake is rare; rather, deficiency is due to inborn errors of metabolism. Biotin deficiency has been induced by experimental feeding of egg white diets and by biotin-free parenteral nutrition in patients with short bowels. In adults, biotin deficiency results in mental changes (depression, hallucinations), paresthesia, anorexia, and nausea. A scaling, seborrheic, and erythematous rash may occur around the eyes, nose, and mouth as well as on the extremities. In infants, biotin deficiency presents as hypotonia, lethargy, and apathy. In addition, infants may develop alopecia and a characteristic rash that includes the ears. The laboratory diagnosis of biotin deficiency can be established on the basis of a decreased concentration of urinary biotin (or its major metabolites), increased urinary excretion of 3-hydroxyisovaleric acid after a leucine challenge, or decreased activity of biotin-dependent enzymes in lymphocytes (e.g., propionyl-CoA carboxylase). Treatment requires pharmacologic doses of biotin–i.e., up to 10 mg/d. No toxicity is known.

PANTOTHENIC ACID (VITAMIN B_5)

Pantothenic acid is a component of coenzyme A and phosphopantetheine, which are involved in fatty acid metabolism and the synthesis of cholesterol, steroid hormones, and all compounds formed from isoprenoid units. In addition, pantothenic acid is involved in the acetylation of proteins. The vitamin is excreted in the urine, and the laboratory diagnosis of deficiency is based on low urinary vitamin levels.

The vitamin is ubiquitous in the food supply. Liver, yeast, egg yolks, whole grains, and vegetables are particularly good sources. Human pantothenic acid deficiency has been demonstrated only by experimental feeding of diets low in pantothenic acid or by administration of a specific pantothenic acid antagonist. The symptoms of pantothenic acid deficiency are nonspecific and include gastrointestinal disturbance, depression, muscle cramps, paresthesia, ataxia, and hypoglycemia. Pantothenic acid deficiency is believed to have caused the "burning feet syndrome" seen in prisoners of war during World War II. No toxicity of this vitamin has been reported.

CHOLINE

Choline is a precursor for acetylcholine, phospholipids, and betaine. Choline is necessary for the structural integrity of cell membranes, cholinergic neurotransmission, lipid and cholesterol metabolism, methyl-group metabolism, and transmembrane signaling. Recently, a recommended adequate intake was set at 550 mg/d for men and 425 mg/d for women, although certain genetic polymorphisms can increase an individual's requirement. Choline is thought to be a "conditionally essential" nutrient in that its de novo synthesis occurs in the liver and results in lesser-than-used amounts only under certain stress conditions (e.g., alcoholic liver disease). The dietary requirement for choline depends on the status of other nutrients involved in methyl-group metabolism (folate, vitamin B_{12}, vitamin B_6, and methionine) and thus varies widely. Choline is widely distributed in food (e.g., egg yolks, wheat germ, organ meat, milk) in the form of lecithin (phosphatidylcholine). Choline deficiency has occurred in patients receiving parenteral nutrition devoid of choline. Deficiency results in fatty liver, elevated aminotransferase levels, and skeletal muscle damage with high creatine phosphokinase values. The diagnosis of choline deficiency is currently based on low plasma levels, although nonspecific conditions (e.g., heavy exercise) may also suppress plasma levels.

Toxicity from choline results in hypotension, cholinergic sweating, diarrhea, salivation, and a fishy body odor. The upper limit for choline intake has been set at 3.5 g/d. Because of its ability to lower cholesterol and homocysteine levels, choline treatment has been suggested for patients with dementia and patients at high risk of cardiovascular disease. However, the benefits of such treatment have not been firmly documented. Choline- and betaine-restricted diets are of therapeutic value in trimethylaminuria ("fish odor syndrome").

FLAVONOIDS

Flavonoids constitute a large family of polyphenols that contribute to the aroma, taste, and color of fruits and vegetables. Major groups of dietary flavonoids include anthocyanidins in berries; catechins in green tea and chocolate; flavonols (e.g., quercitin) in broccoli, kale, leeks, onions, and the skins of grapes and apples; and isoflavones (e.g., genistein) in legumes. Isoflavones have a low bioavailability and are partially metabolized by the intestinal flora. The dietary intake of flavonoids is estimated at 10–100 mg/d; this figure is almost certainly an underestimate attributable to a lack of information on their concentrations in many foods. Several flavonoids have antioxidant activity and affect cell signaling. From observational epidemiologic studies and limited clinical (human and animal) studies, flavonoids have been postulated to play a role in the prevention of several chronic diseases, including neurodegenerative disease, diabetes, and osteoporosis. The ultimate importance and usefulness of these compounds against human disease have not been demonstrated.

VITAMIN A

Vitamin A, in the strictest sense, refers to retinol. However, the oxidized metabolites retinaldehyde and retinoic acid are also biologically active compounds. The term *retinoids* includes all molecules (including synthetic molecules) that are chemically related to retinol. Retinaldehyde (11-*cis*) is the essential form of vitamin A that is required for normal vision, whereas retinoic acid is necessary for normal morphogenesis, growth, and cell differentiation. Retinoic acid does not function in vision and, in contrast to retinol, is not involved in reproduction. Vitamin A also plays a role in iron utilization, humoral immunity, T cell–mediated immunity, natural killer cell activity, and phagocytosis. Vitamin A is commercially available in esterified forms (e.g., acetate, palmitate), which are more stable than other forms.

There are more than 600 carotenoids in nature, ~50 of which can be metabolized to vitamin A. β-Carotene is the most prevalent carotenoid with provitamin A activity in the food supply. In humans, significant fractions of carotenoids are absorbed intact and are stored in liver and fat. It is estimated that ≥12 μg (range, 4–27 μg) of dietary all-*trans* β-carotene is equivalent to 1 μg of retinol activity, whereas the figure is ≥24 μg for other dietary provitamin A carotenoids (e.g., cryptoxanthin, α-carotene). The vitamin A equivalency for a β-carotene supplement in an oily solution is 2:1.

Metabolism

The liver contains ~90% of the vitamin A reserves and secretes vitamin A in the form of retinol, which is bound to retinol-binding protein. Once binding has occurred, the retinol-binding protein complex interacts with a second protein, transthyretin. This trimolecular complex functions to prevent vitamin A from being filtered by the kidney glomerulus, thus protecting the body against the toxicity of retinol and allowing retinol to be taken up by specific cell-surface receptors that recognize retinol-binding protein. A certain amount of vitamin A enters peripheral cells even if it is not bound to retinol-binding protein. After retinol is internalized by the cell, it becomes bound to a series of cellular retinol-binding proteins, which function as sequestering and transporting agents as well as co-ligands for enzymatic reactions. Certain cells also contain retinoic acid–binding proteins, which have sequestering functions but also shuttle retinoic acid to the nucleus and enable its metabolism.

Retinoic acid is a ligand for certain nuclear receptors that act as transcription factors. Two families of receptors (retinoic acid receptors [RARs] and retinoid X receptors [RXRs]) are active in retinoid-mediated gene transcription. Retinoid receptors regulate transcription by binding as dimeric complexes to specific DNA sites—the retinoic acid response elements—in target genes. The receptors can either stimulate or repress gene expression in response to their ligands. RARs bind all-*trans* retinoic acid and 9-*cis*-retinoic acid, whereas RXRs bind only 9-*cis*-retinoic acid.

The retinoid receptors play an important role in controlling cell proliferation and differentiation. Retinoic acid is useful in the treatment of promyelocytic leukemia and also is used in the treatment of cystic acne because it inhibits keratinization, decreases sebum secretion, and possibly alters the inflammatory reaction. RXRs dimerize with other nuclear receptors to function as coregulators of genes responsive to retinoids, thyroid hormone, and calcitriol. RXR agonists induce insulin sensitivity experimentally, perhaps because RXRs are cofactors for the peroxisome proliferator-activated receptors, which are targets for thiazolidinedione drugs such as rosiglitazone and troglitazone.

Dietary sources

The retinol activity equivalent (RAE) is used to express the vitamin A value of food: 1 RAE is defined as 1 μg of retinol (0.003491 mmol), 12 μg of β-carotene, and 24 μg of other provitamin A carotenoids. In older literature, vitamin A often was expressed in international units (IU), with 1 μg of retinol equal to 3.33 IU of retinol and 20 IU of β-carotene, but these units are no longer in scientific use.

Liver, fish, and eggs are excellent food sources for preformed vitamin A; vegetable sources of provitamin A carotenoids include dark green and deeply colored fruits and vegetables. Moderate cooking of vegetables enhances carotenoid release for uptake in the gut. Carotenoid absorption is also aided by some fat in a meal. Infants are particularly susceptible to vitamin A deficiency because neither breast nor cow's milk supplies enough vitamin A to prevent deficiency. In developing countries, chronic dietary deficiency is the main cause of vitamin A deficiency and is exacerbated by infection. In early childhood, low vitamin A status results from inadequate intakes of animal food sources and edible oils, both of which are expensive, coupled with seasonal unavailability of vegetables and fruits and lack of marketed fortified food products. Concurrent zinc deficiency can interfere with the mobilization of vitamin A from liver stores. Alcohol interferes with the conversion of retinol to retinaldehyde in the eye by competing for alcohol (retinol) dehydrogenase. Drugs that interfere with the absorption of vitamin A include mineral oil, neomycin, and cholestyramine.

Deficiency

Vitamin A deficiency is endemic in areas where diets are chronically poor, especially in southern Asia, sub-Saharan Africa, some parts of Latin America, and the western Pacific, including parts of China. Vitamin A status is usually assessed by measuring serum retinol (normal range, 1.05–3.50 μmol/L [30–100 μg/dL]) or blood-spot retinol or by tests of dark adaptation. Stable isotopic or invasive liver biopsy methods are available to estimate total body stores of vitamin A. As judged by deficient serum retinol (<0.70 μmol/L [20 μg/dL]), vitamin A deficiency worldwide is present in >90 million preschool-age children, among whom >4 million have an ocular manifestation of deficiency termed *xerophthalmia*. This condition includes milder stages of night blindness and conjunctival *xerosis* (dryness) with *Bitot's spots* (white patches of keratinized epithelium appearing on the sclera) as well as rare, potentially blinding corneal ulceration and necrosis. *Keratomalacia* (softening of the cornea) leads to corneal scarring that blinds at least a quarter of a million children each year and is associated with fatality rates of 4–25%. However, vitamin A deficiency at any stage poses an increased risk of death from diarrhea, dysentery, measles, malaria, or respiratory disease. Vitamin A deficiency can compromise barrier, innate, and acquired immune defenses to infection. In areas where deficiency is widely prevalent, vitamin A supplementation can markedly reduce the risk of childhood mortality (by 23–34%, on average). About 10% of pregnant women in undernourished settings also develop night blindness (assessed by history) during the latter half of pregnancy, and this moderate vitamin A deficiency is associated with an increased risk of maternal infection and death.

TREATMENT Vitamin A Deficiency

Any stage of xerophthalmia should be treated with 60 mg (or RAE) of vitamin A in oily solution, usually contained in a soft-gel capsule. The same dose is repeated 1 and 14 days later. Doses should be reduced by half for patients 6–11 months of age. Mothers with night blindness or Bitot's spots should be given vitamin A orally–either 3 mg daily or 7.5 mg twice a week for 3 months. These regimens are efficacious, and they are less expensive and more widely available than injectable water-miscible vitamin A. A common approach to prevention is to provide vitamin A supplementation every 4–6 months to young children and infants (both HIV-positive and HIV-negative) in high-risk areas. Infants 6–11 months of age should receive 30 mg vitamin A; children 12–59 months of age, 60 mg. For reasons that are not clear, vitamin A supplementation has not proven useful in high-risk settings for preventing morbidity or death among infants 1–5 months of age.

Uncomplicated vitamin A deficiency is rare in industrialized countries. One high-risk group—extremely low-birth-weight (<1000-g) infants—is likely to be vitamin A–deficient and should receive a supplement of 1500 μg (or RAE) three times a week for 4 weeks. Severe measles in any society can lead to secondary vitamin A deficiency. Children hospitalized with measles should receive two 60-mg doses of vitamin A on two consecutive days. Vitamin A deficiency most often occurs in patients with malabsorptive diseases (e.g., celiac sprue, short-bowel syndrome) who have abnormal dark adaptation or symptoms of night blindness without other ocular changes. Typically, such patients are treated for 1 month with 15 mg/d of a water-miscible preparation of vitamin A. This treatment is followed by a lower maintenance dose, with the exact amount determined by monitoring serum retinol.

No specific signs or symptoms result from carotenoid deficiency. It was postulated that β-carotene would be an effective chemopreventive agent for cancer because numerous epidemiologic studies had shown that diets high in β-carotene were associated with lower incidences of cancers of the respiratory and digestive systems. However, intervention studies in smokers found that treatment with high doses of β-carotene actually resulted in more lung cancers than did treatment with placebo. Non–provitamin A carotenoids such as lutein and zeaxanthin have been suggested to confer protection against macular degeneration, and one large-scale intervention study did not show a beneficial effect except in those with a low lutein status. The use of the non–provitamin A carotenoid lycopene to protect against prostate cancer has been proposed. Again, however, the effectiveness of these agents has not been proved by intervention studies, and the mechanisms underlying these purported biologic actions are unknown.

Selective plant-breeding techniques that lead to a higher provitamin A content in staple foods may decrease vitamin A malnutrition in low-income countries. Moreover, a recently developed genetically modified food (Golden Rice) has an improved β-carotene–to-vitamin A conversion ratio of ~3:1.

Toxicity

The acute toxicity of vitamin A was first noted in Arctic explorers who ate polar bear liver and has also been seen after administration of 150 mg to adults or 100 mg to children. Acute toxicity is manifested by increased intracranial pressure, vertigo, diplopia, bulging fontanels (in children), seizures, and exfoliative dermatitis; it may result in death. Among children being treated for vitamin A deficiency according to the protocols outlined above, transient bulging of fontanels occurs in 2% of infants, and transient nausea, vomiting, and headache occur in 5% of preschoolers. Chronic vitamin A intoxication is largely a concern in industrialized countries and has been seen in otherwise healthy adults who ingest 15 mg/d and children who ingest 6 mg/d over a period of several months. Manifestations include dry skin, cheilosis, glossitis, vomiting, alopecia, bone demineralization and pain, hypercalcemia, lymph node enlargement, hyperlipidemia, amenorrhea, and features of pseudotumor cerebri with increased intracranial pressure and papilledema. Liver fibrosis with portal hypertension and bone demineralization may result from chronic vitamin A intoxication. Provision of vitamin A in excess to pregnant women has resulted in spontaneous abortion and in congenital malformations, including craniofacial abnormalities and valvular heart disease. In pregnancy, the daily dose of vitamin A should not exceed 3 mg. Commercially available retinoid derivatives are also toxic, including 13-*cis*-retinoic acid, which has been associated with birth defects. Thus contraception should be continued for at least 1 year and possibly longer in women who have taken 13-*cis*-retinoic acid.

In malnourished children, vitamin A supplements (30–60 mg), in amounts calculated as a function of age and given in several rounds over 2 years, are considered to amplify nonspecific effects of vaccines. However, for unclear reasons, there may be a negative effect on mortality rates in incompletely vaccinated girls.

High doses of carotenoids do not result in toxic symptoms but should be avoided in smokers due to an increased risk of lung cancer. Very high doses of β-carotene (~200 mg/d) have been used to treat or prevent the skin rashes of erythropoietic protoporphyria. Carotenemia, which is characterized by a yellowing of the skin (in creases of the palms and soles) but not the sclerae, may follow ingestion of >30 mg of β-carotene daily. Hypothyroid patients are particularly susceptible to the development of carotenemia due to impaired breakdown of carotene to vitamin A. Reduction of carotenes in the diet results in the disappearance of skin yellowing and carotenemia over a period of 30–60 days.

VITAMIN D

The metabolism of the fat-soluble vitamin D is described in detail in. The biologic effects of this vitamin are mediated by vitamin D receptors, which are found in most tissues; binding with these receptors potentially expands vitamin D actions on nearly all cell systems and organs (e.g., immune cells, brain, breast, colon, and prostate) as well as exerting classic endocrine effects on calcium metabolism and bone health. Vitamin D is thought to be important for maintaining normal function of many nonskeletal tissues such as muscle (including heart muscle), for immune function, and for inflammation as well as for cell proliferation and differentiation. Studies have shown that vitamin D may be useful as adjunctive treatment for tuberculosis, psoriasis, and multiple sclerosis or for the prevention of certain cancers. Vitamin D insufficiency may increase the risk of type 1 diabetes mellitus, cardiovascular disease (insulin resistance, hypertension, or low-grade inflammation), or brain dysfunction (e.g., depression). However, the exact physiologic roles of vitamin D in these nonskeletal diseases and the importance of these roles have not been clarified.

The skin is a major source of vitamin D, which is synthesized upon skin exposure to ultraviolet B radiation (UV-B; wavelength, 290–320 nm). Except for fish, food (unless fortified) contains only limited amounts of vitamin D. Vitamin D_2 (ergocalciferol) is obtained from plant sources and is the chemical form found in some supplements.

Deficiency

Vitamin D status has been assessed by measuring serum levels of 25-dihydroxyvitamin D ($25[OH]_2$ vitamin D); however, there is no consensus on a uniform assay or on optimal serum levels. The optimal level might, in fact, differ according to the targeted disease entity. Epidemiologic and experimental data indicate that a $25(OH)_2$ vitamin D level of >20 ng/mL (≥50 nmol/L; to convert ng/mL to nmol/L, multiply by 2.496) is sufficient for good bone health. Some experts advocate higher serum levels (e.g., >30 ng/mL) for other desirable endpoints of vitamin D action. There is insufficient evidence to recommend combined vitamin D and calcium supplementation as a primary preventive strategy for reduction of the incidence of fractures in healthy men and premenopausal women.

Risk factors for vitamin D deficiency are old age, lack of sun exposure, dark skin (especially among residents of northern latitudes), fat malabsorption, and obesity. *Rickets* represents the classic disease of vitamin D deficiency. Signs of deficiency are muscle soreness, weakness, and bone pain. Some of these effects are independent of calcium intake.

The U.S. National Academy of Sciences recently concluded that the majority of North Americans are receiving adequate amounts of vitamin D (RDA = 15 μg/d or 600 IU/d; **Chap. 56**). However, for people older than 70 years, the RDA is set at 20 μg/d (800 IU/d). The consumption of fortified or enriched foods as well as suberythemal sun exposure should be encouraged for people at risk for vitamin D deficiency. If adequate intake is impossible, vitamin D supplements should be taken, especially during the winter months. Vitamin D deficiency can be treated by the oral administration of 50,000 IU/week for 6–8 weeks followed by a maintenance dose of 800 IU/d (100 μg/d) from food and supplements once normal plasma levels have been attained.

The physiologic effects of vitamin D_2 and vitamin D_3 are identical when these vitamins are ingested over long periods.

Toxicity

The upper limit of intake has been set at 4000 IU/d. Contrary to earlier beliefs, acute vitamin D intoxication is rare and usually is caused by the uncontrolled and excessive ingestion of supplements or by faulty food fortification practices. High plasma levels of $1,25(OH)_2$ vitamin D and calcium are central features of toxicity and mandate discontinuation of vitamin D and calcium supplements; in addition, treatment of hypercalcemia may be required.

VITAMIN E

Vitamin E is the collective designation for all stereoisomers of tocopherols and tocotrienols, although only the RR tocopherols meet human requirements. Vitamin E acts as a chain-breaking antioxidant and is an efficient pyroxyl radical scavenger that protects low-density lipoproteins and polyunsaturated fats in membranes from oxidation. A network of other antioxidants (e.g., vitamin C, glutathione) and enzymes maintains vitamin E in a reduced state. Vitamin E also inhibits prostaglandin synthesis and the activities of protein kinase C and phospholipase A_2.

Absorption and metabolism

After absorption, vitamin E is taken up from chylomicrons by the liver, and a hepatic α-tocopherol transport protein mediates intracellular vitamin E transport and incorporation into very low density lipoprotein. The transport protein has a particular affinity for the RRR isomeric form of α-tocopherol; thus, this natural isomer has the most biologic activity.

Requirement

Vitamin E is widely distributed in the food supply, with particularly high levels in sunflower oil, safflower oil, and wheat germ oil; γ-tocotrienols are notably present in soybean and corn oils. Vitamin E is also found in meats, nuts, and cereal grains, and small amounts are present in fruits and vegetables. Vitamin E pills containing doses of 50–1000 mg are ingested by ~10% of the U.S. population. The RDA for vitamin E is 15 mg/d (34.9 μmol or 22.5 IU) for all adults. Diets high in polyunsaturated fats may necessitate a slightly higher intake of vitamin E.

Dietary deficiency of vitamin E does not exist. Vitamin E deficiency is seen only in severe and prolonged malabsorptive diseases, such as celiac disease, or after small-intestinal resection or bariatric surgery. Children with cystic fibrosis or prolonged cholestasis may develop vitamin E deficiency characterized by areflexia and hemolytic anemia. Children with abetalipoproteinemia cannot absorb or transport vitamin E and become deficient quite rapidly. A familial form of isolated vitamin E deficiency also exists; it is due to a defect in the α-tocopherol transport protein. Vitamin E deficiency causes axonal degeneration of the large myelinated axons and results in posterior column and spinocerebellar symptoms. Peripheral neuropathy is initially characterized by areflexia, with progression to an ataxic gait, and by decreased vibration and position sensations. Ophthalmoplegia, skeletal myopathy, and pigmented retinopathy may also be features of vitamin E deficiency. A deficiency of either vitamin E or selenium in the host has been shown to increase certain viral mutations and, therefore, virulence. The laboratory diagnosis of vitamin E deficiency is based on low blood levels of α-tocopherol (<5 μg/mL, or <0.8 mg of α-tocopherol per gram of total lipids).

TREATMENT Vitamin E Deficiency

Symptomatic vitamin E deficiency should be treated with 800–1200 mg of α-tocopherol per day. Patients with abetalipoproteinemia may need as much as 5000–7000 mg/d. Children with symptomatic vitamin E deficiency should be treated orally with water-miscible esters (400 mg/d); alternatively, 2 mg/kg per day may be administered intramuscularly. Vitamin E in high doses may protect against oxygen-induced retrolental fibroplasia and bronchopulmonary dysplasia as well as intraventricular hemorrhage of prematurity. Vitamin E has been suggested to increase sexual performance, treat intermittent claudication, and slow the aging process, but evidence for these properties is lacking. When given in combination with other antioxidants, vitamin E may help prevent macular degeneration. High doses (60–800 mg/d) of vitamin E have been shown in controlled trials to improve parameters of immune function and reduce colds in nursing home residents, but intervention studies using vitamin E to prevent cardiovascular disease or cancer have not shown efficacy, and, at doses >400 mg/d, vitamin E may even increase all-cause mortality rates.

Toxicity

All forms of vitamin E are absorbed and could contribute to toxicity; however, the toxicity risk seems to be rather low as long as liver function is normal. High doses of vitamin E (>800 mg/d) may reduce platelet aggregation and interfere with vitamin K metabolism and are therefore contraindicated in patients taking warfarin and antiplatelet agents (such as aspirin or clopidogrel). Nausea, flatulence, and diarrhea have been reported at doses >1 g/d.

VITAMIN K

There are two natural forms of vitamin K: vitamin K_1, also known as *phylloquinone*, from vegetable and animal sources, and vitamin K_2, or *menaquinone*, which is synthesized by bacterial flora and found in hepatic tissue. Phylloquinone can be converted to menaquinone in some organs.

Vitamin K is required for the posttranslational carboxylation of glutamic acid, which is necessary for calcium binding to γ-carboxylated proteins such as prothrombin (factor II); factors VII, IX, and X; protein C; protein S; and proteins found in bone (osteocalcin) and vascular smooth muscle (e.g., matrix Gla protein). However, the importance of vitamin K for bone mineralization and prevention of vascular calcification is not known. Warfarin-type drugs inhibit γ-carboxylation by preventing the conversion of vitamin K to its active hydroquinone form.

Dietary sources

Vitamin K is found in green leafy vegetables such as kale and spinach, and appreciable amounts are also present in margarine and liver. Vitamin K is present in vegetable oils; olive, canola, and soybean oils are particularly rich sources. The average daily intake by Americans is estimated to be ~100 μg/d.

Deficiency

The symptoms of vitamin K deficiency are due to hemorrhage; newborns are particularly susceptible because of low fat stores, low breast milk levels of vitamin K, relative sterility of the infantile intestinal tract, liver immaturity, and poor placental transport. Intracranial bleeding as well as gastrointestinal and skin bleeding can occur in vitamin K–deficient infants 1–7 days after birth. Thus, vitamin K (0.5–1 mg IM) is given prophylactically at delivery.

Vitamin K deficiency in adults may be seen in patients with chronic small-intestinal disease (e.g., celiac disease, Crohn's disease), in those with obstructed biliary tracts, or after small-bowel resection. Broad-spectrum antibiotic treatment can precipitate vitamin K deficiency by reducing numbers of gut bacteria, which synthesize menaquinones, and by inhibiting the metabolism of vitamin K. In patients with warfarin therapy, the anti-obesity drug orlistat can lead to international normalized ratio changes due to vitamin K malabsorption. Vitamin K deficiency usually is diagnosed on the basis of an elevated prothrombin time or reduced clotting factors, although vitamin K may also be measured directly by high-pressure liquid chromatography. Vitamin K deficiency is treated with a parenteral dose of 10 mg. For patients with chronic malabsorption, 1–2 mg/d should be given orally or 1–2 mg per week can be taken parenterally. Patients with liver disease may have an elevated prothrombin time because of liver cell destruction as well as vitamin K deficiency. If an elevated prothrombin time does not improve during vitamin K therapy, it can be deduced that this abnormality is not the result of vitamin K deficiency.

Toxicity

Toxicity from dietary phylloquinones and menaquinones has not been described. High doses of vitamin K can impair the actions of oral anticoagulants.

MINERALS

See also Table 57-2.

CALCIUM

ZINC

Zinc is an integral component of many metalloenzymes in the body; it is involved in the synthesis and stabilization of proteins, DNA, and RNA and plays a structural role in ribosomes and membranes. Zinc is necessary for the binding of steroid hormone receptors and several other transcription factors to DNA. Zinc is absolutely required for normal spermatogenesis, fetal growth, and embryonic development.

Absorption

The absorption of zinc from the diet is inhibited by dietary phytate, fiber, oxalate, iron, and copper as well as by certain drugs, including penicillamine, sodium valproate, and ethambutol. Meat, shellfish, nuts, and legumes are good sources of bioavailable zinc, whereas zinc in grains and legumes is less available for absorption.

Deficiency

Mild zinc deficiency has been described in many diseases, including diabetes mellitus, HIV/AIDS, cirrhosis, alcoholism, inflammatory bowel disease, malabsorption syndromes, and sickle cell disease. In these diseases, mild chronic zinc deficiency can cause stunted growth in children, decreased taste sensation

TABLE 57-2

DEFICIENCIES AND TOXICITIES OF METALS

ELEMENT	DEFICIENCY	TOXICITY	TOLERABLE UPPER (DIETARY) INTAKE LEVEL
Boron	No biologic function determined	Developmental defects, male sterility, testicular atrophy	20 mg/d (extrapolated from animal data)
Calcium	Reduced bone mass, osteoporosis	Renal insufficiency (milk-alkali syndrome), nephrolithiasis, impaired iron absorption, thiazide diuretics	2500 mg/d (milk-alkali)
Copper	Anemia, growth retardation, defective keratinization and pigmentation of hair, hypothermia, degenerative changes in aortic elastin, osteopenia, mental deterioration	Nausea, vomiting, diarrhea, hepatic failure, tremor, mental deterioration, hemolytic anemia, renal dysfunction	10 mg/d (liver toxicity)
Chromium	Impaired glucose tolerance	*Occupational:* Renal failure, dermatitis, pulmonary cancer	Not determined
Fluoride	↑ Dental caries	Dental and skeletal fluorosis, osteosclerosis	10 mg/d (fluorosis)
Iodine	Thyroid enlargement, ↓ T_4, cretinism	Thyroid dysfunction, acne-like eruptions	1100 μg/d (thyroid dysfunction)
Iron	Muscle abnormalities, koilonychia, pica, anemia, ↓ work performance, impaired cognitive development, premature labor, ↑ perinatal maternal death	Gastrointestinal effects (nausea, vomiting, diarrhea, constipation), iron overload with organ damage, acute and chronic systemic toxicity, increased susceptibility to malaria, increased risk association with certain chronic diseases (e.g., diabetes)	45 mg/d of elemental iron (gastrointestinal side effects)
Manganese	Impaired growth and skeletal development, reproduction, lipid and carbohydrate metabolism; upper body rash	*General:* Neurotoxicity, Parkinson-like symptoms *Occupational:* Encephalitis-like syndrome, Parkinson-like syndrome, psychosis, pneumoconiosis	11 mg/d (neurotoxicity)
Molybdenum	Severe neurologic abnormalities	Reproductive and fetal abnormalities	2 mg/d (extrapolated from animal data)
Selenium	Cardiomyopathy, heart failure, striated muscle degeneration	*General:* Alopecia, nausea, vomiting, abnormal nails, emotional lability, peripheral neuropathy, lassitude, garlic odor to breath, dermatitis *Occupational:* Lung and nasal carcinomas, liver necrosis, pulmonary inflammation	400 μg/d (hair, nail changes)
Phosphorus	Rickets (osteomalacia), proximal muscle weakness, rhabdomyolysis, paresthesia, ataxia, seizure, confusion, heart failure, hemolysis, acidosis	Hyperphosphatemia	4000 mg/d
Zinc	Growth retardation, ↓ taste and smell, alopecia, dermatitis, diarrhea, immune dysfunction, failure to thrive, gonadal atrophy, congenital malformations	*General:* Reduced copper absorption, gastritis, sweating, fever, nausea, vomiting *Occupational:* Respiratory distress, pulmonary fibrosis	40 mg/d (impaired copper metabolism)

(*hypogeusia*), and impaired immune function. Severe chronic zinc deficiency has been described as a cause of hypogonadism and dwarfism in several Middle Eastern countries. In these children, hypopigmented hair is also part of the syndrome. Acrodermatitis enteropathica is a rare autosomal recessive disorder characterized by abnormalities in zinc absorption. Clinical manifestations include diarrhea, alopecia, muscle wasting, depression, irritability, and a rash involving the extremities, face, and perineum. The rash is characterized by vesicular and pustular crusting with scaling and erythema. Occasional patients with Wilson's disease have developed zinc deficiency as a consequence of penicillamine therapy.

Zinc deficiency is prevalent in many developing countries and usually coexists with other micronutrient deficiencies (especially iron deficiency). Zinc (20 mg/d until recovery) may be an effective adjunctive therapeutic strategy for diarrheal disease and pneumonia in children ≥ 6 months of age.

The diagnosis of zinc deficiency is usually based on a serum zinc level <12 μmol/L (<70 μg/dL). Pregnancy and birth control pills may cause a slight depression in serum zinc levels, and hypoalbuminemia from any cause can result in hypozincemia. In acute stress situations, zinc may be redistributed from serum into tissues. Zinc deficiency may be treated with 60 mg of elemental zinc taken by mouth twice a day. Zinc gluconate lozenges (13 mg of elemental zinc every 2 h while awake) have been reported to reduce the duration and symptoms of the common cold in adults, but study results are conflicting.

Toxicity

Acute zinc toxicity after oral ingestion causes nausea, vomiting, and fever. Zinc fumes from welding may also be toxic and cause fever, respiratory distress, excessive salivation, sweating, and headache. Chronic large doses of zinc may depress immune function and cause hypochromic anemia as a result of copper deficiency. Intranasal zinc preparations should be avoided because they may lead to irreversible damage of the nasal mucosa and anosmia.

COPPER

Copper is an integral part of numerous enzyme systems, including amine oxidases, ferroxidase (ceruloplasmin), cytochrome c oxidase, superoxide dismutase, and dopamine hydroxylase. Copper is also a component of ferroprotein, a transport protein involved in the basolateral transfer of iron during absorption from the enterocyte. As such, copper plays a role in iron metabolism, melanin synthesis, energy production, neurotransmitter synthesis, and CNS function; the synthesis and cross-linking of elastin and collagen; and the scavenging of superoxide radicals. Dietary sources of copper include shellfish, liver, nuts, legumes, bran, and organ meats.

Deficiency

Dietary copper deficiency is relatively rare, although it has been described in premature infants who are fed milk diets and in infants with malabsorption (Table 57-2). Copper-deficiency anemia (refractory to therapeutic iron) has been reported in patients with malabsorptive diseases and nephrotic syndrome and in patients treated for Wilson's disease with chronic high doses of oral zinc, which can interfere with copper absorption. *Menkes kinky hair syndrome* is an X-linked metabolic disturbance of copper metabolism characterized by mental retardation, hypocupremia, and decreased circulating ceruloplasmin. This syndrome is caused by mutations in the copper-transporting *ATP7A* gene. Children with this disease often die within 5 years because of dissecting aneurysms or cardiac rupture. Aceruloplasminemia is a rare autosomal recessive disease characterized by tissue iron overload, mental deterioration, microcytic anemia, and low serum iron and copper concentrations.

The diagnosis of copper deficiency is usually based on low serum levels of copper (<65 μg/dL) and low ceruloplasmin levels (<20 mg/dL). Serum levels of copper may be elevated in pregnancy or stress conditions since ceruloplasmin is an acute-phase reactant and 90% of circulating copper is bound to ceruloplasmin.

Toxicity

Copper toxicity is usually accidental (Table 57-2). In severe cases, kidney failure, liver failure, and coma may ensue. In Wilson's disease, mutations in the copper-transporting *ATP7B* gene lead to accumulation of copper in the liver and brain, with low blood levels due to decreased ceruloplasmin.

SELENIUM

Selenium, in the form of selenocysteine, is a component of the enzyme glutathione peroxidase, which serves to protect proteins, cell membranes, lipids, and nucleic acids from oxidant molecules. As such, selenium is being actively studied as a chemopreventive agent against certain cancers, such as prostate cancer. Selenocysteine is also found in the deiodinase enzymes, which mediate the deiodination of thyroxine to triiodothyronine. Rich dietary sources of selenium include seafood, muscle meat, and cereals, although the selenium content of cereal is determined by the soil concentration. Countries with low soil concentrations include parts of Scandinavia, China, and New Zealand. *Keshan disease* is an endemic cardiomyopathy found in children and young women residing in regions of China where dietary intake of selenium is low (<20 μg/d). Concomitant deficiencies of iodine and selenium may worsen the clinical manifestations of cretinism. Chronic ingestion of large amounts of selenium leads to selenosis, characterized by hair and nail brittleness and loss, garlic breath odor, skin rash, myopathy, irritability, and other abnormalities of the nervous system.

CHROMIUM

Chromium potentiates the action of insulin in patients with impaired glucose tolerance, presumably by increasing insulin receptor–mediated signaling, although its usefulness in treating type 2 diabetes is uncertain. In addition, improvement in blood lipid profiles has been reported in some patients. The usefulness of chromium supplements in muscle building has not been substantiated. Rich food sources of chromium include yeast, meat, and grain products. Chromium in the trivalent state is found in supplements and is largely nontoxic; however, chromium-6 is a product of stainless steel welding and is a known pulmonary carcinogen as well as a cause of liver, kidney, and CNS damage.

MAGNESIUM

FLUORIDE, MANGANESE, AND ULTRATRACE ELEMENTS

An essential function for fluoride in humans has not been described, although it is useful for the maintenance of structure in teeth and bones. Adult fluorosis results in mottled and pitted defects in tooth enamel as well as brittle bone (skeletal fluorosis).

Manganese and molybdenum deficiencies have been reported in patients with rare genetic abnormalities and in a few patients receiving prolonged total parenteral nutrition. Several manganese-specific enzymes have been identified (e.g., manganese superoxide dismutase). Deficiencies of manganese have been reported to result in bone demineralization, poor growth, ataxia, disturbances in carbohydrate and lipid metabolism, and convulsions.

Ultratrace elements are defined as those needed in amounts <1 mg/d. Essentiality has not been established for most ultratrace elements, although selenium, chromium, and iodine are clearly essential. Molybdenum is necessary for the activity of sulfite and xanthine oxidase, and molybdenum deficiency may result in skeletal and brain lesions.

CHAPTER 58

MALNUTRITION AND NUTRITIONAL ASSESSMENT

Douglas C. Heimburger

Malnutrition can arise from primary or secondary causes, resulting in the former case from inadequate or poor-quality food intake and in the latter case from diseases that alter food intake or nutrient requirements, metabolism, or absorption. *Primary* malnutrition occurs mainly in developing countries and under conditions of political unrest, war, or famine. *Secondary* malnutrition, the main form encountered in industrialized countries, was largely unrecognized until the early 1970s, when it was appreciated that persons with adequate food supplies can become malnourished as a result of acute or chronic diseases that alter nutrient intake or metabolism, particularly diseases that cause acute or chronic inflammation. Various studies have shown that protein-energy malnutrition (PEM) affects one-third to one-half of patients on general medical and surgical wards in teaching hospitals. The consistent finding that nutritional status influences patient prognosis underscores the importance of preventing, detecting, and treating malnutrition.

Definitions for forms of PEM are in flux. Traditionally, the two major types of PEM have been *marasmus* and *kwashiorkor*. These conditions are compared in Table 58-1. Marasmus is the end result of a long-term deficit of dietary energy, whereas kwashiorkor has been understood to result from a protein-poor diet. Although the former concept remains essentially correct, evidence is accumulating that PEM syndromes are distinguished by two main features: insufficient dietary intake and underlying inflammatory processes. Energy-poor diets with minimal inflammation cause gradual erosion of body mass, resulting in classic marasmus. By contrast, inflammation from acute illnesses such as injury or sepsis or from chronic illnesses such as cancer, lung or heart disease, or HIV infection can erode lean body mass even in the presence of relatively sufficient dietary intake, leading to a kwashiorkor-like state. Quite often, inflammatory illnesses impair appetite and dietary intake, producing combinations of the two conditions.

Consensus committees have proposed the following revised definitions. *Starvation–related malnutrition* is suggested for instances of chronic starvation without inflammation, *chronic disease–related malnutrition* when inflammation is chronic and of mild to moderate degree, and *acute disease– or injury–related malnutrition* when inflammation is acute and of a severe degree. However, because distinguishing diagnostic criteria for these conditions have not been universally adopted, this chapter integrates the older and newer terms.

MARASMUS (STARVATION–RELATED MALNUTRITION) AND CACHEXIA (CHRONIC DISEASE–RELATED MALNUTRITION)

Marasmus (starvation–related malnutrition) is a state in which virtually all available body fat stores have been exhausted due to starvation without systemic inflammation. *Cachexia* (chronic disease–related malnutrition) is a state that involves substantial loss of lean body mass in the presence of chronic systemic inflammation. Conditions that produce cachexia tend to be chronic and indolent, such as cancer and chronic pulmonary disease, whereas, in high-income countries, the classic setting for marasmus is in patients with anorexia nervosa. These conditions are relatively easy to detect because of the patient's starved appearance. The diagnosis is based on fat and muscle wastage resulting from prolonged calorie deficiency and/or inflammation. Diminished skinfold thickness reflects the loss of fat reserves; reduced arm muscle circumference with temporal and interosseous muscle wasting reflects the catabolism of protein throughout the body, including in vital organs such as the heart, liver, and kidneys.

Routine laboratory findings in cachexia/marasmus are relatively unremarkable. The creatinine-height index (24-h urinary creatinine excretion compared with normal values based on height) is low, reflecting the loss of muscle mass. Occasionally, the serum albumin level is

TABLE 58-1

COMPARISON OF MARASMUS/CACHEXIA AND KWASHIORKOR/ACUTE MALNUTRITION

FEATURE	MARASMUS (STARVATION–RELATED MALNUTRITION) AND CACHEXIA (CHRONIC DISEASE–RELATED MALNUTRITION)	KWASHIORKOR (ACUTE DISEASE– OR INJURY–RELATED MALNUTRITION)[a]
Clinical setting	Prolonged ↓ energy and protein intake with or without systemic inflammation	Acute ↓ energy and protein intake with substantial systemic inflammation
Time course to develop	Months or years	Weeks
Clinical features	Starved appearance (body mass index <18.5) Reduced triceps skinfold Reduced midarm muscle circumference	Normal body mass index (although loss of body mass may be masked by edema) Easy hair pluckability[b] Edema
Laboratory findings	Serum albumin normal (marasmus, no inflammation) or decreased (cachexia, with inflammation)	Serum albumin <2.8 g/dL Total iron-binding capacity <200 μg/dL Lymphocytes <1500/μL Anergy
Clinical course	Reasonably preserved responsiveness to short-term stress	Infections Poor wound healing, decubitus ulcers, skin breakdown
Mortality risk	Low unless related to underlying disease	High
Diagnostic criteria	Triceps skinfold <3 mm Midarm muscle circumference <15 cm	Serum albumin <2.8 g/dL At least one of the following: Poor wound healing, decubitus ulcers, or skin breakdown Easy hair pluckability[b] Edema

[a]The findings used to diagnose kwashiorkor/acute malnutrition must be unexplained by other causes.
[b]Tested by *firmly* pulling a lock of hair from the top (not the sides or back), grasping with the thumb and forefinger. An average of three or more hairs removed easily and painlessly is considered abnormal hair pluckability.

reduced, but it remains above 2.8 g/dL when systemic inflammation is absent. Despite a morbid appearance, immunocompetence, wound healing, and the ability to handle short-term stress are reasonably well preserved in most patients.

Pure starvation–related malnutrition is a chronic, fairly well adapted form of starvation rather than an acute illness; it should be treated cautiously in an attempt to reverse the downward trend gradually. Although nutritional support is necessary, overly aggressive repletion can result in severe, even life-threatening metabolic imbalances such as hypophosphatemia and cardiorespiratory failure (*refeeding syndrome*). When possible, oral or enteral nutritional support is preferred; treatment started slowly allows readaptation of metabolic and intestinal functions **(Chap. 59)**.

KWASHIORKOR (ACUTE DISEASE– OR INJURY–RELATED MALNUTRITION)

By contrast, *kwashiorkor* (acute disease– or injury–related malnutrition) in developed countries occurs mainly in connection with acute, life-threatening conditions such as trauma and sepsis. The physiologic stress produced by these illnesses increases protein and energy requirements at a time when intake is often limited. A classic scenario is an acutely stressed patient who receives only 5% dextrose solutions for periods as brief as 2 weeks. Although the etiologic mechanisms are not fully known, the protein-sparing response normally seen in starvation is blocked by the stressed state and by carbohydrate infusion.

In its early stages, the physical findings of kwashiorkor/acute malnutrition are few and subtle. Initially unaffected fat reserves and muscle mass give the deceptive appearance of adequate nutrition. Signs that support the diagnosis include easy hair pluckability, edema, skin breakdown, and poor wound healing. The major sine qua non is severe reduction of levels of serum proteins such as albumin (<2.8 g/dL) and transferrin (<150 mg/dL) or of iron-binding capacity (<200 μg/dL). Cellular immune function is depressed, as reflected by lymphopenia (<1500 lymphocytes/μL in adults and older children) and lack of response to skin test antigens (*anergy*).

The prognosis of adult patients with full-blown kwashiorkor/acute malnutrition is not good even with aggressive nutritional support. Surgical wounds often dehisce (fail to heal), pressure sores develop, gastroparesis and diarrhea can occur with enteral feeding, the risk of gastrointestinal bleeding from stress ulcers is increased, host defenses are compromised, and death from overwhelming infection may occur despite antibiotic therapy. Unlike treatment of marasmus, therapy for kwashiorkor entails aggressive nutritional support to restore better metabolic balance rapidly **(Chap. 59)**.

PHYSIOLOGIC CHARACTERISTICS OF HYPOMETABOLIC AND HYPERMETABOLIC STATES

The metabolic characteristics and nutritional needs of hypermetabolic patients who are stressed from injury, infection, or chronic inflammatory illness differ from those of hypometabolic patients who are unstressed but chronically starved. In both cases, nutritional support is important, but misjudgments in selecting the appropriate approach may have serious adverse consequences.

The *hypometabolic* patient is typified by the relatively less stressed but mildly catabolic and chronically starved individual who, with time, will develop cachexia/marasmus. The *hypermetabolic* patient stressed from injury or infection is catabolic (experiencing rapid breakdown of body mass) and is at high risk for developing acute malnutrition/kwashiorkor if nutritional needs are not met and/or the illness does not resolve quickly. As summarized in Table 58-2, the two states are distinguished by differing perturbations of metabolic rate, rates of protein breakdown (*proteolysis*), and rates of gluconeogenesis. These differences are mediated by proinflammatory cytokines and counterregulatory hormones—tumor necrosis factor, interleukins 1 and 6, C-reactive protein, catecholamines (epinephrine and norepinephrine), glucagon, and cortisol—whose levels are relatively reduced in hypometabolic patients and increased in hypermetabolic patients. Although insulin levels are also elevated in stressed patients, insulin resistance in the target tissues blocks insulin-mediated anabolic effects. Physiologic characteristics of patients at risk for chronic disease–related malnutrition are less predictable and likely represent a mixture of the two extremes depicted in Table 58-2.

TABLE 58-2

PHYSIOLOGIC CHARACTERISTICS OF HYPOMETABOLIC AND HYPERMETABOLIC STATES

PHYSIOLOGIC CHARACTERISTICS	HYPOMETABOLIC, NONSTRESSED PATIENT (RISK FOR STARVATION/ MARASMUS)	HYPERMETABOLIC, STRESSED PATIENT (RISK FOR KWASHIORKOR/ ACUTE MALNUTRITION)
Cytokines, catecholamines, glucagon, cortisol, insulin	↓	↑
Metabolic rate, O_2 consumption	↓	↑
Proteolysis, gluconeogenesis	↓	↑
Ureagenesis, urea excretion	↓	↑
Fat catabolism, fatty acid utilization	Relative ↑	Absolute ↑
Adaptation to starvation	Normal	Abnormal

Metabolic rate

In starvation and semistarvation, the resting metabolic rate falls between 10% and 30% as an adaptive response to energy restriction, slowing the rate of weight loss. By contrast, the resting metabolic rate rises in the presence of physiologic stress in proportion to the degree of the insult. The rate may increase by ~10% after elective surgery, 20–30% after bone fractures, 30–60% with severe infections such as peritonitis or gram-negative septicemia, and as much as 110% after major burns.

If the metabolic rate (energy requirement) is not matched by energy intake, weight loss results—slowly in hypometabolism and quickly in hypermetabolism. Losses of up to 10% of body mass are unlikely to be detrimental; however, greater losses in acutely ill hypermetabolic patients may be associated with rapid deterioration in body functions.

Protein catabolism

The rate of endogenous protein breakdown (*catabolism*) to supply energy needs normally falls during uncomplicated energy deprivation. After ~10 days of total starvation, an unstressed individual loses about 12–18 g of protein per day (equivalent to ~60 g of muscle tissue or ~2–3 g of nitrogen). In contrast, in injury and sepsis, protein breakdown accelerates in proportion to the degree of stress, reaching 30–60 g/d after elective surgery, 60–90 g/d with infection, 100–130 g/d with severe sepsis or skeletal trauma, and >175 g/d with major burns or head injuries. These losses are reflected by proportional increases in the excretion of urea nitrogen, the major by-product of protein breakdown.

Gluconeogenesis

The major aim of protein catabolism during a state of starvation is to provide the glucogenic amino acids (especially alanine and glutamine) that serve as substrates for endogenous glucose production (*gluconeogenesis*) in the liver. In the hypometabolic/starved state, protein breakdown for gluconeogenesis is minimized, especially as ketones derived from fatty acids become the substrate preferred by certain tissues. In the hypermetabolic/stress state, gluconeogenesis increases dramatically and in proportion to the degree of the insult to increase the supply of glucose (the major fuel of reparation). Glucose is the only fuel that can be utilized by hypoxemic tissues (*anaerobic glycolysis*), white blood cells, and newly generated fibroblasts. Infusions of glucose partially offset a negative energy balance but do not significantly suppress the high rates of gluconeogenesis in catabolic patients. Hence, adequate supplies of protein are needed to replace the amino acids used for this metabolic response.

In summary, a hypometabolic patient is adapted to starvation and conserves body mass through reduction of the metabolic rate and use of fat as the primary fuel (rather than glucose and its precursor amino acids). A hypermetabolic patient also uses fat as a fuel but rapidly breaks down body protein to produce glucose, with consequent loss of muscle and organ tissue and danger to vital body functions.

MICRONUTRIENT MALNUTRITION

The same illnesses and reductions in nutrient intake that lead to PEM often produce deficiencies of vitamins and minerals as well **(Chap. 57)**. Deficiencies of nutrients that are stored in small amounts (such as the water-soluble vitamins) occur because of loss through external secretions, such as zinc in diarrhea fluid or burn exudate, and are probably more common than is generally recognized.

Deficiencies of vitamin C, folic acid, and zinc are relatively common in sick patients. Signs of scurvy, such as corkscrew hairs on the lower extremities, are found frequently in chronically ill and/or alcoholic patients. The diagnosis can be confirmed by determination of plasma vitamin C levels. Folic acid intakes and blood levels are often less than optimal, even among healthy persons; with illness, alcoholism, poverty, or poor dentition, these deficiencies are common. Low blood zinc levels are prevalent in patients with malabsorption syndromes such as inflammatory bowel disease. Patients with zinc deficiency often exhibit poor wound healing, pressure ulcer formation, and impaired immunity. Thiamine deficiency is a common complication of alcoholism but may be prevented by therapeutic doses of thiamine in patients treated for alcohol abuse.

Patients with low plasma vitamin C levels usually respond to the doses in multivitamin preparations, but patients with deficiencies should be supplemented with 250–500 mg/d. Folic acid is absent from some oral multivitamin preparations; patients with deficiencies should be supplemented with ~1 mg/d. Patients with zinc deficiencies resulting from large external losses sometimes require oral supplementation with 220 mg of zinc sulfate one to three times daily. For these reasons, laboratory assessments of the micronutrient status of patients at high risk are desirable.

Hypophosphatemia develops in hospitalized patients with remarkable frequency and generally results from rapid intracellular shifts of phosphate in underweight or alcoholic patients receiving intravenous glucose **(Chap. 63)**. The adverse clinical sequelae are numerous; some, such as acute cardiopulmonary failure, are collectively called *refeeding syndrome* and can be life-threatening.

GLOBAL CONSIDERATIONS

Many developing countries are still faced with high prevalences of the classic forms of PEM: marasmus and kwashiorkor. *Food insecurity*, which characterizes many poor countries, prevents consistent dietary sufficiency and/or quality and leads to endemic or cyclic malnutrition. Factors threatening food security include marked seasonal variations in agricultural productivity (rainy season–dry season cycles), periodic droughts, political unrest or injustice, and disease epidemics (especially of HIV/AIDS). The coexistence of malnutrition and disease epidemics exacerbates the latter and increases complications and mortality rates, creating vicious cycles of malnutrition and disease.

As economic prosperity improves, developing countries have been observed to undergo an epidemiologic transition, a component of which has been termed the *nutrition transition*. As improved economic resources make greater dietary diversity possible, middle-income populations (e.g., in southern Asia, China, and Latin America) typically begin to adopt lifestyle habits of industrialized nations, with increased consumption of energy and fat and decreased levels of physical activity. These changes lead to rising levels of obesity, metabolic syndrome, diabetes, cardiovascular disease, and cancer, sometimes coexisting in populations with persistent undernutrition.

Micronutrient deficiencies also remain prevalent in many countries of the world, impairing functional status and productivity and increasing mortality rates. Vitamin A deficiency impairs vision and increases morbidity and mortality rates from infections such as measles. Mild to moderate iron deficiency may be prevalent in up to 50% of the world, resulting from poor dietary diversity coupled with periodic blood loss and pregnancies. Iodine deficiency remains prevalent, causing goiter, hypothyroidism, and cretinism. Zinc deficiency is endemic in many populations, producing growth retardation, hypogonadism, and dermatoses and impairing wound healing. Fortunately, public health supplementation programs have substantially improved vitamin A and zinc status in developing countries during the past two decades, reducing mortality rates from measles, diarrheal diseases, and other manifestations. However, with the advancing nutrition transition and a shift toward nutritionally related chronic noncommunicable conditions, it is estimated that nutrition remains one of the three greatest contributors of risk for morbidity and mortality worldwide.

NUTRITIONAL ASSESSMENT

Because interactions between illness and nutrition are complex, many physical and laboratory findings reflect both underlying disease and nutritional status. Therefore, the nutritional evaluation of a patient requires an integration of history, physical examination, anthropometrics, and laboratory studies. This approach helps both to detect nutritional problems and to prevent the conclusion that isolated findings indicate nutritional problems when they do not. For example, hypoalbuminemia caused by an inflammatory illness does not necessarily indicate malnutrition.

Nutritional history

Elicitation of a nutritional history is directed toward the identification of underlying mechanisms that put patients at risk for nutritional depletion or excess. These mechanisms include inadequate intake, impaired absorption, decreased utilization, increased losses, and increased requirements for nutrients.

Individuals with the characteristics listed in Table 58-3 are at particular risk for nutritional deficiencies.

TABLE 58-3

NUTRITIONAL DEFICIENCY: THE HIGH-RISK PATIENT
Underweight (body mass index <18.5) and/or recent loss of ≥10% of usual body mass
Poor intake: anorexia, food avoidance (e.g., psychiatric condition), or NPO[a] status for more than ~5 days
Protracted nutrient losses: malabsorption, enteric fistulas, draining abscesses or wounds, renal dialysis
Hypermetabolic states: sepsis, protracted fever, extensive trauma or burns
Alcohol abuse or use of drugs with antinutrient or catabolic properties: glucocorticoids, antimetabolites (e.g., methotrexate), immunosuppressants, antitumor agents
Impoverishment, isolation, advanced age

[a]Nil per os (nothing by mouth).

Physical examination

Physical findings that suggest vitamin, mineral, and protein-energy deficiencies and excesses are outlined in Table 58-4. Most of the physical findings are not specific for individual nutrient deficiencies and must be integrated with historic, anthropometric, and laboratory findings. For example, follicular hyperkeratosis on the back of the arms is a fairly common, normal finding. However, if it is widespread in a person who consumes few fruits and vegetables and smokes regularly (increasing ascorbic acid requirements), vitamin C deficiency is likely. Similarly, easily pluckable hair may be a consequence of chemotherapy but suggests acute malnutrition/kwashiorkor in a hospitalized patient who has poorly healing surgical wounds and hypoalbuminemia.

Anthropometric measurements

Anthropometric measurements provide information on body muscle mass and fat reserves. The most practical and commonly used measurements are body weight, height, triceps skinfold (TSF), and midarm muscle circumference (MAMC). Body weight is one of the most useful nutritional parameters to follow in patients who are acutely or chronically ill. Unintentional weight loss during illness often reflects loss of lean body mass (muscle and organ tissue), especially if it is rapid and is not caused by diuresis. Such weight loss can be an ominous sign since it indicates use of vital body protein stores for metabolic fuel. The reference standard for normal body weight, body mass index (BMI: weight in kilograms divided by height, in meters, squared), is discussed in **Chap. 61**. BMI values <18.5 are considered underweight; <17, significantly underweight; and <16, severely wasted. Values of 18.5–24.9 are normal; 25–29.9, overweight; and ≥30, obese.

Measurement of skinfold thickness is useful for estimating body fat stores, because ~50% of body fat is normally located in the subcutaneous region. This measurement can also permit discrimination of fat mass from muscle mass. The triceps is a convenient site that is generally representative of the body's overall fat level. A thickness <3 mm suggests virtually complete exhaustion of fat stores. The MAMC can be used to estimate skeletal muscle mass, calculated as follows:

$$\text{MAMC (cm)} = \text{upper arm circumference (cm)} - [0.314 \times \text{TSF (mm)}]$$

Laboratory studies

A number of laboratory tests used routinely in clinical medicine can yield valuable information about a patient's nutritional status if a slightly different

TABLE 58-4

PHYSICAL FINDINGS OF NUTRITIONAL DEFICIENCIES

CLINICAL FINDINGS	POSSIBLE DEFICIENCY OR FORM OF MALNUTRITION	POSSIBLE EXCESS
Hair, nails		
Corkscrew hairs and unemerged coiled hairs	Vitamin C	
Easily pluckable hair	Acute malnutrition	
Flag sign (transverse depigmentation of hair)	Acute malnutrition	
Sparse hair	Biotin, zinc; acute malnutrition	Vitamin A
Transverse ridging of nails	Acute malnutrition	
Skin		
Cellophane appearance	Acute malnutrition	
Cracking ("flaky-paint" or "crazy-pavement" dermatosis)	Acute malnutrition	
Follicular hyperkeratosis	Vitamins A, C	
Petechiae (especially perifollicular)	Vitamin C	
Purpura	Vitamins C, K	
Pigmentation, scaling of sun-exposed areas	Niacin	
Poor wound healing, decubitus ulcers	Vitamin C, zinc; acute malnutrition	
Scaling	Vitamin A, essential fatty acids, biotin	Vitamin A
Yellow pigmentation sparing sclerae (benign)	Zinc (hyperpigmented)	Carotene
Eyes		
Night blindness	Vitamin A	
Papilledema		Vitamin A
Perioral		
Angular stomatitis	Riboflavin, pyridoxine, niacin	
Cheilosis (dry, cracking, ulcerated lips)	Riboflavin, pyridoxine, niacin	
Oral		
Atrophic lingual papillae (slick tongue)	Riboflavin, niacin, folate, vitamin B_{12}, iron; acute malnutrition	
Glossitis (scarlet, raw tongue)	Riboflavin, niacin, pyridoxine, folate, vitamin B_{12}	
Hypogeusesthesia, hyposmia	Zinc	
Swollen, retracted, bleeding gums (if teeth present)	Vitamin C	
Bones, joints		
Beading of ribs, epiphyseal swelling, bowlegs	Vitamin D	
Tenderness, subperiosteal hemorrhage in children	Vitamin C	
Neurologic		
Confabulation, disorientation	Thiamine (Korsakoff's psychosis)	
Drowsiness, lethargy, vomiting		Vitamin A
Dementia	Niacin, vitamin B_{12}, folate	
Headache		Vitamin A
Ophthalmoplegia	Thiamine, phosphorus	
Peripheral neuropathy (e.g., weakness, paresthesias, ataxia, footdrop, and decreased tendon reflexes, fine tactile sense, vibratory sense, and position sense)	Thiamine, pyridoxine, vitamin B_{12}	Pyridoxine
Tetany	Calcium, magnesium	
Other		
Edema	Thiamine; acute malnutrition	
Heart failure	Thiamine ("wet" beriberi), phosphorus	
Hepatomegaly	Acute malnutrition	Vitamin A
Parotid enlargement	Acute malnutrition (consider also bulimia)	
Sudden heart failure, death	Vitamin C	

approach to their interpretation is used. For example, abnormally low serum albumin levels, low total iron-binding capacity, and anergy may have a distinct explanation, but collectively they may represent kwashiorkor. In the clinical setting of a hypermetabolic, acutely ill patient who is edematous and has easily pluckable hair and inadequate protein intake, the diagnosis of acute malnutrition/kwashiorkor is clear-cut. Commonly used laboratory tests for assessing nutritional status are outlined in Table 58-5. The table also provides tips to avoid the assignment of nutritional significance to tests that may be abnormal for nonnutritional reasons.

Assessment of circulating (visceral) proteins

The serum proteins most commonly used to assess nutritional status include albumin, total iron-binding capacity (or transferrin), thyroxine-binding prealbumin (or transthyretin), and retinol-binding protein. Because they have different synthesis rates and half-lives (the half-life of serum albumin is ~21 days, whereas those of prealbumin and retinol-binding protein are ~2 days and ~12 h, respectively), some of these proteins reflect changes in nutritional status more quickly than do others. However, rapid fluctuations can also make shorter-half-life proteins less reliable.

Levels of circulating proteins are influenced by their rates of synthesis and catabolism, "third spacing" (loss into interstitial spaces), and, in some cases, external loss. Although an adequate intake of calories and protein is necessary for optimal circulating protein levels, serum protein levels generally do not reflect protein intake. For example, a drop in the serum level of albumin or transferrin often accompanies significant physiologic stress (e.g., from infection or injury) and is not necessarily an indication of malnutrition or poor intake. A low serum albumin level in a burned patient with both hypermetabolism and increased dermal losses of protein may not indicate malnutrition. However, adequate nutritional support of the patient's calorie and protein needs is critical for returning circulating proteins to normal levels as stress resolves. Thus low values by themselves do not define malnutrition, but they often point to increased risk of malnutrition because of the hypermetabolic stress state. As long as significant physiologic stress persists, serum protein levels remain low, even with aggressive nutritional support. However, if the levels do not rise after the underlying illness improves, the patient's protein and calorie needs should be reassessed to ensure that intake is sufficient.

Assessment of vitamin and mineral status

The use of laboratory tests to confirm suspected micronutrient deficiencies is desirable because the physical findings for those deficiencies are often equivocal or nonspecific. Low blood micronutrient levels can predate more serious clinical manifestations and also may indicate drug-nutrient interactions.

ESTIMATING PROTEIN AND ENERGY REQUIREMENTS

A patient's basal energy expenditure (BEE, measured in kilocalories per day) can be estimated from height, weight, age, and sex with the Harris-Benedict equations:

$$\text{Men: BEE} = 66.47 + 13.75W + 5.00H - 6.76A$$
$$\text{Women: BEE} = 655.10 + 9.56W + 1.85H - 4.68A$$

In these equations, *W* is weight in kilograms, *H* is height in centimeters, and *A* is age in years. After these equations are solved, total energy requirements are estimated by multiplying BEE by a factor that accounts for the stress of illness. Multiplying by 1.1–1.4 yields a range 10–40% above basal that estimates the 24-h energy expenditure of the majority of patients. The lower value (1.1) is used for patients without evidence of significant physiologic stress; the higher value (1.4) is appropriate for patients with marked stress such as sepsis or trauma. The result is used as a 24-h energy goal for feeding.

When it is important to have a more accurate assessment, energy expenditure can be measured at the bedside by indirect calorimetry. This technique is useful in patients who are thought to be hypermetabolic from sepsis or trauma and whose body weight cannot be ascertained accurately. Indirect calorimetry can also be useful in patients who have difficulty weaning from a ventilator and whose energy needs therefore should not be exceeded to avoid excessive CO_2 production. Patients at the extremes of weight (e.g., obese persons) and/or age are good candidates as well, because the Harris-Benedict equations were developed from measurements in adults with roughly normal body weights.

Because urea is a major by-product of protein catabolism, the amount of urea nitrogen excreted each day can be used to estimate the rate of protein catabolism and determine whether protein intake is adequate to offset it. Total protein loss and protein balance can be calculated from urinary urea nitrogen (UUN) as follows:

$$\text{Protein catabolic rate (g/d)} = [\text{24-h UUN (g)} + 4] \times 6.25\ (\text{g protein/g nitrogen})$$

The value of 4 g added to the UUN represents a liberal estimate of the unmeasured nitrogen lost in the urine (e.g., creatinine and uric acid), sweat, hair, skin, and feces. When protein intake is low (e.g., less

TABLE 58-5

LABORATORY TESTS FOR NUTRITIONAL ASSESSMENT

TEST (NORMAL VALUES)	NUTRITIONAL USE	CAUSES OF NORMAL VALUE DESPITE MALNUTRITION	OTHER CAUSES OF ABNORMAL VALUE
Serum albumin (3.5–5.5 g/dL)	2.8–3.5 g/dL: Protein depletion or systemic inflammation Increasing value reflects positive protein balance	Dehydration	**Low**
<2.8 g/dL: Possible acute malnutrition or severe inflammation	Infusion of albumin, fresh-frozen plasma, or whole blood	*Common:* Infection and other stress, especially with poor protein intake Burns, trauma Congestive heart failure Fluid overload Severe liver disease *Uncommon:* Nephrotic syndrome Zinc deficiency Bacterial stasis/overgrowth of small intestine	
Serum prealbumin, also called transthyretin (20–40 mg/dL; lower in prepubertal children)	10–15 mg/dL: Mild protein depletion or inflammation 5–10 mg/dL: Moderate protein depletion or inflammation <5 mg/dL: Severe protein depletion or inflammation Increasing value reflects positive protein balance	Chronic renal failure	Similar to serum albumin
Serum total iron-binding capacity (240–450 μg/dL)	<200 μg/dL: Protein depletion or inflammatory state; possible acute malnutrition Increasing value reflects positive protein balance More labile than albumin	Iron deficiency	**Low** Similar to serum albumin **High** Iron deficiency
Prothrombin time (2.0–15.5 s)	Prolongation: vitamin K deficiency		**Prolonged** Anticoagulant therapy (warfarin) Severe liver disease
Serum creatinine (0.6–1.6 mg/dL)	<0.6 mg/dL: Muscle wasting due to prolonged energy deficit Reflects muscle mass		**High** Despite muscle wasting: Renal failure Severe dehydration
24-h urinary creatinine (500–1200 mg/d, standardized for height and sex)	Low value: muscle wasting due to prolonged energy deficit	>24-h collection Decreasing serum creatinine	**Low** Incomplete urine collection Increasing serum creatinine Neuromuscular wasting
24-h urinary urea nitrogen (UUN; <5 g/d; depends on level of protein intake)	*Determine level of catabolism* (as long as protein intake is ≥10 g below calculated protein loss or <20 g total, and as long as carbohydrate intake has been at least 100 g) 5–10 g/d: Mild catabolism or normal fed state 10–15 g/d: Moderate catabolism >15 g/d: Severe catabolism *Estimate protein balance* Protein balance = protein intake – protein loss where protein loss (protein catabolic rate) = [24-h UUN (g) + 4] × 6.25. Adjustments required in burn patients and others with large nonurinary nitrogen losses and in patients with fluctuating levels of blood urea nitrogen (e.g., in renal failure)		

(*continued*)

TABLE 58-5

LABORATORY TESTS FOR NUTRITIONAL ASSESSMENT (*CONTINUED*)

TEST (NORMAL VALUES)	NUTRITIONAL USE	CAUSES OF NORMAL VALUE DESPITE MALNUTRITION	OTHER CAUSES OF ABNORMAL VALUE
Blood urea nitrogen (8–23 mg/dL)	<8 mg/dL: Possibly inadequate protein intake 12–23 mg/dL: Possibly adequate protein intake >23 mg/dL: Possibly excessive protein intake If serum creatinine is normal, use BUN.		**Low** Severe liver disease Anabolic state Syndrome of inappropriate antidiuretic hormone
	If serum creatinine is elevated, use BUN/creatinine ratio. (Normal range is essentially the same as for BUN.)		**High** Despite poor protein intake: Renal failure (Use BUN/creatinine ratio.) Congestive heart failure Gastrointestinal hemorrhage

than ~20 g/d), the equation indicates both the patient's protein requirement and the severity of the catabolic state (Table 58-5). More substantial protein intakes can raise the UUN because some of the ingested (or intravenously infused) protein is catabolized and converted to UUN. Thus, at lower protein intakes, the equation is useful for estimating *requirements*, and at higher protein intakes it is useful for assessing protein *balance*.

$$\text{Protein balance (g/d)} = \text{protein intake} - \text{protein catabolic rate}$$

CHAPTER 59

ENTERAL AND PARENTERAL NUTRITION THERAPY

Bruce R. Bistrian ■ L. John Hoffer ■ David F. Driscoll

When correctly implemented, specialized nutritional support (SNS) plays a major and often life-saving role in medicine. SNS is used for two main purposes: (1) to provide an appropriate nutritional substrate in order to maintain or replenish the nutritional status of patients unable to voluntarily ingest or absorb sufficient amounts of food, and (2) to maintain the nutritional and metabolic status of adequately nourished patients who are experiencing systemic hypercatabolic effects of severe inflammation, injury, or infection in the course of persistent critical illness. Patients with permanent major loss of intestinal length or function often require lifelong SNS. Many patients who require treatment in chronic-care facilities receive enteral SNS, most often because their voluntary food intake is deemed insufficient or because impaired chewing and swallowing create a high risk of aspiration pneumonia.

Enteral SNS is the provision of liquid formula meals through a tube placed into the gut. *Parenteral* SNS is the direct infusion of complete mixtures of crystalline amino acids, dextrose, triglyceride emulsions, and micronutrients into the bloodstream through a central venous catheter or (rarely in adults) via a peripheral vein. The enteral route is almost always preferred because of its relative simplicity and safety, its low cost, and the benefits of maintaining digestive, absorptive, and immunologic barrier functions of the gastrointestinal tract. Pliable, small-bore feeding tubes make placement relatively easy and acceptable to patients. Constant-rate infusion pumps increase the reliability of nutrient delivery. The chief disadvantage of enteral SNS is that many days may be required to meet the patient's nutrient requirements.

For short-term use, the feeding tube can be placed via the nose into the stomach, duodenum, or jejunum. For long-term use, these sites may be accessed through the abdominal wall by endoscopic or surgical procedures. The chief disadvantage of tube feeding in acute illness is intolerance due to gastric retention, risk of vomiting, or diarrhea. The presence of severe coagulopathy is a relative contraindication to the insertion of a feeding tube. In adults, parenteral nutrition (PN) almost always requires aseptic insertion of a central venous catheter with a dedicated port. Many circumstances can delay or slow the progression of enteral SNS, whereas parenteral SNS can provide a complete substrate mix easily and promptly. This practical advantage is mitigated by the need to infuse relatively large fluid volumes and the real risk of inadvertent toxic overfeeding.

APPROACH TO THE PATIENT: Requirements for Specialized Nutritional Support

INDICATIONS FOR SPECIALIZED NUTRITIONAL SUPPORT Approximately one-fifth to one-quarter of patients in acute-care hospitals suffer from at least moderate protein-energy malnutrition (PEM), the defining features of which are malnutrition-induced weight loss and skeletal muscle atrophy. Usually, but not always, other features further compromise clinical responses; these features include a subnormal adipose tissue mass, with the accompanying adverse consequences of weakness, skin thinning, and breakdown; reduced ventilatory drive; ineffective cough; immunodeficiency; and impaired thermoregulation. Commonly, PEM is already present at the time of hospital admission and remains unimproved or worsens during the ensuing hospital stay. Common reasons for PEM worsening during hospitalization are refusal of food (because of anorexia, nausea, pain, or delirium), communication barriers, an unmet need for hand-feeding of patients with physical or sensory impairment, disordered or ineffective chewing or swallowing, and prolonged periods of physician-ordered fasting—all potentially taking place in a context of caregiver unawareness and inattention. Most patients who are suffering from in-hospital PEM do not, or ought not, to require SNS. A large proportion of these patients can be expected to improve with appropriate management of their primary disease. Others have a terminal disease whose downward course will not be altered by SNS. In yet other cases, the PEM is sufficiently mild that the benefits of SNS are exceeded by its risks. For patients who fall into this last category, the correct approach is to intensify and/or modify the patient's oral nutrition as directed by the unit dietitian.

PEM is often classified as minimal, moderate, or severe on the basis of weight for height (body mass index, BMI) and percentage of body weight recently lost. As shown in Table 59-1, the BMI (when corrected for abnormal extracellular fluid accumulation) is a crude but useful indicator of PEM severity. Note, however, that obesity does not preclude moderate or severe PEM, especially in older or bedridden patients; indeed, obesity can mask the presence of PEM if the patient's muscle mass is not specifically examined.

The decision to implement SNS must be based on the determinations (1) that intensified or modified oral nutrition has failed or is impossible, impractical, or undesirable; and (2) that SNS will increase the patient's rate and likelihood of recovery, reduce the risk of infection, improve healing, or otherwise shorten the hospital stay. In chronic-care situations, the decision to institute SNS is based on the likelihood that the intervention will extend the duration or quality of the patient's life. An algorithm for determining when to use SNS is depicted in Fig. 59-1.

The decision to enhance oral nutrition or—that attempt failing—to resort to SNS is based on the anticipated consequences of non-intervention. The mnemonic "in-in-in" (for inanition-inflammation-inactivity) can serve as a reminder of the three main factors that come into play when deciding whether or not it is acceptable to withhold SNS from a patient with PEM.

Inanition Key issues include whether normal food intake is likely to be impossible for a prolonged period and whether the patient can tolerate prolonged starvation. A previously well-nourished person can tolerate ~7 days of starvation without harm, even in the presence of a moderate systemic response to inflammation (SRI), whereas the degree of tolerance to prolonged starvation is much less in patients whose skeletal muscle mass is already reduced, whether from PEM, from the muscle atrophy of old age (sarcopenia), or from muscle atrophy due to neuromuscular disease. Excess body fat does not exclude the possibility of coexisting muscle atrophy from any of these causes. In general, unintentional weight loss of >10% during the previous 6 months or a weight-to-height ratio that is <90% of standard, when associated with physiologic impairment, crudely predicts that the patient has moderate PEM. Weight loss >20% of usual or <80% of standard makes severe PEM more likely.

Inflammation The anorexia that invariably accompanies the SRI reduces the likelihood that a patient's nutritional goals will be achieved by intensifying or modifying the diet, by providing counseling, or by hand-feeding. Furthermore, the protein-catabolic effects of the SRI accelerate skeletal muscle wasting and substantially block normal protein-sparing adaptation to protein and energy starvation.

Inactivity A nutritional red flag should be raised over every acutely ill patient who remains bedridden or inactive for a prolonged period. Such patients commonly manifest muscle atrophy (due to nutritional deficiencies and disuse) and anorexia with inadequate voluntary food intake.

Once it has been determined that a patient has significant—and, in particular, *progressive*—PEM despite meaningful efforts to reverse it by modifying the diet or the way food is provided, the next step is to decide whether SNS will have a net positive effect on the patient's clinical outcome. The pathway to the end stage of most severe chronic diseases leads through PEM. In most patients with end-stage untreatable cancer or certain end-organ diseases, SNS will neither reverse PEM nor improve the quality of life. Provision of food and water is commonly regarded as an aspect of basic humane care; in contrast, enteral and parenteral SNS is a therapeutic intervention that can cause discomfort and pose risks. As with other life-support interventions, the discontinuation of enteral or parenteral SNS can be psychologically difficult for patients, their families, and their caregivers. Indeed, the difficulty can be greater with SNS than with other life-support interventions because the provision of food and water is often considered equivalent to comfort care. In such difficult, near

TABLE 59-1

BODY MASS INDEX (BMI), MUSCLE MASS, AND PROTEIN ENERGY MALNUTRITION (PEM)

BMI (KG/M²)	SKELETAL MUSCLE MASS	NUTRITIONAL STATUS
>30	Normal	Obese
25–29.9	Normal	Overweight
20–24.9	Normal	Normal
>18.5	Decreased	PEM despite adequate or excessive adipose tissue store
>18.5	Decreased	Moderate PEM
<16	Decreased	Severe PEM
<13	Decreased	Lethal in men
<11	Decreased	Lethal in women

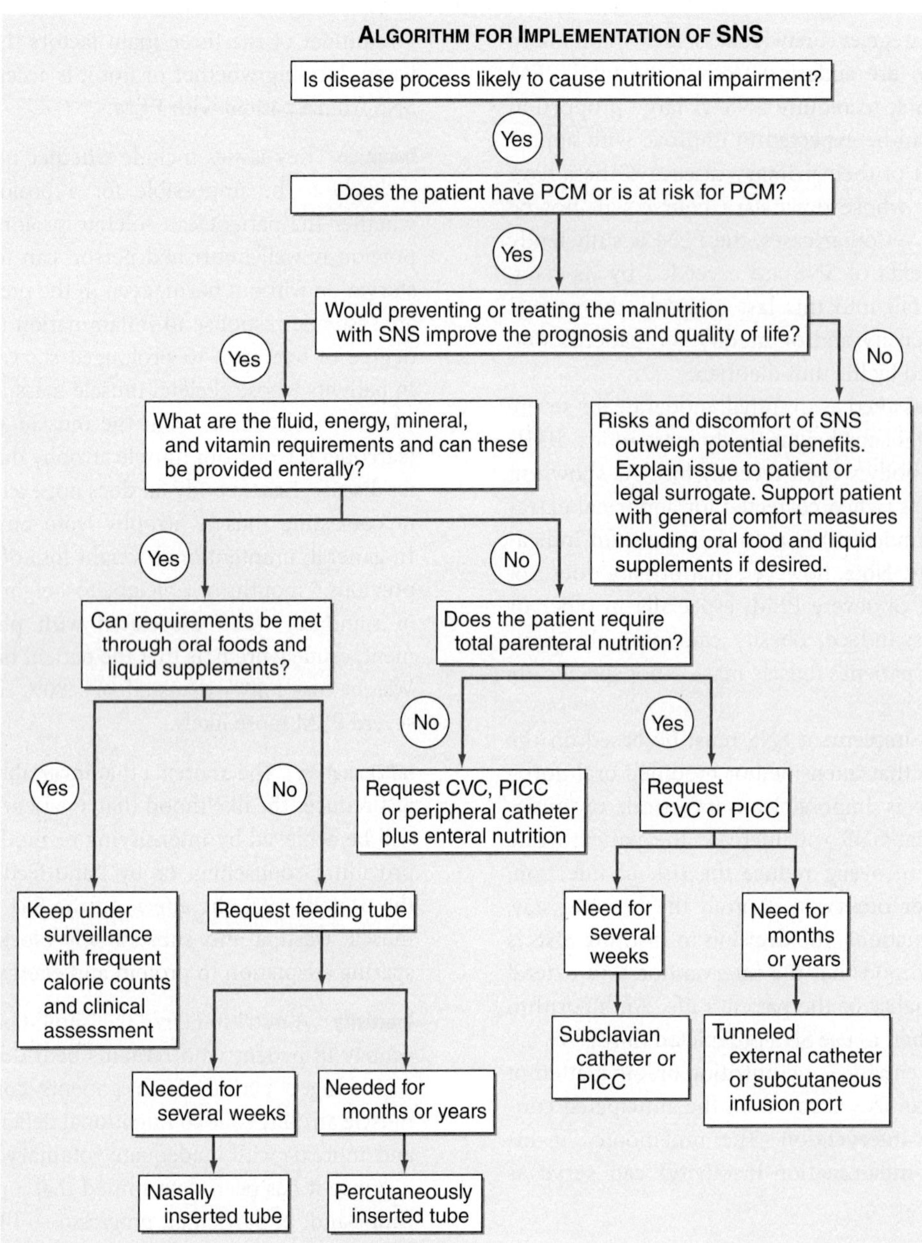

FIGURE 59-1

Decision-making for the implementation of specialized nutritional support (SNS). CVC, central venous catheter; PICC, peripherally inserted central catheter. *(Adapted from the chapter on this topic in Harrison's Principles of Internal Medicine, 16e, by Lyn Howard, MD.)*

end-of-life situations, it is prudent to explicitly state the treatment goals at the outset of a course of SNS therapy. Such clarity can smooth the way for subsequent appropriate discontinuation in those patients whose prognosis has become hopeless.

After the decision has been made that SNS is indeed appropriate, the next determinations are the route of delivery (enteral versus parenteral), timing, and calculation of the patient's nutritional goals. Although enteral SNS is the default option, the choice of optimal route depends on the degree of gut function as well as on available technical resources.

Both the choice of route and the timing of SNS require an evaluation of the patient's current nutritional status, the presence and extent of the SRI, and the anticipated clinical course. Severe SRI is identified on the basis of the standard clinical signs of leukocytosis, tachycardia, tachypnea, and temperature elevation or depression. Serum albumin is a negative acute-phase protein and hence a marker of the SRI. More severe hypoalbuminemia is a crude indicator of greater SRI severity, but this condition is almost certainly worsened by concurrent dietary protein deficiency. Despite the importance of adequate protein provision to patients with the SRI, no amount of SNS will raise serum albumin levels into the normal range as long as the SRI persists.

The SRI can be graded as mild, moderate, or severe. Examples of a severe SRI include (1) sepsis or other major inflammatory diseases (e.g., pancreatitis) that require care in the intensive care unit; (2) multiple trauma with an Injury Severity Score >20–25 or an Acute Physiology and Chronic Health Evaluation II (APACHE II) score >25; (3) closed head injury with a Glasgow Coma Scale <8; and (4) major third-degree burns of >40% of the body surface area. A moderate SRI occurs with less severe infections, injuries, or inflammatory conditions like pneumonia, uncomplicated major surgery, acute hepatic or renal injury, and exacerbations of ulcerative colitis or regional enteritis requiring hospitalization.

Patients with a severe SRI require the initiation of SNS within the first several days of care, for they are highly unlikely to consume an adequate amount of food voluntarily over the next 7 days. On the other hand, a moderate SRI, as is common during the period following major uncomplicated surgery without oral intake, may be tolerated for 5–7 days as long as the patient is initially well nourished. Patients awaiting elective major surgery benefit from preoperative nutritional repletion for 5–10 days but only in the presence of significant PEM. When adequate preoperative nutrition or SNS is impractical, early postoperative SNS is usually indicated. Furthermore, patients with a combination of a moderate SRI and moderate PEM are likely to benefit from early postoperative SNS.

RISKS AND BENEFITS OF SPECIALIZED NUTRITIONAL SUPPORT The risks of enteral SNS are determined primarily by the patient's state of alertness and swallowing competence, the anatomy and function of the gastrointestinal tract, and the experience of the supervising clinical team. The safest and least costly approach is to avoid SNS by close attention to oral food intake; personal encouragement; dietary modifications; hand-feeding, when possible; and, often, the addition of an oral liquid supplement. For this reason, all patients at nutritional risk should be assessed and followed by a nutritionist. There is increasing interest in the use, under selected circumstances and when not contraindicated, of pharmacologic doses of anabolic steroids to stimulate appetite and promote muscle anabolism.

Nasogastric tube insertion is a bedside procedure, but many critically ill patients have impaired gastric emptying and a high risk of aspiration pneumonia. This risk can be reduced by placing the tip of the feeding tube in the jejunum beyond the ligament of Treitz, a procedure that usually requires fluoroscopic or endoscopic guidance. When a laparotomy is planned for a patient who has other surgical conditions likely to necessitate prolonged SNS, it is advantageous to place a jejunal feeding tube at the time of surgery.

A major disadvantage of enteral SNS is that the amounts of protein and calories provided to critically ill patients commonly fail to reach target goals within the first 7–14 days after SNS is initiated. This problem is compounded by the lack of enteral products that allow the provision of the recommended protein target of 1.5–2.0 g/kg without simultaneously inducing potentially harmful caloric overfeeding.

Enteral SNS is often required in patients with anorexia, impaired swallowing, or small-intestinal disease. The bowel and its associated digestive organs derive 70% of their required nutrients directly from nutritional substrates absorbed from the intestinal lumen. Enteral feeding also supports gut function by stimulating splanchnic blood flow, neuronal activity, IgA antibody release, and secretion of gastrointestinal hormones that stimulate gut trophic activity. These factors support the gut as an immunologic barrier against enteric pathogens. For these reasons, current evidence indicates that some luminal nutrition should be provided, even when PN is required to provide most of the nutritional support. The nonessential amino acids arginine and glutamine, short-chain fatty acids, long-chain omega 3 fatty acids, and nucleotides are available in some specialty enteral formulas and appear to have an important role in maintaining immune function. The addition of supplemental PN to enteral feeding (either by mouth or as SNS by enteral tube) may hasten the transition to full enteral feeding, which is usually successful when >50% of requirements can be met enterally. As long as protein and other essential nutrient requirements are met, substantial nutritional benefit can be achieved by providing ~50% of energy needs for periods of up to 10 days. As a rule of thumb, dietary protein provision should be increased by ~25–50% when energy intake is reduced by this amount, since negative energy balance reduces the efficiency of dietary protein retention. For longer periods and in patients who have a normal or increased body fat content, it may be preferable to provide only 75–80% of energy needs (together with increased protein), as the mild energy deficit improves gastrointestinal tolerance, makes glycemic control far easier, and avoids excess fluid administration.

The main risks of PN are related to the placement of a central venous catheter, with its complications of thrombosis and infection, and the relatively large intravenous volumes infused. Less often appreciated are the risks associated with the ease of inadvertently infusing excessive carbohydrate and lipid directly into the bloodstream. These risks include hyperglycemia, inadequate lipid clearance from the circulation, hepatic steatosis and inflammation, and even respiratory failure in patients with borderline pulmonary function. On the other hand, renal dysfunction does not reduce a patient's requirement for protein or amino acids. In cases in which renal function is a limiting factor, appropriate renal replacement therapy must be provided along with SNS.

In the past, bowel rest through PN was the cornerstone of treatment for many severe gastrointestinal disorders. However, the value of providing even minimal amounts of enteral nutrition (EN) is now widely accepted. Protocols to facilitate more widespread use of EN include initiation within 24 h of ICU admission; aggressive use of the head-upright position; use of postpyloric and nasojejunal feeding tubes; use of prokinetic agents; more rapid increases in feeding rates; tolerance of higher gastric residuals; and adherence to nurse-directed algorithms for feeding progression. Parenteral SNS alone is generally necessary only for severe gut dysfunction due to prolonged ileus, intestinal obstruction, or severe hemorrhagic pancreatitis.

In critically ill patients, parenteral SNS can be commenced within the first 24 h of care, with the anticipation of a better clinical outcome and a lower mortality risk than those following delayed or inadequate enteral SNS; however, this point remains controversial. Some evidence suggests that early SNS is associated with a reduced risk of death but also with an increased risk of serious infection. More recent data, obtained in studies of moderately critically ill patients, suggest that early hypocaloric parenteral SNS lessens morbidity and mitigates muscle atrophy without an increased risk of infection, but also without a detectable reduction in mortality risk. Unfortunately, the current clinical-trial evidence fails to address several important unknowns. It is important to note that the level of protein substrate provided in published clinical trials generally falls well below the current recommendation, even in trials of supplemental parenteral SNS. Much of the increase in morbidity associated with parenteral and enteral SNS can be ascribed to hyperglycemia, which can be prevented by appropriately intensive insulin therapy. The level of glycemia necessary to prevent complications, whether <110 mg/dL or <150 mg/dL, remains unclear. Adequately fed surgical patients may benefit from the lower glucose range, but studies of intensive insulin therapy alone, without full feeding, suggest improved morbidity and mortality outcomes with looser control of glucose at <180 mg/dL.

In the early years of its use, PN was relatively expensive, but its components now are often less costly than specialty enteral formulas. Percutaneous placement of a central venous catheter into the subclavian vein or (less desirably) the internal jugular vein with advancement into the superior vena cava can be accomplished at the bedside by trained personnel using sterile techniques. Peripherally inserted central catheters (PICCs) can also be used, although they are usually more appropriate for non-ICU patients. Subclavian or internal jugular catheters carry the risks of pneumothorax or serious vascular damage but are generally well tolerated and, rather than requiring reinsertion, can be exchanged over a wire when catheter infection is suspected.

Although most SNS is delivered in hospitals, some patients require it on a long-term basis. At-home SNS requires a safe home environment, a stable clinical condition, and the patient's ability and willingness to learn appropriate self-care techniques. Other important considerations in determining the appropriateness of at-home parenteral or enteral SNS are that the patient's prognosis indicates survival for longer than several months and that the therapy enhances the patient's quality of life.

DISEASE-SPECIFIC NUTRITIONAL SUPPORT The purpose of SNS is to correct and prevent malnutrition. Certain conditions require special modification of the SNS regimen. Protein intake may need to be limited in many stable patients with renal insufficiency or borderline liver function. In renal disease, except for brief periods, protein intakes should approach the required level for normal adults of at least 0.8 g/kg and should aim for 1.2 g/kg as long as severe azotemia does not occur. Patients with severe renal failure who require SNS need concurrent renal replacement therapy. In hepatic failure, protein intakes of 1.2–1.4 g/kg (up to 1.5 g/kg) should be provided as long as encephalopathy due to protein intolerance does not occur. In the presence of protein intolerance, formulas containing 33–50% branched-chain amino acids are available and can be provided at the 1.2- to 1.4-g/kg level. Cardiac patients and many other severely stressed patients often benefit from fluid and sodium restriction to 1000 mL of PN formula and 5–20 meq of sodium per day. In patients with severe chronic PEM characterized by severe weight loss, it is important to initiate PN gradually because of the profound antinatriuresis, antidiuresis, and intracellular accumulation of potassium, magnesium, and phosphorus that develop as a consequence of the resulting high insulin levels. This modification of parenteral SNS is usually accomplished by limiting daily fluid intake initially to ~1000 mL; limiting carbohydrate intake to 10–20% dextrose; limiting sodium intake; and providing ample potassium, magnesium, and phosphorus, with careful daily assessment of fluid and electrolyte status. Protein need not be restricted.

THE DESIGN OF INDIVIDUAL REGIMENS

FLUID REQUIREMENTS

Normal adults require ~30 mL of fluid/kg of body weight from all sources each day as well as the replacement of abnormal losses such as those caused by diuretic therapy, nasogastric tube drainage, wound output, high rates of perspiration (which can be several liters per day during periods of extreme heat), and diarrhea/ostomy losses. Electrolyte and mineral losses can be estimated or measured and need to be replaced (Table 59-2). Fluid restriction may be necessary in

TABLE 59-2

APPROXIMATE VOLUME AND COMPOSITION OF FLUID SECRETIONS[a]						
SECRETION	VOLUME (L/D)	NA	K	CL	HCO_3	PH
Saliva	1–2	15	30	15	30	6–8
Gastric juice	1–2	50–90	5–30	90–130	0	1.5–3.5
Hepatic bile	0.5–1	130–150	5–10	80–120	30–50	7–9
Pancreas	0.5–1	130–150	5–10	70–100	90–110	8–9
Small intestine	1–3	120–140	10–20	80–120	20–40	7–9
Diarrhea	Varies	30–50	20–30		Varies	

[a]Concentration values are in mmol/L.

patients with fluid overload. Total fluid input can usually be limited to 1200 mL/d as long as urine is the only significant source of fluid output. In severe fluid overload, a 1-L central vein PN solution of 7% crystalline amino acids (70 g) and 21% dextrose (210 g) can temporarily provide an acceptable amount of glucose and protein substrate in the absence of significant catabolic stress.

Patients who require PN or EN in the acute-care setting generally have associated hormonal adaptations to their underlying disease (e.g., increased secretion of antidiuretic hormone, aldosterone, insulin, glucagon, or cortisol), and these signals promote fluid retention and hyperglycemia. In critical illness, body weight is invariably increased due to fluid resuscitation and fluid retention. Lean-tissue accretion is minimal in the acute phase of critical illness, no matter how much protein and or how many calories are provided. Because excess fluid removal can be difficult, limiting fluid intake to allow for balanced intake and output is more effective.

ENERGY REQUIREMENTS

Total energy expenditure comprises resting energy expenditure, activity energy expenditure, and the thermal effect of feeding **(Chap. 58)**. Resting energy expenditure accounts for two-thirds of total energy expenditure, activity energy expenditure for one-fourth to one-third, and the thermal effect of feeding for ~10%. For normally nourished, healthy individuals, the total energy expenditure is ~30–35 kcal/kg. Critical illness increases resting energy expenditure, but this increase is significant only in initially well-nourished individuals with a robust SRI who experience, for example, severe multiple trauma, extensive burns, sepsis, sustained high fever, or closed head injury. In these situations, total energy expenditure can reach 40–45 kcal/kg. The chronically starved patient with adapted PEM has a reduced energy expenditure and is inactive, with a usual total energy expenditure of ~20–25 kcal/kg. Very few patients with adapted PEM require as much as 30 kcal/kg for energy balance. Because providing ~50% of measured energy expenditure as SNS is at least as effective as 100% for the first 10 days of critical illness, actual measurement of energy expenditure generally is not necessary in the early period of SNS. However, in patients who remain critically ill beyond several weeks, in patients with severe PEM for whom estimates of energy expenditure are unreliable, and in patients who are difficult to wean from ventilators, it is reasonable to measure energy expenditure directly when the technique is available, targeting an energy intake of 100–120% of the measured energy expenditure.

Insulin resistance due to the SRI is associated with increased gluconeogenesis and reduced peripheral glucose utilization, with resulting hyperglycemia. Hyperglycemia is aggravated by excessive exogenous carbohydrate administration from SNS. In critically ill patients receiving SNS, normalization of blood glucose levels by insulin infusion reduces morbidity and mortality risk. In mildly or moderately malnourished patients, it is reasonable to provide metabolic support in order to improve protein synthesis and maintain metabolic homeostasis. Hypocaloric nutrition, with provision of ~1000 kcal and 70 g protein per day for up to 10 days, requires less fluid and reduces the likelihood of poor glycemic control, although a higher protein intake would be optimal. During the second week of SNS, energy and protein provision can be advanced to 20–25 kcal/kg and 1.5 g/kg per day, respectively, as metabolic conditions permit. As mentioned above, patients with multiple trauma, closed head injury, and severe burns often have greatly elevated energy expenditures, but there is little evidence that providing >30 kcal/kg daily confers further benefit, and such high caloric intake may well be harmful as it substantially increases the risk of hyperglycemia.

As a rule, amino acids and glucose are provided in an increasing dose until energy provision matches estimated resting energy expenditure. At this point, it becomes beneficial to add fat. A surfeit of glucose merely stimulates de novo lipogenesis—an energy-inefficient process. Polyunsaturated long-chain triglycerides (e.g., in soybean oil) are the chief ingredient in most parenteral fat emulsions and provide the majority of the fat in enteral feeding formulas. These vegetable oil–based emulsions provide essential fatty acids. The fat content of enteral feeding formulas ranges from 3% to 50% of energy. Parenteral fat is provided in separate containers as 20% and 30% emulsions that can be infused separately or mixed in the sterile pharmacy as an all-in-one or total nutrient admixture of amino acids, glucose, lipid, electrolytes, vitamins, and minerals. Although parenteral fat needs to make up only ~3% of the energy requirement in order to meet essential fatty acid requirements, when provided daily as an all-in-one mixture of carbohydrate, fat, and protein, the complete admixture has a fat content of 2–3 g/dL and provides 20–30% of the total energy requirement—an acceptable level that offers the advantage of ensuring emulsion stability. When given as a separate infusion, parenteral fat should not be provided at rates exceeding 0.11 g/kg of body mass or 100 g over 12 h—equivalent to 500 mL of 20% parenteral fat.

Medium-chain triglycerides containing saturated fatty acids with chain lengths of 6, 8, 10, or 12 carbons (>95% of which are C8 and C10) are included in a number of enteral feeding formulas because they are absorbed preferentially. Fish oil contains polyunsaturated fatty acids of the omega 3 family, which improve immune function and reduce the inflammatory response. At this time, fish oil injectable emulsions are available in the United States as an investigational new drug.

PN formulations provide carbohydrate as hydrous glucose (3.4 kcal/g). In enteral formulas, glucose is the carbohydrate source for so-called monomeric diets. These diets provide protein as amino acids and fat in minimal amounts (3%) to meet essential fatty acid requirements. Monomeric formulas are designed to optimize absorption in the seriously compromised gut. These formulas, like immune-enhancing diets, are expensive. In polymeric diets, the carbohydrate source is usually an osmotically less active polysaccharide, the protein is usually soy or casein protein, and fat is present at concentrations of 25–50%. Such formulas are usually well tolerated by patients with normal intestinal length, and some are acceptable for oral consumption.

PROTEIN OR AMINO ACID REQUIREMENTS

The daily protein recommendation for healthy adults is 0.8 g/kg, but body proteins are replenished faster with 1.5 g/kg in patients with PEM, and net protein catabolism is reduced in critically ill patients when 1.5–2.0 g/kg is provided. In patients who are not critically ill but who require SNS in the acute-care setting, at least 1 g of protein/kg is recommended, and larger amounts up to 1.5 g/kg are appropriate when volume, renal, and hepatic tolerances allow. The standard parenteral and enteral formulas contain protein of high biologic value and meet the requirements for the eight essential amino acids when nitrogen needs are met. Parenteral amino acid mixtures and elemental enteral mixtures consist of hydrated individual amino acids. Because of their hydrated status, elemental amino acid solutions deliver 17% less protein substrate than intact proteins. In protein-intolerant conditions such as renal and hepatic failure, modified amino acid formulas may be considered. In hepatic failure, higher branched-chain, amino acid–enriched formulas appear to improve outcomes. Conditionally essential amino acids like arginine and glutamine may also have some benefit in supplemental amounts.

Protein (nitrogen) balance provides a measure of the efficacy of parenteral or enteral SNS. This balance is calculated as protein intake/6.25 (because proteins are, on average, 16% nitrogen) minus the 24-h urine urea nitrogen plus 4 g of nitrogen (the latter reflecting other nitrogen losses). In critical illness, a mild negative nitrogen balance of 2–4 g/d is often achievable. A similarly mild positive nitrogen balance is observed in the nonstressed recuperating patient. Each gram of nitrogen lost or gained represents ~30 g of lean tissue.

MINERAL AND VITAMIN REQUIREMENTS

Parenteral electrolyte, vitamin, and trace mineral requirements are summarized in Tables 59-3, 59-4, and 59-5, respectively. Electrolyte modifications are

TABLE 59-3

USUAL DAILY ELECTROLYTE ADDITIONS TO PARENTERAL NUTRITION

ELECTROLYTE	PARENTERAL EQUIVALENT	USUAL INTAKE
Sodium		1–2 meq/kg + replacement, but can be as low as 5–40 meq/d
Potassium		40–100 meq/d + replacement of unusual losses
Chloride		As needed for acid-base balance, but usually 2:1 to 1:1 with acetate
Acetate		As needed for acid-base balance
Calcium	10 meq	10–20 meq/d
Magnesium	10 meq	8–16 meq/d
Phosphorus	30 mmol	20–40 mmol

TABLE 59-4

PARENTERAL MULTIVITAMIN REQUIREMENTS FOR ADULTS

VITAMIN	REVISED VALUES
Vitamin A	3300 IU
Thiamin (B_1)	6 mg
Riboflavin (B_2)	3.6 mg
Niacin (B_3)	40 mg
Folic acid	600 μg
Pantothenic acid	15 mg
Pyridoxine (B_6)	6 mg
Cyanocobalamin (B_{12})	5 μg
Biotin	60 μg
Ascorbic acid (C)	200 mg
Vitamin D	200 IU[a]
Vitamin E	10 IU
Vitamin K[b]	150 μg

[a]The current vitamin D requirement—a minimum of 600 IU/day—cannot be met with available injectable vitamin formulations. Calcitriol is not equivalent to vitamin D and is not a suitable replacement for it, since it is not a substrate for 25-hydroxyvitamin D biosynthesis.
[b]A product is available without vitamin K. Vitamin K supplementation is recommended at 2–4 mg/week in patients not receiving oral anticoagulation therapy when the vitamin K–free product is used.

TABLE 59-5

PARENTERAL TRACE METAL SUPPLEMENTATION FOR ADULTS[a]

TRACE MINERAL	INTAKE
Zinc[b]	2.5–4 mg/d; an additional 10–15 mg/d per L of stool or ileostomy output
Copper	0.5–1.5 mg/d; possibility of retention in biliary tract obstruction
Manganese	0.1–0.3 mg/d; possibility of retention in biliary tract obstruction
Chromium	10–15 μg/d
Selenium	20–100 μg/d; necessary for long-term PN, optional for short term
Molybdenum	20–120 μg/d; necessary for long-term PN, optional for short term
Iodine	75–150 μg/d; necessary for long-term PN, optional for short term

[a]Commercial products are available with the first four, the first five, and all seven of these metals in recommended amounts.
[b]The basal IV zinc requirement is approximately one-third of the oral requirement, because only approximately one-third of orally ingested zinc is absorbed.
Abbreviation: PN, parenteral nutrition.

necessary with substantial gastrointestinal losses from nasogastric drainage or intestinal losses from fistulas, diarrhea, or ostomy outputs. Such losses also imply extra calcium, magnesium, and zinc losses. Zinc losses are high in secretory diarrhea. Secretory diarrhea contains ~12 mg of zinc/L, and patients with intestinal fistulas or chronic diarrhea require an average of ~12 mg of parenteral zinc/d (equivalent to 30 mg of oral elemental zinc) to maintain zinc balance. Excessive urinary potassium losses with amphotericin or magnesium losses with cisplatin or in renal failure necessitate adjustments in sodium, potassium, magnesium, phosphorus, and acid-base balance. Vitamin and trace element requirements are met by the daily provision of a complete parenteral vitamin supplement and trace elements via PN and by the provision of adequate amounts of enteral feeding formulas that contain these micronutrients.

Iron is a highly reactive catalyst of oxidative reactions and thus is not included in PN mixtures. The parenteral iron requirement is normally only ~1 mg/d. Iron deficiency occurs with considerable frequency in acutely ill hospitalized patients, especially those with PEM and gastrointestinal tract disease, and in patients subjected to frequent blood withdrawals. Iron deficiency is sometimes inadequately considered in hospitalized patients because there are commoner causes: the inflammation-mediated anemia of chronic disease (with an associated increase in serum ferritin, an acute-phase protein) and redistribution of the intravascular fluid volume during prolonged bed rest. Iron deficiency should be considered in every patient receiving SNS. A falling mean red cell volume, even if still in the low-normal range, together with an intermediate serum ferritin concentration is suggestive of iron deficiency. Intravenous iron infusions follow standard guidelines, always with a termination order and never as a standing order because of the risk of inadvertent iron overdosing. Major iron replacement during critical illness is of some concern because of the possibility that a substantial rise in the serum iron concentration may increase susceptibility to some bacterial infections.

PARENTERAL NUTRITION

INFUSION TECHNIQUE AND PATIENT MONITORING

Parenteral feeding through a peripheral vein is limited by osmolarity and volume constraints. Solutions with an osmolarity >900 mOsm/L (e.g., those which contain >3% amino acids and 5% glucose [290 kcal/L]) are poorly tolerated peripherally. Parenteral lipid emulsions (20%) can be given to increase the calories delivered. The total volume required for a marginal amino acid provision rate of 60 g (equivalent to 50 g of protein) and a total of 1680 kcal is 2.5 L. Moreover, the risk of significant morbidity and mortality from incompatibilities of calcium and phosphate salts is greatest in these low-osmolarity, low-glucose regimens. For short-term infusions, calcium may be temporarily limited or even omitted from the mixture. Parenteral feeding via a peripheral vein is generally intended as a supplement to oral feeding; it is not suitable for the critically ill. Peripheral PN may be enhanced by small amounts of heparin (1000 U/L) and co-infusion with parenteral fat to reduce osmolarity, but volume constraints still limit the value of this therapy, especially in critical illness.

PICCs may be used to infuse solutions of 20–25% dextrose and 4–7% amino acids, thus avoiding the traumatic complications of percutaneous central vein catheter placement. With PICC lines, however, flow can be position-related, and the lines cannot be exchanged over a wire for infection monitoring. It is important to withdraw blood samples carefully and appropriately from a dual-port PICC because intermixing of the blood sample with even tiny volumes of nutrient infusate will falsely indicate hyperglycemia and hyperkalemia. For all these reasons, centrally placed catheters are preferred in critical illness. The subclavian approach is best tolerated by the patient and is the easiest to dress. The jugular approach is less likely to cause a pneumothorax. Femoral vein catheterization is strongly discouraged because of the risk of catheter infection. For long-term feeding at home, tunneled catheters and implanted ports are used to reduce infection risk and are more acceptable to patients. Tunneled catheters require placement in the operating room.

Catheters are made of Silastic®, polyurethane, or polyvinyl chloride. Silastic catheters are less thrombogenic and are best for tunneled catheters. Polyurethane is best for temporary catheters. To avoid infection, dressing changes with dry gauze should be performed at regular intervals by nurses skilled in catheter care. Chlorhexidine solution is more effective than alcohol or iodine compounds. Appropriate monitoring for patients receiving PN is summarized in Table 59-6.

TABLE 59-6

MONITORING THE PATIENT RECEIVING PARENTERAL NUTRITION[a]

Clinical Data	
General sense of well-being	
Strength, as evidenced by getting out of bed, walking, and resistance exercise as appropriate	
Vital signs, including temperature, blood pressure, pulse, and respiratory rate	
Fluid balance: weight (recorded at least several times weekly); fluid intake (parenteral and enteral) vs. fluid output (urine, stool, gastric drainage, wound, ostomy)	
Parenteral nutrition delivery equipment: tubing, pump, filter, catheter, dressing	
Nutrient solution composition	
Laboratory Data	
Finger-stick glucose	Three times daily until stable
Blood glucose, Na, K, Cl, HCO_3, BUN	Daily until stable and fully advanced; then twice weekly
Serum creatinine, albumin, PO_4, Ca, Mg, Hb/Hct, WBC count	Baseline; then twice weekly
INR	Baseline; then weekly
Micronutrient tests	As indicated

[a]Parameters are assessed daily unless otherwise specified.
Abbreviations: BUN, blood urea nitrogen; Hb, hemoglobin; Hct, hematocrit; INR, international normalized ratio; WBC, white blood cell.
Source: Adapted from the chapter on this topic in *Harrison's Principles of Internal Medicine*, 16e, by Lyn Howard, MD.

STANDARD VERSUS INDIVIDUALIZED NUTRIENT PROVISION

Even though premixed solutions of crystalline amino acids and dextrose are in common use, the future of evidence-based PN lies in computer-controlled sterile compounders that rapidly and inexpensively generate personalized solutions that meet the specific protein and calorie goals for different patients in different clinical situations. For example, 1 L of a standard mixture of 5% amino acids/25% dextrose solution provides 50 g of amino acids (41.5 g of protein substrate) and 1000 kcal; the use of this solution to meet the 1.5–to 2.0-g/kg protein requirement of an acutely ill 70-kg patient requires the infusion of 2.5–3.4 L of fluid and a potentially excessively high energy dose of 2500-3300 kcal. When the body fat store is adequate, clinical evidence increasingly supports the greater safety and efficacy of high-protein, moderately hypocaloric SNS in such patients. A sterile compounder can accurately generate an appropriate recipe for such a patient. For example, 1 L of a solution including 600 mL of 15% amino acids, 300 mL of 50% dextrose, and 100 mL of electrolyte/micronutrient mix contains 75 g of protein substrate and 800 kcal; thus it is feasible to meet the patient's protein requirement with only 1.4–1.9 L of solution and a more appropriate 1100–1520 kcal; any mild gap in energy provision is easily filled by use of intravenous lipid.

COMPLICATIONS

Mechanical

The insertion of a central venous catheter should be performed by trained and experienced personnel using aseptic techniques to limit the major common complications of pneumothorax and inadvertent arterial puncture or injury. The catheter's position should be radiographically confirmed to be in the superior vena cava distal to the junction with the jugular or subclavian vein and not directly against the vessel wall. Thrombosis related to the catheter may occur at the site of entry into the vein and extend to encase the catheter. Catheter infection predisposes to thrombosis, as does the SRI. The addition of 6000 U of heparin to the daily parenteral formula for hospitalized patients with temporary catheters reduces the risk of fibrin sheath formation and catheter infection. Temporary catheters that develop a thrombus should be removed and, according to clinical findings, treated with anticoagulants. Thrombolytic therapy can be considered for patients with permanent catheters, depending on the ease of replacement and the presence of alternative, reasonably acceptable venous access sites. Low-dose warfarin therapy (1 mg/d) reduces the risk of thrombosis in permanent catheters used for at-home parenteral SNS, but full anticoagulation may be required for patients who have recurrent thrombosis related to permanent catheters. A recent U.S. Food and Drug Administration mandate to reformulate parenteral multivitamins to include vitamin K at a dose of 150 μg/d may affect the efficacy of low-dose warfarin therapy. A "no vitamin K" version is available for patients receiving this therapy. Catheters can become occluded due to mechanical factors; by fibrin at the tip; or by fat, minerals, or drugs intraluminally. These occlusions can be managed with low-dose alteplase for fibrin, with indwelling 70% alcohol for fat, with 0.1 *N* hydrochloric acid for mineral precipitates, and with either 0.1 *N* hydrochloric acid or 0.1 *N* sodium hydroxide for drugs, depending on the pH of the drug.

Metabolic

The most common problems caused by parenteral SNS are fluid overload and hyperglycemia (Table 59-7). Hypertonic dextrose stimulates a much higher insulin level than meal feeding. Because insulin is a potent antinatriuretic and antidiuretic hormone, hyperinsulinemia leads to sodium and fluid retention. Consequently, in the absence of gastrointestinal losses or renal dysfunction, net fluid retention is likely when total fluid intake exceeds 2000 mL/d. Close monitoring of body mass as well as of fluid intake and output is necessary to prevent this complication. In the absence of significant renal impairment, the sodium content of the urine is likely to be <10 meq/L. Provision of sodium in limited amounts (40 meq/d) and the use of both glucose and fat in the PN mixture will reduce serum glucose levels and help reduce fluid retention. The elevated insulin level also increases the intracellular transport of potassium, magnesium, and phosphorus, which can precipitate a dangerous re-feeding syndrome if the total glucose content of the PN solution is advanced too quickly in severely malnourished patients. To assess glucose tolerance, it is generally best to start PN with <200 g of glucose/d. Regular insulin can be added to the PN formula to establish glycemic control, and the insulin doses can be increased proportionately as the glucose content is advanced. As a general rule, patients with insulin-dependent diabetes require about twice their usual at-home insulin dose when receiving PN at 20–25 kcal/kg, largely as a consequence of parenteral glucose administration and some loss of insulin to the formula's container. As a rough estimate, the amount of insulin provided can be proportionately similar to the number of calories provided as total parenteral nutrition (TPN) relative to full feeding, and the insulin can be placed in the TPN formula. Subcutaneous regular insulin can be provided to improve glucose control as assessed by measurements of blood glucose every 6 h. About two-thirds of the total 24-h amount can be added to the next day's order, with SC insulin supplements as needed. Advances in the TPN glucose concentration should be made when reasonable glucose control is established, and the insulin dose can be adjusted proportionately to the calories added as glucose and amino acids. These are general rules, and they are conservative. Given the adverse clinical impact of hyperglycemia, it may be necessary to use intensive insulin therapy as a separate infusion with a standard protocol to initially establish control. Once control is established, this insulin dose can be added to the PN formula. Acid-base imbalance is also common during parenteral SNS. Amino acid formulas are buffered, but critically ill patients are prone to metabolic acidosis, often due to renal tubular impairment. The use of sodium and potassium acetate salts in the PN formula may address this problem. Bicarbonate salts should not be used because they are incompatible with TPN formulations. Nasogastric drainage produces hypochloremic alkalosis that can be managed by attention to chloride balance. Occasionally, hydrochloric acid may be required for a more rapid response or when diuretic therapy limits the ability to provide substantial sodium chloride. Up to 100 meq/L and up to 150 meq of hydrochloric acid per day may be placed in a fat-free TPN formula.

Infectious

Infections of the central access catheter rarely occur in the first 72 h. Fever during this period is usually attributable to infection elsewhere or another cause. Fever that develops during parenteral SNS can be addressed

TABLE 59-7

SELECTED METABOLIC DISTURBANCES CAUSED BY PN AND THEIR CORRECTION

DISTURBANCE	CAUSE	CORRECTIVE ACTION WITH PN
Hyponatremia	Increased total body water or decreased total body sodium	Decrease free water or increase sodium.
Hypernatremia	Occurs commonly with excessive isotonic or hypertonic fluid followed by diuretic administration with free water clearance; can also occur with dehydration and normal total body sodium	Increase free water to produce net positive fluid balance, maintaining sodium and chloride balance.
Hypokalemia	Inadequate intake relative to need	Use supplements.
	Excessive diuresis, tubular dysfunction	Use supplements.
	Magnesium deficiency	Increase PN magnesium.
	Metabolic alkalosis	Correct alkalosis.
	Hyperinsulinemia	Maintain constant PN; increase potassium.
Hyperkalemia	Excessive provision	Reduce supplements.
	Metabolic acidosis	Evaluate acidosis. Treat with PN acetate salt, and decrease potassium.
	Renal deterioration	Evaluate patient and adjust PN as indicated.
Hypocalcemia	Reciprocal response to phosphorus repletion	Increase calcium.
	Critical illness effect	Increase calcium.
	Severe malabsorption	Supplement calcium.
Hypercalcemia	Excessive administration or pathology (cancer, hyperparathyroidism)	Reduce or eliminate calcium.
Hypomagnesemia	Increased requirements due to diuretic use, alcoholism, malabsorption, malnutrition	Supplement magnesium.
	Critical illness	Supplement magnesium.
Hypophosphatemia	Inadequate intake relative to needs related to malnutrition, alcohol use	Supplement phosphorus.
	Increased calcium intake	Use supplements.
Hyperphosphatemia	Excessive administration or worsening renal function	Reduce phosphorus.
Azotemia	Excessive amino acid infusion or worsening renal function	Reduce amino acid level if feasible, but use renal replacement therapy if 1 g of protein/kg cannot be provided for prolonged periods.

Abbreviation: PN, parenteral nutrition.

by checking the catheter site and, if the site looks clean, exchanging the catheter over a wire, with cultures taken through the catheter and at the catheter tip. If these cultures are negative, as they usually are, the new catheter can continue to be used. If a culture is positive for a relatively nonpathogenic bacterium like *Staphylococcus epidermidis*, a second exchange over a wire with repeat cultures or replacement of the catheter can be considered in light of the clinical circumstances. If cultures are positive for more pathogenic bacteria or for fungi like *Candida albicans*, it is generally best to replace the catheter at a new site. Whether antibiotic treatment is required is a clinical decision, but *C. albicans* grown from the blood culture in a patient receiving PN should always be treated with an antifungal drug because the consequences of failure to treat can be dire.

Catheter infections can be minimized by dedicating the feeding catheter to TPN, without blood sampling or medication administration. Central catheter infections are a serious complication, with an attributed mortality rate of 12–25%. Fewer than three infections per 1000 catheter-days should occur in central venous catheters dedicated to feeding. At-home TPN catheter infections may be treated through the catheter without its removal, particularly if the offending organism is *S. epidermidis*. Clearing of the biofilm and fibrin sheath by local treatment of the catheter with indwelling alteplase may increase the likelihood of eradication. Antibiotic lock therapy with high concentrations of antibiotic, with or without heparin in addition to systemic therapy, may improve efficacy. Sepsis with hypotension should precipitate catheter removal in either the temporary or the permanent TPN setting.

ENTERAL NUTRITION

TUBE PLACEMENT AND PATIENT MONITORING

The types of enteral feeding tubes, methods of insertion, their clinical uses, and potential complications are outlined in Table 59-8. The different types of enteral formulas are listed in Table 59-9. Patients receiving EN are at risk for many of the same metabolic complications as those who receive PN and should be monitored in the same manner. EN can be a source of similar problems, but not to the same degree, because the insulin response to EN is about half of that to PN. Enteral feeding formulas have fixed electrolyte compositions that are generally modest in sodium and somewhat higher in potassium. Acid-base disturbances can be addressed to a more limited extent with EN. Acetate salts can be added to the formula to treat chronic metabolic acidosis. Calcium chloride can be added to treat mild chronic metabolic alkalosis. Medications and other additives to enteral feeding formulas can clog the tubes (e.g., calcium chloride may interact with casein-based formulas to form insoluble calcium caseinate products) and may reduce the efficacy of some drugs (e.g., phenytoin). Since small-bore tubes are easily displaced, tube position should be checked at intervals by aspirating and measuring the pH of the gut fluid (normal: <4 in the stomach, >6 in the jejunum).

COMPLICATIONS

Aspiration

The debilitated patient with poor gastric emptying and impairment of swallowing and cough is at risk for aspiration; this complication is particularly common among patients who are mechanically ventilated. Tracheal suctioning induces coughing and gastric regurgitation, and cuffs on endotracheal or tracheostomy tubes seldom protect against aspiration. Preventive measures include elevating the head of the bed to 30°,

TABLE 59-8

ENTERAL FEEDING TUBES

TYPE/INSERTION TECHNIQUE	CLINICAL USES	POTENTIAL COMPLICATIONS
Nasogastric Tube		
External measurement: nostril, ear, xiphisternum; tube stiffened by ice water or stylet; position verified by air injection and auscultation or by x-ray	Short-term clinical situation (weeks) or longer periods with intermittent insertion; bolus feeding is simpler, but continuous drip with pump is better tolerated	Aspiration; ulceration of nasal and esophageal tissues, leading to stricture
Nasoduodenal Tube		
External measurement: nostril, ear, anterior superior iliac spine; tube stiffened by stylet and passed through pylorus under fluoroscopy or with endoscopic loop	Short-term clinical situations where gastric emptying is impaired or proximal leak is suspected; requires continuous drip with pump	Spontaneous pulling back into stomach (position verified by aspirating content, pH >6); diarrhea common, fiber-containing formulas may help
Gastrostomy Tube		
Percutaneous placement endoscopically, radiologically, or surgically; after track is established, can be converted to a gastric "button"	Long-term clinical situations, swallowing disorders, or impaired small-bowel absorption requiring continuous drip	Aspiration; irritation around tube exit site; peritoneal leak; balloon migration and obstruction of pylorus
Jejunostomy Tube		
Percutaneous placement endoscopically or radiologically via pylorus or endoscopically or surgically directly into the jejunum	Long-term clinical situations where gastric emptying is impaired; requires continuous drip with pump; direct endoscopic placement (PEJ) is most comfortable for patient	Clogging or displacement of tube; jejunal fistula if large-bore tube is used; diarrhea from dumping; irritation of surgical anchoring suture
Combined Gastrojejunostomy Tube		
Percutaneous placement endoscopically, radiologically, or surgically; intragastric arm for continuous or intermittent gastric suction; jejunal arm for enteral feeding	Used for patients with impaired gastric emptying and high risk for aspiration or patients with acute pancreatitis or proximal leaks	Clogging, especially of small-bore jejunal tube

Abbreviation: PEJ, percutaneous endoscopic jejunostomy.
Note: All small tubes are at risk for clogging, especially if used for crushed medications. In long-term enteral nutrition patients, gastrostomy and jejunostomy tubes can be exchanged for a low-profile "button" once the track is established.
Source: Adapted from the chapter on this topic in *Harrison's Principles of Internal Medicine*, 16e, by Lyn Howard, MD.

TABLE 59-9

ENTERAL FORMULAS

COMPOSITION CHARACTERISTICS	CLINICAL INDICATIONS
Standard Enteral Formula	
Complete dietary products (+)[a] 1. Caloric density: 1 kcal/mL 2. Protein: ~14% cals (caseinates, soy, lactalbumin) 3. Carbohydrate: ~60% cals (hydrolyzed corn starch, maltodextrin, sucrose) 4. Fat: ~30% cals (corn, soy, safflower oils) 5. Recommended daily intake of all minerals and vitamins in >1500 kcal/d 6. Osmolality: ~300 mosmol/kg	Suitable for most patients requiring tube feeding; some standard formulas can be used orally
Modified Enteral Formulas	
1. Caloric density: 1.5–2 kcal/mL (+)	Fluid-restricted patients
2. Protein	Critically ill patients
a. High protein (~20–25% protein) (+)	Impaired absorption
b. Hydrolyzed protein to small peptides (+)	Immune-enhancing diets
c. ↑ Arginine, glutamine, nucleotides, ω3 fat (+++)	Liver failure patients intolerant of 0.8 g of protein/kg
d. ↑ Branched-chain amino acids, ↓ aromatic amino acids (+++)	Renal failure patients for brief periods if critically ill
e. Low protein of high biologic value	Fat malabsorption
3. Fat	Pulmonary failure with CO_2 retention on standard formula, limited utility
a. Low-fat partial MCT substitution (+)	Improvement in glycemic index control in diabetes
b. ↑ Fat (>40% cals) (++)	Improved ventilation in ARDS
c. ↑ Fat from MUFA (++)	Improved laxation
d. ↑ Fat from ω3 and ↓ fat from ω6 linoleic acid (+++)	
4. Fiber: provided as soy polysaccharide (+)	

[a]Cost: +, inexpensive; ++, moderately expensive; +++, very expensive.

Note: ARDS, acute respiratory distress syndrome; MCT, medium-chain triglyceride; MUFA, monounsaturated fatty acids; ω3 or ω6, polyunsaturated fat with first double bond at carbon 3 (fish oils) or carbon 6 (vegetable oils).

Source: Adapted from the chapter on this topic in *Harrison's Principles of Internal Medicine*, 16e, by Lyn Howard, MD.

using nurse-directed algorithms for formula advancement, combining enteral with parenteral feeding, and using post–ligament of Treitz feeding. Tube feeding should not be discontinued for gastric residuals of <300 mL unless there are other signs of gastrointestinal intolerance, such as nausea, vomiting, or abdominal distention. Continuous feeding using pumps is better tolerated intragastrically than bolus feeding and is essential for feeding into the jejunum. For small-bowel feeding, residuals are not assessed, but abdominal pain and distention should be monitored.

Diarrhea

Enteral feeding often leads to diarrhea, especially if bowel function is compromised by disease or drugs (most often, broad-spectrum antibiotics). Sorbitol used to flavor some medications can also cause diarrhea. Diarrhea may be controlled by the use of a continuous drip, with a fiber-containing formula, or by the addition of an antidiarrheal agent to the formula. However, *Clostridium difficile*, which is a common cause of diarrhea in patients being tube-fed, should be ruled out as the etiology before antidiarrheal agents are used. H2 blockers may help reduce the net volume of fluid presented to the colon. Diarrhea associated with enteral feeding does not necessarily imply inadequate absorption of nutrients other than water and electrolytes. Amino acids and glucose are particularly well absorbed in the upper small bowel except in the most diseased or shortest bowel. Since luminal nutrients exert trophic effects on the gut mucosa, it is often appropriate to persist with tube feeding despite diarrhea, even when this course necessitates supplemental parenteral fluid support. Apart from conditions with drastically diminished small-intestinal absorptive function, there are no established indications for short peptide–based or elemental formulas.

GLOBAL CONSIDERATIONS

In the United States, the only parenteral lipid emulsion available is made with soybean oil, whose constituent fatty acids have been suggested to be immunosuppressive under certain circumstances.

In Europe and Japan, a number of other lipid emulsions are available, including those containing fish oil only; mixtures of fish oil, medium-chain triglycerides, and long-chain triglycerides as olive oil and/or soybean oil; mixtures of medium-chain triglycerides and long-chain triglycerides as soybean oil; and long-chain triglyceride mixtures as olive oil and soybean oil, which may be more beneficial in terms of metabolism and hepatic and immune function. Furthermore, a glutamine-containing dipeptide for inclusion in TPN formulas is available in Europe and may be helpful in terms of immune function and resistance to infection, although a recent study using a larger-than-recommended dose was associated with net harm.

ACKNOWLEDGMENT

The authors acknowledge the contributions of Lyn Howard, MD, the author in earlier editions of HPIM, to material in this chapter.

SECTION XI

OBESITY AND EATING DISORDERS

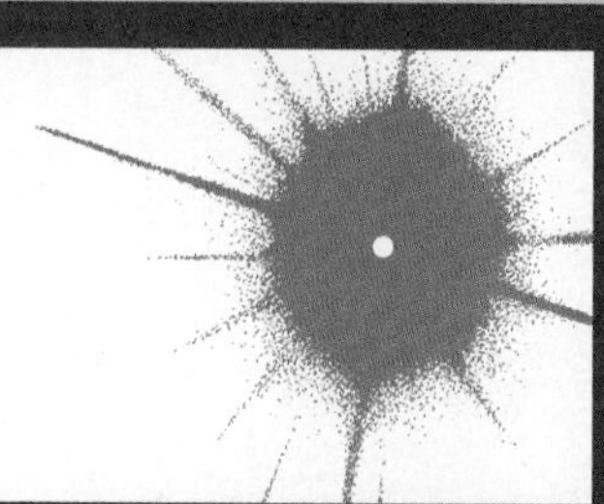

CHAPTER 60

BIOLOGY OF OBESITY

Jeffrey S. Flier ■ Eleftheria Maratos-Flier

In a world where food supplies are intermittent, the ability to store energy in excess of what is required for immediate use is essential for survival. Fat cells, residing within widely distributed adipose tissue depots, are adapted to store excess energy efficiently as triglyceride and, when needed, to release stored energy as free fatty acids for use at other sites. This physiologic system, orchestrated through endocrine and neural pathways, permits humans to survive starvation for as long as several months. However, in the presence of nutritional abundance and a sedentary lifestyle, and influenced importantly by genetic endowment, this system increases adipose energy stores and produces adverse health consequences.

DEFINITION AND MEASUREMENT

Obesity is a state of excess adipose tissue mass. Although often viewed as equivalent to increased body weight, this need not be the case—lean but very muscular individuals may be overweight by numerical standards without having increased adiposity. Body weights are distributed continuously in populations, so that choice of a medically meaningful distinction between lean and obese is somewhat arbitrary. Obesity is therefore defined by assessing its linkage to morbidity or mortality.

Although not a direct measure of adiposity, the most widely used method to gauge obesity is the *body mass index* (BMI), which is equal to weight/height^2 (in kg/m^2) (Fig. 60-1). Other approaches to quantifying obesity include anthropometry (skinfold thickness), densitometry (underwater weighing), computed tomography (CT) or magnetic resonance imaging (MRI), and electrical impedance. Using data from the Metropolitan Life Tables, BMIs for the midpoint of all heights and frames among both men and women range from 19 to 26 kg/m^2; at a similar BMI, women have more body fat than men. Based on data of substantial morbidity, a BMI of 30 is most commonly used as a threshold for obesity in both men and women. Most but not all large-scale epidemiologic studies suggest that all-cause, metabolic, cancer, and cardiovascular morbidity begin to rise (albeit at a slow rate) when BMIs are ≥25. Most authorities use the term *overweight* (rather than obese) to describe individuals with BMIs between 25 and 30. A BMI between 25 and 30 should be viewed as medically significant and worthy of therapeutic intervention in the presence of risk factors that are influenced by adiposity, such as hypertension and glucose intolerance.

The distribution of adipose tissue in different anatomic depots also has substantial implications for morbidity. Specifically, intraabdominal and abdominal subcutaneous fat have more significance than subcutaneous fat present in the buttocks and lower extremities. This distinction is most easily made clinically by determining the waist-to-hip ratio, with a ratio >0.9 in women and >1.0 in men being abnormal. Many of the most important complications of obesity, such as insulin resistance, diabetes, hypertension, hyperlipidemia, and hyperandrogenism in women, are linked more strongly to intraabdominal and/or upper body fat than to overall adiposity **(Chap. 63)**. The mechanism underlying this association is unknown but may relate to the fact that intraabdominal adipocytes are more lipolytically active than those from other depots. Release of free fatty acids into the portal circulation has adverse metabolic actions, especially on the liver. Adipokines and cytokines that are differentially secreted by adipocyte depots may play a role in the systemic complications of obesity.

PREVALENCE

Data from the National Health and Nutrition Examination Surveys (NHANES) show that the percentage of the American adult population with obesity (BMI >30)

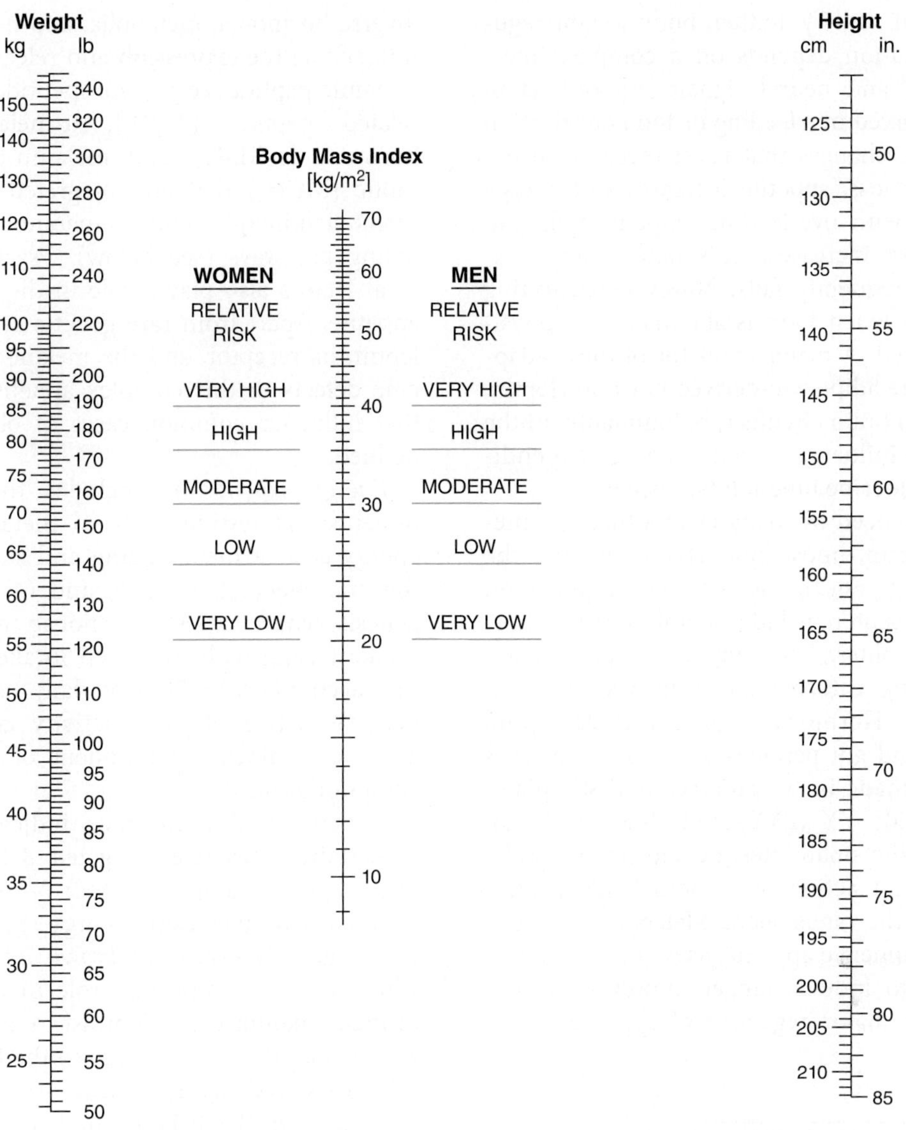

FIGURE 60-1

Nomogram for determining body mass index. To use this nomogram, place a ruler or other straight edge between the body weight (without clothes) in kilograms or pounds located on the left-hand line and the height (without shoes) in centimeters or inches located on the right-hand line. The body mass index is read from the middle of the scale and is in metric units. *(Copyright 1979, George A. Bray, MD; used with permission.)*

has increased from 14.5% (between 1976 and 1980) to 35.7% (between 2009 and 2010). As many as 68% of U.S. adults aged ≥20 years were overweight (defined as BMI >25) between the years of 2007 and 2008. Extreme obesity (BMI ≥40) has also increased and affects 5.7% of the population. The increasing prevalence of medically significant obesity raises great concern. Overall, the prevalence of obesity is comparable in men and women. In women, poverty is associated with increased prevalence. Obesity is more common among blacks and Hispanics. The prevalence in children and adolescents has been rising at a worrisome rate, reaching 15.9% in 2009/2010, but may be leveling off.

PHYSIOLOGIC REGULATION OF ENERGY BALANCE

Substantial evidence suggests that body weight is regulated by both endocrine and neural components that ultimately influence the effector arms of energy intake and expenditure. This complex regulatory system is necessary because even small imbalances between energy intake and expenditure will ultimately have large effects on body weight. For example, a 0.3% positive imbalance over 30 years would result in a 9-kg (20-lb) weight gain. This exquisite regulation of energy balance cannot be monitored easily by calorie-counting in relation to physical activity. Rather, body weight regulation or dysregulation depends on a complex interplay of hormonal and neural signals. Alterations in stable weight by forced overfeeding or food deprivation induce physiologic changes that resist these perturbations: with weight loss, appetite increases and energy expenditure falls; with overfeeding, appetite falls and energy expenditure increases. This latter compensatory mechanism frequently fails, however, permitting obesity to develop when food is abundant and physical activity is limited. A major regulator of these adaptive responses is the adipocyte-derived hormone leptin, which acts through brain circuits (predominantly in the hypothalamus) to influence appetite, energy expenditure, and neuroendocrine function (see below).

Appetite is influenced by many factors that are integrated by the brain, most importantly within the hypothalamus (Fig. 60-2). Signals that impinge on the hypothalamic center include neural afferents, hormones, and metabolites. Vagal inputs are particularly important, bringing information from viscera, such as gut distention. Hormonal signals include leptin, insulin, cortisol, and gut peptides. Among the latter is ghrelin, which is made in the stomach and stimulates feeding, and peptide YY (PYY) and cholecystokinin, which is made in the small intestine and signals to the brain through direct action on hypothalamic control centers and/or via the vagus nerve. Metabolites, including glucose, can influence appetite, as seen by the effect of hypoglycemia to induce hunger; however, glucose is not normally a major regulator of appetite. These diverse hormonal, metabolic, and neural signals act by influencing the expression and release of various hypothalamic peptides (e.g., neuropeptide Y [NPY], Agouti-related peptide [AgRP], α-melanocyte-stimulating hormone [α-MSH], and melanin-concentrating hormone [MCH]) that are integrated with serotonergic, catecholaminergic, endocannabinoid, and opioid signaling pathways (see below). Psychological and cultural factors also play a role in the final expression of appetite. Apart from rare genetic syndromes involving leptin, its receptor, and the melanocortin system, specific defects in this complex appetite control network that influence common cases of obesity are not well defined.

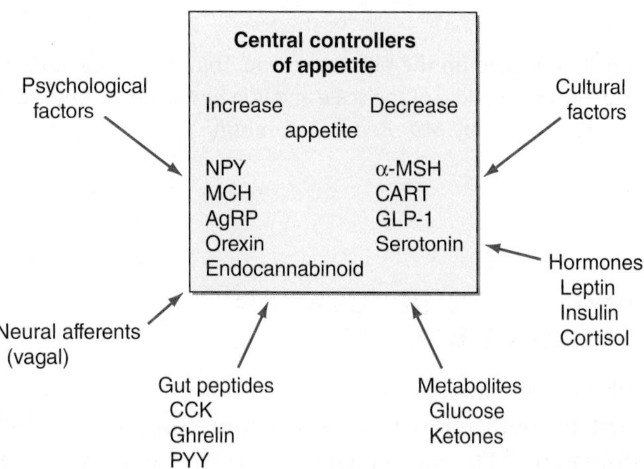

FIGURE 60-2

The factors that regulate appetite through effects on central neural circuits. Some factors that increase or decrease appetite are listed. AgRP, Agouti-related peptide; CART, cocaine- and amphetamine-related transcript; CCK, cholecystokinin; GLP-1, glucagon-related peptide-1; MCH, melanin-concentrating hormone; α-MSH, α-melanocyte-stimulating hormone; NPY, neuropeptide Y.

Energy expenditure includes the following components: (1) resting or basal metabolic rate; (2) the energy cost of metabolizing and storing food; (3) the thermic effect of exercise; and (4) adaptive thermogenesis, which varies in response to long-term caloric intake (rising with increased intake). Basal metabolic rate accounts for ~70% of daily energy expenditure, whereas active physical activity contributes 5–10%. Thus, a significant component of daily energy consumption is fixed.

Genetic models in mice indicate that mutations in certain genes (e.g., targeted deletion of the insulin receptor in adipose tissue) protect against obesity, apparently by increasing energy expenditure. Adaptive thermogenesis occurs in *brown adipose tissue* (BAT), which plays an important role in energy metabolism in many mammals. In contrast to white adipose tissue, which is used to store energy in the form of lipids, BAT expends stored energy as heat. A mitochondrial *uncoupling protein* (UCP-1) in BAT dissipates the hydrogen ion gradient in the oxidative respiration chain and releases energy as heat. The metabolic activity of BAT is increased by a central action of leptin, acting through the sympathetic nervous system that heavily innervates this tissue. In rodents, BAT deficiency causes obesity and diabetes; stimulation of BAT with a specific adrenergic agonist (β_3 agonist) protects against diabetes and obesity. BAT exists in humans (especially neonates), and although its physiologic role is not yet established, identification of functional BAT in many adults using positron emission tomography (PET) imaging has increased interest in the implications of the tissue for pathogenesis and therapy of obesity. Beige fat cells, recently described, resemble BAT cells in expressing UCP-1. They are scattered through white adipose tissue, and their thermogenic potential is uncertain.

THE ADIPOCYTE AND ADIPOSE TISSUE

Adipose tissue is composed of the lipid-storing adipose cell and a stromal/vascular compartment in which cells including preadipocytes and macrophages reside. Adipose mass increases by enlargement of adipose cells through lipid deposition, as well as by an increase in the number of adipocytes. Obese adipose tissue is also characterized by increased numbers of infiltrating macrophages. The process by which adipose cells are derived from a mesenchymal preadipocyte involves an orchestrated series of differentiation steps mediated by a cascade of specific transcription factors. One of the key transcription factors is *peroxisome proliferator-activated receptor γ* (PPARγ), a nuclear receptor that binds the thiazolidinedione class of insulin-sensitizing drugs used in the treatment of type 2 diabetes.

Although the adipocyte has generally been regarded as a storage depot for fat, it is also an endocrine cell that releases numerous molecules in a regulated fashion (Fig. 60-3). These include the energy balance–regulating hormone leptin, cytokines such as tumor necrosis factor (TNF)-α and interleukin (IL)-6, complement factors such as factor D (also known as *adipsin*), prothrombotic agents such as plasminogen activator inhibitor I, and a component of the blood pressure–regulating system, angiotensinogen. Adiponectin, an abundant adipose-derived protein whose levels are reduced in obesity, enhances insulin sensitivity and lipid oxidation and has vascular-protective effects, whereas resistin and RBP4, whose levels are increased in obesity, may induce insulin resistance. These factors, and others not yet identified, play a role in the physiology of lipid homeostasis, insulin sensitivity, blood pressure control, coagulation, and vascular health, and are likely to contribute to obesity-related pathologies.

ETIOLOGY OF OBESITY

Although the molecular pathways regulating energy balance are beginning to be illuminated, the causes of obesity remain elusive. In part, this reflects the fact that obesity is a heterogeneous group of disorders. At one level, the pathophysiology of obesity seems simple: a chronic excess of nutrient intake relative to the level of energy expenditure. However, due to the complexity of the neuroendocrine and metabolic systems that regulate energy intake, storage, and expenditure, it has been difficult to quantitate all the relevant parameters (e.g., food intake and energy expenditure) over time in human subjects.

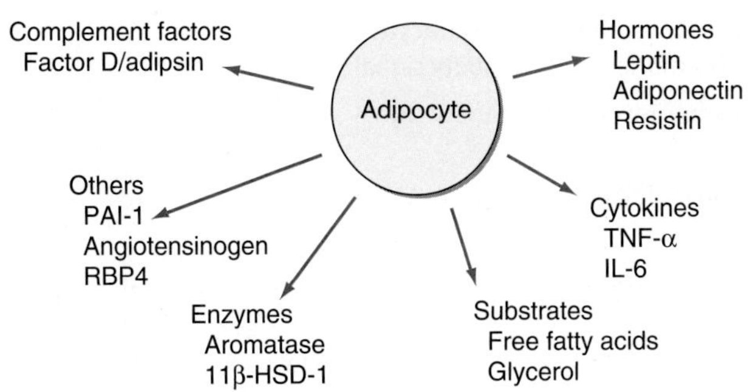

FIGURE 60-3

Factors released by the adipocyte that can affect peripheral tissues. IL-6, interleukin 6; PAI, plasminogen activator inhibitor; RBP4, retinal binding protein 4; TNF, tumor necrosis factor.

Role of genes versus environment

Obesity is commonly seen in families, and the heritability of body weight is similar to that for height. Inheritance is usually not Mendelian, however, and it is difficult to distinguish the role of genes and environmental factors. Adoptees more closely resemble their biologic than adoptive parents with respect to obesity, providing strong support for genetic influences. Likewise, identical twins have very similar BMIs whether reared together or apart, and their BMIs are much more strongly correlated than those of dizygotic twins. These genetic effects appear to relate to both energy intake and expenditure. Currently, identified genetic variants, both common and rare, account for less than 5% of the variance of body weight.

Whatever the role of genes, it is clear that the environment plays a key role in obesity, as evidenced by the fact that famine prevents obesity in even the most obesity-prone individual. In addition, the recent increase in the prevalence of obesity in the United States is far too rapid to be due to changes in the gene pool. Undoubtedly, genes influence the susceptibility to obesity in response to specific diets and availability of nutrition. Cultural factors are also important—these relate to both availability and composition of the diet and to changes in the level of physical activity. In industrial societies, obesity is more common among poor women, whereas in underdeveloped countries, wealthier women are more often obese. In children, obesity correlates to some degree with time spent watching television. Although the role of diet composition in obesity continues to generate controversy, it appears that high-fat diets may, when combined with simple, rapidly absorbed carbohydrates, promote obesity. Specific genes are likely to influence the response to specific diets, but these genes are largely unidentified.

Additional environmental factors may contribute to the increasing obesity prevalence. Both epidemiologic correlations and experimental data suggest that sleep deprivation leads to increased obesity. Changes in gut microbiome with capacity to alter energy balance are receiving experimental support from animal studies, and a possible role for obesigenic viral infections continues to receive sporadic attention.

Specific genetic syndromes

For many years, obesity in rodents has been known to be caused by a number of distinct mutations distributed through the genome. Most of these single-gene mutations cause both hyperphagia and diminished energy expenditure, suggesting a physiologic link between these two parameters of energy homeostasis. Identification of the *ob* gene mutation in genetically obese (ob/ob) mice represented a major breakthrough in the field. The ob/ob mouse develops severe obesity, insulin resistance, and hyperphagia, as well as efficient metabolism (e.g., it gets fat even when ingesting the same number of calories as lean litter mates). The product of the *ob* gene is the peptide leptin, a name derived from the Greek root *leptos*, meaning thin. Leptin is secreted by adipose cells and acts primarily through the hypothalamus. Its level of production provides an index of adipose energy stores (Fig. 60-4). High leptin levels decrease food intake and increase energy expenditure. Another mouse mutant, db/db, which is resistant to leptin, has a mutation in the leptin receptor and develops a similar syndrome. The *ob* gene is present in humans where it is also expressed in fat. Several families with morbid, early-onset obesity caused by inactivating mutations in either leptin or the leptin receptor have been described, thus demonstrating the biologic relevance of the leptin pathway in humans. Obesity in these individuals begins shortly after birth, is severe, and is accompanied by neuroendocrine abnormalities. The most prominent of these is hypogonadotropic hypogonadism, which is reversed by leptin replacement in the leptin-deficient subset. Central hypothyroidism and growth retardation are seen in the mouse model, but their occurrence in leptin-deficient humans is less clear. Mutations in the leptin or leptin receptor genes do not play a prominent role in common forms of obesity.

Mutations in several other genes cause severe obesity in humans (Table 60-1); each of these syndromes is rare. Mutations in the gene encoding proopiomelanocortin

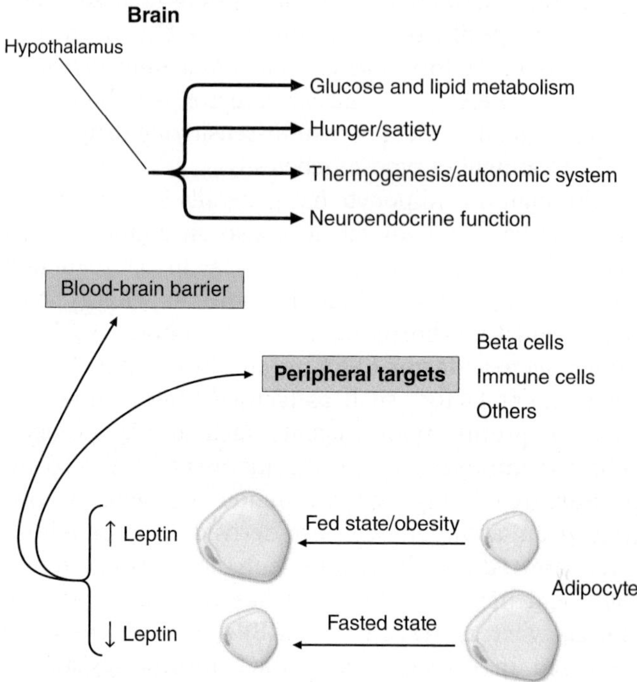

FIGURE 60-4
The physiologic system regulated by leptin. Rising or falling leptin levels act through the hypothalamus to influence appetite, energy expenditure, and neuroendocrine function and through peripheral sites to influence systems such as the immune system.

TABLE 60-1

SELECTED OBESITY GENES IN HUMANS AND MICE

GENE	GENE PRODUCT	MECHANISM OF OBESITY	IN HUMAN	IN RODENT
Lep (ob)	Leptin, a fat-derived hormone	Mutation prevents leptin from delivering satiety signal; brain perceives starvation	Yes	Yes
LepR (db)	Leptin receptor	Same as above	Yes	Yes
POMC	Proopiomelanocortin, a precursor of several hormones and neuropeptides	Mutation prevents synthesis of melanocyte-stimulating hormone (MSH), a satiety signal	Yes	Yes
MC4R	Type 4 receptor for MSH	Mutation prevents reception of satiety signal from MSH	Yes	Yes
AgRP	Agouti-related peptide, a neuropeptide expressed in the hypothalamus	Overexpression inhibits signal through *MC4R*	No	Yes
PC-1	Prohormone convertase 1, a processing enzyme	Mutation prevents synthesis of neuropeptide, probably MSH	Yes	No
Fat	Carboxypeptidase E, a processing enzyme	Same as above	No	Yes
Tub	Tub, a hypothalamic protein of unknown function	Hypothalamic dysfunction	No	Yes
TrkB	TrkB, a neurotrophin receptor	Hyperphagia due to uncharacterized hypothalamic defect	Yes	Yes

(POMC) cause severe obesity through failure to synthesize α-MSH, a key neuropeptide that inhibits appetite in the hypothalamus. The absence of POMC also causes secondary adrenal insufficiency due to absence of adrenocorticotropic hormone (ACTH), as well as pale skin and red hair due to absence of α-MSH. Proenzyme convertase 1 (PC-1) mutations are thought to cause obesity by preventing synthesis of α-MSH from its precursor peptide, POMC. α-MSH binds to the type 4 melanocortin receptor (MC4R), a key hypothalamic receptor that inhibits eating. Heterozygous loss-of-function mutations of this receptor account for as much as 5% of severe obesity. Loss of function of MRAP2, a protein required for normal MC4R signaling, has been found in rare cases of severe obesity. These six genetic defects define a pathway through which leptin (by stimulating POMC and increasing α-MSH) restricts food intake and limits weight (Fig. 60-5). The results of genomewide association studies to identify genetic loci responsible for obesity in the general population have so far been disappointing. More than 40 replicated loci linked to obesity have been identified, but together they account for less than 3% of interindividual variation in BMI. The most replicated of these is a gene named *FTO*, which is of unknown function, but like many of the other recently described candidates, is expressed in the brain. Because the heritability of obesity is estimated to be 40–70%, it is likely that many more loci remain to be identified. It is possible that epistatic interactions between causative loci or unknown gene-environment interactions explain the poor success at identifying causal loci.

In addition to these human obesity genes, studies in rodents reveal several other molecular candidates for hypothalamic mediators of human obesity or

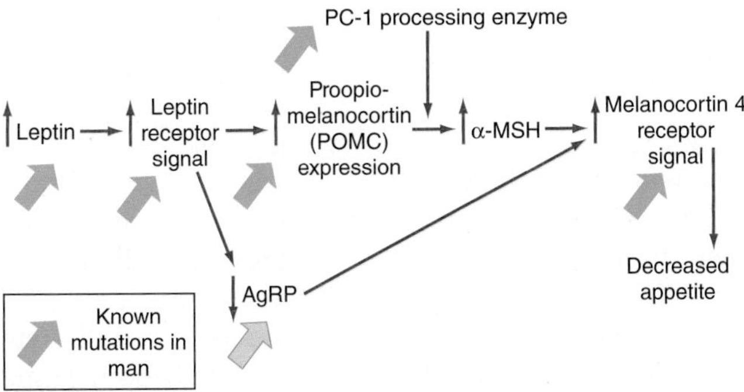

FIGURE 60-5
A central pathway through which leptin acts to regulate appetite and body weight. Leptin signals through proopiomelanocortin (POMC) neurons in the hypothalamus to induce increased production of α-melanocyte-stimulating hormone (α-MSH), requiring the processing enzyme PC-1 (proenzyme convertase 1). α-MSH acts as an agonist on melanocortin-4 receptors to inhibit appetite, and the neuropeptide AgRp (Agouti-related peptide) acts as an antagonist of this receptor. Mutations that cause obesity in humans are indicated by the *solid green arrows*.

leanness. The *tub* gene encodes a hypothalamic peptide of unknown function; mutation of this gene causes late-onset obesity. The *fat* gene encodes carboxypeptidase E, a peptide-processing enzyme; mutation of this gene is thought to cause obesity by disrupting production of one or more neuropeptides. AgRP is coexpressed with NPY in arcuate nucleus neurons. AgRP antagonizes α-MSH action at MC4 receptors, and its overexpression induces obesity. In contrast, a mouse deficient in the peptide MCH, whose administration causes feeding, is lean.

A number of complex human syndromes with defined inheritance are associated with obesity (Table 60-2). Although specific genes have limited definition at present, their identification will likely enhance our understanding of more common forms of human obesity. In the Prader-Willi syndrome, a multigenic neurodevelopmental disorder, obesity coexists with short stature, mental retardation, hypogonadotropic hypogonadism, hypotonia, small hands and feet, fish-shaped mouth, and hyperphagia. Most patients have reduced expression of imprinted paternally inherited genes encoded in the 15q11-13 chromosomal region. Reduced expression of Snord116, a small nucleolar RNA highly expressed in hypothalamus, may be an important cause of defective hypothalamic function in this disorder. Bardet-Biedl syndrome (BBS) is a genetically heterogeneous disorder characterized by obesity, mental retardation, retinitis pigmentosa, diabetes, renal and cardiac malformations, polydactyly, and hypogonadotropic hypogonadism. At least 12 genetic loci have been identified, and most of the encoded proteins form two multiprotein complexes that are involved in ciliary function and microtubule-based intracellular transport. Some evidence suggests that mutations might disrupt leptin receptor trafficking in key hypothalamic neurons, causing leptin resistance.

Other specific syndromes associated with obesity

Cushing's syndrome

Although obese patients commonly have central obesity, hypertension, and glucose intolerance, they lack other specific stigmata of Cushing's syndrome. Nonetheless, a potential diagnosis of Cushing's syndrome is often entertained. Cortisol production and urinary metabolites (17OH steroids) may be increased in simple obesity. Unlike in Cushing's syndrome, however, cortisol levels in blood and urine in the basal state and in response to corticotropin-releasing hormone (CRH) or ACTH are normal; the overnight 1-mg dexamethasone suppression test is normal in 90%, with the remainder being normal on a standard 2-day low-dose dexamethasone suppression test. Obesity may be associated with excessive local reactivation of cortisol in fat by

TABLE 60-2

A COMPARISON OF SYNDROMES OF OBESITY—HYPOGONADISM AND MENTAL RETARDATION

	SYNDROME				
FEATURE	**PRADER-WILLI**	**LAURENCE-MOON-BIEDL**	**AHLSTROM'S**	**COHEN'S**	**CARPENTER'S**
Inheritance	Sporadic; two-thirds have defect	Autosomal recessive	Autosomal recessive	Probably autosomal recessive	Autosomal recessive
Stature	Short	Normal; infrequently short	Normal; infrequently short	Short or tall	Normal
Obesity	Generalized	Generalized	Truncal	Truncal	Truncal, gluteal
	Moderate to severe	Early onset, 1–2 years	Early onset, 2–5 years	Mid-childhood, age 5	
	Onset 1–3 years				
Craniofacies	Narrow bifrontal diameter	Not distinctive	Not distinctive	High nasal bridge	Acrocephaly
	Almond-shaped eyes			Arched palate	Flat nasal bridge
	Strabismus			Open mouth	High-arched palate
	V-shaped mouth			Short philtrum	
	High-arched palate				
Limbs	Small hands and feet	Polydactyly	No abnormalities	Hypotonia	Polydactyly
	Hypotonia			Narrow hands and feet	Syndactyly
					Genu valgum
Reproductive status	1° Hypogonadism	1° Hypogonadism	Hypogonadism in males but not in females	Normal gonadal function or hypogonadotropic hypogonadism	2° Hypogonadism
Other features	Enamel hypoplasia			Dysplastic ears	
	Hyperphagia			Delayed puberty	
	Temper tantrums				
	Nasal speech				
Mental retardation	Mild to moderate		Normal intelligence	Mild	Slight

11β-hydroxysteroid dehydrogenase 1, an enzyme that converts inactive cortisone to cortisol.

Hypothyroidism

The possibility of hypothyroidism should be considered, but it is an uncommon cause of obesity; hypothyroidism is easily ruled out by measuring thyroid-stimulating hormone (TSH). Much of the weight gain that occurs in hypothyroidism is due to myxedema.

Insulinoma

Patients with insulinoma often gain weight as a result of overeating to avoid hypoglycemic symptoms. The increased substrate plus high insulin levels promote energy storage in fat. This can be marked in some individuals but is modest in most.

Craniopharyngioma and other disorders involving the hypothalamus

Whether through tumors, trauma, or inflammation, hypothalamic dysfunction of systems controlling satiety, hunger, and energy expenditure can cause varying degrees of obesity. It is uncommon to identify a discrete anatomic basis for these disorders. Subtle hypothalamic dysfunction is probably a more common cause of obesity than can be documented using currently available imaging techniques. Growth hormone (GH), which exerts lipolytic activity, is diminished in obesity and is increased with weight loss. Despite low GH levels, insulin-like growth factor (IGF) I (somatomedin) production is normal, suggesting that GH suppression may be a compensatory response to increased nutritional supply.

Pathogenesis of common obesity

Obesity can result from increased energy intake, decreased energy expenditure, or a combination of the two. Thus, identifying the etiology of obesity should involve measurements of both parameters. However, it is difficult to perform direct and accurate measurements of energy intake in free-living individuals; and the obese, in particular, often underreport intake. Measurements of chronic energy expenditure are possible using doubly labeled water or metabolic chamber/rooms. In subjects at stable weight and body composition, energy intake equals expenditure. Consequently, these techniques allow assessment of energy intake in free-living individuals. The level of energy expenditure differs in established obesity, during periods of weight gain or loss, and in the pre- or postobese state. Studies that fail to take note of this phenomenon are not easily interpreted.

There is continued interest in the concept of a body weight "set point." This idea is supported by physiologic mechanisms centered around a sensing system in adipose tissue that reflects fat stores and a receptor, or "adipostat," that is in the hypothalamic centers. When fat stores are depleted, the adipostat signal is low, and the hypothalamus responds by stimulating hunger and decreasing energy expenditure to conserve energy. Conversely, when fat stores are abundant, the signal is increased, and the hypothalamus responds by decreasing hunger and increasing energy expenditure. The recent discovery of the *ob* gene, and its product leptin, and the *db* gene, whose product is the leptin receptor, provides important elements of a molecular basis for this physiologic concept (see above).

What is the status of food intake in obesity? (do the obese eat more than the lean?)

This question has stimulated much debate, due in part to the methodologic difficulties inherent in determining food intake. Many obese individuals believe that they eat small quantities of food, and this claim has often been supported by the results of food intake questionnaires. However, it is now established that average energy expenditure increases as individuals get more obese, due primarily to the fact that metabolically active lean tissue mass increases with obesity. Given the laws of thermodynamics, the obese person must therefore eat more than the average lean person to maintain their increased weight. It may be the case, however, that a subset of individuals who are predisposed to obesity have the capacity to become obese initially without an absolute increase in caloric consumption.

What is the state of energy expenditure in obesity?

The average total daily energy expenditure is higher in obese than lean individuals when measured at stable weight. However, energy expenditure falls as weight is lost, due in part to loss of lean body mass and to decreased sympathetic nerve activity. When reduced to near-normal weight and maintained there for a while, (some) obese individuals have lower energy expenditure than (some) lean individuals. There is also a tendency for those who will develop obesity as infants or children to have lower resting energy expenditure rates than those who remain lean. The physiologic basis for variable rates of energy expenditure (at a given body weight and level of energy intake) is essentially unknown.

Another component of thermogenesis, called *nonexercise activity thermogenesis* (NEAT), has been linked to obesity. It is the thermogenesis that accompanies physical activities other than volitional exercise such as the activities of daily living, fidgeting, spontaneous muscle contraction, and maintaining posture. NEAT accounts for about two-thirds of the increased daily energy expenditure induced by overfeeding. The wide variation in fat storage seen in overfed individuals is predicted by the degree to which NEAT is induced. The molecular basis for NEAT and its regulation is unknown.

Leptin in typical obesity

The vast majority of obese persons have increased leptin levels but do not have mutations of either leptin or its receptor. They appear, therefore, to have a form of functional "leptin resistance." Data suggesting that some individuals produce less leptin per unit fat mass than others or have a form of relative leptin deficiency that predisposes to obesity are at present contradictory and unsettled. The mechanism for leptin resistance, and whether it can be overcome by raising leptin levels or combining leptin with other treatments in a subset of obese individuals, is not yet established. Some data suggest that leptin may not effectively cross the blood-brain barrier as levels rise. It is also apparent from animal studies that leptin-signaling inhibitors, such as SOCS3 and PTP1b, are involved in the leptin-resistant state.

PATHOLOGIC CONSEQUENCES OF OBESITY

(See also Chap. 61) Obesity has major adverse effects on health. Obesity is associated with an increase in mortality, with a 50–100% increased risk of death from all causes compared to normal-weight individuals, mostly due to cardiovascular causes. Obesity and overweight together are the second leading cause of preventable death in the United States, accounting for 300,000 deaths per year. Mortality rates rise as obesity increases, particularly when obesity is associated with increased intraabdominal fat (see above). Life expectancy of a moderately obese individual could be shortened by 2–5 years, and a 20- to 30-year-old male with a BMI >45 may lose 13 years of life. It is likely that the degree to which obesity affects particular organ systems is influenced by susceptibility genes that vary in the population.

Insulin resistance and type 2 diabetes mellitus

Hyperinsulinemia and insulin resistance are pervasive features of obesity, increasing with weight gain and diminishing with weight loss **(Chap. 63)**. Insulin resistance is more strongly linked to intraabdominal fat than to fat in other depots. Molecular links between obesity and insulin resistance in fat, muscle, and liver have been sought for many years. Major factors include: (1) insulin itself, by inducing receptor downregulation; (2) free fatty acids that are increased and capable of impairing insulin action; (3) intracellular lipid accumulation; and (4) several circulating peptides produced by adipocytes, including the cytokines TNF-α and IL-6, RBP4, and the "adipokines" adiponectin and resistin, which have altered expression in obese adipocytes and can modify insulin action. Additional mechanisms are obesity-linked inflammation, including infiltration of macrophages into tissues including fat, and induction of the endoplasmic reticulum stress response, which can bring about resistance to insulin action in cells. Despite the prevalence of insulin resistance, most obese individuals do not develop diabetes, suggesting that diabetes requires an interaction between obesity-induced insulin resistance and other factors such as impaired insulin secretion. Obesity, however, is a major risk factor for diabetes, and as many as 80% of patients with type 2 diabetes mellitus are obese. Weight loss and exercise, even of modest degree, increase insulin sensitivity and often improve glucose control in diabetes.

Reproductive disorders

Disorders that affect the reproductive axis are associated with obesity in both men and women. Male hypogonadism is associated with increased adipose tissue, often distributed in a pattern more typical of females. In men whose weight is >160% ideal body weight (IBW), plasma testosterone and sex hormone–binding globulin (SHBG) are often reduced, and estrogen levels (derived from conversion of adrenal androgens in adipose tissue) are increased. Gynecomastia may be seen. However, masculinization, libido, potency, and spermatogenesis are preserved in most of these individuals. Free testosterone may be decreased in morbidly obese men whose weight is >200% IBW.

Obesity has long been associated with menstrual abnormalities in women, particularly in women with upper body obesity. Common findings are increased androgen production, decreased SHBG, and increased peripheral conversion of androgen to estrogen. Most obese women with oligomenorrhea have polycystic ovarian syndrome (PCOS), with its associated anovulation and ovarian hyperandrogenism; 40% of women with PCOS are obese. Most nonobese women with PCOS are also insulin-resistant, suggesting that insulin resistance, hyperinsulinemia, or the combination of the two are causative or contribute to the ovarian pathophysiology in PCOS in both obese and lean individuals. Increasing evidence supports a role for adipokines in mediating a link between obesity and the reproductive dysfunction of PCOS. In obese women with PCOS, weight loss or treatment with insulin-sensitizing drugs often restores normal menses. The increased conversion of androstenedione to estrogen, which occurs to a greater degree in women with lower body obesity, may contribute to the increased incidence of uterine cancer in postmenopausal women with obesity.

Cardiovascular disease

The Framingham Study revealed that obesity was an independent risk factor for the 26-year incidence of cardiovascular disease in men and women (including coronary disease, stroke, and congestive heart failure). The waist-to-hip ratio may be the best predictor of these risks. When the additional effects of hypertension and glucose intolerance associated with obesity are included, the adverse impact of obesity is even more evident. The effect of obesity on cardiovascular mortality in women may be seen at BMIs as low as 25. Obesity, especially abdominal obesity, is associated with an atherogenic lipid profile; with increased low-density lipoprotein cholesterol, very-low-density lipoprotein, and triglyceride; and with decreased high-density lipoprotein cholesterol and decreased levels of the vascular protective adipokine adiponectin. Obesity is also associated with hypertension. Measurement of blood pressure in the obese requires use of a larger cuff size to avoid artifactual increases. Obesity-induced hypertension is associated with increased peripheral resistance and cardiac output, increased sympathetic nervous system tone, increased salt sensitivity, and insulin-mediated salt retention; it is often responsive to modest weight loss.

Pulmonary disease

Obesity may be associated with a number of pulmonary abnormalities. These include reduced chest wall compliance, increased work of breathing, increased minute ventilation due to increased metabolic rate, and decreased functional residual capacity and expiratory reserve volume. Severe obesity may be associated with obstructive sleep apnea and the "obesity hypoventilation syndrome" with attenuated hypoxic and hypercapnic ventilatory responses. Sleep apnea can be obstructive (most common), central, or mixed and is associated with hypertension. Weight loss (10–20 kg) can bring substantial improvement, as can major weight loss following gastric bypass or restrictive surgery. Continuous positive airway pressure has been used with some success.

Hepatobiliary disease

Obesity is frequently associated with nonalcoholic fatty liver disease (NAFLD), and this association represents one of the most common causes of liver disease in industrialized countries. The hepatic fatty infiltration of NAFLD progresses in a subset to inflammatory nonalcoholic steatohepatitis (NASH) and more rarely to cirrhosis and hepatocellular carcinoma. Steatosis typically improves following weight loss, secondary to diet or bariatric surgery. The mechanism for the association remains unclear. Obesity is associated with enhanced biliary secretion of cholesterol, supersaturation of bile, and a higher incidence of gallstones, particularly cholesterol gallstones **(Chap. 47)**. A person 50% above IBW has about a sixfold increased incidence of symptomatic gallstones. Paradoxically, fasting increases supersaturation of bile by decreasing the phospholipid component. Fasting-induced cholecystitis is a complication of extreme diets.

Cancer

Obesity is associated with increased risk of several cancer types, and in addition can lead to poorer treatment outcomes and increased cancer mortality. Obesity in males is associated with higher mortality from cancer of the esophagus, colon, rectum, pancreas, liver, and prostate; obesity in females is associated with higher mortality from cancer of the gallbladder, bile ducts, breasts, endometrium, cervix, and ovaries. Some of the latter may be due to increased rates of conversion of androstenedione to estrone in adipose tissue of obese individuals. Other possible mechanistic links may involve hormones, growth factors, and cytokines whose levels are linked to nutritional state, including insulin, leptin, adiponectin, and IGF-I, as well as activation of signaling pathways linked to both obesity and cancer. It has been estimated that obesity accounts for 14% of cancer deaths in men and 20% in women in the United States.

Bone, joint, and cutaneous disease

Obesity is associated with an increased risk of osteoarthritis, no doubt partly due to the trauma of added weight bearing, but potentially linked as well to activation of inflammatory pathways that could promote synovial pathology. The prevalence of gout may also be increased. One of the skin problems associated with obesity is acanthosis nigricans, manifested by darkening and thickening of the skinfolds on the neck, elbows, and dorsal interphalangeal spaces. Acanthosis reflects the severity of underlying insulin resistance and diminishes with weight loss. Friability of skin may be increased, especially in skinfolds, enhancing the risk of fungal and yeast infections. Finally, venous stasis is increased in the obese.

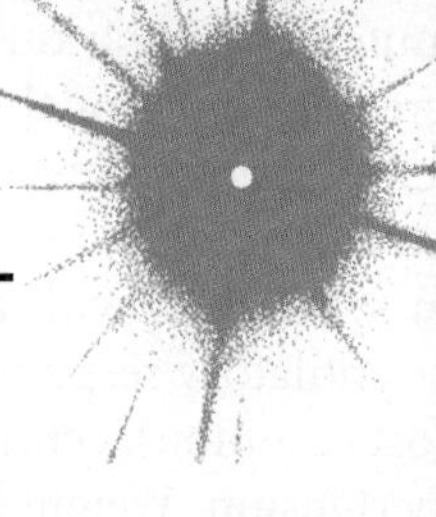

CHAPTER 61

EVALUATION AND MANAGEMENT OF OBESITY

Robert F. Kushner

More than 66% of U.S. adults are categorized as overweight or obese, and the prevalence of obesity is increasing rapidly in most of the industrialized world. Children and adolescents also are becoming more obese, indicating that the current trends will accelerate over time. Obesity is associated with an increased risk of multiple health problems, including hypertension, type 2 diabetes, dyslipidemia, obstructive sleep apnea, nonalcoholic fatty liver disease, degenerative joint disease, and some malignancies. Thus, it is important for physicians to identify, evaluate, and treat patients for obesity and associated comorbid conditions.

EVALUATION

Physicians should screen all adult patients for obesity and offer intensive counseling and behavioral interventions to promote sustained weight loss. The five main steps in the evaluation of obesity, as described below, are (1) a focused obesity-related history, (2) a physical examination to determine the degree and type of obesity, (3) assessment of comorbid conditions, (4) determination of fitness level, and (5) assessment of the patient's readiness to adopt lifestyle changes.

The obesity-focused history

Information from the history should address the following seven questions:

- What factors contribute to the patient's obesity?
- How is the obesity affecting the patient's health?
- What is the patient's level of risk from obesity?
- What does the patient find difficult about managing weight?
- What are the patient's goals and expectations?
- Is the patient motivated to begin a weight management program?
- What kind of help does the patient need?

Although the vast majority of cases of obesity can be attributed to behavioral factors that affect diet and physical activity patterns, the history may suggest secondary causes that merit further evaluation. Disorders to consider include polycystic ovarian syndrome, hypothyroidism, Cushing's syndrome, and hypothalamic disease. Drug-induced weight gain also should be considered. Common causes include medications for diabetes (insulin, sulfonylureas, thiazolidinediones); steroid hormones; psychotropic agents; mood stabilizers (lithium); antidepressants (tricyclics, monoamine oxidase inhibitors, paroxetine, mirtazapine); and antiepileptic drugs (valproate, gabapentin, carbamazepine). Other medications, such as nonsteroidal anti-inflammatory drugs and calcium channel blockers, may cause peripheral edema but do not increase body fat.

The patient's current diet and physical activity patterns may reveal factors that contribute to the development of obesity and may identify behaviors to target for treatment. This type of historic information is best obtained by the combination of a questionnaire and an interview.

Body mass index (BMI) and waist circumference

Three key anthropometric measurements are important in evaluating the degree of obesity: weight, height, and waist circumference. The BMI, calculated as weight (kg)/height (m)^2 or as weight (lbs)/height (inches)^2 × 703, is used to classify weight status and risk of disease (Tables 61-1 and 61-2). BMI provides an estimate of body fat and is related to disease risk. Lower BMI thresholds for overweight and obesity have been

TABLE 61-1

BODY MASS INDEX (BMI)

BMI	19	20	21	22	23	24	25	26	27	28	29	30	31	32	33	34	35
HEIGHT (INCHES)	**BODY WEIGHT (POUNDS)**																
58	91	96	100	105	110	115	119	124	129	134	138	143	148	153	158	162	167
59	94	99	104	109	114	119	124	128	133	138	143	148	153	158	163	168	173
60	97	102	107	112	118	123	128	133	138	143	148	153	158	163	168	174	179
61	100	106	111	116	122	127	132	137	143	148	153	158	164	169	174	180	185
62	104	109	115	120	126	131	136	142	147	153	158	164	169	175	180	186	191
63	107	113	118	124	130	135	141	146	152	158	163	169	175	180	186	191	197
64	110	116	122	128	134	140	145	151	157	163	169	174	180	186	192	197	204
65	114	120	126	132	138	144	150	156	162	168	174	180	186	192	198	204	210
66	118	124	130	136	142	148	155	161	167	173	179	186	192	198	204	210	216
67	121	127	134	140	146	153	159	166	172	178	185	191	198	204	211	217	223
68	125	131	138	144	151	158	164	171	177	184	190	197	203	210	216	223	230
69	128	135	142	149	155	162	169	176	182	189	196	203	209	216	223	230	236
70	132	139	146	153	160	167	174	181	188	195	202	209	216	222	229	236	243
71	136	143	150	157	165	172	179	186	193	200	208	215	222	229	236	243	250
72	140	147	154	162	169	177	184	191	199	206	213	221	228	235	242	250	258
73	144	151	159	166	174	182	189	197	204	212	219	227	235	242	250	257	265
74	148	155	163	171	179	186	194	202	210	218	225	233	241	249	256	264	272
75	152	160	168	176	184	192	200	208	216	224	232	240	248	256	264	272	279
76	156	164	172	180	189	197	205	213	221	230	238	246	254	263	271	279	287

BMI	36	37	38	39	40	41	42	43	44	45	46	47	48	49	50	51	52	53	54
58	172	177	181	186	191	196	201	205	210	215	220	224	229	234	239	244	248	253	258
59	178	183	188	193	198	203	208	212	217	222	227	232	237	242	247	252	257	262	267
60	184	189	194	199	204	209	215	220	225	230	235	240	245	250	255	261	266	271	276
61	190	195	201	206	211	217	222	227	232	238	243	248	254	259	264	269	275	280	285
62	196	202	207	213	218	224	229	235	240	246	251	256	262	267	273	278	284	289	295
63	203	208	214	220	225	231	237	242	248	254	259	265	270	278	282	287	293	299	304
64	209	215	221	227	232	238	244	250	256	262	267	273	279	285	291	296	302	308	314
65	216	222	228	234	240	246	252	258	264	270	276	282	288	294	300	306	312	318	324
66	223	229	235	241	247	253	260	266	272	278	284	291	297	303	309	315	322	328	334
67	230	236	242	249	255	261	268	274	280	287	293	299	306	312	319	325	331	338	344
68	236	243	249	256	262	269	276	282	289	295	302	308	315	322	328	335	341	348	354
69	243	250	257	263	270	277	284	291	297	304	311	318	324	331	338	345	351	358	365
70	250	257	264	271	278	285	292	299	306	313	320	327	334	341	348	355	362	369	376
71	257	265	272	279	286	293	301	308	315	322	329	338	343	351	358	365	372	379	386
72	265	272	279	287	294	302	309	316	324	331	338	346	353	361	368	375	383	390	397
73	272	280	288	295	302	310	318	325	333	340	348	355	363	371	378	386	393	401	408
74	280	287	295	303	311	319	326	334	342	350	358	365	373	381	389	396	404	412	420
75	287	295	303	311	319	327	335	343	351	359	367	375	383	391	399	407	415	423	431
76	295	304	312	320	328	336	344	353	361	369	377	385	394	402	410	418	426	435	443

TABLE 61-2

CLASSIFICATION OF WEIGHT STATUS AND DISEASE RISK

CLASSIFICATION	BODY MASS INDEX (KG/M²)	OBESITY CLASS	DISEASE RISK
Underweight	<18.5	—	—
Healthy weight	18.5–24.9	—	—
Overweight	25.0–29.9	—	Increased
Obesity	30.0–34.9	I	High
Obesity	35.0–39.9	II	Very high
Extreme obesity	≥40	III	Extremely high

Source: Adapted from the National Institutes of Health, National Heart, Lung, and Blood Institute: *Clinical Guidelines on the Identification, Evaluation, and Treatment of Overweight and Obesity in Adults.* U.S. Department of Health and Human Services, U.S. Public Health Service, 1998.

proposed for the Asia-Pacific region since this population appears to be at risk for glucose and lipid abnormalities at lower body weights.

Excess abdominal fat, assessed by measurement of waist circumference or waist-to-hip ratio, is independently associated with a higher risk for diabetes mellitus and cardiovascular disease. Measurement of the waist circumference is a surrogate for visceral adipose tissue and should be performed in the horizontal plane above the iliac crest (Table 61-3).

TABLE 61-3

ETHNIC-SPECIFIC CUTPOINT VALUES FOR WAIST CIRCUMFERENCE

ETHNIC GROUP	WAIST CIRCUMFERENCE
Europeans	
Men	>94 cm (>37 in)
Women	>80 cm (>31.5 in)
South Asians and Chinese	
Men	>90 cm (>35 in)
Women	>80 cm (>31.5 in)
Japanese	
Men	>85 cm (>33.5 in)
Women	>90 cm (>35 in)
Ethnic South and Central Americans	Use South Asian recommendations until more specific data are available.
Sub-Saharan Africans	Use European data until more specific data are available.
Eastern Mediterranean and Middle Eastern (Arab) populations	Use European data until more specific data are available.

Source: From KGMM Alberti et al for the IDF Epidemiology Task Force Consensus Group: Lancet 366:1059, 2005.

Physical fitness

Several prospective studies have demonstrated that physical fitness, reported by questionnaire or measured by a maximal treadmill exercise test, is an important predictor of all-cause mortality rate independent of BMI and body composition. These observations highlight the importance of taking a physical activity and exercise history during examination as well as emphasizing physical activity as a treatment approach.

Obesity-associated comorbid conditions

The evaluation of comorbid conditions should be based on presentation of symptoms, risk factors, and index of suspicion. For all patients, a fasting lipid panel should be performed (total, low-density lipoprotein, and high-density lipoprotein cholesterol and triglyceride levels) and a fasting blood glucose level and blood pressure determined. Symptoms and diseases that are directly or indirectly related to obesity are listed in Table 61-4. Although individuals vary, the number and severity of organ-specific comorbid conditions usually rise with increasing levels of obesity. Patients at very high absolute risk include those with the following: established coronary heart disease; presence of other atherosclerotic diseases, such as peripheral arterial disease, abdominal aortic aneurysm, and symptomatic carotid artery disease; type 2 diabetes; and sleep apnea.

Assessing the patient's readiness to change

An attempt to initiate lifestyle changes when the patient is not ready usually leads to frustration and may hamper future weight-loss efforts. Assessment includes patient motivation and support, stressful life events, psychiatric status, time availability and constraints, and appropriateness of goals and expectations. Readiness can be viewed as the balance of two opposing forces: (1) motivation, or the patient's desire to change; and (2) resistance, or the patient's resistance to change.

A helpful method to begin a readiness assessment is to use the motivational interviewing technique of "anchoring" the patient's interest and confidence to change on a numerical scale. With this technique, the patient is asked to rate—on a scale from 0 to 10, with 0 being not so important (or confident) and 10 being very important (or confident)—his or her level of interest in and confidence about losing weight at this time. This exercise helps establish readiness to change and also serves as a basis for further dialogue.

TABLE 61-4

OBESITY-RELATED ORGAN SYSTEMS REVIEW

Cardiovascular	**Respiratory**
Hypertension	Dyspnea
Congestive heart failure	Obstructive sleep apnea
Cor pulmonale	Hypoventilation syndrome
Varicose veins	Pickwickian syndrome
Pulmonary embolism	Asthma
Coronary artery disease	
Endocrine	**Gastrointestinal**
Metabolic syndrome	Gastroesophageal reflux disease
Type 2 diabetes	Nonalcoholic fatty-liver disease
Dyslipidemia	Cholelithiasis
	Hernias
	Colon cancer
Musculoskeletal	**Genitourinary**
Hyperuricemia and gout	Urinary stress incontinence
Immobility	Obesity-related glomerulopathy
Osteoarthritis (knees and hips)	Hypogonadism (male)
Low back pain	Breast and uterine cancer
Carpal tunnel syndrome	Pregnancy complications
Psychological	**Neurologic**
Depression/low self-esteem	Stroke
Body image disturbance	Idiopathic intracranial hypertension
Social stigmatization	Meralgia paresthetica
Integument	Dementia
Striae distensae	
Stasis pigmentation of legs	
Lymphedema	
Cellulitis	
Intertrigo, carbuncles	
Acanthosis nigricans	
Acrochordons (skin tags)	
Hidradenitis suppurativa	

TREATMENT Obesity

THE GOAL OF THERAPY The primary goals of treatment are to improve obesity-related comorbid conditions and to reduce the risk of developing future comorbidities. Information obtained from the history, physical examination, and diagnostic tests is used to determine risk and develop a treatment plan (Fig. 61-1). The decision of how aggressively to treat the patient and which modalities to use is determined by the patient's risk status, expectations, and available resources. Not all patients who are deemed obese by BMI alone need to be treated, as exemplified by the concepts of obesity paradox or the metabolically healthy obese. However, patients who present with obesity-related comorbidities and who would benefit from weight loss intervention should be managed proactively. Therapy for obesity always begins with lifestyle management and may include pharmacotherapy or surgery, depending on BMI risk category (Table 61-5). Setting an initial weight-loss goal of 8–10% over 6 months is a realistic target.

LIFESTYLE MANAGEMENT Obesity care involves attention to three essential elements of lifestyle: dietary habits, physical activity, and behavior modification. Because obesity is fundamentally a disease of energy imbalance, all patients must learn how and when energy is consumed (diet), how and when energy is expended (physical activity), and how to incorporate this information into their daily lives (behavioral therapy). Lifestyle management has been shown to result in a modest (typically 3–5 kg) weight loss when compared with no treatment or usual care.

Diet Therapy The primary focus of diet therapy is to reduce overall calorie consumption. Guidelines from the National Heart, Lung, and Blood Institute recommend initiating treatment with a calorie deficit of 500–1000 kcal/d compared with the patient's habitual diet. This reduction is consistent with a goal of losing ~1–2 lbs per week. The calorie deficit can be instituted through dietary substitutions or alternatives. Examples include choosing smaller portion sizes, eating more fruits and vegetables, consuming more whole-grain cereals, selecting leaner cuts of meat and skimmed dairy products, reducing consumption of fried foods and other foods with added fats and oils, and drinking water instead of sugar-sweetened beverages. It is important that dietary counseling remain patient centered and that the goals set be practical, realistic, and achievable.

The macronutrient composition of the diet will vary with the patient's preference and medical condition. The 2010 U.S. Department of Agriculture Dietary Guidelines for Americans **(Chap. 56)**, which focus on health promotion and risk reduction, can be applied to treatment of overweight or obese patients. The recommendations include maintaining a diet rich in whole grains, fruits, vegetables, and dietary fiber; consuming two servings (8 oz) of fish high in omega 3 fatty acids per week; decreasing sodium intake to <2300 mg/d; consuming 3 cups of milk (or equivalent low-fat or fat-free dairy products) per day; limiting cholesterol intake to <300 mg/d; and keeping total fat intake at 20–35% of daily calories and saturated fat intake at <10% of daily calories. Application of these guidelines to specific calorie goals can be found on the website *www.choosemyplate.gov*. The revised Dietary Reference Intakes for Macronutrients released by the Institute of Medicine recommends that 45–65% of calories come from carbohydrates, 20–35% from fat, and 10–35% from protein. The guidelines also recommend daily fiber intake of 38 g (men) and 25 g (women) for persons over 50 years of age and 30 g (men) and 21 g (women) for those under age 50.

Since portion control is one of the most difficult strategies for patients to manage, the use of pre-prepared products such as meal replacements is a simple and convenient suggestion. Examples include frozen entrees, canned beverages, and bars.

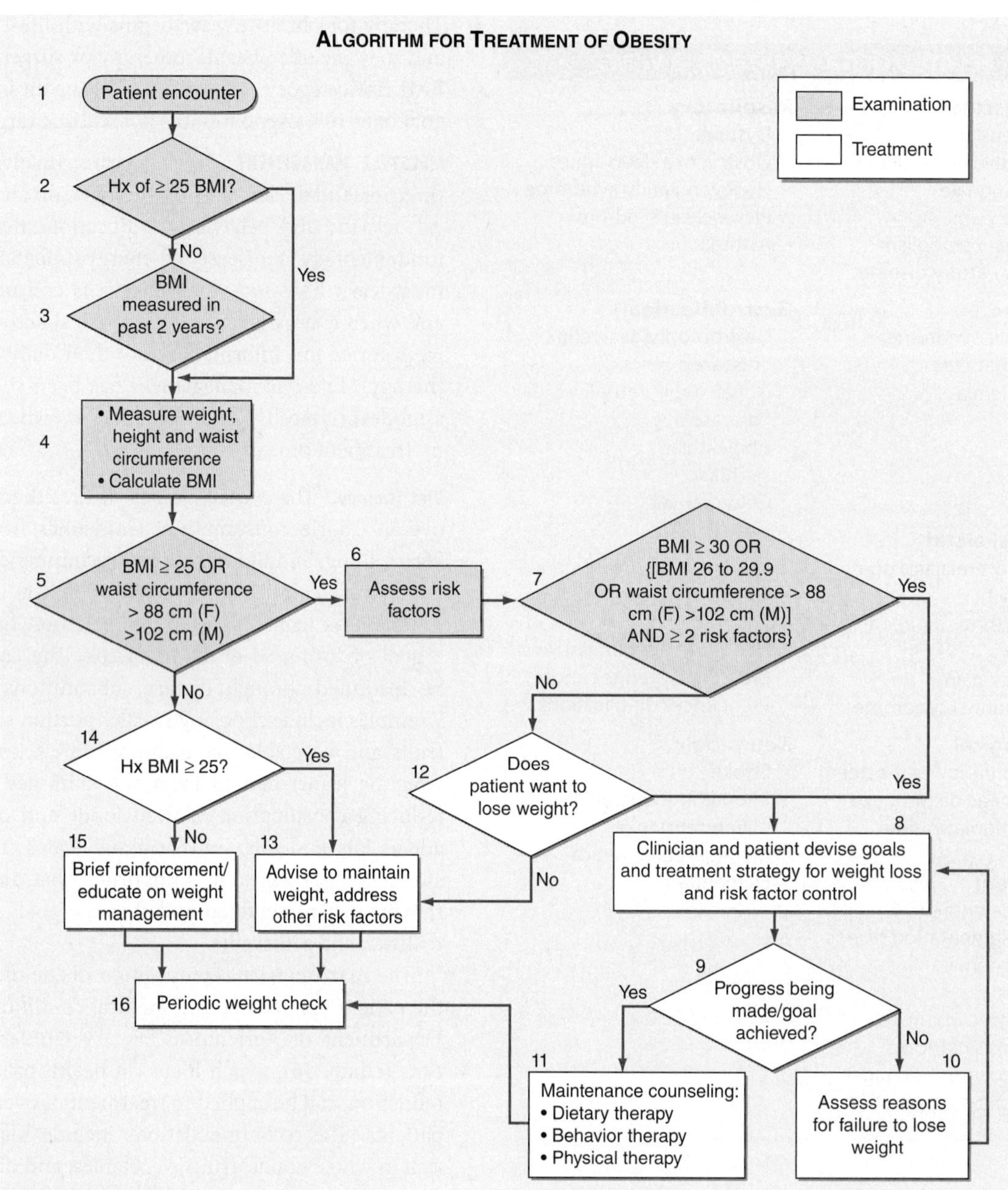

FIGURE 61-1

Algorithm for the treatment of obesity. This algorithm applies only to assessment for overweight and obesity and subsequent decisions based on that assessment. It does not reflect initial overall assessment for other conditions that the physician may wish to perform. BMI, body mass index; Hx, history. *(From the National, Heart, Lung, and Blood Institute: Clinical guidelines on the identification, evaluation, and treatment of overweight and obesity in adults: The evidence report. Washington, DC, US Department of Health and Human Services, 1998.)*

Use of meal replacements in the diet has been shown to result in a 7–8% weight loss.

Numerous randomized trials comparing diets of different macronutrient composition (e.g., low-carbohydrate, low-fat, Mediterranean) have shown that weight loss depends primarily on reduction of total caloric intake and adherence to the prescribed diet, not the specific proportions of carbohydrate, fat, and protein in the diet. The macronutrient composition will ultimately be determined by the patient's taste preferences, cooking style, and culture. However, the patient's underlying medical problems are also important in guiding the recommended dietary composition. The dietary prescription will vary according to the patient's metabolic profile and risk factors. A consultation with a registered dietitian for medical nutrition therapy is particularly useful in considering patient preference and treatment of comorbid diseases.

Another dietary approach to consider is based on the concept of *energy density*, which refers to the number of calories (i.e., amount of energy) a food contains per unit of weight. People tend to ingest a constant volume of food regardless

TABLE 61-5

A GUIDE TO OPTING FOR TREATMENT FOR OBESITY

	BMI CATEGORY (KG/M²)				
Treatment	**25–26.9**	**27–29.9**	**30–34.9**	**35–39.9**	**≥40**
Diet, exercise, behavioral therapy	With comorbidities	With comorbidities	+	+	+
Pharmacotherapy	—	With comorbidities	+	+	+
Surgery	—	—	—	With comorbidities	+

Source: From the National Heart, Lung, and Blood Institute, North American Association for the Study of Obesity (2000).

of caloric or macronutrient content. Adding water or fiber to a food decreases its energy density by increasing weight without affecting caloric content. Examples of foods with low-energy density include soups, fruits, vegetables, oatmeal, and lean meats. Dry foods and high-fat foods such as pretzels, cheese, egg yolks, potato chips, and red meat have a high-energy density. Diets containing low-energy-dense foods have been shown to control hunger and thus to result in decreased caloric intake and weight loss.

Occasionally, very low-calorie diets (VLCDs) are prescribed as a form of aggressive dietary therapy. The primary purpose of a VLCD is to promote a rapid and significant (13- to 23-kg) short-term weight loss over a 3- to 6-month period. The proprietary formulas designed for this purpose typically supply ≤800 kcal, 50–80 g of protein, and 100% of the recommended daily intake for vitamins and minerals. According to a review by the National Task Force on the Prevention and Treatment of Obesity, indications for initiating a VLCD include the involvement of well-motivated individuals who are moderately to severely obese (BMI, >30 kg/m^2), have failed at more conservative approaches to weight loss, and have a medical condition that would be immediately improved with rapid weight loss. These conditions include poorly controlled type 2 diabetes, hypertriglyceridemia, obstructive sleep apnea, and symptomatic peripheral edema. The risk for gallstone formation increases exponentially at rates of weight loss >1.5 kg/week (3.3 lb/week). Prophylaxis against gallstone formation with ursodeoxycholic acid (600 mg/d) is effective in reducing this risk. Because of the need for close metabolic monitoring, VLCDs usually are prescribed by physicians specializing in obesity care.

Physical Activity Therapy Although exercise alone is only moderately effective for weight loss, the combination of dietary modification and exercise is the most effective behavioral approach for the treatment of obesity. The most important role of exercise appears to be in the maintenance of the weight loss. The 2008 Physical Activity Guidelines for Americans (*www.health.gov/paguidelines*) recommend that adults should engage in 150 min of moderate-intensity or 75 min a week of vigorous-intensity aerobic physical activity per week, performed in episodes of at least 10 min and preferably spread throughout the week. Focusing on simple ways to add physical activity into the normal daily routine through leisure activities, travel, and domestic work should be suggested. Examples include walking, using the stairs, doing housework and yard work, and engaging in sports. Asking the patient to wear a pedometer or accelerometer to monitor total accumulation of steps or kcal expended as part of the activities of daily living is a useful strategy. Step counts are highly correlated with activity level. Studies have demonstrated that lifestyle activities are as effective as structured exercise programs for improving cardiorespiratory fitness and weight loss. A high level of physical activity (>300 min of moderate-intensity activity per week) is often needed to lose weight and sustain weight loss. These exercise recommendations are daunting to most patients and need to be implemented gradually. Consultation with an exercise physiologist or personal trainer may be helpful.

Behavioral Therapy Cognitive behavioral therapy is used to help change and reinforce new dietary and physical activity behaviors. Strategies include self-monitoring techniques (e.g., journaling, weighing, and measuring food and activity); stress management; stimulus control (e.g., using smaller plates, not eating in front of the television or in the car); social support; problem solving; and cognitive restructuring to help patients develop more positive and realistic thoughts about themselves. When recommending any behavioral lifestyle change, the patient should be asked to identify what, when, where, and how the behavioral change will be performed. The patient should keep a record of the anticipated behavioral change so that progress can be reviewed at the next office visit. Because these techniques are time-consuming to implement, their supervision is often undertaken by ancillary office staff, such as a nurse-clinician or registered dietitian.

PHARMACOTHERAPY Adjuvant pharmacologic treatments should be considered for patients with a BMI ≥30 kg/m^2 or—for patients who have concomitant obesity-related diseases and for whom dietary and physical activity therapy has not been successful—a BMI ≥27 kg/m^2. When an antiobesity medication is prescribed, patients should be actively engaged in a lifestyle program that provides the strategies and skills needed to use the drug effectively, since such support increases total weight loss.

Medications for obesity have traditionally fallen into two major categories: appetite suppressants (*anorexiants*) and gastrointestinal fat blockers. Appetite-suppressing medications have primarily targeted three monoamine receptor systems in the hypothalamus: noradrenergic, dopaminergic, and serotonergic receptors. Two new appetite suppressants were approved by the U.S. Food and Drug Administration (FDA) in 2012: lorcaserin and phentermine/topiramate (PHEN/TPM) extended release. Gastrointestinal fat blockers reduce the absorption of selective macronutrients, such as fat, from the gastrointestinal tract.

Centrally Acting Anorexiant Medications Anorexiants affect *satiety* (the absence of hunger after eating) and hunger (the biologic sensation that prompts eating). By increasing satiety and decreasing hunger, these agents help patients reduce caloric intake without a sense of deprivation. The target site for the actions of anorexiants is the ventromedial and lateral hypothalamic regions in the central nervous system **(Chap. 60)**. The biologic effect of these agents on appetite regulation is produced by augmentation of the neurotransmission of three monoamines: norepinephrine; serotonin (5-hydroxytryptamine, or 5-HT); and, to a lesser degree, dopamine. The classic sympathomimetic adrenergic agents (benzphetamine, phendimetrazine, diethylpropion, mazindol, and phentermine) function by stimulating norepinephrine release or by blocking its reuptake. Among the anorexiants, phentermine has been the most commonly prescribed; there is limited long-term data on its effectiveness. A 2002 review of six randomized, placebo-controlled trials of phentermine for weight control found that patients lost 0.6–6.0 additional kilograms of weight over 2–24 weeks of treatment. The most common side effects of the amphetamine-derived anorexiants are restlessness, insomnia, dry mouth, constipation, and increased blood pressure and heart rate.

PHEN/TPM is a combination drug that contains a catecholamine releaser (phentermine) and an anticonvulsant (topiramate). Topiramate is approved by the FDA as an anticonvulsant for the treatment of epilepsy and for the prophylaxis of migraine headaches. Weight loss was identified as an unintended side effect of topiramate during clinical trials for epilepsy. The mechanism responsible for weight loss is uncertain but is thought to be mediated through the drug's modulation of γ-aminobutyric acid receptors, inhibition of carbonic anhydrase, and antagonism of glutamate. PHEN/TPM has undergone two 1-year pivotal randomized, placebo-controlled, double-blind trials of efficacy and safety: EQUIP and CONQUER. In a third study, SEQUEL, 78% of CONQUER participants continued to receive their blinded treatment for an additional year. All participants received diet and exercise counseling. Participant numbers, eligibility, characteristics, and weight loss outcomes are displayed in Table 61-6. Intention-to-treat 1-year placebo-subtracted weight loss for the PHEN/TPM 15-mg/92-mg dose was 9.3% and 8.6%, respectively, in the EQUIP and CONQUER trials. Clinical and statistical dose-dependent improvements were seen in selected cardiovascular and metabolic outcome measurements that were related to the weight loss. The most common adverse events experienced by the drug-randomized group were paresthesias, dry mouth, constipation, dysgeusia, and insomnia. Because of an increased risk of congenital fetal oral-cleft formation from topiramate, the FDA approval of PHEN/TPM stipulated a Risk Evaluation and Mitigation Strategies requirement to educate prescribers about the need for active birth control among women of childbearing age and a contraindication for use during pregnancy.

Lorcaserin is a selective 5-HT2C receptor agonist with a functional selectivity ~15 times that of 5-HT2A receptors and 100 times that of 5-HT2B receptors. This selectivity is important, since the drug-induced valvulopathy documented with two other serotonergic agents that were removed from the market—fenfluramine and dexfenfluramine—was due to activation of the 5-HT2B receptors expressed on cardiac valvular interstitial cells. By activating the 5-HT2C receptor, lorcaserin is thought to decrease food intake through the proopiomelanocortin system of neurons.

Lorcaserin has undergone two randomized, placebo-controlled, double-blind trials for efficacy and safety. Participants were randomized to receive lorcaserin (10 mg bid) or placebo in the BLOOM study and to receive lorcaserin (10 mg bid or qd) or placebo in the BLOSSOM study. All participants received diet and exercise counseling. Participant numbers, eligibility, characteristics, and weight loss outcomes are displayed in Table 61-6. Overweight or obese subjects had at least one coexisting condition (hypertension, dyslipidemia, cardiovascular disease, impaired glucose tolerance, or sleep apnea)—medical conditions that are commonly seen in the office setting. Intention-to-treat 1-year placebo-subtracted weight loss was 3.6% and 3.0%, respectively, in the BLOOM and BLOSSOM trials. Echocardiography was performed at the screening visit and at scheduled time points over the course of the studies. There was no difference in the development of FDA-defined valvulopathy between drug-treated and placebo-treated participants at 1 year or 2 years. Modest statistical improvements consistent with the weight loss were seen in selected cardiovascular and metabolic outcome measurements. The most common adverse events experienced by the drug group were headache, dizziness, and nausea.

In approving both PHEN/TPM and lorcaserin, the FDA introduced a new provision with important clinical relevance: a prescription trial period to assess effectiveness. Response to both medications should be assessed after 3 months of treatment. For lorcaserin, the medication should be discontinued if the patient has not lost at least 5% of body weight by that point. For PHEN/TPM, if the patient has not lost at least 3% of body weight at 3 months, the clinician can either escalate the dose and reassess progress at 6 months or discontinue treatment entirely.

Peripherally Acting Medications Orlistat (Xenical™) is a synthetic hydrogenated derivative of a naturally occurring lipase inhibitor, lipostatin, that is produced by the mold *Streptomyces*

TABLE 61-6

CLINICAL TRIALS FOR WEIGHT LOSS MEDICATIONS[a]

	LORCASERIN		PHEN/TPM[d]	
	BLOOM[b]	**BLOSSOM[c]**	**EQUIP**	**CONQUER**
No. of participants (ITT-LOCF)	3182	4008	1230	2448
Age (years)	18–65	18–65	≥35	27–45
BMI (kg/m^2)	27–45	27–45	18–70	18–70
Comorbid conditions (cardiovascular and metabolic)	≥1	≥1	≥1	≥2
Mean weight loss (%) with treatment vs. placebo	5.8 vs. 2.2	4.8 vs. 2.8	11 vs. 1.6	10.4 vs. 1.8
Placebo-subtracted weight loss (%)	3.6	3.0	9.3	8.6
Categorical change in 5% weight loss with treatment vs. placebo	47.5 vs. 20.3	47.2 vs. 25	67 vs. 17	70 vs. 21
Completion rate (%)	Lorcaserin, 55.4; placebo, 45.1	55.5	59.9	62

[a]Table shows a comparison of two 1-year prospective, randomized, double-blind trials of lorcaserin (BLOOM and BLOSSOM) and phentermine-topiramate extended release (EQUIP and CONQUER).
[b]Lorcaserin dose: 10 mg bid.
[c]Lorcaserin dose: 10 mg bid or qd.
[d]Phentermine-topiramate extended release dose: 15 mg/92 mg.
Abbreviations: BMI, body mass index (see Table 61-1); ITT-LOCF, intention to treat, last observation carried forward; PHEN/TPM, phentermine-topiramate extended release.

toxytricini. This drug is a potent, slowly reversible inhibitor of pancreatic, gastric, and carboxylester lipases and phospholipase A_2, which are required for the hydrolysis of dietary fat into fatty acids and monoacylglycerols. Orlistat acts in the lumen of the stomach and small intestine by forming a covalent bond with the active site of these lipases. Taken at a therapeutic dose of 120 mg tid, orlistat blocks the digestion and absorption of ~30% of dietary fat. After discontinuation of the drug, fecal fat content usually returns to normal within 48–72 h.

Multiple randomized, double-blind, placebo-controlled studies have shown that, after 1 year, orlistat produces a weight loss of ~9–10%, whereas placebo recipients have a 4–6% weight loss. Because orlistat is minimally (<1%) absorbed from the gastrointestinal tract, it has no systemic side effects. The drug's tolerability is related to the malabsorption of dietary fat and the subsequent passage of fat in the feces. Adverse gastrointestinal effects, including flatus with discharge, fecal urgency, fatty/oily stool, and increased defecation, are reported in at least 10% of orlistat-treated patients. These side effects generally are experienced early, diminish as patients control their dietary fat intake, and only infrequently cause patients to withdraw from clinical trials. When taken concomitantly, psyllium mucilloid is helpful in controlling orlistat-induced gastrointestinal side effects. Because serum concentrations of the fat-soluble vitamins D and E and β-carotene may be reduced by orlistat treatment, vitamin supplements are recommended to prevent potential deficiencies. Orlistat was approved for over-the-counter use in 2007.

Antiobesity Drugs in Development Two additional medications are currently in development. Bupropion and naltrexone (Contrave™)—a dopamine and norepinephrine reuptake inhibitor and an opioid receptor antagonist, respectively—are theoretically combined to dampen the motivation/reinforcement that food brings (dopamine effect) and the pleasure/palatability of eating (opioid effect). In the COR-1 randomized, double-blind, placebo-controlled trial, 1742 enrolled participants, who were 18–65 years of age and had BMIs of 30–45 kg/m^2, were randomized to receive naltrexone (16 mg/d) plus bupropion (360 mg/d), naltrexone (32 mg/d) plus bupropion (360 mg/d), or placebo. Mean change in body weight for the three groups was 5.0%, 6.1%, and 1.3%, respectively. The most common adverse events were nausea, headache, constipation, dizziness, vomiting, and dry mouth. However, the FDA rejected the drug in 2011 because of cardiovascular concerns and concluded that a large-scale study of the long-term cardiovascular effects of naltrexone would be needed before approval could be considered.

Liraglutide, a glucagon-like peptide 1 receptor agonist currently approved for the treatment of type 2 diabetes, has independent weight loss effects via hypothalamic neural activation causing appetite suppression. In a double-blind, placebo-controlled trial, 564 adults with BMIs of 30–40 kg/m^2 were randomized to receive once-daily SC liraglutide (1.2, 1.8, 2.4, or 3.0 mg), placebo, or open-label orlistat (120 mg tid) for 1 year. The liraglutide and placebo recipients were switched to 2.4 mg of liraglutide during the second year and then to 3.0 mg for an additional year. One-year placebo-subtracted mean weight loss was 5.8 kg for liraglutide and 3.8 kg more than those on orlistat. The most common side effects were nausea, vomiting, and change in bowel habits.

SURGERY Bariatric surgery (Fig. 61-2) can be considered for patients with severe obesity (BMI, ≥40 kg/m^2) or for those with moderate obesity (BMI, ≥35 kg/m^2) associated with a serious medical condition. Weight loss surgeries have traditionally been classified into three categories on the basis of anatomic changes: restrictive, restrictive malabsorptive, and malabsorptive. More recently, however, the clinical benefits of bariatric surgery in achieving weight loss and alleviating metabolic comorbidities have been attributed largely to changes in the physiologic responses of gut hormones and in adipose tissue metabolism. Metabolic effects resulting from bypassing the foregut include altered responses of ghrelin, glucagon-like peptide 1, peptide YY3-36, and oxyntonodulin. Additional effects on food intake and body weight control may be attributed to changes in vagal signaling. The loss of fat mass, particularly visceral fat, is associated with multiple metabolic, adipokine, and inflammatory changes that include improved insulin sensitivity and glucose disposal; reduced free fatty acid flux; increased adiponectin levels; and decreased interleukin 6, tumor necrosis factor α, and high-sensitivity C-reactive protein levels.

Restrictive surgeries limit the amount of food the stomach can hold and slow the rate of gastric emptying. *Laparoscopic adjustable gastric banding* is the prototype of this category. The first banding device, the LAP-BAND, was approved for use in the United States in 2001 and the second, the REALIZE band, in 2007. In contrast to previous devices, these bands have diameters that are adjustable by way of their connection to a reservoir that is implanted under the skin. Injection of saline into the reservoir and removal of saline from

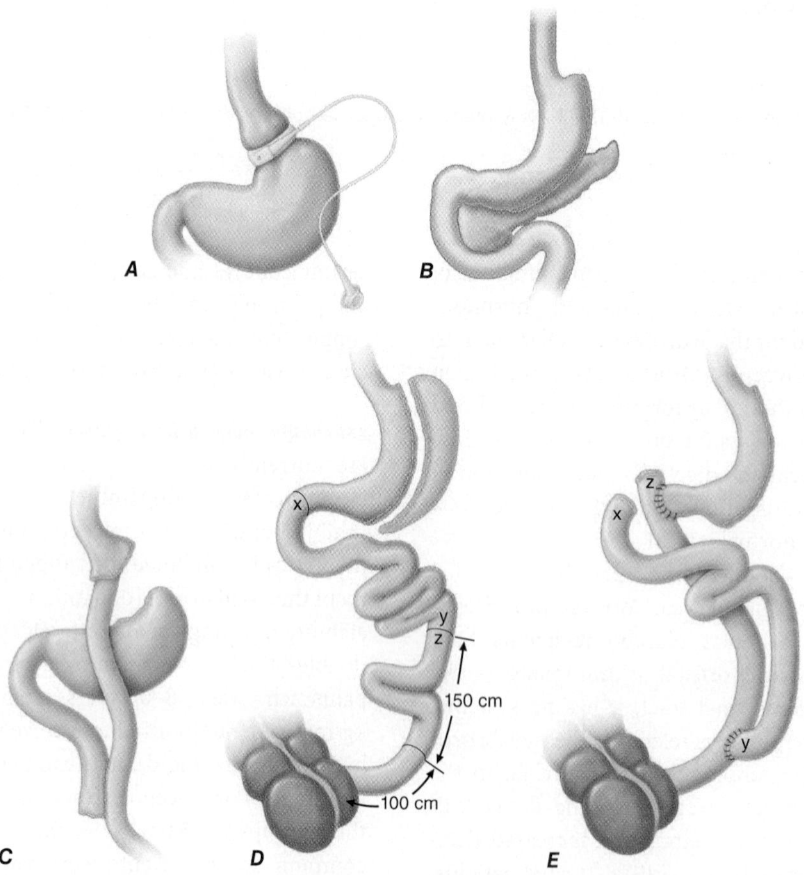

FIGURE 61-2

Bariatric surgical procedures. Examples of operative interventions used for surgical manipulation of the gastrointestinal tract. ***A.*** Laparoscopic adjustable gastric banding. ***B.*** Laparoscopic sleeve gastrectomy. ***C.*** The Roux-en-Y gastric bypass. ***D.*** Biliopancreatic diversion with duodenal switch. ***E.*** Biliopancreatic diversion. *(From ML Kendrick, GF Dakin: Mayo Clin Proc 815:518, 2006; with permission.)*

the reservoir tighten and loosen the band's internal diameter, respectively, thus changing the size of the gastric opening. The mean percentage of total body weight lost at 5 years is estimated at 20–25%. In *laparoscopic sleeve gastrectomy*, the stomach is restricted by stapling and dividing it vertically, removing ~80% of the greater curvature, and leaving a slim banana-shaped remnant stomach along the lesser curvature. Weight loss after this procedure is superior to that after laparoscopic adjustable gastric banding.

The three restrictive-malabsorptive bypass procedures combine the elements of gastric restriction and selective malabsorption. These procedures are Roux-en-Y gastric bypass, biliopancreatic diversion, and biliopancreatic diversion with duodenal switch (Fig. 61-2). Roux-en-Y is the most commonly undertaken and most accepted bypass procedure. It may be performed with an open incision or by laparoscopy.

These procedures generally produce a 30–35% average total body weight loss that is maintained in nearly 60% of patients at 5 years. In general, mean weight loss is greater after the combined restrictive-malabsorptive procedures than after the restrictive procedures. Significant improvement in multiple obesity-related comorbid conditions, including type 2 diabetes, hypertension, dyslipidemia, obstructive sleep apnea, quality of life, and long-term cardiovascular events, has been reported. A meta-analysis of controlled clinical trials comparing bariatric surgery versus no surgery showed that surgery was associated with a reduced odds ratio (OR) risk of global mortality (OR = 0.55), cardiovascular death (OR = 0.58), and all-cause mortality (OR = 0.70).

Among the observed improvements in comorbidities, the prevention and treatment of type 2 diabetes resulting from bariatric surgery has garnered the most attention. Fifteen-year data from the Swedish Obese Subjects study demonstrated a marked reduction (i.e., by 78%) in the incidence of type 2 diabetes development among obese patients who underwent bariatric surgery. Several randomized controlled studies have shown greater weight loss and more improved glycemic control at 1 and 2 years among surgical patients than among patients receiving conventional medical therapy. A retrospective cohort study of more than 4000 adults with diabetes found that, overall, 68.2% of patients experienced an initial complete type 2 diabetes remission within 5 years after surgery. However, among these patients, one-third redeveloped type 2 diabetes within 5 years. The rapid improvement seen in diabetes after restrictive-malabsorptive procedures is thought to be due to surgery-specific, weight-independent effects on glucose homeostasis brought about by alteration of gut hormones.

The mortality rate from bariatric surgery is generally <1% but varies with the procedure, the patient's age and comorbid conditions, and the experience of the surgical team. The most common surgical complications include stomal stenosis or marginal ulcers (occurring in 5–15% of patients) that present as prolonged nausea and vomiting after eating or inability to advance the diet to solid foods. These complications typically are treated by endoscopic balloon dilation and acid suppression therapy, respectively. For patients who undergo laparoscopic adjustable gastric banding, there are no intestinal absorptive abnormalities other than mechanical reduction in gastric size and outflow. Therefore, selective deficiencies are uncommon unless eating habits become unbalanced. In contrast, the restrictive-malabsorptive procedures carry an increased risk for micronutrient deficiencies of vitamin B_{12}, iron, folate, calcium, and vitamin D. Patients with restrictive-malabsorptive procedures require lifelong supplementation with these micronutrients.

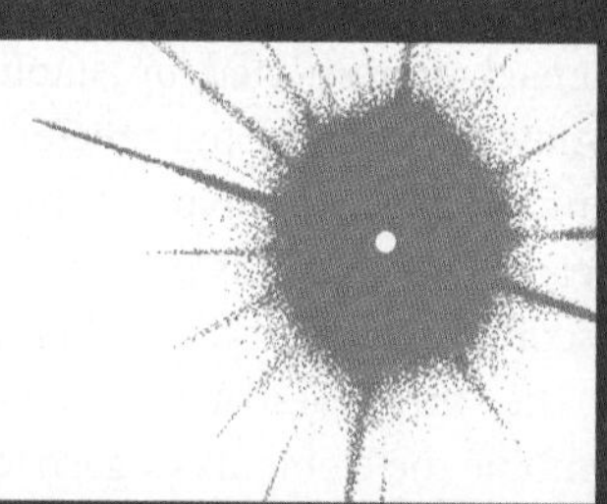

CHAPTER 62

EATING DISORDERS

Victor I. Reus

FEEDING AND EATING DISORDERS

CLINICAL MANIFESTATIONS

Feeding and eating disorders constitute a group of conditions in which there is a persistent disturbance of eating or associated behaviors that significantly impair an individual's physical health or psychosocial functioning. In DSM-5 the described categories (with the exception of pica) are defined to be mutually exclusive in a given episode, based on the understanding that although they are phenotypically similar in some ways, they differ in course, prognosis, and effective treatment interventions. Compared with DSM-IV-TR, three disorders (i.e., avoidant/restrictive food intake disorder, rumination disorder, pica) that were previously classified as disorders of infancy or childhood have been grouped together with the disorders of anorexia and bulimia nervosa. Binge-eating disorder is also now included as a formal diagnosis; the intent of each of these modifications is to encourage clinicians to be more specific in their codification of eating and feeding pathology.

PICA

Pica is diagnosed when the individual, over age 2, eats one or more nonnutritive, nonfood substances for a month or more and requires medical attention as a result. There is usually no specific aversion to food in general but a preferential choice to ingest substances such as clay, starch, soap, paper, or ash. The diagnosis requires the exclusion of specific culturally approved practices and has not been commonly found to be caused by a specific nutritional deficiency. Onset is most common in childhood but the disorder can occur in association with other major psychiatric conditions in adults. An association with pregnancy has been observed, but the condition is only diagnosed when medical risks are increased by the behavior.

RUMINATION DISORDER

In this condition, individuals who have no demonstrable associated gastrointestinal or other medical condition repeatedly regurgitate their food after eating and then either rechew or swallow it or spit it out. The behavior typically occurs on a daily basis and must persist for at least 1 month. Weight loss and malnutrition are common sequelae, and individuals may attempt to conceal their behavior, either by covering their mouth or through social avoidance while eating. In infancy, the onset is typically between 3 to 12 months, and the behavior may remit spontaneously, although in some it appears to be recurrent.

AVOIDANT/RESTRICTIVE FOOD INTAKE DISORDER

The cardinal feature of this disorder is avoidance or restriction of food intake, usually stemming from a lack of interest in or distaste of food and associated with weight loss, nutritional deficiency, dependency on nutritional supplementation, or marked impairment in psychosocial functioning, either alone or in combination. Culturally approved practices, such as fasting, or a lack of available food must be excluded as possible causes. The disorder is distinguished from anorexia nervosa by the presence of emotional factors, such as a fear of gaining weight and distortion of body image in the latter condition. Onset is usually in infancy or early childhood, but avoidant behaviors may persist into adulthood. The disorder is equally prevalent in males and females and is frequently comorbid with anxiety and cognitive and attention-deficit disorders and situations of familial stress. Developmental delay and functional deficits may be significant if the disorder is long-standing and unrecognized.

ANOREXIA NERVOSA

Individuals are diagnosed with anorexia nervosa if they restrict their caloric intake to a degree that their body weight deviates significantly from age, gender, health, and developmental norms and if they also exhibit a fear of gaining weight and an associated disturbance in body image. The condition is further characterized by differentiating those who achieve their weight loss predominantly through restricting intake or by excessive exercise (restricting type) from those who engage in recurrent binge eating and/or subsequent purging, self-induced vomiting, and usage of enemas, laxatives, or diuretics (binge-eating/purging type). Such subtyping is more state than trait specific, as individuals may transition from one profile to the other over time. Determination of whether an individual satisfies the primary criterion of significant low weight is complex and must be individualized, using all available historical information and comparison of body habitus to international body mass norms and guidelines.

Individuals with anorexia nervosa frequently lack insight into their condition and are in denial about possible medical consequences; they often are not comforted by their achieved weight loss and persist in their behaviors despite having met previously self-designated weight goals. Recent research has identified alterations in the circuitry of reward sensitivity and executive function in anorexia and implicated disturbances in frontal cortex and anterior insula regulation of interoceptive awareness of satiety and hunger. Neurochemical findings, including the role of ghrelin, remain controversial.

Onset is most common in adolescence, although onset in later life can occur. Many more females than males are affected, with a lifetime prevalence in women of up to 4%. The disorder appears most prevalent in postindustrialized and urbanized countries and is frequently comorbid with preexisting anxiety disorders. The medical consequences of prolonged anorexia nervosa are multisystemic and can be life-threatening in severe presentations. Changes in blood chemistry include leukopenia with lymphocytosis, elevations in blood urea nitrogen, and metabolic alkalosis and hypokalemia when purging is present. History and physical examination may reveal amenorrhea in females, skin abnormalities (petechiae, lanugo hair, dryness), and signs of hypometabolic function, including hypotension, hypothermia, and sinus bradycardia. Endocrine effects include hypogonadism, growth hormone resistance, and hypercortisolemia. Osteoporosis is a longer-term concern.

The course of the disorder is variable, with some individuals recovering after a single episode, while others exhibit recurrent episodes or a chronic course. Untreated anorexia has a mortality of 5.1/1000, the highest among psychiatric conditions. Maudsley family-based therapy has proven to be an effective therapy in younger individuals, with strict behavioral contingencies used when weight loss becomes critical. No pharmacologic intervention has proven to be specifically beneficial, but comorbid depression and anxiety should be treated. Weight gain should be undertaken gradually with a goal of 0.5 to 1 pound per week to prevent refeeding syndrome. Most individuals are able to achieve remission within 5 years of the original diagnosis.

BULIMIA NERVOSA

Bulimia nervosa describes individuals who engage in recurrent and frequent (at least once a week for 3 months) periods of binge eating and who then resort to compensatory behaviors, such as self-induced purging, enemas, use of laxatives, or excessive exercise to avoid weight gain. Binge eating itself is defined as excessive food intake in a prescribed period of time, usually <2 h. As in anorexia nervosa, disturbances in body image occur and promote the behavior, but unlike in anorexia, individuals are of normal weight or even somewhat overweight. Subjects typically describe a loss of control and express shame about their actions, and often relate that their episodes are triggered by feelings of negative self-esteem or social stresses. The lifetime prevalence in women is approximately 2%, with a 10:1 female-to-male ratio. The disorder typically begins in adolescence and may be persistent over a number of years. Transition to anorexia occurs in only 10–15% of cases. Many of the medical risks associated with bulimia nervosa parallel those of anorexia nervosa and are a direct consequence of purging, including fluid and electrolyte disturbances and conduction abnormalities. Physical examination often results in no specific findings, but dental erosion and parotid gland enlargement may be present. Effective treatment approaches include SSRI antidepressants, usually in combination with cognitive-behavioral, emotion regulation, or interpersonal-based psychotherapies.

BINGE-EATING DISORDER

Binge-eating disorder is distinguished from bulimia nervosa by the absence of compensatory behaviors to prevent weight gain after an episode and by a lack of effort to restrict weight gain between episodes. Other features are similar, including distress over the behavior and the experience of loss of control, resulting in eating more rapidly or in greater amounts than intended or eating when not hungry. The 12-month prevalence in females is 1.6%, with a much lower female-to-male ratio than bulimia nervosa. Little is known about the course of the disorder, given its recent categorization, but its prognosis is markedly better than for other eating disorders, both in terms of its natural course and response to treatment. Transition to other eating disorder conditions is thought to be rare.

CHAPTER 63

THE METABOLIC SYNDROME

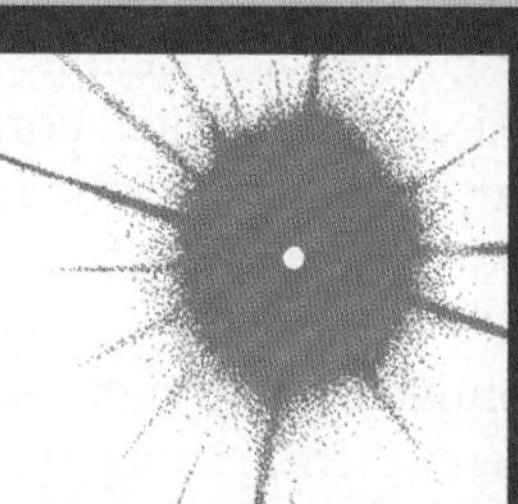

Robert H. Eckel

The metabolic syndrome (syndrome X, insulin resistance syndrome) consists of a constellation of metabolic abnormalities that confer increased risk of cardiovascular disease (CVD) and diabetes mellitus. Evolution of the criteria for the metabolic syndrome since the original definition by the World Health Organization in 1998 reflects growing clinical evidence and analysis by a variety of consensus conferences and professional organizations. The major features of the metabolic syndrome include central obesity, hypertriglyceridemia, low levels of high-density lipoprotein (HDL) cholesterol, hyperglycemia, and hypertension (Table 63-1).

EPIDEMIOLOGY

The most challenging feature of the metabolic syndrome to define is waist circumference. Intraabdominal circumference (visceral adipose tissue) is considered most strongly related to insulin resistance and risk of diabetes and CVD, and for any given waist circumference the distribution of adipose tissue between SC and visceral depots varies substantially. Thus, within and between populations, there is a lesser vs. greater risk at the same waist circumference. These differences in populations are reflected in the

TABLE 63-1

NCEP: ATPIII[a] 2001 AND HARMONIZING DEFINITION CRITERIA FOR THE METABOLIC SYNDROME

<table>
<tr><th>NCEP: ATPIII 2001</th><th colspan="3">HARMONIZING DEFINITION[b]</th></tr>
<tr><td rowspan="6">Three or more of the following:
• Central obesity: waist circumference >102 cm (M), >88 cm (F)
• Hypertriglyceridemia: triglyceride level ≥150 mg/dL or specific medication
• Low HDL[c] cholesterol: <40 mg/dL and <50 mg/dL for men and women, respectively, or specific medication
• Hypertension: blood pressure ≥130 mmHg systolic or ≥85 mmHg diastolic or specific medication
• Fasting plasma glucose level ≥100 mg/dL or specific medication or previously diagnosed type 2 diabetes</td><td colspan="3">Three of the following:
• Waist circumference (cm)</td></tr>
<tr><td>Men</td><td>Women</td><td>Ethnicity</td></tr>
<tr><td>≥94</td><td>≥80</td><td>Europid, sub-Saharan African, Eastern and Middle Eastern</td></tr>
<tr><td>≥90</td><td>≥80</td><td>South Asian, Chinese, and ethnic South and Central American</td></tr>
<tr><td>≥85</td><td>≥90</td><td>Japanese</td></tr>
<tr><td colspan="3">• Fasting triglyceride level >150 mg/dL or specific medication
• HDL cholesterol level <40 mg/dL and <50 mg/dL for men and women, respectively, or specific medication
• Blood pressure >130 mm systolic or >85 mm diastolic or previous diagnosis or specific medication
• Fasting plasma glucose level ≥100 mg/dL (alternative indication: drug treatment of elevated glucose levels)</td></tr>
</table>

[a]National Cholesterol Education Program and Adult Treatment Panel III.

[b]In this analysis, the following thresholds for waist circumference were used: white men, ≥94 cm; African-American men, ≥94 cm; Mexican-American men, ≥90 cm; white women, ≥80 cm; African-American women, ≥80 cm; Mexican-American women, ≥80 cm. For participants whose designation was "other race—including multiracial," thresholds that were once based on Europid cutoffs (≥94 cm for men and ≥80 cm for women) and on South Asian cutoffs (≥90 cm for men and ≥80 cm for women) were used. For participants who were considered "other Hispanic," the International Diabetes Federation thresholds for ethnic South and Central Americans were used.

[c]High-density lipoprotein.

range of waist circumferences considered to confer risk in different geographic locations (Table 63-1).

The prevalence of the metabolic syndrome varies around the world, in part reflecting the age and ethnicity of the populations studied and the diagnostic criteria applied. In general, the prevalence of the metabolic syndrome increases with age. The highest recorded prevalence worldwide is among Native Americans, with nearly 60% of women ages 45–49 and 45% of men ages 45–49 meeting the criteria of the National Cholesterol Education Program and Adult Treatment Panel III (NCEP:ATPIII). In the United States, the metabolic syndrome is less common among African-American men and more common among Mexican-American women. Based on data from the National Health and Nutrition Examination Survey (NHANES) 2003–2006, the age-adjusted prevalence of the metabolic syndrome in U.S. adults without diabetes is 28% for men and 30% for women. In France, studies of a cohort of 30- to 60-year-olds have shown a <10% prevalence for each sex, although 17.5% of people 60–64 years of age are affected. Greater global industrialization is associated with rising rates of obesity, which are expected to increase the prevalence of the metabolic syndrome dramatically, especially as the population ages. Moreover, the rising prevalence and severity of obesity among children is reflected in features of the metabolic syndrome in a younger population.

The frequency distribution of the five components of the syndrome for the U.S. population (NHANES III) is summarized in Fig. 63-1. Increases in waist circumference predominate among women, whereas increases in

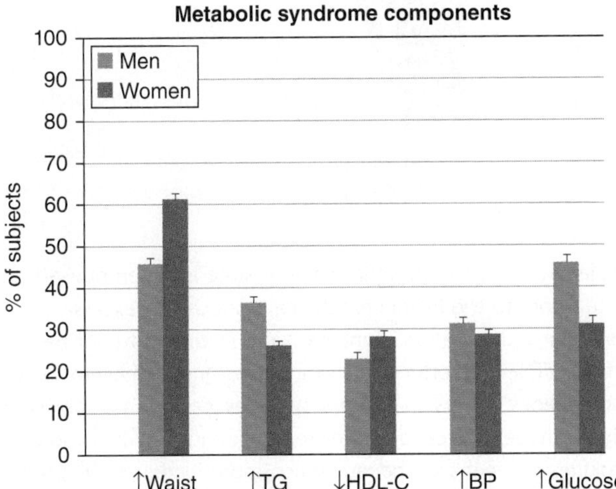

FIGURE 63-1

Prevalence of the metabolic syndrome components, from NHANES 2003–2006. NHANES, National Health and Nutrition Examination Survey; TG, triglyceride; HDL-C, high-density lipoprotein cholesterol; BP, blood pressure. The prevalence of elevated glucose includes individuals with known diabetes mellitus. *(Created from data in ES Ford et al: J Diabetes 2:1753, 2010.)*

fasting plasma triglyceride levels (i.e., to >150 mg/dL), reductions in HDL cholesterol levels, and hyperglycemia are more likely in men.

RISK FACTORS

Overweight/obesity

Although the metabolic syndrome was first described in the early twentieth century, the worldwide overweight/obesity epidemic has recently been the force driving its increasing recognition. Central adiposity is a key feature of the syndrome, and the syndrome's prevalence reflects the strong relationship between waist circumference and increasing adiposity. However, despite the importance of obesity, patients who are of normal weight may also be insulin resistant and may have the metabolic syndrome.

Sedentary lifestyle

Physical inactivity is a predictor of CVD events and the related risk of death. Many components of the metabolic syndrome are associated with a sedentary lifestyle, including increased adipose tissue (predominantly central), reduced HDL cholesterol, and increased triglycerides, blood pressure, and glucose in genetically susceptible persons. Compared with individuals who watch television or videos or use the computer <1 h daily, those who do so for >4 h daily have a twofold increased risk of the metabolic syndrome.

Aging

The metabolic syndrome affects nearly 50% of the U.S. population older than age 50, and at >60 years of age women are more often affected than men. The age dependency of the syndrome's prevalence is seen in most populations around the world.

Diabetes mellitus

Diabetes mellitus is included in both the NCEP and the harmonizing definitions of the metabolic syndrome. It is estimated that the great majority (~75%) of patients with type 2 diabetes or impaired glucose tolerance have the metabolic syndrome. The presence of the metabolic syndrome in these populations relates to a higher prevalence of CVD than in patients who have type 2 diabetes or impaired glucose tolerance but do not have this syndrome.

Cardiovascular disease

Individuals with the metabolic syndrome are twice as likely to die of cardiovascular disease as those who do not, and their risk of an acute myocardial infarction or stroke is threefold higher. The approximate prevalence of the metabolic syndrome among patients with coronary heart disease (CHD) is 50%, with a prevalence of ~35% among patients with premature coronary artery disease (before or at age 45) and a particularly high prevalence among women. With appropriate cardiac rehabilitation and changes in lifestyle (e.g., nutrition, physical activity, weight reduction, and—in some cases—pharmacologic therapy), the prevalence of the syndrome can be reduced.

Lipodystrophy

Lipodystrophic disorders in general are associated with the metabolic syndrome. Both genetic lipodystrophy (e.g., Berardinelli-Seip congenital lipodystrophy, Dunnigan familial partial lipodystrophy) and acquired lipodystrophy (e.g., HIV-related lipodystrophy in patients receiving antiretroviral therapy) may give rise to severe insulin resistance and many of the components of the metabolic syndrome.

ETIOLOGY

Insulin resistance

The most accepted and unifying hypothesis to describe the pathophysiology of the metabolic syndrome is insulin resistance, which is caused by an incompletely understood defect in insulin action. The onset of insulin resistance is heralded by postprandial hyperinsulinemia, which is followed by fasting hyperinsulinemia and ultimately by hyperglycemia.

An early major contributor to the development of insulin resistance is an overabundance of circulating fatty acids (Fig. 63-2). Plasma albumin-bound free fatty

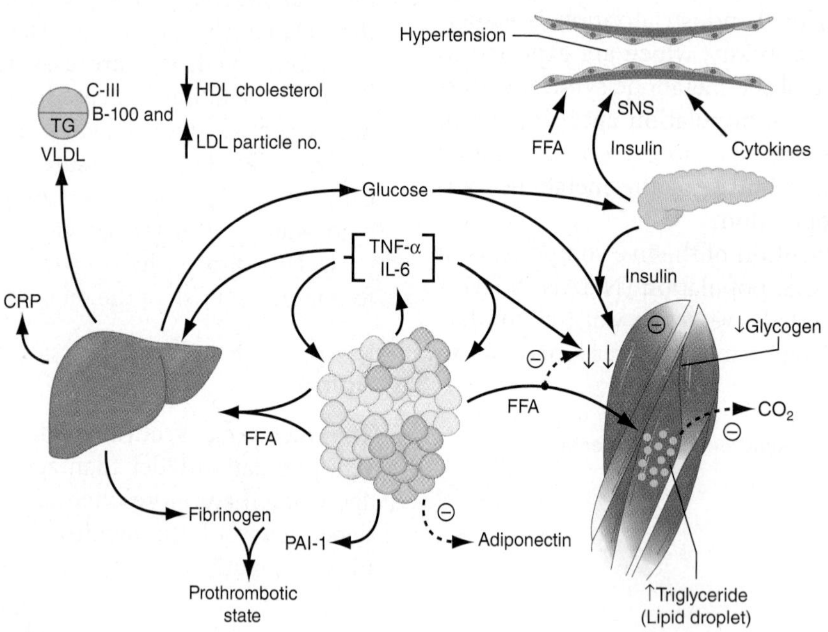

FIGURE 63-2

Pathophysiology of the metabolic syndrome. Free fatty acids (FFAs) are released in abundance from an expanded adipose tissue mass. In the liver, FFAs result in increased production of glucose and triglycerides and secretion of very low density lipoproteins (VLDLs). Associated lipid/lipoprotein abnormalities include reductions in high-density lipoprotein (HDL) cholesterol and an increased low-density lipoprotein (LDL) particle number (no.). FFAs also reduce insulin sensitivity in muscle by inhibiting insulin-mediated glucose uptake. Associated defects include a reduction in glucose partitioning to glycogen and increased lipid accumulation in triglyceride (TG). The increase in circulating glucose, and to some extent FFAs, increases pancreatic insulin secretion, resulting in hyperinsulinemia. Hyperinsulinemia may result in enhanced sodium reabsorption and increased sympathetic nervous system (SNS) activity and contribute to hypertension, as might higher levels of circulating FFAs. The proinflammatory state is superimposed and contributory to the insulin resistance produced by excessive FFAs. The enhanced secretion of interleukin 6 (IL-6) and tumor necrosis factor α (TNF-α) produced by adipocytes and monocyte-derived macrophages results in more insulin resistance and lipolysis of adipose tissue triglyceride stores to circulating FFAs. IL-6 and other cytokines also enhance hepatic glucose production, VLDL production by the liver, hypertension and insulin resistance in muscle. Cytokines and FFAs also increase hepatic production of fibrinogen and adipocyte production of plasminogen activator inhibitor 1 (PAI-1), resulting in a prothrombotic state. Higher levels of circulating cytokines stimulate hepatic production of C-reactive protein (CRP). Reduced production of the anti-inflammatory and insulin-sensitizing cytokine adiponectin is also associated with the metabolic syndrome. *(Modified from RH Eckel et al: Lancet 365:1415, 2005.)*

acids are derived predominantly from adipose-tissue triglyceride stores released by intracellular lipolytic enzymes. Fatty acids are also derived from the lipolysis of triglyceride-rich lipoproteins in tissues by lipoprotein lipase. Insulin mediates both antilipolysis and the stimulation of lipoprotein lipase in adipose tissue. Of note, the inhibition of lipolysis in adipose tissue is the most sensitive pathway of insulin action. Thus, when insulin resistance develops, increased lipolysis produces more fatty acids, which further decrease the antilipolytic effect of insulin. Excessive fatty acids enhance substrate availability and create insulin resistance by modifying downstream signaling. Fatty acids impair insulin-mediated glucose uptake and accumulate as triglycerides in both skeletal and cardiac muscle, whereas increased glucose production and triglyceride accumulation take place in the liver.

Leptin resistance has also been raised as a possible pathophysiologic mechanism to explain the metabolic syndrome. Physiologically, leptin reduces appetite, promotes energy expenditure, and enhances insulin sensitivity. In addition, leptin may regulate cardiac and vascular function through a nitric oxide–dependent mechanism. However, when obesity develops, hyperleptinemia ensues, with evidence of leptin resistance in the brain and other tissues resulting in inflammation, insulin resistance, hyperlipidemia, and a plethora of cardiovascular disorders, such as hypertension, atherosclerosis, CHD, and heart failure.

The oxidative stress hypothesis provides a unifying theory for aging and the predisposition to the metabolic syndrome. In studies of insulin-resistant individuals with obesity or type 2 diabetes, the offspring of patients with type 2 diabetes, and the elderly, a defect in mitochondrial oxidative phosphorylation that leads to the accumulation of triglycerides and related lipid molecules in muscle has been identified.

Recently, the gut microbiome has emerged as an important contributor to the development of obesity and related metabolic disorders, including the metabolic syndrome. Although the mechanism remains uncertain, interaction among genetic predisposition, diet, and the intestinal flora is important.

Increased waist circumference

Waist circumference is an important component of the most recent and frequently applied diagnostic criteria for the metabolic syndrome. However, measuring waist circumference does not reliably distinguish increases in SC adipose tissue from those in visceral fat; this distinction requires CT or MRI. With increases in visceral adipose tissue, adipose tissue–derived free fatty acids are directed to the liver. In contrast, increases in abdominal SC fat release lipolysis products into the systemic circulation and avert more direct effects on hepatic metabolism. Relative increases in visceral versus SC adipose tissue with increasing waist circumference in Asians and Asian Indians may explain the greater prevalence of the syndrome in those populations than in African-American men, in whom SC fat predominates. It is also possible that visceral fat is a marker for—but not the source of—excess postprandial free fatty acids in obesity.

Dyslipidemia

In general, free fatty acid flux to the liver is associated with increased production of ApoB-containing, triglyceride-rich, very low-density lipoproteins (VLDLs). The effect of insulin on this process is complex, but *hypertriglyceridemia* is an excellent marker of the insulin-resistant condition. Not only is hypertriglyceridemia a feature of the metabolic syndrome, but patients with the metabolic syndrome have elevated levels of ApoCIII carried on VLDLs and other lipoproteins. This increase in ApoCIII is inhibitory to lipoprotein lipase, further contributing to hypertriglyceridemia and also associated with more atherosclerotic cardiovascular disease.

The other major lipoprotein disturbance in the metabolic syndrome is a *reduction in HDL cholesterol*. This reduction is a consequence of changes in HDL composition and metabolism. In the presence of hypertriglyceridemia, a decrease in the cholesterol content of HDL is a consequence of reduced cholesteryl ester content of the lipoprotein core in combination with cholesteryl ester transfer protein–mediated alterations in triglyceride that make the particle small and dense. This change in lipoprotein composition also results in increased clearance of HDL from the circulation. These changes in HDL have a relationship to insulin resistance that is probably indirect, occurring in concert with the changes in triglyceride-rich lipoprotein metabolism.

In addition to HDLs, low-density lipoproteins (LDLs) are modified in composition in the metabolic syndrome. With fasting serum triglycerides at >2.0 mM (~180 mg/dL), there is almost always a predominance of small, dense LDLs, which are thought to be more atherogenic although their association with hypertriglyceridemia and low HDLs make their independent contribution to CVD events difficult to assess. Individuals with hypertriglyceridemia often have increases in cholesterol content of both VLDL1 and VLDL2 subfractions and in LDL particle number. Both of these lipoprotein changes may contribute to atherogenic risk in patients with the metabolic syndrome.

Glucose intolerance

Defects in insulin action in the metabolic syndrome lead to impaired suppression of glucose production by the liver and kidney and reduced glucose uptake and metabolism in insulin-sensitive tissues—i.e., muscle and adipose tissue. The relationship between impaired fasting glucose or impaired glucose tolerance and insulin resistance is well supported by studies of humans, nonhuman primates, and rodents. To compensate for defects in insulin action, insulin secretion and/or clearance must be modified so that euglycemia is sustained. Ultimately, this compensatory mechanism fails, usually because of defects in insulin secretion, resulting in progression from impaired fasting glucose and/or impaired glucose tolerance to diabetes mellitus.

Hypertension

The relationship between insulin resistance and hypertension is well established. Paradoxically, under normal physiologic conditions, insulin is a vasodilator with secondary effects on sodium reabsorption in the kidney. However, in the setting of insulin resistance, the vasodilatory effect of insulin is lost but the renal effect on sodium reabsorption is preserved. Sodium reabsorption is increased in whites with the metabolic syndrome but not in Africans or Asians. Insulin also increases the activity of the sympathetic nervous system, an effect that may be preserved in the setting of insulin resistance. Insulin resistance is characterized by pathway-specific impairment in phosphatidylinositol-3-kinase signaling. In the endothelium, this impairment may cause an imbalance between the production of nitric oxide and the secretion of endothelin 1, with a consequent decrease in blood flow. Although these mechanisms are provocative, evaluation of insulin action by measurement of fasting insulin levels or by homeostasis model assessment shows that insulin resistance contributes only partially to the increased prevalence of hypertension in the metabolic syndrome.

Another possible mechanism underlying hypertension in the metabolic syndrome is the vasoactive role of perivascular adipose tissue. Reactive oxygen species released by NADPH oxidase impair endothelial function and result in local vasoconstriction. Other paracrine effects could be mediated by leptin or other proinflammatory cytokines released from adipose tissue, such as tumor necrosis factor α.

Hyperuricemia is another consequence of insulin resistance and is commonly observed in the metabolic syndrome. There is growing evidence not only that uric acid is associated with hypertension but also that reduction of uric acid normalizes blood pressure in hyperuricemic adolescents with hypertension. The mechanism appears to be related to an adverse effect of uric acid on nitric acid synthase in the macula densa of the kidney and stimulation of the renin-angiotensin aldosterone system.

Proinflammatory cytokines

The increases in proinflammatory cytokines—including interleukins 1, 6, and 18; resistin; tumor necrosis factor α; and the systemic biomarker C-reactive protein—reflect overproduction by the expanded adipose tissue mass (Fig. 63-2). Adipose tissue–derived macrophages may be the primary source of proinflammatory cytokines locally and in the systemic circulation. It remains unclear, however, how much of the insulin resistance is caused by the paracrine effects of these cytokines and how much by the endocrine effects.

Adiponectin

Adiponectin is an anti-inflammatory cytokine produced exclusively by adipocytes. Adiponectin enhances insulin sensitivity and inhibits many steps in the inflammatory process. In the liver, adiponectin inhibits the expression of gluconeogenic enzymes and the rate of glucose production. In muscle, adiponectin increases glucose transport and enhances fatty acid oxidation, partially through the activation of AMP kinase. Adiponectin levels are reduced in the metabolic syndrome. The relative contributions of adiponectin deficiency and overabundance of the proinflammatory cytokines are unclear.

CLINICAL FEATURES

Symptoms and signs

The metabolic syndrome typically is not associated with symptoms. On physical examination, waist circumference may be expanded and blood pressure elevated. The presence of either or both of these signs should prompt the clinician to search for other biochemical abnormalities that may be associated with the metabolic syndrome. Less frequently, lipoatrophy or acanthosis nigricans is found on examination. Because these physical findings characteristically are associated with severe insulin resistance, other components of the metabolic syndrome should be expected.

Associated diseases

Cardiovascular disease

The relative risk for new-onset CVD in patients with the metabolic syndrome who do not have diabetes averages 1.5–3 fold. However, an 8-year follow-up of middle-aged participants in the Framingham Offspring Study documented that the population-attributable CVD risk in the metabolic syndrome was 34% among men and only 16% among women. In the same study, both the metabolic syndrome and diabetes predicted ischemic stroke, with greater risk among patients with the metabolic syndrome than among those with diabetes alone (19% vs. 7%) and a particularly large difference among women (27% vs. 5%). Patients with the metabolic syndrome are also at increased risk for peripheral vascular disease.

Type 2 diabetes

Overall, the risk for type 2 diabetes among patients with the metabolic syndrome is increased three- to fivefold. In the Framingham Offspring Study's 8-year follow-up of middle-aged participants, the population-attributable risk for developing type 2 diabetes was 62% among men and 47% among women.

Other associated conditions

In addition to the features specifically associated with the metabolic syndrome, other metabolic alterations accompany insulin resistance. Those alterations include increases in ApoB and ApoCIII, uric acid, prothrombotic factors (fibrinogen, plasminogen activator inhibitor 1), serum viscosity, asymmetric dimethylarginine, homocysteine, white blood cell count, proinflammatory cytokines, C-reactive protein, microalbuminuria, nonalcoholic fatty liver disease and/or nonalcoholic steatohepatitis, polycystic ovary syndrome, and obstructive sleep apnea.

Nonalcoholic fatty liver disease

Fatty liver is a relatively common condition, affecting 25–45% of the U.S. population **(see also Chap. 46)**. However, in nonalcoholic steatohepatitis, triglyceride accumulation and inflammation coexist. Nonalcoholic steatohepatitis is now present in 3–12% of the population of the United States and other Western countries. Of patients with the metabolic syndrome, ~25–60% have nonalcoholic fatty liver disease and up to 35% have nonalcoholic steatohepatitis. As the prevalence of overweight/obesity and the metabolic syndrome increases, nonalcoholic steatohepatitis may become one of the more common causes of end-stage liver disease and hepatocellular carcinoma.

Hyperuricemia

Hyperuricemia reflects defects in insulin action on the renal tubular reabsorption of uric acid and may contribute to hypertension through its effect on the endothelium. An increase in asymmetric dimethylarginine, an endogenous inhibitor of nitric oxide synthase, also relates to endothelial dysfunction. In addition, microalbuminuria may be caused by altered endothelial pathophysiology in the insulin-resistant state.

Polycystic ovary syndrome

Polycystic ovary syndrome is highly associated with insulin resistance (50–80%) and the metabolic syndrome, with a prevalence of the syndrome between 40% and 50%. Women with polycystic ovary syndrome are two to four times more likely to have the metabolic syndrome than are women without polycystic ovary syndrome.

Obstructive sleep apnea

Obstructive sleep apnea is commonly associated with obesity, hypertension, increased circulating cytokines, impaired glucose tolerance, and insulin resistance. With these associations, it is not surprising that individuals with obstructive sleep apnea frequently have the metabolic syndrome. Moreover, when biomarkers of insulin resistance are compared between patients with obstructive sleep apnea and weight-matched controls, insulin resistance is found to be more severe in those with apnea. Continuous positive airway pressure treatment improves insulin sensitivity in patients with obstructive sleep apnea.

DIAGNOSIS

The diagnosis of the metabolic syndrome relies on fulfillment of the criteria listed in Table 63-1, as assessed using tools at the bedside and in the laboratory. The medical history should include evaluation of symptoms for obstructive sleep apnea in all patients and polycystic ovary syndrome in premenopausal women. Family history will help determine risk for CVD and diabetes mellitus. Blood pressure and waist circumference measurements provide information necessary for the diagnosis.

Laboratory tests

Measurement of fasting lipids and glucose is needed in determining whether the metabolic syndrome is present. The measurement of additional biomarkers associated with insulin resistance can be individualized. Such tests might include those for ApoB, high-sensitivity C-reactive protein, fibrinogen, uric acid, urinary microalbumin, and liver function. A sleep study should be performed if symptoms of obstructive sleep apnea are present. If polycystic ovary syndrome is suspected on the basis of clinical features and anovulation, testosterone, luteinizing hormone, and follicle-stimulating hormone should be measured.

TREATMENT The Metabolic Syndrome

LIFESTYLE Obesity is the driving force behind the metabolic syndrome **(see also Chap. 61)**. Thus, weight reduction is the primary approach to the disorder. With weight reduction, improvement in insulin sensitivity is often accompanied by favorable modifications in many components of the metabolic syndrome. In general, recommendations for weight loss include a combination of caloric restriction, increased physical activity, and behavior modification. Caloric restriction is the most important component, whereas increases in physical activity are important for maintenance of weight loss. Some but not all evidence suggests that the addition of exercise to caloric restriction may promote greater weight loss from the visceral depot. The tendency for weight regain after successful weight reduction underscores the need for long-lasting behavioral changes.

Diet Before prescribing a weight-loss diet, it is important to emphasize that it has taken the patient a long time to develop an expanded fat mass; thus, the correction need not occur quickly. Given that ~3500 kcal = 1 lb of fat, ~500-kcal restriction daily equates to weight reduction of 1 lb per week. Diets restricted in carbohydrate typically provide a rapid initial weight loss. However, after 1 year, the amount of weight reduction is minimally reduced or no different from that with caloric restriction alone. Thus, adherence to the diet is more important than which diet is chosen. Moreover, there is concern about low-carbohydrate diets enriched in saturated fat, particularly for patients at risk for CVD. Therefore, a high-quality dietary pattern—i.e., a diet enriched in fruits, vegetables, whole grains, lean poultry, and fish—should be encouraged to maximize overall health benefit.

Physical Activity Before a physical activity recommendation is provided to patients with the metabolic syndrome, it is important to ensure that the increased activity does not incur risk. Some high-risk patients should undergo formal cardiovascular evaluation before initiating an exercise program. For an inactive participant, gradual increases in physical activity should be encouraged to enhance adherence and avoid injury. Although increases in physical activity can lead to modest weight reduction, 60–90 min of daily activity is required to achieve this goal. Even if an overweight or obese adult is unable to undertake this level of activity, a significant health benefit will follow from at least 30 min of moderate-intensity activity daily. The caloric value of 30 min of a variety of activities can be found at *www.heart.org/HEARTORG/GettingHealthy/WeightManagement/LosingWeight/Losing-Weight_UCM_307904_Article.jsp*. Of note, a variety of routine activities, such as gardening, walking, and housecleaning, require moderate caloric expenditure. Thus, physical activity need not be defined solely in terms of formal exercise such as jogging, swimming, or tennis.

Behavior Modification Behavioral treatment typically includes recommendations for dietary restriction and more physical activity, resulting in weight loss that benefits metabolic health. The subsequent challenge is the duration of the program because weight regain so often follows successful weight reduction. Long-term outcomes may be enhanced by a variety of methods, such as the Internet, social media, and telephone follow-up to maintain contact between providers and patients.

Obesity In some patients with the metabolic syndrome, treatment options need to extend beyond lifestyle intervention (**see also Chap. 61**). Weight-loss drugs come in two major classes: appetite suppressants and absorption inhibitors. Appetite suppressants approved by the U.S. Food and Drug Administration include phentermine (for short-term use [3 months] only) as well as the more recent additions phentermine/topiramate and lorcaserin, which are approved without restrictions on the duration of therapy. In clinical trials, the phentermine/topiramate combination has resulted in ~10% weight loss in 50% of patients. Side effects include palpitations, headache, paresthesias, constipation, and insomnia. Lorcaserin results in less weight loss—typically ~5% beyond placebo—but can cause headache and nasopharyngitis. Orlistat inhibits fat absorption by ~30% and is moderately effective compared with placebo (~5% more weight loss). Orlistat has been shown to reduce the incidence of type 2 diabetes, an effect that was especially evident among patients with impaired glucose tolerance at baseline. This drug is often difficult of take because of oily leakage per rectum.

Metabolic or bariatric surgery is an option for patients with the metabolic syndrome who have a body mass index >40 kg/m^2, or >35 kg/m^2 with comorbidities. An evolving application for metabolic surgery includes patients with a body mass index as low as 30 kg/m^2 and type 2 diabetes. Gastric bypass or vertical sleeve gastrectomy results in dramatic weight reduction and improvement in the features of the metabolic syndrome. A survival benefit with gastric bypass has also been realized.

LDL CHOLESTEROL The rationale for the NCEP:ATPIII's development of criteria for the metabolic syndrome was to go beyond LDL cholesterol in identifying and reducing the risk of CVD. The working assumption by the panel was that LDL cholesterol goals had already been achieved and that increasing evidence supports a linear reduction in CVD events as a result of progressive lowering of LDL cholesterol with statins. For patients with the metabolic syndrome and diabetes, a statin should be prescribed. For those patients with diabetes and known CVD, the current evidence supports a maximum of penultimate dose of a potent statin (e.g., atorvastatin or rosuvastatin). For those patients with the metabolic syndrome but without diabetes, a score that predicts a 10-year CVD risk exceeding 7.5% should also take a statin. With a 10-year risk of <7.5%, use of statin therapy is not evidence based.

Diets restricted in saturated fats (<7% of calories) and *trans*-fats (as few as possible) should be applied aggressively. Although less evidence exists, dietary cholesterol should also be restricted. If LDL cholesterol remains elevated, pharmacologic intervention is needed. Treatment with statins, which lower LDL cholesterol by 15–60%, is evidence based and is the first-choice medication intervention. Of note, for each doubling of the statin dose, LDL cholesterol is further lowered by only ~6%. Hepatotoxicity (more than a threefold increase in hepatic aminotransferases) is rare, and myopathy is seen in ~10% of patients. The cholesterol absorption inhibitor ezetimibe is well tolerated and should be the second-choice medication intervention. Ezetimibe typically reduces LDL cholesterol by 15–20%. The bile acid sequestrants cholestyramine, colestipol, and colesevalam may be more effective than ezetimibe but, because they can increase triglyceride levels, must be used with caution in patients with the metabolic syndrome. In general, bile sequestrants should not be administered when fasting triglyceride levels are >250 mg/dL. Side effects include gastrointestinal symptoms (palatability, bloating, belching, constipation, anal irritation). Nicotinic acid has modest LDL cholesterol–lowering capabilities (<20%). Fibrates are best employed to lower LDL cholesterol when both LDL cholesterol and triglycerides are elevated. Fenofibrate may be more effective than gemfibrozil in this setting.

TRIGLYCERIDES The NCEP: ATPIII has focused on non-HDL cholesterol rather than on triglycerides. However, a fasting triglyceride value of <150 mg/dL is recommended. In general, the response of fasting triglycerides relates to the amount of weight reduction achieved: a weight reduction of >10% is necessary to lower fasting triglyceride levels.

A fibrate (gemfibrozil or fenofibrate) is the drug of choice to lower fasting triglyceride levels, which are typically reduced by 30–45%. Concomitant administration with drugs metabolized by the 3A4 cytochrome P450 system (including some statins) increases the risk of myopathy. In these cases, fenofibrate may be preferable to gemfibrozil. In the Veterans Affairs HDL Intervention Trial, gemfibrozil was administered to men with known CHD and levels of HDL cholesterol <40 mg/dL. A coronary disease event and mortality rate benefit was experienced predominantly among men with hyperinsulinemia and/or diabetes, many of whom were identified retrospectively as having the metabolic syndrome. Of note, the degree of triglyceride lowering in this trial did not predict benefit. Although levels of LDL cholesterol did not change, a decrease in LDL particle number correlated with benefit. Several additional clinical trials have not shown clear evidence that fibrates reduce CVD risk; however, post hoc analyses of several studies demonstrated that patients with baseline triglyceride levels >200 mg/dL and HDL cholesterol levels <35 mg/dL did benefit.

Other drugs that lower triglyceride levels include statins, nicotinic acid, and—in high doses—omega-3 fatty acids. For this purpose, an intermediate or high dose of the "more potent" statins (atorvastatin, rosuvastatin) is needed. The effect of nicotinic acid on fasting triglycerides is dose related and ~20–35%, an effect that is less pronounced than that of fibrates. In patients with the metabolic syndrome and diabetes, nicotinic acid may increase fasting glucose levels. Omega-3 fatty acid preparations that include high doses of docosahexaenoic acid plus eicosapentaenoic acid (~1.5–4.5 g/d) or eicosapentaenoic acid alone lower fasting triglyceride levels by ~30–40%. No drug interactions with fibrates or statins occur, and the main side effect of their use is eructation with a fishy taste. This taste can be partially blocked by ingestion of the nutraceutical after freezing. Clinical trials of nicotinic acid or high-dose omega-3 fatty acids in patients with the metabolic syndrome have not been reported.

HDL CHOLESTEROL Very few lipid-modifying compounds increase HDL cholesterol levels. Statins, fibrates, and bile acid sequestrants have modest effects (5–10%), whereas ezetimibe and omega-3 fatty acids have no effect. Nicotinic acid is the only currently available drug with predictable HDL cholesterol-raising properties. The response is dose related, and nicotinic acid can increase HDL cholesterol by ~30% above baseline. After several trials of nicotinic acid versus placebo in statin-treated patients, there is still no evidence that raising HDL with nicotinic acid beneficially affects CVD events in patients with or without the metabolic syndrome.

BLOOD PRESSURE The direct relationship between blood pressure and all-cause mortality rate has been well established in studies comparing patients with hypertension (>140/90 mmHg), patients with pre-hypertension (>120/80 mmHg but <140/90 mmHg), and individuals with normal blood pressure (<120/80 mmHg). In patients who have the metabolic syndrome without diabetes, the best choice for the initial antihypertensive medication is an angiotensin-converting enzyme (ACE) inhibitor or an angiotensin II receptor blocker, as these two classes of drugs appear to reduce the incidence of new-onset type 2 diabetes. In all patients with hypertension, a sodium-restricted dietary pattern enriched in fruits and vegetables, whole grains, and low-fat dairy products should be advocated. Home monitoring of blood pressure may assist in maintaining good blood-pressure control.

IMPAIRED FASTING GLUCOSE In patients with the metabolic syndrome and type 2 diabetes, aggressive glycemic control may favorably modify fasting levels of triglycerides and/or HDL cholesterol. In patients with impaired fasting glucose who do not have diabetes, a lifestyle intervention that includes weight reduction, dietary fat restriction, and increased physical activity has been shown to reduce the incidence of type 2 diabetes. Metformin also reduces the incidence of diabetes, although the effect is less pronounced than that of lifestyle intervention.

INSULIN RESISTANCE Several drug classes (biguanides, thiazolidinediones [TZDs]) increase insulin sensitivity. Because insulin resistance is the primary pathophysiologic mechanism for the metabolic syndrome, representative drugs in these classes reduce its prevalence. Both metformin and TZDs enhance insulin action in the liver and suppress endogenous glucose production. TZDs, but not metformin, also improve insulin-mediated glucose uptake in muscle and adipose tissue. Benefits of both drugs have been seen in patients with nonalcoholic fatty liver disease and polycystic ovary syndrome, and the drugs have been shown to reduce markers of inflammation.

REVIEW AND SELF-ASSESSMENT*

Charles M. Wiener ■ Cynthia D. Brown ■ Brian Houston

QUESTIONS

DIRECTIONS: Choose the one best response to each question.

1. The advantages of endoscopy over barium radiography in the evaluation of dysphagia include all of the following EXCEPT:

   A. Ability to assess function and morphology
   B. Ability to intervene as well as diagnose
   C. Ability to obtain biopsy specimens
   D. Increased sensitivity for the detection of abnormalities identified by color, e.g. Barrett metaplasia
   E. Increased sensitivity for the detection of mucosal lesions

2. A 47-year-old man is evaluated in the emergency department for chest pain that developed at a restaurant after swallowing a piece of steak. He reports intermittent episodes of meat getting stuck in his lower chest over the past 3 years, but none as severe as this event. He denies food regurgitation outside of these episodes or heartburn symptoms. He is able to swallow liquids without difficulty and has not had any weight loss. Which of the following is the most likely diagnosis?

   A. Achalasia
   B. Adenocarcinoma of the esophagus
   C. Esophageal diverticula
   D. Plummer-Vinson syndrome
   E. Schatzki ring

3. Which of the following has a well-established association with gastroesophageal reflux?

   A. Chronic sinusitis
   B. Dental erosion
   C. Pulmonary fibrosis
   D. Recurrent aspiration pneumonia
   E. Sleep apnea

4. A 36-year-old woman with acquired immunodeficiency syndrome (AIDS) and a CD4 count of 35/μL presents with odynophagia and progressive dysphagia. The patient reports daily fevers and a 20-lb

4. (*Continued*)
   weight loss. The patient has been treated with clotrimazole troches without relief. On physical examination, the patient is cachectic with a body mass index (BMI) of 16 and a weight of 86 lbs. The patient has a temperature of 38.2°C (100.8°F). She is noted to be orthostatic by blood pressure and pulse. Examination of the oropharynx reveals no evidence of thrush. The patient undergoes esophagogastroduodenoscopy (EGD), which reveals serpiginous ulcers in the distal esophagus without vesicles. No yellow plaques are noted. Multiple biopsies are taken that show intranuclear and intracytoplasmic inclusions in large endothelial cells and fibroblasts. What is the best treatment for this patient's esophagitis?

   A. Ganciclovir
   B. Glucocorticoids
   C. Fluconazole
   D. Foscarnet
   E. Thalidomide

5. A 43-year-old man presents with 6 months of worsening dysphagia and postprandial regurgitation. He reports difficulty and pain with swallowing both liquids and solids. He has no difficulty with the initial components of swallowing but reports pain in the midchest region. He will frequently regurgitate undigested food 20–60 minutes after eating or drinking. In the past 2 months, he has lost 15 lbs. He also has had one episode of presumed pneumonia 4 months ago notable for a right lower lobe infiltrate. He has no significant past medical history, takes no medications, and does not smoke cigarettes. He works as a service representative at a major electronics store and has never left the United States. Other than signs of recent weight loss, his physical examination is unremarkable. A barium swallow is performed and is shown in Figure 5. Which of the following is the most likely cause of his disease?

   A. Autoimmune reaction to latent herpes virus
   B. Diffuse spasm on smooth muscle

*Questions and answers were taken from Wiener CM et al. (eds). *Harrison's Principles of Internal Medicine Self-Assessment and Board Review*. 19th ed. New York: McGraw-Hill; 2017.

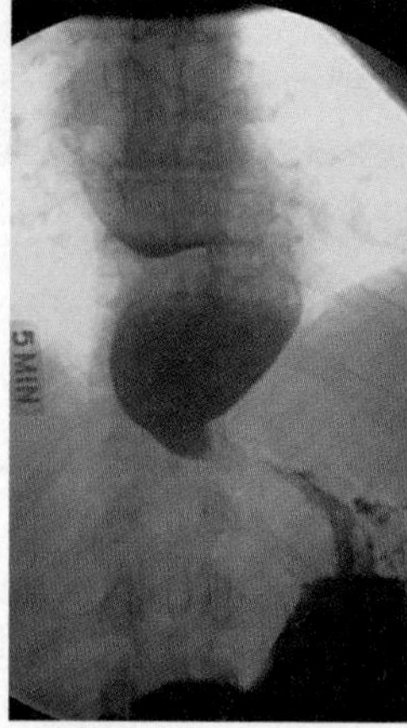

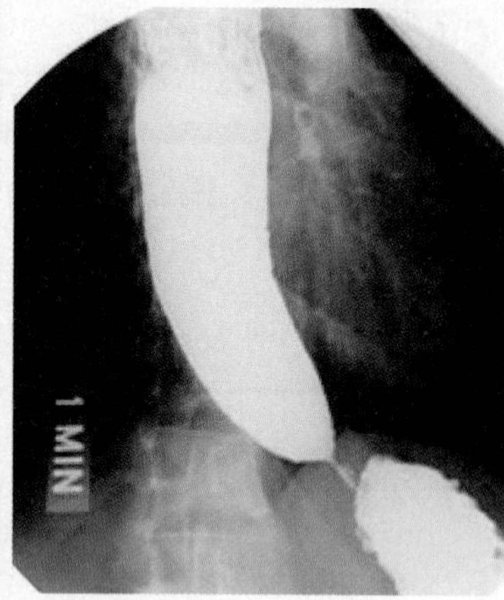

FIGURE 5

5. *(Continued)*
   C. Infection by *Trypanosoma cruzi*
   D. Malignant growth of columnar epithelial cells
   E. Malignant growth squamous epithelial cells

6. In the patient described in Question 5, which of the following is the most efficacious therapy?

   A. Botulinum toxin
   B. Calcium channel blocker
   C. Esophagectomy
   D. Nitroglycerine
   E. Radiation therapy

7. A 64-year-old man with a long history of abdominal pain, heartburn, and dyspepsia has an EGD to evaluate for peptic ulcer disease. No gastric or duodenal ulcers are found, but there are tongues of reddish mucosa extending proximally from the gastroesophageal junction into the esophagus. Biopsies of these areas demonstrate columnar metaplasia. All of the following statements regarding this diagnosis are true EXCEPT:

   A. Finding high-grade dysplasia mandates further intervention.
   B. High-dose proton pump inhibitor therapy will likely cause regression of the mucosal abnormalities.
   C. The incidence of these lesions has increased in the era of potent acid suppression.
   D. The patient has a high risk of coexisting cancer.
   E. The patient is at significant risk of esophageal adenocarcinoma.

8. A 57-year-old man is evaluated with an EGD after an episode of hematemesis. The patient reports a history of tobacco use and hypercholesterolemia but is otherwise healthy. He has had lower back pain for the past month and has been intermittently using acetaminophen 1000 mg for relief. His endoscopy shows a 3-cm duodenal ulcer. Which of the following statements is correct regarding this finding?

   A. The lesion should be biopsied because duodenal ulcers have an elevated risk of being due to carcinoma.
   B. First-line therapy should be discontinuation of acetaminophen use.
   C. The patient is not at risk for any associated cancers.
   D. Poor socioeconomic status is a risk factor for development of this condition.
   E. Antral gastritis is rarely found with this condition.

9. A 58-year-old man is evaluated for abdominal pain by his primary care physician. He reports severe stress at the job for the last 3 months and has since noted that he has epigastric pain that is relieved by eating and drinking milk. He has not had food regurgitation, dysphagia, or bloody emesis or bowel movements. He denies any symptoms in his chest. Peptic ulcer disease is suspected. Which of the following statements regarding noninvasive testing for *Helicobacter pylori* is true?

   A. There is no reliable noninvasive method to detect *H. pylori*.
   B. Stool antigen testing is appropriate for both diagnosis of and proof of cure after therapy for *H. pylori*.
   C. Plasma antibodies to *H. pylori* offer the greatest sensitivity for diagnosis of infection.
   D. Expose to low-dose radiation is a limitation to urea breath test.
   E. False-negative test results using the urea breath test may occur with recent use of nonsteroidal anti-inflammatory drugs (NSAIDs).

10. A 44-year-old woman complains of 6 months of epigastric pain that is worst between meals. She also reports symptoms of heartburn. The pain is typically relieved by over-the-counter antacid medications. She comes to clinic after noting her stools darkening. She has no significant past medical history and takes no medications. Her physical examination is normal except for diffuse mid-epigastric pain. Her stools are heme positive. She undergoes EGD, which demonstrates a well-circumscribed, 2-cm duodenal ulcer that is positive for *H. pylori*. Which of the following is the recommended initial therapy given these findings?

    A. Lansoprazole, clarithromycin, and metronidazole for 14 days

10. (*Continued*)
   B. Pantoprazole and amoxicillin for 21 days
   C. Pantoprazole and clarithromycin for 14 days
   D. Omeprazole, bismuth, tetracycline, and metronidazole for 14 days
   E. Omeprazole, metronidazole, and clarithromycin for 7 days

11. A 57-year-old man with peptic ulcer disease experiences transient improvement with *H. pylori* eradication. However, 3 months later, symptoms recur despite acid-suppressing therapy. He does not take NSAIDs. Stool analysis for *H. pylori* antigen is negative. Upper gastrointestinal (GI) endoscopy reveals prominent gastric folds together with the persistent ulceration in the duodenal bulb previously detected and the beginning of a new ulceration 4 cm proximal to the initial ulcer. Fasting gastrin levels are elevated, and basal acid secretion is 15 mEq/hr. What is the best test to perform to make the diagnosis?

   A. No additional testing is necessary.
   B. Blood sampling for gastrin levels following a meal
   C. Blood sampling for gastrin levels following secretin administration
   D. Endoscopic ultrasonography of the pancreas
   E. Genetic testing for mutations in the *MEN1* gene

12. A 65-year-old man presented to the hospital 2 weeks ago with an acute abdomen, hypotension, anemia, and respiratory failure. His past medical history was notable for hypertension and hypercholesterolemia for which he took enalapril and atorvastatin. At laparotomy, he was found to have a perforated duodenal ulcer with peritonitis and hemoperitoneum. A vagotomy and Billroth I anastomosis were performed. He has improved gradually and is increasing his oral intake and ambulation. His white blood cell (WBC) count and hemoglobin are normal. This afternoon approximately 3 hours after lunch, he reported the acute onset of lightheadedness, confusion, palpitations, and diaphoresis. His temperature is 36.0°C, heart rate is 110 bpm, blood pressure is 120/70 mmHg, and oxygen saturation is 95% on room air. Which of the following is most likely present?

   A. Anemia
   B. Hypoglycemia
   C. Pulmonary embolism on helical chest computed tomography (CT)
   D. Seizure focus on electroencephalogram (EEG)
   E. ST elevation on electrocardiogram (ECG)

13. In the patient described in Question 12, which of the following is the most likely diagnosis?

   A. Acute GI bleed
   B. Diabetes mellitus
   C. Dumping syndrome
   D. Inferior wall myocardial infarction
   E. Pulmonary embolism

14. A 23-year-old woman is evaluated by her primary care physician for diffuse, crampy abdominal pain. She reports that she has had abdominal pain for the last several years, but it is getting worse and is now associated with intermittent diarrhea without flatulence. This does not waken her at night. Stools do not float and are not hard to flush. She has not noted any worsening with specific foods, but she does have occasional rashes on her lower legs. She has lost about 10 pounds over the last year. She is otherwise healthy and takes no medications. Which of the following is the most appropriate recommendation at this point?

   A. Increased dietary fiber intake
   B. Measurement of antiendomysial antibody
   C. Measurement of 24-hour fecal fat
   D. Referral to gastroenterologist for endoscopy
   E. Trial of lactose-free diet

15. All of the following are direct complications of short bowel syndrome EXCEPT:

   A. Cholesterol gallstones
   B. Coronary artery disease
   C. Gastric acid hypersecretion
   D. Renal calcium oxalate calculi
   E. Steatorrhea

16. A 54-year-old man is evaluated by a gastroenterologist for diarrhea that has been present for approximately 1 month. He reports stools that float and are difficult to flush down the toilet; these can occur at any time of day or night but seem worsened by fatty meals. In addition, he reports pain in many joints lasting days to weeks and not relieved by ibuprofen. His wife notes that the patient has had difficulty with memory for the last few months. He has lost 30 pounds and reports intermittent low-grade fevers. He takes no medications and is otherwise healthy. Endoscopy is recommended. Which of the following is the most likely finding on small bowel biopsy?

   A. Dilated lymphatics
   B. Flat villi with crypt hyperplasia
   C. Mononuclear cell infiltrate in the lamina propria

16. (*Continued*)
    D. Normal small bowel biopsy
    E. Periodic acid–Schiff (PAS)–positive macrophages containing small bacilli

17. A 54-year-old man presents with 1 month of diarrhea. He states that he has 8–10 loose bowel movements a day. He has lost 8 pounds during this time. Vital signs and physical examination are normal. Serum laboratory studies are normal. A 24-hour stool collection reveals 500 g of stool with a measured stool osmolality of 200 mOsmol/L and a calculated stool osmolality of 210 mOsmol/L. Based on these findings, what is the most likely cause of this patient's diarrhea?

    A. Celiac sprue
    B. Chronic pancreatitis
    C. Lactase deficiency
    D. Vasoactive intestinal peptide tumor
    E. Whipple disease

18. Which of the following GI disorders is characterized by increased absorption from the GI tract into the portal circulation?

    A. Celiac disease
    B. Crohn disease
    C. Hemochromatosis
    D. Pernicious anemia
    E. Whipple disease

19. Which of the following statements regarding the epidemiology of inflammatory bowel disease is correct?

    A. Monozygotic twins are highly concordant for ulcerative colitis.
    B. Oral contraceptive use decreases the incidence of Crohn disease.
    C. Persons of Asian descent have the highest rates of ulcerative colitis and Crohn disease.
    D. Smoking may decrease the incidence of ulcerative colitis.
    E. Typical age of onset for Crohn disease is 40–50 years old.

20. A 24-year-old woman is admitted to the hospital with a 1-year history of severe abdominal pain and chronic diarrhea that has been bloody for the past 2 months. She reports a 20-lb weight loss, frequent fevers, and night sweats. She denies vomiting. Her abdominal pain is crampy and primary involves her right lower quadrant. She is otherwise healthy. Examination is concerning for an acute abdomen with rebound and guarding present. CT shows free air in the peritoneum. She is urgently taken to the operating room for surgical exploration, where she is found to have multiple strictures and a perforation of her bowel in the terminal ileum. The rectum was spared, and a fissure from the duodenum to the jejunum is found. The perforated area is resected and adhesions lysed. Which of the following findings on pathology of her resected area confirms her diagnosis?

    A. Crypt abscesses
    B. Flat villi
    C. Noncaseating granuloma throughout the bowel wall
    D. Special stain for *Clostridium difficile* toxin
    E. Transmural acute and chronic inflammation

21. A 45-year-old man with ulcerative colitis has been treated for the past 5 years with infliximab with excellent resolution of his bowel symptoms and endoscopic evidence of normal colonic mucosa. He is otherwise healthy. He is evaluated by a dermatologist for a lesion that initially was a pustule over his right lower extremity but has since progressed in size with ulceration. The ulcer is moderately painful. He does not recall any trauma to the area. On examination, the ulcer measures 15 × 7 cm, and central necrosis is present. The edges of the ulcer are violaceous. No other lesions are identified. Which of the following is the most likely diagnosis?

    A. Erythema nodosum
    B. Metastatic Crohn disease
    C. Psoriasis
    D. Pyoderma gangrenosum
    E. Pyoderma vegetans

22. Inflammatory bowel disease (IBD) may be caused by exogenous factors. GI flora may promote an inflammatory response or may inhibit inflammation. Probiotics have been used to treat IBD. Which of the following organisms has been used in the treatment of IBD?

    A. *Campylobacter* spp.
    B. *C. difficile*
    C. *Escherichia* spp.
    D. *Lactobacillus* spp.
    E. *Shigella* spp.

23. Your 33-year-old patient with Crohn disease has had a disappointing disease response to glucocorticoids and 5-aminosalicylic acid (5-ASA) agents.

23. *(Continued)*
He is interested in glucocorticoid-sparing agents. He has no liver or renal disease. You prescribe once-weekly methotrexate injections. In addition to monitoring hepatic function and complete blood count, what other complication of methotrexate therapy do you advise the patient of?

A. Disseminated histoplasmosis
B. Lymphoma
C. Pancreatitis
D. Pneumonitis
E. Primary sclerosing cholangitis

24. All of the following statements regarding the risk of cancer in patients with IBD are correct EXCEPT:

A. Patients with Crohn disease are at greater risk for hematologic malignancies than the general population.
B. Patients with Crohn disease are at lower risk of GI malignancies than patients with ulcerative colitis.
C. Patients with long-standing ulcerative colitis are at increased risk of developing carcinoma of the colon.
D. Screening colonoscopy is recommended every 1–2 years in patients with an >8- to 10-year history of extensive ulcerative colitis regardless of age.
E. Ulcerative colitis patients with high-grade dysplasia found on colonoscopy should undergo immediate colectomy.

25. Which of the following patients requires no further testing before making the diagnosis of irritable bowel syndrome and initiating treatment?

A. A 76-year-old woman with 6 months of intermittent crampy abdominal pain that is worse with stress and associated with bloating and diarrhea.
B. A 25-year-old woman with 6 months of abdominal pain, bloating, and diarrhea that has worsened steadily and who now awakes from sleep at night to move her bowels.
C. A 30-year-old man with 6 months of lower abdominal crampy pain relieved with bowel movements, usually loose. Symptoms are worse during the daytime at work and better on the weekend. Weight loss is not present.
D. A 19-year-old female college student with 2 months of diarrhea and worsening abdominal pain with occasional blood in her stool.
E. A 27-year-old woman with 6 months of intermittent abdominal pain, bloating, and diarrhea without associated weight loss. Crampy pain and diarrhea persist after a 48-hour fast.

26. A 29-year-old woman comes to see you in clinic because of abdominal discomfort. She feels abdominal discomfort on most days of the week, and the pain varies in location and intensity. She notes constipation as well as diarrhea, but diarrhea predominates. Compared to 6 months ago, she has more bloating and flatulence than she has had before. She identifies eating and stress as aggravating factors, and her pain is relieved by defecation. You suspect irritable bowel syndrome. Laboratory data include: WBC count 8000/μL, hematocrit 32%, platelets 210,000/μL, and erythrocyte sedimentation rate (ESR) 44 mm/hr. Stool studies show the presence of lactoferrin but no blood. Which intervention is appropriate at this time?

A. Antidepressants
B. Ciprofloxacin
C. Colonoscopy
D. Reassurance and patient counseling
E. Stool bulking agents

27. After a careful history and physical and a cost-effective workup, you have diagnosed a 24-year-old female patient with irritable bowel syndrome. What other condition would you reasonably expect to find in this patient?

A. Abnormal brain anatomy
B. Autoimmune disease
C. History of sexually transmitted diseases
D. Psychiatric diagnosis
E. Sensory hypersensitivity to peripheral stimuli

28. A 24-year-old woman has had 2 years of abdominal complaints characterized by episodic abdominal pain that is relieved by stooling. She reports that she has frequent small stools often soon after eating. She does not wake at night to use the bathroom. She has treated herself with various over-the-counter medications. She reports that she has tried a variety of diets recommended by daytime television that have occasionally but not consistently helped her symptoms. Her past medical history is notable for mild depression for which she takes fluoxetine. Her physical examination is completely normal, as are her basic metabolic panel, thyroid function, and complete blood count. A diet low in which of the following has been shown to be beneficial in patients such as her?

A. Animal protein
B. Capsaicin

28. *(Continued)*

C. Fermentable oligosaccharides, disaccharides, monosaccharides, and polyols
D. Rice and rice products
E. Vegetable protein

29. A 78-year-old woman is admitted to the hospital with fever, loss of appetite, and left lower quadrant pain. She is not constipated but has not moved her bowels recently. Laboratory examination is notable for an elevated WBC count. These symptoms began approximately 3 days ago and have steadily worsened. Which of the following statements regarding the use of radiologic imaging to evaluate her condition is true?

A. Air-fluid levels are commonly seen on plain abdominal films.
B. Less than 25% of patients present with peritoneal signs.
C. Lower GI bleeding will likely be visualized on CT angiography.
D. Thickened colonic wall is not required on CT for the diagnosis of her likely condition.
E. Ultrasound of the pelvis is the best modality to visualize the likely pathologic process.

30. Which of the following patients is MOST appropriate for surgical management of the their acute diverticulitis?

A. A 45-year-old woman with rheumatoid arthritis treated with infliximab and prednisone.
B. A 63-year-old woman with diverticulitis in the descending colon and a distal stricture.
C. A 70-year-old woman with end-stage renal disease and colonic wall thickening of 8 mm on CT scan.
D. A 77-year-old man with two episodes of diverticulitis in the past 2 years.

31. A 67-year-old man is evaluated by the emergency department for blood in the toilet bowel after moving his bowels. Blood was also present on the toilet paper after wiping. He does report straining and recent constipation. He has a history of systemic hypertension and hyperlipidemia. Vital signs are normal, and he is not orthostatic. Anoscopy shows external hemorrhoids, hematocrit is normal, and bleeding does not recur during his 6-hour emergency department stay. Which of the following is the most appropriate management?

31. *(Continued)*

A. Ciprofloxacin and metronidazole
B. Cortisone suppositories and fiber supplementation
C. Hemorrhoidal banding
D. Operative hemorrhoidectomy
E. Upper endoscopy

32. Which of the following statements regarding anorectal abscess is true?

A. Anorectal abscess is more common in diabetic patients.
B. Anorectal abscess is more common in women.
C. Difficulty voiding is uncommon and should prompt further evaluation of anorectal abscess.
D. Examination in the operating room under anesthesia is required for adequate exploration in most cases.
E. The peak incidence is in the seventh decade of life.

33. An 88-year-old woman is brought to your clinic by her family because she has become increasingly socially withdrawn. The patient lives alone and has been reluctant to visit or be visited by her family. Family members, including seven children, also note a foul odor in her apartment and on her person. She has not had any weight loss. Alone in the examining room, she only complains of hemorrhoids. On mental status examination, she does have signs of depression. Which of the following interventions is most appropriate at this time?

A. Head CT scan
B. Treatment with an antidepressant medication
C. Physical examination including genitourinary and rectal examination
D. Screening for occult malignancy
E. Serum thyroid-stimulating hormone

34. An 85-year-old woman is brought to a local emergency department by her family. She has been complaining of abdominal pain off and on for several days, but this morning, she states that this is the worst pain of her life. She is able to describe a sharp, stabbing pain in her abdomen. Her family reports that she has not been eating and seems to have no appetite. She has a past medical history of atrial fibrillation and hypercholesterolemia. She has had two episodes of vomiting, and in the emergency department experiences diarrhea that is hemoccult positive. On examination, she is afebrile, with a heart rate of 105 bpm and blood pressure of 111/69 mmHg. Her abdomen is mildly distended, and she has hypoactive bowel sounds. She does not exhibit

34. (*Continued*)
rebound tenderness or guarding. She is admitted for further management. Several hours after admission, she becomes unresponsive. Blood pressure is difficult to obtain and at best approximation is 60/40 mmHg. She has a rigid abdomen. Surgery is called, and the patient is taken for emergent laparotomy. She is found to have acute mesenteric ischemia. Which of the following statements is true regarding this diagnosis?

A. Mortality for this condition is >50%.
B. Risk factors include low-fiber diet and obesity.
C. The "gold standard" for diagnosis is CT scan of the abdomen.
D. The lack of acute abdominal signs in this case is unusual for mesenteric ischemia.
E. The splanchnic circulation is poorly collateralized.

35. A 63-year-old man with a history of diabetes and myocardial infarction was admitted to the medical intensive care unit (ICU) 1 day ago with sepsis due to pneumococcal pneumonia with bacteremia. He was started on antibiotics immediately but initially required high doses of noradrenaline and fluids to stabilize his blood pressure. The noradrenaline was weaned off approximately 12 hours ago. Over the past 2 hours, he has had increasing abdominal pain, distension, and bloody stools. His physical examination is notable for blood pressure of 100/50 mmHg, regular heart rate of 100 bpm, respiratory rate of 22 breaths/min, and oxygen saturation of 93% on high-flow nasal oxygen. He has a diffusely tender abdomen with no audible bowel sounds. An abdominal radiograph shows multiple small bowel air-fluid levels. Which of the following is the most likely diagnosis?

A. Arterial embolus
B. *C. difficile* colitis
C. Inflammatory bowel disease
D. Nonocclusive mesenteric ischemia
E. Venous thrombosis

36. A 74-year-old woman is 2 days status post hip surgery for a fracture after a fall. Her only medication prior to admission was a calcium supplement, and she has no prior surgical history. Over the past 24 hours, she has had increasing abdominal discomfort and distension. She received a dose of cefazolin prior to surgery but no other antibiotics. On physical examination, she is afebrile with blood pressure of 140/80 mmHg, heart rate of 110 bpm, respiratory rate of 16 breaths/min, and oxygen saturation of 100% on 2 L of nasal oxygen. She has a distended tympanic abdomen with absent bowel sounds. There is no rebound tenderness. Her upright abdominal film is shown in Figure 36. Which of the following is the most likely diagnosis?

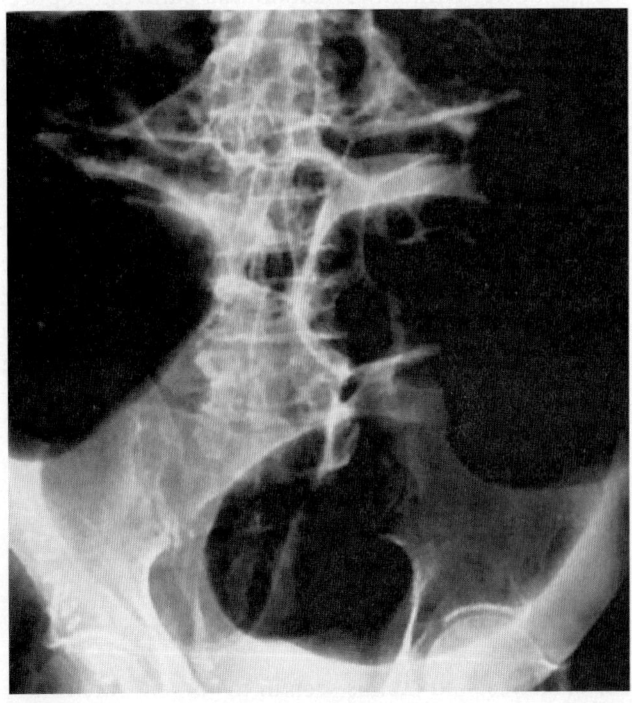

FIGURE 36
Reproduced, with permission, from Bongard FS, Sue DY [eds]. *Current Critical Care Diagnosis & Treatment*. Originally published by Appleton & Lange. Copyright © 1994 by The McGraw-Hill Companies, Inc., Fig. 13-18A.

A. Acalculous cholecystitis
B. Colonic pseudo-obstruction
C. Perforated duodenal ulcer
D. Small bowel obstruction
E. Small bowel ileus

37. Which of the following is the next recommended therapy for the patient described in Question 36?

A. Atropine
B. Laparotomy
C. Morphine
D. Neostigmine
E. Vancomycin

38. All of the following are potential causes of appendix obstruction and appendicitis EXCEPT:

A. *Ascaris* infection
B. Carcinoid tumor

38. (*Continued*)
C. Cholelithiasis
D. Fecalith
E. Measles infection

39. A 32-year-old woman is evaluated in the emergency department for abdominal pain. She reports a vague loss of appetite for the past day and has had progressively severe abdominal pain, initially at her umbilicus, but now localized to her right lower quadrant. The pain is crampy. She has not moved her bowels or vomited. She reports that she is otherwise healthy and has had no sick contact. Exam is notable for a temperature of 100.7°F and heart rate of 105 bpm, but otherwise, vital signs are normal. Her abdomen is tender in the right lower quadrant, and pelvic examination is normal. Urine pregnancy test is negative. Which of the following imaging modalities is most likely to confirm her diagnosis?

A. CT of the abdomen without contrast
B. Colonoscopy
C. Pelvic ultrasound
D. Plain film of the abdomen
E. Ultrasound of the abdomen

40. A 38-year-old man is seen in the urgent care center with several hours of severe abdominal pain. His symptoms began suddenly, but he reports several months of pain in the epigastrium after eating, with a resultant 10-lb weight loss. He takes no medications besides over-the-counter antacids and has no other medical problems or habits. On physical examination, temperature is 38.0°C (100.4°F), pulse is 130 bpm, respiratory rate is 24 breaths/min, and blood pressure is 110/50 mmHg. His abdomen has absent bowel sounds and is rigid with involuntary guarding diffusely. A plain film of the abdomen is obtained and shows free air under the diaphragm. Which of the following is most likely to be found in the operating room?

A. Necrotic bowel
B. Necrotic pancreas
C. Perforated duodenal ulcer
D. Perforated gallbladder
E. Perforated gastric ulcer

41. Which of the following is the mostly likely source of peritonitis in the patient in Question 40?

A. Bile
B. Blood
C. Foreign body
D. Gastric contents
E. Pancreatic enzymes

42. A 61-year-old man is admitted to your service for swelling of the abdomen. You detect ascites on clinical examination and perform a paracentesis. The results show a WBC count of 300 leukocytes/μL with 35% polymorphonuclear cells. The peritoneal albumin level is 1.2 g/dL, protein is 2.0 g/dL, and triglycerides are 320 mg/dL. Peritoneal cultures are pending. Serum albumin is 2.6 g/dL. Which of the following is the most likely diagnosis?

A. Congestive heart failure
B. Peritoneal tuberculosis
C. Peritoneal carcinomatosis
D. Chylous ascites
E. Bacterial peritonitis

43. Which of the following is the most common symptom or sign of liver disease?

A. Fatigue
B. Itching
C. Jaundice
D. Nausea
E. Right upper quadrant pain

44. In women, what is the average amount of reported daily alcohol intake that is associated with the development of chronic liver disease?

A. 1 drink
B. 2 drinks
C. 3 drinks
D. 6 drinks
E. 12 drinks

45. All of the following are CAGE questions, which should be a component of the medical history focusing on alcohol abuse and dependence, EXCEPT:

A. Do you feel like you have a greater tolerance for alcohol than your friends?
B. Have you ever felt you ought to cut down on your drinking?
C. Have people annoyed you by criticizing your drinking?
D. Have you ever felt guilty or bad about your drinking?
E. Have you ever had a drink first thing in the morning to steady your nerves or get rid of a hangover?

46. Elevation in all of the following laboratory studies would be indicative of liver disease EXCEPT:

A. 5′-Nucleotidase
B. Aspartate aminotransferase
C. Conjugated bilirubin
D. Unconjugated bilirubin
E. Urine bilirubin

47. All of the following statements regarding liver function tests are true EXCEPT:

A. Alanine aminotransferase (ALT) is found in liver, cardiac muscle, skeletal muscle, and kidney.
B. Elevation of aspartate aminotransferase (AST) and ALT to >1000 IU/L is typical of ischemic hepatitis.
C. Elevation of AST is more specific for liver dysfunction than elevation of ALT.
D. Increased AST and ALT with an AST:ALT ratio of >3 is typical of acute viral hepatitis.
E. The magnitude of elevated AST and ALT has important prognostic significance in acute hepatitis.

48. A 26-year-old male resident is noticed by his attending physician to have yellow eyes after his 24-hour call period. When asked, the resident states he has no medical history, but on occasion he has thought he might have mild jaundice when he is stressed or has more than four to five alcoholic drinks. He never sought medical treatment because he was uncertain, and his eyes would return fully to normal within 2 days. He denies nausea, abdominal pain, dark urine, light-colored stools, pruritus, or weight loss. On examination, he has a BMI of 20.1 kg/m^2, and his vital signs are normal. Scleral icterus is present. There are no stigmata of chronic liver disease. The patient's abdomen is soft and nontender. The liver span is 8 cm to percussion. The liver edge is smooth and palpable only with deep inspiration. The spleen is not palpable. Laboratory examinations are normal except for a total bilirubin of 3.0 mg/dL. Direct bilirubin is 0.2 mg/dL. AST, ALT, and alkaline phosphatase are normal. Hematocrit, lactate dehydrogenase, and haptoglobin are normal. Which of the following is the most likely diagnosis?

A. Autoimmune hemolytic anemia
B. Crigler-Najjar syndrome type 1
C. Choledocholithiasis
D. Dubin-Johnson syndrome
E. Gilbert syndrome

49. What is the next step in the evaluation and management of the patient in Question 48?

49. (*Continued*)
A. Genotype studies
B. Peripheral blood smear
C. Prednisone
D. Reassurance
E. Right upper quadrant ultrasound

50. Which of the following statements regarding the hyperbilirubinemia seen in patients with significant intravascular hemolysis is true?

A. Bilirubin values <4 mg/dL imply concomitant gallbladder or biliary dysfunction.
B. Bilirubin values >4 mg/dL (68 μmol/L) imply concomitant liver dysfunction.
C. It is typically composed of 50% conjugated and 50% unconjugated bilirubin.
D. Prolonged hemolysis may result in the development of nephrolithiasis due to bile pigment stones.

51. A 34-year-old man presents to the physician complaining of yellow eyes. For the past week, he has felt ill, with decreased oral intake, low-grade fevers (~100°F), fatigue, nausea, and occasional vomiting. With the onset of jaundice, he has noticed pain in his right upper quadrant. He currently uses marijuana and ecstasy and has a prior history of injection drug use with cocaine. He has no other past medical history, but he was unable to donate blood for reasons that he cannot recall 4 years previously. His social history is remarkable for working as a veterinary assistant. On sexual history, he reports five male sexual partners over the past 6 months. He does not consistently use condoms. On physical examination, he appears ill and has obvious jaundice with scleral icterus. His liver is 15 cm to percussion, palpable 6 cm below the right costal margin. The edge is smooth and tender to palpation. The spleen is not enlarged. There are no stigmata of chronic liver disease. His AST is 1232 IU/L, ALT is 1560 IU/L, alkaline phosphatase is 394 IU/L, total bilirubin is 13.4 mg/dL, and direct bilirubin is 12.2 mg/dL. His international normalized ratio (INR) is 2.3, and activated partial thromboplastin time (aPTT) is 52 seconds. Hepatitis serologies are sent and reveal the following:

Hepatitis A IgM	negative
Hepatitis A IgG	negative
Hepatitis B core IgM	positive
Hepatitis B core IgG	negative
Hepatitis B surface antigen	positive
Hepatitis B surface antibody	negative
Hepatitis B e antigen	positive

51. (*Continued*)

Hepatitis B e antibody	negative
Hepatitis C antibody	positive

What is the cause of the patient's current clinical presentation?

A. Acute hepatitis A infection
B. Acute hepatitis B infection
C. Acute hepatitis C infection
D. Chronic hepatitis B infection
E. Drug-induced hepatitis

52. In the patient described in Question 51, what would be the best approach to prevent development of chronic hepatitis?

A. Administration of anti-hepatitis A virus immunoglobulin (Ig) G
B. Administration of lamivudine
C. Administration of pegylated interferon-α plus ribavirin
D. Administration of prednisone beginning at a dose of 1 mg/kg daily
E. Do nothing and observe, as 99% of individuals with this disease recover

53. Which of the following viral causes of acute hepatitis is most likely to cause fulminant hepatitis in a pregnant woman?

A. Hepatitis A
B. Hepatitis B
C. Hepatitis C
D. Hepatitis D
E. Hepatitis E

54. A 16-year-old girl had visited your clinic 1 month ago with jaundice, vomiting, malaise, and anorexia. Two other family members were ill with similar symptoms. Based on viral serologies, including a positive anti-hepatitis A virus IgM, a diagnosis of hepatitis A was made. The patient was treated conservatively, and 1 week after first presenting, she appeared to have made a full recovery. She returns to your clinic today complaining of the same symptoms she had 1 month ago. She is jaundiced, and an initial panel of laboratory tests returns elevated transaminases. Which of the following offers the best explanation of what has occurred in this patient?

A. Co-infection with hepatitis C
B. Inappropriate treatment of initial infection
C. Incorrect initial diagnosis; this patient likely has hepatitis B

54. (*Continued*)

D. Reinfection with hepatitis A
E. Relapse of hepatitis A

55. A 26-year-old woman presents to your clinic and is interested in getting pregnant. She seeks your advice regarding vaccines she should obtain, and in particular asks about the hepatitis B vaccine. She works as a receptionist for a local business, denies alcohol or illicit drug use, and is in a monogamous relationship. Which of the following is true regarding hepatitis B vaccination?

A. Hepatitis B vaccine consists of two intramuscular doses 1 month apart.
B. Only patients with defined risk factors need to be vaccinated.
C. Pregnancy is not a contraindication to the hepatitis B vaccine.
D. This patient's hepatitis serologies should be checked prior to vaccination.
E. Vaccination should not be administered to children under 2 years old.

56. An 18-year-old man presents to a rural clinic with nausea, vomiting, anorexia, abdominal discomfort, myalgias, and jaundice. He describes occasional alcohol use and is sexually active. He describes using heroin and cocaine "a few times in the past." He works as a short-order cook in a local restaurant. He has lost 15.5 kg (34 lbs) since his last visit to clinic and appears emaciated and ill. On examination, he is noted to have icteric sclerae and a palpable, tender liver below the right costal margin. In regard to acute hepatitis, which of the following is true?

A. A distinction between viral etiologies cannot be made using clinical criteria alone.
B. Based on age and risk factors, he is likely to have hepatitis B infection.
C. He does not have hepatitis E virus, as this infects only pregnant women.
D. This patient cannot have hepatitis C because his presentation is too acute.
E. This patient does not have hepatitis A because his presentation is too fulminant.

57. A 36-year-old man presents with fatigue and tea-colored urine for 5 days. Physical examination reveals jaundice and tender hepatomegaly but is otherwise unremarkable. Laboratories are remarkable for an AST of 2400 IU/L and an ALT of 2640 IU/L. Alkaline phosphatase is 210 IU/L. Total bilirubin is 8.6 mg/dL. Which of the following diagnoses

57. *(Continued)*
is least likely to cause this clinical picture and these laboratory abnormalities?

A. Acute hepatitis A infection
B. Acute hepatitis B infection
C. Acute hepatitis C infection
D. Acetaminophen ingestion
E. Budd-Chiari syndrome

58. Which of the following drugs has a direct toxic effect on hepatocytes?

A. Acetaminophen
B. Chlorpromazine
C. Halothane
D. Isoniazid
E. Rosuvastatin

59. A 32-year-old woman is admitted to the ICU following an overdose of acetaminophen with co-ingestion of alcohol. She was known to be alert and interactive about 4 hours prior to her presentation when she had a fight with her boyfriend who then left the home. When he returned 6 hours later, he found an empty bottle of acetaminophen 500-mg capsules as well as an empty vodka bottle. The exact number of pills in the bottle is unknown, but the full bottle held as many as 50 capsules. The patient was unresponsive and had vomited, so her boyfriend called 911. Upon arrival to the emergency department, the patient is stuporous. Her vital signs are: pulse 109 bpm, respiratory rate 20 breaths/min, blood pressure 96/52 mmHg, and oxygen saturation 95% on room air. Her examination shows mild nonspecific abdominal pain with palpation. The liver is not enlarged. Her initial laboratory values show a normal complete blood count, normal electrolytes, and kidney function. The AST is 68 IU/L, ALT is 46 IU/L, alkaline phosphatase is 110 IU/L, and total bilirubin is 1.2 mg/dL. Glucose and coagulation studies are normal. The serum alcohol level is 210 g/dL. The acetaminophen level is 350 μg/mL. What is the most appropriate next step in the treatment of this patient?

A. Administration of activated charcoal or cholestyramine
B. Administration of *N*-acetylcysteine 140 mg/kg followed by 70 mg/kg every 4 hours for a total of 15–20 doses
C. Continued monitoring of liver function, glucose, and coagulation studies every 4 hours with administration of *N*-acetylcysteine if these begin to change

59. *(Continued)*
D. Do nothing, as normal liver function tests and coagulation studies are indicative of only a minor ingestion
E. Initiate hemodialysis for toxin clearance

60. A 31-year-old healthcare worker is found to have a newly positive tuberculin skin test 6 weeks after an exposure to a patient with active pulmonary tuberculosis. He is asymptomatic and has a normal chest radiograph. Which of the following statements regarding initiation of isoniazid (INH) prophylactic therapy is true?

A. Acute hepatocellular injury due to INH is an idiosyncratic reaction that will manifest within the first 2 months of initiation of therapy.
B. Controlled trials have demonstrated that monthly monitoring of aminotransferase levels reduces morbidity in U.S. healthcare workers receiving INH prophylaxis.
C. Elevation of aminotransferase levels in the first 2 months of therapy is an indication to stop INH and switch to another drug.
D. The patient has a 50%–70% chance of transient elevation of his aminotransferase levels in the first 2 months of treatment.
E. The frequency of acute hepatocellular injury due to INH is age-dependent, increasing in patients >35 years of age.

61. You are caring for a 48-year-old former drug user with chronic hepatitis C who is currently on no medications and whose most recent cardiovascular risk profile suggests he would benefit from initiation of statin therapy. His most recent liver function tests reveal high normal AST and ALT, normal alkaline phosphatase, and normal INR. He has not initiated antiviral therapy because of insurance issues with the new expensive curative therapies. Which of the following statements regarding statin therapy is true?

A. Monitoring of aminotransferase levels should be initiated in patients starting statin therapy.
B. Overall, between 5% and 10% of patients receiving statins develop mild reversible elevations in aminotransferase levels.
C. Statins are not contraindicated in patients with chronic hepatitis C.
D. Statins should be discontinued in asymptomatic patients who develop an isolated elevation in aminotransferase activity.

62. All of the following are likely causes of chronic hepatitis EXCEPT:

A. Autoimmune hepatitis
B. Hepatitis A virus
C. Hepatitis B virus
D. Hepatitis C virus
E. Hepatitis D virus

63. A 38-year-old woman is evaluated for elevated transaminase levels that were identified during routine laboratory testing for life insurance. She is originally from Thailand and immigrated to the United States 10 years previously. She has been married to an American for the past 12 years, having met him while he was living abroad for business. She previously worked in Thailand as a deputy tourism minister for the government but is not currently employed. She has no significant past medical history. She had one uncomplicated pregnancy at the age of 22. When queried about risk factors for liver disease, she denies alcohol intake or drug abuse. She has never had a blood transfusion. She recalls an episode of jaundice that she did not seek evaluation for about 15 years ago. It resolved spontaneously. She currently feels well, and her husband wished to have her added to his life insurance policy. There is no stigmata of chronic liver disease. Her laboratory studies reveal an AST of 346 IU/L, ALT of 412 IU/L, alkaline phosphatase of 98 IU/L, and total bilirubin 1.5 of mg/dL. Further workup includes the following viral studies: hepatitis A IgG positive, hepatitis B surface antigen positive, hepatitis B e antigen positive, anti-hepatitis B virus core IgG positive, and hepatitis C IgG negative. The HBV DNA level is 4.8×10^4 IU/mL. Which of the following medications is indicated for this patient?

A. Acyclovir
B. Entecavir
C. Ritonavir
D. Simeprevir
E. No treatment is necessary

64. A 46-year-old man is known to have chronic hepatitis C virus (HCV) infection. He is a former intravenous drug user for more than 20 years who has been abstinent from drug use for 1 year. He was treated for tricuspid valve endocarditis 3 years previously. He does not know when he acquired HCV. His laboratory studies show a positive HCV IgG antibody with a viral load of greater than 1 million copies. The virus is genotype 2. His AST is 82 IU/L, and his ALT is 74 IU/L. He undergoes liver biopsy, which

64. (*Continued*)
demonstrates a moderate degree of bridging fibrosis. Which of the following is the most predictive of the development of cirrhosis?

A. Abnormal transaminases
B. Bridging fibrosis on liver biopsy
C. Genotype 2
D. History of bacterial endocarditis
E. History of intravenous drug use

65. A 34-year-old woman is evaluated for fatigue, malaise, arthralgias, and a 10-lb weight loss over the past 6–8 weeks. She has no past medical history. Since feeling poorly, she has taken approximately one or two tablets of acetaminophen 500 mg daily. On physical examination, her temperature is 100.2°F, respiratory rate is 18 breaths/min, blood pressure is 100/48 mmHg, heart rate is 92 bpm, and oxygen saturation is 96% on room air. She has scleral icterus. Her liver edge is palpable 3 cm below the right costal margin. It is smooth and tender. The spleen is not enlarged. She has mild synovitis in the small joints of her hands. Her AST is 542 IU/L, ALT is 657 IU/L, alkaline phosphatase is 102 IU/L, total bilirubin is 5.3 mg/dL, and direct bilirubin is 4.8 mg/dL. Which of the following tests would be LEAST likely to be positive in this diagnosis?

A. Antinuclear antibodies in a homogeneous pattern
B. Anti-liver/kidney microsomal antibodies
C. Antimitochondrial antibodies
D. Hypergammaglobulinemia
E. Rheumatoid factor

66. In chronic hepatitis B virus infection, presence of hepatitis B e antigen signifies which of the following?

A. Development of liver fibrosis leading to cirrhosis
B. Dominant viral population is less virulent and less transmissible
C. Increased likelihood of an acute flare in the next 1–2 weeks
D. Ongoing viral replication
E. Resolving infection

67. All of the following statements regarding alcoholic liver disease are true EXCEPT:

A. Fatty liver is present in >90% of daily and binge drinkers.
B. Hepatitis C infection worsens the prognosis of alcoholic liver disease.
C. Over 50% of alcoholics will develop alcoholic hepatitis.

67. (*Continued*)
   D. Quantity and duration of alcohol consumption are the most important risk factors for the development of alcoholic liver disease.
   E. The pathologic hallmarks of alcoholic liver disease are fatty liver, hepatitis, and cirrhosis.

68. A 32-year-old woman is admitted to the hospital with fever, abdominal pain, and jaundice. She drinks approximately 6 beers daily and has recently increased her alcohol intake to more than 12 beers daily. She has no other substance abuse history and has no prior history of alcoholic liver disease or pancreatitis. She is not taking any medications. On physical examination, she appears ill and disheveled with a fruity odor to her breath. Her vital signs are: heart rate 122 bpm, blood pressure 95/56 mmHg, respiratory rate 22 breaths/min, temperature 101.2°F, and oxygen saturation 98% on room air. She has scleral icterus, and spider angiomata are present on the trunk. The liver edge is palpable 10 cm below the right costal margin. The liver is smooth and tender to palpation. The spleen is not palpable. No ascites or lower extremity edema is present. Laboratory studies demonstrate as AST of 431 IU/L, ALT of 198 IU/L, bilirubin of 8.6 mg/dL, alkaline phosphatase of 201 IU/L, amylase of 88 U/L, and lipase of 50 U/L. Total protein is 6.2 g/dL, and albumin is 2.8 g/dL. The prothrombin time is 29 seconds (control, 13 seconds) with INR of 2.2. What is the best approach to treatment of this patient?

   A. Administer intravenous fluids, thiamine, and folate and observe for improvement in laboratory tests and clinical condition.
   B. Administer intravenous fluids, thiamine, folate, and imipenem while awaiting blood culture results.
   C. Administer prednisone 40 mg daily for 4 weeks before beginning a taper.
   D. Consult surgery for management of acute cholecystitis.
   E. Perform an abdominal CT with intravenous contrast to assess for necrotizing pancreatitis.

69. Which of the following statements regarding nonalcoholic fatty liver disease (NAFLD) is true?

   A. Imaging studies suggest that fatty liver is present to some degree in 10% of adult Americans.
   B. NAFLD does not occur in lean individuals.
   C. NAFLD is more common in African Americans than Hispanic Americans.
   D. NAFLD is strongly associated with obesity and insulin resistance.
   E. While common in the United States, NAFLD is uncommon in other countries.

70. A 44-year-old man seeks evaluation for an abnormal finding on ultrasonography. He has a history of type 2 diabetes mellitus and is on insulin therapy. Last week, he was evaluated in the emergency department for mid-epigastric pain likely due to NSAID therapy for muscle aches (he recently started exercising because his wife told him to lose weight). During the evaluation, an abdominal ultrasound showed marked fatty infiltration of the liver. Laboratory studies show his transaminases are 2× normal with normal alkaline phosphatase, bilirubin, and prothrombin time. Other than insulin, he takes no medications, does not consume alcohol or illicit drugs, and has no family history of liver disease. On physical examination, he is obese (BMI, 32 kg/m^2) with normal vital signs and no other abnormalities. You think he likely has NAFLD. All of the following statements regarding his potential therapy are true EXCEPT:

   A. Bariatric surgery is safe in patients with NAFLD.
   B. Exercise may reduce hepatic steatosis.
   C. Statins may worsen inflammation in NAFLD.
   D. There are no Food and Drug Administration–approved therapies for NAFLD.
   E. Vitamin E may reduce aminotransferase levels and hepatic steatosis.

71. All of the following statements regarding alcohol-induced liver disease are true EXCEPT:

   A. Alcohol-induced cirrhosis is characterized by predominantly large (>2 cm) nodules.
   B. Alcohol use is the most common cause of cirrhosis in the United States.
   C. Chronic alcohol use can cause liver fibrosis in the absence of accompanying inflammation.
   D. Excessive alcohol use can cause acute hepatitis.
   E. Excessive alcohol use can worsen liver disease due to hemochromatosis.

72. A 64-year-old man is admitted to the ICU with a large GI bleed. EGD reveals esophageal varices. He is confused and unable to provide any history. His physical examination is notable for abnormal hand findings as shown in Figures 72A and 72B. Ultrasound demonstrates a small liver consistent with cirrhosis. Which of the following is the most likely cause of his cirrhosis?

   A. Alcoholism
   B. Autoimmune hepatitis
   C. Chronic hepatitis C infection
   D. Hemochromatosis
   E. Primary biliary cirrhosis

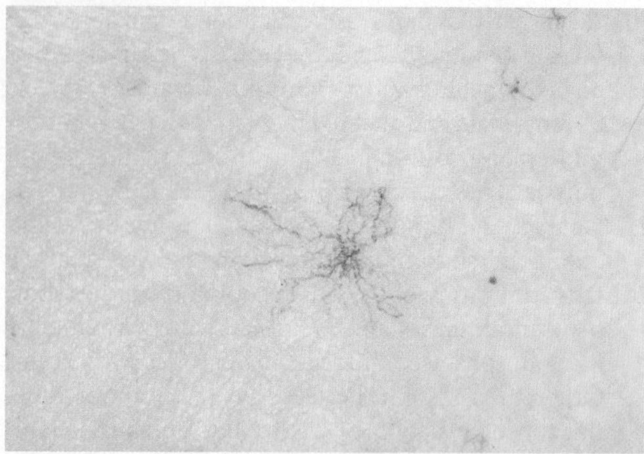

A

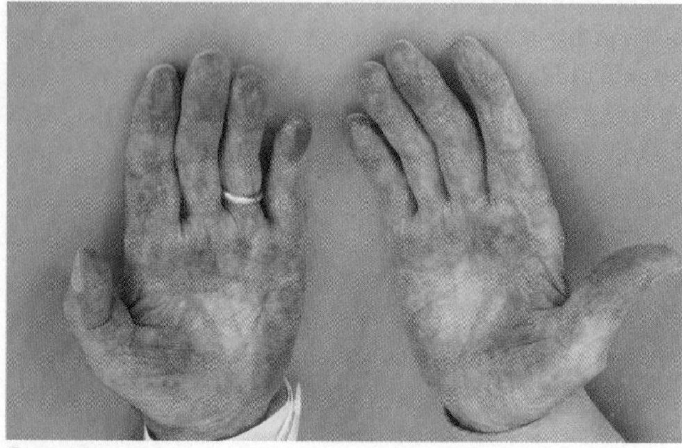

B

FIGURE 72

73. In the patient described in Question 72, all of the following may be used to control his variceal bleeding EXCEPT:

A. Endoscopic sclerotherapy
B. Endoscopic variceal ligation
C. Octreotide
D. Propranolol
E. Transjugular intrahepatic portosystemic shunt

74. You are following a 44-year-old woman with cirrhosis due to chronic hepatitis C infection. To date, she has no evidence of portal hypertension, and her disease is well controlled on her current medical regimen. All of the following new findings on a diagnostic study are suggestive of the development of portal hypertension EXCEPT:

A. 15-cmHg gradient between wedged and free hepatic vein pressures
B. Ascites on ultrasound
C. Enlarged spleen on physical examination
D. Left atrial dilation on echocardiogram
E. Thrombocytopenia

75. A 63-year-old man with cirrhosis and portal hypertension due to hemochromatosis presents with altered mental status. He has chronic ascites controlled with diet and spironolactone. He has a history of one esophageal bleed but none since starting propranolol. His family reports that over the last 2 days, he has become more confused, but he has had no melena or hematemesis. He is afebrile with normal vital signs, and physical examination is notable for ascites, asterixis, and being oriented only to person. His laboratory examination is notable for a hemoglobin of 10.1 (baseline, 9.5), creatinine of 1.4 (baseline, 1.4), and blood urea nitrogen of 45 (baseline, 18). A paracentesis is performed that yields reveals clear fluid with 800 WBC (40% neutrophils). Which of the following is the most indicated therapy?

A. Ampicillin, ceftriaxone, vancomycin
B. Cefotaxime
C. EGD with banding
D. Hemodialysis
E. Lactulose

76. A 48-year-old woman presents complaining of fatigue and itching. She has been tired for the past 6 months and recently has developed itching diffusely. It is worse in the evening hours but is intermittent. She does not note it to be worse following hot baths or showers. Her past medical history is significant only for hypothyroidism for which she takes levothyroxine 125 μg daily. On physical examination, she has mild jaundice and scleral icterus. The liver is enlarged to 15 cm on palpation and is palpable 5 cm below the right costal margin. Xanthomas are seen on both elbows. Hyperpigmentation is noticeable on the trunk and arms where the patient has excoriations. Laboratory studies demonstrate the following: WBC 8900/μL, hemoglobin 13.3 g/dL, hematocrit 41.6%, and platelets 160,000/μL. The creatinine is 1.2 mg/dL. The AST is 52 IU/L, ALT is 62 IU/L, alkaline phosphatase is 216 IU/L, total bilirubin is 3.2 mg/dL, and direct bilirubin is 2.9 mg/dL. The total protein is 8.2 g/dL, and albumin is 3.9 U/L. The thyroid-stimulating hormone is 4.5 U/mL. Antimitochondrial antibodies are positive. Perinuclear antineutrophil cytoplasmic antibodies (ANCA) and cytoplasmic ANCA are negative. What is the most likely cause of the patient's symptoms?

A. Lymphoma
B. Polycythemia vera
C. Primary biliary cirrhosis
D. Primary sclerosis cholangitis
E. Uncontrolled hypothyroidism

77. A 42-year-old man with cirrhosis related to hepatitis C and alcohol abuse has ascites requiring frequent large-volume paracentesis. All of the following therapies would be indicated for this patient EXCEPT:

A. Fluid restriction to less than 2 L daily
B. Furosemide 40 mg daily
C. Sodium restriction to less than 2 g daily
D. Spironolactone 100 mg daily
E. Transjugular intrahepatic portosystemic shunt if medical therapy fails

78. Which of the following statements about cardiac cirrhosis is true?

A. AST and ALT levels may mimic the very high levels seen in acute viral hepatitis.
B. Budd-Chiari syndrome cannot be distinguished clinically from cardiac cirrhosis.
C. Echocardiography is the gold standard for diagnosing constrictive pericarditis as a cause of cirrhosis.
D. Prolonged passive congestion from right-sided heart failure results in congestion and necrosis of portal triads, resulting in subsequent fibrosis.
E. Veno-occlusive disease can be confused with cardiac cirrhosis and is a major cause of morbidity and mortality in patients undergoing liver transplantation.

79. You are asked to consult on a 62-year-old white woman with pruritus for 4 months. She has noted progressive fatigue and a 5-lb weight loss. She has intermittent nausea but no vomiting and denies changes in her bowel habits. There is no history of prior alcohol use, blood transfusions, or illicit drug use. The patient is widowed and has had two heterosexual partners in her lifetime. Her past medical history is significant only for hypothyroidism, for which she takes levothyroxine. Her family history is unremarkable. On examination, she is mildly icteric. She has spider angiomata on her torso. You palpate a nodular liver edge 2 cm below the right costal margin. The remainder of the examination is unremarkable. A right upper quadrant ultrasound confirms your suspicion of cirrhosis. You order a complete blood count and a comprehensive metabolic panel. What is the most appropriate next test?

A. 24-Hour urine copper
B. Antimitochondrial antibodies
C. Endoscopic retrograde cholangiopancreatography
D. Hepatitis B serologies
E. Serum ferritin

80. All of the following are potential indications for liver transplantation EXCEPT:

A. Autoimmune hepatitis
B. Cholangiocarcinoma
C. Primary biliary cirrhosis
D. Primary hepatocellular carcinoma
E. Primary sclerosing cholangitis

81. Which of the following patients is highest priority for liver transplantation?

A. A 24-year-old woman with cirrhosis due to autoimmune hepatitis. She has been on the transplant list for 2 months and now has an elevated bilirubin, INR, and creatinine.
B. A 38-year-old woman with chronic hepatitis C and normal bilirubin and INR.
C. A 49-year-old man with alcoholic cirrhosis who has been on the transplant list for 6 months. He has had two esophageal variceal bleeds.
D. A 59-year-old man with a history of hyperlipidemia who was admitted to the ICU 2 days ago with fulminant hepatic failure due to mistakenly ingesting *Amanita* mushrooms from his lawn.
E. A 64-year-old woman with primary hepatocellular carcinoma admitted to the hospital with acute renal failure.

82. A 44-year-old woman is evaluated for complaints of abdominal pain. She describes the pain as a postprandial burning pain. It is worse with spicy or fatty foods and is relieved with antacids. She is diagnosed with a gastric ulcer and is treated appropriately for *H. pylori*. During the course of her evaluation for her abdominal pain, the patient had a right upper quadrant ultrasound that demonstrated the presence of gallstones. Following treatment of *H. pylori*, her symptoms have resolved. She is requesting your opinion regarding whether treatment is required for the finding of gallstone disease. Upon review of the ultrasound report, there were numerous stones in the gallbladder, including in the neck of the gallbladder. The largest stone measures 2.8 cm. What is your advice to the patient regarding the risk of complications and the need for definitive treatment?

A. Given the size and number of stones, prophylactic cholecystectomy is recommended.
B. No treatment is necessary unless the patient develops symptoms of biliary colic frequent and severe enough to interfere with the patient's life.
C. The only reason to proceed with cholecystectomy is development of gallstone pancreatitis or cholangitis.

82. (*Continued*)

D. The risk of developing acute cholecystitis is about 5%–10% per year.
E. Ursodeoxycholic acid should be given at a dose of 10–15 mg/kg daily for a minimum of 6 months to dissolve the stones.

83. A 62-year-old man has been hospitalized in intensive care for the past 3 weeks following an automobile accident resulting in multiple long bone fractures and acute respiratory distress syndrome. He has been slowly improving but remains on mechanical ventilation. He is now febrile and hypotensive requiring vasopressors. He is being treated empirically with cefepime and vancomycin. Multiple blood cultures are negative. He has no new infiltrates or increasing secretions on chest radiograph. His laboratory studies demonstrated a rise in his liver function tests, bilirubin, and alkaline phosphatase. Amylase and lipase are normal. A right upper quadrant ultrasound shows sludge in the gallbladder but no stones. The bile duct is not dilated. What is the next best step in the evaluation and treatment of this patient?

A. Discontinue cefepime
B. Initiate treatment with clindamycin
C. Initiate treatment with metronidazole
D. Perform hepatobiliary scintigraphy
E. Refer for exploratory laparotomy

84. All the following are associated with an increased risk for cholesterol stone cholelithiasis EXCEPT:

A. Gallbladder sludge on ultrasound
B. High-protein diet
C. Oral contraceptives
D. Pregnancy
E. Rapid weight loss

85. All of the following conditions are associated with an increased risk of pigment stone cholelithiasis EXCEPT:

A. Alcoholic cirrhosis
B. Chronic biliary tract infection
C. Chronic hemolytic anemia
D. Cystic fibrosis
E. Primary biliary cirrhosis

86. A 41-year-old woman presents to your clinic with a week of jaundice. She notes pruritus, icterus, and dark urine. She denies fever, abdominal pain, or weight loss. The examination is unremarkable except for yellow discoloration of the skin. Total bilirubin is 6.0 mg/dL, and direct bilirubin is 5.1 mg/dL. AST is 84 IU/L, and ALT is 92 IU/L. Alkaline phosphatase is 662 IU/L. CT scan of the abdomen is unremarkable. Right upper quadrant ultrasound shows a normal gallbladder but does not visualize the common bile duct. What is the most appropriate next management step?

A. Antibiotics and observation
B. Endoscopic retrograde cholangiopancreatography
C. Hepatitis serologies
D. Hepatobiliary iminodiacetic acid (HIDA) scan
E. Serologies for antimitochondrial antibodies

87. A 32-year-old woman is being evaluated for her second episode of acute-onset right upper quadrant pain and jaundice. She has noticed worsening jaundice over the last 2 weeks and now complains of diffuse itchiness. She has a 10-year history of ulcerative colitis treated with sulfasalazine. She is found to have a markedly elevated serum bilirubin and alkaline phosphatase. Her aminotransferases and prothrombin time are normal. Ultrasound shows no gallstones. Magnetic resonance cholangiopancreatography reveals a beaded appearance of her intrahepatic and extrahepatic bile ducts due to multiple discrete strictures. All of the following statements regarding her diagnosis are true EXCEPT:

A. Cyclosporine A is the most effective medical therapy.
B. Median survival with medical therapy is approximately 10 years.
C. She may be a candidate for liver transplantation.
D. Surgical therapy is rarely indicated.
E. The biliary disease is associated with her ulcerative colitis.

88. Which of the following is the most important ion secreted by the pancreas?

A. Bicarbonate
B. Chloride
C. Magnesium
D. Potassium
E. Sodium

89. A 45-year-old woman with known history of cholelithiasis is admitted to the hospital with severe mid-epigastric pain, fever to 38.5°C, tachycardia to 110 bpm, and a blood pressure of 100/50 mmHg. Her examination shows a diffusely tender abdomen with guarding. Radiographs show an abdominal ileus with no free air. Laboratories are notable for

89. (*Continued*)
a hemoglobin of 15 g/dL and elevations or amylase and lipase. Which of the following statements regarding this patient's likely diagnosis is true?

A. Elevated lipase is more specific than elevated amylase for the diagnosis of acute pancreatitis.
B. Hypercalcemia occurs in >75% of cases of acute pancreatitis.
C. Magnitude of lipase elevation above normal is correlated with the severity of acute pancreatitis.
D. Serum amylase levels will remain elevated for up to 30 days after the resolution of acute pancreatitis.
E. The combination of elevated serum amylase and metabolic acidosis (pH <7.32) has a >90% positive predictive value for acute pancreatitis.

90. A 27-year-old woman is admitted to the hospital with acute-onset severe right upper quadrant pain that radiates to the back. The pain is constant and not relieved with eating or bowel movements. Her labs show marked elevation in amylase and lipase, and acute pancreatitis is diagnosed. Which of the following is the best first test to demonstrate the etiology of her pancreatitis?

A. Right upper quadrant ultrasound
B. Serum alcohol level
C. Serum triglyceride level
D. Technetium HIDA scan
E. Urine drug screen

91. A 58-year-old man with severe alcoholism is admitted to the hospital with acute pancreatitis. His symptoms have been present for 3 days, and he has continued to drink heavily. He now has persistent vomiting and feels dizzy upon standing. On examination, he has severe epigastric and right upper quadrant tenderness and decreased bowel sounds, and he appears uncomfortable. A faint blue discoloration is present around the umbilicus. What is the significance of this finding?

A. A CT of the abdomen is likely to show severe necrotizing pancreatitis.
B. Abdominal plain film is likely to show pancreatic calcification.
C. Concomitant appendicitis should be ruled out.
D. He likely has a pancreatico-aortic fistula.
E. Pancreatic pseudocyst is likely present.

92. A 36-year-old man is admitted to the hospital with acute pancreatitis. In order to determine the severity of disease and risk of mortality, the Bedside Index of Severity in Acute Pancreatitis (BISAP) is calculated. All of the following variables are used to calculate this score EXCEPT:

A. Age >60 years
B. Blood urea nitrogen >35
C. Impaired mental status
D. Pleural effusion
E. Serum lipase >3× normal

93. A 54-year-old man is admitted to the ICU with severe pancreatitis. His BMI is ≥30 kg/m^2, and he has a prior history of diabetes mellitus. A CT of the abdomen is obtained and shows severe necrotizing pancreatitis. He is presently afebrile. Which of the following medications has been shown to be effective in the treatment of acute necrotizing pancreatitis?

A. Calcitonin
B. Cimetidine
C. Glucagon
D. Imipenem
E. None of the above

94. Which of the following statements regarding enteral feeding in acute pancreatitis is true?

A. A patient with persistent evidence of pancreatic necrosis on CT 2 weeks after acute presentation should be maintained on bowel rest.
B. All patients with elevations of amylase and lipase and CT evidence of pancreatitis should be fasted until amylase and lipase normalize.
C. Enteral feeding has been demonstrated to have fewer infectious complications than total parenteral nutrition in the management of patients with acute pancreatitis.
D. Patients requiring surgical removal of infected pancreatic pseudocysts should be treated with total parental nutrition.
E. Total parenteral nutrition has been shown to maintain integrity of the intestinal tract in acute pancreatitis.

95. A 47-year-old woman presents to the emergency department with severe mid-abdominal pain radiating to her back. The pain began acutely and is sharp. She denies cramping or flatulence. She has had two episodes of emesis of bilious material since the pain began, but this has not lessened the pain. She currently rates the pain as a 10 out of 10 and feels the pain is worse in the supine position. For the past few months, she has had intermittent episodes of right upper and mid-epigastric pain that occur after

95. (*Continued*)
eating but subside over a few hours. These are associated with a feeling of excess gas. She denies any history of alcohol abuse. She has no medical history of hypertension or hyperlipidemia. On physical examination, she is writhing in distress and slightly diaphoretic. Vital signs are: heart rate 127 bpm, blood pressure 92/50 mmHg, respiratory rate 20 breaths/min, temperature 37.9°C, oxygen saturation 88% on room air. Her BMI is 29 kg/m^2. The cardiovascular examination reveals a regular tachycardia. The chest examination shows dullness to percussion at bilateral bases with a few scattered crackles. On abdominal examination, bowel sounds are hypoactive. There is no rash or bruising evident on inspection of the abdomen. There is voluntary guarding on palpation. The pain with palpation is greatest in the periumbilical and epigastric area without rebound tenderness. There is no evidence of jaundice, and the liver span is about 10 cm to percussion. Amylase level is 750 IU/L, and lipase level is 1129 IU/L. Other laboratory values include: AST 168 IU/L, ALT 196 IU/L, total bilirubin 2.3 mg/dL, alkaline phosphatase 268 IU/L, lactate dehydrogenase 300 U/L, and creatinine 1.9 mg/dL. The hematocrit is 43%, and WBC count is 11,500/μL with 89% neutrophils. An arterial blood gas shows a pH of 7.32, PCO2 of 32 mmHg, and PO2 of 56 mmHg. An ultrasound confirms a dilated common bile duct with evidence of pancreatitis manifested as an edematous and enlarged pancreas. A CT scan shows no evidence of necrosis. After 3 L of normal saline, her blood pressure comes up to 110/60 mmHg with a heart rate of 105 bpm. Which of the following best describes the pathophysiology of this disease?

A. Intrapancreatic activation of digestive enzymes with autodigestion and acinar cell injury
B. Chemoattraction of neutrophils with subsequent infiltration and inflammation
C. Distant organ involvement and systemic inflammatory response syndrome related to release of activated pancreatic enzymes and cytokines
D. All of the above

96. A 25-year-old woman with cystic fibrosis is diagnosed with chronic pancreatitis. She is at risk for all of the following complications EXCEPT:

A. Vitamin B_{12} deficiency
B. Vitamin A deficiency
C. Pancreatic carcinoma
D. Niacin deficiency
E. Steatorrhea

97. A 64-year-old man seeks evaluation from his primary care physician because of chronic diarrhea. He reports that he has two or three large loose bowel movements daily. He describes them as markedly foul smelling, and they often leave an oily ring in the toilet. He also notes that the bowel movements often follow heavy meals, but if he fasts or eats low-fat foods, the stools are more formed. Over the past 6 months, he has lost about 18 kg (40 lbs). In this setting, he reports intermittent episodes of abdominal pain that can be quite severe. He describes the pain as sharp and in a mid-epigastric location. He has not sought evaluation of the pain previously, but when it occurs, he will limit his oral intake and treat the pain with nonsteroidal anti-inflammatory drugs. He notes the pain has not lasted for >48 hours and is not associated with meals. His past medical history is remarkable for peripheral vascular disease and tobacco use. He currently smokes one pack of cigarettes daily. In addition, he drinks two to six beers daily. He has stopped all alcohol intake for up to a week at a time in the past without withdrawal symptoms. His current medications are aspirin 81 mg daily and albuterol metered-dose inhaler on as needed basis. On physical examination, the patient is thin but appears well. His BMI is 18.2 kg/m^2. Vital signs are normal. Cardiac and pulmonary examinations are normal. The abdominal examination shows mild epigastric tenderness without rebound or guarding. The liver span is 12 cm to percussion and palpable 2 cm below the right costal margin. There is no splenomegaly or ascites present. There are decreased pulses in the lower extremities bilaterally. An abdominal radiograph demonstrates calcifications in the epigastric area, and CT scan confirms that these calcifications are located within the body of the pancreas. No pancreatic ductal dilatation is noted. An amylase level is 32 U/L, and lipase level is 22 U/L. What is the next most appropriate step in diagnosing and managing this patient's primary complaint?

A. Advise the patient to stop all alcohol use and prescribe pancreatic enzymes.
B. Advise the patient to stop all alcohol use and prescribe narcotic analgesia and pancreatic enzymes.
C. Perform angiography to assess for ischemic bowel disease.
D. Prescribe prokinetic agents to improve gastric emptying.
E. Refer the patient for endoscopic retrograde cholangiopancreatography for sphincterotomy.

Answers

1. The answer is A.
(Chap. 14) Endoscopy, also known as esophagogastroduodenoscopy (EGD) is the best test for evaluation of the proximal gastrointestinal tract. Because of high-quality images, disorders of color such as Barrett metaplasia and mucosal irregularities are easily demonstrated. Sensitivity of endoscopy is superior to that of barium radiography for mucosal lesions. Because the endoscope has an instrumentation channel, biopsy specimens are easily obtained, and dilation of strictures can also be performed. The sensitivity of radiography compared with endoscopy for detecting reflux esophagitis reportedly ranges from 22%–95%, with higher grades of esophagitis (i.e., ulceration or stricture) exhibiting greater detection rates. Conversely, the sensitivity of barium radiography for detecting esophageal strictures is greater than that of endoscopy, especially when the study is done in conjunction with barium-soaked bread or a 13-mm barium tablet. Barium studies also provide an assessment of esophageal function and morphology that may be undetected on endoscopy. The major shortcoming of barium radiography is that it rarely obviates the need for endoscopy. Barium radiography does not require sedation, which in some populations at risk for conscious sedation is an important consideration.

2. The answer is E.
(Chap. 14) Intermittent solid food dysphagia is a classic symptom in Schatzki ring in which a distal esophageal ring occurs at the squamocolumnar mucosal junction. The origin of these rings is unknown, and smaller rings with a lumen of greater than 13 mm are common in the general population (up to 15%). When the lumen is less than 13 mm, dysphagia may occur. Schatzki rings typically occur in persons older than 40 years and often cause "steakhouse syndrome" from meat getting stuck at the ring. The rings are easily treated with dilation. Plummer-Vinson syndrome also includes esophageal rings, but typically, the rings occur in the proximal esophagus, are associated with iron-deficiency anemia, and occur in middle-aged women. Achalasia involves both solid and liquid dysphagia, often with regurgitation. Adenocarcinoma often includes solid and liquid dysphagia at later stages. Most esophageal diverticulae are asymptomatic.

3. The answer is B.
(*Chap. 14*) Aside from the discomfort and local complications of gastroesophageal reflux disease (GERD), a number of other, non–gastrointestinal (GI)-related sites may have complications related to GERD. Syndromes with well-established association with GERD include chronic cough, laryngitis, asthma, and dental erosions. Other diseases have implicated GERD as potentially contributory, but the role of GERD is less well established. These include pharyngitis, pulmonary fibrosis, chronic sinusitis, cardiac arrhythmias, sleep apnea, and recurrent aspiration pneumonia.

4. The answer is A.
(Chap. 14) This patient has symptoms of esophagitis. In patients with human immunodeficiency virus (HIV), various infections can cause this disease, including herpes simplex virus (HSV), cytomegalovirus (CMV), varicella-zoster virus (VZV), *Candida*, and HIV itself. The lack of thrush does not rule out *Candida* as a cause of esophagitis, and EGD is necessary for diagnosis. CMV classically causes serpiginous ulcers in the distal esophagus that may coalesce to form large ulcers. Brushings alone are insufficient for diagnosis, and biopsies must be performed. Biopsies reveal intranuclear and intracytoplasmic inclusions with enlarged nuclei in large fibroblasts and endothelial cells. Given this patient's notable swallowing symptoms, intravenous ganciclovir is the treatment of choice. Valganciclovir is an effective oral preparation. Foscarnet is useful in treating ganciclovir-resistant CMV. HSV manifests as vesicles and punched-out lesions in the esophagus with the characteristic finding on biopsy of ballooning degeneration with ground-glass changes in the nuclei. It can be treated with acyclovir or foscarnet in resistant cases. Candida esophagitis has the appearance of yellow nodular plaques with surrounding erythema. Treatment usually requires fluconazole therapy. Finally, HIV alone can cause esophagitis that can be quite resistant to therapy. On EGD, these ulcers appear deep and linear. Treatment with thalidomide or oral glucocorticoids is employed, and highly active antiretroviral therapy should be considered.

5. and 6. The answers are A and A, respectively.
(Chap. 14) The barium swallow image demonstrates achalasia with esophageal dilation narrowing at the gastroesophageal junction and an air-fluid level in the mid-esophagus. Achalasia is a rare disease caused by loss of ganglion cells within the esophageal myenteric plexus with a population incidence of about 1:100,000; it usually presents between age 25 and 60. With long-standing disease, aganglionosis is noted. The disease involves both

excitatory (cholinergic) and inhibitory (nitric oxide) ganglionic neurons. This leads to impaired deglutitive lower esophageal sphincter (LES) relaxation and absent peristalsis. Increasing evidence suggests that the ultimate cause of ganglion cell degeneration in achalasia is an autoimmune process attributable to a latent infection with human HSV-1 combined with genetic susceptibility. Long-standing achalasia is characterized by progressive dilatation and sigmoid deformity of the esophagus with hypertrophy of the LES. Clinical manifestations may include dysphagia, regurgitation, chest pain, and weight loss. Most patients report solid and liquid food dysphagia. Regurgitation occurs when food, fluid, and secretions are retained in the dilated esophagus. Patients with advanced achalasia are at risk for bronchitis, pneumonia, or lung abscess from chronic regurgitation and aspiration. The differential diagnosis of achalasia includes diffuse esophageal spasm, Chagas disease, and pseudoachalasia. Chagas disease is endemic in areas of central Brazil, Venezuela, and northern Argentina and spread by the bite of the reduviid (kissing) bug that transmits the protozoan *Trypanosoma cruzi*. The chronic phase of the disease develops years after infection and results from destruction of autonomic ganglion cells throughout the body, including the heart, gut, urinary tract, and respiratory tract. Tumor infiltration, most commonly seen with carcinoma in the gastric fundus or distal esophagus, can mimic idiopathic achalasia. The resultant "pseudoachalasia" accounts for up to 5% of suspected cases and is more likely with advanced age, abrupt onset of symptoms (<1 year), and weight loss. Hence, endoscopy is a necessary part of the evaluation of achalasia. When the clinical suspicion for pseudoachalasia is high and endoscopy nondiagnostic, computed tomography (CT) scanning or endoscopic ultrasound may be of value. There is no known way of preventing or reversing achalasia. Therapy is directed at reducing LES pressure so that gravity and esophageal pressurization promote esophageal emptying. Peristalsis rarely, if ever, recovers. Botulinum toxin, injected into the LES under endoscopic guidance, inhibits acetylcholine release from nerve endings and improves dysphagia in about 66% of cases for at least 6 months. The only durable therapies for achalasia are pneumatic dilatation and Heller myotomy. Pneumatic dilatation, with a reported efficacy ranging from 32%–98%, is an endoscopic technique using a noncompliant, cylindrical balloon dilator positioned across the LES and inflated to a diameter of 3–4 cm. The major complication is perforation, with a reported incidence of 0.5%–5%.

7. The answer is B.

(Chap. 14) Barrett metaplasia is the most serious complication of GERD. It has a strong association with the subsequent development of esophageal adenocarcinoma. The incidence of these lesions has increased, not decreased, in the era of potent acid suppression. Barrett metaplasia is endoscopically recognized by tongues of reddish mucosa extending proximally from the gastroesophageal junction or histopathologically identified by the finding of specialized columnar metaplasia. Barrett metaplasia can progress to adenocarcinoma through the intermediate stages of low- and high-grade dysplasia. Due to this risk, areas of Barrett metaplasia and especially any included areas of mucosal irregularity should be extensively biopsied. No high-level evidence confirms that aggressive antisecretory therapy or antireflux surgery causes regression of Barrett esophagus or prevents adenocarcinoma. Although the management of Barrett esophagus remains controversial, the finding of dysplasia in Barrett esophagus, particularly high-grade dysplasia, mandates further intervention. In addition to the high rate of progression to adenocarcinoma, there is also a high prevalence of unrecognized coexisting cancer with high-grade dysplasia. Nonetheless, treatment remains controversial. Esophagectomy, intensive endoscopic surveillance, and mucosal ablation have all been advocated. Currently, esophagectomy is the gold standard treatment for high-grade dysplasia in an otherwise healthy patient with minimal surgical risk. However, esophagectomy has a mortality ranging from 3%–10%, along with substantial morbidity. As a result of these factors and the increasing evidence of the effectiveness of endoscopic therapy with purpose-built radiofrequency ablation devices, many now favor this therapy as a preferable management strategy.

8. The answer is D.

(Chap. 15) The patient has a duodenal ulcer, which is almost universally due to *Helicobacter pylori* infection, although in a minority of cases, nonsteroidal anti-inflammatory drug (NSAID) use may either facilitate development or be the only identified cause. The patient was taking acetaminophen and not a traditional NSAID, making *H. pylori*–associated peptic ulcer disease the most likely cause of the findings. *H. pylori* infection is closely correlated with advancing age, low socioeconomic status, and low education levels. After initial infection, antral gastritis is common, and in a portion of patients, duodenal or gastric ulcers form. Associated with these conditions

is the development of gastric cancer or mucosa-associated lymphoid tissue (MALT) lymphoma. Duodenal ulcers are rarely cancerous, whereas this is a not an uncommon finding in gastric ulcers. After discovery of the ulcer, first-line therapy is eradication of *H. pylori* in addition to acid suppression.

9. The answer is D.
(Chap. 15) Noninvasive testing for *H. pylori* infection is recommended in patients with suggestive symptoms and no other indication for endoscopy (e.g., GI bleeding, atypical symptoms). Several tests have good sensitivity and specificity, including plasma serology for *H. pylori*, ^{14}C- or ^{13}C-urea breath test, and the fecal *H. pylori* antigen test (Table 9). Sensitivity and specificity are >80% and >90%, respectively for serology, whereas the sensitivity and specificity of the urea breath test and fecal antigen testing are >90% for both. Serology is not useful for early follow-up after therapy completion because antibody titers will take several weeks to months to fall. The urea breath test, which relies on the presence of urease secreted by *H. pylori* to digest the swallowed radioactive urea and liberate ^{14}C or ^{13}C as part of ammonia, is simple and rapid. It is useful for early follow-up because it requires living bacteria to secrete urease and produce a positive test. The limitations to the test include requirement for ingestion of radioactive materials, albeit low dose, and false-negative results with recent use of proton pump inhibitors, antibiotics, or bismuth compounds. Stool antigen testing is cheap and convenient but is not established for proof of eradication.

TABLE 9

TESTS FOR DETECTION OF *H PYLORI*

TEST	SENSITIVITY/ SPECIFICITY, %	COMMENTS
Invasive (Endoscopy/Biopsy Required)		
Rapid urease	80–95/95–100	Simple, false negative with recent use of PPIs, antibiotics, or bismuth compounds
Histology	80–90/>95	Requires pathology processing and staining; provides histologic information
Culture	—/—	Time-consuming, expensive, dependent on experience; allows determination of antibiotic susceptibility
Noninvasive		
Serology	>80/>90	Inexpensive, convenient; not useful for early follow-up
Urea breath test	>90/>90	Simple, rapid; useful for early follow-up; false negatives with recent therapy (see rapid urease test); exposure to low-dose radiation with ^{14}C test
Stool antigen	>90/>90	Inexpensive, convenient

Abbreviation: PPIs, proton pump inhibitors.

10. The answer is A.
(Chap. 15) Documented eradication of *H. pylori* in patients with peptic ulcer disease (PUD) is associated with a dramatic decrease in ulcer recurrence to <10%–20% as compared to 59% in gastric ulcer patients and 67% in duodenal ulcer patients when the organism is not eliminated. Eradication of the organism may lead to diminished recurrent ulcer bleeding. The effect of its eradication on ulcer perforation is unclear. Extensive effort has been made in determining who of the many individuals with *H. pylori* infection should be treated. The common conclusion arrived at by multiple consensus conferences around the world is that *H. pylori* should be eradicated in patients with documented PUD. This holds true independent of time of presentation (first episode or not), severity of symptoms, presence of confounding factors such as ingestion of NSAIDs, or whether the ulcer is in remission. Multiple drugs have been evaluated in the therapy of *H. pylori*. No single agent is effective in eradicating the organism. Combination therapy for 14 days provides the greatest efficacy, although regimens based on sequential administration of antibiotics also appear promising. A shorter administration course (7–10 days), although attractive, has not proved as successful as the 14-day regimens. Suggested treatment regimens for *H. pylori* are outlined in Table 10. Choice of a particular regimen will be influenced by several factors, including efficacy, patient tolerance, existing antibiotic resistance, and cost of the drugs. The aim for initial eradication rates should be 85%–90%. Dual therapy (proton pump inhibitor [PPI] plus amoxicillin, PPI plus clarithromycin, ranitidine bismuth citrate [Tritec] plus clarithromycin) is not recommended in view of studies demonstrating

TABLE 10

REGIMENS RECOMMENDED FOR ERADICATION OF *H. PYLORI* INFECTION

DRUG	DOSE
Triple Therapy	
1. Bismuth subsalicylate *plus*	2 tablets qid
Metronidazole *plus*	250 mg qid
Tetracycline[a]	500 mg qid
2. Ranitidine bismuth citrate *plus*	400 mg bid
Tetracycline *plus*	500 mg bid
Clarithromycin or metronidazole	500 mg bid
3. Omeprazole (lansoprazole) *plus*	20 mg bid (30 mg bid)
Clarithromycin *plus*	250 or 500 mg bid
Metronidazole[b] *or*	500 mg bid
Amoxicillin[c]	1 g bid
Quadruple Therapy	
Omeprazole (lansoprazole)	20 mg (30 mg) daily
Bismuth subsalicylate	2 tablets qid
Metronidazole	250 mg qid
Tetracycline	500 mg qid

[a]Alternative: use *prepacked* Helidac (see text).
[b]Alternative: use prepacked Prevpac (see text).
[c]Use either metronidazole or amoxicillin, not both.

eradication rates of <80%–85%. Addition of acid suppression assists in providing early symptom relief and enhances bacterial eradication. Triple therapy, although effective, has several drawbacks, including the potential for poor patient compliance and drug-induced side effects. Compliance is being addressed by simplifying the regimens so that patients can take the medications twice a day. Simpler (dual therapy) and shorter regimens (7 and 10 days) are not as effective as triple therapy for 14 days. Two anti–*H. pylori* regimens are available in prepackaged formulation: Prevpac (lansoprazole, clarithromycin, and amoxicillin) and Helidac (bismuth subsalicylate, tetracycline, and metronidazole). The contents of the Prevpac are to be taken twice per day for 14 days, whereas Helidac constituents are taken four times per day with an antisecretory agent (PPI or H_2 blocker), also taken for at least 14 days. Clarithromycin-based triple therapy should be avoided in settings where *H. pylori* resistance to this agent exceeds 15%–20%. Quadruple therapy should be reserved for patients with failure to eradicate *H. pylori* after an effective initial course.

11. The answer is C.

(Chap. 15) Fasting gastrin levels can be elevated in a variety of conditions, including atrophic gastritis with or without pernicious anemia, G-cell hyperplasia, and acid suppressive therapy (gastrin levels increase as a consequence of loss of negative feedback). The diagnostic concern in a patient with persistent ulcers following optimal therapy is Zollinger-Ellison syndrome (ZES). The result is not sufficient to make a diagnosis because gastrin levels may be elevated in a variety of conditions. Elevated basal acid secretion also is consistent with ZES, but up to 12% of patients with PUD may have basal acid secretion as high as 15 mEq/hr. Thus, additional testing is necessary. Gastrin levels may go up with a meal (>200%), but this test does not distinguish G-cell hyperfunction from ZES. The best test in this setting is the secretin stimulation test. An increase in gastrin levels >200 pg within 15 minutes of administering 2 μg/kg of secretin by intravenous bolus has a sensitivity and specificity of >90% for ZES. Endoscopic ultrasonography is useful in locating the gastrin-secreting tumor once the positive secretin test is obtained. Genetic testing for mutations in the gene that encodes the menin protein can detect the fraction of patients with gastrinomas that are a manifestation of multiple endocrine neoplasia type 1 (Wermer syndrome). Gastrinoma is the second most common tumor in this syndrome after parathyroid adenoma, but its peak incidence is generally in the third decade.

12 and 13. The answers are B and C, respectively.

(Chap. 15) Surgical intervention in PUD can be viewed as being either elective, for treatment of medically refractory disease, or as urgent/emergent, for the treatment of an ulcer-related complication. The development of pharmacologic and endoscopic approaches for the treatment of PUD and its complications has led to a substantial decrease in the number of operations needed for this disorder, with a decrease of over 90% for elective ulcer surgery over the last four decades. Refractory ulcers are an exceedingly rare occurrence. Surgery is more often required for treatment of an ulcer-related complication. Free peritoneal perforation occurs in ~2%–3% of DU patients. As in the case of bleeding, up to 10% of these patients will not have antecedent ulcer symptoms. Concomitant bleeding may occur in up to 10% of patients with perforation, with mortality being increased substantially. The procedure that provides the lowest rates of ulcer recurrence (1%) but has the highest complication rate is vagotomy (truncal or selective) in combination with antrectomy. Antrectomy is aimed at eliminating an additional stimulant

of gastric acid secretion, gastrin. Two principal types of reanastomoses are used after antrectomy: gastroduodenostomy (Billroth I) and gastrojejunostomy (Billroth II). Dumping syndrome consists of a series of vasomotor and GI signs and symptoms and occurs in patients who have undergone vagotomy and drainage (especially Billroth procedures). Two phases of dumping, early and late, can occur. Early dumping takes place 15–30 minutes after meals and consists of crampy abdominal discomfort, nausea, diarrhea, belching, tachycardia, palpitations, diaphoresis, light-headedness, and, rarely, syncope. These signs and symptoms arise from the rapid emptying of hyperosmolar gastric contents into the small intestine, resulting in a fluid shift into the gut lumen with plasma volume contraction and acute intestinal distention. Release of vasoactive GI hormones (vasoactive intestinal polypeptide, neurotensin, motilin) is also theorized to play a role in early dumping. The late phase of dumping typically occurs 90 minutes to 3 hours after meals. Vasomotor symptoms (light-headedness, diaphoresis, palpitations, tachycardia, and syncope) predominate during this phase. This component of dumping is thought to be secondary to hypoglycemia from excessive insulin release. Dumping syndrome is most noticeable after meals rich in simple carbohydrates (especially sucrose) and high osmolarity. Ingestion of large amounts of fluids may also contribute. Up to 50% of postvagotomy and drainage patients will experience dumping syndrome to some degree early on. Signs and symptoms often improve with time, but a severe protracted picture can occur in up to 1% of patients. Although this patient is certainly at risk of pulmonary embolism and myocardial infarction, his symptoms are typical of hypoglycemia due to dumping syndrome.

14. The answer is B.

(Chap. 16) The patient presents with nonspecific GI symptoms, but the presence of weight loss does suggest malabsorption syndrome. Patients with lactose intolerance are usually able to relate symptoms to consumption of milk-based products and also report a strong history of crampy pain and flatulence. Therefore, a lactose-free diet is unlikely to be helpful. The patient does not have nocturnal diarrhea, which is commonly a feature of steatorrhea along with floating stools. In the absence of symptoms suggesting fat malabsorption, the first test should not be fecal fat measurement. Because the patient has weight loss, irritable bowel syndrome is less likely, and increased dietary fiber is unlikely to be useful. Finally, the patient's symptoms may be consistent with celiac disease. The widespread availability of antibodies to gliadin, endomysium, and tissue transglutaminase can be easily measured in peripheral blood. Antiendomysial antibody has a 90%–95% sensitivity and equal specificity, making it a reasonable first test in symptomatic individuals. The presence of the antibody is not diagnostic, however, and duodenal biopsy is recommended. Duodenal biopsy will show villous atrophy, absence or reduced height of villi, cuboidal appearance of surface epithelial cells, and increased lymphocytes and plasma cells in the lamina propria. These changes regress with complete removal of gluten from the diet.

15. The answer is B.

(Chap. 16) Short bowel syndrome is a descriptive term referring to the many clinical complications that may occur after resection of varying lengths of the small bowel. Rarely, these complications may be due to congenital abnormalities of the small bowel. Most commonly, in adults, short bowel syndrome occurs in mesenteric vascular disease, primary mucosal or submucosal disease (Crohn disease), and operations without preexisting small bowel disease such as trauma. Multiple factors contribute to diarrhea and steatorrhea including gastric acid hypersecretion, increased bile acids in the colon due to absent or decreased reabsorption in the small bowel, and lactose intolerance due to increased gastric acid secretion. Nonintestinal symptoms may include renal calcium oxalate calculi due to an increase in oxalate absorption by the large intestine with subsequent hyperoxaluria. This may be due to increased fatty acids in the colon that bind calcium, and therefore calcium in the gut is not free to bind oxalate, and free oxalate is thus absorbed in the large intestine. Increased bile acid pool size results in the generation of cholesterol gallstones from supersaturation in gallbladder bile. Gastric hypersecretion of acid is well described and thought to be due to loss of inhibition of gastric acid secretion because of absent short bowel, which secretes inhibitory hormones. Coronary artery disease is not described as a complication of short bowel syndrome.

16. The answer is E.

(Chap. 16) The patient presents with symptoms suggestive of Whipple disease, a chronic multisystem disease often including diarrhea/steatorrhea, migratory arthralgias, weight loss, and central nervous system (CNS) or cardiac problems. Generally the presentation is of insidious onset, and dementia is a late finding and poor prognostic sign. The disease primarily occurs in middle-aged white males. The diagnosis requires small bowel biopsy

and demonstration of periodic acid–Schiff (PAS)–positive macrophages within the small bowel. Small bacilli are often present and suggest the diagnosis of Whipple disease. Similar macrophages may be found in other affected organs (e.g., the CNS). Dilated lymphatics are present in patients with intestinal lymphangiectasia. Mononuclear cell infiltrate in the lamina propria is often demonstrated in patients with tropical sprue, and flat villi with crypt hyperplasia is the hallmark of celiac disease.

17. The answer is D.
(Chap. 16) This patient has a stool osmolality gap (measured stool osmolality – calculated stool osmolality) of 10 mOsmol/L, suggesting a secretory rather than an osmotic cause for diarrhea. Secretory causes of diarrhea include toxin-mediated diarrhea (cholera, enterotoxigenic *Escherichia coli*) and intestinal peptide–mediated diarrhea in which the major pathophysiology is a luminal or circulating secretagogue. The distinction between secretory diarrhea and osmotic diarrhea aids in forming a differential diagnosis. Secretory diarrhea will not decrease substantially during a fast and has a low osmolality gap. Osmotic diarrhea will generally decrease during a fast and has a high (>50 mOsmol/L) osmolality gap. Celiac sprue, chronic pancreatitis, lactase deficiency, and Whipple disease all cause an osmotic diarrhea. A low stool osmolality (<290 mOsmol/kg H_2O) reflects the addition of either dilute urine or water, indicating either collection of urine and stool together or so-called factitious diarrhea, a form of Münchausen syndrome.

18. The answer is C.
(Chap. 16) Almost all GI malabsorption clinical problems are associated with *diminished* intestinal absorption of one or more dietary nutrients and are often referred to as malabsorption syndrome. Most malabsorption syndromes are associated with steatorrhea, an increase in stool fat excretion to >6% of dietary fat intake. The only clinical conditions in which absorption is *increased* are hemochromatosis and Wilson disease, in which absorption of iron and copper, respectively, is elevated. Celiac disease may cause significant malabsorption of multiple nutrients, with diarrhea, steatorrhea, weight loss, and the consequences of nutrient depletion (i.e., anemia and metabolic bone disease) or depletion of a single nutrient (e.g., iron or folate deficiency, osteomalacia, edema from protein loss). Malabsorption of bile salts and vitamins is common in Crohn disease due to ileal involvement. The magnitude of malabsorption is dependent on the extent of disease. Whipple disease is a chronic multisystemic disease associated with diarrhea, steatorrhea, weight loss, arthralgia, and CNS and cardiac problems; it is caused by the bacterium *Tropheryma whipplei*.

19. The answer is D.
(Chap. 18) The incidence of inflammatory bowel disease is highly influenced by ethnicity, location, and environmental factors. Both conditions have their highest incidence in the United Kingdom and North America, and the peak incidence has a bimodal distribution of age of presentation: 15–30 years and 60–80 years of age. Incidence of both ulcerative colitis and Crohn disease is highest among persons of Ashkenazi Jewish population. Prevalence decreases progressively in non-Jewish white, African American, Hispanic, and Asian populations. Cigarette smoking is associated with a decreased incidence of ulcerative colitis but may cause Crohn disease. Oral contraceptive use is associated with a slightly higher incidence of Crohn disease but not ulcerative colitis. Monozygotic twins are highly concordant for Crohn disease but not ulcerative colitis.

20. The answer is C.
(Chap. 18) Chronic, bloody diarrhea associated with weight loss and systemic symptoms in a young person is highly suggestive of inflammatory bowel disease. The patient's surgical findings suggest discontinuous lesions, which is typical of Crohn disease. Ulcerative colitis, in contrast, typically affects the rectum and proceeds caudally from there without normal mucosa until the area of inflammation terminates. The presence of strictures and fissures further supports the diagnosis of Crohn disease, as these are not features of ulcerative colitis. Microscopically, both ulcerative colitis and Crohn disease may have crypt abscess, and although Crohn disease is more often transmural, full-thickness disease may be present in ulcerative colitis. The hallmark of Crohn disease is granulomas that may be present throughout the bowel wall and involve the lymph nodes, mesentery, peritoneum, liver, and pancreas. Although pathognomonic for Crohn disease, granulomas are only found in about half of surgical resections. Flat villi are not always present in either disease and are more commonly found in isolation with celiac disease.

21. The answer is D.
(Chap. 18) There are a number of dermatologic manifestations of inflammatory bowel disease (IBD), and each type of IBD has a particular predilection for different dermatologic conditions. This patient has

pyoderma gangrenosum. Pyoderma gangrenosum can occur in up to 12% of patients with ulcerative colitis and is characterized by a lesion that begins as a pustule and progresses concentrically to surrounding normal skin. The lesions ulcerate with violaceous, heaped margins and surrounding erythema. They are typically found on the lower extremities. Often the lesions are difficult to treat and respond poorly to colectomy; similarly, pyoderma gangrenosum is not prevented by colectomy. Treatment commonly includes intravenous antibiotics, glucocorticoids, dapsone, infliximab, and other immunomodulatory agents. Erythema nodosum is more common in Crohn disease and attacks correlate with bowel symptoms. The lesions are typically multiple, red hot, tender nodules measuring 1–5 cm and are found on the lower legs and arms. Psoriasis is more common in ulcerative colitis. Finally, pyoderma vegetans is a rare disorder in intertriginous areas reported to be a manifestation of IBD in the skin.

22. **The answer is D.**
(*Chap. 18 and Cochrane Database Syst Rev 2007 Oct 17; [4]*) Despite being described as a clinical entity for over a century, the etiology of IBD remains cryptic. Current theory is related to an interplay between inflammatory stimuli in genetically predisposed individuals. Recent studies have identified a group of genes or polymorphisms that confer risk of IBD. Multiple microbiologic agents, including some that reside as "normal" flora, may initiate IBD by triggering an inflammatory response. Anaerobic organisms (e.g., *Bacteroides* and *Clostridia* spp.) may be responsible for the induction of inflammation. Other organisms, for unclear reasons, may have the opposite effect. These "probiotic" organisms include *Lactobacillus* spp., *Bifidobacterium* spp., *Taenia suis*, and *Saccharomyces boulardii*. *Shigella*, *Escherichia*, and *Campylobacter* spp. are known to promote inflammation. Studies of probiotic therapy in adults and children with IBD have shown potential benefit for reducing disease activity.

23. **The answer is D.**
Methotrexate, azathioprine, cyclosporine, tacrolimus, and anti–tumor necrosis factor (TNF) antibody are reasonable options for patients with Crohn disease, depending on the extent of macroscopic disease. Pneumonitis is a rare but serious complication of methotrexate therapy. Primary sclerosing cholangitis is an extraintestinal manifestation of IBD. Pancreatitis is an uncommon complication of azathioprine, and IBD patients treated with azathioprine are at fourfold increased risk of developing a lymphoma. Anti-TNF antibody therapy is associated with an increased risk of tuberculosis, disseminated histoplasmosis, and a number of other infections.

24. **The answer is B.**
(*Chap. 18*) Patients with long-standing ulcerative colitis (UC) are at increased risk for developing colonic epithelial dysplasia and carcinoma. The risk of neoplasia in chronic UC increases with duration and extent of disease. From one large meta-analysis, the risk of cancer in patients with UC is estimated at 2% after 10 years, 8% after 20 years, and 18% after 30 years of disease. Data from a 30-year surveillance program in the United Kingdom calculated the risk of colorectal cancer to be 7.7% at 20 years and 15.8% at 30 years of disease. The rates of colon cancer are higher than in the general population, and colonoscopic surveillance is the standard of care. Annual or biennial colonoscopy with multiple biopsies is recommended for patients with >8–10 years of extensive colitis (greater than one-third of the colon involved) or 12–15 years of proctosigmoiditis (less than one-third but more than just the rectum). The cancer risks in Crohn disease and UC are probably equivalent for similar extent and duration of disease. Thus, the same endoscopic surveillance strategy used for UC is recommended for patients with chronic Crohn colitis. If flat high-grade dysplasia is encountered on colonoscopic surveillance, the usual treatment is colectomy for UC and either colectomy or segmental resection for Crohn disease. If flat low-grade dysplasia is found, most investigators recommend immediate colectomy. Patients with Crohn disease may have an increased risk of non-Hodgkin lymphoma, leukemia, and myelodysplastic syndromes.

25. **The answer is C.**
(*Chap. 19*) Irritable bowel syndrome (IBS) is characterized by the following: recurrence of lower abdominal pain with altered bowel habits over a period of time without progressive deterioration, onset of symptoms during periods of stress or emotional upset, absence of other systemic symptoms such as fever and weight loss, and small-volume stool without evidence of blood. Warning signs that the symptoms may be due to something other than IBS include presentation for the first time in old age, progressive course from the time of onset, persistent diarrhea after a 48-hour fast, and presence of nocturnal diarrhea or steatorrheal stools. Each patient, except for patient C, has "warning" symptoms that should prompt further evaluation.

26. The answer is C.

(Chap. 19) Although this patient has signs and symptoms consistent with IBS, the differential diagnosis is large. Few tests are required for patients who have typical IBS symptoms and no alarm features. In this patient, alarm features include anemia, an elevated erythrocyte sedimentation rate, and evidence of white blood cells in the stool. Alarm features warrant further investigation to rule out other GI disorders such as colonic pathology including diverticular disease or IBD. In this case, colonoscopy to evaluate for luminal lesions and mucosal characteristics would be the logical first step. At this point, with the warning signs, empiric therapy for IBS is premature. Reassurance, stool-bulking agents, and antidepressants are all therapies to consider if a patient does indeed have IBS.

27. The answer is D.

(Chap. 19) Up to 80% of patients with IBS also have abnormal psychiatric features; however, no single psychiatric diagnosis predominates. The mechanism is not well understood but may involve altered pain thresholds. Although these patients are hypersensitive to colonic stimuli, this does not carry over to the peripheral nervous system. Functional brain imaging shows disparate activation in, for example, the mid-cingulate cortex, but brain anatomy does not discriminate IBS patients from those without IBS. An association between a history of sexual abuse and IBS has been reported. There is no reported association with sexually transmitted diseases. Patients with IBS do not have an increased risk of autoimmunity.

28. The answer is C.

(Chap. 19) This patient has a diarrhea-predominant form of IBS. Alteration in bowel habits is the most consistent clinical feature in IBS. The most common pattern is constipation alternating with diarrhea, usually with one of these symptoms predominating. At first, constipation may be episodic, but eventually, it becomes continuous and increasingly intractable to treatment with laxatives. Patients whose predominant symptom is constipation may have weeks or months of constipation interrupted with brief periods of diarrhea. In other patients, diarrhea may be the predominant symptom. Diarrhea resulting from IBS usually consists of small volumes of loose stools. Most patients have stool volumes of <200 mL. Nocturnal diarrhea does not occur in IBS. Diarrhea may be aggravated by emotional stress or eating. Stool may be accompanied by passage of large amounts of mucus. Bleeding is not a feature of IBS unless hemorrhoids are present, and malabsorption or weight loss does not occur.

Bowel pattern subtypes are highly unstable, with patients frequently alternating between constipation, diarrhea, or a mixed pattern. A diet low in fermentable oligosaccharides, disaccharides, monosaccharides, and polyols (FODMAPs) has been shown to be helpful in IBS patients (Table 28). FODMAPs are poorly absorbed by the small intestine and fermented by bacteria in the colon to produce gas and osmotically active carbohydrates. A randomized controlled study showed that a diet low in FODMAPs reduced symptoms in IBS patients.

29. The answer is B.

(Chap. 20) The patient presents with classic signs of diverticulitis with fever, abdominal pain that is usually left lower quadrant, anorexia or obstipation, and leukocytosis. This most commonly occurs in older individuals. Patients may present with acute abdomen due to perforation, although this occurs in <25% of cases. Plain radiographs of the abdomen are seldom helpful but may show the presence of an air-fluid level in the left lower quadrant indicating a giant diverticulum with impending perforation. CT with oral contrast is the diagnostic modality of choice with the following findings: sigmoid diverticula, thickened colonic wall >4 mm, and inflammation within the pericolic space with or without the collection of contrast material or fluid. In 16% of patients, an abdominal abscess may be present. Symptoms of IBS may mimic those of diverticulitis. Therefore, suspected diverticulitis that does not meet CT criteria or is not associated with a leukocytosis or fever is not diverticular disease. Other conditions that can mimic diverticular disease include an ovarian cyst, endometriosis, acute appendicitis, and pelvic inflammatory disease. Although the benefit of colonoscopy in the evaluation of patients with diverticular disease has been called into question, its use is still considered important in the exclusion of colorectal cancer. The parallel epidemiology of colorectal cancer and diverticular disease provides enough concern for an endoscopic evaluation before operative management. Therefore, a colonoscopy should be performed ~6 weeks after an attack of diverticular disease. Although diverticular disease may result in hematochezia, these are generally not temporally linked to diverticulitis.

30. The answer is B.

(Chap. 20) Medical management is appropriate for many patients with uncomplicated diverticular disease. Uncomplicated disease involves fever,

TABLE 28

SOME COMMON FOOD SOURCES OF FODMAPs

FOOD TYPE	FREE FRUCTOSE	LACTOSE	FRUCTANS	GALACTO-OLIGOSACCHARIDES	POLYOLS
Fruits	Apple, cherry, mango, pear, watermelon		Peach, persimmon, watermelon		Apple, apricot, pear, avocado, blackberries, cherry, nectarine, plum, prune
Vegetables	Asparagus, artichokes, sugar snap peas		Artichokes, beetroot, Brussels sprouts, chicory, fennel, garlic, leeks, onions, peas		Cauliflower, mushroom, snow peas
Grains and cereals			Wheat, rye, barley		
Nuts and seeds			Pistachios		
Milk and milk products		Milk, yogurt, ice cream, custard, soft cheeses			
Legumes			Legumes, lentils, chickpeas	Legumes, chickpeas, lentils	
Other	Honey, high-fructose corn syrup		Chicory drinks		
Food additives			Inulin, FOS		Sorbitol, mannitol, maltitol, xylitol, isomalt

Abbreviations: FODMAPs, fermentable oligosaccharides, disaccharides, monosaccharides, and polyols; FOS, fructo-oligosaccharides.
Source: Adapted from PR Gibson et al: *Am J Gastroenterol* 107:657, 2012.

abdominal pain, leukocytosis, and anorexia/obstipation, whereas complicated disease is characterized by abscess formation, perforation, strictures, or fistulae. Uncomplicated disease accounts for at least 75% of cases. Medical therapy generally involves bowel rest and antibiotics, usually trimethoprim/sulfamethoxazole or ciprofloxacin and metronidazole targeting aerobic gram-negative rods and anaerobic bacteria. Patients with more than two attacks of diverticulitis were previously thought to require surgical therapy, but newer data suggest that these patients do not have an increased risk of perforation and can continue medical management. Patients with immunosuppressive therapy, chronic renal failure, or collagen vascular disease have a fivefold higher risk of perforation during recurrent attacks. Surgical therapy is indicated for surgical low-risk patients with complicated disease, such as a stricture.

31. The answer is B.

(Chap. 20) Hemorrhoids can be internal or external; however, they are normally internal and may prolapse to the external position. Hemorrhoids are staged in the following manner: stage I, enlargement with bleeding; stage II, protrusion with spontaneous reduction; stage III, protrusion requiring manual reduction; and stage IV, irreducible protrusion. Stage I, which this patient has, is treated with fiber supplementation, cortisone suppositories, and/or sclerotherapy. Stage II is treated with fiber and cortisone suppositories. Stage III is offered the prior three therapies and banding or operative hemorrhoidectomy. Stage IV patients benefit from fiber and cortisone therapy as well as operative hemorrhoidectomy. Although substantial upper GI bleeding may result in hematochezia, the absence of suggestive signs/symptoms and the consistent findings of hemorrhoids do not indicate the need for upper endoscopy.

32. The answer is A.

(Chap. 20) An anorectal abscess is an abnormal fluid-containing cavity in the anorectal region. Anorectal abscess results from an infection involving the glands surrounding the anorectal canal. The disease

is more common in males, with a peak incidence in the third to fifth decades. Patients with diabetes, with IBD, or who are immunocompromised are at increased risk for this condition. Perianal pain with defecation and fever are common presenting symptoms.

33. The answer is C.

(Chap. 20) This patient has symptoms (social isolation), signs (foul odor), and risk factors (multiparity) for procidentia (rectal prolapse) and fecal incontinence. Procidentia is far more common in women than men and is often associated with pelvic floor disorders. It is not uncommon for these patients to become socially withdrawn and suffer from depression because of the associated fecal incontinence. The foul odor is a result of poor perianal hygiene due to the prolapsed rectum. Although depression in the elderly is an important medical problem, it is too premature in the evaluation to initiate medical therapy for depression. Occult malignancy and thyroid abnormalities may cause fecal incontinence and depression, but a physical examination would be diagnostic and avoid costly tests. Often patients are concerned they have a rectal mass or carcinoma. Examination after an enema often makes the prolapse apparent. Medical therapy is limited to stool-bulking agents or fiber. Surgical correction is the mainstay of therapy.

34. The answer is A.

(Chap. 21) Mesenteric ischemia is a relatively uncommon and highly morbid illness. Acute mesenteric ischemia is usually due to arterial embolus (usually from the heart) or to thrombosis in a diseased vascular bed. Major risk factors include age, atrial fibrillation, valvular disease, recent arterial catheterization, and recent myocardial infarction. Ischemia occurs when the intestines are inadequately perfused by the splanchnic circulation. This blood supply has extensive collateralization and can receive up to 30% of the cardiac output, making poor perfusion an uncommon event. Patients with acute mesenteric ischemia will frequently present with pain out of proportion to their initial physical examination. As ischemia persists, peritoneal signs and cardiovascular collapse will follow. Mortality is >50%. While radiographic imaging can suggest ischemia, the gold standard for diagnosis is laparotomy.

35. The answer is D.

(Chap. 21) This patient with a history of atherosclerotic cardiovascular disease and diabetes is at high risk for nonocclusive mesenteric ischemia in the setting of sepsis, hypotension, and administered vasoconstrictors. Intestinal ischemia is further classified based on etiology, which dictates management (Table 35): (1) arteria-occlusive mesenteric ischemia, (2) nonocclusive mesenteric ischemia, and (3) mesenteric venous thrombosis. Risk factors for arteria-occlusive mesenteric ischemia are generally acute in onset and include atrial fibrillation, recent myocardial infarction, valvular heart disease, and recent cardiac or vascular catheterization, all of which result in embolic clots reaching the mesenteric circulation. Nonocclusive mesenteric ischemia, also known as "intestinal angina," is generally more insidious and most often seen in the aging population affected by atherosclerotic disease. Nonocclusive mesenteric ischemia is also seen in patients receiving high-dose vasopressor infusions, patients with cardiogenic or septic shock, and patients with cocaine overdose. Nonocclusive mesenteric ischemia is the most prevalent GI disease complicating cardiovascular surgery. Mesenteric venous thrombosis is less common and is associated with the presence of a hypercoagulable state including protein C or S deficiency, anti–thrombin III deficiency, polycythemia vera, and carcinoma. In the absence of atrial fibrillation, nonocclusive mesenteric ischemia is more likely in this patient. There is no reason to suspect IBD as a cause of the bloody stools in this critically ill patient with known bacteremic sepsis, and the patient has only been on antibiotics for 1 day and is unlikely to have *Clostridium difficile* colitis at this point.

36 and 37. The answers are B and D, respectively.

(Chap. 22) The radiograph shows massively dilated colon extending to the rectum. This radiograph is consistent with colonic pseudo-obstruction or Ogilvie syndrome. Ogilvie syndrome may be seen in elderly patients after nonabdominal surgery or in patients with underlying autonomic dysfunction. The presence of gas in the colon makes small bowel obstruction unlikely. There is no extraintestinal air that would be suggestive of small or large bowel perforation. Small bowel ileus is characterized by multiple small bowel air–fluid levels on radiograph. The differential for extensive colonic dilation includes toxic megacolon due to *C. difficile* infection. In this case, that is less likely given the recent surgery and lack of antibiotic treatment. Neostigmine is an acetylcholinesterase inhibitor that increases cholinergic (parasympathetic) activity and can stimulate colonic motility. Some studies have shown it to be moderately effective in alleviating acute colonic

TABLE 35

OVERVIEW OF THE MANAGEMENT OF ACUTE INTESTINAL ISCHEMIA

CONDITION	KEY TO EARLY DIAGNOSIS	TREATMENT OF UNDERLYING CAUSE	TREATMENT OF SPECIFIC LESION	TREATMENT OF SYSTEMIC CONSEQUENCE
Arterio-occlusive mesenteric ischemia				
1. Arterial embolus	Computed tomography (CT) angiography Early laparotomy	Anticoagulation Cardioversion Proximal thrombectomy	Laparotomy Embolectomy Vascular bypass Assess viability and resect dead bowel	Ensure hydration Give antibiotics Reverse acidosis Optimize oxygen delivery Avoid vasoconstrictors
2. Arterial thrombosis	Duplex ultrasound Angiography	Anticoagulation Hydration	Endovascular approach: thrombolysis, angioplasty, and stenting Endarterectomy/thrombectomy or vascular bypass Assess viability and resect dead bowel	Give antibiotics Reverse acidosis Optimize oxygen delivery Support cardiac output Avoid vasoconstrictors
Mesenteric venous thrombosis	Spiral CT	Anticoagulation	Anticoagulation ± laparotomy/thrombectomy/catheter-directed thrombolysis	Give antibiotics Reverse acidosis Optimize oxygen delivery
Venous thrombosis	Angiography with venous phase	Massive hydration	Assess viability and resect dead bowel	Support cardiac output Avoid vasoconstrictors
Nonocclusive mesenteric ischemia	Vasospasm: Angiography Hypoperfusion: Spiral CT or colonoscopy	Ensure hydration Support cardiac output Avoid vasoconstrictors	Vasospasm: Intra-arterial vasodilators Hypoperfusion: Delayed laparotomy Assess viability and resect dead bowel	Ensure hydration Give antibiotics Reverse acidosis Optimize oxygen delivery Support cardiac output Avoid vasoconstrictors

Source: Modified from GB Bulkley, in JL Cameron (ed): *Current Surgical Therapy*, 2nd ed. Toronto: BC Decker, 1986.

pseudo-obstruction. It is the most common therapeutic approach and can be used once it is certain that there is no mechanical obstruction. Cardiac monitoring is required, and atropine should be immediately available for symptomatic bradycardia. Intravenous administration induces defecation and flatus within 10 minutes in the majority of patients who will respond. Surgical therapy may be necessary in cases of bowel perforation or impending perforation. Morphine, with its anticholinergic side effects, may worsen small or large bowel pseudo-obstruction. Oral vancomycin is the treatment for *C. difficile* infection.

38. The answer is C.
(Chap. 23) Obstruction of the appendiceal lumen is believed to typically result in appendicitis. Although obstruction is most commonly caused by fecalith, which results from accumulation and inspissation of fecal matter around vegetable fibers, other causes have been described. These other potential causes include enlarged lymphoid follicles associated with viral infection (e.g., measles), inspissated barium, worms (e.g., pinworms, *Ascaris*, and *Taenia*), and tumors such as carcinoma or carcinoid. Cholelithiasis is a common cause of acute pancreatitis.

39. The answer is A.
(Chap. 23) The patient presents with typical findings for acute appendicitis with anorexia, progressing to vague periumbilical pain, followed by localization to the right lower quadrant. Low-grade fever and leukocytosis are frequently present. Although acute appendicitis is primarily a clinical diagnosis, imaging modalities are frequently employed because the symptoms are not always classic. Plain radiographs are rarely helpful except when an opaque fecalith is found in the right lower quadrant (<5% of cases). Ultrasound may demonstrate an enlarged appendix

with a thick wall but is most useful to rule out ovarian pathology, tubo-ovarian abscess, or ectopic pregnancy. The effectiveness of ultrasonography as a tool to diagnose appendicitis is highly operator dependent. Even in very skilled hands, the appendix may not be visualized. Its overall sensitivity is 0.86, with a specificity of 0.81. Nonenhanced and contrast-enhanced CT are superior to ultrasound or plain radiograph in the diagnosis of acute appendicitis with sensitivity of 0.94 and specificity of 0.95. Findings often include a thickened appendix with periappendiceal stranding and often the presence of a fecalith (Figure 39). Free air is uncommon, even in the case of a perforated appendix. Nonvisualization of the appendix on CT is associated with surgical findings of a normal appendix 98% of the time. Colonoscopy has no role in the diagnosis of acute appendicitis.

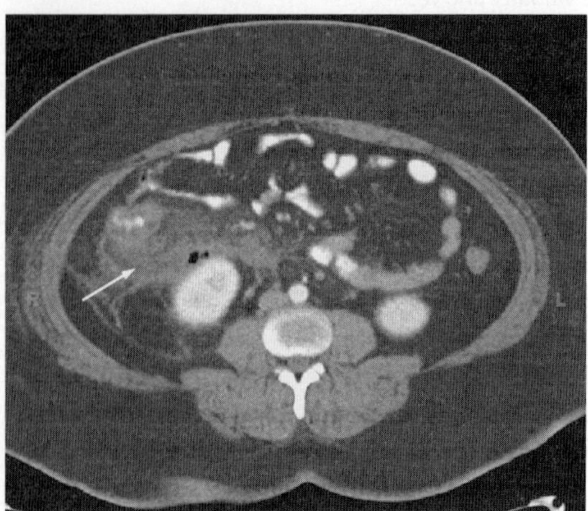

FIGURE 39

40 and 41. The answers are C and D, respectively.
(Chap. 23) The patient presents with several months of epigastric abdominal pain that is worse after eating. His symptoms are highly suggestive of peptic ulcer disease, with the worsening pain after eating suggesting a duodenal ulcer. The current presentation with acute abdomen and free air under the diaphragm points to a diagnosis of perforated viscus. Perforated gallbladder is less likely in light of the duration of symptoms and the absence of the significant systemic symptoms that often accompany this condition. Because the patient is relatively young with no risk factors for mesenteric ischemia, necrotic bowel from an infarction is highly unlikely. Pancreatitis can have a similar presentation, but a pancreas cannot perforate and liberate free air. Peritonitis is most commonly associated with bacterial infection, but it can be caused by the abnormal presence of physiologic fluids; for example, gastric contents, bile, pancreatic enzymes, blood, or urine, or by foreign bodies. In this case, peritonitis is most likely due to the presence of gastric juice in the peritoneal cavity after perforation of a duodenal ulcer has allowed these juices to leave the gut lumen.

42. The answer is A.
(Chaps. 9 and 36) Diagnostic paracentesis is part of the routine evaluation in a patient with ascites. Fluid should be examined for its gross appearance, protein content, cell count and differential, and albumin. Cytologic and culture studies should be performed when one suspects infection or malignancy. The serum-ascites albumin gradient (SAG) offers the best correlation with portal pressure. A high gradient (>1.1 g/dL) is characteristic of uncomplicated cirrhotic ascites and differentiates ascites caused by portal hypertension from ascites not caused by portal hypertension in more than 95% of cases. Conditions that cause a low gradient include more "exudative" processes such as infection, malignancy, and inflammatory processes. Similarly, congestive heart failure and nephrotic syndrome cause high gradients. In this patient, the SAG is 1.5 g/dL, indicating a high gradient. The low number of leukocytes and polymorphonuclear cells makes bacterial or tubercular infection unlikely. Chylous ascites often is characterized by an opaque milky fluid with a triglyceride level greater than 1000 mg/dL in addition to a low SAG.

43. The answer is A.
(Chap. 36) The most common and most characteristic symptom of liver disease is fatigue. Unfortunately, it is also very nonspecific, with little specific diagnostic utility. The fatigue in liver disease seems to improve in the morning and worsen throughout the day, but it can be intermittent. Jaundice is the hallmark of liver disease and is much more specific. Jaundice, however, is typically a sign of more advanced disease. Itching is also typically a symptom of more advanced disease and is more common in cholestatic causes of liver disease. Nausea often occurs in severe disease and can be accompanied by vomiting. Right upper quadrant pain is a less common symptom and indicates stretching of the liver capsule.

44. The answer is B.
(Chap. 36) Women are more susceptible to the effects of alcohol on the liver. On average, drinking about two drinks daily can lead to chronic liver disease in women, whereas men report drinking about three drinks daily. However, in individuals with

alcoholic cirrhosis, the average daily alcohol intake is usually much higher, and heavy levels of drinking for more than 10 years are typical prior to the onset of liver disease.

45. The answer is A.
(Chap. 36) In assessing alcohol intake, the history should also focus on whether alcohol abuse or dependence is present. Alcoholism is usually defined by the behavioral patterns and consequences of alcohol intake, not by the amount. *Abuse* is defined by a repetitive pattern of drinking alcohol that has adverse effects on social, family, occupational, or health status. *Dependence* is defined by alcohol-seeking behavior, despite its adverse effects. Many alcoholics demonstrate both dependence and abuse, and dependence is considered the more serious and advanced form of alcoholism. A clinically helpful approach to diagnosis of alcohol dependence and abuse is the use of the CAGE questionnaire, which is recommended for all medical history taking. One "yes" response should raise suspicion of an alcohol use problem, and more than one "yes" response is a strong indication of abuse or dependence.

46. The answer is D.
(Chap. 37) It is important to understand the patterns of laboratory abnormalities that indicate liver disease is present. One way to consider laboratory evaluation of liver disease is to consider three general categories of tests: tests based on excretory function of the liver, tests of biosynthetic activity of the liver, and coagulation factors. The most common tests of liver function fall under the category of tests based on the detoxification and excretory function of the liver. These include serum bilirubin, urine bilirubin, ammonia, and enzyme levels. Bilirubin can exist as a conjugated and an unconjugated form. The unconjugated form is often referred to as the indirect fraction. Isolated elevation in the unconjugated form of bilirubin is typically not related to liver disease but is most commonly seen in hemolysis and a number of benign genetic conditions such as Gilbert syndrome. In contrast, conjugated hyperbilirubinemia almost always indicates disease of the liver or biliary tract. Conjugated bilirubin is water soluble and excreted in the urine, but unconjugated bilirubin is not. Rather, it binds to albumin in the blood. Therefore, bilirubinuria implies liver disease as well. Among the serum enzymes, it is useful to consider enzymes as those that are associated with hepatocellular injury or those that reflect cholestasis. Alanine and aspartate aminotransferases are the primary enzymes that indicate hepatocyte injury. Alkaline phosphatase is the most common enzyme elevated in cholestasis, but bone disease also causes increased alkaline phosphatase. In some cases, one needs additional information to determine whether the alkaline phosphatase is liver or bone in origin. Other tests that would be elevated in cholestatic liver disease are 5′-nucleotidase and γ-glutamyl transferase. The primary test of synthetic function is measurement of serum albumin. Coagulation factors can be directly measured, but impaired production of coagulation factors in liver disease is primarily inferred from elevations in prothrombin time.

47. The answer is B.
(Chap. 37) The aminotransferases are sensitive indicators of liver cell injury and are most helpful in recognizing acute hepatocellular diseases such as hepatitis. They include aspartate aminotransferase (AST) and alanine aminotransferase (ALT). AST is found in the liver, cardiac muscle, skeletal muscle, kidneys, brain, pancreas, lungs, leukocytes, and erythrocytes in decreasing order of concentration. ALT is found primarily in the liver and is therefore a more specific indicator of liver injury. The aminotransferases are normally present in the serum in low concentrations. These enzymes are released into the blood in greater amounts when there is damage to the liver cell membrane, resulting in increased permeability. Liver cell necrosis is not required for the release of the aminotransferases, and there is a poor correlation between the degree of liver cell damage and the level of the aminotransferases. Thus, the absolute elevation of the aminotransferases is of no prognostic significance in acute hepatocellular disorders.

Any type of liver cell injury can cause modest elevations in the serum aminotransferases. Levels of up to 300 IU/L are nonspecific and may be found in any type of liver disorder. Minimal ALT elevations in asymptomatic blood donors rarely indicate severe liver disease; studies have shown that fatty liver disease is the most likely explanation. Striking elevations—i.e., aminotransferases >1000 IU/L—occur almost exclusively in disorders associated with extensive hepatocellular injury such as viral hepatitis, ischemic liver injury (prolonged hypotension or acute heart failure), or toxin- or drug-induced liver injury.

The pattern of the aminotransferase elevation can be helpful diagnostically. In most acute hepatocellular disorders, the ALT is higher than or equal to the AST. Whereas the AST:ALT ratio is typically <1 in patients with chronic viral hepatitis and nonalcoholic fatty liver disease, a number of groups have noted that as cirrhosis develops, this ratio rises to >1. An AST:ALT ratio >2:1 is suggestive, whereas a ratio >3:1 is highly suggestive, of alcoholic liver disease. The AST in alcoholic liver disease is rarely >300 IU/L, and the ALT is often normal. The aminotransferases are usually not greatly elevated in obstructive jaundice.

48 and 49. The answers are E and D, respectively. *(Chap. 38)* This patient is presenting with an asymptomatic and mild elevation in unconjugated hyperbilirubinemia that has occurred during a time of increased stress, fatigue, and likely decreased caloric intake. This presentation is characteristic of Gilbert syndrome, an inherited disorder of bilirubin conjugation. In Gilbert syndrome, there is a mutation of the *UGT1A1* gene that encodes bilirubin UDP-glucuronosyltransferase, which leads to a reduction in activity on the enzyme to 10%–35% of normal. This enzyme is of critical importance in the conjugation of bilirubin. Most of the time, there is no apparent jaundice because the reduced ability to conjugate bilirubin is not reduced to a degree that leads to an elevation of bilirubin. However, during times of stress, fatigue, alcohol use, decreased caloric intake, or intercurrent illness, the enzyme can become overwhelmed, leading to a mild hyperbilirubinemia. Typical bilirubin levels are less than 4.0 mg/dL unless the individual is ill or fasting. Diagnosis usually occurs during young adulthood, and episodes are self-limited and benign. If a liver biopsy were to be performed, hepatic histology would be normal. No treatment is necessary because there are no long-term consequences of Gilbert syndrome, and patient reassurance is recommended. Other inherited disorders of bilirubin conjugation are Crigler-Najjar syndromes types 1 and 2. Crigler-Najjar syndrome type 1 is a congenital disease characterized by more dramatic elevations in bilirubin as high as 20–45 mg/dL that is first diagnosed in the neonatal period and is present throughout life. This rare disorder was once fatal in early childhood due to the development of kernicterus. However, with phototherapy, individuals are now able to survive into adulthood, although neurologic deficits are common. Crigler-Najjar syndrome type 2 is similar to type 1, but the elevations in bilirubin are not as great. Kernicterus is rare. This is due to the fact that there is some residual function of the bilirubin UDP-glucuronosyltransferase enzyme (<10%) that is totally absent in type 1 disease. Hemolysis is another frequent cause of elevated unconjugated bilirubin. Hemolysis can be caused by many factors including medications, autoimmune disorders, and inherited disorders, among others. However, the normal hematocrit, lactate dehydrogenase, and haptoglobin eliminate hemolysis as a possibility. Dubin-Johnson syndrome is another congenital hyperbilirubinemia. However, it is a predominantly conjugated hyperbilirubinemia caused by a defect in biliary excretion from hepatocytes. Obstructive choledocholithiasis is characterized by right upper quadrant pain that is often exacerbated by fatty meals. The absence of symptoms or elevation in other liver function tests, especially alkaline phosphatase, also makes this diagnosis unlikely.

50. The answer is B. *(Chap. 38)* Increased destruction of erythrocytes leads to increased bilirubin turnover and unconjugated hyperbilirubinemia; the hyperbilirubinemia is usually modest in the presence of normal liver function. Hemolysis alone cannot result in a sustained hyperbilirubinemia of more than 4 mg/dL (~68 μmol). Higher values imply concomitant hepatic dysfunction. When hemolysis is the only abnormality in an otherwise healthy individual, the result is a purely unconjugated hyperbilirubinemia, with the direct-reacting fraction as measured in a typical clinical laboratory being ≤15% of the total serum bilirubin. In the presence of systemic disease, which may include a degree of hepatic dysfunction, hemolysis may produce a component of conjugated hyperbilirubinemia in addition to an elevated unconjugated bilirubin concentration. Prolonged hemolysis may lead to the precipitation of bilirubin salts within the gallbladder or biliary tree, resulting in the formation of gallstones in which bilirubin, rather than cholesterol, is the major component. Such pigment stones may lead to acute or chronic cholecystitis, biliary obstruction, or any other biliary tract consequence of calculous disease.

51. The answer is B. *(Chap. 39)* This patient presents with acute hepatitis, which has numerous etiologies. These include viruses, toxins/drugs, autoimmune diseases, metabolic disease, alcohol, ischemia, pregnancy, and other infectious etiologies including rickettsial diseases and leptospirosis. In this clinical scenario, the patient does have risk factors for hepatitis A, B, and C infection, including being a man who has sex with men and a prior history of injection drug use. All acute viral hepatitis presents with a similar clinical pattern, although incubation periods vary after exposure. The most common initial symptoms are fatigue, anorexia, nausea, vomiting, myalgias, and headache. These symptoms precede the onset of jaundice by about 1–2 weeks. Once jaundice develops, the prodromal symptoms regress. On physical examination, there is usually obvious icterus with an enlarged and tender liver. Splenomegaly can occur. AST and ALT are elevated with peak levels that are quite variable between 400 and 4000 IU/L, and alkaline phosphatase levels are increased to a much lesser degree. Hyperbilirubinemia (levels 5–20 mg/dL) occurs with primarily increased levels of conjugated bilirubin. Thus, it is important to recognize the patterns of antibody production in the viral hepatitides. Hepatitis A is an RNA virus that presents with acute hepatitis and is transmitted by the fecal-oral route. In the acute state, the immunoglobulin (Ig) M would be elevated, which is not seen in this scenario. Hepatitis B virus is a DNA virus with three common antigens that are tested serologically to determine the time course of the illness. These antigens are the surface antigen, the core antigen, and the e antigen, which is a nucleocapsid protein produced from the same gene as the core antigen but immunologically distinct. Several distinct patterns can be observed. In acute hepatitis B, the core IgM, surface antigen, and e antigen are all positive, which is what is seen in this case. At this point, the patient is highly infectious, with viral shedding in body fluids, including saliva. In a late acute infection, core IgG may be positive at the same time as surface and e antigen positivity. In chronic hepatitis B, this same pattern of serologies is seen. If a patient has a prior infection without development of chronic hepatitis, the core IgG and surface antibody is positive. However, when immunity is obtained via vaccination, only the surface antibody (SAb) is positive; the e antigen and surface antigen will be negative since the patient was never infected. The variety of antigen-antibody positivities that can result are outlined in Table 51. Acute hepatitis C often is detectable with contemporary immunoassays early during the disease when the aminotransferases are positive. Thus, a positive HCV antibody could indicate acute hepatitis C in this individual. However, given his clinical history of prior injection drug use and inability to donate blood, this likely indicates chronic hepatitis C infection. In some instances, ecstasy has been reported to cause drug-induced hepatitis, but given the viral serologies in this patient, this would be unlikely.

52. The answer is E.

(Chap. 39) No treatment is recommended for acute hepatitis B in most individuals because 99% of infected individuals recover without assistance. Therefore, it would not be expected that an individual would derive any particular benefit from treatment. In severe acute hepatitis B, nucleoside analogues, including lamivudine, have been used successfully, although there are no clinical trial data to support such an approach. Hepatitis A is an acute and self-limited illness that does not progress to chronic liver disease. Thus, no treatment is required. Anti–hepatitis A virus immunoglobulin can be given prophylactically following a known exposure to prevent development of disease, but it is not helpful in established disease. There is no role for oral or intravenous glucocorticoids in the treatment of acute viral hepatitis of any etiology. It has demonstrated no clinical benefit and may increase the risk of developing chronic disease.

53. The answer is E.

(Chap. 39) In most instances, patients with any form of acute viral hepatitis do not succumb to fulminant liver failure. However, pregnant women are highly susceptible to fulminant hepatic failure in the setting of acute hepatitis E infection. This RNA virus is an enteric virus that is endemic in India, Asia, Africa, the Middle East, and Central America and is spread via contaminated water supplies. Person-to-person spread is rare. Generally, the clinical course of hepatitis E infection is mild and the rate of fulminant hepatitis is only 1%–2%. However, in pregnant women, this is as high as 10%–20%. For hepatitis A and C, the rate of fulminant hepatic failure is about 0.1% or less. It is slightly higher for hepatitis B, at around 0.1%–1%. Hepatitis D occurs as a coinfection with hepatitis B virus. When the two viruses are acquired simultaneously, the rate of fulminant hepatitis is about 5% or less. When hepatitis D is acquired in the setting of chronic hepatitis B infection, this number rises to 20%.

54. The answer is E.

(Chap. 39) Hepatitis A virus (HAV) is an acute, self-limited virus that is acquired almost exclusively via the fecal-oral route. It is classically a disease of poor hygiene and overcrowding. Outbreaks have been traced to contaminated water, milk, frozen raspberries and strawberries, green onions, and shellfish. Infection occurs mostly in children and young adults. It almost invariably resolves spontaneously and results in lifelong immunity. Fulminant disease occurs in ≤0.1% of cases, and there is no chronic form (in contrast to hepatitis B and C). Diagnosis is made by demonstrating a positive IgM antibody to HAV, as described earlier. An IgG antibody to HAV indicates immunity, obtained by previous infection or vaccination. A small proportion of patients will experience relapsing hepatitis weeks to months after a full recovery from HAV infection. This too is self-limited. There is no approved antiviral therapy for

TABLE 51

ANTIGEN AND ANTIBODY PROFILES IN VIRAL HEPATITIS

HEPATITIS TYPE	VIRUS PARTICLE, NM	MORPHOLOGY	GENOME[a]	CLASSIFICATION	ANTIGEN(S)	ANTIBODIES	REMARKS
HAV	27	Icosahedral nonenveloped	7.5-kb RNA, linear, ss, +	Hepatovirus	HAV	Anti-HAV	Early fecal shedding Diagnosis: IgM anti-HAV Previous infection: IgG anti-HAV
HBV	42	Double-shelled virion (surface and core) spherical	3.2-kb DNA, circular, ss/ds	Hepadnavirus	HBsAg HBcAg HBeAg	Anti-HBs Anti-HBc Anti-HBe	Bloodborne virus; carrier state Acute diagnosis: HBsAg, IgM anti-HBc Chronic diagnosis: IgG anti-HBc, HBsAg Markers of replication: HBeAg, HBV DNA
	27	Nucleocapsid core			HBcAg HBeAg	Anti-HBc Anti-HBe	Liver, lymphocytes, other organs Nucleocapsid contains DNA and DNA polymerase; present in hepatocyte nucleus; HBcAg does not circulate; HBeAg (soluble, nonparticulate) and HBV DNA circulate—correlate with infectivity and complete virions
	22	Spherical and filamentous; represents excess virus coat material			HBsAg	Anti-HBs	HBsAg detectable in >95% of patients with acute hepatitis B; found in serum, body fluids, hepatocyte cytoplasm; anti-HBs appears following infection—protective antibody
HCV	Approximately 50–80	Enveloped	9.4-kb RNA, linear, ss, +	Hepacivirus	HCV C100-3 C33c C22-3 NS5	Anti-HCV	Bloodborne agent, formerly labeled non-A, non-B hepatitis Acute diagnosis: Anti-HCV (C33c, C22-3, NS5), HCV RNA Chronic diagnosis: Anti-HCV (C100-3, C33c, C22-3, NS5) and HCV RNA; cytoplasmic location in hepatocytes
HDV	35–37	Enveloped hybrid particle with HBsAg coat and HDV core	1.7-kb RNA, circular, ss, –	Resembles viroids and plant satellite viruses (genus *Deltavirus*)	HBsAg HDAg	Anti-HBs Anti-HDV	Defective RNA virus, requires helper function of HBV (hepadnaviruses); HDV antigen (HDAg) present in hepatocyte nucleus Diagnosis: Anti-HDV, HDV RNA; HBV/HDV co-infection—IgM anti-HBc and anti-HDV; HDV superinfection—IgG anti-HBc and anti-HDV
HEV	32–34	Nonenveloped icosahedral	7.6-kb RNA, linear, ss, +	Hepevirus	HEV antigen	Anti-HEV	Agent of enterically transmitted hepatitis; rare in United States; occurs in Asia, Mediterranean countries, Central America Diagnosis: IgM/IgG anti-HEV (assays not routinely available); virus in stool, bile, hepatocyte cytoplasm

[a]ss, single-strand; ss/ds, partially single-strand, partially double-strand; –, minus-strand; +, plus-strand.

Abbreviations: HAV, hepatitis A virus; HBV, hepatitis B virus; HCV, hepatitis C virus; HDV, hepatitis D virus; HEV, hepatitis E virus; Ig, immunoglobulin.

HAV. An inactivated vaccine has decreased the incidence of the disease, and it is recommended for all U.S. children, for high-risk adults, and for travelers to endemic areas. Passive immunization with immunoglobulin is also available, and it is effective in preventing clinical disease before exposure or during the early incubation period.

55. The answer is C.
(Chap. 39) The current hepatitis B vaccine is a recombinant vaccine consisting of yeast-derived hepatitis B surface antigen particles. A strategy of vaccinating only high-risk individuals in the United States has been shown to be ineffective, and universal vaccination against hepatitis B is now recommended. Pregnancy is not a contraindication to vaccination. Vaccination should ideally be performed in infancy. Routine evaluation of hepatitis serologies is not cost-effective and is not recommended. The vaccine is given in three divided intramuscular doses at 0, 1, and 6 months.

56. The answer is A.
(Chap. 39) A clear distinction between viral etiologies of acute hepatitis cannot be made on clinical or epidemiologic features alone. This patient is at risk of many forms of hepatitis due to his lifestyle. Given his occupation in food services, from a public health perspective, it is important to make an accurate diagnosis. Serologies must be obtained to make a diagnosis. Although hepatitis C virus typically does not present as an acute hepatitis, this is not absolute. Hepatitis E virus infects men and women equally and resembles hepatitis A virus in clinical presentation. This patient should be questioned regarding IV drug use, and in addition to hepatitis serologies, an HIV test should be performed.

57. The answer is C.
(Chaps. 37 and 39) Causes of extreme elevations in serum transaminases generally fall into a few major categories, including viral infections, toxic ingestions, and vascular/hemodynamic causes. Both acute hepatitis A and hepatitis B infections may be characterized by high transaminases. Fulminant hepatic failure may occur, particularly in situations in which acute hepatitis A occurs on top of chronic hepatitis C infection or if hepatitis B and hepatitis D are co-transmitted. Most cases of acute hepatitis A or B infection in adults are self-limited. Hepatitis C is an RNA virus that does not typically cause acute hepatitis. However, it is associated with a high probability of chronic infection. Therefore, progression to cirrhosis and hepatoma is increased in patients with chronic hepatitis C infection. Extreme transaminitis is highly unlikely with acute hepatitis C infection. Acetaminophen remains one of the major causes of fulminant hepatic failure and is managed by prompt administration of *N*-acetylcysteine. Budd-Chiari syndrome is characterized by posthepatic thrombus formation. It often presents with jaundice, painful hepatomegaly, ascites, and elevated transaminases.

58. The answer is A.
(Chap. 40) The liver is the primary site for metabolism of many drugs and, as such, is susceptible to injury related to drugs and toxins. Indeed, the most common cause of acute hepatic failure is drug-induced liver injury. In general, it is useful to think of chemical hepatotoxicity within two broad categories: direct toxic effects or idiosyncratic reactions. Drugs or toxins that cause a direct toxic effect on liver are either poisons themselves or are metabolized to toxic substances. With agents that cause a direct toxic effect on hepatocytes, there is a predictable, dose-related pattern of injury, and the time to effect is relatively short. The most common drug or toxin causing direct hepatocyte toxicity is acetaminophen. In therapeutic doses, acetaminophen does not cause liver injury. However, in higher doses, one of the metabolites of acetaminophen, *N*-acetyl-*p*-benzoquinone imine (NAPQI), can overwhelm the glutathione stores of the liver that are necessary to convert NAPQI to a nontoxic metabolite and lead to hepatocyte necrosis. Other medications or toxins that cause direct hepatocyte injury are carbon tetrachloride, trichloroethylene, tetracycline, and the *Amanita phalloides* mushroom. More commonly known as the death cap mushroom, ingestion of a single *A. phalloides* mushroom can contain enough hepatotoxin to be lethal. Idiosyncratic reactions are infrequent and unpredictable. There is no dose dependency, and the timing of hepatic injury has little association with the duration of drug treatment. Many drugs produce idiosyncratic reactions, and it is difficult to know when an idiosyncratic reaction will lead to more serious liver failure. Often, mild increases in transaminase levels will occur, but over time, adaptation leads to a return of liver enzymes to normal levels. In other instances, idiosyncratic reactions can lead to fulminant hepatic failure. Although rare, serious hepatic reactions can lead to medications being removed from the market. It is now recognized that many idiosyncratic reactions are related to metabolites that cause liver injury. However, it is likely that individual genetic variations in liver metabolism are the primary cause, and these are not predictable effects of the drug given

our current state of knowledge. Common medications that can lead to idiosyncratic drug reactions include halothane, isothane, isoniazid, 3-hydroxy-3-methylglutaryl–coenzyme A (HMG-CoA) reductase inhibitors, and chlorpromazine.

59. The answer is B.

(Chap 40) Acetaminophen overdose is the most common cause of acute liver failure and the most common cause of drug-induced liver failure that leads to transplantation. Acetaminophen is metabolized in the liver through two pathways. The primary pathway is a phase II reaction that produces nontoxic sulfate and glucuronide metabolites. The minor pathway occurs through a phase I reaction leading to production of NAPQI. This metabolite is directly toxic to liver cells and can lead to hepatocyte necrosis. With therapeutic use of acetaminophen, glutathione in the liver rapidly converts NAPQI to a nontoxic metabolite that is excreted in the urine. However, glutathione stores can become depleted in the setting of a large acute ingestion, chronic alcoholism, or chronic ingestion of increased acetaminophen. In addition, alcohol upregulates the first enzyme in the metabolic pathway, causing NAPQI to accumulate more quickly in alcoholics. Given the known hepatotoxicity of acetaminophen, the U.S. Food and Drug Administration has recommended a maximum daily dose of no more than 3.25 g, with lower doses in individuals with chronic alcohol use. Acute ingestions of 10–15 g of acetaminophen are sufficient to cause clinical evidence of liver injury, and doses higher than 25 g can lead to fatal hepatic necrosis. The course of illness with acute acetaminophen ingestion follows a predictable pattern. Nausea, vomiting, abdominal pain, and shock occur within 4–12 hours after ingestion. Liver enzymes and synthetic function are normal at this time. Within 24–48 hours, these symptoms subside and are followed by evidence of hepatic injury. Maximal levels of aminotransferases can reach more than 10,000 IU/L and may not occur until 4–6 days after ingestion. These patients must be followed carefully for fulminant hepatic failure with serious complications including encephalopathy, cerebral edema, marked coagulopathy, renal failure, metabolic acidosis, electrolyte abnormalities, and refractory shock. Levels of acetaminophen are predictive of the development of hepatotoxicity. The first level should be measured no sooner than 4 hours after a known ingestion. Levels should be plotted on a nomogram that relates levels to the time after ingestion. If, at 4 hours, the acetaminophen level is greater than 300 μg/mL, significant hepatotoxicity is likely. In the setting of overdose, it may be difficult to know the exact quantity and timing of an ingestion. For the patient presenting in the clinical scenario in this question, her level of greater than 300 μg/mL is quite concerning for a large ingestion, and treatment should be initiated immediately. The primary treatment for acetaminophen overdose is *N*-acetylcysteine. *N*-Acetylcysteine acts to replete glutathione levels in the liver and also provides a reservoir of sulfhydryl groups to bind to the toxic metabolites. The typical regimen of *N*-acetylcysteine is 140 mg/kg given as a loading dose, followed by 70 mg/kg every 4 hours for a total of 15–20 doses. This drug can also be given by continuous infusion. Activated charcoal or cholestyramine should only be given if the patient presents within 30 minutes after ingestion. Hemodialysis will not accelerate clearance of acetaminophen and will not protect the liver. Most patients with fulminant hepatic failure develop acute renal failure, often requiring hemodialysis. If a patient survives an acetaminophen overdose, there is usually no chronic liver injury.

60. The answer is E.

(Chap. 40) Isoniazid (INH) remains central to most antituberculous prophylactic and therapeutic regimens, despite its long-standing recognition as a hepatotoxin. In 10% of patients treated with INH, elevated serum aminotransferase levels develop during the first few weeks of therapy; however, these elevations in most cases are self-limited, mild (values for ALT <200 IU/L), and resolve despite continued drug use. This adaptive response allows continuation of the agent if symptoms and progressive enzyme elevations do not follow the initial elevations. Acute hepatocellular drug-induced liver injury secondary to INH is evident with a variable latency period up to 6 months and is more frequent in alcoholics and patients taking certain other medications, such as barbiturates, rifampin, and pyrazinamide. If the clinical threshold of encephalopathy is reached, severe hepatic injury is likely to be fatal or to require liver transplantation. Liver biopsy reveals morphologic changes similar to those of viral hepatitis or bridging hepatic necrosis. Substantial liver injury appears to be age-related, increasing substantially after age 35; the highest frequency is in patients over age 50. Even for patients >50 years of age monitored carefully during therapy, hepatotoxicity occurs in only ~2%, well below the risk estimate derived from earlier experiences. Many public health programs that require INH prophylaxis for a positive tuberculin skin test or Quantiferon test include monthly monitoring of aminotransferase levels, although this practice has been called into question. Even more effective in limiting

serious outcomes may be encouraging patients to be alert for symptoms such as nausea, fatigue, or jaundice, because most fatalities occur in the setting of continued INH use despite clinically apparent illness.

61. The answer is C.
(Chap. 40) HMG-COA reductase inhibitors, or statins, may cause an idiosyncratic mixed hepatocellular and cholestatic reaction. Between 1% and 2% of patients taking lovastatin, simvastatin, pravastatin, fluvastatin, or one of the newer statin drugs for the treatment of hypercholesterolemia experience asymptomatic, reversible elevations (greater than threefold) of aminotransferase activity. Acute hepatitis-like histologic changes, centrilobular necrosis, and centrilobular cholestasis have been described in a very small number of cases. In a larger proportion, minor aminotransferase elevations appear during the first several weeks of therapy. Careful laboratory monitoring can distinguish between patients with minor, transitory changes, who may continue therapy, and those with more profound and sustained abnormalities, who should discontinue therapy. Because clinically meaningful aminotransferase elevations are so rare after statin use and do not differ in meta-analyses from the frequency of such laboratory abnormalities in placebo recipients, the National Lipid Association's Safety Task Force concluded that liver test monitoring was not necessary in patients treated with statins and that statin therapy need not be discontinued in patients found to have asymptomatic isolated aminotransferase elevations during therapy. Statin hepatotoxicity is not increased in patients with chronic hepatitis C, hepatic steatosis, or other underlying liver diseases, and statins can be used safely in these patients.

62. The answer is B.
(Chap. 41) Chronic hepatitis represents a series of liver disorders of varying causes and severity in which hepatic inflammation and necrosis continue for at least 6 months. Milder forms are nonprogressive or only slowly progressive, whereas more severe forms may be associated with scarring and architectural reorganization, which, when advanced, lead ultimately to cirrhosis. Several categories of chronic hepatitis have been recognized. These include chronic viral hepatitis, drug-induced chronic hepatitis, and autoimmune chronic hepatitis. In many cases, clinical and laboratory features are insufficient to allow assignment into one of these three categories; these "idiopathic" cases are also believed to represent autoimmune chronic hepatitis (Table 62). Finally, clinical and laboratory features

TABLE 62 CLINICAL AND LABORATORY FEATURES OF CHRONIC HEPATITIS

TYPE OF HEPATITIS	DIAGNOSTIC TEST(s)	AUTOANTIBODIES	THERAPY
Chronic hepatitis B	HBsAg, IgG anti-HBc, HBeAg, HBV DNA	Uncommon	IFN-α, PEG IFN-α Oral agents First-line: entecavir, tenofovir Second-line: lamivudine, adefovir, telbivudine
Chronic hepatitis C	Anti-HCV, HCV RNA	Anti-LKM1[a]	PEG IFN-α plus ribavirin Telaprevir[b] Boceprevir[b]
Chronic hepatitis D	Anti-HDV, HDV RNA, HBsAg, IgG anti-HBc	Anti-LKM3	IFN-α, PEG IFN-α[c]
Autoimmune hepatitis	ANA[d] (homogeneous), anti-LKM1 (±) Hyperglobulinemia	ANA, anti-LKM1, anti-SLA[e]	Prednisone, azathioprine
Drug-associated	—	Uncommon	Withdraw drug
Cryptogenic	All negative	None	Prednisone (?), azathioprine (?)

[a]Antibodies to liver-kidney microsomes type 1 (autoimmune hepatitis type II and some cases of hepatitis C).
[b]Administered as a triple-drug combination with PEG IFN and ribavirin. Recently, two additional drugs were approved for hepatitis C, simeprevir and sofosbuvir (see *www.hcvguidelines.org*).
[c]Early clinical trials suggested benefit of IFN-α therapy; PEG IFN-α is as effective, if not more so, and has supplanted standard IFN-α.
[d]Antinuclear antibody (autoimmune hepatitis type I).
[e]Antibodies to soluble liver antigen (autoimmune hepatitis type III).
Abbreviations: HBc, hepatitis B core; HBeAg, hepatitis B e antigen; HBsAg, hepatitis B surface antigen; HBV, hepatitis B virus; HCV, hepatitis C virus; HDV, hepatitis D virus; IFN-α, interferon-α; IgG, immunoglobulin G; LKM, liver-kidney microsome; PEG IFN-α, pegylated interferon-α; SLA, soluble liver antigen.

of chronic hepatitis are observed occasionally in patients with such hereditary/metabolic disorders as Wilson disease (copper overload), α_1-antitrypsin deficiency (Chaps. 44), and nonalcoholic fatty liver disease (Chap. 46), and even occasionally in patients with alcoholic liver injury (Chap. 42). Both of the enterically transmitted forms of viral hepatitis, hepatitis A and E, are self-limited and do not cause chronic hepatitis.

63. The answer is B.
(Chap. 41) The patient in this scenario has evidence of chronic active hepatitis B virus (HBV) infection. The presence of hepatitis B e antigen (HBeAg) is indicative of ongoing viral replication, and individuals with HBeAg positivity typically have high levels of HBV DNA on testing. The spectrum of clinical infection in chronic hepatitis B is quite variable, and often, individuals are asymptomatic with elevated liver enzymes identified on testing for other reasons. Thus, the decision to treat chronic HBV infection should not be based on clinical features. Most experts recommend treatment of HBeAg-positive chronic HBV infection with HBV DNA levels $>2 \times 10^4$ IU/mL if the ALT is elevated greater than twice the upper limit of normal (Table 63). To date, seven drugs have been approved for treatment of chronic HBV: injectable interferon (IFN) α; pegylated IFN (long-acting IFN bound to polyethylene glycol [PEG IFN]); and the oral agents lamivudine, adefovir dipivoxil, entecavir, telbivudine, and tenofovir. PEG IFN, entecavir, or tenofovir is recommended as first-line therapy. Simeprevir is a protease inhibitor that is approved for the treatment of hepatitis C virus infection. Acyclovir is used to treat herpes simplex viral infections, and ritonavir is a protease inhibitor used to treat HIV infection. The patient's husband should also be screened for HBV given the continued viremia.

64. The answer is B.
(Chap. 41) Chronic hepatitis develops in about 85% of all individuals affected with hepatitis C virus (HCV), and 20%–25% of these individuals will progress to cirrhosis over about 20 years. Among those infected with HCV, about one-third of individuals will have normal or near-normal levels of aminotransferases, although liver biopsy demonstrates active hepatitis in as many as one-half of patients. Moreover, about 25% of individuals with normal aminotransferase levels at one point in time will develop elevations in these enzymes later and can develop progressive liver disease. Thus, normal aminotransferase levels at a single point in time do not definitively rule out the possibility that cirrhosis can develop. Progression to end-stage liver disease in individuals with chronic HCV hepatitis is more likely in older individuals and in patients with longer duration of infection, advanced histologic stage and grade, genotype 1 infection, more complex quasi-species diversity, concomitant other liver disease, HIV infection, and obesity. Among these factors, the best prognostic indicator for the development of progressive liver disease is liver histology. Specifically, patients who have moderate to severe inflammation or necrosis, including septal or bridging fibrosis, have the greatest risk of developing cirrhosis over the course of 10–20 years.

65. The answer is C.
(Chap. 41) Three types of autoimmune hepatitis have been identified based on clinical and laboratory characteristics. Type I autoimmune hepatitis is typically a disorder seen in young women. The clinical characteristics can be variable from those of chronic hepatitis to fulminant hepatic failure, and many of the features are difficult to distinguish from other causes of chronic hepatitis. In some individuals, extrahepatic manifestations, including fatigue, malaise, weight loss, anorexia, and arthralgias, can be quite prominent. Liver enzymes are elevated but may not correlate with the clinical severity of disease. In more severe cases, elevations in serum bilirubin between 3 and 10 mg/dL can be seen. Hypoalbuminemia occurs in advanced disease, and hypergammaglobulinemia (>2.5 g/dL) is common. The circulating antibody profile in autoimmune hepatitis depends to some extent on the type of hepatitis. Antinuclear antibodies are positive in a homogeneous staining pattern almost invariably in the disease, and rheumatoid factor is also common. Perinuclear antineutrophilic cytoplasmic antibody may be positive, but in an atypical fashion. Anti–smooth muscle antibodies and anti-liver/kidney microsomal antibodies are frequently seen, but these are nonspecific because other causes of chronic hepatitis can lead to positivity of these enzymes. Because of the lack of a specific autoimmune profile, the diagnostic criteria for autoimmune hepatitis incorporate a variety of clinical and laboratory features. Specific features that argue against this diagnosis include prominent alkaline phosphatase elevation, presence of mitochondrial antibodies, markers of viral hepatitis, history of hepatotoxic drugs or excess alcohol intake, histologic evidence of bile duct injury, or atypical biopsy features including excess hepatic iron, fatty infiltration, and viral inclusions. Antimitochondrial

TABLE 63

RECOMMENDATIONS FOR TREATMENT OF CHRONIC HEPATITIS B[a]

HBEAG STATUS	CLINICAL	HBV DNA (IU/ML)	ALT	RECOMMENDATION
HBeAg-reactive[b]	Chronic hepatitis Cirrhosis compensated Cirrhosis decompensated	$>2 \times 10^4$ $>2 \times 10^4$[d] $>2 \times 10^3$ $<2 \times 10^3$ Detectable Undetectable	≤2 × ULN[c,d] >2 × ULN[d] < or > ULN >ULN < or > ULN < or > ULN	No treatment; monitor In patients >40 with family history of hepatocellular carcinoma and/or ALT persistently at the high end of the twofold range, liver biopsy may help in decision to treat Treat[e] Treat[e] with oral agents, not PEG IFN Consider treatment[f] Treat[e] with oral agents,[g] not PEG IFN; refer for liver transplantation Observe; refer for liver transplantation
HBeAg-negative[b]	Chronic hepatitis Chronic hepatitis Cirrhosis compensated Cirrhosis decompensated	$\leq 2 \times 10^3$ $>10^3$ $>10^4$ $>2 \times 10^3$ $<2 \times 10^3$ Detectable Undetectable	≤ULN 1 to >2 × ULN[d] >2 × ULN[d] < or > ULN >ULN < or > ULN < or > ULN	Inactive carrier; treatment not necessary Consider liver biopsy; treat[h] if biopsy shows moderate to severe inflammation or fibrosis Treat[h,i] Treat[e] with oral agents, not PEG IFN Consider treatment[f] Treat[h] with oral agents,[g] not PEG IFN; refer for liver transplantation Observe; refer for liver transplantation

[a]Based on practice guidelines of the AASLD. Except as indicated in footnotes, these guidelines are similar to those issued by the EASL.
[b]Liver disease tends to be mild or inactive clinically; most such patients do not undergo liver biopsy.
[c]This pattern is common during the early decades of life in Asian patients infected at birth.
[d]According to the EASL guidelines, treat if HBV DNA is $>2 \times 10^3$ IU/mL and ALT is >ULN.
[e]One of the potent oral drugs with a high barrier to resistance (entecavir or tenofovir) or PEG IFN can be used as first-line therapy (see text). These oral agents, but not PEG IFN, should be used for IFN-refractory/intolerant and immunocompromised patients. PEG IFN is administered weekly by subcutaneous injection for a year; the oral agents are administered daily for at least a year and continued indefinitely or until at least 6 months after HBeAg seroconversion.
[f]According to EASL guidelines, patients with compensated cirrhosis and detectable HBV DNA at any level, even with normal ALT, are candidates for therapy. Most authorities would treat indefinitely, even in HBeAg-positive disease after HBeAg seroconversion.
[g]Because the emergence of resistance can lead to loss of antiviral benefit and further deterioration in decompensated cirrhosis, a low-resistance regimen is recommended—entecavir or tenofovir monotherapy or combination therapy with the more resistance-prone lamivudine (or telbivudine) plus adefovir. Therapy should be instituted urgently.
[h]Because HBeAg seroconversion is not an option, the goal of therapy is to suppress HBV DNA and maintain a normal ALT. PEG IFN is administered by subcutaneous injection weekly for a year; caution is warranted in relying on a 6-month posttreatment interval to define a sustained response, because the majority of such responses are lost thereafter. Oral agents, entecavir or tenofovir, are administered daily, usually indefinitely or until, as very rarely occurs, virologic and biochemical responses are accompanied by HBsAg seroconversion.
[i]For older patients and those with advanced fibrosis, consider lowering the HBV DNA threshold to $>2 \times 10^3$ IU/mL.
Abbreviations: AASLD, American Association for the Study of Liver Diseases; ALT, alanine aminotransferase; EASL, European Association for the Study of the Liver; HBeAg, hepatitis B e antigen; HBsAg, hepatitis B surface antigen; HBV, hepatitis B virus; PEG IFN, pegylated interferon; ULN, upper limit of normal.

antibodies are typically seen in primary biliary cirrhosis.

66. The answer is D.
(Chaps. 39 and 41) In the course of acute hepatitis B, HBeAg positivity is common and usually transient. Persistence of HBeAg in the serum for >3 months indicates an increased likelihood of development of chronic hepatitis B. In chronic hepatitis B, presence of HBeAg in the serum indicates ongoing viral replication and increased infectivity. It is also a surrogate for inflammatory liver injury but not fibrosis. The development of antibody to HBeAg (anti-HBe) is indicative of the nonreplicative phase of HBV infection. During this phase, intact virions do not circulate and infectivity is less. Currently, quantification of HBV DNA with polymerase chain reaction allows risk stratification because $<10^3$ virions/μL is the approximate threshold for liver injury and infectivity.

67. The answer is C.

(Chap. 42) The pathology of alcoholic liver disease consists of three major lesions, with the progressive injury rarely existing in a pure form: (1) fatty liver, (2) alcoholic hepatitis, and (3) cirrhosis. Fatty liver is present in >90% of daily as well as binge drinkers. A much smaller percentage of heavy drinkers will progress to alcoholic hepatitis, thought to be a precursor to cirrhosis. The prognosis of severe alcoholic liver disease is dismal; the mortality of patients with alcoholic hepatitis concurrent with cirrhosis is nearly 60% at 4 years. Although alcohol is considered a direct hepatotoxin, only between 10% and 20% of alcoholics will develop alcoholic hepatitis. The explanation for this apparent paradox is unclear but involves the complex interaction of facilitating factors, such as drinking patterns, diet, obesity, and gender. There are no diagnostic tools that can predict individual susceptibility to alcoholic liver disease. Quantity and duration of alcohol intake are the most important risk factors involved in the development of alcoholic liver disease. The roles of beverage type(s) (i.e., wine, beer, or spirits) and pattern of drinking (daily versus binge drinking) are less clear. Chronic infection with hepatitis C virus (HCV) is an important comorbidity in the progression of alcoholic liver disease to cirrhosis. Even moderate alcohol intake of 20–50 g/d increases the risk of cirrhosis and hepatocellular cancer in HCV-infected individuals. Patients with both alcoholic liver injury and HCV infection develop decompensated liver disease at a younger age and have poorer overall survival.

TABLE 67

RISK FACTORS FOR ALCOHOLIC LIVER DISEASE

RISK FACTOR	COMMENT
Quantity	In men, 40–80 g/d of ethanol produces fatty liver; 160 g/d for 10–20 years causes hepatitis or cirrhosis. Only 15% of alcoholics develop alcoholic liver disease.
Gender	Women exhibit increased susceptibility to alcoholic liver disease at amounts >20 g/d; two drinks per day is probably safe.
Hepatitis C	HCV infection concurrent with alcoholic liver disease is associated with younger age for severity, more advanced histology, and decreased survival.
Genetics	Patatin-like phospholipase domain-containing protein 3 (PNPLA3) has been associated with alcoholic cirrhosis.
Fatty liver	Alcohol injury does not require malnutrition, but obesity and nonalcoholic fatty liver are risk factors. Patients should receive vigorous attention to nutritional support.

68. The answer is C.

(Chap. 42) This patient presents with severe acute alcoholic hepatitis. In its earliest form, alcoholic liver disease is marked by fatty infiltration of the liver. In more acute alcoholic hepatitis, there is hepatocyte injury with balloon degeneration and necrosis. Many cases of alcoholic hepatitis are asymptomatic. However, as in this case, the severe manifestations can include fever, jaundice, spider nevi, and abdominal pain that can mimic an acute abdomen in its severity. On laboratory examination, the AST is typically elevated more than the ALT, although the total transaminase levels are rarely greater than 400 IU/L. Hyperbilirubinemia can be quite marked with lesser elevation in alkaline phosphatase. Hypoalbuminemia and coagulopathy are poor prognostic indicators. A discriminate function (DF) can be calculated as follows: (4.6 × the prolongation of prothrombin time above control) + serum bilirubin. A DF >32 is associated with poor prognosis and is an indication for treatment of acute alcoholic hepatitis. The Model for End-Stage Liver Disease (MELD) score can also be used for prognostication in acute alcoholic hepatitis, with a score greater than 21 being an indication for treatment as well. This patient has a DF of >80, indicating very severe disease and a poor prognosis. Complete abstinence from alcohol is imperative. Treatment with prednisone 40 mg daily (or prednisolone 32 mg daily) for 4 weeks should be initiated. Following the initial period, a taper should be achieved over a period of 4 weeks. The role of tumor necrosis factor (TNF)-α expression and receptor activity in alcoholic liver injury has led to an examination of TNF inhibition as an alternative to glucocorticoids for severe alcoholic hepatitis. The nonspecific TNF inhibitor pentoxifylline (400 mg three times daily for 4 weeks) demonstrated improved survival in the therapy of severe alcoholic hepatitis, primarily due to a decrease in hepatorenal syndrome. Monoclonal antibodies that neutralize serum TNF-α should not be used in alcoholic hepatitis because of studies reporting increased deaths secondary to infection and renal failure. Liver transplantation is an accepted indication for treatment in selected and motivated patients with end-stage cirrhosis. Outcomes are equal or superior to other indications for transplantation.

69. The answer is D.

(Chap. 43) Nonalcoholic fatty liver disease (NAFLD) is the most common chronic liver disease in many parts of the world, including the United States.

Population-based abdominal imaging studies have demonstrated fatty liver in at least 25% of American adults. Because the vast majority of these subjects deny hazardous levels of alcohol consumption (defined as greater than one drink per day in women or two drinks per day in men), they are considered to have NAFLD. NAFLD is strongly associated with overweight/obesity and insulin resistance. However, it can also occur in lean individuals and is particularly common in those with a paucity of adipose depots (i.e., lipodystrophy). Ethnic/racial factors also appear to influence liver fat accumulation; the documented prevalence of NAFLD is lowest in African Americans (~25%), highest in Americans of Hispanic ancestry (~50%), and intermediate in American whites (~33%).

70. The answer is C.

(Chap. 43) At present, there are no Food and Drug Administration–approved therapies for the treatment of NAFLD. Thus, the current approach to NAFLD management focuses on treatment to improve the risk factors for nonalcoholic steatohepatitis (NASH; i.e., obesity, insulin resistance, metabolic syndrome, dyslipidemia). Based on our understanding of the natural history of NAFLD, only patients with NASH or those with features of hepatic fibrosis on liver biopsy are considered currently for targeted pharmacologic therapies. Lifestyle changes and dietary modification are the foundation for NAFLD treatment. Many studies indicate that lifestyle modification can improve serum aminotransferases and hepatic steatosis, with loss of at least 3%–5% of body weight improving steatosis, but greater weight loss (up to 10%) necessary to improve steatohepatitis. The benefits of different dietary macronutrient contents (e.g., low-carbohydrate vs. low-fat diets, saturated vs. unsaturated fat diets) and different intensities of calorie restriction appear to be comparable. In adults with NAFLD, exercise regimens that improve fitness may be sufficient to reduce hepatic steatosis, but their impact on other aspects of liver histology remains unknown. Antioxidants have also been evaluated for the treatment of NAFLD because oxidant stress is thought to contribute to the pathogenesis of NASH. Vitamin E, an inexpensive yet potent antioxidant, has been examined in several small pediatric and adult studies with varying results. In all of those studies, vitamin E was well tolerated, and most showed modest improvements in aminotransferase levels, radiographic features of hepatic steatosis, and/or histologic features of NASH. Statins are an important class of agents to treat dyslipidemia and decrease cardiovascular risk. There is no evidence to suggest that statins cause liver failure in patients with any chronic liver disease, including NAFLD. The incidence of liver enzyme elevations in NAFLD patients taking statins is also no different than that of healthy controls or patients with other chronic liver diseases. Moreover, several studies have suggested that statins may improve aminotransferases and histology in patients with NASH. However, there is continued reluctance to use statins in patients with NAFLD. The lack of evidence that statins harm the liver in NAFLD patients, combined with the increased risk for cardiovascular morbidity and mortality in NAFLD patients, warrants the use of statins to treat dyslipidemia in patients with NAFLD/NASH. Although interest in bariatric surgery as a treatment for NAFLD exists, a recently published Cochrane review concluded that lack of randomized clinical trials or adequate clinical studies prevents definitive assessment of benefits and harms of bariatric surgery as a treatment for NASH. Most studies of bariatric surgery have shown that it is generally safe in individuals with well-compensated chronic liver disease and improves hepatic steatosis and necroinflammation (i.e., features of NAFLD/NASH); however, effects on hepatic fibrosis have been variable.

71. The answer is A.

(Chap. 44) Alcohol is the most commonly used drug in the United States, and more than two-thirds of adults drink alcohol each year. Thirty percent have had a binge within the past month, and over 7% of adults regularly consume more than two drinks per day. Unfortunately, more than 14 million adults in the United States meet the diagnostic criteria for alcohol abuse or dependence. In the United States, chronic liver disease is the 10th most common cause of death in adults, and alcoholic cirrhosis accounts for approximately 40% of deaths due to cirrhosis. Excessive chronic alcohol use can cause several different types of chronic liver disease, including alcoholic fatty liver, alcoholic hepatitis, and alcoholic cirrhosis. Furthermore, use of excessive alcohol can contribute to liver damage in patients with other liver diseases, such as hepatitis C, hemochromatosis, and fatty liver disease related to obesity. Chronic alcohol use can produce fibrosis in the absence of accompanying inflammation and/or necrosis. Fibrosis can be centrilobular, pericellular, or periportal. When fibrosis reaches a certain degree, there is disruption of the normal liver architecture and replacement of liver cells by regenerative nodules. In alcoholic cirrhosis, the nodules are usually <3 mm in diameter; this form of cirrhosis is referred to as

micronodular. With cessation of alcohol use, larger nodules may form, resulting in a mixed micronodular and macronodular cirrhosis.

72. The answer is A.
(Chap. 44) The patient's hands show palmar erythema typical of alcoholic cirrhosis. This finding and the gynecomastia and testicular atrophy make alcoholic cirrhosis the most likely diagnosis. The testicular atrophy may be due to either a direct toxic effect of alcohol or hormonal effects. All of the other items may also cause liver cirrhosis (Table 72).

TABLE 72

CAUSES OF CIRRHOSIS	
Alcoholism	Cardiac cirrhosis
Chronic viral hepatitis	Inherited metabolic liver disease
Hepatitis B	Hemochromatosis
Hepatitis C	Wilson disease
Autoimmune hepatitis	α_1-Antitrypsin deficiency
Nonalcoholic steatohepatitis	Cystic fibrosis
Biliary cirrhosis	Cryptogenic cirrhosis
Primary biliary cirrhosis	
Primary sclerosing cholangitis	
Autoimmune cholangiopathy	

73. The answer is D.
(Chap. 44) The approach to patients once they have had a variceal bleed is first to treat the acute bleed, which can be life-threatening, and then to prevent further bleeding. The medical management of acute variceal hemorrhage includes the use of vasoconstricting agents, usually somatostatin or octreotide. Balloon tamponade (Sengstaken-Blakemore tube or Minnesota tube) can be used in patients who cannot receive endoscopic therapy immediately or who need stabilization prior to endoscopic therapy. Endoscopic intervention is used as first-line treatment to control bleeding acutely. Some endoscopists will use variceal injection therapy (sclerotherapy) as initial therapy, particularly when bleeding is vigorous. Variceal band ligation is used to control acute bleeding in over 90% of cases and should be repeated until obliteration of all varices is accomplished. When esophageal varices extend into the proximal stomach, band ligation is less successful. In these situations, when bleeding continues from gastric varices, consideration for a transjugular intrahepatic portosystemic shunt (TIPS) should be made. This offers an alternative to surgery for acute decompression of portal hypertension. Encephalopathy can occur in as many as 20% of patients after TIPS and is particularly problematic in elderly patients and in patients with preexisting encephalopathy. TIPS should be reserved for individuals who fail endoscopic or medical management or who are poor surgical risks. TIPS can sometimes be used as a bridge to transplantation. Prevention of further bleeding is usually accomplished with repeated variceal band ligation until varices are obliterated. Beta blockers, such as propranolol and nadolol, have been shown to decrease the risk of recurrent variceal bleeding and reduce mortality from a subsequent bleed but should not be used in the setting of the acutely bleeding patient.

74. The answer is D.
(Chap. 44) In patients with cirrhosis who are being followed chronically, the development of portal hypertension is usually revealed by the presence of thrombocytopenia, the appearance of an enlarged spleen, or the development of ascites, encephalopathy, and/or esophageal varices with or without bleeding. In previously undiagnosed patients, any of these features should prompt further evaluation to determine the presence of portal hypertension and liver disease. Varices should be identified by endoscopy. Abdominal imaging, either by CT or magnetic resonance imaging (MRI), can be helpful in demonstrating a nodular liver and in finding changes of portal hypertension with intra-abdominal collateral circulation. If necessary, interventional radiologic procedures can be performed to determine wedged and free hepatic vein pressures that will allow for the calculation of a wedged-to-free gradient, which is equivalent to the portal pressure. The average normal wedged-to-free gradient is 5 mmHg, and patients with a gradient >12 mmHg are at risk for variceal hemorrhage. While dilation of the right atrium may be found in cases of cardiac cirrhosis, dilation of the left atrium is characteristic of left ventricular failure.

75. The answer is B.
(Chap. 44) Spontaneous bacterial peritonitis (SBP) is a common and severe complication of ascites characterized by spontaneous infection of the ascitic fluid without an intra-abdominal source. In patients with cirrhosis and ascites severe enough for hospitalization, SBP can occur in up to 30% of individuals and can have a 25% in-hospital mortality rate. Bacterial translocation is the presumed mechanism

for development of SBP, with gut flora traversing the intestine into mesenteric lymph nodes, leading to bacteremia and seeding of the ascitic fluid. The most common organisms are *E. coli* and other gut bacteria; however, gram-positive bacteria, including *Streptococcus viridans*, *Staphylococcus aureus*, and *Enterococcus* spp. can also be found. If more than two organisms are identified, secondary bacterial peritonitis due to a perforated viscus should be considered. The diagnosis of SBP is made when the fluid sample has an absolute neutrophil count >250/μL. In this case, the patient has an absolute neutrophil count of 320/μL (800 × 0.4). Patients with ascites may present with fever, altered mental status, elevated white blood cell count, and abdominal pain or discomfort, or they may present without any of these features. Therefore, it is necessary to have a high degree of clinical suspicion, and peritoneal taps are important for making the diagnosis. Treatment is with a second-generation cephalosporin, with cefotaxime being the most commonly used antibiotic. In patients with variceal hemorrhage, the frequency of SBP is significantly increased, and prophylaxis against SBP is recommended when a patient presents with upper GI bleeding. Furthermore, in patients who have had an episode(s) of SBP and recovered, once-weekly administration of antibiotics is used as prophylaxis for recurrent SBP. There is no indication for hemodialysis with the normal serum creatine or EGD with no history of bleeding and a stable hemoglobin. Blood urea nitrogen (BUN) may increase as a result of the infection. Similarly, although the BUN is elevated and the patient has altered mental status, lactulose would not treat the primary disorder causing the altered mental status. Given the likely diagnosis of SBP, empiric therapy for meningitis is not warranted at this time.

76. The answer is C.

(Chap. 44) The clinical presentation is consistent with a cholestatic picture, which can present with painless jaundice and pruritus. The pruritus can be prominent and is present in 50% of individuals at the time of diagnosis. The pruritus is typically intermittent and worse in the evening. There is no other prominent association, such as following hot baths or showers, which occurs in polycythemia vera. Other causes of pruritus outside of cholestasis include lymphoma and uncontrolled hypo- or hyperthyroidism. However, the laboratory studies in this patient clearly represent cholestasis with an elevation in alkaline phosphatase and bilirubin. The clinical characteristics are more commonly seen in primary biliary cirrhosis compared to primary sclerosis cholangitis, as the patient is a middle-aged female with positive antimitochondrial antibodies. In contrast, primary sclerosing cholangitis is associated with positive perinuclear antineutrophil cytoplasmic antibodies in 65% of patients, and 50% of individuals with primary sclerosing cholangitis have a history of ulcerative colitis.

77. The answer is A.

(Chap. 44) The cornerstone of the management of ascites is sodium restriction to less than 2 g daily. A common misconception is to institute a fluid restriction as well. However, this is neither effective nor necessary. With a sodium restriction to 2 g daily, most mild ascites can be managed quite well. If sodium restriction alone fails to correct ascites, then initiation of diuretics is required. Spironolactone at a dose of 100–200 mg daily is the initial diuretic used for ascites and can be titrated as high as 400–600 mg daily if tolerated. Loop diuretics can be added to spironolactone. The typical agent is furosemide beginning at 40–80 mg daily with maximum doses of about 120–160 mg daily. Care must be taken to avoid renal dysfunction with loop diuretics, and higher doses may not be tolerated. If ascites is refractory to these treatments, TIPS can be considered. This procedure creates a direct portocaval shunt by introducing an expandable metal stent from the hepatic veins through the substance of the liver into the portal veins. Thus, TIPS decreases portal pressures, which in turn decrease ascites and the risk of variceal bleeding. However, hepatic encephalopathy typically worsens following TIPS.

78. The answer is A.

(Chap. 44) Severe right-sided heart failure may lead to chronic liver injury and cardiac cirrhosis. Elevated venous pressure leads to congestion of the hepatic sinusoids and of the central vein and centrilobular hepatocytes. Centrilobular fibrosis develops, and fibrosis extends outward from the central vein, not the portal triads. Gross examination of the liver shows a pattern of "nutmeg liver." Although transaminases are typically mildly elevated, severe congestion, particularly associated with hypotension, may result in dramatic elevation of AST and ALT 50- to 100-fold above normal. Budd-Chiari syndrome, or occlusion of the hepatic veins or inferior vena cava, may be confused with congestive hepatopathy. However, the signs and symptoms of congestive heart failure are absent in patients with Budd-Chiari syndrome, and these patients can be easily distinguished clinically from those with heart failure. Veno-occlusive disease

may result from hepatic irradiation and high-dose chemotherapy in preparation for hematopoietic stem cell transplantation. It is not a typical complication of liver transplantation. Although echocardiography is a useful tool for assessing left and right ventricular function, findings may be unimpressive in patients with constrictive pericarditis. A high index of suspicion for constrictive pericarditis (e.g., prior episodes of pericarditis, mediastinal irradiation) should lead to a right-sided heart catheterization with demonstration of the "square root sign," limitation of right heart filling pressure in diastole that is suggestive of restrictive cardiomyopathy. Cardiac MRI may also be helpful in determining which patients should proceed to cardiac surgery.

79. The answer is B.

(Chap. 44) The presence of cirrhosis in an elderly woman with no prior risk factors for viral or alcoholic cirrhosis should raise the possibility of primary biliary cirrhosis (PBC). PBC is characterized by chronic inflammation and fibrous obliteration of intrahepatic ductules. The cause is unknown, but autoimmunity is assumed because there is an association with other autoimmune disorders, such as autoimmune thyroiditis, CREST syndrome, and sicca syndrome. The vast majority of patients with symptomatic disease are women. The antimitochondrial antibody (AMA) test is positive in over 90% of patients with PBC and only rarely is positive in other conditions. This makes it the most useful initial test in the diagnosis of PBC. Because there are false-positive results, if AMA is positive, a liver biopsy is performed to confirm the diagnosis. The 24-hour urine copper collection is useful in the diagnosis of Wilson disease. Hepatic failure from Wilson disease typically occurs before age 50 years. Hemochromatosis may result in cirrhosis. It is associated with lethargy, fatigue, loss of libido, discoloration of the skin, arthralgias, diabetes, and cardiomyopathy. Ferritin levels are usually increased, and the most suggestive laboratory abnormality is an elevated transferrin saturation percentage. Although hemochromatosis is a possible diagnosis in this case, PBC is more likely in light of the clinical scenario. Although chronic hepatitis B and hepatitis C are certainly in the differential diagnosis and must be ruled out, they are unlikely because of the patient's history and lack of risk factors.

80. The answer is B.

(Chap. 48) Liver transplantation is indicated in adults for end-stage cirrhosis of all causes. Routine candidates for liver transplantation are patients with alcoholic cirrhosis, chronic viral hepatitis, and primary hepatocellular malignancies. Although all three of these categories are considered to be high risk, liver transplantation can be offered to carefully selected patients. Currently, chronic hepatitis C and alcoholic liver disease are the most common indications for liver transplantation, accounting for over 40% of all adult candidates who undergo the procedure. Patients with alcoholic cirrhosis can be considered as candidates for transplantation if they meet strict criteria for abstinence and reform; however, these criteria still do not prevent recidivism in up to a quarter of cases. In sclerosing cholangitis and Caroli disease (multiple cystic dilatations of the intrahepatic biliary tree), recurrent infections and sepsis associated with inflammatory and fibrotic obstruction of the biliary tree may be an indication for transplantation. Because prior biliary surgery complicates and is a relative contraindication for liver transplantation, surgical diversion of the biliary tree has been all but abandoned for patients with sclerosing cholangitis. Patients with chronic hepatitis C have early allograft and patient survival comparable to those of other subsets of patients after transplantation; however, reinfection in the donor organ is universal, recurrent hepatitis C is insidiously progressive, allograft cirrhosis develops in 20%–30% at 5 years, and cirrhosis and late organ failure occur at a higher frequency beyond 5 years. With the introduction of highly effective direct-acting antiviral agents targeting hepatitis C, it is expected that allograft outcomes will improve significantly in the coming years. In patients with chronic hepatitis B, in the absence of measures to prevent recurrent hepatitis B, survival after transplantation is reduced by approximately 10%–20%; however, prophylactic use of hepatitis B immune globulin (HBIg) during and after transplantation increases the success of transplantation to a level comparable to that seen in patients with nonviral causes of liver decompensation. Specific oral antiviral drugs can be used both for prophylaxis against and for treatment of recurrent hepatitis B. Patients with primary hepatocellular carcinoma with a single tumor <5 cm or three or fewer tumors of <3 cm have 5-year recurrence-free survival rates similar to those with nonmalignant disease. Because of the high rate of recurrent disease after transplantation, patients with cholangiocarcinoma are not transplantation candidates.

81. The answer is D.

(Chap. 48) Currently in the United States, all donor livers are distributed through a nationwide organ-sharing network (United Network for Organ Sharing

[UNOS]) designed to allocate available organs based on regional considerations and recipient acuity. Recipients who have the highest disease severity generally have the highest priority, but allocation strategies that balance highest urgency against best outcomes continue to evolve to distribute cadaver organs most effectively. Allocation is based on the MELD score, which is based on a mathematical model that includes bilirubin, creatinine, and international normalized ratio. Neither waiting time (except as a tie breaker between two potential recipients with the same MELD scores) nor posttransplantation outcome is taken into account. Use of the MELD score has been shown to reduce waiting list mortality, to reduce waiting time prior to transplantation, and to be the best predictor of pretransplantation mortality. The highest priority (status 1) for liver transplantation continues to be reserved for patients with fulminant hepatic failure or primary graft nonfunction.

82. The answer is B.
(Chap. 47) In the National Health and Nutrition Examination Survey, the prevalence of gallstone disease in the United States was 7.9% in men and 16.6% in women. Although the disease is quite prevalent, not all patients with gallstone disease require cholecystectomy. It is estimated that 1%–2% of patients with asymptomatic gallstone disease will develop complications that will require surgery yearly. Therefore, it is important to know which patients with asymptomatic gallstones require referral for surgery. The first factor to consider is whether the patient has symptoms that are caused by gallstones and are frequent enough and severe enough to necessitate surgery. Commonly called biliary colic, the classic symptoms of gallstone disease are right upper quadrant pain and fullness that begins suddenly and can last as long as 5 hours. Nausea and vomiting can accompany the episode. Vague symptoms of epigastric fullness, dyspepsia, and bloating following meals should not be considered biliary colic. A second factor that would be considered in recommending a patient for cholecystectomy is whether the patient has a prior history of complications of gallstone disease such as pancreatitis or acute cholecystitis. A final factor that would lead to the recommendation for cholecystectomy is the presence of anatomical factors that would increase the likelihood of complications such as a porcelain gallbladder or congenital abnormalities of the biliary tract. Individuals with very large stones (>3 cm) would also need to be considered carefully for cholecystectomy. Ursodeoxycholic acid can be used in some instances to dissolve gallstones. It acts to decrease the cholesterol saturation of bile and also allows dispersion of cholesterol from stones by producing a lamellar crystalline phase. However, it is only effective in individuals with radiolucent stones measuring less than 10 mm.

83. The answer is D.
(Chap. 47) A practitioner needs to have a high index of suspicion for acalculous cholecystitis in critically ill patients who develop decompensation during the course of treatment for the underlying disease and have no other apparent source of infection. Some predisposing conditions for the development of acalculous cholecystitis include serious trauma or burns, postpartum following prolonged labor, prolonged parenteral hyperalimentation, and during the postoperative period following orthopedic and other major surgical procedures. The clinical manifestations of acalculous cholecystitis are identical to calculous disease, but the disease is more difficult to diagnose. Ultrasonography and CT scanning typically only show biliary sludge, but they may demonstrate large and tense gallbladders. Hepatobiliary scintigraphy often shows delayed or absent gallbladder emptying. Successful management relies on accurate and early diagnosis. In critically ill patients, a percutaneous cholecystostomy may be the safest immediate procedure to decompress an infected gallbladder. Once the patient is stabilized, early elective cholecystectomy should be considered. Metronidazole to provide anaerobic coverage should be added, but this would not elucidate or adequately treat the underlying condition.

84. The answer is B.
(Chap. 47) Gallstones are very common, particularly in Western countries, with cholesterol stones being responsible for >90% of cases of cholelithiasis and pigment stones account for the remaining <10%. Cholesterol is essentially water-insoluble. Stone formation occurs in the setting of factors that upset cholesterol balance. Obesity, cholesterol-rich diets, high-calorie diets, and certain medications affect biliary secretion of cholesterol. Intrinsic genetic mutations in certain populations may affect the processing and secretion of cholesterol in the liver. Pregnancy results in both an increase in cholesterol saturation during the third trimester and changes in gallbladder contractility. Although rapid weight loss and low-calorie diets are associated with gallstones, there is no evidence that a high-protein diet confers an added risk of cholelithiasis.

85. The answer is E.
(Chap. 47) Pigment stone cholelithiasis may be black or brown stones. Black pigment stones are composed of either pure calcium bilirubinate or polymer-like complexes with calcium and mucin glycoproteins. They are more common in patients who have chronic hemolytic states (with increased conjugated bilirubin in bile), liver cirrhosis, Gilbert syndrome, or cystic fibrosis. Gallbladder stones in patients with ileal diseases, ileal resection, or ileal bypass generally are also black pigment stones. Enterohepatic recycling of bilirubin in ileal disease states contributes to their pathogenesis. Brown pigment stones are composed of calcium salts of unconjugated bilirubin with varying amounts of cholesterol and protein. They are caused by the presence of increased amounts of unconjugated, insoluble bilirubin in bile that precipitates to form stones. Sometimes the enzyme is also produced when bile is chronically infected by bacteria, and such stones are brown. Pigment stone formation is frequent in Asia and is often associated with infections in the gallbladder and biliary tree, including parasitic infections. Primary biliary cirrhosis is associated with cholesterol stones because of decreased bile acid secretion.

86. The answer is B.
(Chaps. 8 and 47) The clinical presentation is consistent with a cholestatic picture. Painless jaundice always requires an extensive workup, as many of the underlying pathologies are ominous and early detection and intervention often offers the only hope for a good outcome. The gallbladder showed no evidence of stones, and the patient shows no evidence of clinical cholecystitis, and so a hepatobiliary iminodiacetic acid (HIDA) scan is not indicated. Similarly, antibiotics are not necessary at this point. The cholestatic picture without significant elevation of the transaminases on the liver function tests makes acute hepatitis unlikely. Antimitochondrial antibodies are elevated in cases of PBC, which may present in a similar fashion. However, PBC is far more common in women than in men, and the average age of onset is the fifth or sixth decade. The lack of an obvious lesion on CT scan does not rule out a source of the cholestasis in the biliary tree. Malignant causes, such as cholangiocarcinoma and tumor of the ampulla of Vater, and nonmalignant causes, such as sclerosing cholangitis and Caroli disease, may be detected only by direct visualization with endoscopic retrograde cholangiopancreatography (ERCP). ERCP is useful both diagnostically and therapeutically as stenting procedures may be done to alleviate the obstruction.

87. The answer is A.
(Chap. 47) Primary or idiopathic sclerosing cholangitis (PSC) is characterized by a progressive, inflammatory, sclerosing, and obliterative process affecting the extrahepatic and/or the intrahepatic bile ducts. The disorder occurs in up to 75% of patients with inflammatory bowel disease, especially ulcerative colitis. It may also be associated with autoimmune pancreatitis; multifocal fibrosclerosis syndromes such as retroperitoneal, mediastinal, and/or periureteral fibrosis; Riedel struma; or pseudotumor of the orbit. Immunoglobulin G4 (IgG4)–associated cholangitis is a recently described biliary disease of unknown etiology that presents with biochemical and cholangiographic features indistinguishable from PSC, is often associated with autoimmune pancreatitis and other fibrosing conditions, and is characterized by elevated serum IgG4 and infiltration of IgG4-positive plasma cells in bile ducts and liver tissue. In contrast to PSC, it is not associated with inflammatory bowel disease and should be suspected if associated with increased serum IgG4 and unexplained pancreatic disease. Patients with PSC often present with signs and symptoms of chronic or intermittent biliary obstruction: right upper quadrant abdominal pain, pruritus, jaundice, or acute cholangitis. Late in the course, complete biliary obstruction, secondary biliary cirrhosis, hepatic failure, or portal hypertension with bleeding varices may occur. The diagnosis is usually established by finding multifocal, diffusely distributed strictures with intervening segments of normal or dilated ducts, producing a beaded appearance on cholangiography. Patients are at higher risk of cholangiocarcinoma. Therapy with cholestyramine may help control symptoms of pruritus, and antibiotics are useful when cholangitis complicates the clinical picture. Glucocorticoids, methotrexate, and cyclosporine have not been shown to be efficacious in PSC. In cases where high-grade biliary obstruction (dominant strictures) has occurred, balloon dilatation or stenting may be appropriate. Only rarely is surgical intervention indicated. The prognosis is unfavorable, with a median survival of 9–12 years following the diagnosis, regardless of therapy. Four variables (age, serum bilirubin level, histologic stage, and splenomegaly) predict survival in patients with PSC and serve as the basis for a risk score. PSC is a common indication for liver transplantation.

88. The answer is A.
(Chap. 50) Bicarbonate is the ion of primary physiologic importance within pancreatic secretion.

The ductal cells secrete bicarbonate predominantly derived from plasma (93%) more than from intracellular metabolism (7%). Bicarbonate enters the duct lumen through the sodium bicarbonate cotransporter with depolarization caused by chloride efflux through the cystic fibrosis transmembrane conductance regulator (CFTR). Secretin and vasoactive intestinal peptide bind at the basolateral surface and cause an increase in secondary messenger intracellular cyclic adenosine monophosphate, and act on the apical surface of the ductal cells, opening the CFTR and promoting secretion. CCK, acting as a neuromodulator, markedly potentiates the stimulatory effects of secretin. Acetylcholine also plays an important role in ductal cell secretion. Intraluminal bicarbonate secreted from the ductal cells helps neutralize gastric acid and creates the appropriate pH for the activity of pancreatic enzymes and bile salts on ingested food.

89. The answer is A.
(Chap. 50) In combination with a consistent clinical story and radiographic findings, serum amylase and lipase values threefold or more above normal virtually clinch the diagnosis of acute pancreatitis. Gut perforation, ischemia, and infarction should be excluded. Serum lipase is the preferred test and has a higher specificity than serum amylase. There is no correlation between the severity of pancreatitis and the degree of serum lipase and amylase elevations. After 3–7 days, even with continuing evidence of pancreatitis, total serum amylase values tend to return toward normal. However, pancreatic isoamylase and lipase levels may remain elevated for 7–14 days. Elevation of serum amylase is not specific for acute pancreatitis; notably, patients with metabolic acidemia (e.g., diabetic ketoacidosis) may have spurious elevation of serum amylase without pancreatitis. Hypocalcemia occurs in approximately 25% of cases of acute pancreatitis, whereas hypercalcemia is not a feature.

90. The answer is A.
(*Chap. 50*) The most common cause of acute pancreatitis in the United States is gallstones causing common bile duct obstruction. Although bile duct obstruction may be demonstrated on technetium HIDA scan, right upper quadrant ultrasound is preferred for ease, demonstration of gallstones in the gallbladder, and demonstration of obstructed bile duct. Alcohol is the second most common cause, followed by complications of ERCP. Hypertriglyceridemia accounts for 1%–4% of cases with triglyceride levels usually >1000 mg/dL. Other potential common causes include trauma, surgery, drugs such as valproic acid, anti-HIV medications, estrogens, and sphincter of Oddi dysfunction. Additionally, a number of rare causes have been described. The most judicious first step in evaluation is to test for gallstones and pursue more rare causes after the most common cause has been ruled out.

91. The answer is A.
(Chap. 50) Physical examination in acute pancreatitis commonly shows an uncomfortable patient, often with low-grade fever, tachycardia, and hypotension. Abdominal tenderness and muscle rigidity are often present to varying degrees. Cullen sign is a faint blue discoloration around the umbilicus that may occur as the result of hemoperitoneum. Turner sign is blue-red-purple or green-brown discoloration of the flanks from tissue catabolism of hemoglobin. Both of these signs indicate the presence of severe necrotizing pancreatitis.

92. The answer is E.
The BISAP (Bedside Index of Severity in Acute Pancreatitis) score has recently replaced Ranson's criteria and Acute Physiology and Chronic Health Evaluation II (APACHE II) severity scores as the recommended modality to assess severity of pancreatitis due to the cumbersome nature of the prior scores and the requirement of prior scores to collect a large amount of clinical and laboratory data over time. Severity of acute pancreatitis should be determined in the emergency department to assist in patient triage to a regular hospital ward or step-down unit or direct admission to an intensive care unit. BISAP incorporates five clinical and laboratory parameters obtained within the first 24 hours of hospitalization—BUN >25 mg/dL, impaired mental status (Glasgow coma score <15), systemic inflammatory response syndrome, age >60 years, and pleural effusion on radiography—that can be useful in assessing severity (Table 92). The presence of three or more of these factors was associated with substantially increased risk for in-hospital mortality among patients with acute pancreatitis. In addition, an elevated hematocrit >44% and admission BUN >22 mg/dL are also associated with more severe acute pancreatitis. Incorporating these indices with the overall patient response to initial fluid resuscitation in the emergency ward can be useful at triaging patients to the appropriate hospital acute care setting. Elevation of serum lipase is important for establishing the diagnosis of acute

pancreatitis, but the degree of elevation is not correlated with severity of disease.

TABLE 92

SEVERE ACUTE PANCREATITIS
Risk Factors for Severity
• Age >60 years
• Obesity, BMI >30
• Comorbid disease (Charlson comorbidity index)
Markers of Severity at Admission or Within 24 Hours
• SIRS—defined by presence of 2 or more criteria:
• Core temperature <36°C or >38°C
• Heart rate >90 bpm
• Respirations >20/min or PCO_2 <32 mmHg
• White blood cell count >12,000/μL, <4000/μL, or 10% bands
• APACHE II
• Hemoconcentration (hematocrit >44%)
• Admission BUN (>22 mg/dL)
• BISAP score
• (B) BUN >25 mg/dL
• (I) Impaired mental status
• (S) SIRS: ≥2 of 4 present
• (A) Age >60 years
• (P) Pleural effusion
• Organ failure (Modified Marshall score)
• Cardiovascular: systolic BP <90 mmHg, heart rate >130 bpm
• Pulmonary: PaO_2 <60 mmHg
• Renal: serum creatinine >2.0 mg/dL
Markers of Severity During Hospitalization
• Persistent organ failure
• Pancreatic necrosis

Abbreviations: APACHE II, Acute Physiology and Chronic Health Evaluation II; BMI, body mass index; BISAP, Bedside Index of Severity in Acute Pancreatitis; BP, blood pressure; BUN, blood urea nitrogen; SIRS, systemic inflammatory response syndrome.

93. The answer is E.

(Chap. 50) Several trials over the last several decades have demonstrated that there is no role for prophylactic antibiotics in the management of either interstitial or necrotizing pancreatitis. Antibiotics are only recommended for patients who appear septic at presentation while awaiting the results of culture data. If cultures are negative, antibiotics should be discontinued to decrease the risk of development of fungal superinfection. Similarly, several drugs have been evaluated in the treatment of acute pancreatitis and found to be of no benefit. These drugs include H^2 blockers, glucagon, protease inhibitors such as aprotinin, glucocorticoids, calcitonin, nonsteroidal anti-inflamatory drugs, and lexipafant, a platelet-activating factor inhibitor. A recent meta-analysis of somatostatin, octreotide, and the antiprotease gabexate mesylate in the therapy of acute pancreatitis suggested reduced mortality rate but no change in complications with octreotide and no effect on mortality but reduced pancreatic damage with gabexate.

94. The answer is C.

(Chap. 50) A low-fat solid diet can be administered to subjects with mild acute pancreatitis after the abdominal pain has resolved. Persistent inflammatory changes in the pancreas may remain for weeks to months after an episode of acute pancreatitis. Similarly, there may be prolonged elevation of amylase and lipase. In this regard, persistent changes on CT or persistent pancreatic enzyme elevation should not discourage clinicians from feeding hungry patients with acute pancreatitis. Although there had been prior concern that feeding patients with pancreatitis may exacerbate pancreatic inflammation, this has not been demonstrated. Enteral feeding maintains gut barrier integrity, limits bacterial translocation, is less expensive, and has fewer complications than total parenteral nutrition. The choice of gastric versus nasojejunal enteral feeding is currently under investigation.

95. The answer is D.

(Chap. 50) The pathophysiology of acute pancreatitis evolves in three phases. During the initial phase, pancreatic injury leads to intrapancreatic activation of digestive enzymes with subsequent autodigestion and acinar cell injury. Acinar injury is primarily attributed to activation of zymogens (proenzymes), particularly trypsinogen, by lysosomal hydrolases. Once trypsinogen is converted to trypsin, the activated trypsin further perpetuates the process by activating other zymogens to further autodigestion. The inflammation initiated by intrapancreatic activation of zymogens leads to the second phase of acute pancreatitis, with local production of chemokines that causes activation and sequestration of neutrophils in the pancreas. Experimental evidence suggests that neutrophilic inflammation can also cause further activation of trypsinogen, leading to a cascade of increasing acinar injury. The third phase of acute pancreatitis reflects the systemic processes that are caused by release of inflammatory cytokines and activated proenzymes into the systemic circulation. This process can lead to the systemic inflammatory response syndrome with acute respiratory distress syndrome, extensive third-spacing of fluids, and multiorgan failure. The morphologic features of acute pancreatitis are provided in Table 95.

TABLE 95

REVISED ATLANTA DEFINITIONS OF MORPHOLOGIC FEATURES OF ACUTE PANCREATITIS

MORPHOLOGIC FEATURE	DEFINITION	COMPUTED TOMOGRAPHY CRITERIA
Interstitial pancreatitis	Acute inflammation of the pancreatic parenchyma and peripancreatic tissues, but without recognizable tissue necrosis.	Pancreatic parenchyma enhancement by IV contrast agent No findings of peripancreatic necrosis
Necrotizing pancreatitis	Inflammation associated with pancreatic parenchymal necrosis and/or peripancreatic necrosis.	Lack of pancreatic parenchymal enhancement by IV contrast agent and/or presence of findings of peripancreatic necrosis (see below—ANC and WON)
Acute pancreatic fluid collection	Peripancreatic fluid associated with interstitial edematous pancreatitis with no associated peripancreatic necrosis. This term applies only to areas of peripancreatic fluid seen within the first 4 weeks after onset of interstitial edematous pancreatitis and without the features of a pseudocyst.	Occurs in the setting of interstitial edematous pancreatitis Homogeneous collection with fluid density Confined by normal peripancreatic fascial planes No definable wall encapsulating the collection Adjacent to pancreas (no intrapancreatic extension)
Pancreatic pseudocyst	An encapsulated collection of fluid with a well-defined inflammatory wall usually outside the pancreas with minimal or no necrosis. This entity usually occurs >4 weeks after onset of interstitial edematous pancreatitis.	Well circumscribed, usually round or oval Homogeneous fluid density No nonliquid component Well-defined wall; i.e., completely encapsulated Maturation usually requires >4 weeks after onset of acute pancreatitis; occurs after interstitial edematous pancreatitis
Acute necrotic collection (ANC)	A collection containing variable amounts of both fluid and necrosis associated with necrotizing pancreatitis; the necrosis can involve the pancreatic parenchyma and/or the peripancreatic tissues.	Occurs only in the setting of acute necrotizing pancreatitis Heterogeneous and nonliquid density of varying degrees in different locations (some appear homogeneous early in their course) No definable wall encapsulating the collection Location—intrapancreatic and/or extrapancreatic
Walled-off necrosis (WON)	A mature, encapsulated collection of pancreatic and/or peripancreatic necrosis that has developed a well-defined inflammatory wall. WON usually occurs >4 weeks after onset of necrotizing pancreatitis.	Heterogeneous with liquid and nonliquid density with varying degrees of loculations (some may appear homogeneous) Well-defined wall; i.e., completely encapsulated Location—intrapancreatic and/or extrapancreatic Maturation usually requires 4 weeks after onset of acute necrotizing pancreatitis

Source: Modified from P Banks et al: *Gut* 62:102, 2013.

96. The answer is D.

(Chap. 50) Chronic pancreatitis is a common disorder in any patient population with relapsing acute pancreatitis, especially patients with alcohol dependence, pancreas divisum, and cystic fibrosis. The disorder is notable for both endocrine and exocrine dysfunction of the pancreas. Often, diabetes ensues as a result of loss of islet cell function; although insulin-dependent, it is generally not as prone to diabetic ketoacidosis or coma as are other forms of diabetes mellitus. Because pancreatic enzymes are essential to fat digestion, their absence leads to fat malabsorption and steatorrhea. In addition, the fat-soluble vitamins (A, D, E, and K) are not absorbed. Vitamin A deficiency can lead to neuropathy. Vitamin B_{12}, or cobalamin, is often deficient. This deficiency is hypothesized to be due to excessive binding of cobalamin by cobalamin-binding proteins other than intrinsic factor that are normally digested by pancreatic enzymes. Replacement of pancreatic enzymes orally with meals will correct the vitamin deficiencies and steatorrhea. The incidence of pancreatic adenocarcinoma is increased in patients with chronic pancreatitis, with a 20-year cumulative incidence of 4%. Chronic abdominal pain is nearly ubiquitous in this disorder, and narcotic dependence is common. Niacin is a water-soluble vitamin, and absorption is not affected by pancreatic exocrine dysfunction.

97. The answer is A.

(Chap. 50) This patient likely has chronic pancreatitis related to long-standing alcohol use, which is

the most common cause of chronic pancreatitis in adults in the United States. Chronic pancreatitis can develop in individuals who consume as little as 50 g of alcohol daily (equivalent to ~30–40 ounces of beer). The patient's description of his loose stools is consistent with steatorrhea, and the recurrent bouts of abdominal pain are likely related to his pancreatitis. In most patients, abdominal pain is the most prominent symptom. However, up to 20% of individuals with chronic pancreatitis present with symptoms of maldigestion alone. The evaluation for chronic pancreatitis should allow one to characterize the pancreatitis as large- versus small-duct disease. Large-duct disease is more common in men and is more likely to be associated with steatorrhea. In addition, large-duct disease is associated with the appearance of pancreatic calcifications and abnormal tests of pancreatic exocrine function. Women are more likely to have small-duct disease, with normal tests of pancreatic exocrine function and normal abdominal radiography. In small-duct disease, the progression to steatorrhea is rare, and the pain is responsive to treatment with pancreatic enzymes. The findings on CT and abdominal radiograph of this patient are characteristic of chronic pancreatitis, and no further workup should delay treatment with pancreatic enzymes. Treatment with pancreatic enzymes orally will improve maldigestion and lead to weight gain, but they are unlikely to fully resolve maldigestive symptoms. Narcotic dependence can frequently develop in individuals with chronic pancreatitis due to recurrent and severe bouts of pain. However, because this individual's pain is mild, it is not necessary to prescribe narcotics at this point in time. An ERCP or magnetic resonance cholangiopancreatography (MRCP) may be considered to evaluate for a possible stricture that is amenable to therapy. However, sphincterotomy is a procedure performed via ERCP that may be useful in treating pain related to chronic pancreatitis and is not indicated in the patient. Angiography to assess for ischemic bowel disease is not indicated because the patient's symptoms are not consistent with intestinal angina. Certainly, weight loss can occur in this setting, but the patient usually presents with complaints of abdominal pain after eating and pain that is out of proportion with the clinical examination. Prokinetic agents would likely only worsen the patient's malabsorptive symptoms and are not indicated.

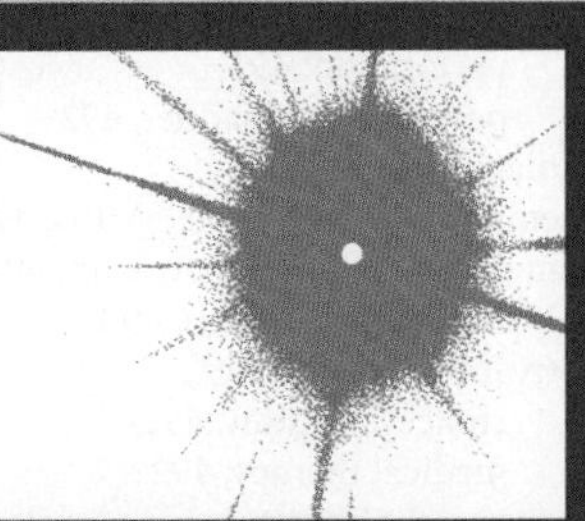

INDEX

Bold numbers indicate the start of the main discussion of the topic; numbers with "f" and "t" refer to figure and table pages, respectively.

INDEX

INDEX

INDEX

INDEX

INDEX

INDEX